Eighth Edition

SHERRIS & RYAN'S
MEDICAL MICROBIOLOGY

EDITOR
KENNETH J. RYAN, MD

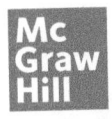

McGraw Hill

New York   Chicago   San Francisco   Athens   London   Madrid
Mexico City   Milan   New Delhi   Singapore   Sydney   Toronto

Sherris & Ryan's Medical Microbiology, Eighth Edition

1 2 3 4 5 6 7 8 9 0   LWI   26 25 24 23 22 21

ISBN 978-1-260-46428-3
MHID 1-260-46428-8

NOTICE

Medicine is an ever-changing science. As new research and clinical experience broaden our knowledge, changes in treatment and drug therapy are required. The authors and the publisher of this work have checked with sources believed to be reliable in their efforts to provide information that is complete and generally in accord with the standards accepted at the time of publication. However, in view of the possibility of human error or changes in medical sciences, neither the authors nor the publisher nor any other party who has been involved in the preparation or publication of this work warrants that the information contained herein is in every respect accurate or complete, and they disclaim all responsibility for any errors or omissions or for the results obtained from use of the information contained in this work. Readers are encouraged to confirm the information contained herein with other sources. For example and in particular, readers are advised to check the product information sheet included in the package of each drug they plan to administer to be certain that the information contained in this work is accurate and that changes have not been made in the recommended dose or in the contraindications for administration. This recommendation is of particular importance in connection with new or infrequently used drugs.

This book was set in Minion Pro by KnowledgeWorks Global Ltd.
The editors were Michael Weitz and Peter J. Boyle.
The production supervisor was Richard Ruzycka.
Production management was provided by Tasneem Kauser, KnowledgeWorks Global Ltd.
The cover designer was W2 Design.
The designer was Alan Barnett.

Cataloging-in-publication data for this book is on file at the Library of Congress.

McGraw Hill books are available at special quantity discounts to use as premiums and sales promotions or for use in corporate training programs. To contact a representative, please visit the Contact Us pages at www.mhprofessional.com.

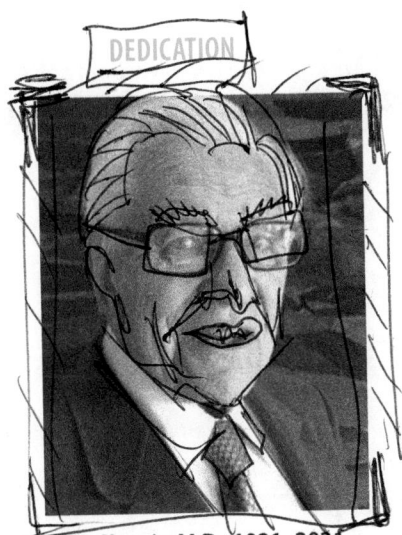

John C. Sherris, M.D., 1921–2021

(Reproduced, with permission, from McAdam AJ. John C. Sherris, M.D, *J Clin Microbiol* 2012 Nov;50(11):3416–3417.)

John Sherris was one of the most respected and admired microbiologists of his time. Trained in London and Oxford he was recruited by the University of Washington School of Medicine in 1959 to develop clinical microbiology laboratories, research, and the first clinical microbiology postdoctoral training program (PhDs and MDs) outside the Center for Disease Control and Prevention (CDC). John's best-known research accomplishment was leading the development and standardization of accurate yet practical antimicrobial susceptibility testing methods for pathogenic bacteria. The single disk diffusion technique was the most celebrated of these, but equally important were the underlying principles of interpreting individual bacterial strain results in relation to known pharmacologic and clinical data. These have turned out to be enduring. Even automated instruments, which now turn out results by the hundreds in a matter of hours, follow John's rules. An excellent teacher, John's motivation in developing this book was to strictly limit the text to material relevant to students of medicine and other health professions, and to explain it well. Stepping down as editor after the second edition he remained involved until literally weeks before his death. John Sherris' work and leadership have been recognized worldwide including presidency of the American Society for Microbiology, chair of the American Board of Medical Microbiology, and an honorary doctorate from Sweden's Karolinska Institute (see reference below the portrait above for many more). Amid all this success John Sherris and his wife Elizabeth were the most kind, witty, and downright enjoyable people one could ever hope to know.

Kenneth J. Ryan

Key Features

Based on recommendations from our Student Advisory Group a number of changes in chapter presentation have been implemented in the 8th edition of *Sherris Medical Microbiology*. These changes are particularly evident in the 40 chapters which describe the microbiology, disease (epidemiology, pathogenesis, immunity), and clinical aspects (manifestations, diagnosis, treatment, prevention) of the viral, bacterial, fungal, and parasitic human pathogens. These features are designed to highlight the most important elements for both course study and preparation for USMLE examinations. Examples of each are demonstrated below.

PATHOGEN LIST

Immediately below the title the pathogens for which at least a paragraph of discussion is included in the chapter are listed.

chapter 27

Mycobacteria

Mycobacterium tuberculosis · Mycobacterium leprae · Mycobacterium kansasii · Mycobacterium avium-intracellulare

Mycobacterium scrofulaceum · Mycobacterium fortuitum · Mycobacterium marinum · Mycobacterium ulcerans

---

MYCOBACTERIUM TUBERCULOSIS (MTB)

Overview

Like other mycobacteria, MTB cells are bacilli with a Gram-positive cell wall structure requiring the acid-fast stain for demonstration. Tuberculosis (TB) is a systemic infection, the most common form of which is a chronic pneumonia with fever, cough, bloody sputum, and weight loss. The natural history follows a course of chronic fever and a wasting to death aptly labeled "consumption" in the 19th century. Disease outside the lung also occurs and is particularly devastating when MTB reaches the central nervous system causing tuberculous meningitis. Most of those infected never develop disease, manifesting infection only by the presence of a skin test or other evidence of an immune response. Although disease may appear immediately following primary infection, in most instances it is delayed following a latent period lasting, months, years, even decades. MTB is not known to produce any classic virulence factors such as toxins. The tissue injury is due to the destructive effects of unremitting delayed-type hypersensitivity in a host whose Th1 cellular immune responses are unable to restrict growth of MTB. Methods for culture diagnosis are sensitive but require specialized expertise. Effective antimicrobial therapy has long been available but multiple drugs are required. The treatment course is prolonged and thus expensive. Together these make TB curable but only in countries that can afford it. TB is the leading infectious cause of premature death in the world.

OVERVIEW

The chapter opens with a boxed narrative paragraph explaining the big picture of the organism and disease features. If the chapter contains more than one major pathogen, an OVERVIEW is given for each.

MARGINAL NOTES

Marginal notes, a feature of *Sherris Medical Microbiology* since the first edition, give a brief statement of the text material in the immediately opposite paragraph. For the 8th edition this has been enhanced by highlighting those items likely to be the subject of USMLE Step 1 questions.

IMMUNITY

Innate immunity high

Humans have a high innate immunity to the development of disease. This was tragically illustrated in the Lübeck disaster of 1926, in which infants were administered wild-type MTB instead of an intended vaccine strain. Despite the large dose, only 76 of 249 died. As stated earlier, over 90% of immunocompetent persons infected with MTB never develop active disease. There is epidemiologic and historic evidence for differences in the immunity in certain population groups and between identical and nonidentical twins.

* Th1 immunity most important

* CD8+ lymphocytes participate

Adaptive immunity to TB is primarily related to the development of reactions mediated through CD4+ T lymphocytes via Th1 pathways. Intracellular killing of MTB by macrophages activated by INF-γ and the CD8+ mediated killing of infected macrophages are the essential steps. The specific components of MTB that are important in initiating these reactions are not known. Although antibodies to MTB are formed in the course of disease, there is no evidence they play any role in immunity.

■ Reactivation Tuberculosis

The times of life when persons infected with MTB are most likely to develop clinical disease are infancy (primary), young adult (primary or reactivation), or old age (reactivation). In Western countries, reactivation of previous quiescent lesions occurs most often after age 50 and is more common in men. Reactivation is associated with a period of immunosuppression precipitated by malnutrition, alcoholism, diabetes, old age, or a dramatic change in the individual's life, such as loss of a spouse. In areas in which tuberculosis is most prevalent, reactivation is more frequently seen in young adults experiencing the immunosuppression that accompanies puberty and pregnancy. Recently, reactivation and progressive primary TB among younger adults have increased as a complication of AIDS.

How can it take this long for disease to develop?

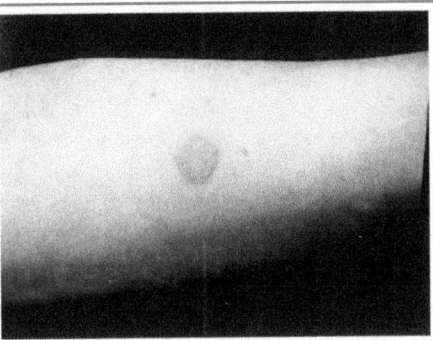

FIGURE 27–6. **Tuberculin skin test.** The purified protein derivative tuberculoprotein was injected intradermally at this site 48 hours previously. The erythema and induration (>15 mm) that are present indicate the development of delayed-type (type IV) hypersensitivity. (Reproduced with permission from Nester EW, Anderson DG, Roberts CE Jr, et al: *Microbiology: A Human Perspective*, 6th ed. New York, NY: McGraw Hill; 2008.)

Think ▸▸ Apply 27-1: **This is due to the long survival of the cells that enter the state of latency. The MTB have been inert but "alive" all this time.**

THINK → APPLY

At random points the author interrupts the text to pose a question. These are designed to challenge the student to think about what they have read earlier in the chapter and apply it to the question much as might be done during a lecture. The answer is given at the bottom of the page.

KEY CONCLUSIONS

At the end of each chapter or major section of a chapter, a bulleted list of sentences giving the major conclusions the student should be able to draw from that section is displayed. This includes microbiologic, disease, and clinical features of the pathogen and is particularly intended for review during preparation for exams.

KEY CONCLUSIONS

- High-lipid mycobacterial cell wall contains mycolic acids and lipoarabinomannan (LAM) which are responsible for the staining property called acid-fastness.
- Infection is by inhalation of respiratory droplets coughed up by human cases.
- Primary pulmonary infection leads to systemic spread of *Mycobacterium tuberculosis* (MTB).
- MTB interferes with killing mechanisms of alveolar macrophages.
- MTB-specific macrophage activation by IFN-γ leads to resolution in most infected persons.
- Incomplete macrophage activation leads to progressive disease (tuberculosis).
- Delayed-type hypersensitivity (DTH) is the sole known cause of injury.
- Entry of MTB into inactive latent state creates risk of reactivation disease in the lung or other sites (much less often) years to decades later.
- DTH response to tuberculin skin test (TST) indicates previous infection but not active disease.
- Definitive diagnosis is by acid-fast bacilli (AFB) smear, culture, or nucleic acid amplification (NAA) procedures on sputum or other tissues.
- Bacillus Calmette-Guérin (BCG) vaccine offers childhood protection but does not prevent reactivation. It also causes a DTH response to TST.
- Antimicrobial chemotherapy of tuberculosis is effective, but few agents able to penetrate the MTB cell wall are available. Cost and compliance limit worldwide effectiveness.
- Up to four drugs are used simultaneously to prevent expression of resistant mutants.

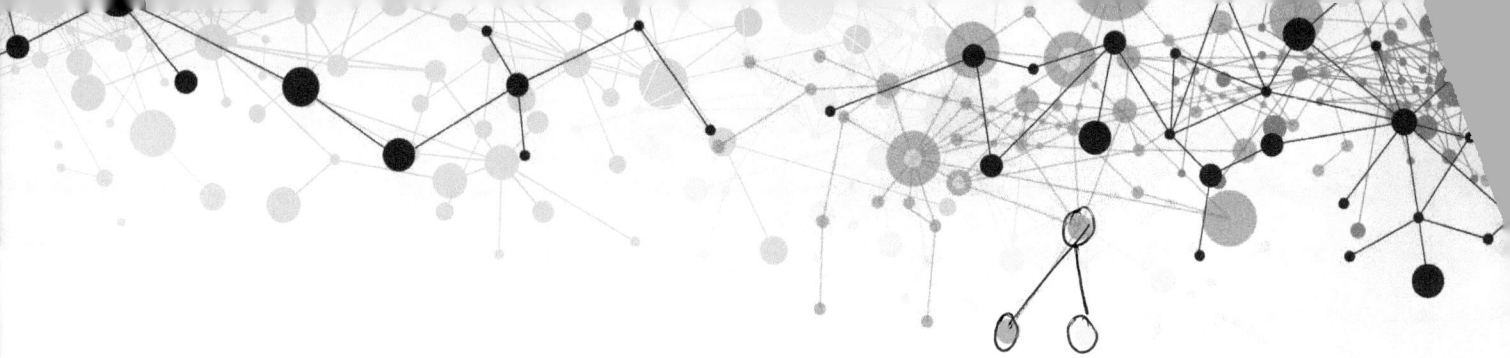

Contents

PART IV • Pathogenic Fungi   713

J. Andrew Alspaugh and Julie M. Steinbrink

PART V • Pathogenic Parasites   775

Paul Pottinger and Charles R. Sterling

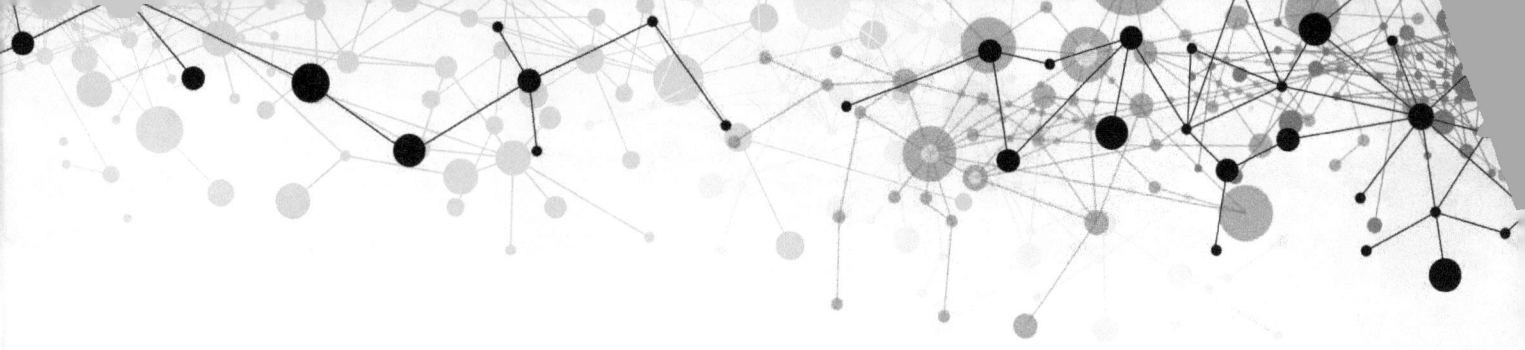

Contributors

Editor

KENNETH J. RYAN, MD
Emeritus Professor of Pathology and Microbiology
University of Arizona College of Medicine
Tucson, Arizona

AUTHORS

NAFEES AHMAD, PhD
Professor of Immunobiology
Director, Immunity and Infection
University of Arizona College of Medicine
Tucson, Arizona

J. ANDREW ALSPAUGH, MD
Professor of Medicine, Molecular Genetics
  and Microbiology
Duke University School of Medicine
Durham, North Carolina

W. LAWRENCE DREW, MD, PhD
Emeritus Professor of Laboratory Medicine
  and Medicine
University of California, San Francisco School
  of Medicine
Mount Zion Medical Center
San Francisco, California

PAUL POTTINGER, MD
Associate Professor of Medicine
Division of Allergy and Infectious Diseases
University of Washington School of Medicine
Seattle, Washington

L. BARTH RELLER, MD
Professor of Pathology and Medicine
Duke University School of Medicine
Durham, North Carolina

MEGAN E. RELLER, MD, PhD, MPH
Associate Professor of Medicine
Duke University School of Medicine
Durham, North Carolina

JULIE M. STEINBRINK, MD
Assistant Professor of Medicine
Duke University School of Medicine
Durham, North Carolina

CHARLES R. STERLING, PhD
Professor Emeritus
School of Animal and Comparative
  Biomedical Sciences
University of Arizona
Tucson, Arizona

GAYATRI VEDANTAM, PhD
Professor
School of Animal and Comparative
  Biomedical Sciences
University of Arizona
Research Career Scientist, US Department
  of Veterans Affairs
Tucson, Arizona

SCOTT WEISSMAN, MD
Associate Professor of Pediatrics
University of Washington School of Medicine
Seattle Children's
Seattle, Washington

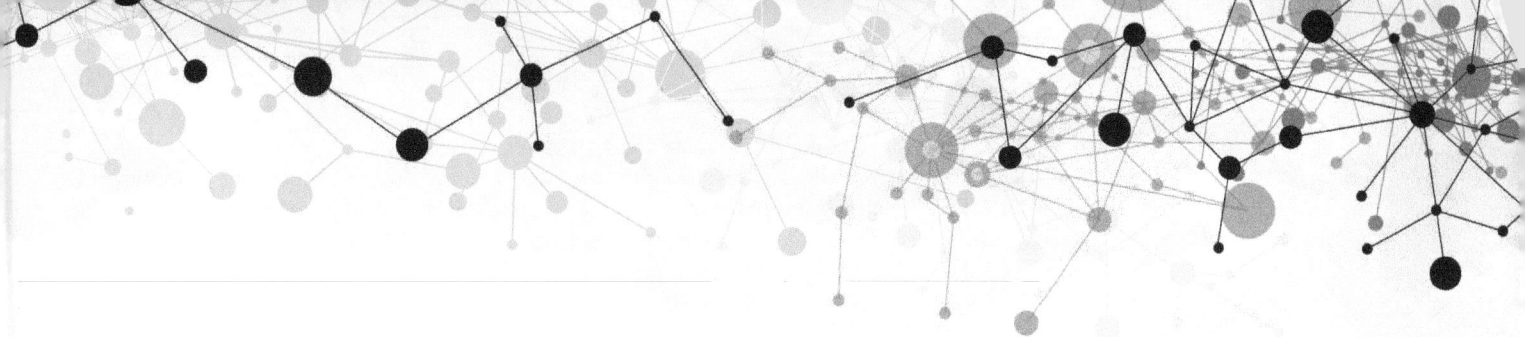

Preface

With this eighth edition, *Sherris Medical Microbiology* will enter its fifth decade as *Sherris & Ryan's Medical Microbiology*. We are pleased to welcome new authors Julie M. Steinbrink and Gayatri Vedantam from Duke University and the University of Arizona. John Sherris, the founding editor, continues to act as an inspiration to all of us (see Dedication).

BOOK STRUCTURE

The goal of *Sherris & Ryan's Medical Microbiology* remains unchanged from that of the first edition (1984). This book is intended to be the primary text for students of medicine and medical science who are encountering microbiology and infectious diseases for the first time. **Part I** opens with a chapter that explains the nature of infection and the infectious agents at the level of a general reader. The following four chapters give more detail on the immunologic, diagnostic, and epidemiologic nature of infection with minimal detail about the agents themselves. **Parts II** through **V** form the core of the text with chapters on the major viral, bacterial, fungal, and parasitic diseases, and each begins with its own chapters on basic biology, pathogenesis, and antimicrobial agents.

CHAPTER STRUCTURE

In the specific organism/disease chapters, the same presentation sequence is maintained throughout the book. First, features of the **Organism** (structure, metabolism, genetics, etc.) are described; then mechanisms of the **Disease** (epidemiology, pathogenesis, immunity) the organism causes are explained; the sequence concludes with the **Clinical Aspects** (manifestations, diagnosis, treatment, prevention) of these diseases. A clinical **Case Study** followed by questions in USMLE format concludes each of these chapters. In *Sherris & Ryan's Medical Microbiology,* the emphasis is on the text narrative, which is designed to be read comprehensively, not as a reference work. Considerable effort has been made to supplement this text with other learning aids such as the above-mentioned cases and questions as well as tables, photographs, and illustrations.

STUDENT-DRIVEN STUDY AIDS

This edition continues a number of new study aids first seen in the seventh edition. These were the product of a **Student Advisory** Group conceived and led by Laura Bricklin, MD then a second-year medical student at the University of Arizona College of Medicine. They include a boxed narrative **OVERVIEW** opening each disease-oriented chapter or major section, highlighted **MARGINAL NOTES** judged to be "high yield" for USMLE Step 1 preparation, and bulleted lists of **KEY CONCLUSIONS** at the end of major sections. A **THINK → APPLY** feature randomly inserts thought-provoking questions into the body of the text, which are answered at the bottom of the page. These new features are explained in detail and illustrated on pages iv and v. **Practice Questions** in USMLE format are also included. In the online version of this book the case-based, and other USMLE type questions are presented independent of the narrative text.

For any textbook, dealing with the onslaught of new information is a major challenge. In this edition, much new material has been included, but to keep the student from being overwhelmed, older or less important information has been deleted to keep the size of this book no larger than of the seventh edition. As a rule of thumb, material on classic microbial structures, toxins, and the like in the Organism section has been trimmed unless its role is clearly explained in the Disease section.

At the same time, we have tried not to eliminate detail to the point of becoming synoptic and uninteresting. Genetics is one of the greatest challenges in this regard. Without doubt this is where major progress is being made in understanding infectious diseases, but a coherent discussion may require using the names and abbreviations of genes, their products, and multiple regulators to tell the complete story. Whenever possible we have tried to tell the story without all the code language. We have also tried to fully describe the major genetic mechanisms in general chapters and then refer to them again when that mechanism is deployed by a pathogen. For example, *Neisseria gonorrhoeae* is used to explain the genetic mechanisms for antigenic variation in a general chapter on bacterial pathogenesis (Chapter 22), but how it influences its disease, gonorrhea, is taken up with its genus *Neisseria* (Chapter 30).

A saving grace is that our topic is important, dynamic, and fascinating—not just to us but to the public at large. Newspapers, radio, television, and now social media reports of infectious diseases are now filled daily with details of the Covid-19 pandemic. Resistance to antimicrobial agents and the havoc created by antivaccine movements remain regular topics on the evening news. It is not all bad news. We sense a new optimism that deeper scientific understanding of worldwide scourges like Covid-19, HIV/AIDS, tuberculosis, and malaria will lead to their control. We are hopeful that the basis for understanding these changes is clearly laid out in the pages of this book.

Kenneth J. Ryan
Editor

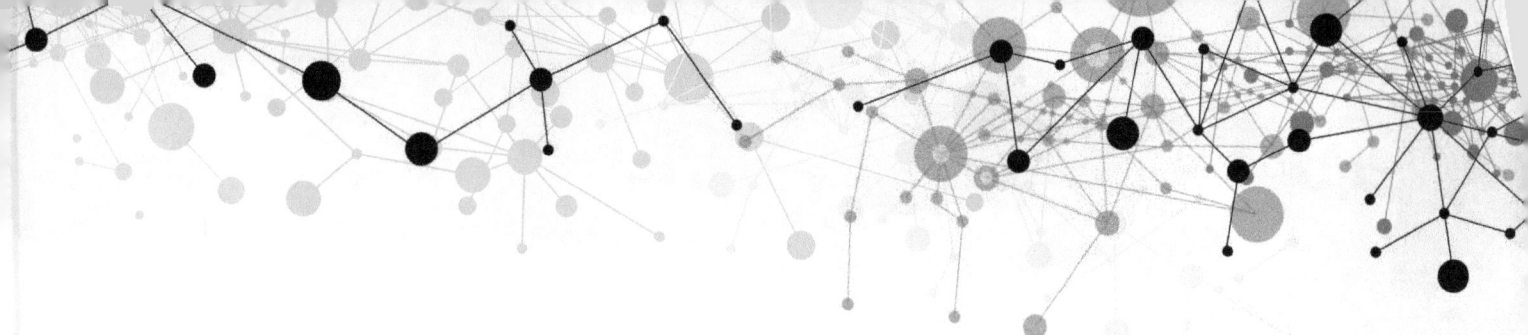

PART I
Infection

L. Barth Reller · Megan E. Reller · Kenneth J. Ryan · Gayatri Vedantam

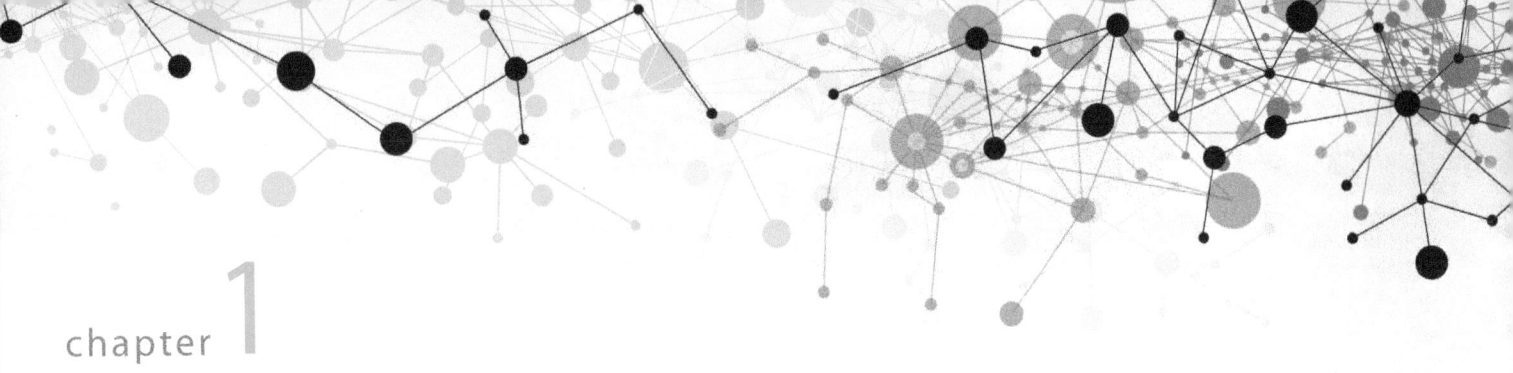

chapter 1

Infection—Basic Concepts

Humanity has but three great enemies: fever, famine, and war; of these by far the greatest, by far the most terrible, is fever.

—Sir William Osler, 1896*

When Sir William Osler, the great physician/humanist, wrote these words, fever (infection) was indeed the scourge of the world. Tuberculosis and other forms of pulmonary infection were the leading causes of premature death among the well-to-do and the less fortunate. The terror was due to the fact that, although some of the causes of infection were being discovered, little could be done to prevent or alter the course of disease. In the 20th century, advances in public sanitation and the development of vaccines and antimicrobial agents changed this (**Figure 1–1**), but only for the nations that can afford these interventions. As we move through the second decade of the 21st century, the world is divided into countries in which heart attacks, cancer, and stroke have surpassed infection as causes of premature death and those in which infection is still the leader. That is, unless there is a pandemic causing infection to again become the leading killer everywhere.

A new uneasiness that is part evolutionary, part discovery, and part diabolic has taken hold. Infectious agents once conquered have shown resistance to established therapy, such as multiresistant *Mycobacterium tuberculosis*, and diseases, such as acquired immunodeficiency syndrome (AIDS), have emerged. The spectrum of infection has widened, with discoveries that organisms earlier thought to be harmless can cause disease under certain circumstances. Who could have guessed that *Helicobacter pylori*, not even mentioned in the first edition of this book (1984), would be the major cause of gastric and duodenal ulcers and an officially declared carcinogen? Bioterrorist forces have unearthed two previously controlled infectious diseases—anthrax and smallpox—and threatened their distribution as agents of biological warfare. Finally, our current COVID-19 pandemic caused by the emergence of a new member of the well-known *Coronavirus* genus threatens to become the leading killer, not just in a century but ever. For students of medicine, understanding the fundamental basis of infectious diseases has more relevance than ever.

BACKGROUND

The science of medical microbiology dates back to the pioneering studies of Pasteur and Koch, who isolated specific agents and proved that they could cause disease by introducing the experimental method. The methods they developed lead to the first golden age of microbiology (1875-1910), when many bacterial diseases and the organisms responsible for them were defined. These efforts, combined with epidemiologic work begun by Semmelweis and Lister, which showed how these diseases spread, led to the great advances in public health that initiated the

---

*Osler W. *JAMA*. 1896;26:999.

FIGURE 1-1. Death rates for infectious disease in the United States in the 20th century. Note the steady decline in death rates related to the introduction of public health, immunization, and antimicrobial interventions.

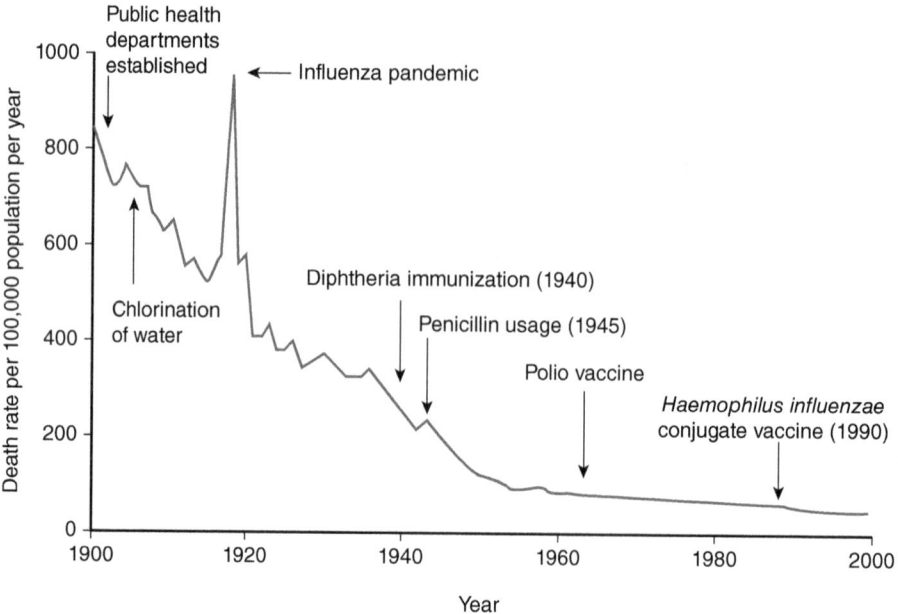

decline in disease and death. In the first half of the 20th century, scientists studied the structure, physiology, and genetics of microbes in detail and began to answer questions relating to the links between specific microbial properties and disease. By the end of the 20th century, the sciences of molecular biology, genetics, genomics, and proteomics extended these insights to the molecular level. Genetic advances have reached the point at which it is possible to know not only the genes involved but also to understand how they are regulated and mutated. The discoveries of penicillin by Fleming in 1929 and of sulfonamides by Domagk in 1935 opened the way to great developments in chemotherapy. These gradually extended from bacterial diseases to fungal, parasitic, and finally viral infections. Almost as quickly, virtually all categories of infectious agents developed resistance to all categories of antimicrobial agents to counter these chemotherapeutic agents.

● INFECTIOUS AGENTS: THE MICROBIAL WORLD

Microbes are small

Microbiology is a science defined by smallness. Its creation was made possible by the invention of the microscope (Gr. *micro,* small + *skop,* to look, see), which allowed visualization of structures too small to see with the naked eye. This definition of microbiology as the study of microscopic living forms still holds if one can accept that some organisms can reproduce only within other cells (eg, all viruses and some bacteria) and that others include macroscopic forms in their life cycle (eg, fungal molds, parasitic worms). The relative sizes of some microorganisms are shown in **Figure 1-2.**

Most play benign roles in the environment

Microorganisms are responsible for much of the breakdown and natural recycling of organic material in the environment. Some synthesize nitrogen-containing compounds that contribute to the nutrition of living things that lack this ability; others (oceanic algae) contribute to the atmosphere by producing oxygen through photosynthesis. Because microorganisms have an astounding range of metabolic and energy-yielding abilities, some can exist under conditions that are lethal to other life forms. For example, some bacteria can oxidize inorganic compounds such as sulfur and ammonium ions to generate energy. Others can survive and multiply in hot springs at temperatures higher than 75°C.

Products of microbes contribute to the atmosphere

Some microbial species have adapted to a symbiotic relationship with higher forms of life. For example, bacteria that can fix atmospheric nitrogen colonize root systems of legumes and of a few trees, such as alders, and provide the plants with their nitrogen requirements. When these plants die or are plowed under, the fertility of the soil is enhanced by nitrogenous compounds originally derived from the metabolism of the bacteria. Ruminants can use grasses as their prime source of

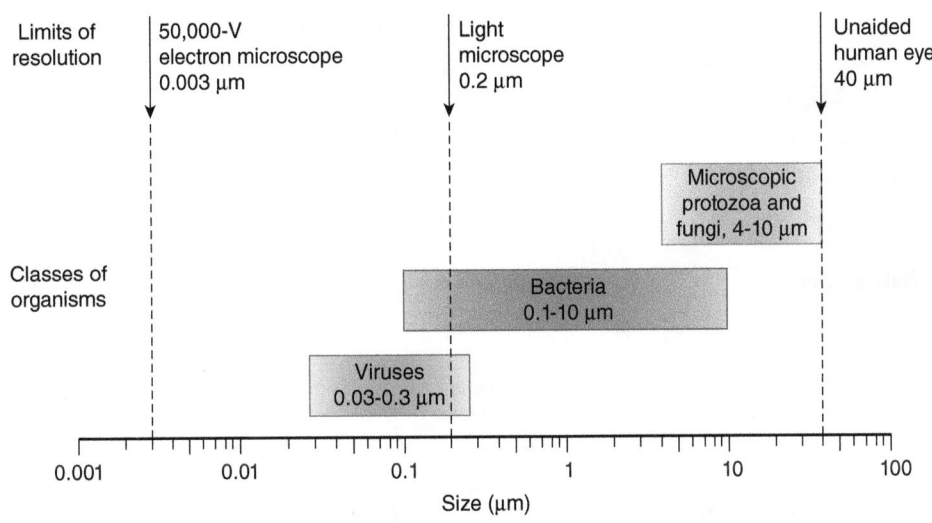

FIGURE 1–2. Relative size of microorganisms.

nutrition because the abundant flora of anaerobic bacteria in the rumen break down cellulose and other plant compounds into usable carbohydrates and amino acids. They can synthesize essential nutrients including some amino acids and vitamins. These few examples illustrate the protean nature of microbial life and their essential place in our ecosystem.

The major classes of microorganisms in terms of ascending size and complexity are viruses, bacteria, fungi, and parasites. Parasites exist as single or multicellular structures with the same compartmentalized eukaryotic cell plan of our own cells including a nucleus and cytoplasmic organelles like mitochondria. Fungi are also eukaryotic, but they have a rigid external wall that makes them seem more like plants than animals. Bacteria also have a cell wall, but with a cell plan called "prokaryotic" that lacks the organelles of eukaryotic cells. Viruses are not cells at all. They have a genome and some structural elements, but must take over the machinery of another living cell (eukaryotic or prokaryotic) to replicate. The four classes of infectious agents are summarized in **Table 1–1,** and generic examples of each are shown in **Figure 1–3.**

Increasing complexity: viruses → bacteria → fungi → parasites

VIRUSES

Viruses are strict intracellular parasites of other living cells, not only of mammalian and plant cells but also of simple unicellular organisms, including bacteria (the bacteriophages). Viruses are simple forms of replicating, biologically active particles that carry genetic information in either DNA or RNA molecules. Most mature viruses have a protein coat over their nucleic acid and, sometimes, a lipid surface membrane derived from the cell they infect. Because viruses lack the protein-synthesizing enzymes and structural apparatus necessary for their own replication, they bear essentially no resemblance to a true eukaryotic or prokaryotic cell.

Viruses contain little more than DNA or RNA

TABLE 1–1	Features of Infectious Agents			
	VIRUSES	**BACTERIA**	**FUNGI**	**PARASITES**
Size (μm)	<1	2-8	4+	2+
Cell wall	No	Yes	Yes	No/Yes[a]
Cell plan	None	Prokaryotic	Eukaryotic	Eukaryotic
Free living	No	Yes[b]	Yes	Yes
Intracellular	Yes	No/Yes	No	No/Yes[c]

[a]Parasitic cysts have cell walls.
[b]A few bacteria grow only within cells.
[c]The life cycle of some parasites includes intracellular multiplication.

FIGURE 1–3. **Infectious agents. A.** Virus. **B.** Bacterium. **C.** Fungus. **D.** Parasite. (Reproduced with permission from Willey JM: *Prescott, Harley, & Klein's Microbiology*, 7th ed. New York, NY: McGraw Hill; 2008.)

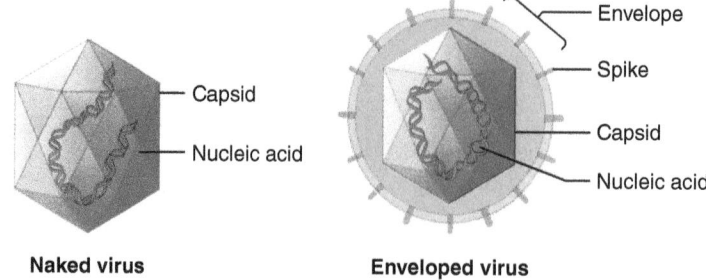

Naked virus   **Enveloped virus**

A

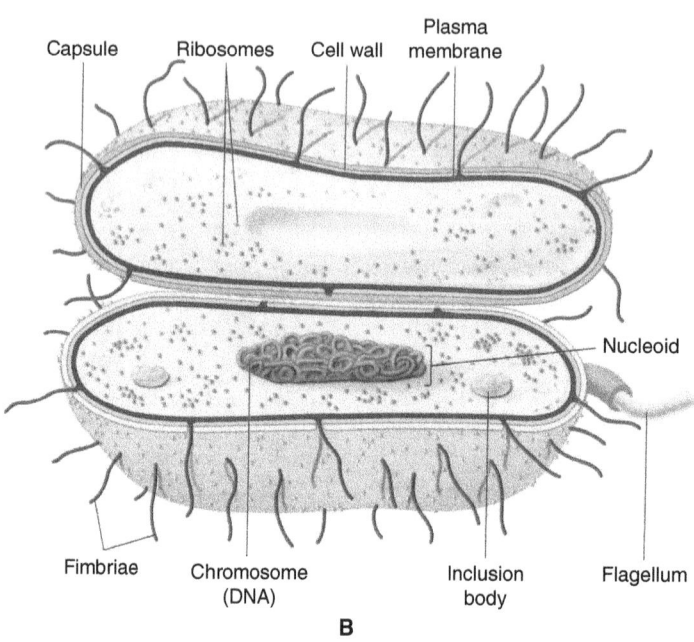

B

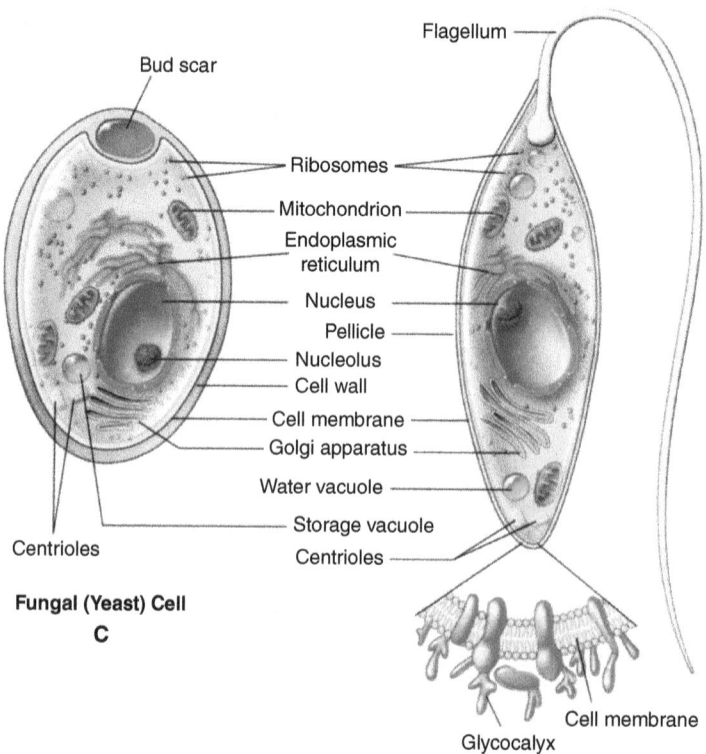

Fungal (Yeast) Cell
C

Protozoan Cell
D

Viruses replicate by using their own genes to direct the metabolic activities of the cell they infect to bring about the synthesis and reassembly of their component parts. A cell infected with a single viral particle may, thus, yield thousands of viral particles, which can be assembled almost simultaneously under the direction of the viral nucleic acid. Infection of other cells by the newly formed viruses occurs either by seeding from or lysis of the infected cells. Sometimes, viral and cell reproduction proceed simultaneously without cell death, although cell physiology may be affected. The close association of the virus with the cell sometimes results in the integration of viral nucleic acid into the functional nucleic acid of the cell, producing a latent infection that can be transmitted intact to the progeny of the cell.

Replication by control of the host cell metabolic machinery

Some integrate into genome

BACTERIA

Bacteria are the smallest (0.1-0 µm) independently living agents known. They have a cytoplasmic membrane surrounded by a cell wall; a unique interwoven polymer called peptidoglycan makes the wall rigid. The simple prokaryotic cell plan includes no mitochondria, lysosomes, endoplasmic reticulum, or other organelles (**Table 1–2**). In fact, most bacteria are approximately the size of mitochondria. Their cytoplasm contains only ribosomes and a single, double-stranded DNA chromosome. Bacteria have no nucleus, but all the chemical elements of nucleic acid and protein synthesis are present. Although their nutritional requirements vary greatly, most bacteria are free living if given an appropriate energy source. Tiny metabolic factories, they divide by binary fission and can be grown in artificial culture, producing progeny sometimes in a matter of hours. The Archaea are similar to bacteria but evolutionarily distinct. They are prokaryotic, but they differ in the chemical structure of their cell walls and other features. The Archaea (archebacteria) can live in environments humans consider hostile (eg, hot springs, high salt areas) but are not associated with disease.

Smallest living cells

Prokaryotic plan lacks nucleus, organelles

FUNGI

Fungi exist in either yeast or mold forms. The smallest of yeasts are similar in size to bacteria, but most are larger (2-12 µm) and multiply by budding. Molds form tubular extensions called hyphae, which, when linked together in a branched network, form the fuzzy structure seen on neglected bread slices. Fungi are eukaryotic, and both yeasts and molds have a rigid external cell wall composed of their own unique polymers, called glucan, mannan, and chitin. Their genome may exist in a diploid or haploid state and replicate by meiosis or simple mitosis. Most fungi are free living and widely distributed in nature. Generally, fungi grow more slowly than bacteria, although their growth rates sometimes overlap.

Yeasts and molds surrounded by cell wall

PARASITES

Parasites are the most diverse of all microorganisms. They range from unicellular amoebas of 10 to 12 µm to multicellular tapeworms 1 m long. The individual cell plan is eukaryotic, but organisms such as worms are highly differentiated and have their own organ systems. Most worms have

Range from tiny amoebas to meter-long worms

TABLE 1–2	Distinctive Features of Prokaryotic and Eukaryotic Cells	
CELL COMPONENT	**PROKARYOTES**	**EUKARYOTES**
Nucleus	No membrane, single circular chromosome	Membrane bounded, a number of individual chromosomes
Extrachromosomal DNA	Often present in form of plasmid(s)	In organelles
Organelles in cytoplasm	None	Mitochondria (and chloroplasts in photosynthetic organisms)
Cytoplasmic membrane	Contains enzymes of respiration; active secretion of enzymes; site of phospholipid and DNA synthesis	Semipermeable layer not possessing functions of prokaryotic membrane
Cell wall	Rigid layer of peptidoglycan (absent in Mycoplasma)	No peptidoglycan (in some cases cellulose present)
Sterols	Absent (except in Mycoplasma)	Usually present
Ribosomes	70 S in cytoplasm	80 S in cytoplasmic reticulum

a microscopic egg or larval stage, and part of their life cycle may involve multiple vertebrate and invertebrate hosts. Most parasites are free living, but some depend on combinations of animal, arthropod, or crustacean hosts for their survival.

● THE HUMAN MICROBIOTA

Before moving on to discuss how, when, and where the previously mentioned agents cause human disease, we should note that the presence of microbes on or in humans is not, by itself, abnormal. In fact, from shortly after birth onward, it is universal; we harbor 10 times more microbial cells than human cells. This population, formerly called the normal flora, is now referred to as our **microbiota** or **microbiome**. These microorganisms, which are overwhelmingly bacteria, are frequently found colonizing various body sites in healthy individuals. The constituents and numbers of the microbiota vary in different areas of the body and, sometimes, at different ages and physiologic states. Their names are mostly unfamiliar because they have not (yet) been associated with disease. They comprise microorganisms whose morphologic, physiologic, and genetic properties allow them to colonize and multiply under the conditions that exist in particular sites, to coexist with other colonizing organisms, and to inhibit competing intruders. Thus, each accessible area of the body presents a particular ecologic niche, colonization of which requires a particular set of properties of the colonizing microbe.

Organisms of the microbiota may have a symbiotic relationship that benefits the host or may simply live as commensals with a neutral relationship to the host. A parasitic relationship that injures the host would not be considered "normal," but, in most instances, not enough is known about the organism–host interactions to make such distinctions. Some have been characterized by genomic methods but not yet grown in culture. Like houseguests, the members of the microbiota may stay for highly variable periods. **Residents** are strains that have an established niche at one of the many body sites, which they occupy indefinitely. **Transients** are acquired from the environment and establish themselves briefly, but they tend to be excluded by competition from residents or by the host's innate or immune defense mechanisms. The term **carrier state** is used when organisms known to be potentially pathogenic are involved, although its implication of risk is not always justified. For example, *Streptococcus pneumoniae,* a cause of pneumonia, and *Neisseria meningitidis,* a cause of meningitis, may be isolated from the throat of 5% to 40% of healthy people. Whether these bacteria represent transient flora, resident flora, or carrier state is largely semantic. The possibility that their presence could be the prelude to disease is presently impossible to determine in advance.

It is important for students of medical microbiology and infectious disease to understand the role of the microbiota because of its significance both as a defense mechanism against infection and as a source of potentially pathogenic organisms. In addition, it is important for physicians to know the typical composition of the microbiota at various sites to avoid confusion when interpreting laboratory culture results. The following excerpt indicates that the English poet W.H. Auden understood the need for balance between the microbiota and its host. He was stimulated by a 1969 article by Mary J. Marples in *Scientific American* about the microbial flora of the skin.

> On this day tradition allots
>   to taking stock of our lives,
> my greetings to all of you, Yeasts,
>   Bacteria, Viruses,
> Aerobics and Anaerobics:
>   A Very Happy New Year
> to all for whom my ectoderm
>   is as Middle Earth to me.
>
> For creatures your size I offer
>   a free choice of habitat,
> so settle yourselves in the zone
>   that suits you best, in the pools

> of my pores or the tropical
>   forests of arm-pit and crotch,
> in the deserts of my fore-arms,
>   or the cool woods of my scalp.
>
> Build colonies: I will supply
>   adequate warmth and moisture,
> the sebum and lipids you need,
>   on condition you never
> do me annoy with your presence,
>   but behave as good guests should,
> not rioting into acne
>   or athlete's-foot or a boil.

—W.H. Auden, "A New Year Greeting"

Flora may stay for short or extended periods

If pathogens involved, the relationship is called the carrier state

ORIGIN AND NATURE

The healthy fetus is sterile until the birth membranes rupture. During and after birth, the infant is exposed to the flora of the mother's vagina and to other organisms in the environment. During the infant's first few days of life, the microbiota reflects chance exposure to organisms that can colonize particular sites in the absence of competitors. Subsequently, as the infant is exposed to a broader range of organisms, those best adapted to colonize particular sites become predominant. Thereafter, the flora generally resembles that of other individuals in the same age group and cultural milieu.

Local physiologic and ecologic conditions determine the microbial makeup of the microbiota. These conditions are sometimes highly complex, differing from site to site, and sometimes with age. Conditions include the amounts and types of nutrients available, pH, oxidation–reduction potentials, and resistance to local antibacterial substances, such as bile and lysozyme. Many bacteria have adhesin-mediated affinity for receptors on specific types of epithelial cells; this facilitates colonization and multiplication and prevents removal by the flushing effects of surface fluids and peristalsis. Various microbial interactions also determine their relative prevalence in the flora. These interactions include competition for nutrients and inhibition by the metabolic products of other organisms.

Initial flora acquired during and immediately after birth

Physiologic conditions influence colonization

Adherence counteracts mechanical flushing

Must compete for nutrients

MICROBIOTA AT DIFFERENT SITES

At any one time, the microbiota of a single person contains thousands of species of microorganisms, mostly bacteria. The major members known to be important in preventing or causing disease, as well as those that may be confused with etiologic agents of local infections, are summarized in **Table 1–3** and are described in greater detail in subsequent chapters.

■ Blood, Body Fluids, and Tissues

In health, the blood, body fluids, and tissues are sterile. Occasional organisms may be displaced across epithelial barriers as a result of trauma or during childbirth; they may be briefly

TABLE 1–3	Predominant and Potentially Pathogenic Microbiota of Various Body Sites	
BODY SITE	**POTENTIAL PATHOGENS (CARRIER)**	**LOW VIRULENCE (RESIDENT)**
Blood	None	None[a]
Tissues	None	None
Skin	*Staphylococcus aureus*	*Propionibacterium, Corynebacterium* (diphtheroids), coagulase-negative staphylococci
Mouth	*Candida albicans*	*Neisseria* spp., viridans streptococci, *Moraxella, Peptostreptococcus*
Nasopharynx	*Streptococcus pneumoniae, Neisseria meningitidis, Haemophilus influenzae,* group A streptococci, *Staphylococcus aureus* (anterior nares)	*Neisseria* spp., viridans streptococci, *Moraxella, Peptostreptococcus*
Stomach	None	Streptococci, *Peptostreptococcus,* others from mouth
Small intestine	None	Scanty, variable
Colon	*Bacteroides fragilis, E coli, Pseudomonas, Candida, Clostridium (C perfringens, C difficile)*	*Eubacterium, Lactobacillus, Bacteroides, Fusobacterium,* Enterobacteriaceae, *Enterococcus, Clostridium*
Vagina		
Prepubertal and postmenopausal	*Candida albicans*	Diphtheroids, staphylococci, Enterobacteriaceae
Childbearing	Group B streptococci, *C albicans*	*Lactobacillus,* streptococci

[a]Organisms such as viridans streptococci may be transiently present after disruption of a mucosal site.

recoverable from the bloodstream before they are filtered out in the pulmonary capillaries or removed by cells of the reticuloendothelial system. Such transient bacteremia may be the source of infection when structures such as damaged heart valves and foreign bodies (prostheses) are in the bloodstream.

Tissues, body fluids, blood are sterile

■ Skin

The skin surface provides a dry, slightly acidic, aerobic environment. It plays host to an abundant flora that varies according to the presence of its appendages (hair, nails) and the activity of sebaceous and sweat glands. The flora is more abundant on moist skin areas (axillae, perineum, and between toes). Staphylococci and members of the *Propionibacterium* genus occur all over the skin, and facultative *Corynebacterium* species are found in moist areas. *Propionibacterium* species are slim, anaerobic, or microaerophilic Gram-positive rods that grow in subsurface sebum and break down skin lipids to fatty acids. Thus, they are most numerous in the ducts of hair follicles and of the sebaceous glands that drain into them. Even with antiseptic scrubbing, it is difficult to eliminate bacteria from skin sites, particularly those bearing pilosebaceous units. Organisms of the skin flora are resistant to the bactericidal effects of skin lipids and fatty acids, which inhibit or kill many extraneous bacteria. The conjunctivae have a very scanty flora derived from the skin. The low bacterial count is influenced by the high lysozyme content of lachrymal secretions and the flushing effect of tears.

Propionibacteria, staphylococci dominant bacteria

Skin flora is not easily removed

■ Intestinal Tract

The **mouth** and **pharynx** contain large numbers of facultative and anaerobic bacteria. Different species of streptococci predominate on the buccal and tongue mucosa because of different specific adherence characteristics. Other genera include *Actinomyces*, *Bacteroides*, *Fusobacterium*, and *Corynebacterium*. Strict anaerobes and microaerophilic organisms of the oral cavity have their niches in the depths of the gingival crevices surrounding the teeth and in sites such as tonsillar crypts, where anaerobic conditions can develop readily. The role of the oral microbiome in dental infections is addressed in Chapter 41.

Oropharynx has streptococci and anaerobes

The total number of organisms in the oral cavity is very high, and it varies from site to site. Saliva usually contains a mixed flora of about 10^8 organisms per milliliter, derived mostly from the various epithelial colonization sites. The genera include *Actinomyces*, *Bacteroides*, *Prevotella*, *Streptococcus*, and others. The stomach contains few, if any, resident organisms in health because of the lethal action of gastric hydrochloric acid and peptic enzymes on bacteria. One species, *H pylori*, long thought to be a common resident, is now known to be the primary cause of ulcers. The small intestine has a scanty resident flora, except in the lower ileum, where it begins to resemble that of the colon.

H pylori turned out to be a stomach pathogen

Small intestinal flora is scanty but increases toward lower ileum

The colon carries the most abundant and diverse microbiota in the body. In the adult, feces are 25% or more bacteria by weight (about 10^{10} organisms per gram). More than 90% are anaerobes, predominantly members of the genera *Bacteroides*, *Fusobacterium*, *Eubacterium*, and *Clostridium*. The remainder of the flora is composed of facultative organisms, such as *Escherichia coli*, enterococci, yeasts, and numerous other species. There are considerable differences in adult flora depending on the diet of the host. Those whose diets include substantial amounts of meat have more *Bacteroides* and other anaerobic Gram-negative rods in their stools than those on a predominantly vegetable or fish diet. Due to its ability to form spores, *Clostridioides difficile* is able to survive and multiply in association with antimicrobial therapy, causing a life-threatening colitis. Recent studies have suggested the composition of the colonic microbiota could play a role in obesity.

Colonic flora predominantly anaerobic

C difficile causes colitis

■ Respiratory Tract

The external 1 cm of the anterior nares has a flora similar to that of the skin. This is the primary site of carriage of a major pathogen, *Staphylococcus aureus*. Approximately 25% to 30% of healthy people carry this organism as either resident or transient flora at any given time. The nasopharynx has a flora similar to that of the mouth; however, it is often the site of carriage of potentially pathogenic organisms, such as pneumococci, *Neisseria*, and *Haemophilus* species.

S aureus is carried in anterior nares

The respiratory tract below the level of the larynx is protected in health by the action of the epithelial cilia and by the movement of the mucociliary blanket; thus, only transient inhaled organisms are encountered in the trachea and larger bronchi. The accessory sinuses are normally sterile and are protected in a similar fashion, as is the middle ear by the epithelium of the eustachian tubes.

Lower tract is protected by mucociliary action

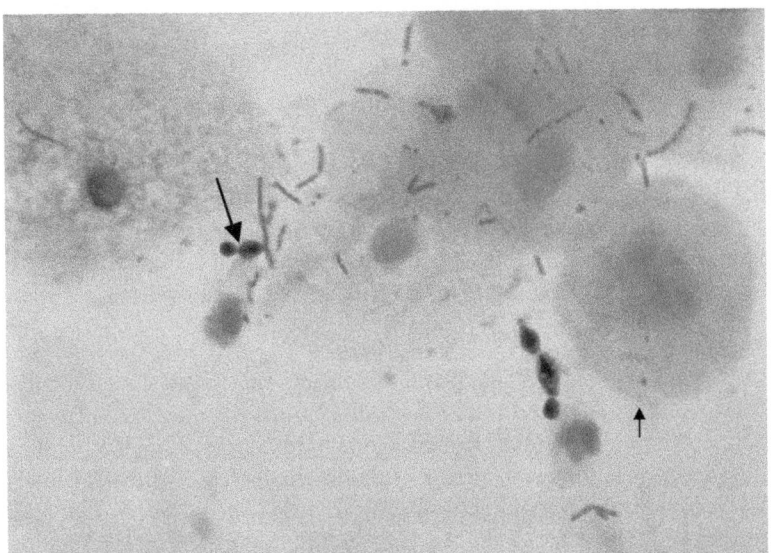

FIGURE 1–4. **Vaginal flora.** Vaginal Gram smear showing budding yeast (long arrow), epithelial cells (short arrow), and a mixture of other bacterial morphologies. The long Gram-positive rods are most likely lactobacilli. (Reproduced with permission from Centers for Disease Control and Prevention [CDC].)

■ Genitourinary Tract

The urinary tract is sterile in health above the distal 1 cm of the urethra, which has a scanty flora derived from the perineum. Thus, in health, the urine in the bladder, ureters, and renal pelvis is sterile. The vagina has a flora that varies according to hormonal influences at different ages. Before puberty and after menopause, it is mixed, nonspecific, and relatively scanty, and it contains organisms derived from the flora of the skin and colon. During the childbearing years, it is composed predominantly of anaerobic and microaerophilic members of the genus *Lactobacillus,* with smaller numbers of anaerobic Gram-negative rods, Gram-positive cocci, and yeasts (**Figure 1–4**) that can survive under the acidic conditions produced by the lactobacilli. These conditions develop because glycogen is deposited in vaginal epithelial cells under the influence of estrogenic hormones and metabolized to lactic acid by lactobacilli. This process results in a vaginal pH of 4 to 5, which is optimal for growth and survival of the lactobacilli but inhibits many other organisms.

Hormonal changes affect the vaginal flora

Use of epithelial glycogen by lactobacilli produces low pH

Bacterial Vaginosis

Bacterial vaginosis (BV) is a long known and unfortunately common syndrome which is still poorly understood. Its dominant feature is an uncomfortable vaginal discharge with a "fishy" odor, which contains epithelial cells coated with bacteria (clue cells). This change is associated with a shift in the vaginal microbiota away from the acidic *Lactobacillus* flora to one with a higher pH and a greater mixture of species including more anaerobes. Over the years, several of these newcomers have been tagged as the cause of BV, particularly *Gardnerella vaginalis* and *Mobiluncus.* The BV situation appears to be more complex than this, involving complex interactions of the vaginal microbiota.

BV is associated with a shift in vaginal microbiota

ROLES IN HEALTH AND DISEASE

■ Opportunistic Infection

Many species among the microbiota are opportunists in that they can cause infection when they reach protected areas of the body in sufficient numbers. For example, certain strains of *E coli* can reach the urinary bladder by ascending the urethra and cause acute urinary tract infection. Perforation of the colon from a ruptured diverticulum or a penetrating abdominal wound releases feces into the peritoneal cavity; this contamination may be followed by peritonitis or intraabdominal abscesses caused by members of the flora which have virulence factors allowing them to exploit this situation. There are now examples of the microbiota supplying a step in the pathogenesis of a classic pathogen. Attachment of *Neisseria gonorrhoeae* to the cervix has been shown to be enhanced when an enzyme produced by the cervicovaginal microbiota unmasks a crucial receptor. Caries and periodontal disease are caused by organisms that are members of the oral microbiota (see Chapter 41).

Flora that reach sterile sites may cause disease

Virulence factors increase opportunity for invasion

■ Exclusionary Effect

Balancing the prospect of opportunistic infection is the tendency of the resident microbiota to produce conditions that compete with extraneous newcomers who happen to be pathogens and thus reduce their ability to establish a niche in the host. The microbiota in the colon of the breast-fed infant produces an environment inimical to colonization by enteric pathogens, as does a vaginal flora dominated by lactobacilli. The benefit of this exclusionary effect has been demonstrated by what happens when it is removed. Antibiotic therapy, particularly with broad-spectrum agents, may so alter the microbiota of the gastrointestinal tract that antibiotic-resistant organisms multiply in the ecologic vacuum as in the *C difficile* toxic colitis discussed above.

■ Priming of Immune System

Organisms of the microbiota play an important role in the development of immunologic competence. Animals delivered and raised under completely aseptic conditions ("sterile" or gnotobiotic animals) have a poorly developed reticuloendothelial system, low serum levels of immunoglobulins, and lack antibodies to antigens that often confer a degree of protection against pathogens. There is evidence of immunologic differences between children who are raised under usual conditions and those whose exposure to diverse flora is minimized. Some studies have found a higher incidence of immunopathologic states, such as asthma in the more isolated children.

PROMOTING A GOOD MICROBIOTA

The field of probiotics is based on the notion that we can manipulate the microbiota by promoting colonization with "good" bacteria. Elie Metchnikoff originally suggested this in his observation that the longevity of Bulgarian peasants was attributable to their consumption of large amounts of yogurt; the live lactobacilli in the yogurt presumably replaced the colonic flora to the general benefit of their health. This notion persists today in capsules containing freeze-dried lactobacilli sold by the sizable probiotics industry and by promotion of the health benefit of natural (unpasteurized) yogurt, which contains live lactobacilli. Because these lactobacilli are adapted to food and not the intestine, they are unlikely to persist, much less replace, the typical microbiota of the adult colon. In some clinical studies, administration of preparations containing a particular strain of *Lactobacillus* (*Lactobacillus rhamnosus* strain GG, LGG) has been shown to reduce the duration of rotavirus diarrhea in children. The use of similar preparations to prevent relapses of antibiotic-associated diarrhea caused by *C difficile* has shown little success, but fecal transplant (a whole new microbiota) has blocked recurrences of pseudomembranous colitis, the most serious form of this disease.

Research into the role of the microbiota in health and disease is one of the most exciting topics in science. The Human Microbiome Project funded by the US National Institutes of Health is by no means limited to topics related to infectious disease. Currently, the most active areas involve mechanisms of obesity, autoimmune disorders (arthritis, asthma), and more subjective subjects like human cravings. Much of the work involves the interactions between multiple species many of which can only be detected by genomic methods. Obviously, it is going to take considerable time to sort these relationships out.

● INFECTIOUS DISEASE

Of the thousands of species of viruses, bacteria, fungi, and parasites, only a tiny portion is involved in disease of any kind. These are called **pathogens.** There are plant pathogens, animal pathogens, and fish pathogens, as well as the subject of this book, human pathogens. Among pathogens, there are degrees of potency called **virulence,** which sometimes makes drawing the dividing line between benign and virulent microorganisms difficult. Pathogens are associated with disease with varying frequency and severity. *Yersinia pestis,* the cause of plague, causes fulminant disease and death in 50% to 75% of persons who come in contact with it. Therefore, it is highly virulent. Understanding the basis of these differences in virulence is a fundamental goal of this book. The better students of medicine understand how a pathogen causes disease, the better they will be prepared to intervene and help their patients.

For any pathogen, the basic aspects of how it interacts with the host to produce disease can be expressed in terms of its epidemiology, pathogenesis, and immunity. Usually, our knowledge of one or more of these topics is incomplete. It is the task of the physician to relate these topics to the clinical aspects of disease and be prepared for new developments which clarify, or in some cases, alter them. We do not know everything, and not all of what we believe we know is correct.

Competing with pathogens has a protective effect

Antibiotic therapy may provide advantage for pathogens

Sterile animals have little immunity

Low exposure correlates with asthma

Intestinal lactobacilli may protect against diarrheal agents

Pathogens are rare

Virulence varies greatly

EPIDEMIOLOGY

Epidemiology is the "who, what, when, and where" of infectious diseases. The power of the science of epidemiology was first demonstrated by Semmelweis, who by careful analysis of statistical data alone determined how streptococcal puerperal fever is transmitted. He even devised a means to prevent transmission (handwashing) decades before the organism itself (*Streptococcus pyogenes*) was discovered. Since then, each organism has built its own profile of vital statistics. Some agents are transmitted by air, some by food, and others by insects; many spread by the person-to-person route. **Figure 1–5** presents some of the variables in this regard. Some agents occur worldwide, and others only in certain geographic locations or ecologic circumstances. Knowing how an organism gains access to its victim and spreads is crucial to understanding the disease. It is also essential in discovering the emergence of "new" diseases, whether they are truly new (HIV, COVID-19) or just recently discovered (Legionnaires disease). Solving mysterious outbreaks or recognizing new epidemiologic patterns have often pointed the way to the isolation of new agents.

Each agent has its own mode of spread

Epidemic spread and disease are facilitated by malnutrition, poor socioeconomic conditions, natural disasters, and hygienic inadequacy. Epidemics, caused by the introduction of new organisms of unusual virulence, often result in high morbidity and mortality rates. We are currently witnessing a new and extended COVID-19 pandemic, but the prospect of recurrence of old pandemic infections (influenza, cholera) remains. Modern times and technology have introduced new wrinkles to epidemiologic spread. Air travel has allowed diseases to leap continents even when they have very short incubation periods. The efficiency of the food industry has sometimes backfired when the distributed products are contaminated with infectious agents. The outbreaks of hamburger-associated *E coli* O157:H7 bloody diarrhea and hemolytic uremic syndrome are examples. The nature of massive meat-packing facilities allowed organisms from infected cattle on isolated farms to be mixed with other meat and distributed rapidly and widely. By the time outbreaks were recognized, cases of disease were widespread, and tons of meat had to be recalled. In simpler times, local outbreaks from the same source might have been detected and contained more quickly.

Poor socioeconomic conditions foster infection

Modern society may facilitate spread

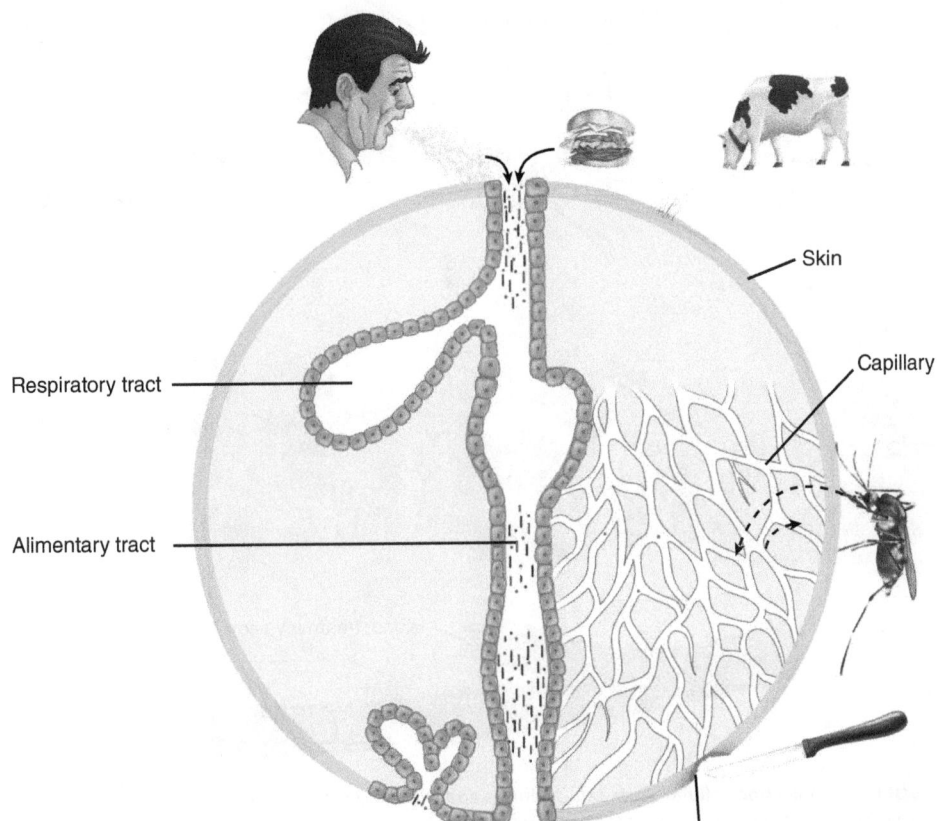

FIGURE 1–5. **Infection overview.** The sources and potential sites of infection are shown. Infection may be endogenous from the internal flora or exogenous from the sources shown around the outside.

Skin

Capillary

Respiratory tract

Alimentary tract

Scratch, injury

Of course, the most ominous and uncertain epidemiologic threat of these times is not amplification of natural transmission but the specter of unnatural, deliberate spread. Anthrax is a disease uncommonly transmitted by direct contact with animals or animal products. Under natural conditions, it produces a nasty, but not usually life-threatening, ulcer. The inhalation of human-produced aerosols of anthrax spores could produce a lethal pneumonia on a massive scale. Smallpox is the only disease officially eradicated from the world. It took place sufficiently long ago that most of the population has never been exposed or immunized and is, thus, vulnerable to its reintroduction. We do not know whether infectious bioterrorism will work on the scale contemplated by its perpetrators; however, in the case of anthrax, we do know that sophisticated systems have been designed to attempt it. We hope never to learn whether bioterrorism will work on a large scale.

Anthrax and smallpox are new bioterrorism threats

PATHOGENESIS

When a potential pathogen reaches its host, features of the organism determine whether or not disease ensues. The primary reason pathogens are so few in relation to the microbial world is that being successful at producing disease is a very complicated process. Multiple features, called virulence factors, are required to persist, cause disease, and escape to repeat the cycle. The variations are many, but the mechanisms used by many pathogens have now been dissected at the molecular level.

Pathogenicity is multifactorial

The first step for any pathogen is to attach and persist at whatever site it gains access. This usually involves specialized surface molecules or structures that correspond to receptors on human cells. Because human cells were not designed to receive the microorganisms, the pathogens are often exploiting some molecule important for some other essential function of the cell. For some toxin-producing pathogens, this attachment alone may be enough to produce disease. For most pathogens, it just allows them to persist long enough to proceed to the next stage—invasion into or beyond the surface mucosal cells. For viruses, invasion of cells is essential, because they cannot replicate on their own. Invading pathogens must also be able to adapt to a new milieu. For example, the nutrients and ionic environment of the cell surface differ from those inside the cell or in the submucosa. Some of the steps in pathogenesis at the cellular level are illustrated in **Figure 1–6.**

Pathogens have molecules that bind to host cells

Invasion requires adaptation to new environments

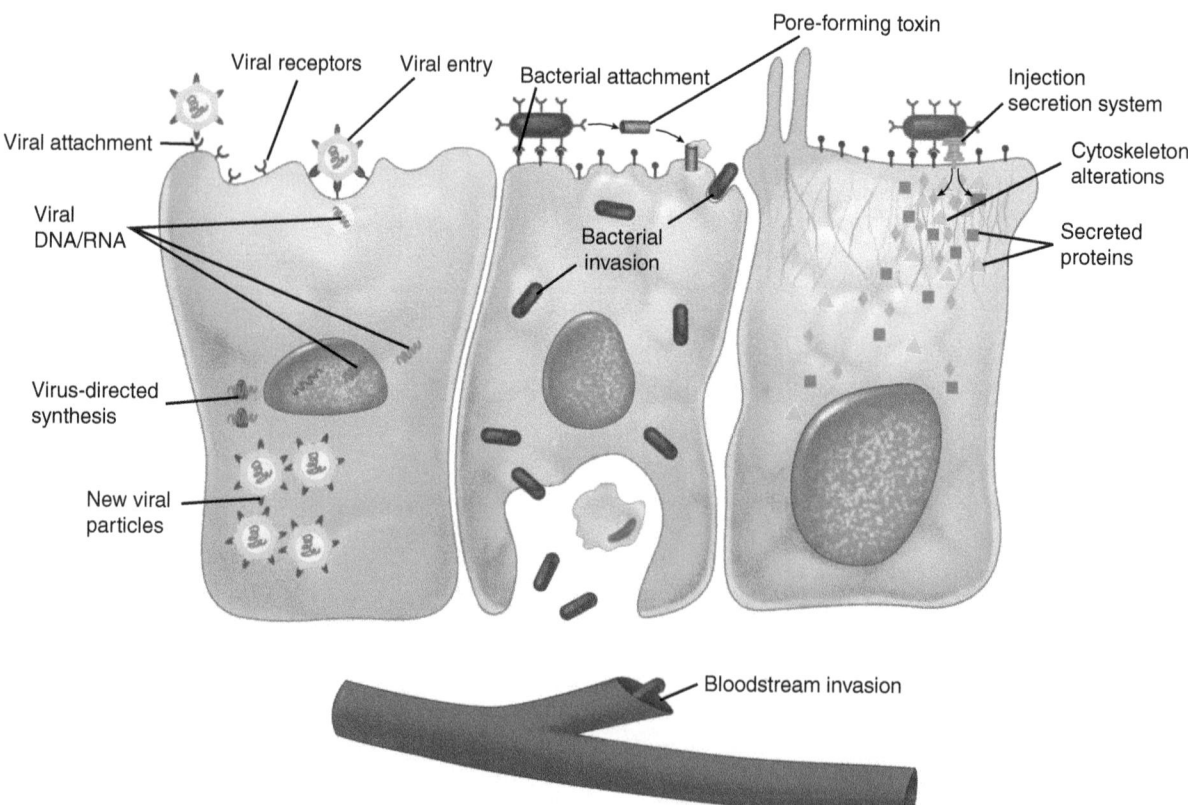

FIGURE 1–6. Infection cellular view. *Left.* A virus is attaching to the cell surface but can replicate only within the cell. *Middle.* A bacterial cell attaches to the surface, invades, and spreads through the cell to the bloodstream. *Right.* A bacterial cell attaches and injects proteins into the cell. The cell is disrupted while the organism remains on the surface.

Persistence and even invasion do not necessarily translate immediately to disease. The invading organisms must disrupt function in some way. For some, the inflammatory response they stimulate is enough. For example, a lung alveolus filled with neutrophils responding to the presence of *S pneumoniae* loses its ability to exchange oxygen. The longer a pathogen can survive in the face of the host response, the greater the compromise in host function. Most pathogens do more than this. Destruction of host cells through the production of digestive enzymes, toxins, or intracellular multiplication is among the more common mechanisms. Other pathogens operate by altering the function of a cell without injury. Diphtheria is caused by a bacterial toxin that blocks protein synthesis inside the host cell. Details of the molecular mechanism for this action are illustrated in **Figure 1–7.** Some viruses cause the insertion of molecules in the host cell membrane, which causes other host cells to attack it. The variations are diverse and fascinating.

Inflammation alone can result in injury

Cells may be destroyed or their function altered

IMMUNITY

Although the science of immunology is beyond the scope of this book, understanding the immune response to infection (see Chapter 2) is an important part of appreciating pathogenic mechanisms. In fact, one of the most important virulence attributes any pathogen can have

Evading the immune response is a major feature of virulence

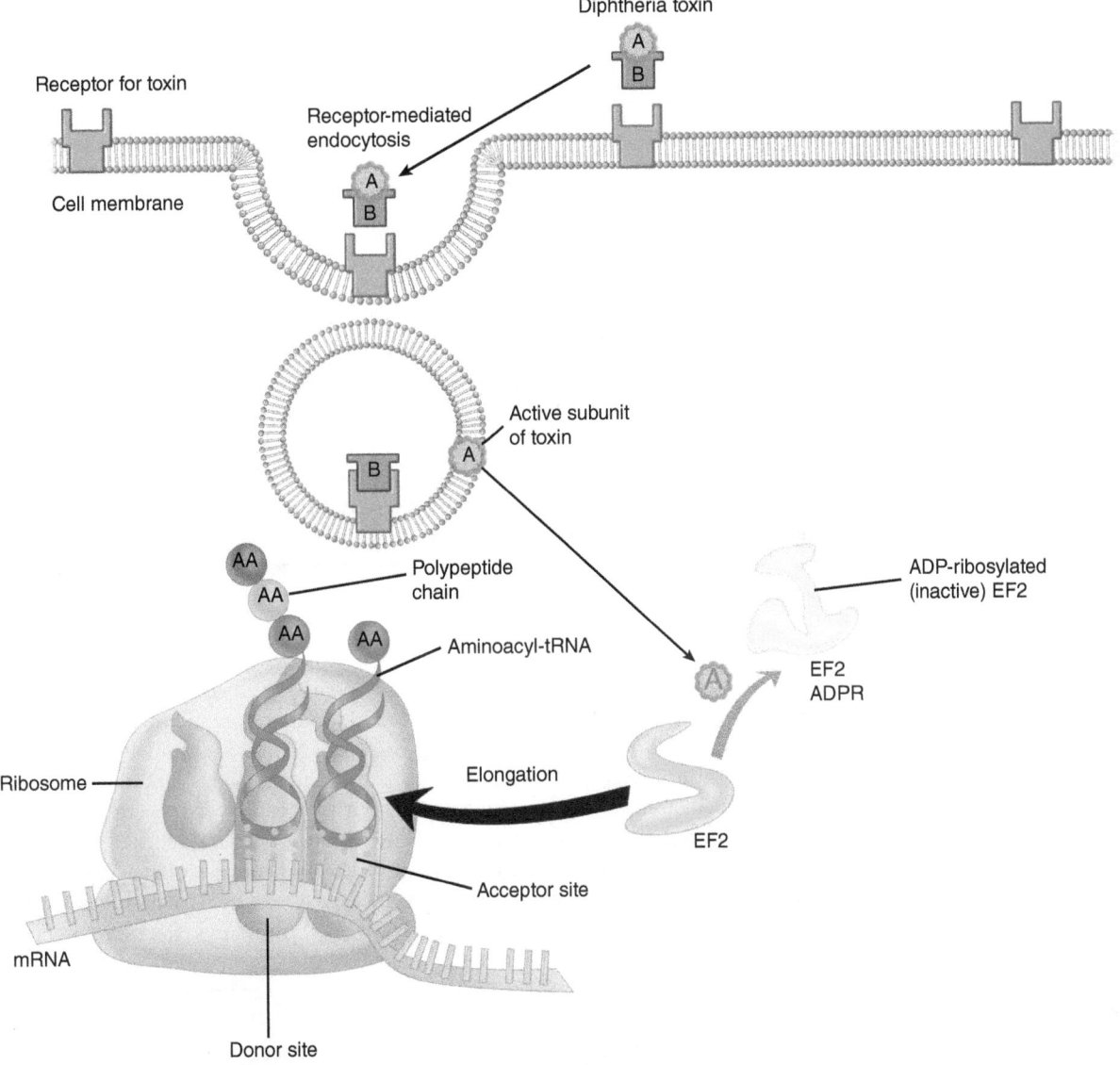

FIGURE 1–7. Action of diphtheria toxin, molecular view. The toxin-binding (B) portion attaches to the cell membrane, and the complete molecule enters the cell. In the cell, the A subunit dissociates and catalyzes a reaction that ADP-ribosylates (ADPR) and, thus, inactivates elongation factor 2 (EF-2). This factor is essential for ribosomal reactions at the acceptor and donor sites, which transfer triplet code from messenger RNA (mRNA) to amino acid sequences via transfer RNA (tRNA). Inactivation of EF-2 stops building of the polypeptide chain.

is an ability to neutralize the immune response to it in some way. Some pathogens attack the immune effector cells, and others undergo changes that evade the immune response. The old observation that there seems to be no immunity to gonorrhea turns out to be an example of the latter mechanism. *Neisseria gonorrhoeae*, the causative agent of gonorrhea, undergoes antigenic variation of important surface structures so rapidly that antibodies directed against the bacteria become irrelevant.

Antibody or cell-mediated mechanisms may be protective

For each pathogen, the primary interest is whether there is natural immunity and, if so, whether it is based on cell-mediated (T_H1, CMI) or humoral (T_H2, antibody) mechanisms. Humoral and CMI responses are broadly stimulated with most infections, but the specific response to a particular molecular structure is usually dominant in mediating immunity to reinfection. For example, the repeated nature of strep throat (group A *streptococcus*) in childhood is not due to antigenic variation as described above for gonorrhea. The antigen against which protective antibodies are directed (M protein) is stable, but naturally exists in more than 80 types. Each type requires its own specific antibody. Thus, even with a strong immune response the gauntlet is great. Identifying the specific molecular structure against which the protective immune response is directed is particularly important for devising preventive vaccines.

CLINICAL ASPECTS OF INFECTIOUS DISEASE

■ Manifestations

Fever, pain, and swelling are the universal signs of infection. Beyond this, the particular organs involved and the speed of the process dominate the signs and symptoms of disease. Cough, diarrhea, and mental confusion represent disruption of three different body systems. On the basis of clinical experience, physicians have become familiar with the range of behavior of the major pathogens. However, signs and symptoms overlap considerably. Skilled physicians use this knowledge to begin a deductive process leading to a list of suspected pathogens and a strategy to make a specific diagnosis and provide patient care. Through the probability assessment, an understanding of how the diseases work is a distinct advantage in making the correct decisions.

Body system(s) involved dictate clinical approach

■ Diagnosis

A major difference between infectious and other diseases is that the probabilities just described can be specifically resolved, often overnight. Most microorganisms can be isolated from the patient, grown in artificial culture, and identified. Others can be seen microscopically or detected by measuring the specific immune response to the pathogen. Preferred modalities for diagnosis of each agent have been developed and are available in clinics, hospitals, and public health laboratories all over the world. Empiric diagnosis made on the basis of clinical findings can be confirmed and the treatment plan modified accordingly. New methods which detect molecular or genomic markers of the agent are now realizing much greater application for rapid, specific diagnosis.

Disease-causing microbes can be identified by culture or genomics

■ Treatment

Over the past 80+ years, therapeutic tools of remarkable potency and specificity have become available for the treatment of bacterial infections. These include all the antibiotics and an array of synthetic chemicals that kill or inhibit the infecting organism but have minimal or acceptable toxicity for the host. Antibacterial agents exploit the structural and metabolic differences between microbial and human eukaryotic cells to provide the selectivity necessary for good antimicrobial therapy. Penicillin, for example, interferes with the synthesis of the bacterial cell wall, a structure that has no analog in human cells. There are fewer antifungal and antiprotozoal agents because the eukaryotic cells of the host and those of the parasite have metabolic and structural similarities. Nevertheless, hosts and parasites do have some significant differences, and effective therapeutic agents have been discovered or developed to exploit them.

Antibiotics are directed at structures of bacteria not present in host

Specific therapeutic attack on viral disease has posed more complex problems, because of the intimate involvement of viral replication with the metabolic and replicative activities of the cell. However, recent advances in molecular virology have identified specific viral targets that can be attacked. Scientists have developed successful antiviral agents, including those that interfere with viral attachment, the liberation of viral nucleic acid from its protective protein coat, or with the processes of viral nucleic acid synthesis and replication. The successful development of new agents for human immunodeficiency virus has involved targeting enzymes coded by the virus genome.

Antivirals target unique virus-coded enzymes

The success of the "antibiotic era" has been clouded by the development of resistance by the organisms. The mechanisms involved are varied but, most often, involve a mutational alteration in the enzyme, ribosome site, or other target against which the antimicrobial is directed. In some instances, organisms acquire new enzymes or block entry of the antimicrobial to the cell. Many bacteria produce enzymes that directly inactivate antibiotics. To make the situation worse, the genes involved are readily spread by promiscuous genetic mechanisms. New agents that are initially effective against resistant strains have been developed, but resistance by new mechanisms usually follows. The battle is by no means lost, but it has become a never-ending policing action.

Resistance complicates therapy

Mechanisms include mutation and inactivation

■ Prevention

The goal of the scientific study of any disease is its prevention. In the case of infectious diseases, this has involved public health measures and immunization. The public health measures depend on knowledge of transmission mechanisms and on interfering with them. Water disinfection, food preparation, insect control, handwashing, and a myriad of other measures prevent humans from coming in contact with infections agents. Immunization relies on knowledge of immune mechanisms and designing vaccines that stimulate protective immunity.

Public health and immunization are primary preventive measures

Immunization follows two major strategies—live vaccines and inactivated vaccines. The former uses live organisms that have been modified (attenuated) so they do not produce disease, but still stimulate a protective immune response. Such vaccines have been effective, but they carry the risk that the vaccine strain itself may cause disease. This event has been observed with the live oral polio vaccine. Although this rarely occurs, it has caused a shift back to the original Salk inactivated vaccine. This issue has reemerged with a debate over strategies for the use of smallpox immunization to protect against bioterrorism. This vaccine uses vaccinia virus, a cousin of smallpox, and its potential to produce disease on its own has been recognized since its original use by Jenner in 1798. Serious disease would be expected primarily in immunocompromised individuals (eg, from cancer chemotherapy or AIDS), who represent a significantly larger part of the population than when smallpox immunization was stopped in the 1970s. Could immunization cause more disease than it prevents? Despite the claims of those who oppose the use of all vaccines as "unnatural," the risk/benefit ratio of all currently licensed vaccines is greatly on the positive side.

Attenuated strains stimulate immunity

Live vaccines rarely cause disease

The safest immunization strategy is the use of organisms that have been killed or, better yet, killed and purified to contain only the immunizing component. This approach requires much better knowledge of pathogenesis and immune mechanisms. Vaccines for meningitis use the polysaccharide capsule of the bacterium, and vaccines for diphtheria and tetanus use only a formalin-inactivated protein toxin. Pertussis (whooping cough) immunization has undergone a transition in this regard. The original killed whole-cell vaccine was effective, but it caused a significant incidence of side effects. A purified vaccine containing pertussis toxin and a few surface components has reduced side effects, but its efficacy compared with the previous vaccine is now in question.

Purified components are safe vaccines

The newest approaches for vaccines require neither live organisms nor killed, purified ones. As the entire genomes of more and more pathogens are being reported, an entirely genetic strategy is emerging. Armed with knowledge of molecular pathogenesis and immunity and the tools of genomics and proteomics, scientists can now synthesize an immunogenic protein without ever growing the organism itself. Two of the most successful new COVID-19 vaccines use coded messenger RNA (mRNA) which instructs human cells to produce the immunogen. Such ideas would have astonished even the great microbiologists of the last two centuries.

Vaccines can be genetically engineered

SUMMARY

Infectious diseases remain as important and fascinating as ever. Where else do we find the emergence of new diseases, together with improved understanding of the old ones? At a time when the revolution in molecular biology and genetics has brought us to the threshold of new and novel means of infection control, the perpetrators of bioterrorism threaten us with diseases we have already conquered. Meeting this challenge requires a secure knowledge of the pathogenic organisms and how they produce disease, as well as an understanding of the clinical aspects of these diseases. In the collective judgment of the authors, this book presents the principles and facts required for students of medicine to understand the most important infectious diseases.

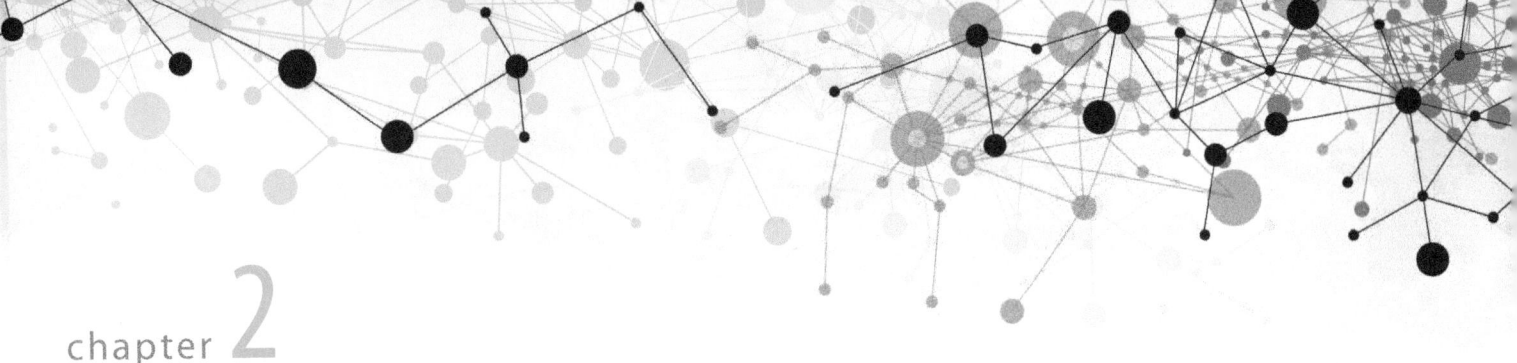

chapter 2

Immune Response to Infection

Within a very short period immunity has been placed in possession not only of a host of medical ideas of the highest importance, but also of effective means of combating a whole series of maladies of the most formidable nature in man and domestic animals.

—Elie Metchnikoff, 1905

The "maladies" Metchnikoff and the other pioneers of immunology were fighting were infections and, for decades, their field was defined in terms of the immune response to infection. We now understand that the immune system is as much a part of everyday human biologic function as the cardiovascular or renal systems. In its adaptive and disordered states, infectious diseases are only one of the major players along with cancer and autoimmune diseases. Students of medicine study immunology as a separate unit with its own textbook covering the field broadly. This chapter is not intended to fulfill that function, or, indeed, to be a shortened but comprehensive version of those sources. It is included as an overview of aspects related to infection for other students and as an internal reference for topics that reappear in later pages of this book. These include some of the greatest successes of medical science. The early and continuing development of vaccines that prevent and potentially eliminate diseases is but one example. In addition, knowledge of the immune response to infection is integral to understanding the pathogenesis of infectious diseases. It turns out that one of the main attributes of a successful pathogen is evading or confounding the immune system.

The immune response to infection is presented as two major components—innate immunity and adaptive immunity. The primary effectors of both are cells that are members of the white blood cell series derived from hematopoietic stem cells in the bone marrow (**Figure 2–1**). Innate immunity includes the role of physical, cellular, and chemical systems that are in place and that respond to all aspects of "foreignness." These include mucosal barriers, phagocytic cells, and the action of circulating glycoproteins such as complement. The adaptive side is sometimes called specific immunity because it has the ability to develop new responses that are highly specific to molecular components of infectious agents, called **antigens.** These encounters trigger the development of new cellular responses and production of circulating antibodies, which have a component of memory if the invader returns. Artificially creating this memory is, of course, the goal of vaccines.

● INNATE (NATURAL) IMMUNITY

Innate immunity acts through a series of specific and nonspecific mechanisms, all working to create a series of hurdles for the pathogen to navigate (**Table 2–1**). The first are mechanical barriers such as the tough multilayered skin or the softer but fused mucosal layers of internal surfaces. As discussed in Chapter 1, the microbiota on these surfaces present formidable competition for space and nutrients. Turbulent movement of the mucosal surfaces and enzymes or acid secreted

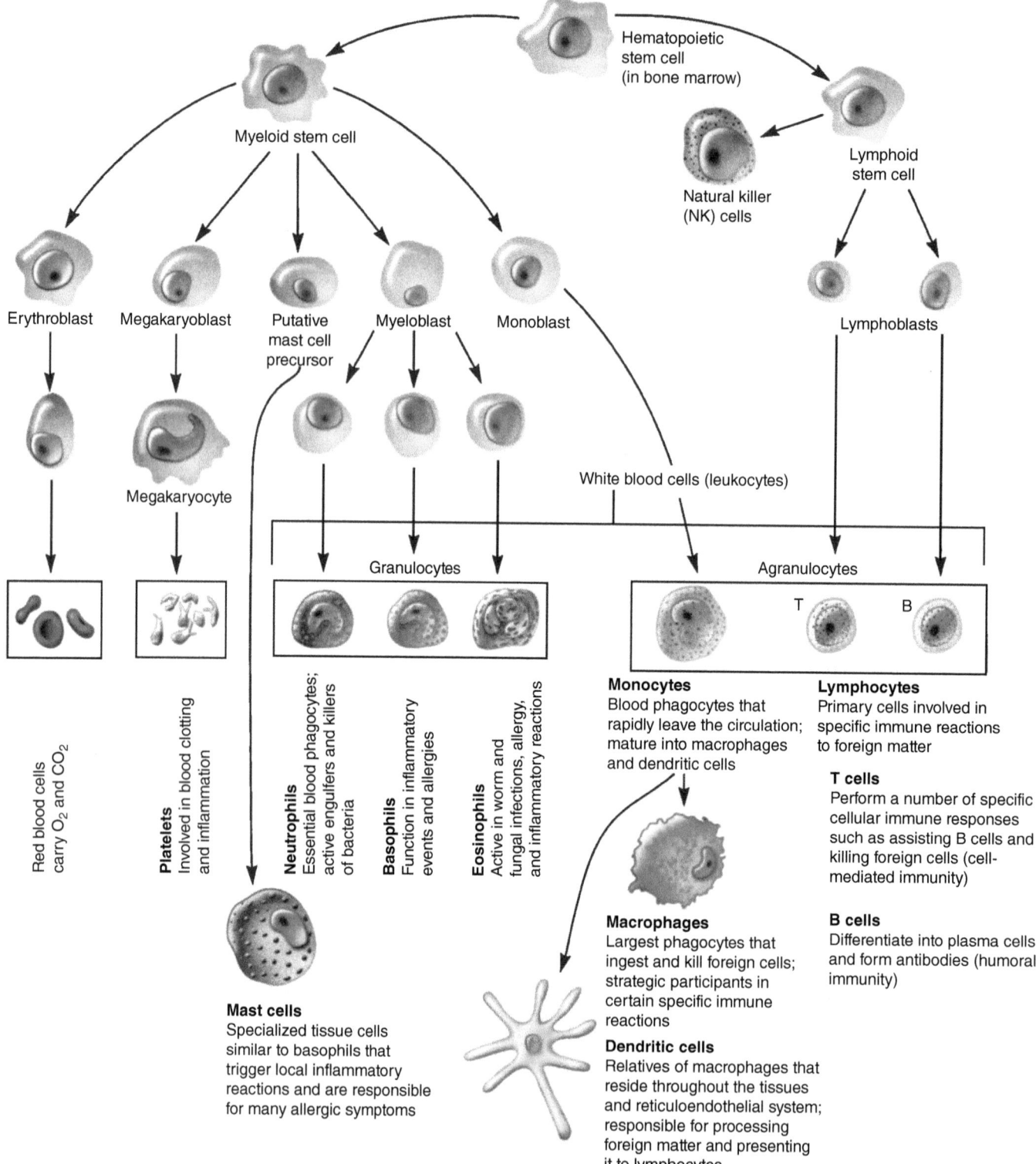

FIGURE 2-1. **Human blood cells.** Stem cells in the bone marrow divide to form two blood cell lineages: **(1)** the lymphoid stem cell gives rise to B cells that become antibody-secreting plasma cells, T cells that become activated T cells, and natural killer cells. **(2)** The common myeloid progenitor cell gives rise to granulocytes and monocytes that give rise to macrophages and dendritic cells. (Reproduced with permission from Willey JM: *Prescott, Harley, & Klein's Microbiology*, 7th ed. New York, NY: McGraw Hill; 2008.)

The following labels appear within the figure:

Hematopoietic stem cell (in bone marrow)

Myeloid stem cell

Natural killer (NK) cells

Lymphoid stem cell

Erythroblast

Megakaryoblast

Putative mast cell precursor

Myeloblast

Monoblast

Lymphoblasts

Megakaryocyte

White blood cells (leukocytes)

Granulocytes

Agranulocytes

T   B

Red blood cells carry O_2 and CO_2

Platelets
Involved in blood clotting and inflammation

Neutrophils
Essential blood phagocytes; active engulfers and killers of bacteria

Basophils
Function in inflammatory events and allergies

Eosinophils
Active in worm and fungal infections, allergy, and inflammatory reactions

Monocytes
Blood phagocytes that rapidly leave the circulation; mature into macrophages and dendritic cells

Lymphocytes
Primary cells involved in specific immune reactions to foreign matter

T cells
Perform a number of specific cellular immune responses such as assisting B cells and killing foreign cells (cell-mediated immunity)

B cells
Differentiate into plasma cells and form antibodies (humoral immunity)

Macrophages
Largest phagocytes that ingest and kill foreign cells; strategic participants in certain specific immune reactions

Dendritic cells
Relatives of macrophages that reside throughout the tissues and reticuloendothelial system; responsible for processing foreign matter and presenting it to lymphocytes

Mast cells
Specialized tissue cells similar to basophils that trigger local inflammatory reactions and are responsible for many allergic symptoms

TABLE 2–1	Features of Innate Immunity in Infection	
	LOCATION	**ACTIVITY AGAINST PATHOGENS**
Cells		
Macrophage	Circulation, tissues	Phagocytosis, digestion
Dendritic cell	Tissues	Phagocytosis, digestion
Polymorphonuclear neutrophil (PMN)	Circulation, tissues (by migration)	Phagocytosis, digestion
M cell	Mucous membranes	Endocytosis and delivery to phagocytes
Surface Receptors		
Lectin	Phagocyte	Recognize carbohydrates
Arginine-glycine-arginine (RGD)	Phagocyte	Recognize arginine-glycine-aspartic acid sequence
Toll-like receptor (TLR)	Phagocyte	Recognizes PAMP, such as bacterial LPS (TLR-4), peptidoglycan[a] (TLR-2)
Inflammation		
Selectins	Endothelium	Attract and attach PMNs
Integrins	PMNs	Attach to selectins
Kallikrein	Extracellular fluid	Release bradykinin, prostaglandins
Chemical Mediators		
Cathelicidin	PMNs, macrophages, epithelial cells	Ionic membrane pores
Defensins	PMN granules	Ionic membrane pores
Complement (classical, alternative, lectin)	Serum, extracellular fluid	Membrane pores, phagocyte receptors

LPS, of gram-negative bacterial outer membrane; PAMP, pathogen-associated molecular pattern.
[a]Cell wall component of gram-positive and gram-negative bacteria.

on their surface make it difficult for an organism to efficiently colonize. Organisms that are able to pass the mucosa encounter a population of cells with the ability to engulf and destroy them. In addition, body fluids contain chemical agents such as complement, which can directly injure the microbe. The entire process has cross-links to the adaptive immune system. The endpoint of phagocytosis and digestion in a macrophage is the presentation of the antigen on its surface, the first step in specific immune recognition.

Skin, mucosa are barriers

Cells engulf, digest, and present antigens from microbes

PHYSICAL BARRIERS

The thick layers of the skin containing insoluble keratins present the most formidable barrier to infection. The mucosal membranes of the alimentary and urogenital tract are not as tough but, often, are bathed in secretions inhospitable to invaders. Lysozyme is an enzyme that digests peptidoglycan—a unique structural component of the bacterial cell wall. Lysozyme is secreted onto many surfaces and is particularly concentrated in conjunctival tears. The acid pH of the vagina and particularly the stomach makes colonization difficult for most organisms. Only small particles (5-10 μm) can be inhaled deep into the lung alveoli because the lining of the respiratory tract includes cilia that trap and move them back toward the pharynx.

Lysozyme digests bacterial walls

Cilia move particles away from pulmonary alveoli

The skin and mucosal surfaces of the intestinal and respiratory tract also contain concentrations of lymphoid tissue within or just below their surfaces, which provide a next-level defense for invaders surviving the above-described barriers. These lymphoid collections are designed to entrap and deliver invaders to some of the phagocytes described in the following text. For example, in the intestine, M cells (**Figure 2–2**) that lack the villous brush border of their neighbors endocytose bacteria and then release them into a pocket containing macrophages and lymphocytic components (T and B cells) of the adaptive immune system. The enteric pathogen *Shigella flexneri* exploits this receptiveness of the M cell to attack the adjacent enterocytes from the side.

M cells deliver to macrophages and lymphocytes

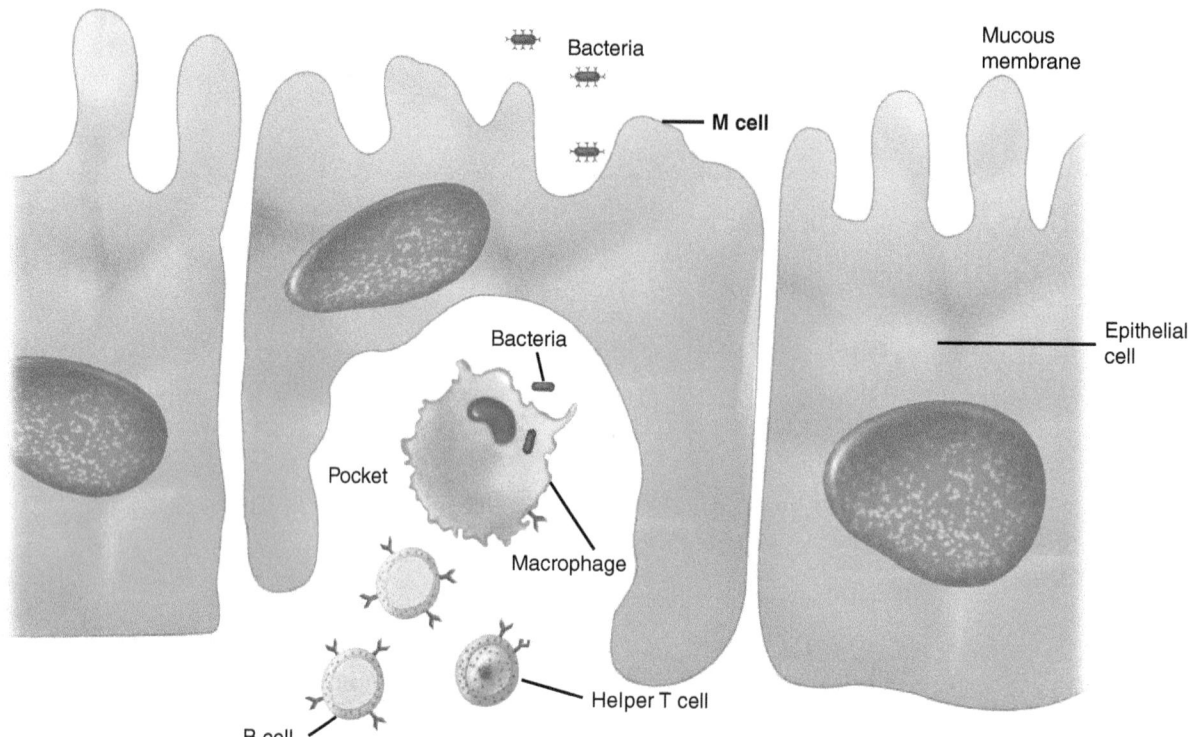

FIGURE 2–2. M cell. An M cell is shown between two epithelial cells in a mucous membrane. It has endocytosed a pathogen and released it into a pocket containing macrophages and other immune cells.

IMMUNORESPONSIVE CELLS AND ORGANS

Not all the cells shown in Figure 2–1 are involved in the immune system; of those that are, not all respond to infection. What the immune-responsive cells have in common is derivation from hematopoietic stem cells in the bone marrow, which create the myeloid and lymphoid series followed by further differentiation into their mature cell types. Of the types shown, the erythroblast and megakaryocyte do not participate in immune reactions. In the myeloid series, basophils and mast cells are primarily involved in allergic reactions rather than infection. Immuno-responsive cells are found throughout the body in the circulation or at fixed locations in tissues. They are concentrated in the lymph nodes and spleen, and form a unified filtration network designed as a sentinel warning system. In the lymphoid series, cells destined to become T cells mature in the thymus (the source of their name). Thus, the thymus, spleen, and lymph nodes might be thought of as the organs of the immune system. These are collectively referred to as the lymphoid tissues.

Stem cells differentiate to myeloid and lymphoid series

Thymus, spleen, and lymph nodes are immune organs

■ Cellular Receptors for Microbes

Fixed and circulating phagocytes express surface receptors which recognize a limited array of uniquely microbial structures based on the pattern of their molecular structure. These Pathogen-Associated Molecular Patterns (PAMPs) include bacterial cell wall peptidoglycan, the lipopolysaccharide (LPS, also called endotoxin) of Gram-negative bacteria, mannose and other glycoproteins, lipids, and polysaccharides. Nucleic acids are also recognized such as the double-stranded RNA found in many viruses. These PAMP-recognizing receptors may be found on the surface of phagocytes, dendritic cells, and specialized compartments called toll-like receptors (TLRs), of which 10 types have been described in humans and 12 in mice. The engagement of TLR receptors potentiates a signaling cascade that ultimately elicits the production of diverse antimicrobial cytokines specific to the TLR type.

Surface receptors recognize uniquely microbial PAMPs

Cytokine production triggered by TLRs

■ Antimicrobial Peptides

Antimicrobial peptides (AMPs) are small peptide molecules with natural antimicrobial effects. In mammals there are two major families of AMPs called cathelicidins and defensins. They are produced by multiple cell types including leukocytes, mast cells, dendritic cells, and platelets in response to tissue damage. They exhibit broad-spectrum activity against bacteria, fungi, parasites, and some enveloped viruses. Their antimicrobial action is by electrostatic interaction with microbial outer membranes, cytoplasmic membranes, and cell walls; these interactions result in membrane rupture, electrostatic potential disruption, and consequently, cell death. Some AMPs may also disrupt metabolic processes like nucleic acid and protein synthesis.

Cathelicidins and defensins bind and disrupt microbial surfaces

■ Cells Responding to Infection

Monocytes

Monocyte is a general morphologic term for cells that include or quickly (within hours) differentiate into macrophages or dendritic cells. These are the cells of the immune system that both phagocytose invaders and process them for presentation to the adaptive immune system. **Macrophages** are found in the circulation and tissues, where they are sometimes given regional names such as alveolar macrophage. They possess surface receptors rich in mannose and fructose, which nonspecifically recognize components commonly found on pathogens and more specialized receptors able to recognize unique components of microbes such as the LPS of Gram-negative bacteria. They also have receptors that recognize antibody and complement.

Macrophages in circulation or tissues

Surface receptors recognize pathogens

Dendritic cells have a distinctive star-like morphology, and are present in the skin and in the mucous membranes of the respiratory and intestinal tracts. Similar to macrophages, they phagocytose and present foreign antigens. They can also recognize PAMPs. After binding and phagocytosis, dendritic cells migrate to lymphoid tissues where specific adaptive immune responses are triggered. This interaction involving lymphocytes and T cells functions as a bridge between the innate and adaptive immune systems.

Star-like tissue phagocytes recognize PAMPs

In lymphoid tissues interact with adaptive immunity

Granulocytes

Of the cells in the granulocyte series, the most active is the **polymorphonuclear neutrophil** or **PMN.** These cells have a distinctive multilobed nucleus and cytoplasmic granules that contain lytic enzymes and antimicrobial substances including peroxidase, lysozyme, defensins, collagenase, and cathelicidins. PMNs have surface receptors for antibody and complement and are active phagocytes. In addition to the digestive enzymes, PMNs have other oxygen-dependent and oxygen-independent pathways for killing microorganisms. Unlike macrophages, they are largely circulatory and are not present in tissues except via migration as part of an acute inflammatory response.

PMNs have digestive and killing pathways

In circulation unless they migrate in inflammation

Eosinophils are nonphagocytic cells that participate in allergic reactions along with **basophils** and **mast cells.** Eosinophils are also involved in the defense against infectious parasites by releasing peptides and toxic reactive oxygen intermediates into the extracellular fluid, which are postulated to be damaging to parasite membranes.

Eosinophils damage parasites

Lymphocytes

Lymphocytes are the primary effector cells of the adaptive immune system. They are produced from a lymphocyte stem cell in the bone marrow and leave in a static state marked to become T, B, or null cells after further differentiation (**Figure 2–3**). This requires activation mediated by surface binding, which then stimulates further replication and differentiation.

T, B, and null cells initially static

B cells mature in the bone marrow and then circulate in the blood to lymphoid organs. At these sites, they may become activated to a form called a plasma cell, which produces antibodies. **T cells** mature in the thymus and then circulate awaiting activation. Their activation results in production of cytokines, which are effector molecules for multiple immunocytes and somatic cells. Some of the uncommitted null cells become **natural killer (NK) cells,** which have the capacity to directly kill cells infected with viruses by secreting IFN-γ.

B cells make antibody

T cells secrete cytokines

Phagocytosis

Phagocytosis is one of the most important defenses against microbial invaders (**Figure 2–4**). The major cells involved are PMNs, macrophages, and dendritic cells. For all, the process begins with surface–pathogen recognition mechanisms, which may be either dependent on opsonization of the organism with complement or antibody or independent of opsonization. At this point, only the opsonin-independent mechanisms are considered. These use the nonspecific mechanisms already described and hydrophobic interactions between bacteria and the phagocyte surface. More powerful killing mechanisms are mediated by **lectins,** which bind carbohydrate moieties, and protein–protein interactions based on a specific peptide sequence (arginine-glycine-aspartic-acid or RGD). These **RGD receptors** are present on virtually all phagocytes.

Opsonization not required

Carbohydrate and peptide sequence recognized

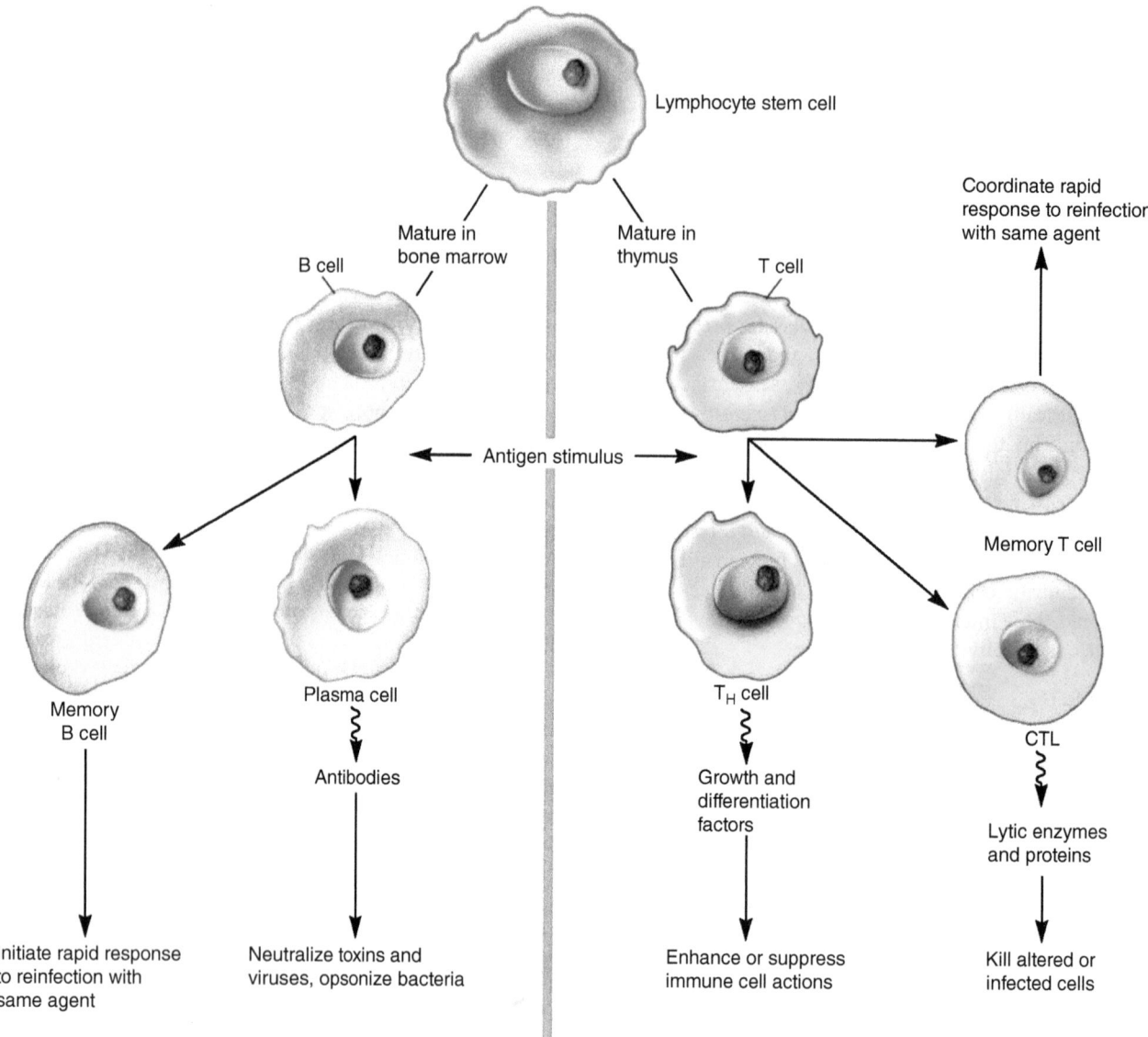

Lymphocyte stem cell

Mature in bone marrow

Mature in thymus

B cell

T cell

Coordinate rapid response to reinfection with same agent

Antigen stimulus

Memory T cell

Memory B cell

Plasma cell

T_H cell

CTL

Antibodies

Growth and differentiation factors

Lytic enzymes and proteins

Initiate rapid response to reinfection with same agent

Neutralize toxins and viruses, opsonize bacteria

Enhance or suppress immune cell actions

Kill altered or infected cells

FIGURE 2–3. B and T lymphocytes. B cells and T cells arise from the same cell lineage but diverge into two functional types. Immature B cells and T cells are indistinguishable by morphology. (Reproduced with permission from Willey JM: *Prescott, Harley, & Klein's Microbiology*, 7th ed. New York, NY: McGraw Hill; 2008.)

Bound organisms are taken inside the phagocyte in a membrane-bound phagosome destined to fuse with lysosomes inside to form a **phagolysosome.** This is the main killing ground of the phagocyte. The lysosomal enzymes include hydrolases and proteases that have maximum activity at the acidic pH inside the phagolysosome. In addition, the hostile intra-phagocyte environment includes oxidative killing mechanisms generated by enzymes that produce **reactive oxygen intermediates** (superoxide, hydrogen peroxide, singlet oxygen) driven by metabolic respiratory bursts in the cell cytoplasm. These mechanisms are particularly used for killing bacteria. Bacterial pathogens whose pathogenesis involves multiplication rather than destruction inside the phagocyte have mechanisms to block one or more of the preceding steps. For example, some pathogens (eg, *M tuberculosis* or *Brucella* sp) are able to block fusion of the phagosome with the lysosome; others (*Listeria* sp) interfere with the acidification of the phagolysosome, and many organisms employ both mechanisms.

Another mechanism effective with some viruses, fungi, and parasites is the formation of **reactive nitrogen intermediates** (nitric oxide, nitrate, and nitrite) delivered into a vacuole or in the cytoplasm. PMN granules contain a variety of other antimicrobial substances, including peptides called **defensins.** Defensins act by permeabilizing membranes and, in addition to bacteria, are active against enveloped viruses.

Enzymes digest in acidic phagolysosome

Reactive oxygen driven by respiratory burst

Reactive nitrogen affects viruses

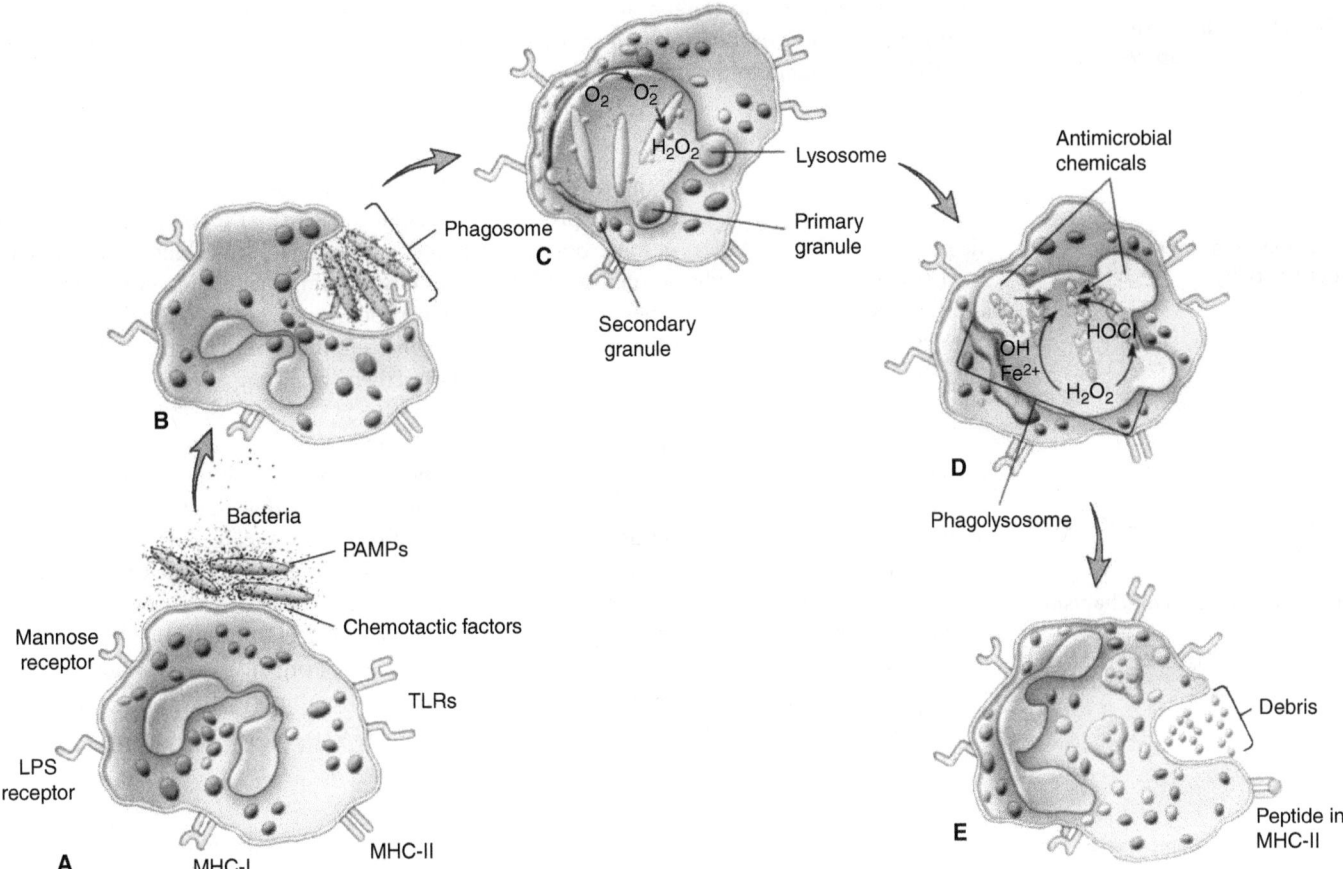

FIGURE 2–4. Phagocytosis. A. Drawing shows receptors on a phagocytic cell, such as a macrophage, and the corresponding PAMPs participating in phagocytosis. The schematic depicts the process of phagocytosis showing ingestion. **B.** Participation of primary and secondary granules. **C.** O_2-dependent killing events. **D.** Intracellular digestion. **E.** Endocytosis LPS receptor, lipopolysaccharide receptor; TLRs, toll-like receptors; MHCI, class I major histocompatibility protein; MHC II, class II major histocompatibility protein; PAMPs, pathogen-associated molecular patterns. (Reproduced with permission from Willey JM: *Prescott, Harley, & Klein's Microbiology*, 7th ed. New York, NY: McGraw Hill; 2008.)

INFLAMMATION

Inflammation encompasses a series of events in which the above-mentioned cells are deployed in response to an injury—such as a new microbial invader. At the first insult, chemical signals mobilize cells, fluids, and other mediators to the site to contain, combat, and heal. In acute inflammation, the first events may be noticed in minutes, and the entire process resolved over a matter of days to a couple of weeks. Chronic inflammation may follow the incomplete resolution of an acute process or arise as a slow insidious process of its own. The natural history of infections such as tuberculosis, which follow this pattern, runs for months, years, even decades.

Acute = hours to days

Chronic = weeks to months

The first event in **acute inflammation** is the release of chemical signals (chemokines) that act on adhesion molecules (selectins) in local capillaries. This slows the movement of passing PMNs and activates adhesive integrins on their surface. This leads to tight adhesion to the endothelium followed by squeezing past the endothelial wall to the tissues below. There, chemotactic factors released by the bacteria lead them to the primary site. Increasing acidity of local fluids releases enzymes (kallikrein, bradykinin) that open junctions in capillary walls and allow increased flow of fluids and more leukocytes. Histamine (from mast cells), arachidonic acid, and prostaglandin release complete the phenotype of swelling and pain.

PMNs migrate from capillaries

Enzymes and chemical mediators facilitate swelling

Chronic inflammation bridges the innate and adaptive immune responses. An acute phase, if present, is usually not noticed, and the cellular infiltrate is composed of lymphocytes and macrophages with relatively few PMNs. It is generally associated with slower-growing pathogens such as mycobacteria, fungi, and parasites in which cell-mediated immunity is the primary adaptive defense. Many of these pathogens have mechanisms that allow them to multiply in nonactivated macrophages. If the macrophages are effectively activated by T cells, the multiplication ceases

Lymphocytes and macrophages predominate

Granulomas indicate failure to resolve by adaptive cellular mechanisms

and the inflammation and injury are minimal. If not, multiplication and chronic inflammation continue sometimes in the form of a **granuloma,** which is an indication of a destructive hypersensitivity component to the inflammation.

CHEMICAL MEDIATORS

Peptides alter membrane permeability

Chemical mediators of innate immunity that have direct antimicrobial activity include cationic proteins and complement. The cationic proteins (cathelicidin, defensins) act on bacterial plasma membranes by the formation of ionic pores, which alter membrane permeability. The complement system is a series of glycoproteins, which can directly insert in bacterial membranes or act as receptors for antibody. Cytokines are proteins or glycoproteins released by one cell population that act as signaling molecules for another. They are generally thought of in the context of the adaptive immune system, but they can be stimulated directly by microorganisms.

■ The Complement System

Multiple components activated in cascade

Differ in initiation mechanism

Opsonization is serum coating of pathogens

The complement system consists of more than 30 distinct components and several other precursors. All are in the plasma of healthy individuals in inactive forms that must be enzymatically cleaved to become active. When this happens, a cascade of reactions is triggered, which activates the various components in a fixed sequence (**Figure 2–5**). The difference between the pathways is in the mechanisms for their initiation. Once started, any pathway can produce the same effects on pathogens, which include enhancing phagocytosis, activation of leukocytes, and lysis of bacterial cell walls. An important step in the process is coating of the organism with serum components, a process called **opsonization.** The coatings may be mannose-binding proteins, complement components, or antibody. There is no immunologic specificity in complement activation or in its effects.

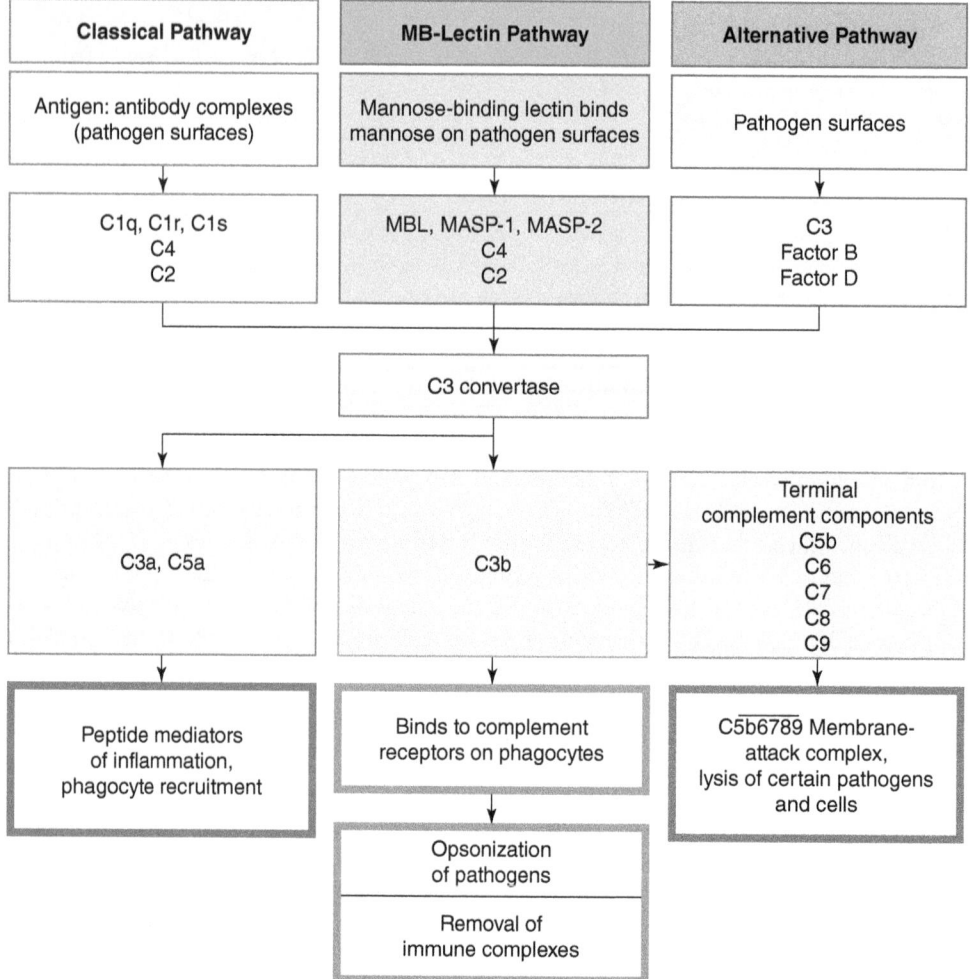

FIGURE 2–5. **Components and action of complement.** Complement activation involves a series of enzymatic reactions that culminate in the formation of C3 convertase, which cleaves complement component C3 into C3b and C3a. The production of the C3 convertase is where the three pathways converge. C3a is a peptide mediator of local inflammation. C3b binds covalently to the bacterial cell membrane and opsonizes the bacteria, enabling phagocytes to internalize them. C5a and C5b are generated by the cleavage of C5 by a C5 convertase. In addition, C5a is a powerful peptide mediator of inflammation. C5b promotes the terminal components complement to assemble into a membrane-attack complex. (Reproduced with permission from Willey JM: *Prescott, Harley, & Klein's Microbiology,* 7th ed. New York, NY: McGraw Hill; 2008.)

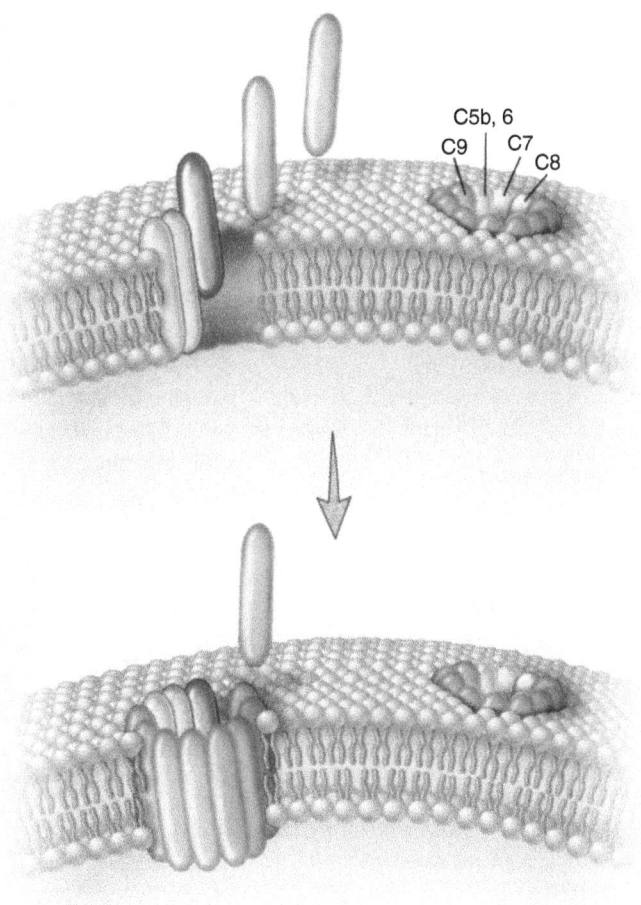

C5b, 6
C9 | C7
         C8

FIGURE 2-6. **Complement membrane-attack complex.** The membrane-attack complex (MAC) is a tubular structure that forms a transmembrane pore in the target cell's plasma membrane. The subunit architecture of the MAC shows that the transmembrane channel is formed by multiple polymerized molecules. (Reproduced with permission from Willey JM: *Prescott, Harley, & Klein's Microbiology*, 7th ed. New York, NY: McGraw Hill; 2008.)

Alternative Pathway

The alternative pathway is activated by bacterial cell wall components with repetitive surface structures such as LPS. The multiple components come together in the formation of the **membrane-attack complex,** which inserts directly into bacterial membranes (**Figure 2–6**), particularly the outer membrane of Gram-negative bacteria. This not only injures the organism but also enhances phagocytosis because the other end of the molecule has receptors for phagocytes. Gram-positive bacteria are less affected because they have no exposed membrane (see Chapter 21). These actions are particularly important for the effectiveness of innate immunity in the early stages of acute infections before the adaptive immune system has time to act. The key complement component for alternate pathway activity is C3b. C3b activation and degradation are regulated by a number of serum factors (factors B, D, and H) that can modulate its activity. A major mechanism for pathogens to block alternate pathway attack is by binding factor H to their surface. This is accomplished by bacterial capsules and surface proteins. This concentration of factor H causes local degradation of C3b (see Chapter 22, Figure 22–4).

Activation by pathogen surfaces

Membrane-attack complex inserts, provides phagocyte receptors

Factor H binding accelerates C3b degradation

Lectin Pathway

Another means of activating the complement system is based on the carbohydrate building of lectins. In this case, the lectins bind to mannose—a common surface component of bacteria, fungi, and some virus envelopes. This binding opsonizes the pathogen and enhances phagocytosis. Thus, as in the alternative pathway, the activation comes from pathogen surfaces and proceeds through the same C3 convertase (Figure 2–5).

Lectins bind mannose on pathogens

Classic Pathway

The classic complement pathway is initiated by the binding of antibodies formed during the adaptive immune response (as described further) with their specific antigens on the surface of a pathogen. This binding is highly specific but amounts to another case of opsonization activating the complement cascade. In this case, specific sites on the Fc portion of immunoglobulin molecules bind and activate the C1 component of complement to start the process. The pathway and

Antigen–antibody reaction exposes complement sites

TABLE 2–2	Some Cytokines Acting in Infection	
	CELL SOURCE	**FUNCTIONS**
Interleukins (IL)		
IL-1	Macrophages, endothelium, fibroblasts, epithelial	Differentiation and function of immune effectors, PMN response (T_H17)
IL-2	T cells (T_H1)	T-cell proliferation, cytolytic activity of natural killer (NK) cells
IL-4	T cells (T_H2), macrophages, B cells	Differentiation of naïve T cells to helper T cells, proliferation of B cells
IL-5	T cells (T_H2)	Eosinophil activation
IL-8	Macrophages, endothelial, T cells, keratinocytes, PMNs	Chemoattractant for PMNs and T cells, PMN degranulation, migration of PMNs
IL-17	T cells (T_H17)	Inflammation, PMN response
IL-22	T cells (T_H17)	Antimicrobial peptides
Interferons (IFN)		
IFN-α/β	T cells, B cells, macrophages, fibroblasts	Antiviral activity, stimulates macrophages, MHC class I expression
IFN-γ	T cells (T_H1, CTLs), NK cells	T-cell activation, macrophage activation, PMNs, NK cells, antiviral, MHC class I and II expression
Tumor Necrosis Factor (TNF)		
TNF-α	T cells, macrophages, NK cells	Expression of multiple cytokines, (growth and transcription factors), stimulates inflammatory response, cytotoxic for tumor cells
TNF-β	T cells, B cells	Same as TNF-α

MHC, major histocompatibility complex; PMN, polymorphonuclear neutrophil.

C3b has phagocyte receptors

sequence of individual complements are characteristics of the classic pathway, but it still reaches C3b, the common point for microbial-directed action. As with the alternative pathway, this creates the membrane-attack complex, the mediators of inflammation, and receptors for phagocytes on C3b.

■ Cytokines

Cytokine is a broad term referring to molecules released from one cell population destined to have an effect on another cell population (**Table 2–2**). As these proteins and glycoproteins have been discovered, they have been named and classified in relation to biologic effects observed initially only to discover that they have multiple other actions. For infectious diseases, the operative subcategories are **chemokines,** which are cytokines chemotactic for inflammatory cell migration, and **interleukins (IL-1, 2, 3,** etc), which regulate growth and differentiation between monocytes and lymphocytes. **Tumor necrosis factor (TNF),** so named for its cytotoxic effect on tumor cells, can also induce apoptosis (programmed cell death) in phagocytes—a useful feature for pathogens they have taken in. **Interferons (INF-α, -β, and -γ)** were originally named for their interference with viral replication (**Figure 2–7**), but are now known to be central to activation of T cells and macrophages. Unless commanded to understand specific situations, cytokine is used to represent all these mediators in these pages.

ILs, IFNs, TNF, chemokines are all cytokines

● THE ADAPTIVE (SPECIFIC) IMMUNE SYSTEM

The adaptive immune system differs from the innate immune response in its discrimination between self and nonself and in the magnitude and diversity of the highly specific immune responses that are engendered (**Table 2–3**). In addition, it has a **memory** function, which is able to mount an accelerated response if an invader returns. The adaptive system operates via two broad arms—**humoral immunity** and **cell-mediated immunity**. Humoral immunity comes from bone marrow-derived **B cells** and is exemplified by antibodies that are produced to bind foreign

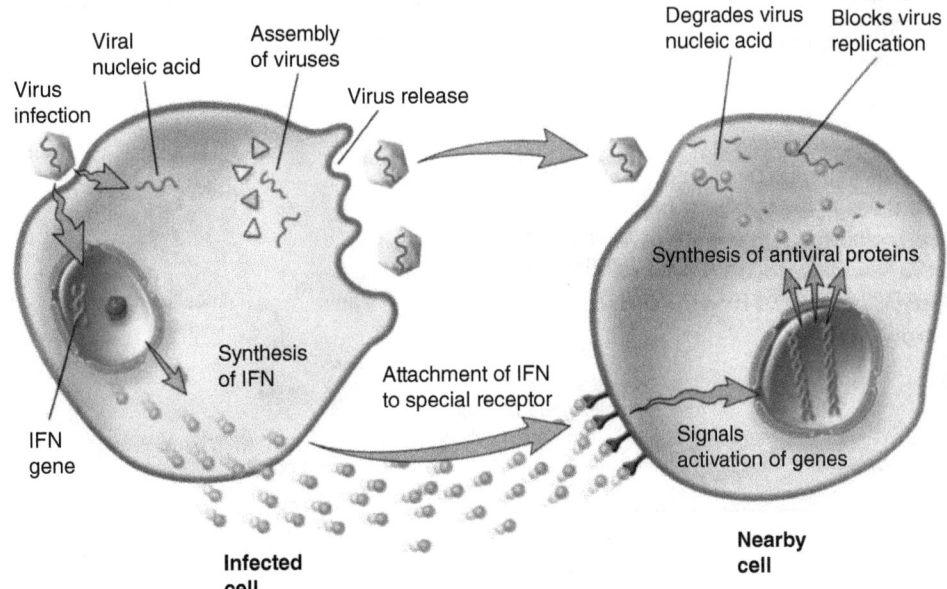

FIGURE 2–7. **Antiviral action of interferon.** Interferon (IFN) synthesis and release are often induced by a virus infection. IFN binds to a ganglioside receptor on the plasma membrane of a second cell and triggers the production of enzymes that render the cell resistant to virus infection. The two most important such enzymes are oligo (A) synthetase and a special protein kinase. When an IFN-stimulated cell is infected, viral protein synthesis is inhibited by an active endoribonuclease that degrades viral RNA. An active protein kinase phosphorylates and inactivates the initiation factor elf-2 required for viral protein. (Reproduced with permission from Willey JM: *Prescott, Harley, & Klein's Microbiology*, 7th ed. New York, NY: McGraw Hill; 2008.)

molecules called antigens. Cell-mediated (cellular) immunity is mediated through **T cells** that mature in the thymus and respond to antigens by directly attacking infected cells or by secreting cytokines to activate other cells. As shown in **Figure 2–8,** B-cell and T-cell systems are interactive.

■ Antigens and Epitopes

An antigen is any substance (usually foreign) with the ability to stimulate an immune response when presented in an effective fashion. They are usually large structurally complex molecules, such as proteins, polysaccharides, or glycolipids. Each antigen can contain many sub-regions that are the actual antigenic determinants or epitopes. These epitopes can consist of separate peptides, carbohydrates, or lipids of the correct size and three-dimensional configuration to fit the combining site of an antibody molecule or a T-cell receptor (TCR) (**Figure 2–9**). Approximately six amino acids or monosaccharide units provide a correctly sized epitope. Antigens presented by

Antigens stimulate immune response

TABLE 2–3	Cells Involved in the Adaptive Immune System			
CELL	FUNCTION	SPECIFIC RECEPTORS FOR ANTIGEN	CHARACTERISTIC CELL-SURFACE MARKER	SPECIAL CHARACTERISTICS
B cells	Production of antibody	Surface immunoglobulin (IgM monomer)	Fc and complement C3d receptors; MHC class II	Differentiate into plasma cells
Helper T lymphocytes (T$_H$)	Stimulate macrophages, eosinophils, PMNs, IgE production, B cells	α/β T-cell receptor (TCR)	CD4+	Presented by MHC class II, Three subsets (T$_H$1, T$_H$2, T$_H$17)
Cytotoxic T lymphocytes (CTLs)	Lyse antigen-expressing cells such as virally infected cells or allografts	α/β TCR	CD8+	Presented by MHC class I
Natural killer (NK) cells	Spontaneous lysis of tumor and infected cells	Inhibitory; activating	Fc receptor for IgG	Recognize MHC class I
Macrophages (monocytes)	Phagocytosis, secretion of cytokines to activate T cells (eg, IL-1) or other accessory cells such as polymorphonuclear neutrophils (PMNs)^c	None, but can be "armed" by antibodies binding to Fc receptors	Macrophage surface antigens	Express surface receptors for the activated third component of complement (C3), kill ingested bacteria by oxidative bursts
Polymorphonuclear leukocytes (neutrophils, eosinophils)	Phagocytosis killing	None, but can be "armed" by antibodies		Protective in bacterial and parasitic (eosinophils) infections

MHC, major histocompatibility complex.

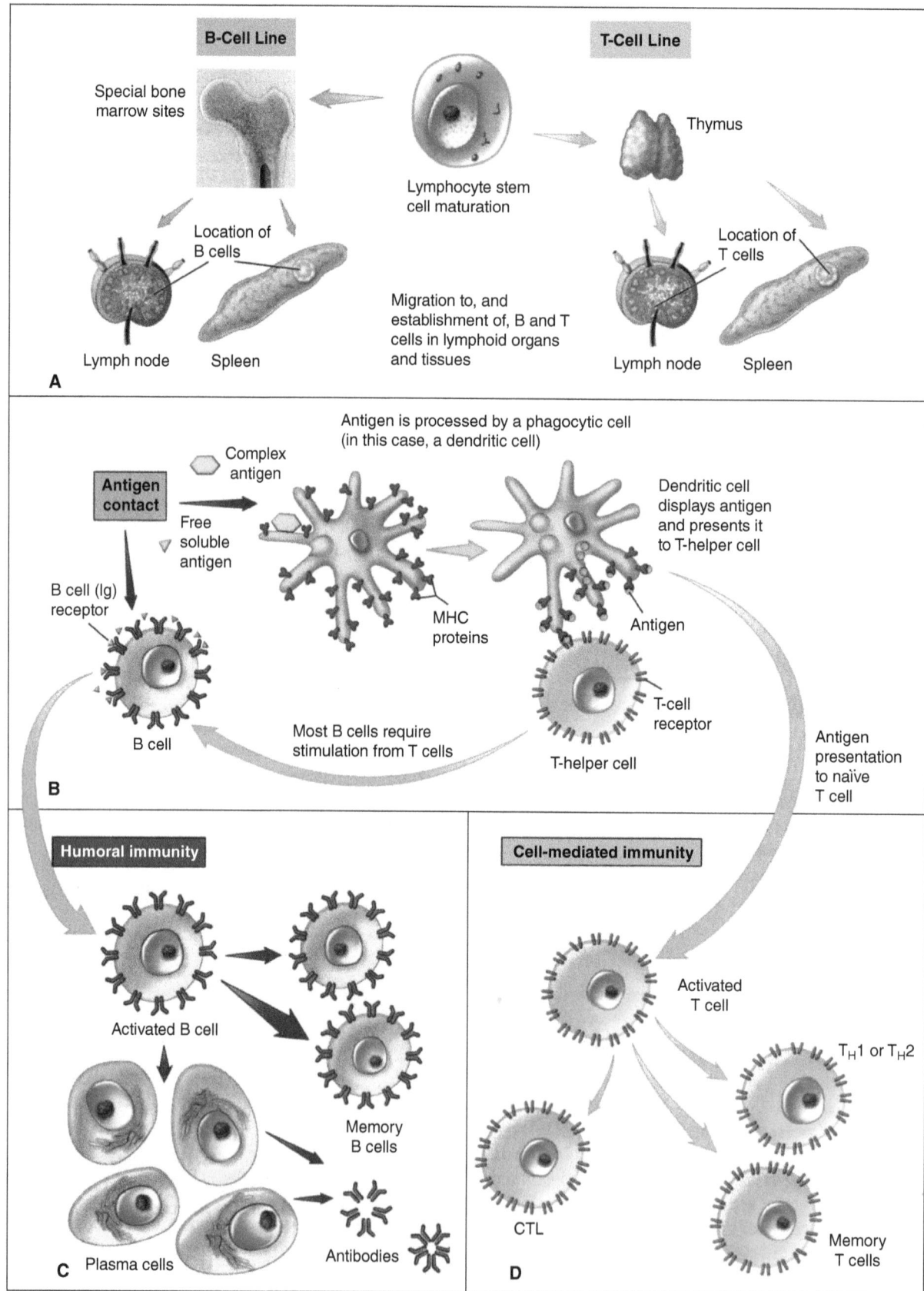

FIGURE 2–8. **Acquired immune system development. A.** Lymphocyte stem cells develop into B- and T-cell precursors that migrate to the bone marrow or thymus, respectively. Mature B and T cells seed secondary lymphoid tissues. **B.** Lymphocyte receptor binding of antigen activates B and T cells to become effector cells. **C.** B lymphocytes develop into memory cells and antibody-secreting plasma cells. **D.** T cells develop into memory cells, helper T cells, and cytotoxic T cells. (Reproduced with permission from Willey JM: *Prescott, Harley, & Klein's Microbiology*, 7th ed. New York, NY: McGraw Hill; 2008.)

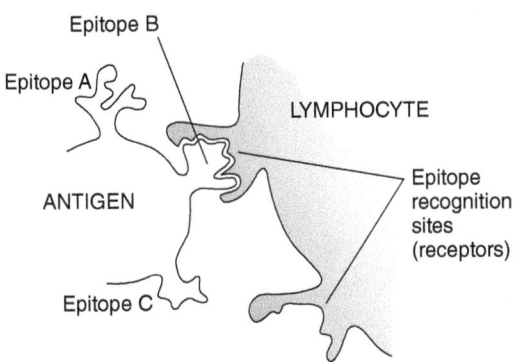

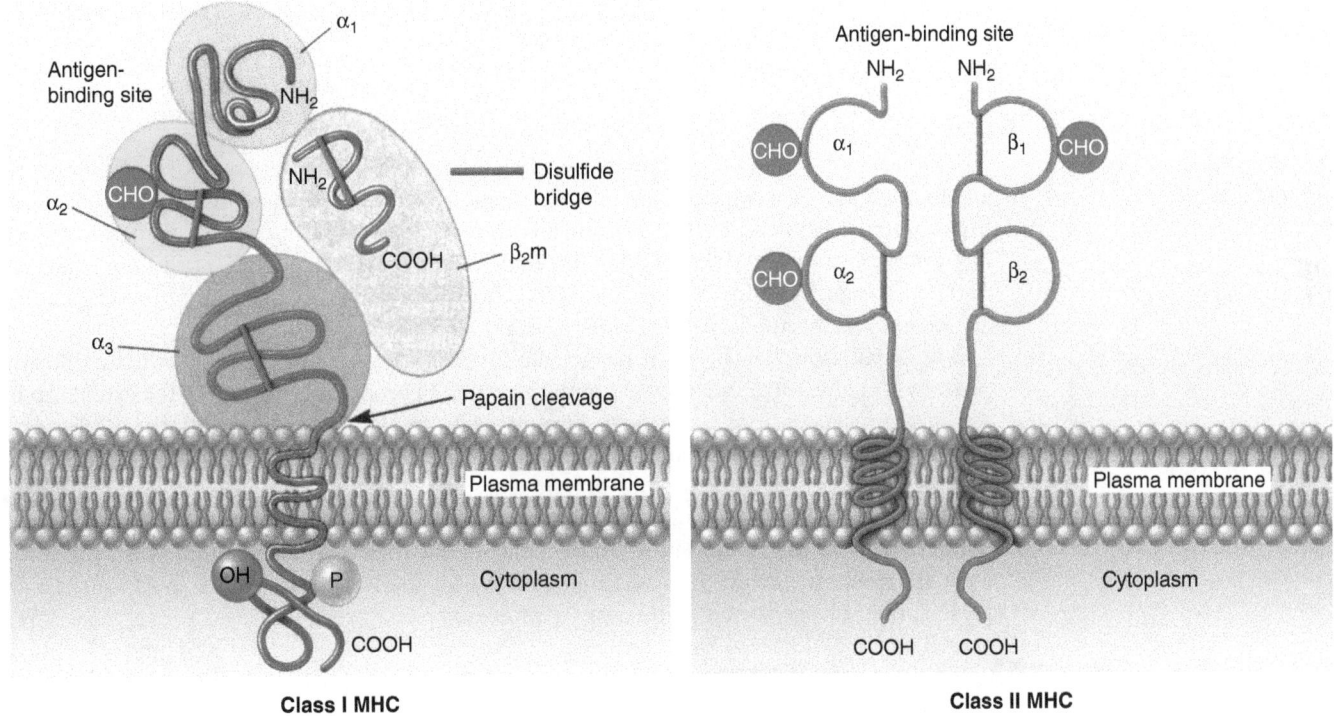

FIGURE 2–9. **Epitopes.** Schematic of epitope recognition by an immunoresponsive lymphocyte. Epitope B on the antigen binds to a complementary recognition site on the surface of the immunoresponsive cell. Antigens may have many different epitopes, but an immunoresponsive lymphocyte has receptors of only one specificity. In most cases, epitopes are recognized on the surface of macrophages that have processed the antigen. The receptor for antigens on B cells is the combining site of the surface immunoglobulin.

infectious agents typically contain multiple epitopes, including copies of the same epitope. Thus, a single microbially derived molecule presents multiple opportunities for diverse antibody binding. Other, smaller molecules that may ordinarily not stimulate an immune response (haptens) may do so if bound to a larger carrier, such as a protein. The specificity of the immune response may be generated for both the hapten and its larger carrier.

Epitopes fit to the combining site of TCR and antibodies

A foreign antigen entering a human host may, by chance, encounter a B cell whose surface antibody is able to bind it. This interaction stimulates the B cell to multiply, differentiate, and produce more surface and soluble antibodies of the same specificity. Eventually, the process leads to production of enough antibody to bind more of the antigen. This mechanism is most likely to operate with antigens such as polysaccharides that have repeating subunits, thus improving the possibility that exposed epitopes are recognized.

B cells multiply and produce antibody

Large, complex antigens such as proteins and viruses must be processed before their epitopes can be effectively recognized by the immune system. This processing takes place in macrophages or specialized epithelial cells found in the skin and lymphoid organs, where they are adjacent to other immunoresponsive cells. The ingested antigen is degraded to peptides of 10 to 20 amino acids that are presented by major histocompatibility molecules on the host cell surface to be recognized by T cells (**Figures 2–10, 2–11**).

Protein antigens must be processed first

FIGURE 2–10. **MHC class I and II molecules. A.** The class I molecule is a heterodimer composed of the alpha protein, which is divided into three domains: α_1, α_2, and α_3, and the protein β_2 microglobulin. **B.** The class II molecule is a heterodimer composed of two distinct proteins called alpha and beta. Each is divided into two domains α_1, α_2 and β_1, β_2, respectively. (Reproduced with permission from Willey JM: *Prescott, Harley, & Klein's Microbiology*, 7th ed. New York, NY: McGraw Hill; 2008.)

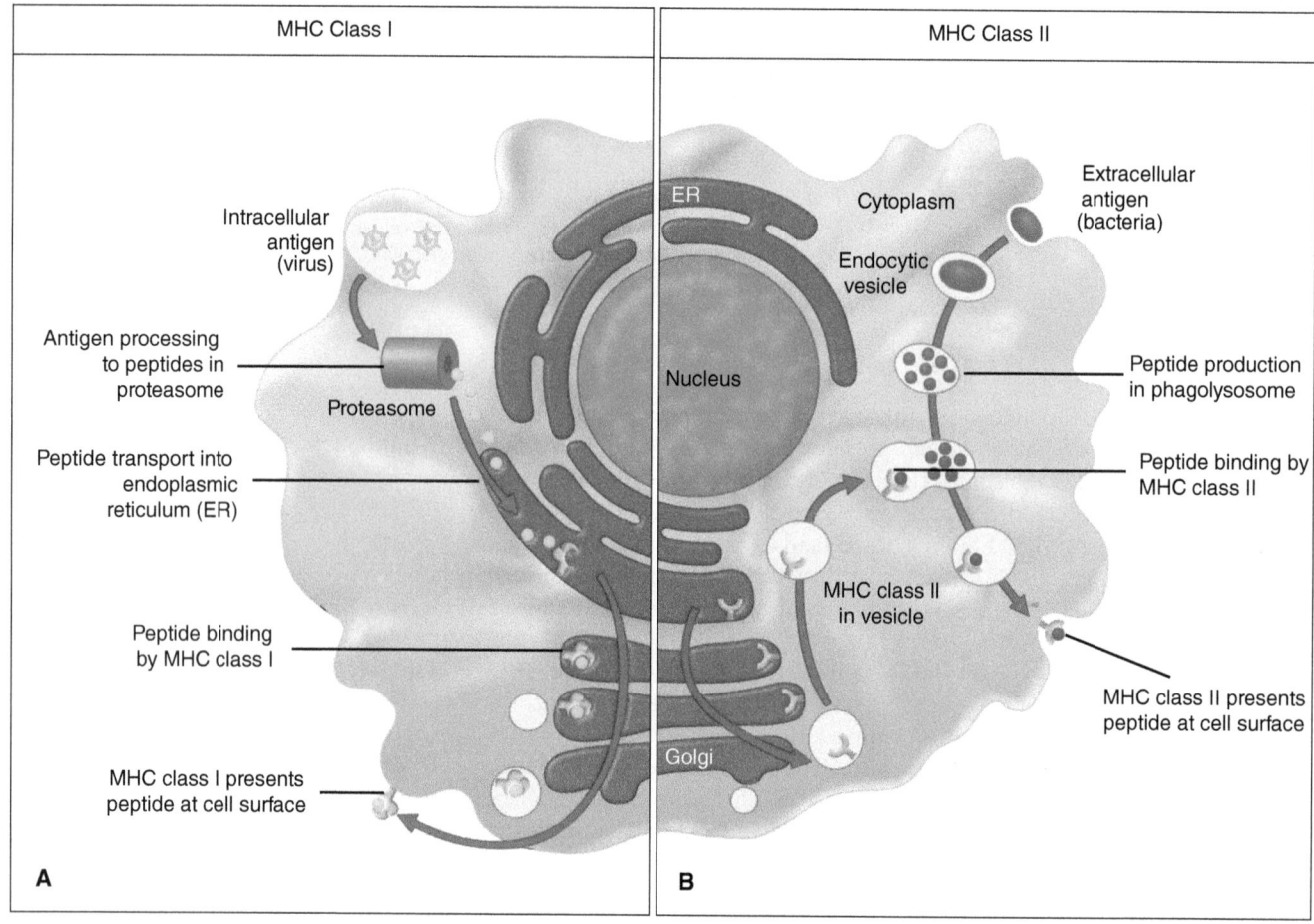

FIGURE 2–11. **Antigen processing and presentation. A.** Antigens originating in the cytoplasm are digested by the proteasome to peptides. The peptides are bound to the MHC class I molecules in the endoplasmic reticulum (ER) and transported to the surface for presentation. **B.** Antigens originating outside the cell are endocytosed and digested in the phagolysosome. The digested peptides are bound to MHC class II molecules in the ER and transported to the surface for presentation. MHC, major histocompatibility complex.

Recognition of Foreignness

Distinguishing between self and nonself is obviously essential to maintaining organism integrity and homeostasis. The compendium of molecules that control these functions is called the **major histocompatibility complex (MHC),** and it is present on the surface of almost all human cells. Of interest in infection are MHC class I and II molecules (Figure 2–10). **MHC class I** molecules are in the membrane of almost all cells, but **MHC class II** molecules are present only on certain leukocytes such as macrophages, dendritic cells, and some T and B cells.

Both MHC class I and class II participate in antigen processing but by distinctly different pathways (Figure 2–11). MHC class I molecules bind to products generated in the cytoplasm by a natural process or a viral infection. Viral proteins are digested to peptides in a cytoplasmic structure called the **proteasome,** and delivered to the endoplasmic reticulum. Here they find the binding site of the class I molecule and are transported to the surface for presentation of the peptide. MHC class II molecules bind to fragments that originally come from outside the cell, but have been taken into the endocytic vacuole of a phagocyte. After digestion in the phagolysosome, peptide fragments are combined with class II molecules and move to the surface for presentation. The presented MHC class I peptides are recognized by CD8+ T cells and the MHC class II by CD4+ T cells.

MHC gene complex codes surface molecules

MHC II on macrophages, dendritic cells

MHC I presents cytoplasmic peptides to CD8+

MHC II presents foreign peptides to CD4+

THE T-CELL RESPONSE

T cells originate in the bone marrow and migrate to the thymus for differentiation. Those that recognize self are destroyed. Those that survive are mature but require activation. T cells have specific **TCRs** on their surface, with binding sites extending to the external milieu (**Figure 2–12**).

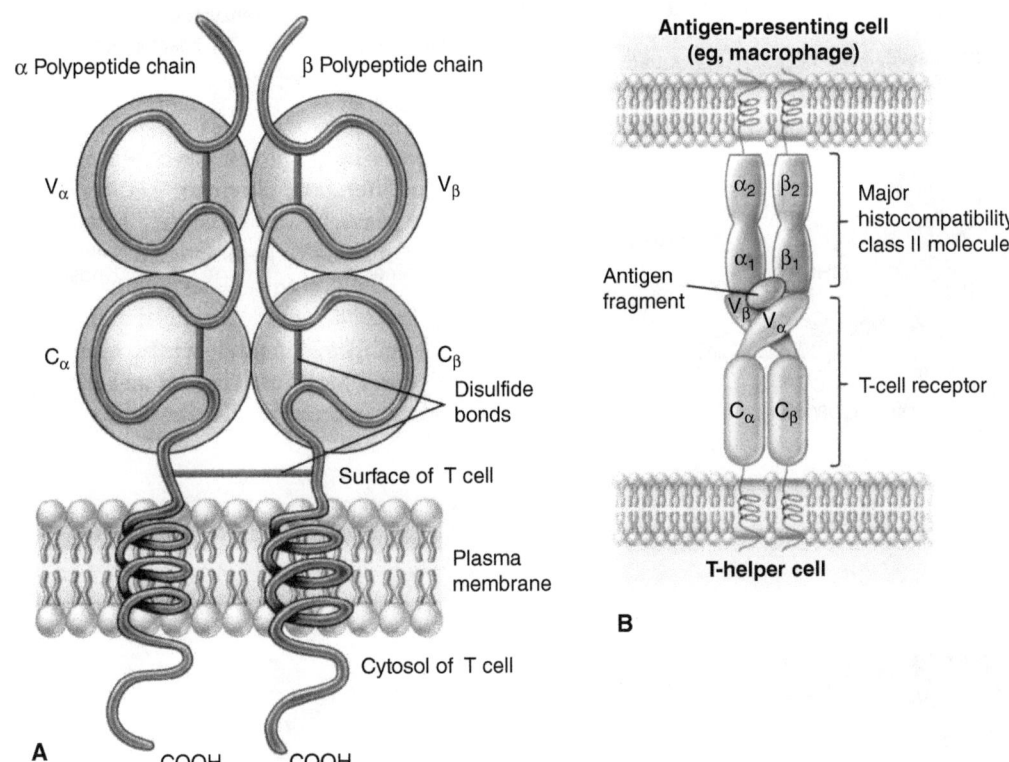

α Polypeptide chain   β Polypeptide chain

V_α V_β

C_α C_β

Disulfide bonds

Surface of T cell

Plasma membrane

Cytosol of T cell

A   COOH   COOH

Antigen-presenting cell (eg, macrophage)

α_2 β_2 Major histocompatibility class II molecule

α_1 β_1

Antigen fragment V_β V_α

C_α C_β T-cell receptor

T-helper cell

B

FIGURE 2–12. **T-cell receptor and helper T activation. A.** Structure of the T-cell antigen receptor. **B.** An antigen-presenting cell begins the activation process by displaying a peptide antigen fragment in its MHC class II molecule. A helper T cell is activated after the variable region of its receptor (Vα, Vβ) reacts with the fragment. (Reproduced with permission from Willey JM: *Prescott, Harley, & Klein's Microbiology*, 7th ed. New York, NY: McGraw Hill; 2008.)

The two major types of T cells are helper T (CD4+) and cytotoxic (CD8+) T cells. The major roles of T cells in the immune response are as follows:

1. Recognition of peptide epitopes presented by MHC molecules on cell surfaces. This is followed by activation and clonal expansion of T cells in the case of epitopes associated with class II MHC molecules.
2. Production of cytokines that act as intercellular signals and mediate the activation and modulation of various aspects of the immune response and of nonspecific host defenses.
3. Direct killing of foreign cells, of host cells bearing foreign surface antigens along with class I MHC molecules (eg, some virally infected cells), and of some immunologically recognized tumor cells.

CD4+ Helper T Lymphocytes

Helper T cells are stimulated by antigen in the context of MHC class II presentation and are further marked by the presence of the CD4 cell surface antigen. If T cells are of the proper MHC background to recognize the antigen specifically, T-cell activation occurs. The antigen–MHC complex presented to a specific T cell by the macrophage is the specific signal that induces the T cell to become activated and divide. At this point, the T helper (Th) cells differentiate into three major subsets of effector cells each with characteristic cytokines, target cells, and typical microbial pathogen profiles. Th1 cells produce IFN-γ, target macrophages, and are effective against intracellular pathogens like *Mycobacterium tuberculosis*. Th2 cells produce multiple IL, and promote IgE, mast cell, and eosinophil-mediated destruction of parasites. Th17 cells also produce IL including IL-17, stimulate neutrophils, and are active against extracellular bacterial and fungal pathogens.

Helper T cells activated by specific antigens

Subsets active against intracellular, extracellular, and parasitic pathogens

CD8+ Cytotoxic T Lymphocytes

CD8+ cytotoxic T lymphocytes (CTLs) are a second class of effector T cells. They are lethal to cells expressing the epitope against which they are directed when the epitope is presented by class I MHC molecules. They too have specific epitope recognition sites, but they are characterized by the CD8 cell surface marker; thus, they are referred to as CD8+ cytotoxic T cells. These cells recognize the association of antigenic epitopes with class I MHC molecules on a wide variety of cells

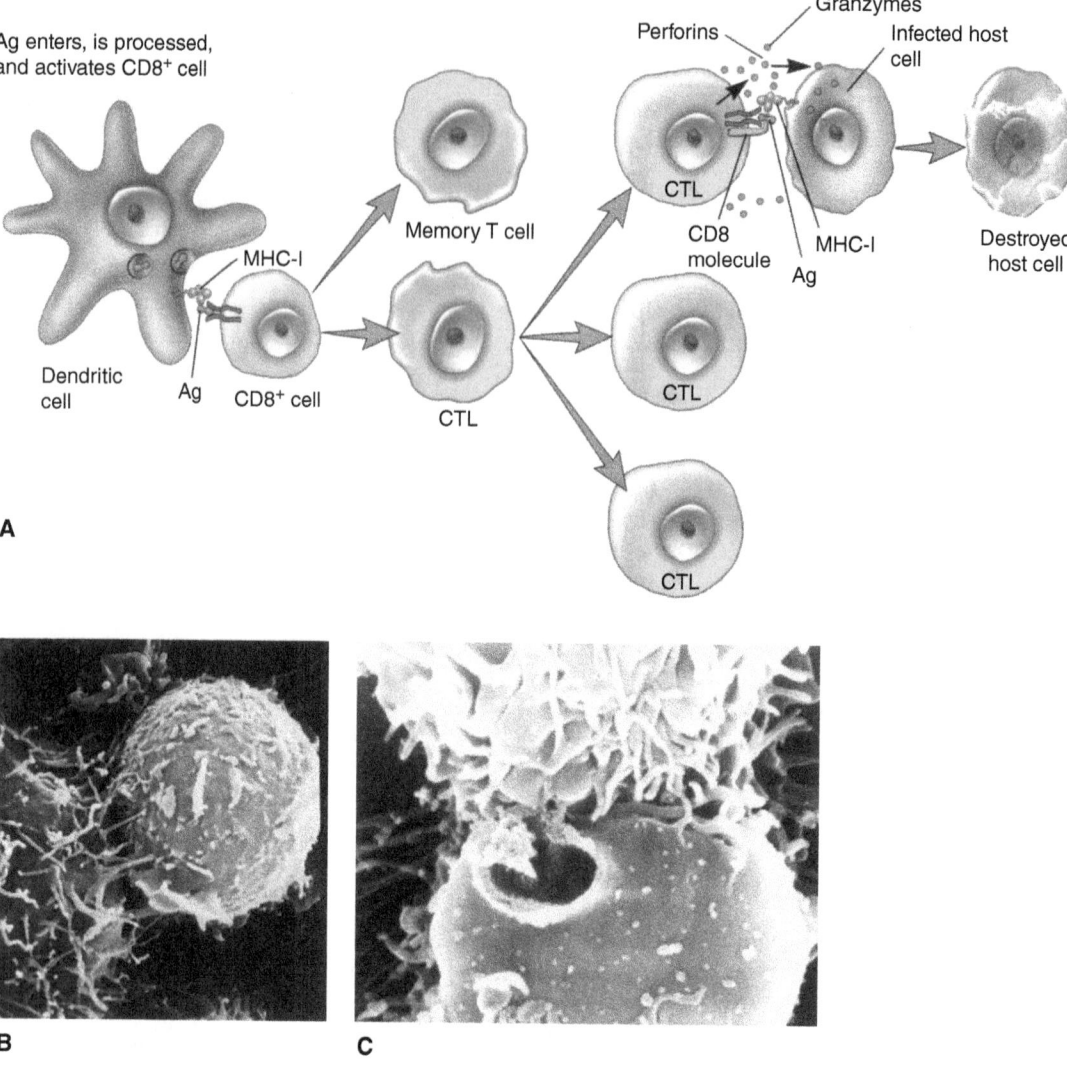

FIGURE 2–13. **Cytotoxic T-cell (CTL) destruction virus-infected cells. A.** Naïve CD8+ T cells are activated when they are exposed to antigen within a class I MHC molecule on an antigen-presenting cell. Antigen activation leads to development of effector CTL and memory cells. Effector CTLs and their memory cells subsequently react with antigen expressed in class I MHC molecules of any host cell to destroy it. T-cell cytotoxicity often involves the perforin pathway and leads to apoptosis or cytolysis. MHC, major histocompatibility complex. **B.** CTL (left) contacting target cell (right). **C.** Perforins form pores in target cell membrane. (Reproduced with permission from Willey JM: *Prescott, Harley, & Klein's Microbiology,* 7th ed. New York, NY: McGraw Hill; 2008.)

CD8+ lymphocytes react with MHC I

Eliminate virally infected cells

of the body. In the case of virally infected cells, cytotoxic CD8+ cells prevent viral production and release by eliminating the host cell before viral synthesis or assembly is complete (**Figure 2–13**). The destruction of the virally infected cell is accomplished through a complement-like action mediated by perforins, which also facilitates entry into the cell of enzymes (granzymes) that activate apoptosis.

■ Superantigens

A group of antigens have been termed superantigens because they stimulate a much larger number of T cells than would be predicted based on the specificity of combining site diversity. This causes a massive cytokine release. The action of superantigens is based on their ability to bind directly to MHC proteins and to particular Vβ regions of the TCR without involving the antigen-combining site. Individual superantigens recognize exposed portions defined by framework of residues that are common to the structure of one or more Vβ regions. Any T cells bearing those Vβ sites may be directly stimulated. A variety of microbial products have been identified as superantigens. Superantigens are discussed further in Chapter 22 (see Figure 22–7) and in Chapters 24 and 25, describing their role in **toxic shock syndromes** caused by *Staphylococcus aureus* and group A streptococci.

Superantigens bind directly to MHC proteins and TCR Vβ region

Higher proportion of T cells are stimulated

■ Cell-Mediated Immunity

In the control of infection, cell-mediated immunity is most important in response to obligate facultative intracellular pathogens. These include some slow-growing bacteria, such as the mycobacteria and fungi against which antibody responses appear to be ineffective. The mechanisms are complex and involve a number of cytokines with amplifying feedback mechanisms for their production. After the initial processing of antigen to stimulate activation of the antigen-recognizing CD4+ T cell, cytokine feedback from the CD4+ T cells to macrophages further increases their clonal expansion (including memory cells) and activates CD8+ (cytotoxic) T lymphocytes. Other cytokines from CD4+ T cells attract macrophages to the site of infection, and activate them to greatly enhance microbiocidal activity. The sum of the individual and collaborative activities of T cells, macrophages, and their products is a progressive mobilization of a range of host defenses to the site of infection and greatly enhanced macrophage activity. In the case of tuberculosis, IFN-γ inhibits the replication of the mycobacteria inside macrophages. In viral infections, CD8+ cytotoxic lymphocytes destroy their cellular habitat leaving already assembled virions accessible to circulating antibody.

Of primary importance with intracellular pathogens

Helper and CTL interact

Macrophages are mobilized and enhanced

B CELLS AND ANTIBODY RESPONSES

B lymphocytes are the cells responsible for antibody responses. They develop from precursor cells in the bone marrow before migrating to other lymphoid tissues. Each mature cell of this series carries a specific epitope recognition site on its surface. This B-cell receptor is actually a monomer of one form of antibody (IgM) oriented with its binding sites facing outward. Upon binding antigen, the receptor-antigen complex is internalized for initiation of antibody production by the stimulated B cell. In this process, the B lymphocytes multiply, differentiating into either **memory** or **plasma cells.** Plasma cells are end cells adapted for secretion of large amounts of antibodies. In addition to their essential role in antibody production, B cells can present antigen to T cells.

B cells carry epitope recognition sites on their surface

Stimulated cells differentiate to form memory, plasma cells

There are two broad types of antigen triggering: T-dependent and T-independent. **T-dependent** reactions are those that use collaboration between helper T cells and B cells to initiate the process of antibody production. This is the mechanism evoked by proteins and haptens bound to proteins. The response is strong and includes memory cells; therefore, it can be boosted in the case of immunization.

T-dependent has memory

T-independent responses are those that do not require help from T cells to stimulate B-cell antibody production. It is evoked by large molecules with many repeating units such as polysaccharides which cannot bind to MHC molecules. At first glance, this independence may seem to be an advantage, but T-independent responses are not the same as T-dependent responses. The antibody generally has a lower affinity for its antigen and a shorter duration in circulation. Memory cells are not produced, and T-independent responses mature more slowly than T-dependent responses. This delay in maturation may contribute to the increased susceptibility to some bacterial infections in early life. It certainly contributed to the failure of the first batch of purified polysaccharide vaccines to effectively immunize children younger than 2 years. For use in children, these vaccines have been replaced with a hapten approach in which the polysaccharide is conjugated to protein. In this form, antibody generated by the T-dependent mechanism (protein carrier) still has specificity for the polysaccharide epitopes.

T-cell independent responses are weaker and lack memory

Poor response under 2 years of age

After challenge with foreign antigen, there is a lag period of 4 to 6 days before antibody can be detected in serum. This period reflects the events involved in the recognition of the antigen, its processing, and the specific activation of the cells of the immune system. The first event is the clearance of antigen from the circulation by what is essentially a metabolic process in which the antigen is recognized in a nonspecific sense and ingested. The vast preponderance of antigen ends up in circulating phagocytes or in stationary macrophages. The macrophages process the antigen; therefore, those immunogenic moieties can be presented to T cells, which then cause the B cells to produce immunoglobulins. The antibody-forming system is a learning system that responds to challenge by foreign molecules by producing large amounts of specific antibody. In addition, the affinity of its binding to the specifically recognized antigen often increases with time or secondary challenge.

Antigen processing causes delay in antibody response

Learning system increases affinity with time or secondary challenge

■ Antibody Structure

Antibodies belong to the **immunoglobulin** family of proteins, which appear in quantity in serum and on the surfaces of B cells. Of the five known structural types, three (IgG, IgM, and IgA) are involved in the defense against infection. The basic structure of an immunoglobulin is illustrated

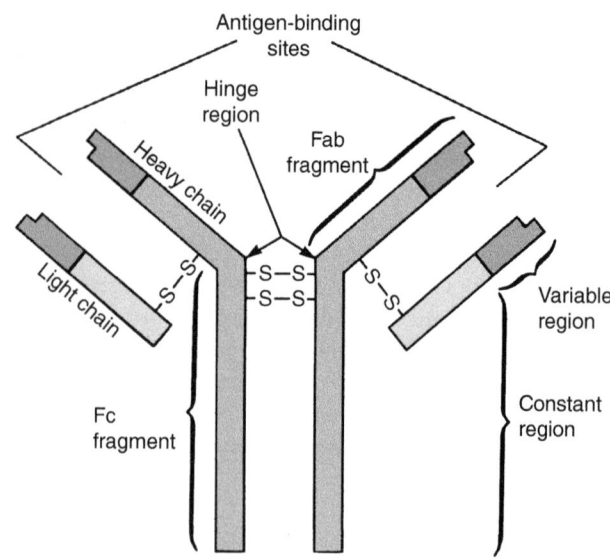

FIGURE 2–14. **Immunoglobulin G structure.** The IgG molecule consists of two identical light chains and two identical heavy chains held together by disulfide bonds. (Reproduced with permission from Willey JM: *Prescott, Harley, & Klein's Microbiology*, 7th ed. New York, NY: McGraw Hill; 2008.)

Immunoglobulin structure combines light and heavy chains

Isotypes defined by type of heavy chain

Fab sites bind antigen

Fc fragment recognized by complement, phagocytes

Combining site is idiotype

in **Figure 2–14,** which depicts an **IgG** molecule. Immunoglobulins have a basic tetrameric structure consisting of two light polypeptide chains and two heavy chains usually associated as light/heavy pairs by disulfide bonds. The two light/heavy pairs are covalently associated by disulfide bonds to form the tetramer. There are two types of light chains, κ and λ, which are the products of distinct genetic loci. The class or isotype of the immunoglobulin is defined by the type of heavy chain expressed.

The Y-shaped structure includes two **antigen binding sites (Fab)** formed by interaction of the **variable domains** of the heavy chain and the light chain. The stalk is called the **Fc fragment.** Antibodies carry out two broad sets of functions: the recognition function is the property of the Fab sites for antigen, and the effector functions are mediated by the constant regions of the heavy chains. Variations in the hypervariable region of the Fab-combining site due to mutations are called **idiotypes.** Antibodies combine with foreign antigens, but the actual destruction or removal of antigen requires the interaction of portions of the Fc fragment with other molecules such as complement components and phagocytes which have **Fc receptors.**

Figure 2–15 shows a schematic representation of a serum **IgM** immunoglobulin. This molecule consists of five subunits of the typical IgG molecule. The molecule occurs as a cyclic pentamer, and a J (joining) chain links the intact structure. When IgM is present on the surface of

FIGURE 2–15. **Immunoglobulin M structure.** The pentameric structure has disulfide bonds linking peptide chains shown in black; carbohydrate side chains are in red. The J chain links the molecule together. (Reproduced with permission from Willey JM: *Prescott, Harley, & Klein's Microbiology*, 7th ed. New York, NY: McGraw Hill; 2008.)

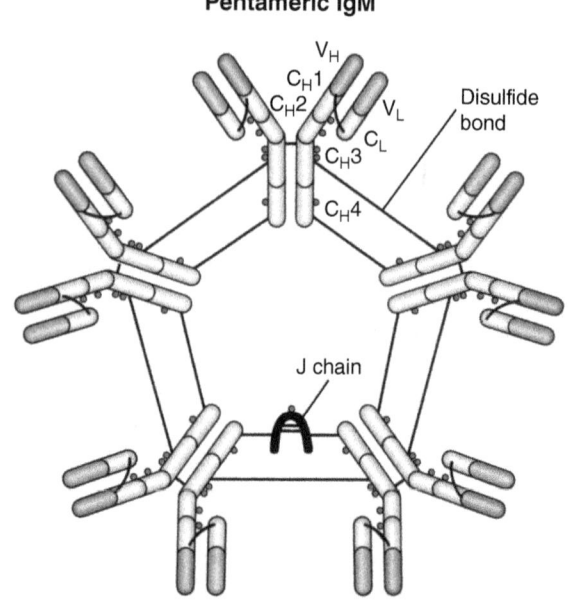

B cells where it serves as a primary receptor for antigen, it is present as a monomer. Other immunoglobulins showing a difference in arrangement from the typical IgG model are the **IgA** immunoglobulins. In serum, these immunoglobulins can occur as a monomer, but they can also occur in dimers in which the joining chain is required to stabilize the dimer. IgA molecules in the gut occur as dimers in which both the J chain and an additional polypeptide, termed the **secretory component,** are present in the complex.

Fab is antigen-binding region

IgM has five subunits

IgA a monomer or dimer

■ Functional Properties of Immunoglobulins

Immunoglobulin G

Immunoglobulin G (IgG) is the most abundant immunoglobulin in health and provides the most extensive and long-lived antibody response to the various microbial and other antigens that are encountered throughout life. Although at least four subclasses of IgG have been characterized, they are grouped together for the purpose of this chapter. The IgG molecule is bivalent with two identical and specific combining sites. The Fc region does not vary with differences in specificity of combining sites of different antibody molecules. The Fc fragment binding sites for phagocytic cells are made available when the variable region of the antibody molecule has reacted with specific antigen, leaving the Fc facing outward.

Bivalent with specific combining site and constant region

Constant region binds phagocytes

IgG antibody is characteristically formed in large amounts during the secondary response to an antigenic stimulus, and usually follows production of IgM (see Immunoglobulin M) in the course of a viral or bacterial infection. Memory cells are programmed for rapid IgG response when another antigenic stimulus of the same type occurs later. IgG antibodies are the most significant antibody class for neutralizing bacterial exotoxins and viruses often by blocking their attachment to cell receptors. Accelerated IgG responses from memory cell expansion frequently confer lifelong immunity when directed against microbial antigens that are determinants of virulence. IgG is the only immunoglobulin class able to cross the placental barrier and, thus, it provides passive immune protection to the newborn in the form of maternal antibody.

Secondary response antibodies neutralize toxins, viruses

Binding may block attachment receptor

Immunoglobulin M

Monomers of immunoglobulin M (IgM) constitute the specific epitope recognition sites on B cells that ultimately give rise to plasma cells producing one or another of the different immunoglobulin classes of antibody. Because of its many specific combining sites, IgM is particularly effective in agglutinating particles carrying epitopes against which it is directed. It also contains many sites for binding the first component of complement. These sites become available once the IgM molecule has reacted with antigen. IgM is particularly active in bringing about complement-mediated cytolytic damage to foreign antigen-bearing cells. It is less effective as an opsonizing antibody because its Fc portion is not available to phagocytes.

Effective agglutinating antibody

Binds complement at multiple sites

Immunoglobulin A

Immunoglobulin A (IgA) has a special role as a major determinant of so-called local immunity in protecting epithelial surfaces from colonization and infection. Certain B cells in lymphoid tissues adjacent to, or draining surface epithelia of the intestines, respiratory tract, and genitourinary tract, are encoded for specific IgA production. After antigenic stimulus, the clone expands locally, and some of the IgA-producing cells also migrate to other viscera and secretory glands. At the epithelia, two IgA molecules combine with another protein, termed the **secretory piece,** which is present on the surface of local epithelial cells. The complex, then termed **secretory IgA** (sIgA), passes through the cells into the mucous layer on the epithelial surface or into glandular secretions, where it exerts its protective effect. The secretory piece not only mediates secretion but also protects the molecule against proteolysis by enzymes such as those present in the intestinal tract.

sIgA is produced at mucosal surfaces

Secretory piece combines molecules, resists proteolysis

The major role of sIgA is to prevent attachment of antigen-carrying particles to receptors on mucous membrane epithelia. Thus, in the case of bacteria and viruses, it reacts with surface antigens that mediate adhesion and colonization and prevents the establishment of local infection or invasion of the subepithelial tissues. sIgA can agglutinate particles but has no Fc domain for activating the classic complement pathway; however, it can activate the alternative pathway. Reaction of IgA with antigen within the mucous membrane initiates an inflammatory reaction that helps mobilize other immunoglobulin and cellular defenses to the site of invasion. IgA response to an antigen is shorter lived than the IgG response.

Interferes with attachment of microbes to mucosal surfaces

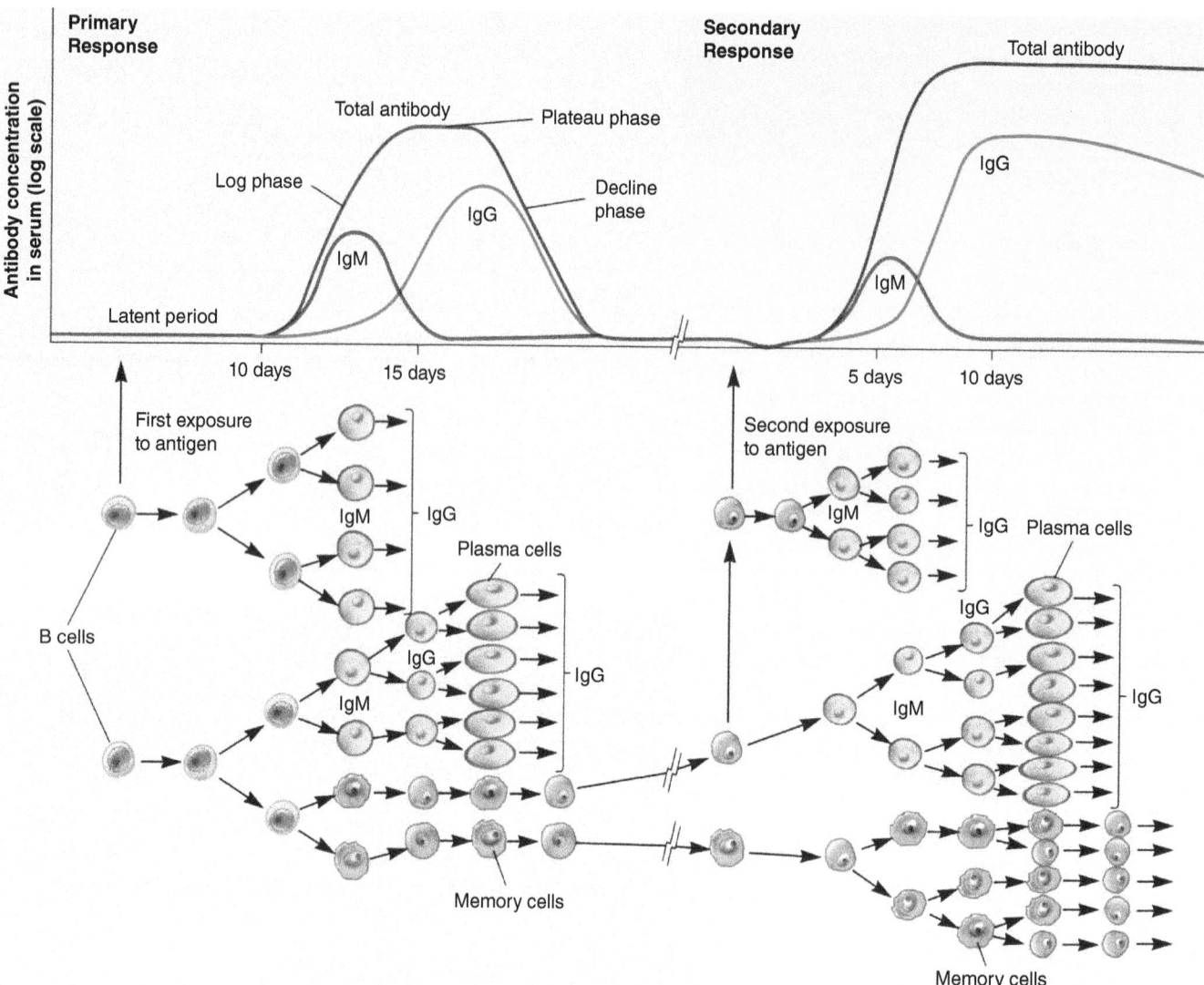

FIGURE 2–16. **Antibody production and kinetics.** The four phases of a primary antibody response correlate to the clonal expansion of the activated B cell, differentiation into plasma cells, and secretion of the antibody protein. The secondary response is much more rapid, and total antibody production is nearly 1000 times greater than that of the primary response. (Reproduced with permission from Willey JM: *Prescott, Harley, & Klein's Microbiology*, 7th ed. New York, NY: McGraw Hill; 2008.)

■ Antibody Production

The major events characterizing the time course of antibody production are illustrated in **Figure 2–16** and summarized as follows: Initial contact with a new antigen evokes the **primary response,** which is characterized by a lag phase of approximately 1 week between the challenge and the detection of circulating antibodies. In general, the length of the lag phase depends on the immunogenicity of the stimulating antigen and the sensitivity of the detection system for the antibodies produced. Once antibody is detected in serum, the levels rise exponentially to attain a maximal steady state in approximately 3 weeks. These levels then decline gradually with time if no further antigenic stimulation is given. The first antibodies synthesized in the primary immune response are IgM and, then in the latter phase, IgG antibodies arise and eventually predominate. This transition is termed the **IgM/IgG switch.**

After a subsequent exposure or booster injection of the same antigen, a different sequence called the **secondary response** or **anamnestic response** ensues. This response involves memory. In the secondary response, the lag time between the immunization and the appearance of antibody is shortened, the rate of exponential increase to the maximum steady-state level is more rapid, and the steady-state level itself is higher, representing a larger amount of antibody. Another key factor of the secondary response is that the antibodies formed are predominantly of the IgG

After lag, primary response lasts for weeks, then declines

IgM response switches to IgG

Secondary response is primarily IgG

class. In addition to higher levels, the secondary IgG antibodies have a higher affinity for their antigen. Figure 2–16 shows the participation of memory T cells created during the primary response in these reactions.

Affinity for antigen is greater

● ADVERSE EFFECTS OF IMMUNOLOGIC REACTIONS

The immune system is no different from any other human system. In balance, we do not even know it is there, but in an exaggerated state called **hypersensitivity,** it can cause injury and even chronic disease. Hypersensitivity reactions have been placed into four classes on the basis of their mechanism of immunologic injury. Type I or allergic reactions relate to the action of IgE and the release of powerful mediators, such as histamine from mast cells. Type II or cytotoxic reactions are created when IgG or IgM antibodies are misdirected to host cells. Type III or immune complex reactions are created when an excess of antigen–antibody complexes are deposited and followed by complement-mediated inflammation. Type IV reactions are cell-mediated and often called delayed-type hypersensitivity (DTH) because of the time delay in invoking the T_H1 response. The hypersensitivity diseases include allergy, anaphylaxis, asthma, transfusion reactions, rheumatoid arthritis, and type 1 diabetes. Infectious diseases are a relatively small part of this spectrum, but involve three of the four mechanisms (II, III, and IV).

Mechanisms I-IV involve antibody and cell-mediated injury

Allergy, asthma, and diabetes due to hypersensitivity

Infection a small part

ANTIBODY-MEDIATED (TYPE II) HYPERSENSITIVITY

Type II hypersensitivity is antibody-dependent cytotoxicity that occurs when antibody binds to antigens on host cells, leading to phagocytosis, cytotoxic T-cell activity, or complement-mediated lysis. The cells to which the antibody is specifically bound, as well as the surrounding tissues, are damaged because of the inflammatory amplification. In the best-understood situations related to infection, the mechanism of antibody stimulation is **molecular mimicry.** That is, the antibody stimulated by an epitope on the pathogen, unfortunately, also binds to a similar epitope on host cells. In rheumatic fever, the infectious epitope is in a surface protein of the group A streptococcus and the host epitope in the myocardium of the heart (see Chapter 25). The streptococcal protein and cardiac myosin share similar amino acid sequences; therefore, it is a cross-reaction. The result is acute myocarditis.

Antibody against microbe epitope also reacts with host cells

Rheumatic fever is caused by molecular mimicry

IMMUNE COMPLEX (TYPE III) HYPERSENSITIVITY

When IgG is mixed in appropriate proportions with multivalent antigen molecules (ie, bearing multiple epitopes), aggregates of many antigen and antibody molecules may form. These antigen–antibody complexes can occur in infection when sufficient amounts of specific antibody and free antigen from an infecting microorganism combine to form an immune complex. These complexes are usually removed by cells of the monocyte-macrophage system, but, in excess, can circulate and become deposited in blood vessels, kidneys, or joints. When deposited, they bind complement and stimulate an inflammatory reaction that may injure the local tissue. This is postulated to be the mechanism of poststreptococcal acute glomerulonephritis (see Chapter 25), and is suspected to be responsible for some of the manifestations when microorganisms circulate in the bloodstream.

Excess antigen–antibody complexes are deposited in tissues

In the past, an immune complex disease called **serum sickness** used to follow the infusion of antibodies (antisera) produced in horses to combat infection. Human antibody to the foreign horse immunoglobulin was formed. These diseases (diphtheria, tetanus) are now prevented by vaccines that stimulate antibody against the same epitopes in humans. When passive immunization is used, human sources of antibody are now available.

Complement-mediated inflammation causes injury

Serum sickness is reaction to animal immunoglobulin

DELAYED-TYPE (TYPE IV) HYPERSENSITIVITY

Type IV DTH is a cell-mediated immune reaction. The delay is the time required after initiation of a T_H1 response for antigen to be processed, cytokines produced, and T cells to migrate and accumulate at the antigen site. At the site, cytotoxic T cells, macrophages, and other inflammatory mediators directed at cells containing the antigen also produce injury in the surrounding tissue. The purest form of DTH is the intradermal skin test for tuberculosis. In persons already sensitized to the antigens of *M tuberculosis,* it takes 1 to 2 days for induration to be produced at the site of inoculation of a standardized antigen called tuberculin. This is a useful diagnostic test, but, in infectious disease, DTH is also the hypersensitivity mechanism that causes the most injury.

DTH requires time for T_H1 response to develop

Inflammation causes continuing local injury

This occurs in diseases in which immunity is cell-mediated with little or no effective antibody component. If these responses are successful in containing the infection at an early stage, there is little destruction. If they are not successful enough to contain growth of the pathogen, increasing amounts of antigen stimulate continuing DTH-mediated destructive inflammation. This is the primary mechanism of injury in tuberculosis, fungal infections, and many parasitic diseases.

● FAVORABLE USE OF THE IMMUNE RESPONSE

NATURAL IMMUNITY TO INFECTION

Natural infection often confers life-long immunity

Clinical disease is not required

The majority of encounters with microorganisms including pathogens end favorably for the host. The heightened immunologic responses following infection usually provide immunity, often for life. This is called natural immunity. In some instances, the gauntlet is long because a pathogen of the same name may exhibit diverse antigenic profiles. Because of the specificity of the adaptive immune response, immunity must be developed individually for each antigenic type. Development of natural immunity need not require a clinical infection. There is ample evidence from population studies that individuals with no history or recollection of infection have evidence of immunity in the form of specific antibody. From the time of birth forward, we have many encounters with infectious agents, most of which lead to immunity without disease.

PASSIVE IMMUNITY

Transplacental IgG protects the fetus

Passive immunity is the transfer of antibodies from one person to another. Because the antibody was not made by the recipient, this antibody is transient and lasts only a few weeks or months. This is a natural process in the case of IgG transferred transplacentally from mother to fetus. The protection provided by this antibody is limited to the immunologic experience of the mother, but covers a particularly vulnerable time in life, lasting as long as 6 months after birth. Passive immunity can also be provided as a therapeutic product in which specific antibodies are infused. Such antisera are available for only a limited number of diseases such as rabies, botulism, and tetanus.

VACCINES

Live vaccines use attenuated strains

Killed vaccines may require purification

Vaccines artificially stimulate immunity through exposure to an antigenic substance. The early vaccines such as Jenner's for smallpox and Pasteur's for anthrax (in animals) were live attenuated strains with the ability to produce a true, if mild, infection. We later learned how to kill the agent in a way that retained its antigenicity. These killed vaccines are practical if the number of antigens present is limited as with a virus (polio) or bacterial toxin (diphtheria), but usually too crude if whole bacteria are used. Progress with killed bacterial vaccines required knowledge of just which antigenic component provides protective immunity. This allowed inactivation followed by purification of the selected component. This approach with bacterial polysaccharide capsules has produced a dramatic reduction (>95%) in childhood meningitis. Genomic approaches are now aimed at producing a protective antigen without growth of the organism itself. For each of the 57 chapters in this book devoted to specific infectious agents, vaccines and the immunologic mechanisms involved are carefully examined.

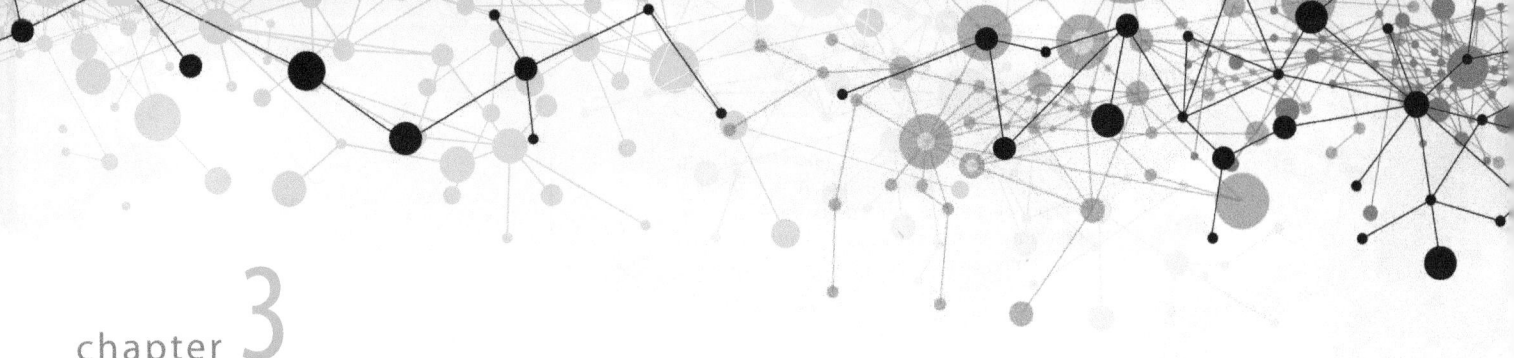

chapter 3

Sterilization, Disinfection, and Infection Control

From the time of debates about the germ theory of disease, killing microbes before they reach patients has been a major strategy for preventing infection. In fact, Ignaz Semmelweis successfully applied disinfection principles decades before bacteria were first isolated. This chapter discusses the most important methods used for this purpose in modern medical practice. Understanding how these methods work has become of increasing importance in an environment that includes immunocompromised patients, transplantation, indwelling devices, and COVID-19.

DEFINITIONS

Death/killing as it relates to microbial organisms is defined in terms of how we detect them in culture. Operationally, it is a loss of ability to multiply under any known conditions. This is complicated by the fact that organisms that appear to be irreversibly inactivated may, sometimes, recover when appropriately treated. For example, mechanisms exist for repair of the damage done by things like ultraviolet light. Such considerations are of great significance in the preparation of safe vaccines from inactivated virulent organisms.

Absence of growth may not indicate sterility

Sterilization is an absolute term. It means complete killing, or removal, of all living organisms from a particular location or material. It can be accomplished by incineration, nondestructive heat treatment, certain gases, exposure to ionizing radiation, some liquid chemicals, and filtration.

✳ **Sterilization is killing of all living forms**

Pasteurization is the use of heat at a temperature sufficient to inactivate important pathogenic organisms in liquids such as water or milk, but at a temperature lower than that needed to ensure sterilization. For example, heating milk at a temperature of 74°C for 3 to 5 seconds or 62°C for 30 minutes kills the vegetative forms of most pathogenic bacteria that may be present without altering its quality. Obviously, spores are not killed at these temperatures.

✳ **Heat kills vegetative bacteria**

Disinfection is a less precise term. It implies the destruction of pathogenic microorganisms by processes that fail to meet the criteria for sterilization. Pasteurization is a form of disinfection, but the term is most commonly applied to the use of liquid chemical agents known as disinfectants, which usually have some degree of selectivity. Bacterial spores, organisms with waxy coats (eg, mycobacteria), and some viruses may show considerable resistance to the common disinfectants. **Antiseptics** are disinfecting agents that can be used on body surfaces, such as the skin or vaginal tract, to reduce the numbers of pathogenic agents in the local microbiota. They have lower toxicity than disinfectants used environmentally, but are usually less active in killing vegetative organisms. **Sanitization** is an even less precise term with a meaning somewhere between disinfection and cleanliness. It is used primarily in housekeeping and food preparation contexts.

Chemical agents kill pathogens with varying efficiency

Spores particularly resistant

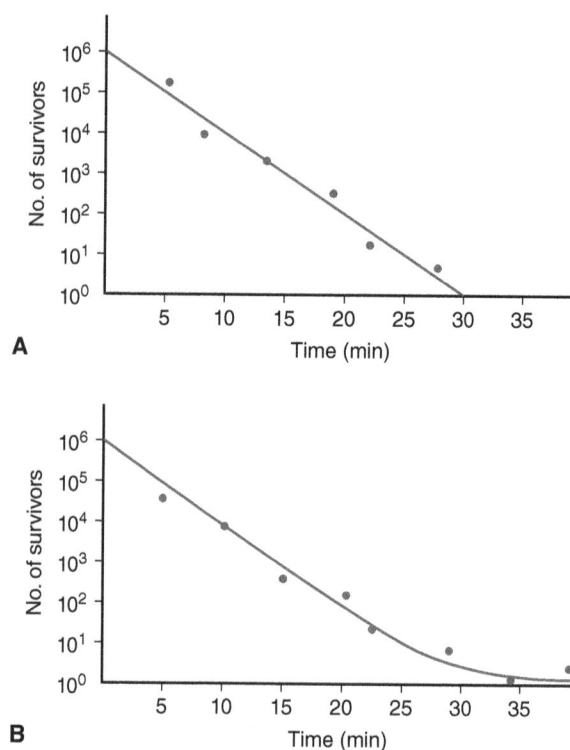

FIGURE 3–1. **Kinetics of bacterial killing.**
A. Exponential killing is shown as a function
of population size and time. **B.** Deviation from
linearity, as with a mixed population, extends
the time.

Asepsis describes working systems designed to prevent microorganisms from reaching a protected environment. It is manifest in the multiple procedures used in the operating room, in the preparation of therapeutic agents, and in technical manipulations in the microbiology laboratory. An essential component of aseptic techniques is the prior sterilization of all materials and equipment to be used.

Applies sterilization and disinfection

MICROBIAL KILLING

Killing of bacteria by heat, radiation, or chemicals is usually exponential with time; that is, a fixed proportion of survivors are killed during each time increment. Thus, plots of the logarithm of the number of survivors against time are linear (**Figure 3–1A**); however, the slope of the curve varies with the effectiveness of the killing process. In general, the rate of killing increases exponentially with arithmetic increases in temperature or in concentrations of disinfectant. If the microbial population includes a small proportion of more resistant forms (spores), the later stages of the curve may be flattened (**Figure 3–1B**), and extrapolations from the exponential phase of killing may underestimate the time needed for achieving complete sterility.

Killing follows exponential kinetics

STERILIZATION

The availability of reliable methods of sterilization has made possible the major developments in surgery and intrusive medical techniques that have helped to revolutionize medicine since the latter part of the 19th century. Furthermore, sterilization procedures form the basis of many food preservation procedures, particularly in the canning industry. The various modes of sterilization described in the text are summarized in **Table 3–1.**

■ Heat

The simplest method of sterilization is to expose the surface to be sterilized to a naked flame, as is done with the wire loop used in microbiology laboratories. It can be used equally effectively for emergency sterilization of a knife blade or a needle. Of course, disposable material is rapidly and effectively decontaminated by incineration. Carbonization of organic material and destruction of microorganisms, including spores, occur after exposure to dry heat of 160°C for 2 hours in a sterilizing oven. This method is applicable to metals, glassware, and some heat-resistant oils and waxes that are immiscible in water and therefore cannot be sterilized in the autoclave. A major use of the dry-heat sterilizing oven is in preparation of laboratory glassware.

Incineration rapid, effective

✳ **Dry heat requires 2 hours to kill**

TABLE 3–1	Methods of Disinfection and Sterilization		
METHOD	ACTIVITY LEVEL	SPECTRUM	USES/COMMENTS
Heat			
Autoclave	Sterilizing	All	General
Boiling	High	Most pathogens, some spores	General
Pasteurization	Intermediate	Vegetative bacteria	Beverages, plastic hospital equipment
Ethylene oxide gas	Sterilizing	All	Potentially explosive; aeration required
Radiation			
Ultraviolet	Sterilizing	All	Poor penetration
Ionizing	Sterilizing	All	General, food
Chemicals			
Alcohol	Intermediate	Vegetative bacteria, fungi, some viruses	
Hydrogen peroxide	High	Viruses, vegetative bacteria, fungi	Contact lenses; inactivated by organic matter
Chlorine	High	Viruses, vegetative bacteria, fungi	Water; inactivated by organic matter
Iodophors	Intermediate	Viruses, vegetative bacteria[a] fungi	Skin disinfection; inactivated by organic matter
Phenolics	Intermediate	Some viruses, vegetative bacteria, fungi	Handwashing
Glutaraldehyde	High	All	Endoscopes, other equipment
Quaternary ammonium compounds	Low	Most bacteria and fungi, lipophilic viruses	General cleaning; inactivated by organic matter

[a]Variable results with *Mycobacterium tuberculosis*.

Moist heat in the form of water or steam is far more rapid and effective in sterilization than dry heat because reactive water molecules denature protein irreversibly by disrupting hydrogen bonds between peptide groups at relatively low temperatures. Most vegetative bacteria are killed within a few minutes at 70°C or less, although some bacterial spores can resist boiling for prolonged periods.

Moisture aids protein denaturation

In effect, the **autoclave** is a sophisticated pressure cooker (**Figure 3–2**). In its simplest form, it consists of a chamber in which the air can be replaced with pure saturated steam under pressure. Air is removed either by evacuation of the chamber before filling it with steam or by displacement through a valve at the bottom of the autoclave, which remains open until all air has drained out. The latter, which is termed a **downward displacement autoclave,** capitalizes on the heaviness of air compared with saturated steam. When the air has been removed, the temperature in the chamber is proportional to the pressure of the steam; autoclaves are usually operated at 121°C. Under these conditions, spores directly exposed are killed in less than 5 minutes, although the normal sterilization time is 10 to 15 minutes to account for variation in the ability of steam to penetrate different materials and to allow a wide margin of safety.

Autoclave = steam under pressure

The effectiveness of autoclaves depends on the absence of air, pure saturated steam, and access of steam to the material to be sterilized. Pressure per se plays no role in sterilization other than to ensure the increased temperature of the steam. **"Flash" autoclaves,** which are used in operating rooms, often use saturated steam at a temperature of 134°C for 3 minutes. Air and steam are removed mechanically before and after the sterilization cycle to ensure that metal instruments may be available rapidly.

Steam required for sterilization

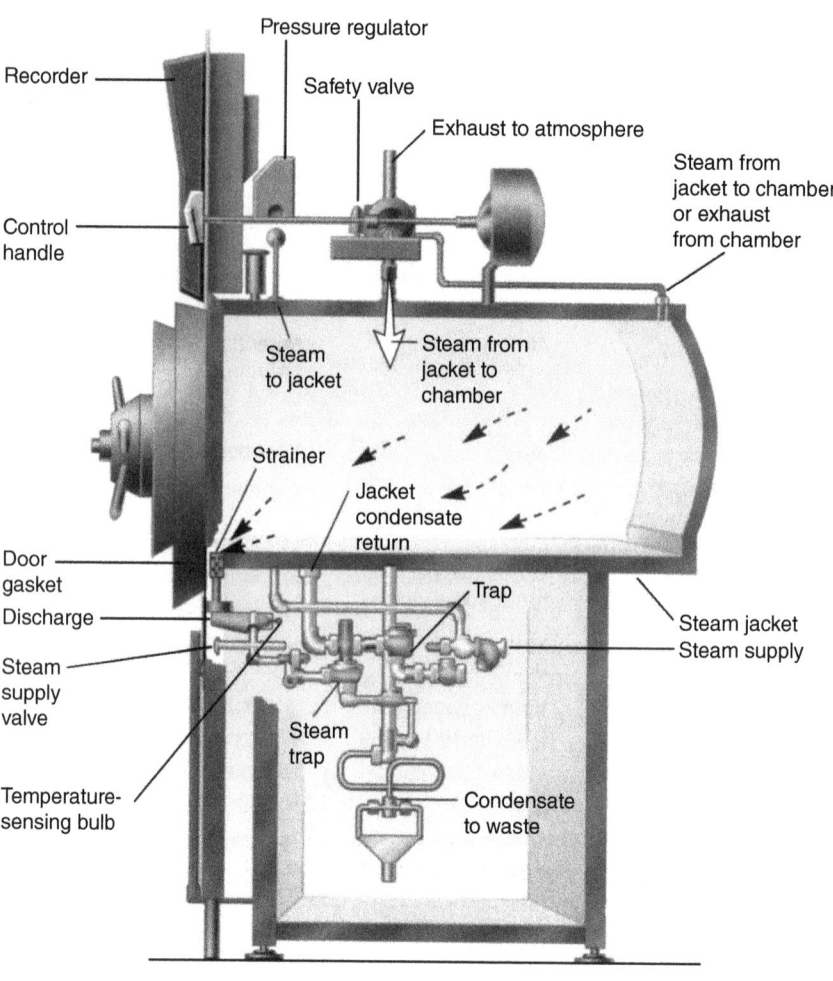

■ Gas

✳ Ethylene oxide used for heat-labile materials

A number of articles, particularly certain plastics and lensed instruments that are damaged by autoclaving, can be sterilized with gases. **Ethylene oxide** is an inflammable and potentially explosive gas. It is an alkylating agent that inactivates microorganisms by replacing labile hydrogen atoms in DNA. Exposure times must be followed by a prolonged period of aeration to allow the gas to diffuse out of substances that have absorbed it. Ethylene oxide is an effective sterilizing agent for heat-labile devices such as artificial heart valves that cannot be treated at the temperature of the autoclave. Other alkylating agents such as **formaldehyde** vapor can be used without pressure to decontaminate larger areas such as rooms.

■ Ultraviolet Light and Ionizing Radiation

UV light damages DNA

Ultraviolet (UV) light is absorbed by nucleic acids and causes genetic damage. The practical value of UV sterilization is limited by its poor ability to penetrate. Its main application has been in irradiation of air in the vicinity of critical hospital sites and as an aid in the decontamination of the air in facilities used for handling particularly hazardous organisms.

Ionizing radiation used for surgical supplies

Ionizing radiation carries far greater energy than UV light. It, too, causes direct damage to DNA and produces toxic-free radicals and hydrogen peroxide from water within the microbial cells. Cathode and gamma rays are widely used in industrial processes, including the sterilization of many disposable surgical supplies such as gloves, plastic syringes, specimen containers, some foodstuffs, and the like, because they can be packaged before exposure to the penetrating radiation.

DISINFECTION

■ Physical Methods

Filtration

Both live and dead microorganisms can be removed from liquids by positive- or negative-pressure filtration. Membrane filters are available commercially with variable pore sizes (0.005-1 μm).

For removal of bacteria, a pore size of 0.2 μm is effective for disinfection of large volumes of fluid, especially fluid containing heat-labile components such as serum. Filtration is not considered effective for removing viruses.

Pasteurization

Pasteurization involves exposure of liquids to temperatures in the range of 55°C to 75°C to remove all vegetative bacteria. Spores are unaffected by the pasteurization process. Pasteurization is used commercially to render milk safe and to extend its storage quality. With the outbreaks of infection due to contamination with enterohemorrhagic *Escherichia coli* (see Chapter 33); this has been extended (reluctantly) to fruit drinks. To the dismay of some of his compatriots, Pasteur proposed application of the process to wine-making to prevent microbial spoilage and vinegarization. Pasteurization in water at 70°C for 30 minutes has been effective and inexpensive when used to render plastics, such as those used in inhalation therapy equipment, free of organisms that may, otherwise, multiply in mucus and humidifying water.

Microwaves

The use of microwaves in the form of microwave ovens or specially designed units is another method of disinfection. These systems are not under pressure, but they can achieve temperatures near boiling if moisture is present. In some situations, they are being used as a practical alternative to incineration for disinfection of hospital waste. These procedures are not considered sterilization because heat-resistant spores may survive the process.

■ Chemical Methods

Given access and sufficient time, chemical disinfectants cause the death of pathogenic vegetative bacteria. Some disinfectants such as the quaternary ammonium compounds, alcohol, and the iodophors reduce the superficial flora and can eliminate contaminating pathogenic bacteria from the skin surface. Other agents such as the phenolics are valuable only for treating inanimate surfaces or for rendering contaminated materials safe. All are bound and inactivated to varying degrees by protein and dirt, and they lose considerable activity when applied to other than clean surfaces.

Alcohol

The alcohols are protein denaturants that rapidly kill vegetative bacteria when applied as aqueous solutions in the range of 70% to 95% alcohol. They are inactive against bacterial spores and many viruses. Solutions of 100% alcohol dehydrate organisms rapidly but fail to kill, because the lethal process requires water molecules. Isopropyl alcohol (90-95%) is widely used for skin decontamination before simple invasive procedures such as venipuncture.

Halogens

Iodine is an effective disinfectant that acts by iodinating or oxidizing essential components of the microbial cell. Tincture of iodine in alcohol has now been largely replaced by preparations in which iodine is combined with carriers (povidone) or nonionic detergents. These agents, termed **iodophors,** gradually release small amounts of iodine. They cause less skin staining and dehydration than tinctures, and are widely used in preparation of skin before surgery.

Chlorine exists as hypochlorous acid in aqueous solutions that dissociate to yield free chlorine over a wide pH range, particularly under slightly acidic conditions. In concentrations of less than one part per million, chlorine is lethal within seconds to most vegetative bacteria and inactivates most viruses; this efficacy accounts for its use in rendering supplies of drinking water safe and in chlorination of water in swimming pools. Chlorine is the agent of choice for decontaminating surfaces and glassware that have been contaminated with viruses or spores of pathogenic bacteria. For these purposes, it is usually applied as a 5% solution called **hypochlorite.**

Hydrogen Peroxide

Hydrogen peroxide is a powerful oxidizing agent that attacks membrane lipids and other cell components. Hydrogen peroxide has been useful in disinfecting items such as contact lenses, which are not susceptible to its corrosive effect. A newer version containing surfactants acts more rapidly.

Surface-Active Compounds

Surfactants are compounds with hydrophobic and hydrophilic groups that attach to and solubilize various compounds or alter their properties. Anionic detergents such as soaps are highly

---

Membrane filters remove bacteria

✳ **Kills vegetative bacteria but not spores**

Kill by generating heat

✳ **Inactivated by organic material**

Alcohols require water

✳ **Iodophors combine iodine with detergents**

Oxidative action rapid

Oxidizes cell components

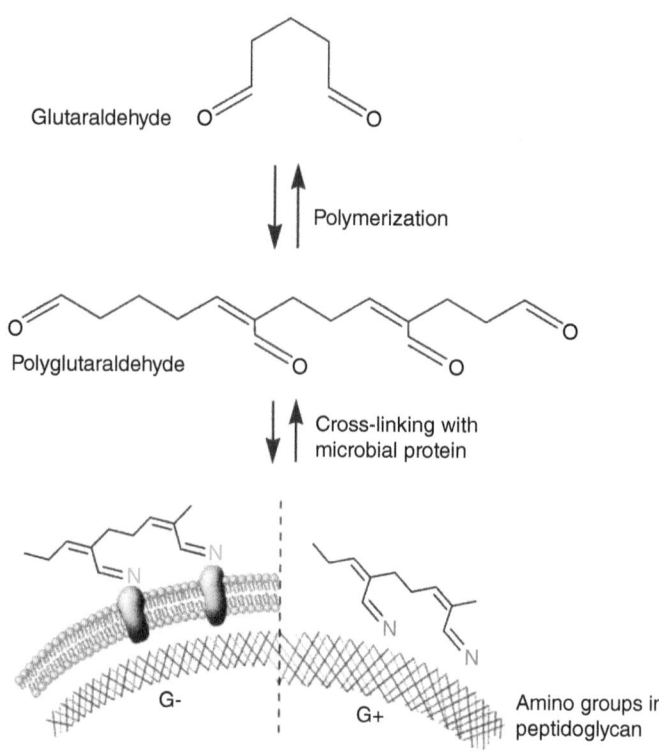

FIGURE 3–3. **Action of glutaraldehyde.** Glutaraldehyde polymerizes and then interacts with amino acids in proteins (*left*) or in bacterial peptidoglycan (*right*). As a result, they are alkylated and inactivated. (Reproduced with permission from Willey JM: *Prescott, Harley, & Klein's Microbiology*, 7th ed. New York, NY: McGraw Hill; 2008.)

Surfactants act on lipids

Quats adsorb to surfaces, cotton

effective cleansers, but have little direct antibacterial effect, probably because their charge is similar to that of most microorganisms. Cationic detergents, particularly the **quaternary ammonium compounds** ("quats") such as benzalkonium chloride, are highly bactericidal in the absence of contaminating organic matter. Their hydrophobic and lipophilic groups react with the lipid of the cell membrane of the bacteria, alter the membrane's surface properties and its permeability, and lead to loss of essential cell components and death. They are inactive against spores and most viruses.

Phenolics

Phenol is a potent protein denaturant and bactericidal agent. Phenolics are too toxic to skin and tissues to be used as antiseptics, although brief exposures can be tolerated.

Chlorhexidine persists in skin

Chlorhexidine is used as a routine hand and skin disinfectant. It has the ability to bind to the skin and produce a persistent antibacterial effect. It is cationic and, thus, its action is neutralized by soaps and anionic detergents.

Glutaraldehyde and Formaldehyde

Glutaraldehyde for equipment

Glutaraldehyde and formaldehyde are alkylating agents highly lethal to essentially all microorganisms (**Figure 3–3**). Formaldehyde gas has irritative, allergenic, and unpleasant—properties that limit its use. Glutaraldehyde is an effective high-level disinfecting agent for apparatus that cannot be heat-treated, such as some lensed instruments and equipment for respiratory therapy.

INFECTION CONTROL AND NOSOCOMIAL INFECTIONS

Some risk of infection exists in all healthcare settings. Hospitalized patients are particularly vulnerable, and the hospital environment is complex. Infection control is the proper matching of the principles and procedures described here to general and specialized situations, together with aseptic practices to reduce these risks. "Nosocomial" is a medical term for "hospital-associated." Nosocomial infections are complications that arise during hospitalizations. The morbidity, mortality, and costs associated with these infections are preventable to a substantial degree. The purpose of hospital infection control is prevention of nosocomial infections by application of epidemiologic concepts and methods.

■ History: Semmelweis and Childbed Fever

The shining example of the fundamental importance of epidemiology in detection and control of nosocomial infections is the work of Ignaz Semmelweis, which preceded the microbiologic

TABLE 3–2	Childbed Fever at the Vienna General Hospital					
	DIVISION I (TEACHING UNIT)			**DIVISION II (MIDWIFE UNIT)**		
YEAR	**BIRTHS**	**MATERNAL DEATHS**	**PERCENTAGE**	**BIRTHS**	**MATERNAL DEATHS**	**PERCENTAGE**
1846[a]	4010	459	11.4	3754	105	2.7
1848[b]	3556	45	1.3	3219	43	1.3

[a]No handwashing.
[b]First full year of chlorine handwashing.

discoveries of Pasteur and Koch by a decade. Semmelweis was an obstetrician at the Vienna General Hospital, where childbed fever (puerperal endometritis), which we now know is caused by group A streptococci, was a major problem. The cases were primarily in the physician not the midwife delivery unit. Semmelweis postulated that the key feature was the transmission of "invisible cadaver particles" by direct contact between the mother and physicians' hands contaminated performing autopsies. As a countermeasure he required handwashing with a chlorine solution. The result was the dramatic drop in maternal mortality shown in **Table 3-2**. Handwashing is still considered the most important infection control measure.

Childbed fever reversed by handwashing

NOSOCOMIAL INFECTIONS AND THEIR SOURCES

Infections occurring during any hospitalization could be either community-acquired or nosocomial. Community-acquired infections are defined as those present or incubating at the time of hospital admission. All others are considered nosocomial. For example, a hospital case of chickenpox could be community-acquired if it erupted on the fifth hospital day (incubating) or nosocomial if hospitalization was beyond the limits of the known incubation period (20 days). Infections appearing shortly after discharge (2 weeks) are considered nosocomial, although some could have been acquired at home.

Nosocomial infections acquired in hospital

The infectious agents responsible for nosocomial infections arise from various sources, including patients' own microbiota. In addition to any immunocompromising disease or therapy, the hospital may impose additional risks by treatments that breach the normal defense barriers. Surgery, urinary or intravenous catheters, and invasive diagnostic procedures all may provide opportunistic microbes with access to usually sterile sites. Infections in which the source of organisms is the hospital rather than the patient include those derived from hospital personnel, the environment, and medical equipment.

■ Hospital Personnel

Physicians, nurses, students, therapists, and any others who come in contact with the patient may transmit infection. Transmission from one patient to another is called **cross-infection.** The vehicle of transmission is most often the inadequately washed hands of a medical attendant. Another source is the actively infected medical attendant. Many hospital outbreaks have been traced to hospital personnel, particularly physicians, who continue to care for patients despite an overt infection. Transmission is usually by direct contact, although airborne transmission is also possible. A third source is the person who is not ill, but asymptomatically carrying a virulent strain. For *Staphylococcus aureus* and group A streptococci, nasal carriage is most important, but sites such as the perineum have also been involved in outbreaks. An occult carrier is less often the source of nosocomial infection than a physician covering up a boil or a nurse minimizing "the flu."

＊Cross-infection by direct contact

＊Infected attendants dangerous

■ Environment

With the exception of the immediate vicinity of an infected individual or a carrier, transmission through the air or on fomites is much less important than that caused by personnel or equipment. Notable exceptions are when the environment becomes contaminated with *Mycobacterium tuberculosis* from a patient or *Legionella pneumophila* in the water supply. These events are most likely to result in disease when the organisms are numerous or the patient is particularly vulnerable (eg, after heart surgery or bone marrow transplantation).

M tuberculosis and Legionella are risks

■ Medical Devices

Much of the success of modern medicine is related to medical devices that support or monitor basic body functions. By their very nature, devices such as catheters, implants, and respirators carry a risk of nosocomial infection because they bypass normal defense barriers, providing microorganisms access to normally sterile fluids and tissues. Most of the recognized causes are bacterial or fungal. The risk of infection is related to the degree of debilitation of the patient and various factors concerning the design and management of the device. Any device that crosses the skin or a mucosal barrier may allow microbes in the patient or environment to gain access to deeper sites beyond the outside surface. Possible access inside the device (eg, in the lumen) adds another and, sometimes, greater risk. In some devices, such as urinary catheters, contamination is avoidable; in others, such as respirators, complete sterility is either impossible or impractical to achieve.

The risk of contamination leading to infection is increased if organisms that gain access can multiply within the system. The availability of water, nutrients, and a suitable temperature largely determine which organism will survive and multiply. Many of the gram-negative rods such as *Pseudomonas*, *Acinetobacter*, and members of Enterobacteriaceae can multiply in an environment containing water and little else. Gram-positive bacteria generally require more physiologic conditions.

Even with proper growth conditions, many hours are required before contaminating organisms multiply to numbers sufficient to cause disease. Detailed studies of catheters and similar devices show that the risk of infection begins to increase after 24 to 48 hours of use and is cumulative even if the device is changed or disinfected at intervals. It is, thus, important to discontinue transcutaneous procedures as soon as medically indicated. The medical devices most frequently associated with nosocomial infections are listed in the following text. The infectious risk of others can be estimated from the principles discussed previously. New devices are constantly being introduced into medical care, occasionally, without adequate consideration of their potential to cause nosocomial infection.

Urinary Catheters

Urinary tract infection (UTI) accounts for 40% to 50% of all nosocomial infections, and at least 80% of these are associated with catheterization. The infectious risk of a single urinary catheterization has been estimated at 1%, and indwelling catheters carry a risk that may be as high as 10%. The major preventive measure is maintenance of a completely closed system through the use of valves and aspiration ports designed to prevent bacterial access to the inside of the catheter or collecting bag. Unfortunately, breaks in closed systems eventually occur when the system is in place for more than 30 days. The urine itself serves as an excellent culture medium once bacteria gain access.

Vascular Catheters

Needles and plastic catheters placed in veins for fluid administration, monitoring vital functions, or diagnostic procedures are a leading cause of nosocomial bacteremia. These sites should always be suspected as a source of organisms whenever blood cultures are positive with no apparent primary site for the bacteremia. Contamination at the insertion site is generally staphylococcal, with continued growth in the catheter tip. Organisms may gain access somewhere in the lines, valves, bags, or bottles of intravenous solutions proximal to the insertion site. The latter circumstance usually involves gram-negative rods. Preventive measures include aseptic insertion technique and appropriate care of the lines, including changes at regular intervals.

Respirators

Machines that assist or control respiration by pumping air directly into the trachea have a great potential for causing nosocomial pneumonia if the aerosol they deliver becomes contaminated. Bacterial growth is significant only in the parts of the device that contain water; in systems using nebulizers, bacteria can be suspended in water droplets small enough to reach the alveoli. The organisms involved include *Pseudomonas*, Enterobacteriaceae, and a wide variety of environmental bacteria such as *Acinetobacter*. The primary control measure is periodic changing and disinfection of the tubing, reservoirs, and nebulizer jets.

※ Equipment provides microbial access

Conditions for bacterial growth increase risk

Indwelling devices should be changed

Urinary drainage systems violated

※ Skin primary source for IVs

Changing controls nebulizer contamination

Blood and Blood Products

Infections related to contact with blood and blood products are generally more a risk for healthcare workers rather than patients. Manipulations ranging from phlebotomy and hemodialysis to surgery carry the varying risks of blood containing an infectious agent reaching mucous membranes or skin of the healthcare worker. The major agents transmitted in this manner are hepatitis B, hepatitis C, and HIV. Control requires meticulous attention to procedures that prevent direct contact with blood, such as the use of gloves, eyewear, and gowns. Cuts and needle sticks among healthcare workers carry a risk approaching 2%. Identification of hepatitis virus and HIV carriers is a part of a protective process that must be balanced by patient privacy considerations. Healthcare facilities all have established policies concerning serologic surveillance of patients and the procedures to follow (eg, testing, prophylaxis) when blood-related accidents occur. Similarly, products for transfusion undergo extensive screening to protect the recipient.

Risk of hepatitis, HIV related to blood manipulation

INFECTION CONTROL

Infection control is the sum of all the means used to prevent nosocomial infections. Historically, such methods have been developed as an integral part of the study of infectious diseases, often serving as key elements in the proof of infectious etiology. In the 19th century, Joseph Lister achieved a dramatic reduction in surgical wound infections by infusion of a phenolic antiseptic into wounds. This local destruction of organisms was known as **antisepsis.** As it became recognized that contamination of wounds was not inevitable, the emphasis gradually shifted to preventing contact between microorganisms and susceptible sites—a concept called **asepsis.** Asepsis, which combines containment with the methods of sterilization and disinfection previously discussed, is the central approach of infection control. The measures taken to achieve asepsis vary, depending on whether the circumstances and environment are the operating room, hospital ward, or outpatient clinic.

✳ **Asepsis prevents contamination**

■ Asepsis

Operating Room

The surgical suite and operating room represent the most controlled and rigid application of aseptic principles. The procedure begins with the use of an antiseptic scrub of the skin over the operative site and the hands and forearms of all who will have contact with the patient. The use of sterile drapes, gowns, and instruments serves to prevent spread through direct contact, and caps and face masks reduce airborne spread from personnel to the wound. The level of bacteria in the air is generally increased by the number of persons and amount of movement in the operating room more than any change in the incoming air. The net effect of these procedures is to draw a sterile curtain around the operative site, thus minimizing contact with microorganisms. Surgical asepsis is also used in other areas where invasive special procedures such as cardiac catheterization are carried out.

Sterile drapes prevent organism contact

✳ **Personnel generate airborne bacteria**

Hospital Ward

Although theoretically desirable, strict aseptic procedures as used in the operating room are impractical in the ward setting. Asepsis is practiced by the use of sterile needles, medications, dressings, and other items that could serve as transmission vehicles if contaminated. A "no touch" technique for examining wounds and changing dressings eliminates direct contact with any nonsterile item. Invasive procedures such as catheter insertion and lumbar punctures are carried out under aseptic precautions similar to those used in the operating room. In all circumstances, handwashing between patient contacts is the single most important aseptic precaution.

✳ **Handwashing most important**

Outpatient Clinic

The general aseptic practices used on the hospital ward are also appropriate to the outpatient situation as preventive measures. Patients who may be infected should be segregated whenever possible using techniques similar to those of hospital ward isolation. The examining room may be used in a manner analogous to the private rooms on a hospital ward. Although this approach is difficult because of patient turnover, it should be attempted for infections that would require strict or respiratory isolation in the hospital.

Waiting areas a risk

TABLE 3–3		Precautions for Prevention of Nosocomial Infections				
PRECAUTION	ROOM	HANDWASHING[a]	GLOVES	GOWNS	MASK[b]	TYPICAL DISEASES
Standard		After removing gloves, between patients	Blood, fluid contact, touching skin	Blood, fluid contact, during procedures	During procedures	All
Transmission-based						
Airborne	Private, negative pressure[c]	After removing gloves, between patients	Room entry	Room entry	Room entry or respirator[d]	Measles, chicken-pox, tuberculosis[d]
Droplet	Private[e]	After removing gloves, between patients	Blood, fluid contact	Blood, fluid contact	Within 3 ft of patient	Meningitis, pertussis, plague, influenza
Contact	Private[e]	After removing gloves, between patients	Room entry	Patient contact	—	Infectious diarrhea,[f] Staphylococcus aureus wounds

[a]Using a disinfectant soap.
[b]Standard surgical mask, goggles.
[c]Room pressure must be negative in relation to surrounding area and the circulation exhausted outside the building.
[d]For patients with diagnosed or suspect tuberculosis, a specially filtered respirator/mask must be worn.
[e]Door may be left open and patients with the same organism may share a room.
[f]Particularly Clostridium difficile, Escherichia coli O:157, Shigella, and incontinent patients shedding rotavirus or hepatitis A.

■ Isolation Procedures

Patients with infections pose special problems because they may transmit their infections to other patients either directly or by contact with a staff member. This additional risk is managed by the techniques of isolation, which place barriers between the infected patient and others on the ward. Because not every infected patient presents with suspect signs and/or symptoms, some precautions should be taken with all patients. In the system recommended by the Centers for Disease Control and Prevention, these are called **standard precautions** and include the use of gowns and gloves when in contact with patient blood or secretions. These are particularly directed at protecting healthcare workers from HIV and hepatitis infection. For those with suspected or proven infection, additional precautions are taken, the nature of which is determined by the known mode of transmission of the organism. These **transmission-based precautions** are divided into those directed at airborne, droplet, and contact routes. The **airborne** transmission precautions are for infections known to be transmitted by extremely small (<5 μm) particles suspended in the air. This requires that the room air circulation be maintained with negative pressure relative to the surrounding area and be exhausted to the outside. Those entering the room must wear surgical masks, and in the case of tuberculosis, specially designed respirators. **Droplet** precautions are for infections in which the organisms are suspended in larger droplets, which may be airborne, but generally do not travel more than 3 ft from the patient who generates them. These can be contained by the use of gowns, gloves, and masks when working close to the patient. **Contact** precautions are used for infections that require direct contact with organisms on or that pass in secretions of the patient. Diarrheal infections are of special concern because of the extent to which they contaminate the environment. Details of the precautions and examples of the typical infectious agents are summarized in **Table 3–3.**

* Transmission precautions block airborne, droplet, contact routes

■ Prevention

The prevention of nosocomial infections is contingent on basic and applied knowledge drawn from all parts of this book. Applied with common sense, these principles can both prevent disease and reduce the costs of medical care.

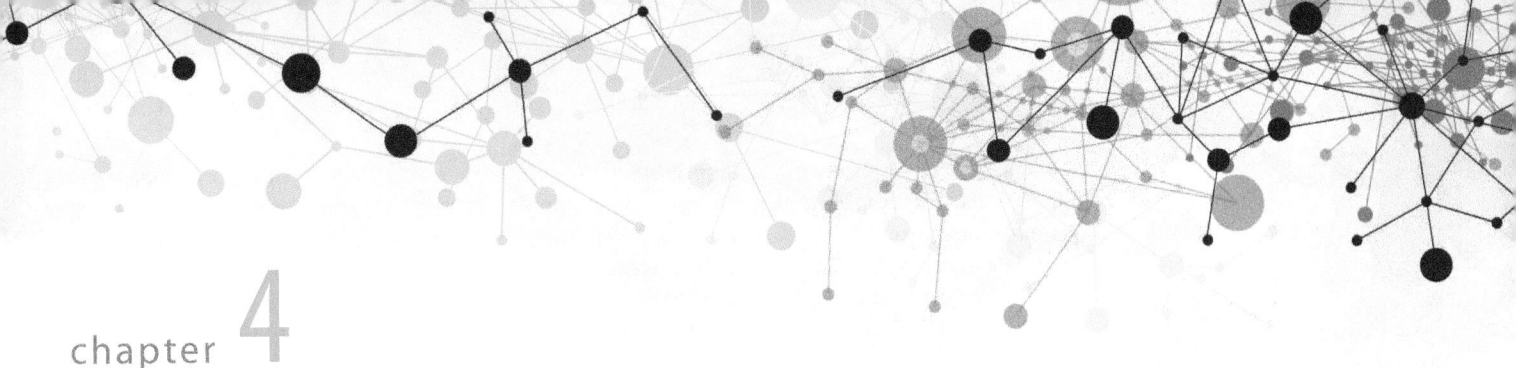

4

Principles of
Laboratory Diagnosis
of Infectious Diseases

The diagnosis of a microbial infection begins with an assessment of the clinical and epidemiologic features and formulation of a diagnostic hypothesis. Anatomic localization of the infection depends on physical and radiologic findings (eg, right lower lobe pneumonia, subphrenic abscess). This **clinical diagnosis** suggests a number of possible etiologic agents based on knowledge of infectious syndromes and their courses. The specific cause or **etiologic diagnosis** is then established by the application of methods described in this chapter. A combination of science and art on the part of both the clinician and laboratory worker is required: The clinician must select the appropriate tests and specimens to be processed and, where appropriate, suggest the suspected etiologic agents to the laboratory. The laboratory scientist must use the methods that will demonstrate the probable agents and be prepared to explore other possibilities suggested by the clinical situation or by the findings of the laboratory examinations. The best results are obtained when communication between the clinician and laboratory is optimal.

※ Clinical diagnosis guides approach to etiologic diagnosis

Behind every clinical specimen submitted to the diagnostic laboratory should be a question. Does my patient have, can I exclude, does the result confirm the disease? Answers to such questions depend on understanding, whether articulated specifically or not, the characteristics of the tests ordered and performed. These characteristics are **sensitivity** (the test's ability to rule out [sn**out**] a disease because there are few false-negative results and thus fewer cases missed) and **specificity** (the test's ability to rule in [sp**in**] or confirm an etiology because there are few false-positive results). Ideally, a test would have both excellent sensitivity and specificity, but traditional methods often involved a trade-off between the two, which only emphasizes the need to know the clinical question or reason for ordering a test. Molecular methods, however, tend to have improved sensitivity as well as specificity, which is dramatically so for viral etiologic diagnoses.

※ Sensitivity is capacity of test to rule OUT a diagnosis

※ Specificity is ability of test to rule IN or confirm diagnosis

Predictive value of a test is determined by its sensitivity and specificity and the prevalence of disease in a population or the likelihood thereof in a patient based on the history, clinical findings, and epidemiology of the infectious disease agent being considered. The more sensitive a test, the greater its negative predictive value (NPV), thus a patient with a negative test is very unlikely to have the disease. A positive result with a more specific test makes a diagnosis more likely or has a higher positive predictive value (PPV) and basically confirms an etiologic diagnosis. When the prevalence of a disease is exceedingly low or the likelihood is virtually nil based on the history, clinical findings, and epidemiology, even tests with high sensitivity and specificity may have a low PPV. This reality highlights the importance of the clinical diagnosis in guiding the approach to making an etiologic diagnosis based on the question(s) posed to the diagnostic microbiology laboratory.

The general approaches to laboratory diagnosis vary with different microorganisms and infectious diseases. However, the types of methods are usually some combination of direct microscopic examinations, culture, antigen detection, and antibody detection (serology). Nucleic acid amplification (NAA) assays that enable direct detection of genomic components of pathogens are now essential in clinical microbiology laboratories, especially for viral infections. Multiplexed polymerase chain reaction (PCR) platforms that enable rapid, direct detection of multiple potential pathogens in appropriate specimens are now available for respiratory, gastrointestinal, and central nervous system pathogens and for identification of positive blood cultures. Despite such progress, however, traditional methods remain important and complementary, since isolation of microorganisms by culture is needed for most antimicrobial susceptibility testing. Not all pathogens are detected in these panels, and only known pathogens are sought. Therefore, this chapter considers the principles of infectious disease laboratory diagnosis and the methods available with an emphasis on bacterial and fungal infections. Details about particular agents are discussed in the relevant chapters and in the section about infectious disease syndromes and etiologies at the back of the book. All diagnostic approaches begin with some kind of specimen collected from the patient.

✳ Microscopic, culture, antigen, antibody detection classic

✳ NAA foremost for viral pathogens

THE SPECIMEN

The primary connection between the clinical encounter and the diagnostic laboratory is the specimen submitted for processing. If it is not appropriately chosen and/or collected, no degree of laboratory skill can rectify the error. Failure at the level of specimen collection is the most common reason for failing to establish an etiologic diagnosis, or worse, for suggesting a wrong diagnosis. In the case of bacterial infections, the primary problem lies in distinguishing resident or contaminating normal floral organisms from those causing the infection. The three specimen categories illustrated in **Figure 4–1A-C** are discussed in the text that follows.

✳ Quality of specimen crucial

■ Direct Tissue or Fluid Samples

Direct specimens (**Figure 4–1A**) are collected from normally sterile tissues (lung, liver) and body fluids (cerebrospinal fluid, blood). The methods range from needle aspiration of an abscess to surgical biopsy. In general, such collections require the direct involvement of a physician and may carry some risk for the patient. The results are always useful because positive findings are diagnostic and negative findings can exclude infection at the suspected site.

✳ Direct samples highest quality and risk

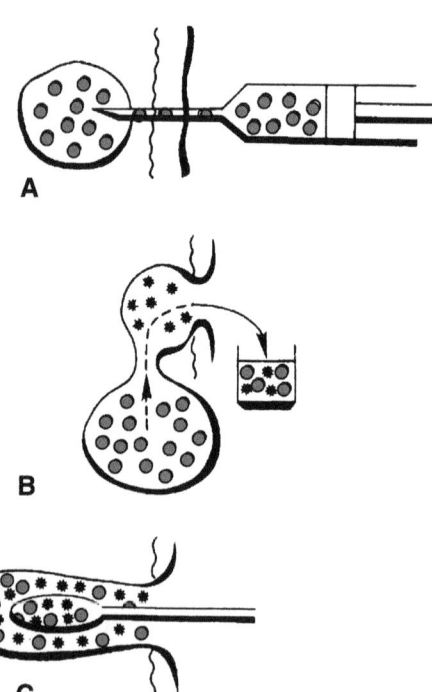

FIGURE 4–1. **Specimens for the diagnosis of infection. A.** Direct specimen. The pathogen is localized in an otherwise sterile site, and a barrier such as the skin must be passed to sample it. This may be done surgically or by needle aspiration as shown. The specimen collected contains only the pathogen. Examples are deep abscess and cerebrospinal fluid. **B.** Indirect sample. The pathogen is localized as in A but must pass through a site containing normal flora in order to be collected. The specimen contains the pathogen, but is contaminated with the nonpathogenic flora. The degree of contamination is often related to the skill with which the normal floral site was "bypassed" in specimen collection. Examples are expectorated sputum and voided urine. **C.** Sample from site with normal flora. The pathogen and nonpathogenic flora are mixed at the site of infection. Both are collected and the nonpathogen is either inhibited by the use of selective culture methods or discounted in interpretation of culture results. Examples are throat and stool.

■ Indirect Samples

Indirect samples (**Figure 4–1B**) are specimens of inflammatory exudates (expectorated sputum, voided urine) that have passed through sites known to be colonized with the resident microbiota. The site of origin is usually sterile in healthy persons; however, some assessment of the probability of contamination with resident microbiota during collection is necessary in interpretation of the results. This assessment requires knowledge of the potential contaminating flora as well as the probable pathogens to be sought. Indirect samples are usually more convenient for both physician and patient, but carry a higher risk of misinterpretation. For some specimens, such as expectorated sputum, guidelines to assess specimen quality have been developed by correlation of clinical and microbiologic findings.

Bypassing microbiota requires effort

Assessment of contamination required

■ Samples from Microbiota Sites

Frequently, the primary site of infection is in an area known to be colonized with many organisms (pharynx and large intestine) (**Figure 4–1C**). This is primarily an issue with bacterial diagnosis because they dominate the makeup of the microbiota. In such instances, examinations are made selectively for organisms known to cause infection that are not normally found at the infected site. For example, the enteric pathogens *Salmonella*, *Shigella*, and *Campylobacter* may be sought selectively in a stool specimen or only β-hemolytic streptococci in a throat culture. In these instances, selective media that inhibit growth of the other bacteria are used or, if growing, they are simply ignored. Molecular methods that target the specific pathogens in these specimens are becoming more widely used in place of the selective cultures.

Strict pathogens sought specifically

The selection of specimens for viral diagnosis is easier because there is usually little resident viral flora to confuse interpretation. This allows selection guided by knowledge of which sites are most likely to yield the suspected etiologic agent. For example, enteroviruses are the most common viruses involved in acute infection of the central nervous system. Moreover, NAA tests have replaced viral cultures in virtually all clinical microbiology laboratories owing to their rapidity, sensitivity, and specificity in detecting viral pathogens.

Lack of viral microbiota simplifies interpretation

■ Specimen Collection and Transport

The **sterile swab** is often used for specimen collection; however, it provides the poorest conditions for survival of bacterial pathogens, can only absorb a small volume of inflammatory exudate, and is easily contaminated with adjacent microbiota. The worst possible specimen is a dried-out swab; the best is a collection of 5 to 10 mL or more of the infected fluid or tissue when possible. The volume is important because infecting organisms that are present in small numbers may not be detected in a small sample. Throat swabs suffice for detection of group A streptococci by culture or antigen testing. Multiplex panels targeting respiratory viruses are validated for use with special (flocked) nasopharyngeal (NP) swabs, because these swabs collect some host epithelial cells in which the pathogenic viruses grow and thereby increase sensitivity of detection.

Swabs limit volume, survival, and may mislead

Specimens should be transported to the laboratory as soon after collection as possible because some microorganisms survive only briefly outside the body. In contrast, some bacteria survive well and may even multiply after the specimen is collected. The growth of enteric Gram-negative rods in specimens awaiting culture may, in fact, compromise specimen interpretation or interfere with the isolation of more fastidious organisms. Significant changes are associated with delays of more than 3 to 4 hours.

Viability lost if specimen is delayed

Various **transport media** have been developed to minimize the effects of the delay between specimen collection and laboratory processing. In general, they are buffered fluid or semisolid media containing minimal nutrients and are designed to prevent drying, maintain a neutral pH, and minimize growth of bacterial contaminants. Other features may be required to meet special requirements, such as an oxygen-free atmosphere for obligate anaerobes or specific (validated) collection-transport systems for molecular assays.

Transport media stabilize

DIRECT EXAMINATION

Of the infectious agents discussed in this book, only some of the parasites are large enough to be seen with the naked eye. Bacteria and fungi can be seen clearly with the light microscope when appropriate methods are used, whereas individual viruses are too small. Various stains are used to visualize and differentiate microorganisms in smears and histologic sections.

Parasites require microscopy

■ Light (Bright-field) Microscopy

Direct examination of stained or unstained preparations by light microscopy is particularly useful for detection of bacteria, fungi, and parasites. Even the smallest bacteria (1-2 μm wide) can be visualized, although all require staining and some require special lighting techniques. Since the resolution limit of the light microscope is near 0.2 μm, the optics must be ideal if small organisms are to be seen clearly by direct microscopy.

Bacteria may be stained by a variety of dyes, including methylene blue, crystal violet, carbol-fuchsin (red), and safranin (red). The two most important methods, the Gram and acid-fast techniques, use staining, decolorization, and counterstaining in a manner that helps to classify as well as stain the organism.

The Gram Stain

The differential staining procedure described in 1884 by the Danish physician Hans Christian Gram has proved one of the most useful in microbiology and medicine. The procedure (**Figure 4–2A**) involves the application of a solution of iodine in potassium iodide to cells previously stained with an acridine dye, such as crystal violet. This treatment produces a mordanting action in which purple insoluble complexes are formed with ribonuclear protein in the cell. The difference between Gram-positive and Gram-negative bacteria is in the permeability of the cell wall to these complexes on treatment with mixtures of acetone and alcohol solvents. This extracts the purple

Bacteria visible if optics maximized

Bacteria must be stained

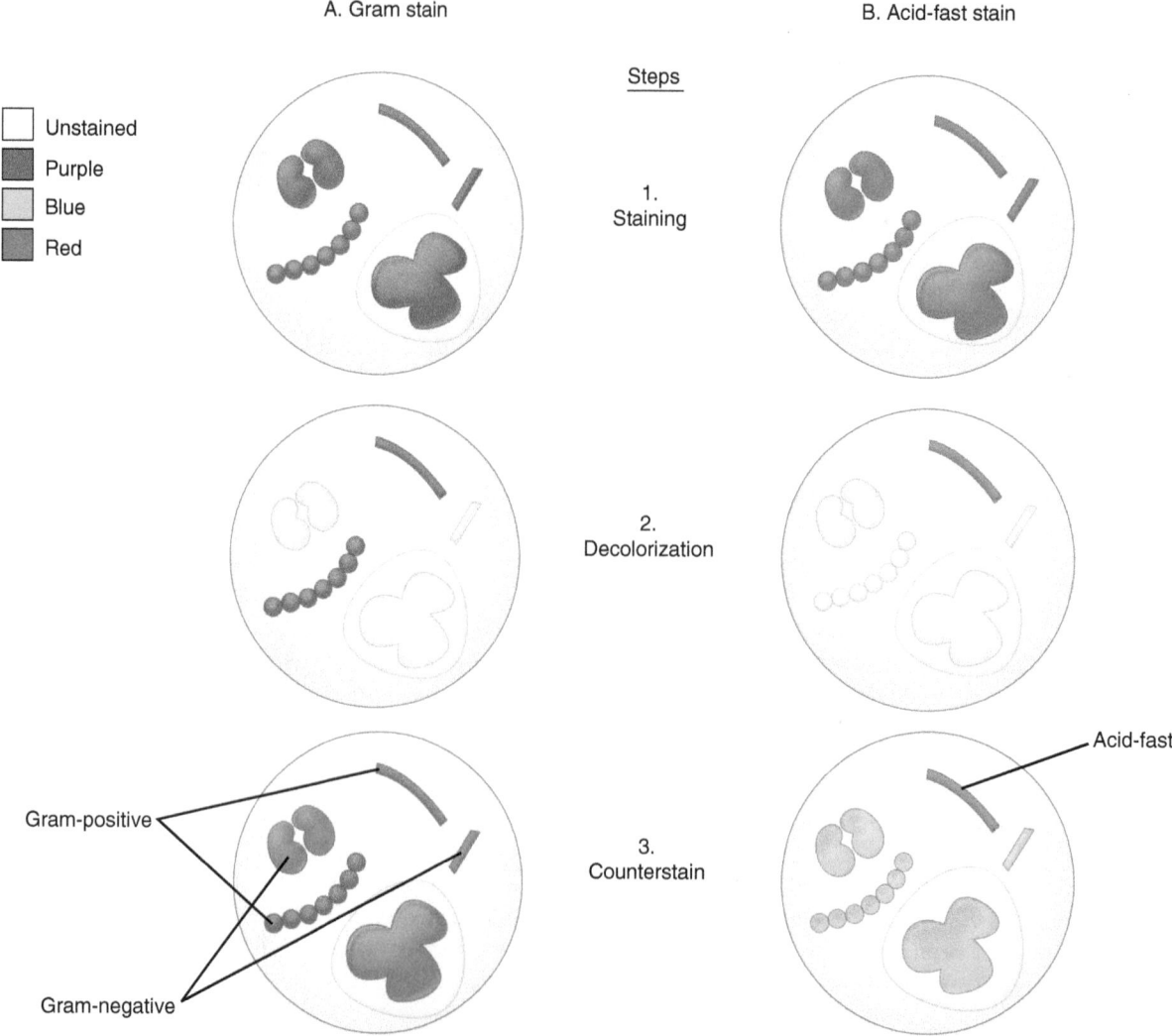

FIGURE 4–2. Gram and acid-fast stains. Four bacteria and a polymorphonuclear neutrophil are shown at each stage. All are initially stained purple by the crystal violet and iodine of the Gram stain (A1) and red by the carbol fuch-sin of the acid-fast stain (B1). After decolorization, Gram-positive and acid-fast organisms retain their original stain. Others are unstained (A2, B2). The safranin of the Gram counterstain stains the Gram-negative bacteria and makes the background red (A3), and the methylene blue leaves a blue background for the contrasting red acid-fast bacillus (B3).

iodine-dye complexes from Gram-negative cells, whereas Gram-positive bacteria retain them. An intact cell wall is necessary for a positive reaction, and Gram-positive bacteria may fail to retain the stain if the organisms are old, dead, or damaged by antimicrobial agents. The stain is completed by the addition of a red counter-stain such as safranin, which is taken up by bacteria that have been decolorized. Thus, cells stained purple are Gram positive, and those stained red are Gram negative. As indicated in **Chapter 21,** Gram positivity and negativity correspond to major structural differences in the cell wall.

In many bacterial infections, the etiologic agents are readily seen on stained Gram smears of pus or fluids. The purple or red bacteria are seen against a Gram-negative (red) background of leukocytes, exudate, and debris (**Figures 4–2A1-3** and **4–3C**). This information, combined with

✳ Gram positive (purple) retain purple iodine-dye complexes

✳ Gram negative (pink-red) do not retain

Simple Stains

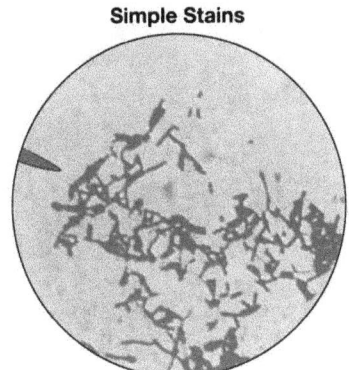

A Crystal violet stain of *Escherichia coli*

Differential Stains

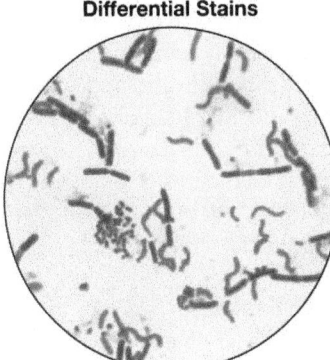

C Gram stain
Purple cells are Gram positive.
Red cells are Gram negative.

Special Stains

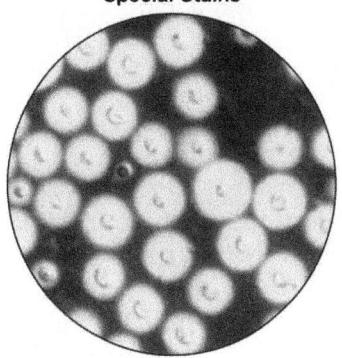

F India ink capsule stain of *Cryptococcus neoformans*

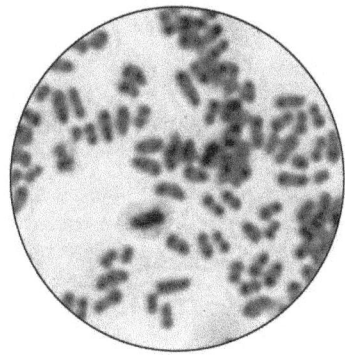

B Methylene blue stain of *Corynebacterium*

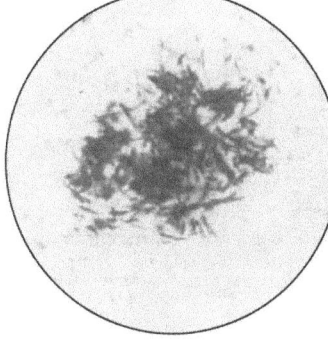

D Acid-fast stain
Red cells are acid-fast.
Blue cells are nonacid-fast.

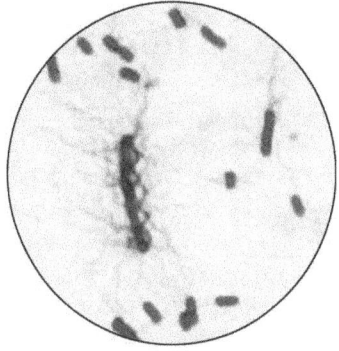

G Flagellar stain of *Proteus vulgaris*.
A basic stain was used to build up the flagella.

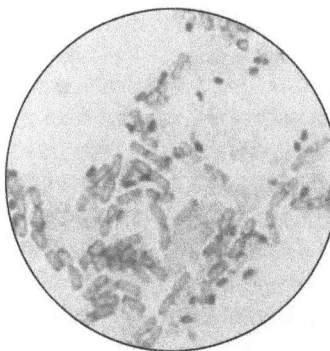

E Endospore stain, showing endospores (red) and vegetative cells (blue)

FIGURE 4–3. **Types of microbiologic stains.** (Reproduced with permission from Willey JM: *Prescott, Harley, & Klein's Microbiology*, 7th ed. New York, NY: McGraw Hill; 2008.)

the clinical findings, may guide the management of infection before culture results are available. For example, paired Gram-positive cocci and polymorphonuclear leucocytes (PMNs) in a quality sputum specimen devoid of squamous epithelial cells denote a pneumococcal etiology in a patient with the clinical diagnosis of pneumonia, whereas small, pleomorphic Gram-negative rods suggest *Haemophilus influenzae* as the culprit. Done well the Gram-stained smear can achieve sensitivities of 70% to 80% and specificities of 90% to 95% for pneumococcal and *H influenzae* pneumonia, respectively, in a patient with pulmonary infiltrates and disease acquired in the community. Interpretation requires considerable experience and knowledge of probable causes, of their morphology and Gram reaction, and of any organisms normally present in health at the infected site.

The Acid-fast Stain

Acid fastness is a property of the mycobacteria (eg, *Mycobacterium tuberculosis*) and related organisms. Acid-fast organisms generally stain very poorly with dyes, including those used in the Gram stain. However, they can be stained by prolonged application of more concentrated dyes, by penetrating agents, or by heat treatment. Their unique feature is that when stained, acid-fast bacteria resist decolorization by concentrations of mineral acids and ethanol that remove the same dyes from other bacteria. This combination of weak initial staining and strong retention once stained is related to the high lipid content of the mycobacterial cell wall. Acid-fast stains are completed with a counterstain to provide a contrasting background for viewing the stained bacteria (**Figures 4–2B1-3** and **4–3D**).

In the acid-fast procedure, the slide is flooded with carbol-fuchsin (red) and decolorized with hydrochloric acid in alcohol. When counterstained with methylene blue, acid-fast organisms appear red against a blue background (**Figure 4–3D**). A variant is the **fluorochrome stain,** which uses a fluorescent dye (auramine, or an auramine–rhodamine mixture), followed by decolorization with acid–alcohol. Acid-fast organisms retain the fluorescent stain, which allows their visualization by fluorescence microscopy. The fluorochrome stain is more sensitive and allows rapid screening and, therefore, has become the method of choice in most laboratories performing testing for acid-fast organisms.

Stains used in the diagnostic laboratory can be classified as simple, differential, or special as depicted in (**Figure 4–3**). Some are rarely used, but can be instructive. For example, **Figure 4–3A** shows the appearance of the Gram stain if the decolorization and counter-stain steps are omitted. Historically, the one-step methylene blue satin (**4-3B**) was used for *Corynebacterium diphtheriae*. The endospore stain (**4-3E**) delineates the presence and location of spores as in **Bacillus** spp. (**Chapter 26**) and **Clostridia** spp. (**Chapter 29**) and the flagellar stain (**4-3G**) show the peritrichous flagella of *Proteus* spp. and some other Enterobacteriacae (**Chapter 33**) or unipolar as with *Vibrio cholerae* (**Chapter 32**).

Fungal and Parasitic Stains

The smallest fungi are the size of large bacteria, and all parasitic forms are larger. This allows detection in simple wet mount preparations, often without staining. Fungi in sputum or body fluids can be seen by mixing the specimen with a potassium hydroxide solution (to dissolve debris) and viewing with a medium power lens. The use of simple stains or the fluorescent calcofluor white reagent improves the sensitivity of detection. Another technique is to mix the specimen with India ink, which outlines the fungal cells (**Figure 4–3F**). Detection of the cysts and eggs of parasites requires a concentration procedure if the specimen is stool, but once done they can be visualized with a simple iodine stain (**Figure 4–4**).

CULTURE

Despite widespread use of nucleic acid diagnostic procedures, cultures remain essential in clinical diagnostic laboratories. Isolation in pure culture is required for identification and most phenotypic antimicrobial susceptibility testing.

Growth on artificial media, isolation, and identification of the infecting agent is usually the most sensitive and specific means for an etiologic diagnosis of common bacterial and fungal pathogens. Theoretically, the presence of a single live organism in the specimen can yield a positive result. Most bacteria and fungi can be grown in a variety of artificial media, but strictly intracellular microorganisms (eg, *Chlamydia*, *Rickettsia*, and viruses) can be isolated only in cultures of living eukaryotic cells. Consequently, molecular methods have replaced culture for these pathogens.

Decolorized background should be pink-red

Gram reaction, morphology guide clinical decisions

Acid-fast bacteria take stains poorly

Once stained, they retain it strongly

There are multiple variants of the acid-fast stain

Fungi and parasites visible with simple stains

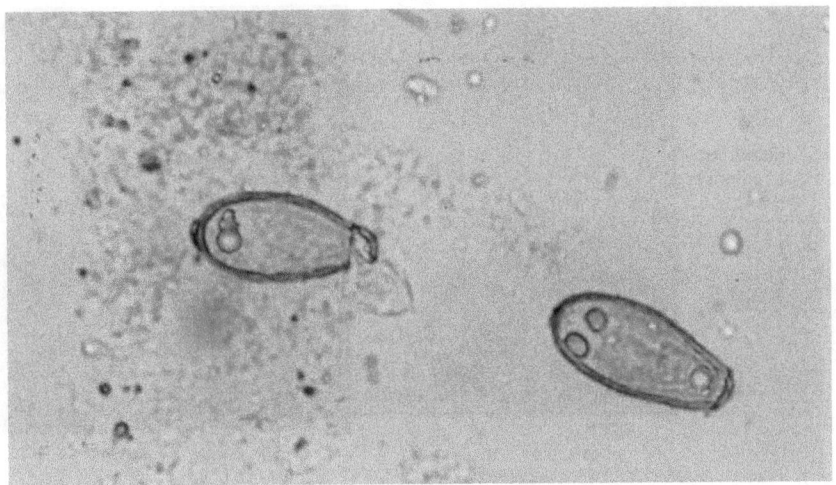

FIGURE 4–4. **Iodine-stained parasite eggs.** Two eggs of the intestinal fluke *Clonorchis sinensis* are present in this stool specimen. (Reproduced with permission from Connor DH, Chandler FW, Schwartz DQ, et al: *Pathology of Infectious Diseases.* Stamford CT: Appleton & Lange; 1997.)

■ Isolation and Identification of Bacteria and Fungi

Almost all medically important bacteria can be cultivated outside the host in artificial culture media. A single bacterium placed in the proper culture conditions multiplies to quantities sufficient to be seen by the naked eye. Bacteriologic media are broth recipes prepared from digests of animal or vegetable protein supplemented with nutrients such as glucose, yeast extract, serum, or blood to meet the metabolic requirements of the organism. Their chemical composition is complex, and their success depends on matching the nutritional requirements of most heterotrophic living things. The same approaches are used for growing fungi.

Bacteria grow in broth and on solid media

Growth in media prepared in the fluid state (broth) is apparent when bacterial numbers are sufficient to produce turbidity or macroscopic clumps. Turbidity results from reflection of transmitted light by the bacteria; depending on the size of the organism, from 10^5 to 10^6 bacteria per milliliter of broth are required. The addition of a gelling agent to a broth medium allows its preparation in solid form in Petri dishes. The universal gelling agent for diagnostic bacteriology is **agar**—a polysaccharide extracted from seaweed. Agar has the convenient property of becoming liquid at approximately 95°C but not returning to the solid gel state until cooled to less than 50°C. This allows the addition of a heat-labile substance such as blood to the medium before it sets. At temperatures used in the diagnostic laboratory (37°C or lower), broth–agar exists as a smooth, solid, nutrient gel. This medium, usually termed agar, may be qualified with a description of any supplement (eg, blood agar).

Large numbers of bacteria produce turbidity

Agar is used to solidify media

A useful feature of agar plates is that the bacteria can be separated by spreading a small sample of the specimen over the surface. Bacterial cells that are well separated from others grow as isolated colonies, often reaching 2 to 3 mm in diameter after overnight incubation. This allows isolation of bacteria in pure culture because the colony is assumed to arise from a single organism (**Figure 4–5**). Colonies vary greatly in size, shape, texture, color, and other features called **colonial morphology.** Colonies from different species or genera often differ substantially, whereas those derived from the same strain are usually consistent. Differences in colonial morphology are very useful for separating bacteria in mixtures and as clues to their identity.

Bacteria separated in isolated colonies

Colonies may have characteristic features

Culture Media

Over the last 100 years, countless media have been developed by microbiologists to aid in the isolation and identification of medically important bacteria and fungi. Only a few have found their way into routine use in clinical laboratories. These may be classified as nutrient, selective, or indicator media.

Nutrient Media. The nutrient component of a medium is designed to satisfy the growth requirements of the organism to permit isolation and propagation. For medical purposes, the ideal medium would allow rapid growth of all agents. No such medium exists; however, several suffice for good growth of most medically important bacteria and fungi. These media are prepared with enzymatic or acid digests of animal or plant products, such as muscle, milk, or soybeans. The digest reduces the native protein to a mixture of polypeptides and amino acids that also includes

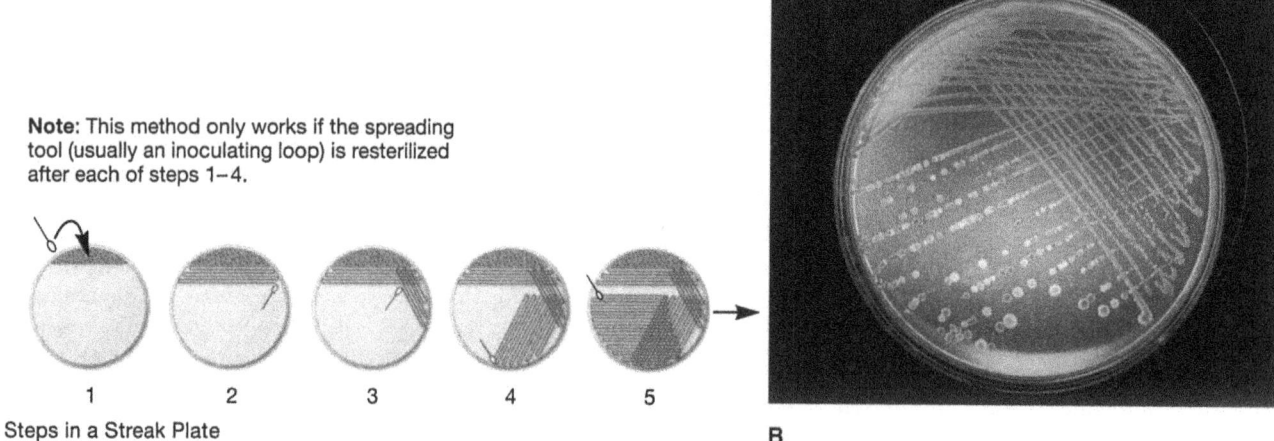

Note: This method only works if the spreading tool (usually an inoculating loop) is resterilized after each of steps 1–4.

1 2 3 4 5

A Steps in a Streak Plate

B

FIGURE 4–5. **Bacteriologic plate streaking.** Plate streaking is essentially a dilution procedure. **A.** (1) The specimen is placed on the plate with a swab, loop, or pipette and evenly spread over approximately part of plate surface with a sterilized bacteriologic loop (2-5). The loop is flamed to remove residual bacteria, and a series of overlapping streaks are made flaming the loop between each one. **B.** After overnight incubation, heavy growth is seen in the primary areas followed by isolated colonies. More than one organism is present because both a red and a clear colony are seen. (Reproduced with permission from Willey JM: *Prescott, Harley, & Klein's Microbiology*, 7th ed. New York, NY: McGraw Hill; 2008.)

Media are prepared from animal or plant products

trace metals, coenzymes, and various undefined growth factors. For example, one common broth contains a digest of casein (milk curd) and a digest of soybean meal. To this nutrient base, salts, vitamins, or body fluids such as serum may be added to provide pathogens with the conditions needed for optimum growth. All cultures of blood use this type of medium.

Selective Media. Selective media are used when specific pathogenic organisms are sought in sites with an extensive microbiota (eg, *Campylobacter* species in fecal specimens). In these cases, other bacteria may overgrow the suspected etiologic species in simple nutrient media, either because the pathogen grows more slowly or because it is present in much smaller numbers. Selective media usually contain dyes, other chemical additives, or antimicrobial agents at concentrations designed to inhibit contaminating flora but not the suspected pathogen.

Contaminants inhibited with chemicals or antimicrobials

Indicator Media. Indicator media contain substances designed to demonstrate biochemical or other features characteristic of specific pathogens or organism groups. The addition to the medium of one or more carbohydrates and a **pH indicator** is frequently used. A color change in a colony indicates the presence of acid products and thus of fermentation or oxidation of the carbohydrate by the organism. The addition of red blood cells (RBCs) to plates allows the **hemolysis** produced by some organisms to be used as a differential feature. In practice, nutrient, selective, and indicator properties are often combined to various degrees in the same medium. It is possible to include an indicator system in a highly nutrient medium and also make it selective by adding appropriate antimicrobials. Some examples of culture media commonly used in diagnostic microbiology are listed in **Appendix 4-1,** and more details of their constitution and application are provided in **Appendix 4-2.**

Metabolic properties demonstrated by indicator systems

Atmospheric Conditions

Aerobic. After inoculation, cultures of most aerobic bacteria are placed in an incubator with temperature maintained at 35°C to 37°C. Slightly higher or lower temperatures are used occasionally to selectively favor a certain organism or organism group. Most bacteria that are not obligate anaerobes grow in air; however, CO_2 is required by some and enhances the growth of others. Incubators that maintain a 2% to 5% concentration of CO_2 in air are frequently used for primary isolation, because this level is not harmful to any bacteria and improves isolation of some. Some bacteria (eg, *Campylobacter*) require a microaerophilic atmosphere with reduced oxygen (5%) and increased CO_2 (10%) levels to grow. This can be achieved by using a commercially available packet that is placed in a jar which is then sealed similar to the anaerobic system described further.

Incubation temperature, atmosphere vary

Anaerobic. Strictly anaerobic bacteria do not grow under the conditions just described, and many die when exposed to atmospheric oxygen or high oxidation–reduction potentials. Most medically important anaerobes grow in the depths of liquid or semisolid media containing any of a variety of **reducing agents,** such as cysteine, thioglycollate, ascorbic acid, or even iron filings. An anaerobic environment for incubation of plates can be achieved by replacing air with a gas mixture containing hydrogen, CO_2, and nitrogen and allowing the hydrogen to react with residual oxygen on a catalyst to form water. A convenient commercial system accomplishes this chemically in a packet that is added before the jar is sealed. Specimens suspected to contain significant anaerobes should be processed under conditions designed to minimize exposure to atmospheric oxygen at all stages.

Anaerobes require reducing conditions, no oxygen

Clinical Microbiology Procedures

Routine laboratory procedures for processing specimens from various sites are needed because no single medium or atmosphere is ideal for all bacteria. Combinations of broth and solid-plated media and aerobic, CO_2, and anaerobic incubation must be matched to the organisms expected at any particular site or clinical circumstance. Examples of such routines are shown in **Table 4–1.** In general, it is not practical to routinely include specialized media for isolation of rare organisms, such as *C diphtheriae* or *Legionella pneumophila*. For detection of these and other uncommon organisms, the laboratory must be specifically informed of their possible presence by the physician. Appropriate media and special procedures can then be included.

Designed to detect the most common organisms

Identification

When growth is detected in any medium, the process of identification begins. Identification involves methods for obtaining pure cultures from single colonies, followed by tests designed to characterize and identify the isolate. The exact tests and their sequences vary with different groups of organisms, and the taxonomic level (genus, species, subspecies, etc.) of identification needed varies according to the medical usefulness of the information. In some cases, only a general description or the exclusion of particular organisms is important. For example, a report of "mixed oral flora" in a sputum specimen or "No *Salmonella*, *Shigella*, or *Campylobacter* isolated" in a fecal specimen may provide all the information needed. MALDI-TOF (matrix-assisted laser desorption ionization-time of flight) mass spectroscopy has become the foremost tool used for the rapid identification of microorganisms already isolated in pure culture and has reduced time to identification and reporting substantially from a day or more to minutes. Although a major advance, MALDI-TOF complements but does not replace fully the need for traditional methods.

Extent of identification is linked to medical relevance

TABLE 4–1	Routine Use of Gram Smear and Isolation Systems for Selected Clinical Specimens[a]							
	SPECIMEN							
MEDIUM (INCUBATION)	**BLOOD**	**CEREBROSPINAL FLUID**	**WOUND, PUS**	**GENITAL, CERVIX**	**THROAT**	**SPUTUM**	**URINE**	**STOOL**
Gram smear		×	×	×		×		
Soybean–casein digest broth $(CO_2)^a$	×							
Blood agar (CO_2)		×	×		×[b]	×	×	
Chocolate agar (CO_2)		×	×	× PCR preferred		×		
Blood agar (anaerobic)			×					
MacConkey agar (air)			×			×	×	×
Hektoen agar (air)								×
Selenite F broth (air)								×
Campylobacter agar $(CO_2, 42°C)^c$								×
Martin–Lewis agar (CO_2)				× PCR preferred				

[a]The added sensitivity of a nutrient broth is used only when contamination by normal flora is unlikely. Exact media and protocols may vary between laboratories.
[b]Anaerobic incubation used to enhance hemolysis by β-hemolytic streptococci.
[c]Incubation in a reduced oxygen atmosphere.

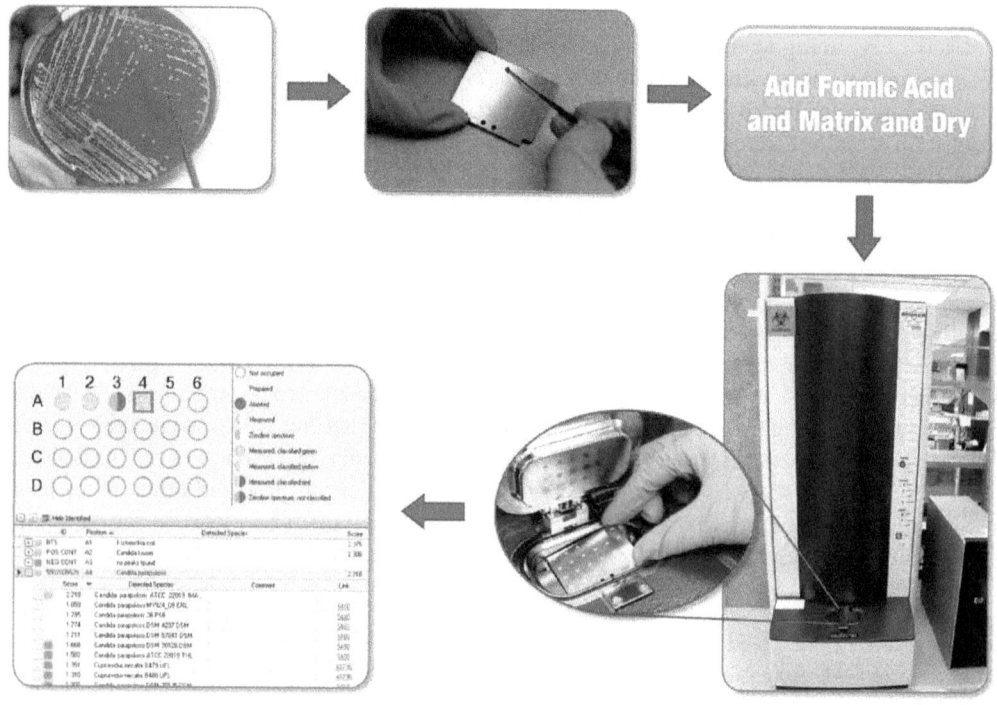

The scope and accuracy of MALDI-TOF depend on the quality of the data based used for comparisons. As depicted schematically in **Figure 4-6**, ionized microorganisms are separated by mass-charge-ratio (effectively by molecular weight), collide under vacuum with an ion detector, and thereby generate a mass spectrum for comparative analysis. The net result is rapid identification of bacterial or fungal, especially yeasts, isolates.

■ Features Used to Classify Bacteria and Fungi

Cultural Characteristics

Growth under various conditions

Cultural characteristics include the demonstration of properties such as unique nutritional requirements, pigment production, and the ability to grow in the presence of certain substances (sodium chloride, bile) or on certain media (MacConkey, nutrient agar). Demonstration of the ability to grow at a particular temperature or to cause hemolysis on blood agar plates is also used. For fungi, growth as a yeast colony or a mold is the primary separator. For molds, the morphology of the mold structures (hyphae, conidia, etc.) is the primary means of identification.

Biochemical Characteristics

Biochemical reactions give identification probability

Toxin production and pathogenicity

Traditionally, the ability to attack various substrates or to produce particular metabolic products has broad application to the identification of bacteria and yeast. The most common properties examined are listed in **Appendix 4–3**. Biochemical and cultural tests for bacterial identification are analyzed by reference to tables that show the reaction patterns characteristic of individual species. In fact, advances in computer analysis have now been applied to identification of many bacterial and fungal groups. These systems use the same biochemical principles together with computerized databases to determine the most probable identification from the observed test pattern. In many laboratories, MALDI-TOF mass spectrometry has replaced these biochemical approaches except for a few rapid colorimetric spot tests, eg, indole and PYR. When identification of bacteria remains elusive after biochemical and MALDI-TOF have been attempted, the isolates usually are sent to reference laboratories for 16S rRNA or other sequencing methods if the clinical importance warrants.

Detection of specific toxin may define disease

Molecular assays have been developed for some toxins (eg, *Clostridioides difficile* as an alternative to enzyme immunoassay [EIA]) for use in the clinical laboratory. Neutralization of a toxic effect in a test animal with specific antitoxin is the method used to confirm the identity of *Clostidium botulinum* (**Chapter 29**) toxin and is available only in public health reference laboratories.

Antigenic Structure

Viruses, bacteria, fungi, and parasites possess many antigens, such as capsular polysaccharides, surface proteins, and cell wall components. Serology involves the use of antibodies of known specificity to detect antigens present on whole organisms or free in extracts (soluble antigens). The methods used for demonstrating antigen–antibody reactions are discussed in **Antibody Detection (Serology)**.

Antigenic structure demonstrated with antisera

Genomic Structure

Nucleic acid–sequence relatedness as determined by homology and direct sequence comparisons have become a primary determinant of taxonomic decisions. They are discussed later in the section on Methods of Nucleic Acid Analysis.

■ Isolation and Identification of Viruses

Cell and Organ Culture

Virtually no clinical microbiology laboratory still retains the capacity to do viral isolation by cell or organ culture. The classical techniques are done, if at all, in research or public health laboratories. The extensive repertoire of molecular assays now available for most human viral pathogens has far better sensitivity and specificity than traditional methods. The appropriate use of these NAATs in viral diagnosis is discussed for each virus in **Chapters 9** through **20** in PART II, Pathogenic Viruses.

IMMUNOLOGIC SYSTEMS

Diagnostic microbiology makes great use of the specificity of the binding between antigen and antibody. Antisera of known specificity are used to detect their homologous antigen in cultures, or more recently, directly in body fluids. Conversely, known antigen preparations are used to detect circulating antibodies as evidence of a current or previous infection with that agent. Many methods are in use to demonstrate the antigen–antibody binding. The greatly improved specificity of **monoclonal antibodies** has had a major impact on the quality of methods where they have been applied. Before discussing their application to diagnosis, the principles involved in the methods most often used in clinical laboratories are discussed.

■ Methods for Detecting an Antigen–Antibody Reaction

Precipitation

The amount of antigen or antibody necessary to produce a visible immunologic reaction can be reduced if either is on the surface of a relatively large particle. This condition can be produced by fixing soluble antigens or antibody onto the surface of microscopic latex or charcoal particles on a card/slide or RBCs suspended in a microtiter plate well. Whole bacteria are large enough to serve as the particle if the antigen is present on the microbial surface. The relative proportions of antigen and antibody thus become less critical, and antigen–antibody reactions are detectable by agglutination when immune serum and particulate antigen, or particle-associated antibody and soluble antigen, are mixed on a slide. The process is termed slide agglutination, hemagglutination, or latex agglutination depending on the nature of the sensitized particle. Agglutination tests are commonly used, especially with latex particles (eg, Lancefield typing of β-hemolytic streptococci, detection of cryptococcal antigen in CSF or serum) or charcoal particles (eg, RPR test for syphilis).

Particles coated with antigen or antibody enhance demonstration

Antibody mixing on slide causes agglutination

Immunofluorescence. One of the most common labeling methods in diagnostic microbiology is immunofluorescence in which antibody labeled with a fluorescent dye, usually **fluorescein isothiocyanate (FITC),** is applied to a slide of material that may contain the antigen sought. Under fluorescence microscopy, binding of the labeled antibody can be detected as a bright green halo surrounding bacterium or, in the case of viruses, as a fluorescent clump in or on an infected cell. The method is called direct if the FITC is conjugated directly to the antibody with the desired specificity. In indirect immunofluorescence, the specific antibody is not labeled, but its binding to an antigen is detected in an additional step using an FITC-labeled anti-immunoglobulin antibody that binds to the specific antibody. Choice between the two approaches involves purely technical considerations.

Light halo enhances visualization

Indirect methods use second antibody

Enzyme immunoassay (EIA) or **enzyme-linked immunoassay (ELISA).** These methods are more suitable for liquid phase assays and are amenable to batch testing and automated methods. They are also used in direct and indirect methods and many other ingenious variations such as the

FIGURE 4-7 **The ELISA or EIA test. A.** The direct or double antibody–sandwich method for the detection of antigens. **B.** The indirect assay for detecting antibodies. (Reproduced with permission from Willey JM: *Prescott, Harley, & Klein's Microbiology*, 7th ed. New York, NY: McGraw Hill; 2008.)

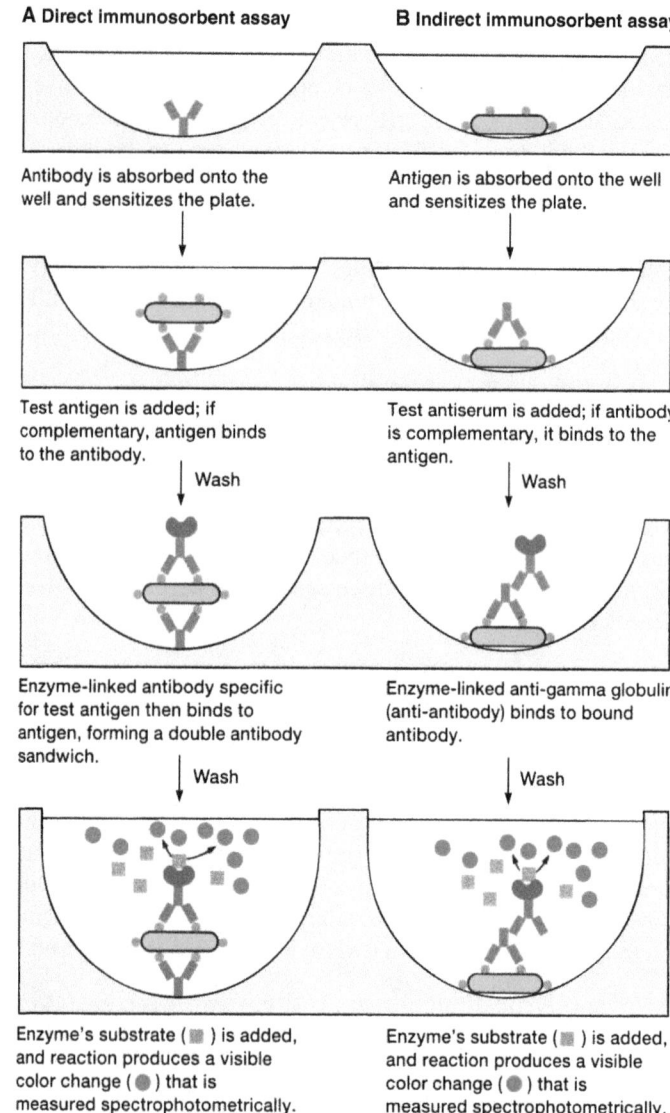

A Direct immunosorbent assay

Antibody is absorbed onto the well and sensitizes the plate.

Test antigen is added; if complementary, antigen binds to the antibody.

Wash

Enzyme-linked antibody specific for test antigen then binds to antigen, forming a double antibody sandwich.

Wash

Enzyme's substrate (▨) is added, and reaction produces a visible color change (●) that is measured spectrophotometrically.

B Indirect immunosorbent assay

Antigen is absorbed onto the well and sensitizes the plate.

Test antiserum is added; if antibody is complementary, it binds to the antigen.

Wash

Enzyme-linked anti-gamma globulin (anti-antibody) binds to bound antibody.

Wash

Enzyme's substrate (▨) is added, and reaction produces a visible color change (●) that is measured spectrophotometrically.

"sandwich" methods, so called because the antigen of interest is "trapped" between two antibodies (**Figure 4–7**). These extremely sensitive techniques are discussed further with regard to antibody detection. Related and complementary techniques used in surgical pathology are immunohistochemistry and immunoperoxidase methods (Figure 40–1). They can be a powerful adjunct to molecular methods, especially for viral pathogens in severely immunocompromised patients (eg, those after solid organ or bone marrow transplantation).

Liquid phase EIA and ELISA methods have many variants

■ Serologic Classification

For most important antigens of diagnostic significance, antisera are commercially available. The most common test methods for bacteria are agglutination and immunofluorescence, and, for viruses, neutralization. In most cases, these methods subclassify organisms below the species level and, thus, are primarily of value for epidemiologic and research purposes. The terms "serotype" and "serogroup" are used together with numbers, letters, or Roman numerals with no apparent logic other than historical precedent. For a few genera, the most fundamental taxonomic differentiation is serologic. This is the case with the streptococci, in which an existing classification based on biochemical and cultural characteristics was superseded because a serologic classification scheme developed by Rebecca Lancefield correlated better with disease.

Antigenic systems classify below the species level

Serology primarily of epidemiologic value

Before these techniques can be applied to the diagnosis of specific infectious diseases, considerable study of the causative agent(s) is required. Antigen–antibody systems may vary in complexity from a single epitope to scores of epitopes on several macromolecular antigens, whose chemical nature may or may not be known. The cause of the original 1976 outbreak of

Legionnaires disease (caused by *L pneumophila*) was proved through the development of immune reagents that detected the bacteria in tissue and antibodies directed against the bacteria in the serum of patients. Now, more than 40 years later, there are more than a dozen serotypes and many additional species, each requiring specific immunologic reagents for antigen or antibody detection for diagnosis.

■ Antibody Detection (Serology)

During infection—viral, bacterial, fungal, or parasitic—the host usually responds with the formation of antibodies, which can be detected by modification of any of the methods used for antigen detection. The formation of antibodies and their time course depend on the antigenic stimulation provided by the infection. The precise patterns vary depending on the antigens used, the classes of antibody detected, and the method. An example of temporal patterns of development and increase and decline in specific antiviral antibodies measured by different tests is illustrated in responses can be used to detect evidence of recent or past infection. The test methods do not inherently indicate immunoglobulin class, but can be modified to do so, usually by pretreatment of the serum to remove IgG to differentiate the IgM and IgG responses. Several basic principles must be emphasized

1. In an acute infection, the antibodies usually appear early in the illness, and then rise sharply over the next 10 to 21 days. Thus, a serum sample collected shortly after the onset of illness (acute serum), and another collected 2 to 3 weeks later (convalescent serum) can be compared quantitatively for changes in specific antibody content.

2. Antibodies can be quantitated by several means. The most common method is to dilute the serum serially in appropriate media and determine the maximal dilution that will still yield detectable antibody in the test system (eg, serum dilutions of 1:4, 1:8, and 1:16). The highest dilution that retains specific activity is called the antibody titer.

3. The interpretation of significant antibody responses (evidence of specific, recent infection) is most reliable when definite evidence of seroconversion is demonstrated; that is, detectable specific antibody is absent from the acute serum but present in the convalescent serum. Alternatively, a fourfold or greater increase in antibody titer supports a diagnosis of recent infection; for example, an acute serum titer of 1:4 or less and a convalescent serum titer of 1:16 or greater would be considered significant.

4. In instances in which the average antibody titers of a population to a specific agent are known, a single convalescent antibody titer significantly greater than the expected mean may be used as a supportive or presumptive evidence of recent infection. However, this finding is considerably less valuable than those obtained by comparing responses of acute and convalescent serum samples. An alternative and somewhat more complex method of serodiagnosis is to determine which major immunoglobulin subclass constitutes the major proportion of the specific antibodies. In primary infections, the IgM-specific response is often dominant during the first days or weeks after onset, but is replaced progressively by IgG-specific antibodies; thus, by 1 to 6 months after infection, the predominant antibodies belong to the IgG subclass. Consequently, serum containing a high titer of antibodies of the IgM subclass would suggest a recent, primary infection.

The immunologic methods used to identify bacterial or viral antigens are applied to serologic diagnosis by simply reversing the detection system: that is, using a known antigen to detect the presence of an antibody. The methods of serologic diagnosis to be used are selected on the basis of their convenience and applicability to the antigen in question. Of the methods for measuring antigen–antibody interaction discussed previously, those now used most frequently for serologic diagnosis are agglutination and EIA (ELISA).

Another approach to detecting antigens is to detect free antigen released by the organism into body fluids. This offers the possibility of bypassing direct examination, culture, and identification tests to achieve a diagnosis. Success requires a highly specific antibody, a sensitive detection method, and the presence of the homologous antigen in an accessible body fluid. The latter is an important limitation, because not all organisms release free antigen in the course of infection. At present, diagnosis by antigen detection is limited to some bacteria with polysaccharide capsules (eg, *Streptococcus pneumoniae*, *H influenzae*) and fungi

Soluble antigens may be
detected in body fluids

Rapid detection can replace
culture if positive

(eg, *Cryptococcus neoformans*). The techniques of agglutination with antibody bound to latex particles or EIA are used to detect free antigen in serum, cerebrospinal fluid, joint fluid, and urine. Live organisms are not required for antigen detection, and these tests may still be positive when the causative organism has been eliminated by antimicrobial therapy (eg, urinary antigen tests for pneumococci and *L pneumophila* serotype 1). The procedures can yield results within 1 or 2 hours, sometimes within a few minutes. Several commercial products detect group A streptococcal antigen in throat swabs with 70% to 90% sensitivity. Although highly specific (95% or greater), these tests are less sensitive than culture; negative results must still be confirmed by culture to rule out streptococcal infection and the need for rheumatic fever prophylaxis (**Chapter 25**).

NUCLEIC ACID ANALYSIS

As with the human genome, the genome sequence of the major human pathogens has or soon will be determined. These data are placed in widely available computer databases and have already been used for applications ranging from taxonomy to detection of antimicrobial resistance genes. Some of the methods and applications relevant to the study of infectious diseases are briefly summarized in the following discussion. The student is referred to textbooks of molecular biology for more complete coverage.

■ Methods of Nucleic Acid Analysis

DNA Hybridization and Probes

If the DNA double helix is opened, leaving single-stranded (denatured) DNA, the nucleotide bases are exposed and, thus, are available to interact with other single-stranded nucleic acid molecules. If complementary sequences of a second DNA molecule are brought into physical contact with the first, they hybridize to it, forming a new double-stranded molecule in that area. A probe is a cloned DNA fragment that has been labeled so that it can be detected if it hybridizes to complementary sequences in such a test system (**Figure 4–8**). The probe may be derived from the gene for a known protein of the pathogen or be empirically derived just for diagnostic purposes. The methods that allow the hybridization to take place include those that immobilize the single-stranded target DNA on a membrane or liquid-phase assays, which can be rapid and automated. The concept is analogous to immunologic methods, but nucleic acid complementarity rather than antibody-antigen specificity is the basis for detection of pathogens, including selected viruses, bacteria, and yeasts as well as some intracellular microorganisms.

✳ DNA hybridization methods
are used to detect target
pathogens

Nucleic Acid Amplification

Nucleic acid amplification (NAA) methods such as the PCR allow the detection and selective replication of a targeted portion of the genome (**Figure 4–9A**). The basic PCR technique uses synthetic oligonucleotide primers and special DNA polymerases in a way that allows repeated cycles of synthesis of only a segment of a targeted DNA molecule that may be as large as an entire genome. The specificity is provided by the sequence of approximately 20 nucleotides in each primer pair, which are crafted to flank the desired segment of the genome. The DNA polymerases used are ones that operate at unusually high temperatures. This enables the use of temperature to control shifts between separation of the complementary DNA strands (so primers can bind) and replication of the DNA sequence that lies between the two primers. Because each strand generates a new fragment, the increase is exponential. In an instrument called a thermocycler, the targeted DNA can be amplified 1 million to 1 billion times in 20 to 30 cycles (**Figure 4–9B**). Other NAA methods use the same principles.

NAA replicates a genome
segment

✳ PCR uses temperature to
manipulate primers and
polymerases

■ Application of Nucleic Acid Methods to Infectious Diseases

DNA Probes

Probes may be recovered from NAA procedures or more commonly synthesized as a single chain of nucleotides (oligonucleotide probe) from known sequence data. They may contain a gene of known function or simply sequences empirically found to be useful for the application in question. When labeled with a fluorescent or chromogenic marker and used in hybridization reactions, they can detect the homologous sequences in unknown specimens (**Figure 4–8**).

The diagnostic use of DNA probes is to detect or identify microorganisms by hybridization of the probe to homologous sequences in DNA extracted from the entire organism. A number of

Probes may be cloned or
synthesized from known
sequences

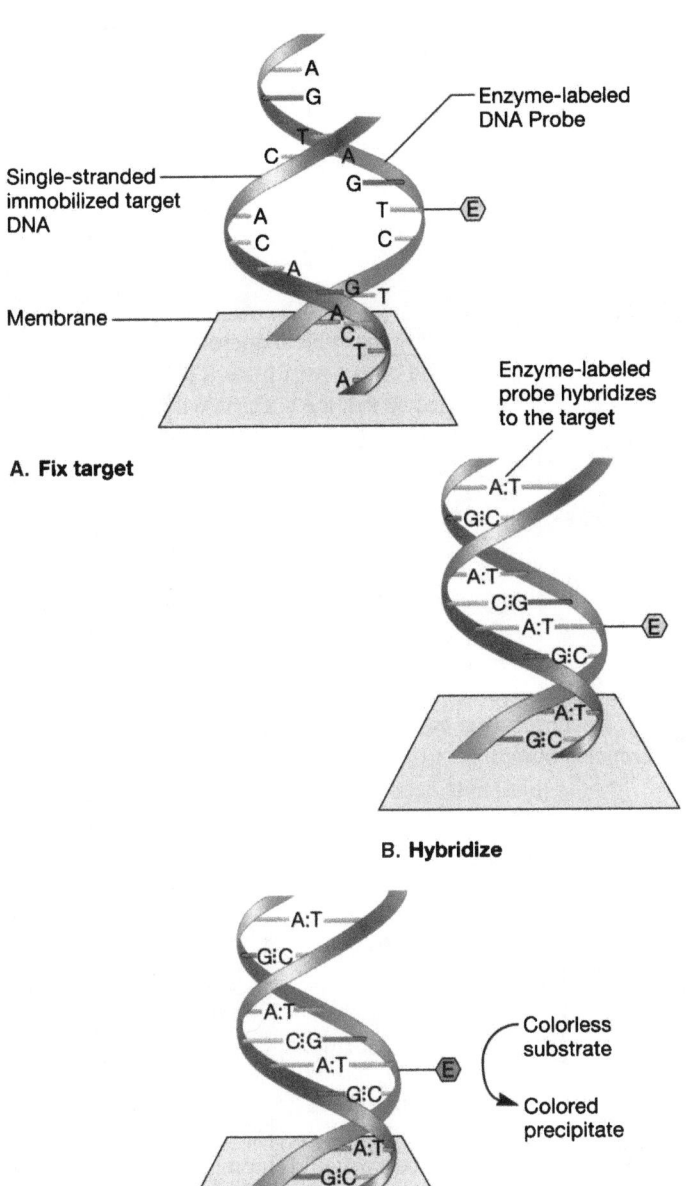

Single-stranded immobilized target DNA

Membrane

Enzyme-labeled DNA Probe

Ⓔ

A. Fix target

Enzyme-labeled probe hybridizes to the target

A:T
G:C
A:T
C:G
A:T —Ⓔ
G:C
A:T
G:C

B. Hybridize

A:T
G:C
A:T
C:G
A:T —Ⓔ ⟶ **Colorless substrate**
G:C   ⟶ **Colored precipitate**
A:T
G:C

C. Detect: Substrates are added

FIGURE 4–8. DNA probe hybridization. A. A single-stranded (denatured) target nucleic acid is bound to a membrane. A DNA probe with attached enzyme (E) is also employed. **B.** If the probe finds complementary sequences, it hybridizes to the target DNA forming a double-stranded hybrid. **C.** A colorless substrate is added, which in the presence of the enzyme is converted to a colored substrate. Measuring the color development quantitates the amount of probe bound to the original target. (Reproduced with permission from Willey JM: *Prescott, Harley, & Klein's Microbiology,* 7th ed. New York, NY: McGraw Hill; 2008.)

probes have been developed that can quickly and reliably identify organisms already isolated in culture. The application of probes for detection of infectious agents directly in clinical specimens such as blood, urine, and sputum is more difficult because only a small number of organisms may be present. This problem of sensitivity can be overcome by combining probes with NAA methods (see further text). This approach offers the potential for rapid diagnosis and the detection of characteristics not possible by routine methods. For example, a bacterial toxin gene probe can demonstrate both the presence of the related organism and its toxigenicity without the need for culture.

Probes can detect DNA of pathogen directly in clinical specimens

■ Applications of Polymerase Chain Reaction

The amplification power of the PCR offers a solution for the sensitivity problems inherent in the direct application of probes in clinical specimens. The nucleic acid segment amplified by PCR can be detected by direct hybridization with the probe (**Figure 4–9C, D2**) or for greater specificity after electrophoresis and Southern transfer (**Figure 4–9D3,4**). This approach has been successful for a wide range of infectious agents and awaits only further resolution of practical problems for wider use.

PCR plus probes gives greatest sensitivity

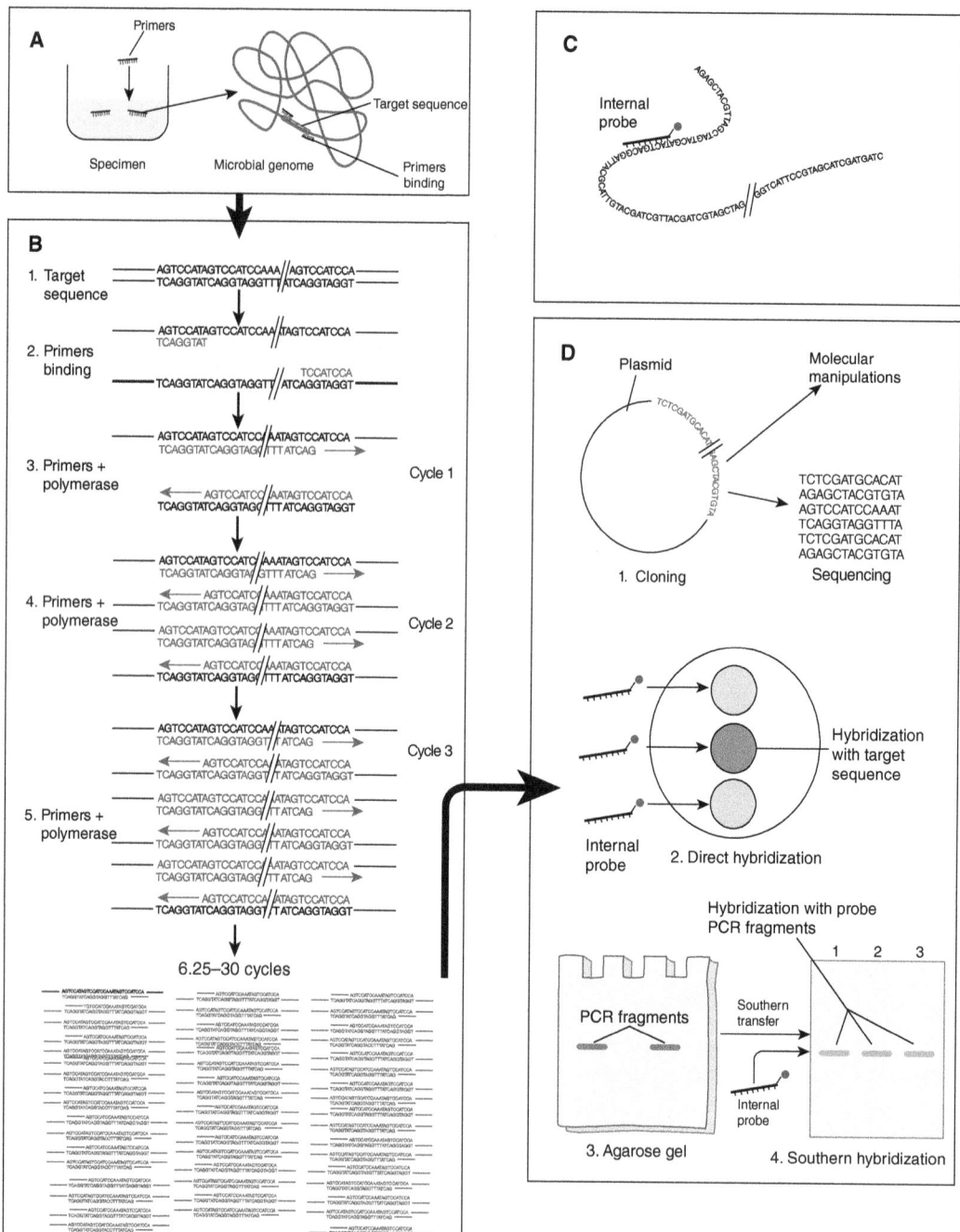

FIGURE 4–9. Diagnostic applications of the polymerase chain reaction (PCR). A. A clinical specimen (eg, pus, tissue) contains DNA from many sources as well as the chromosome of the organism of interest. If the DNA strands are separated (denatured), the PCR primers can bind to their target sequences in the specimen itself. **B.** Amplification of the target sequence by PCR. (1) The target sequence is shown in its native state. (2) The DNA is denatured, allowing the primers to bind where they find the homologous sequence. (3) In the presence of the special DNA polymerase, new DNA is synthesized from both strands in the region between the primers. (4-6) Additional cycles are added by temperature control of the polymerase with each new sequence acting as the template for another. The DNA doubles with each cycle. After 25 to 30 cycles, enough DNA is present to analyze diagnostically. **C.** Internal probe. The amplified target sequence is shown. A probe can be designed to bind to a sequence located between (internal to) the primers. **D.** Analysis of PCR amplified DNA. (1) The amplified sequence can be cloned into a plasmid vector. In this form, a variety of molecular manipulations or sequencing may be carried out. (2) Direct hybridizations usually make use of an internal probe. The example shows three specimens, each of which went through steps **A** and **B**. After amplification, each was bound to a separate spot on a filter (dot blot). The filter is then reacted with the internal probe to detect the PCR-amplified DNA. The result shows that only the middle specimen contained the target sequence. (3) The amplified DNA may be detected directly by agarose gel electrophoresis. The example shows detection of amplified fragments in two of three lanes on the gel. (4) The sensitivity of detection may be increased by use of the internal probe after Southern transfer. The example shows detection of a third fragment of the same size that was not seen on the original gel because the amount of DNA was too small.

Another creative use of PCR has been in the study of infectious agents seen in tissue but not grown in culture. PCR primers derived from sequences known to be highly conserved among bacteria, such as ribosomal RNA, have been applied to tissue specimens. The amplification produces enough DNA to clone and sequence. This sequence can then be compared with sequences published for other organisms using computers. Thus, taxonomic relationships can be inferred for an organism that has never been isolated in culture.

PCR allows study of organisms that cannot be cultured

SUMMARY

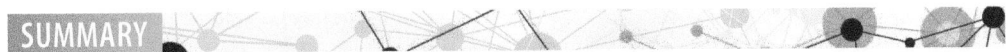

The application of some combination of the principles described in this chapter is appropriate to the diagnosis of any infectious disease. The recognition of specific etiologic agents as the causes of common infectious diseases and their detection in the laboratory in the last quarter of the 19th and early 20th centuries laid the foundation for the practice of medical microbiology for the next 100 years. The number of agents and their disease correlates continued to expand as did improved method for detection. The watershed discovery of the double helix twisted ladder structure of DNA by Watson and Crick in 1953 transformed future practice. The pace of change accelerated with discovery of PCR by Mullis in 1983. Contemporarily, a totally novel disease (AIDS) was recognized as subsequently was its cause (HIV-1) and methods for diagnosis (EIA/ELISA). Classic bacteriology as described in this chapter is still the bedrock of infectious disease diagnosis, but it too has been changed dramatically by the widespread use of NAA tests and MALDI-TOF MS in the past decade. All of the above (double helix, PCR, HIV-1, and MALDI-TOF) as well as below (HBV and HCV) resulted in Nobel Prizes for their discoverers. The advances molecular technologies have enabled in the past 40 years are nothing short of astounding: consider the discovery, methods for diagnosis, and therapeutic agents for HIV, HBV, and HCV despite their having never been grown in culture. There is no basis for expecting the pace of change to slow. There is every prospect that 16S rRNA gene cycle sequencing will become routine for identification of bacteria in the diagnostic laboratory. Whole-genome sequence typing has already supplanted previous methods for outbreak investigations of pathogens old and new. Metagenomic next-generation sequencing (mNGS) is on the way. Lest anyone doubt the need for continued research, education, and support in and of medical microbiology, consider the latest and ongoing pandemic with **SARS-CoV-2 (Chapter 5)**. The quest continues.

APPENDIX 4–1	Some Media Used for Isolation of Bacterial Pathogens
MEDIUM	**USES**
General-purpose Media	
Nutrient broths (eg, soybean–casein digest broth)	Most bacteria, particularly when used for blood culture
Thioglycolate broth	Anaerobes, facultative bacteria
Blood agar	Most bacteria (demonstrates hemolysis) and fungi
Chocolate agar	Most bacteria, including fastidious species (eg, *Haemophilus*) and fungi
Selective Media	
MacConkey agar	Nonfastidious Gram-negative rods
Hektoen enteric agar	*Salmonella* and *Shigella*
Selenite F broth	*Salmonella* enrichment
Sabouraud agar	Isolation of fungi, particularly dermatophytes
Special-purpose Media	
Löwenstein–Jensen medium, Middlebrook agar	*M tuberculosis* and other mycobacteria (selective)
Martin–Lewis medium	*Neisseria gonorrhoeae* and *Neisseria meningitidis* (selective)
Tinsdale agar	*C diphtheriae* (selective)
Regan-Lowe charcoal agar	*Bordetella pertussis* (selective)
Buffered charcoal–yeast extract agar	*Legionella* species (nonselective)
Campylobacter blood agar	*Campylobacter jejuni* (selective)
Thiosulfate-citrate-bile-sucrose agar (TCBS)	*Vibrio cholerae* and *Vibrio parahaemolyticus* (selective)

APPENDIX 4–2   Characteristics of Commonly Used Bacteriologic Media

1. **Nutrient broths.** Some form of nutrient broth is used for culture of blood and all direct tissue samples from sites that are normally sterile to obtain the maximum culture sensitivity. Selective or indicator agents are omitted to prevent inhibition of more fastidious organisms.

2. **Blood agar.** The addition of defibrinated blood to a nutrient agar base enhances the growth of some bacteria, such as streptococci. This often yields distinctive colonies and provides an indicator system for hemolysis. Two major types of hemolysis are seen: β-hemolysis, a complete clearing of red cells from a zone surrounding the colony; and α-hemolysis, which is incomplete (ie, intact red cells are still present in the hemolytic zone), but shows a green color caused by hemoglobin breakdown products. The net effect is a hazy green zone extending 1 to 2 mm beyond the colony. A third type, α'-hemolysis, produces a hazy, incomplete hemolytic zone similar to that caused by α-hemolysis, but without the green coloration.

3. **Chocolate agar.** If blood is added to molten nutrient agar at approximately 80°C and maintained at this temperature, the red cells are gently lysed, hemoglobin products are released, and the medium turns a chocolate brown color. The nutrients released permit the growth of some fastidious organisms such as *H influenzae,* which fail to grow on blood or nutrient agars. This quality is particularly pronounced when the medium is further enriched with vitamin supplements. Given the same incubation conditions, any organism that grows on blood agar also grows on chocolate agar.

4. **Martin–Lewis medium.** A variant of chocolate agar, Martin–Lewis medium is a solid medium selective for the pathogenic *Neisseria* (*N gonorrhoeae* and *N meningitidis*). Growth of most other bacteria and fungi in the genital or respiratory flora is inhibited by the addition of antimicrobial agents. One formulation includes vancomycin, colistin, trimethoprim, and anisomycin.

5. **MacConkey agar.** This agar is both a selective and an indicator medium for Gram-negative rods, particularly members of the family Enterobacteriaceae and the genus *Pseudomonas.* In addition to a peptone base, the medium contains bile salts, crystal violet, lactose, and neutral red as a pH indicator. The bile salts and crystal violet inhibit Gram-positive bacteria and the more fastidious Gram-negative organisms, such as *Neisseria* and *Pasteurella.* Gram-negative rods that grow and ferment lactose produce a red (acid) colony, often with a distinctive colonial morphology.

6. **Hektoen enteric agar.** The Hektoen medium is one of many highly selective media developed for the isolation of *Salmonella* and *Shigella* species from stool specimens. It has both selective and indicator properties. The medium contains a mixture of bile, thiosulfate, and citrate salts that inhibits not only Gram-positive bacteria, but members of Enterobacteriaceae other than *Salmonella* and *Shigella* that appear among the normal flora of the colon. The inhibition is not absolute; recovery of *Escherichia coli* is reduced 1000- to 10,000-fold relative to that on nonselective media, but there is little effect on growth of *Salmonella* and *Shigella.* Carbohydrates and a pH indicator are also included to help to differentiate colonies of *Salmonella* and *Shigella* from those of other enteric Gram-negative rods.

7. **Anaerobic media.** In addition to meeting atmospheric requirements, isolation of some strictly anaerobic bacteria on blood agar is enhanced by reducing agents such as L-cysteine and by vitamin enrichment. Sodium thioglycolate, another reducing agent, is often used in broth media. Plate media are made selective for anaerobes by the addition of aminoglycoside antibiotics, which are active against many aerobic and facultative organisms but not against anaerobic bacteria. The use of selective media is particularly important with anaerobes because they grow slowly and are commonly mixed with facultative bacteria in infections.

8. **Highly selective media.** Media specific to the isolation of almost every important pathogen have been developed. Many allow only a single species to grow from specimens with a rich normal flora (eg, stool). The most common of these media are listed in **Appendix 4–1;** they are discussed in greater detail in following chapters.

APPENDIX 4–3   Common Biochemical Tests for Microbial Identification

1. **Carbohydrate breakdown.** The ability to produce acidic metabolic products, fermentatively or oxidatively, from a range of carbohydrates (eg, glucose, sucrose, and lactose) has been applied to the identification of most groups of bacteria. Such tests are crude and imperfect in defining mechanisms, but have proved useful for taxonomic purposes. More recently, gas chromatographic identification of specific short-chain fatty acids produced by fermentation of glucose has proved useful in classifying many anaerobic bacteria.

2. **Catalase production.** The enzyme catalase catalyzes the conversion of hydrogen peroxide to water and oxygen. When a colony is placed in hydrogen peroxide, liberation of oxygen as gas bubbles can be seen. The test is particularly useful in differentiation of staphylococci (positive) from streptococci (negative), but also has taxonomic application to Gram-negative bacteria.

3. **Citrate utilization.** An agar medium that contains sodium citrate as the sole carbon source may be used to determine ability to use citrate. Bacteria that grow on this medium are termed **citrate-positive.**

4. **Coagulase.** The enzyme coagulase acts with a plasma factor to convert fibrinogen to a fibrin clot. It is used to differentiate *Staphylococcus aureus* from other, less pathogenic staphylococci.

5. **Decarboxylases and deaminases.** The decarboxylation or deamination of the amino acids lysine, ornithine, and arginine is detected by the effect of the amino products on the pH of the reaction mixture or by the formation of colored products. These tests are used primarily with Gram-negative rods.

6. **Hydrogen sulfide.** The ability of some bacteria to produce H_2S from amino acids or other sulfur-containing compounds is helpful in taxonomic classification. The black color of the sulfide salts formed with heavy metals such as iron is the usual means of detection.

7. **Indole.** The indole reaction tests the ability of the organism to produce indole, a benzopyrrole, from tryptophan. Indole is detected by the formation of a red dye after addition of a benzaldehyde reagent. A spot test can be done in seconds using isolated colonies.

8. **Nitrate reduction.** Bacteria may reduce nitrates by several mechanisms. This ability is demonstrated by detection of the nitrites and/or nitrogen gas formed in the process.

9. **O-Nitrophenyl-β-D-galactoside (ONPG) breakdown.** The ONPG test is related to lactose fermentation. Organisms that possess the β-galactoside necessary for lactose fermentation but lack a permease necessary for lactose to enter the cell are ONPG-positive and lactose-negative.

10. **Oxidase production.** The oxidase tests detect the *c* component of the cytochrome–oxidase complex. The reagents used change from clear to colored when converted from the reduced to the oxidized state. The oxidase reaction is commonly demonstrated in a spot test, which can be done quickly from isolated colonies.

11. **Proteinase production.** Proteolytic activity is detected by growing the organism in the presence of substrates, such as gelatin or coagulated egg.

12. **Pyrrolidonyl arylamidase activity (PYR test)** is a rapid colorimetric test for preliminary identification and screening of certain Gram-positive bacteria (eg, group A streptococci, enterococci, and *Staphylococcus lugdenensis*). A positive PYR test is color change from pink to red.

13. **Urease production.** Urease hydrolyzes urea to yield two molecules of ammonia and one of CO_2. This reaction can be detected by the increase in medium pH caused by ammonia production. Urease-positive species vary in the amount of enzyme produced; bacteria can thus be designated as positive, weakly positive, or negative.

14. **Voges–Proskauer test.** The Voges–Proskauer test detects acetylmethylcarbinol (acetoin), an intermediate product in the butene glycol pathway of glucose fermentation.

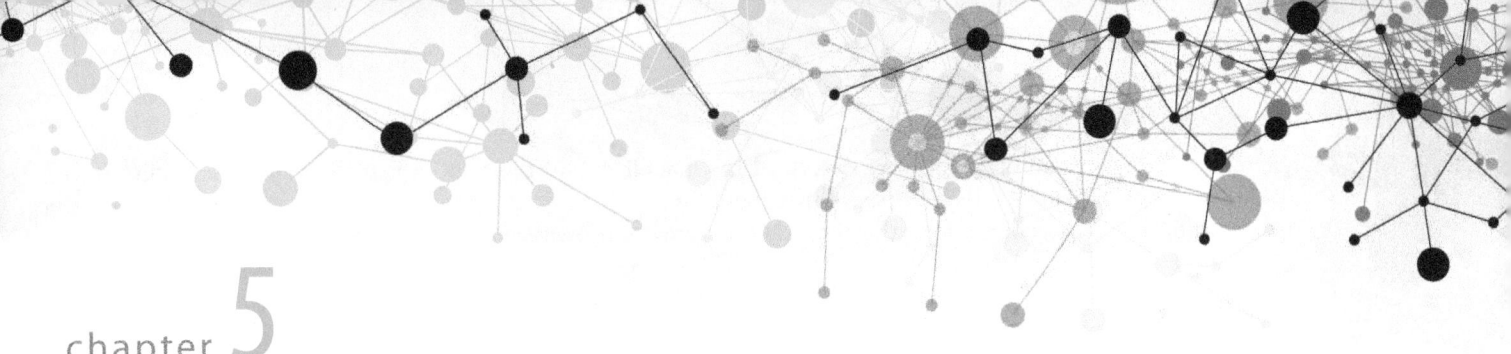

chapter 5

Emerging and Reemerging Infectious Diseases: Emergence and Global Spread of Infection

OVERVIEW

Epidemiology is the study of the distribution and determinants of disease, both infectious and noninfectious, and other perturbations in health. Most epidemiologic studies of infectious diseases have focused on the factors that influence acquisition and spread with the goal of identifying methods for prevention and control. Epidemiologic studies have informed public health measures and thereby have been critical to the control of epidemics, such as those due to cholera, plague, smallpox, yellow fever, and typhus. Knowledge of the principles and practice of epidemiology is essential for clinicians (those treating individual patients) and public health practitioners (those focused on the health of the community) alike. Care of patients with suspected infections requires consideration of the likelihood of possible exposures **in** the community (acquisition) and **to** the community (spread to others). For example, what infections, especially viral, are currently circulating in the community? Has the patient traveled recently to an area where other infections are present? Is a nosocomial or other healthcare-associated infection possible because the patient has been hospitalized recently or resides in a long-term care facility? Does the patient's infection pose a risk to his/her family, school- or workmates, or friends?

EMERGING INFECTIOUS DISEASES

An emerging disease is an infectious disease whose incidence has increased in the past two decades and/or that threatens to increase soon. Emerging infectious diseases reflect the arrival of a new pathogen (newly emerging) or an old pathogen that is increasing in incidence, clinical or laboratory characteristics, or geographic range (re-emerging or resurging). An unusual third group is "deliberately emerging" infections, such as anthrax bioterrorism. The appearance of novel coronaviruses (eg, the severe acute respiratory syndrome [SARS] coronavirus and now SARS-CoV-2 [the cause of COVID-19]) are examples of new pathogens, multidrug-resistant *Mycobacterium tuberculosis* represents an old pathogen with new characteristics, and cholera and Zika in the Americas are examples of old pathogens with a new geographic range (Asia to South America). New methods of detection (eg, molecular) and surveillance (eg, global) have greatly improved our ability to detect and characterize emerging and reemerging infectious diseases. The fundamental methodologies of **molecular**

epidemiology are described in Chapter 4, and their specific applications are discussed in many other chapters throughout this book.

Some factors that increase emergence or reemergence of infectious pathogens include:

- Human and animal demographics and population movement with intrusion into new habitats (particularly tropical forests)
- Irrigation, especially primitive irrigation systems, which fail to control arthropods and enteric organisms
- Uncontrolled urbanization, with vector populations breeding in stagnant water
- Increased international commerce and travel with contact or transport of vectors and pathogens (globalization)
- Breakdown in public health measures, including sanitation, vector control, immunization programs related to social unrest, civil wars, and major natural disasters
- Ecological changes, including global climate change and deforestation, with farmers and their animals exposed to new arthropods, floods, and drought
- Microbial evolution whether related to indiscriminate use of anti-infective agents that leads to selection of multidrug-resistant strains (eg, methicillin-resistant staphylococci or carbapenem-resistant *Enterobacteriaceae*) or pathogens that mutate readily (eg, virulent strains of influenza A and HIV-1)

Zoonotic infections are disproportionately common as emerging pathogens. New, often unexpected, infectious diseases continue to emerge or reemerge despite public health efforts. Although mortality rates declined dramatically during much of the 20th century in the United States due to improved sanitation and the development of vaccines, the mortality rate from infectious diseases increased dramatically in the early 1980s with the introduction of HIV. The development of effective antiretroviral medications in the mid-1990s subsequently reversed HIV-AIDS-specific mortality in the United States that has persisted to the present; however, mortality from other infections, such as vector-borne diseases, drug-resistant pathogens, and *Clostridioides* (formerly *Clostridium) difficile* has increased over the same period such that overall infectious disease–related mortality in the United States is strikingly similar to 25 years ago.

Emerging and resurging infections on the rise globally include bacteria, viruses, and fungi that have outpaced us (antimicrobial resistance); emerging and resurging zoonotic and vector-borne diseases (including those newly emerging with global warming and human encroachment into previously uninhabited areas); global scourges that have eluded vaccine development (malaria and HIV); and infections for which action has trailed science (control measures exist but have not been effectively deployed). Tragically, much of the world has yet to experience the reduction in infectious diseases–related mortality enjoyed by wealthier countries owing to improved sanitation and the development and provision of effective vaccines. Measles has persisted in poor countries and reemerged in wealthy ones when deployment of effective vaccines is inadequate, or acceptance resisted. Control of HIV globally has been stymied not only by lack of a vaccine but also by inability to deploy known preventive measures and provide access to proven therapies. The global distribution of newly emerging and reemerging (resurging) infectious diseases is illustrated in **Figure 5–1.**

SOURCES OF INFECTION AND COMMUNICABILITY

Infectious diseases of humans may be caused by exclusively human pathogens such as *Shigella*, by environmental organisms such as *Legionella pneumophila*, or by organisms that have their primary reservoir in animals such as *Salmonella*.

Noncommunicable infections are those that are not transmitted from human to human and include: (1) infections related to the patient's microbiota gaining access to a previously sterile site, such as peritonitis after rupture of the appendix; (2) infections caused by the ingestion of preformed toxins, such as botulism; and (3) infections caused by organisms found in the environment, such as clostridial gas gangrene. Some diseases transmitted from animals to humans (**zoonotic** infections), such as rabies and brucellosis, are not transmitted between humans, but others such as plague may be. Noncommunicable infections may still occur as common-source outbreaks, such as food poisoning from an enterotoxin-producing

Global Examples of Emerging and Re-Emerging Infectious Diseases

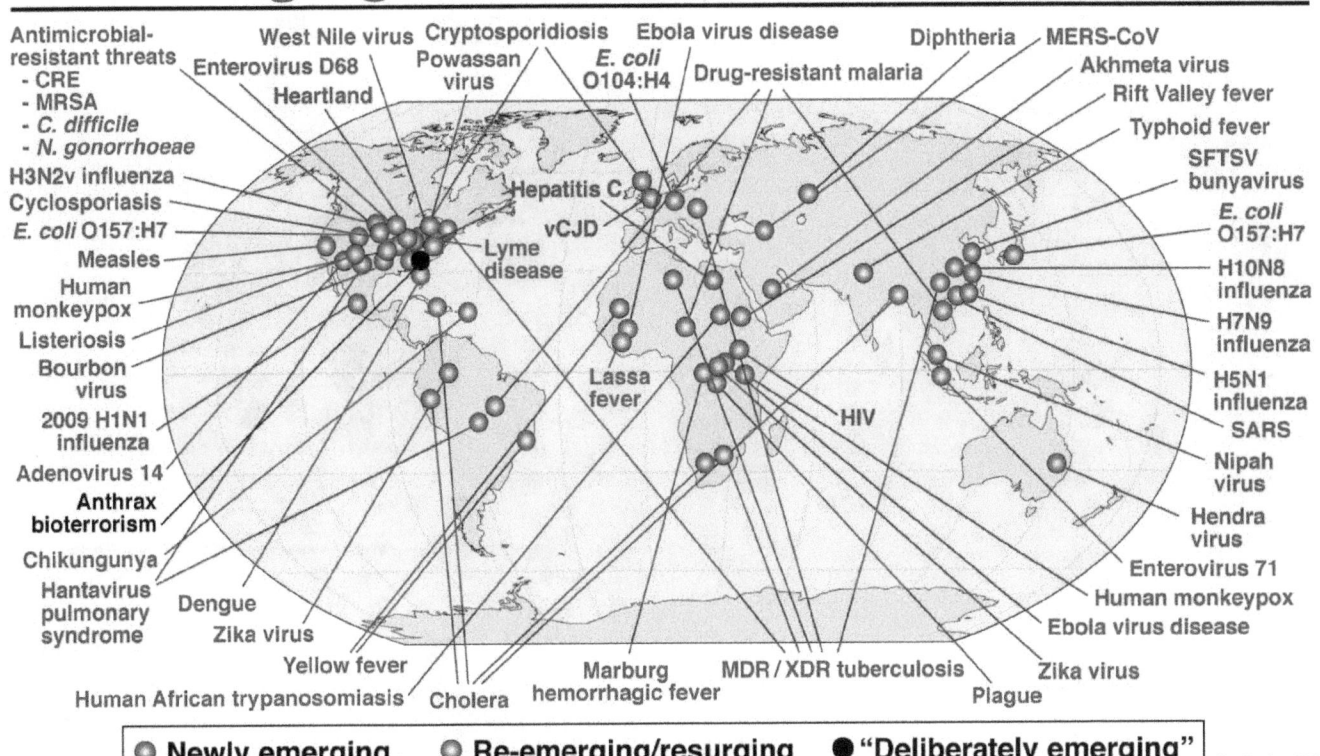

Antimicrobial-resistant threats
- CRE
- MRSA
- *C. difficile*
- *N. gonorrhoeae*

H3N2v influenza
Cyclosporiasis
E. coli O157:H7
Measles
Human monkeypox
Listeriosis
Bourbon virus
2009 H1N1 influenza
Adenovirus 14
Anthrax bioterrorism
Chikungunya
Hantavirus pulmonary syndrome
Dengue
Zika virus
Yellow fever
Human African trypanosomiasis
Cholera

West Nile virus
Enterovirus D68
Heartland
Cryptosporidiosis
Powassan virus
Hepatitis C
vCJD
Lassa fever
Marburg hemorrhagic fever

Ebola virus disease
E. coli O104:H4
Drug-resistant malaria
HIV
MDR/XDR tuberculosis

Diphtheria
MERS-CoV
Akhmeta virus
Rift Valley fever
Typhoid fever
SFTSV bunyavirus
E. coli O157:H7
H10N8 influenza
H7N9 influenza
H5N1 influenza
SARS
Nipah virus
Hendra virus
Enterovirus 71
Human monkeypox
Ebola virus disease
Zika virus
Plague

Lyme disease

⬤ **Newly emerging**   ⬤ **Re-emerging/resurging**   ● **"Deliberately emerging"**   September 2017

FIGURE 5–1. Global examples of emerging and re-emerging infectious diseases. *C difficile, Clostridioides difficile*; CRE, carbapenem-resistant *Enterobacteriaceae*; *E coli, Escherichia coli*; H3N2v, H3N2 variant; MRSA, multidrug-resistant *Staphylococcus aureus*; *N. gonorrhoeae, Neisseria gonorrhoeae*; SARS, severe acute respiratory syndrome; SFTSV, severe fever with thrombocytopenia syndrome virus; vCJD, variant Creutzfeldt-Jakob disease; XDR, extensively drug-resistant. (Reproduced with permission from Fauci AS. Infectious diseases: considerations for the 21st century, *Clin Infect Dis* 2001 Mar 1;32(5):675-685.)

Staphylococcus aureus–contaminated chicken salad or multiple cases of pneumonia from extensive dissemination of *Legionella* through an air-conditioning system. Because these diseases are not transmissible to others, they do not lead to secondary spread.

Communicable infections require an organism to leave the body in a form that is either directly infectious or able to become so after development in a suitable environment. The respiratory spread of influenza virus is an example of direct communicability. In contrast, the malarial parasite requires a developmental cycle in a blood-feeding female anopheline mosquito before it can infect another human. Communicable infections can be **endemic,** present in the population at a low and constant level, or **epidemic,** present at a level of infection higher than that usually found in the community or population. With some infections, such as influenza, the infection can be endemic and persist at a low level from season to season; however, introduction of a new strain may result in epidemics, as illustrated in **Figure 5–2.** Communicable infections that are both widespread, for example, worldwide, and have high attack rates are termed **pandemic.** Pandemics have occurred throughout history, as illustrated in **Figure 5–2**, but have become increasingly frequent. Four new pandemics, three viruses with respiratory spread and one transmitted sexually were experienced in the 20th century. Just 20 years into the 21st century, we have now had five new pandemics, the latest and deadliest (SARS-CoV-2) of which has resulted in over 1 million deaths worldwide in its first 6 months and is still far from being controlled.

Noncommunicable infections not spread person to person can occur as common-source outbreaks

＊ Endemic = constant presence

＊ Epidemic = localized outbreak

＊ Pandemic = widespread regional or global epidemic

INFECTION VERSUS DISEASE

An important consideration in the study of the epidemiology of communicable organisms is the distinction between infection and disease. **Infection** involves multiplication of the organism in or on the host and may be clinically inapparent, such as during the incubation period or latency

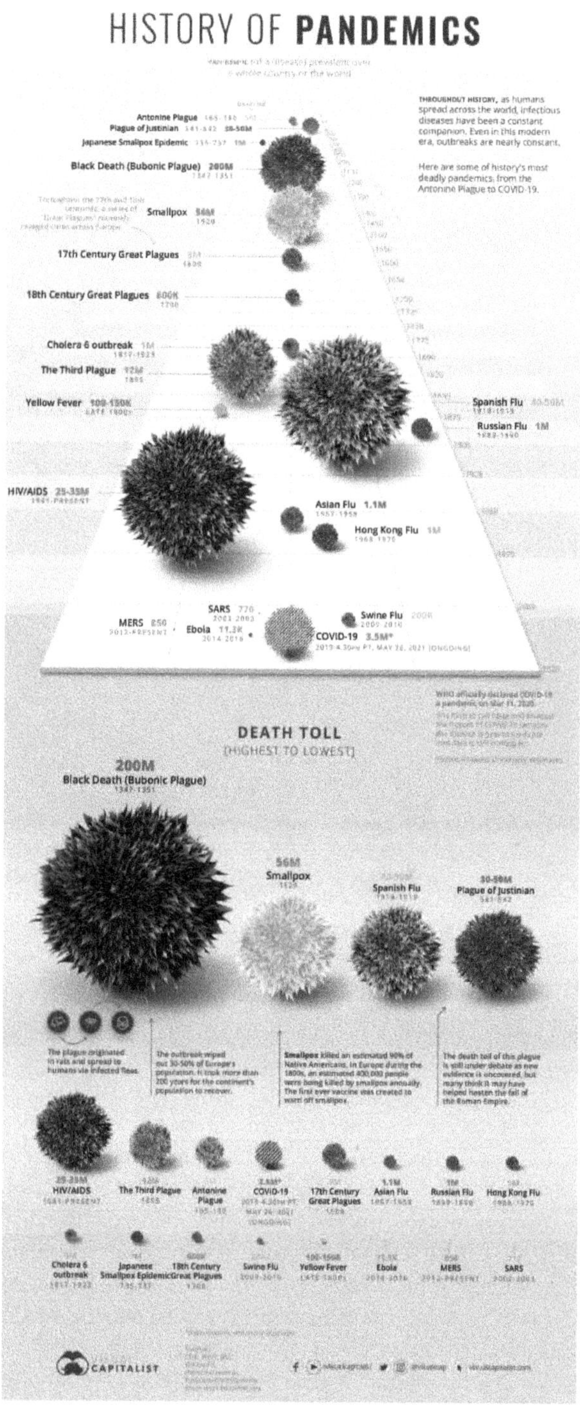

FIGURE 5–2. **History of pandemics**. (Reproduced with permission from Visual Capitalists.www.visualcapitalist.com/history-of-pandemics-deadliest/).

(when little or no replication is occurring, eg, with herpesviruses). **Disease** occurs when the infection becomes clinically apparent, that is, there is evidence of injury to the host as a result of the infection. With many communicable organisms, infection is much more common than disease, and asymptomatic infected individuals are important for propagation of the infectious agent. A recent example is Zika infection, which during the most recent epidemic was found to be nearly always clinically inapparent or mild, except for a developing fetus. Inapparent infections are termed **subclinical,** and the individual is sometimes referred to as a **carrier.** The latter term is also applied to situations in which an infectious agent establishes itself as part of a patient's microbiota or causes low-grade chronic disease after an acute infection. For example, the clinically inapparent presence of *S aureus* in the anterior nares is termed **carriage,** as is chronic gallbladder infection with *Salmonella* serotype Typhi that can follow an attack of typhoid fever and result in fecal excretion of the organism for years. *C difficile* can colonize the gastrointestinal tract but cause severe disease only when associated with the production of a toxin.

With some infectious diseases such as measles, infection is almost invariably accompanied by clinical manifestations of the disease itself. These manifestations facilitate epidemiologic detection and control, because the existence and extent of infection in a community are readily apparent. Organisms associated with long incubation periods or high frequencies of subclinical infection, such as the human immunodeficiency virus (HIV-1), hepatitis B virus, or human papillomaviruses, may propagate and spread in a population for long periods before the extent of the problem is recognized. This makes epidemiologic control more difficult.

The severity of infection reflects biologic characteristics of the organism as well as the host's response. Infectivity reflects the secondary attack rate or the number of ill per number exposed. Pathogenicity reflects the ability of the agent to induce disease. Virulence is the severity of the disease after infection occurs. The expected severity of infection reflects pathogen factors (including infectivity, pathogenicity, and virulence) and host factors (eg, immune status, obesity, underlying illness, and age). Immunogenicity is the ability of a pathogen to produce a durable immune response to protect against reinfection with the same or a related organism. Some pathogens induce lifelong immunity whereas others are weakly immunogenic, so reinfections commonly occur.

> ✳ Infection can result in little or no illness
>
> ✳ Carriers can be asymptomatic, but infectious to others
>
> **Illness severity reflects pathogen and host factors**

INCUBATION PERIOD AND COMMUNICABILITY

The incubation period is the time between the exposure to the organism/infection and the appearance of the first clinical manifestations of the disease. Organisms that multiply rapidly and produce local or systemic infections, such as gonorrhea and influenza, are associated with short incubation periods (eg, 2-4 days). Diseases such as typhoid fever, which depend on hematogenous spread and multiplication of the organism in distant target organs to produce symptoms, often have longer incubation periods (eg, 10 days to 3 weeks). Some diseases have even more prolonged incubation periods because of slow passage of the infecting organism to the target organ, as in rabies, or with slow growth of the organism, as in tuberculosis or leprosy. Incubation periods for one agent may also vary widely depending on route of acquisition and infecting dose; for example, the incubation period of hepatitis B virus infection may vary from a few weeks to several months.

> ✳ Incubation periods range from a few days to several months

Communicability of a disease in which the organism is shed in secretions may occur primarily during the incubation period. In other infections, the disease course is short but the organisms can be excreted from the host for extended periods. In yet other cases, the symptoms are related to host immune response rather than the organism's action and, thus, the disease process may extend far beyond the period in which the etiologic agent can be isolated or spread. Some viruses can integrate into the host genome or survive by replicating very slowly in the presence of an immune response. Such dormancy or latency is exemplified by the herpesviruses, and the organism may emerge long after the original infection and potentially infect others.

> ✳ Transmission to others can occur before illness onset

The inherent infectivity and virulence of an agent are also important determinants of attack rates of disease in a community. In general, organisms of high infectivity spread more easily, and those of greater virulence are more likely to cause disease than subclinical infection. The infecting dose of an organism also varies with different organisms and, thus, influences the chance of infection and development of disease.

ROUTES OF TRANSMISSION

Various transmissible infections may be acquired from others by direct contact, indirectly through contaminated inanimate objects or materials, or by aerosol transmission of infectious secretions. Some infections, such as malaria, dengue, and chikungunya, involve an animate insect vector. These routes of spread are often referred to as **horizontal transmission,** in contrast to **vertical or perinatal transmission**—from mother to fetus or infant.

◼ Vertical or Perinatal Transmission

Some infections can spread from mother to fetus through the placenta, during childbirth, or during breastfeeding. For example, rubella virus may cause birth defects when transmitted from the mother's bloodstream across the placenta during the first trimester of pregnancy. Neonatal infections with group B streptococci, *Chlamydia trachomatis*, and *Neisseria gonorrhoeae* can occur

TABLE 5–1	Common Routes of Transmission of Infection[a]	
ROUTE OF EXIT	**ROUTE OF TRANSMISSION**	**EXAMPLE**
Respiratory	Aerosol droplet inhalation	Influenza virus; tuberculosis
	Nose or mouth → hand or object → nose	Common cold (rhinovirus)
Salivary	Direct salivary transfer (eg, kissing)	Oral-labial herpes; Epstein-Barr virus, cytomegalovirus
	Animal bite	Rabies
Eye	Conjunctival	Adenovirus
Skin	Skin discharge → air → respiratory tract	Varicella, smallpox, or monkeypox
	Skin to skin	Human papillomavirus (warts); syphilis
Genital secretions	Urethral or cervical secretions	Gonorrhea; herpes simplex; *Chlamydia*
	Semen	Cytomegalovirus
Gastrointestinal	Fecal–oral (Stool → hand → mouth and/or stool → object, water or food → mouth)	Enterovirus; hepatitis A
	Stool → water or food → mouth	Salmonellosis; shigellosis
Blood	Transfusion or needle prick	Hepatitis B; cytomegalovirus infection; malaria; HIV
	Mosquito bite	Malaria; arboviruses
Urine	Urine → hand → catheter	Hospital-acquired urinary tract infections
Zoonotic	Animal bite	Rabies
	Contact with carcasses	Tularemia
	Tick bite	Rickettsia; Lyme disease

[a]The examples cited are incomplete, and, in some cases, more than one route of transmission exists. An alternative classification is airborne (respiratory), food- or waterborne (fecal–oral), contact (skin, genital, eye, saliva), zoonotic or vector-borne, bloodborne, and perinatal.

Vertical transmission = mother to fetus

following passage through the birth canal. Cytomegalovirus (CMV) can be acquired prenatally (across the placenta) or perinatally (from passage through an infected cervix, contact with blood, or through breast milk).

Important effects of perinatal infection include prematurity, intrauterine growth retardation (IUGR) and low birth weight, developmental abnormalities, congenital disease, and persistent perinatal infection. Historically, the acronym TORCH was used to describe five clinically similar perinatal infections, including toxoplasmosis, other (syphilis), rubella, CMV, and herpes simplex. Now, however, the category "other" should include varicella-zoster virus, enteroviruses, parvovirus B19, and newly described Zika virus, the latter of which is unique in that it is transmitted by mosquitos (*Aedes*).

✳ TORCH perinatal infections

✳ Horizontal transmission = direct or indirect person to person

The major routes of horizontal transmission of infectious diseases are summarized in **Table 5–1** and discussed in the following text.

■ Respiratory Spread: Airborne, Droplet, or Contact with Respiratory Secretions

Many infections are transmitted by the respiratory route, often by **aerosolization** of respiratory secretions with subsequent inhalation by other persons. The efficiency of this process depends in part on the extent and method of propulsion of discharges from the mouth and nose, the size of the aerosol droplets, and the resistance of the infectious agent to desiccation and inactivation by ultraviolet light. The classic teaching is that in still air a particle 100 µm in diameter requires only seconds to fall the height of a room, a 10 m particle remains airborne for about 20 minutes, and smaller particles remain suspended even longer. When inhaled, particles with a diameter of 6 µm or more are usually trapped by the mucosa of the nasal turbinates, whereas particles of 0.6 to 5.0 µm attach to mucous sites at various levels along the upper and lower respiratory tract and may initiate infection. These "droplet nuclei" are most important in transmitting many respiratory pathogens (eg, *M tuberculosis*). Newer data suggest that humans with respiratory infections produce infectious aerosols comprising a wide range of particle sizes. SARS-CoV-2 coronavirus-2 is transmitted by both small and large particle aerosols; hence, surgical masks and physical "social" distancing (≥6 feet) are complementary approaches to preventing human-to-human transmission.

Respiratory secretions are often transferred on hands or inanimate objects (fomites) and risk of spread in these instances can be reduced best by handwashing. For example, spread of the common cold may involve transfer of infectious secretions from nose to hand by the infected individual, with transfer to others by hand-to-hand contact and then from hand to nose. Transmission of infectious secretions by direct contact with the nasal mucosa or conjunctiva often accounts for the rapid dissemination of agents, such as respiratory syncytial virus and adenovirus.

Droplet nuclei usually less than 6 μm in size

Handwashing is especially important to decrease transmission of the common cold

■ Salivary Spread: Kissing or Bite

Some infections, such as herpes simplex and infectious mononucleosis, can be transferred directly by contact with infectious saliva by drooling small children or through kissing. Saliva containing rabies virus can transmit rabies when the rabid animal bites.

■ Eye-to-Eye Transmission

Infections of the conjunctiva may occur in epidemic or endemic form. Epidemics of adenovirus and *Haemophilus* conjunctivitis may occur and are highly contagious. The major endemic disease is trachoma, caused by *Chlamydia*, which remains a common cause of blindness in developing countries. These diseases may be spread by direct contact via ophthalmologic equipment or by secretions passed manually or through fomites such as towels.

Fomites and unsterile ophthalmologic instruments are associated with transmission

■ Skin-to-Skin Transfer

Skin-to-skin transfer occurs with a variety of infections in which the skin is the portal of entry such as the spirochete of syphilis (*Treponema pallidum*), strains of group A streptococci that cause impetigo, and the dermatophyte fungi that cause ringworm and athlete's foot. In most cases, an unapparent break in the epithelium is involved in infection. Other diseases may be spread indirectly from skin-to-skin through fomites such as shared towels and inadequately cleansed shower and bath floors. Skin-to-skin transfer usually occurs through abrasions of the epidermis, which may be unnoticed.

Syphilis, ringworm, and impetigo are examples

■ Genital Transmission

Disease transmission through the genital tract has been and remains one of the most common infections worldwide. Spread can occur between sexual partners or from the mother to the infant at birth. Major factors related to the persistence of these infections are high rates of asymptomatic carriage and the frequency of recurrence of organisms, such as *C trachomatis*, CMV, herpes simplex virus, and *N gonorrhoeae*.

Asymptomatic carriage and recurrence common

■ Foodborne or Waterborne Transmission: Fecal–Oral Spread

Fecal–oral spread involves direct or finger-to-mouth spread, the use of human feces as a fertilizer, or fecal contamination of food or water. Food handlers who are infected with an organism transmissible by this route constitute a special hazard, especially when they fail to wash their hands. Some viruses disseminated by the fecal–oral route infect and multiply in cells of the oropharynx and then disseminate to other body sites to cause infection. However, organisms that are spread in this way commonly multiply in the intestinal tract and may cause intestinal infections. They must, therefore, be able to resist the acid in the stomach, the bile, and the gastric and small intestinal enzymes. Many bacteria and enveloped viruses are rapidly killed by these conditions, but members of the Enterobacteriaceae and unenveloped viral intestinal pathogens (eg, enteroviruses) are more likely to survive. Even with these organisms, the infecting dose in patients with reduced or absent gastric hydrochloric acid is often much smaller than in those with normal stomach acidity.

✳ Reduced gastric hydrochloric acid can facilitate the spread of enteric infections

■ Blood or Transfusion-Borne

Bloodborne transmission of infection through insect vectors requires a period of multiplication or alteration within an insect vector before the organism can infect another human host, as occurs with the female *Anopheles* mosquito and the malarial parasite. Direct transmission from human to human through blood has become increasingly important because of the use of blood transfusions and blood products and the increased self-administration of illicit drugs by intravenous or subcutaneous routes using shared nonsterile equipment. Hepatitis B and C viruses, as well as HIV, were frequently transmitted in this way before the institution of universal screening of blood.

■ Vector-borne and Zoonotic

Zoonotic infections are spread from animals, where they have their natural reservoir, to humans. Some zoonotic infections such as rabies are directly contracted from the bite of the infected animal, whereas others are transmitted by vectors, especially arthropods (eg, ticks, mosquitoes). Many infections contracted by humans from animals are dead-ended in humans, whereas others may be transferred between humans once the disease is established in a population. Plague, for example, has a natural reservoir in rodents. Human infections contracted from the bites of rodent fleas may produce pneumonia, which may then spread to other humans by the respiratory droplet route. Humans can contract Zika virus from the bite of a mosquito, vertically (from mother to fetus), or horizontally (sexual transmission).

Classically the term vector was restricted to arthropods like ticks and mosquitoes; however, it is often used to refer to any animal that can transmit a pathogen to a human host. The probability of **vector-borne transmission** depends on the biology of the vector (mosquito, tick, snail, etc) and the infectivity of organism.

EPIDEMICS

■ Epidemic Propensity

The likelihood and characterization of epidemics and their recognition in a community involve several quantitative measures and some specific epidemiologic definitions. **Infectivity,** in epidemiologic terms, equates to attack rate and is measured as the frequency with which an infection is transmitted when there is contact between the agent and a susceptible individual. The **disease index** of an infection can be expressed as the number of persons who develop the disease divided by the total number infected. The **virulence** of an agent can be estimated as the number of fatal or severe cases per total number of cases. **Incidence,** the number of new cases of a disease within a specified period, is described as a rate in which the number of cases is the numerator and the number of people in the population under surveillance is the denominator. This is usually normalized to reflect a percentage of the population that is affected. **Prevalence,** which can also be described as a rate, is primarily used to indicate the total number of cases existing in a population at risk at a point in time. Diseases are more prevalent if they are especially common or less common but persist for a long time.

The prerequisites for propagation of an epidemic from person to person are: (1) a sufficient degree of infectivity to allow the organism to spread; (2) sufficient virulence for an increased incidence of disease to become apparent; and (3) sufficient level of susceptibility in the host population to permit transmission and amplification of the infecting organism. Thus, the extent of an epidemic and its degree of severity are determined by complex interactions between infectious agent and host. Host factors such as age, genetic predisposition, and immune status can dramatically influence the manifestations of an infectious disease. Together with differences in infecting dose, these factors are largely responsible for the wide spectrum of disease manifestations that may be seen during an epidemic.

The effect of age can be dramatic. For example, in an epidemic of measles in an isolated population in 1846, the attack rate for all ages averaged 75%; however, mortality rate was 90 times higher in children less than 1 year of age (28%) than in those 1 to 40 years of age (0.3%). Conversely, in one outbreak of poliomyelitis, the attack rate of paralytic polio was 4% in children 0 to 4 years of age, and 20% to 40% in those 5 to 50 years of age. Sex may be a factor in disease manifestations; for example, the likelihood of becoming a chronic carrier of hepatitis B is twice as high for males as for females.

Prior exposure of a population to an organism may alter immune status and the frequency of acquisition, severity of clinical disease, and duration of an epidemic. For example, measles is highly infectious and attacks most susceptible members of an exposed population. However, infection gives solid lifelong immunity. Thus, in unimmunized populations in which the disease is maintained in endemic form, epidemics occur at approximately 3-year intervals when a

---

Margin notes:

❋ Parenteral drug abuse, transfusion a major risk factor

❋ Zoonotic = animals or vectors to humans

❋ Vectorborne = vectors (e.g., mosquitos, ticks, snails) to humans

❋ Incidence and prevalence rates usually are expressed as number of cases per 100,000 population

❋ Prevalence = Incidence × Duration

Interaction between host and infectious agent determines extent and severity

Attack rates, disease severity vary by age and immune status

sufficient number of nonimmune hosts has been born to permit rapid transmission between them. When a sufficient immune population is reestablished, epidemic spread is blocked and the disease again becomes endemic. When immunity is short-lived or incomplete, epidemics can continue for decades if the mode of transmission is unchecked, which accounts for the present epidemic of gonorrhea.

Population immune status influences epidemic behavior

Prolonged and extensive exposure to a pathogen during previous generations selects for a higher degree of innate genetic immunity in a population. For example, extensive exposure of Western urbanized populations to tuberculosis during the 18th and 19th centuries conferred a degree of resistance greater than that among the progeny of rural or geographically isolated populations. The disease spread rapidly and in severe form, for example, when it was first encountered by Native Americans. An even more dramatic example concerns the resistance to the most serious form of malaria that is conferred on people of West African descent by the sickle cell trait. These instances are clear cases of natural selection—a process that accounts for many differences in immunity in different races and populations.

✳ **Immunity in population influences spread**

Occasionally, an epidemic arises from an agent for which immunity is essentially absent in a population, is of enhanced virulence, or appears to be of enhanced virulence because of the lack of immunity. When such an organism is highly infectious, the disease caused may become pandemic and worldwide. An example is the appearance of a new major antigenic variant of influenza A virus against which there is little, if any, cross-immunity from recent epidemics with other strains. The 1918 to 1919 pandemic of influenza was responsible for more deaths than World War I (>20 million). Subsequent, but less serious, pandemics have occurred periodically owing to the development of strains of influenza virus with major antigenic shifts (see Chapter 9). Another example, human immunodeficiency virus/acquired immunodeficiency syndrome (HIV/AIDS), illustrates the same principles but also reflects changes in human ecologic and social behavior.

✳ **Sudden appearance of "new" agents can result in pandemic spread**

A major feature of serious epidemic diseases is their frequent association with poverty, malnutrition, disaster, and war. The association is multifactorial and includes overcrowding, contaminated food and water, an increase in arthropod vectors, and the reduced immunity that can accompany severe malnutrition and overwhelming stress. Overcrowding and understaffing in day-care centers or institutions for the mentally impaired, the aged, or the infirmed can similarly be associated with epidemics of infections, such as *C difficile* and, more recently, COVID-19.

Social, ecologic factors determine epidemic aspects

In recent years, increasing attention has been given to healthcare-associated infections, including central-line-associated bloodstream infections, catheter-associated urinary tract infections, and ventilator-associated pneumonia that are associated in turn with intravascular catheters and intraurethral or intratracheal tubes. Unusually susceptible institutionalized individuals (whether because of age, chronic disease, or immunosuppressive therapy) are also at increased mortality when exposed to infected individuals from the community. Societal injustices are amplified in the setting of a pandemic, wherein those more susceptible often are also more vulnerable. As an example, non-Hispanic persons of American Indian, Alaska Native, Asian, and African American heritage, as well as Hispanic or Latino persons, have higher rates of infection, hospitalization, and death from COVID-19 compared with White, non-Hispanic Americans. Race and ethnicity are risk markers for multiple underlying conditions that impact health, including socioeconomic status, access to care, and increased exposure due to occupation (eg, frontline, essential, and critical infrastructure workers) or living conditions (crowded with close physical contact). Furthermore, despite scientific evidence, persons in positions of authority across the globe have not uniformly reinforced public health measures.

Healthcare-associated infections include nosocomial/hospital-acquired

■ Control of Epidemics

The first principle of control is recognition of the existence of an epidemic. This recognition is sometimes immediate because of the high incidence of disease but, often, the evidence is obtained from ongoing surveillance activities, such as routine disease reports to health departments and records of school and work absenteeism. The causative agent must be identified, and studies to determine route of transmission (eg, food poisoning) must be initiated.

Surveillance key to recognition of an epidemic

 Measures must then be adopted to control the spread and development of further infection. These methods include: (1) blocking the route of transmission, if possible (eg, improved food hygiene, arthropod control, or masks/handwashing/physical distancing); (2) identifying, treating, and, if necessary, isolating infected individuals and carriers (quarantine); (3) raising the level of immunity in the uninfected population by immunization when vaccines are available; (4) making selective use of chemoprophylaxis for subjects or populations at particular risk of infection, as in

Control measures can vary widely

epidemics of meningococcal infection; and (5) correcting conditions such as overcrowding or contaminated water supplies that have led to the epidemic or facilitated transfer.

KEY CONCLUSIONS

- Epidemiology, the study of the distribution and determinants of disease, is critical for recognition and control of emerging infectious diseases.
- Emerging infectious diseases are those that are increasing in incidence, whether due to the appearance of a new agent, pattern of resistance, or geographic spread.
- Communicable diseases differ from noncommunicable diseases in their propensity to cause both endemic disease and pandemics.
- Infections may be clinically inapparent or may cause disease. Those with subclinical disease can be important propagators of the infectious agent.
- Transmission can be vertical (mother to fetus or infant) or horizontal (direct or indirect person to person). Routes of horizontal transmission include respiratory, salivary, eye, skin, genital, fecal-oral, bloodborne, and vector-borne or zoonotic.
- The propensity for epidemic spread of an infection depends on agent, host, and environmental factors. Surveillance is a key to recognition and thereby to control.

Epidemiologic study is essential to identify, characterize, and control infectious diseases. Combating emerging infections requires recognizing new agents and patterns of disease, understanding their nature and spread, and then instituting control measures. The latter may involve prompt treatment of cases, prevention through selective chemoprophylaxis or immunization, implementation of environmental controls, and public education, depending on the specific agent. However, application of epidemiologic principles is essential for the health of both individuals and communities.

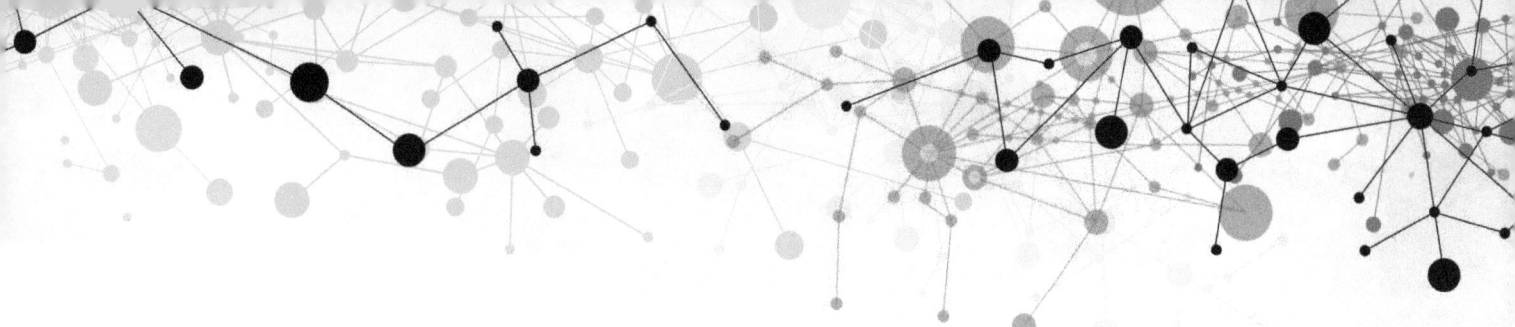

PART II
Pathogenic Viruses

Nafees Ahmad · W. Lawrence Drew

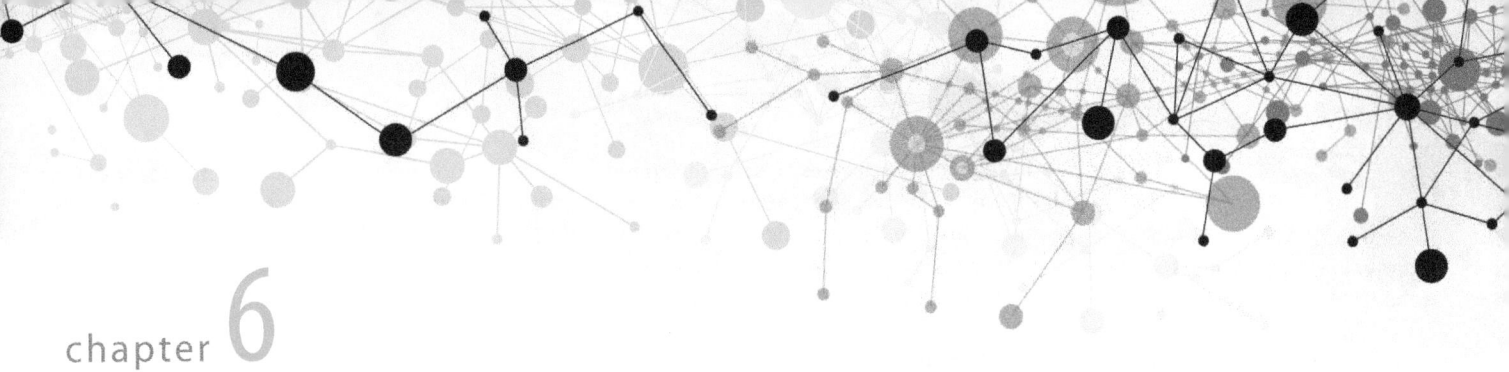

chapter 6

Viruses—Basic Concepts

(A virus is) "a piece of bad news wrapped in a protein coat."

—Peter Medawar

OVERVIEW

Viruses are the smallest form of replicating intracellular microorganisms that are comprised of sets of genes either DNA (DNA viruses) or RNA (RNA viruses) packaged in a protein coat, capsid (naked capsid viruses) or in a nucleocapsid/capsid, and an outer lipid bilayer envelope (enveloped viruses). Viruses have spikes on their outer surface that bind to the receptors on host cells and antibodies generated against the spikes neutralize the virus. Viruses are dependent upon host structural components and metabolic functions. DNA viruses replicate in the nucleus by using host RNA polymerase for transcription and either host or viral DNA polymerase for replication (exception are poxviruses that replicate in the cytoplasm). On the other hand, RNA viruses replicate in the cytoplasm using its own viral RNA-dependent RNA polymerase for both transcription and replication (exception are influenza viruses and retroviruses that replicate in the nucleus). Naked capsid viruses are assembled inside the cell and released upon cell death, whereas enveloped viruses acquire lipid bilayer membrane mainly from plasma membrane and in some cases from nuclear or cytoplasmic membranes. Viral-infected cells may result in cell death and tissue damage (pathology) generally seen in acute infections; however in many cases, the viral infection persists in hosts causing a chronic or latent infection with little or no pathologic changes in target cells or tissues. Since most viruses use their own enzymes (RNA or DNA polymerases) which could be a target for antivirals, they are prone to genetic changes due to lack of proofreading ability of these enzymes. The major genetic changes that viruses undergo are mutation and recombination that allow viruses to escape the immune response and cause damage or persist in the host. During viral latency, viral genome persists in host and may not be eliminated by antiviral drugs. It is difficult to develop strategies to eliminate latent viral infections by antiviral drugs.

A virus is a set of genes, composed of either DNA or RNA, packaged in a protein-containing coat called a **capsid.** Some viruses also have an outer lipid bilayer membrane external to the capsid called an **envelope.** The resulting complete virus particle is called a **virion.** Viruses have an obligate requirement for intracellular growth and a heavy dependence on host cell structural and metabolic components. Therefore, viruses are also referred to as obligate intracellular parasites or microorganisms. Viruses do not have a nucleus, cytoplasm, mitochondria, or other cell organelles. Viruses that infect humans are called **human viruses,** but are considered along with the general class of **animal viruses;** viruses that infect bacteria are referred to as **bacteriophages** (phages for short), and viruses that infect plants are called **plant viruses.**

Virus reproduction requires that a virus particle infect an appropriate host cell and program the cellular machinery to synthesize the viral components required for the assembly of new virions, generally termed as **progeny virions** or **daughter viruses.** The infected host cell may produce hundreds to hundreds of thousands of new virions, usually accompanied by cell death. Tissue damage as a result of cell death accounts for the pathology of many viral diseases in humans. Many of these viruses cause **acute viral infection** followed by viral clearance. In some cases, the infected cells survive, resulting in **persistent virus production,** either a **chronic or latent infection** that can remain asymptomatic, produce a chronic disease state, or lead to relapse of an infection.

Intracellular microorganism containing DNA or RNA genome, a protein coat, and, in some cases, a lipoprotein envelope

Cause acute infection followed by immune clearance

Following acute infection some cause chronic infection with little to no symptoms

In some circumstances, a virus fails to reproduce itself and, instead, enters a **latent state** (called **lysogeny** in the case of bacteriophages), from which there is the potential for reactivation at a later time. A possible consequence of the presence of viral genome in a latent state is a new genotype for the cell. Some determinants of bacterial virulence and some malignancies of animal cells are examples of the genetic effects of latent viruses. Apparently, vertebrates have had to coexist with viruses for a long time because they have evolved the special nonspecific interferon system, which operates in conjunction with the highly specific immune system to combat virus infections.

Two classes of infectious agents exist that are structurally simpler than viruses, namely, viroids and prions. **Viroids** are infectious circular RNA molecules that lack protein shells; they are responsible for a variety of plant diseases. **Prions,** which apparently lack any genes, are composed only of protein, and appear to be responsible for some transmissible and inherited spongiform encephalopathies, such as scrapie in sheep; bovine spongiform encephalopathy in cattle; and kuru, Creutzfeldt-Jakob disease, and Gerstmann-Sträussler-Scheinker syndrome in humans.

VIRUS STRUCTURE

Viruses are approximately 100- to 1000-fold smaller than the cells they infect. The smallest viruses, **virion size** (parvoviruses), are approximately 20 nm in diameter (1 nm = 10^{-9} m), whereas the largest human viruses (poxviruses) have a diameter of approximately 300 nm (**Figure 6–1**) and overlap the size of the smallest bacterial cells (*Chlamydia* and *Mycoplasma*). Therefore, viruses generally pass through filters designed to trap bacteria, and this property can, in principle, be used as evidence of a viral etiology. Viruses were initially described as filterable agents.

The basic structure of all viruses places the nucleic acid genome (DNA or RNA) on the inside of a protein shell called a **capsid.** These viruses have a defined external capsid and are referred to as **naked capsid viruses.** Some human viruses are further packaged into a lipid membrane, or **envelope,** which is usually acquired from the plasma or cytoplasmic membrane of the infected cell during release from the cell. The genomes of enveloped viruses form a protein complex and a structure called a **nucleocapsid,** which is often surrounded by a **matrix** protein that serves as a bridge between the nucleocapsid and the inside of the viral membrane or envelope. Some enveloped viruses also have capsids between nucleocapsid and matrix protein. Protein or glycoprotein structures called **spikes,** which often protrude from the surface of virus particles, are involved in the initial contact with receptor on host cells. These basic design features (naked capsid-icosahedral, enveloped-helical nucleocapsid, and enveloped-icosahedral capsid) are illustrated schematically in **Figure 6–2. Examples of representatives of human/animal viruses** electron micrographs are shown in **Figure 6–3.**

The protein shell forming the capsid or the nucleocapsid assumes one of two basic shapes: cylindrical (**helical**) or spherical (**icosahedral**). Examples of these structural categories can be seen in the electron micrographs in Figure 6–3.

The outer capsid or envelope of viruses functions (1) to protect the nucleic acid genome from damage during the extracellular passage of the virus from one cell to another, (2) to aid in the process of entry into the cell, and (3) in some cases, to package viral enzymes essential for the early steps of the infection process.

In general, the nucleic acid genome of a virus is hundreds of times longer than the longest dimension of the complete virion. It follows that the viral genome must be extensively condensed during the process of virion assembly. For naked capsid viruses, this condensation is achieved by the association of the viral nucleic acid with basic proteins encoded by the virus to form the **core** of the virus (Figure 6–2). For enveloped viruses, the formation of the nucleocapsid serves to condense the viral nucleic acid genome. The virion may also contain certain virus-encoded essential enzymes and/or accessory/regulatory proteins.

GENOME STRUCTURE

Viral genomes can be made of either RNA or DNA and also can be either single-stranded or double-stranded. The RNA viruses can be either positive sense (indicated by a +) (polarity of mRNA) or negative sense (−) (complementary to or antisense of mRNA), double-stranded (one strand + and the second strand −) or ambisense (both + and − polarity on the same strand). Although the RNA genomes of most viruses are linear, some RNA viruses such as influenza and reoviruses have segmented genomes (several segments or pieces of RNA), with each segment responsible for encoding a protein.

Marginal notes (left column):

Some after acute infection enter into latency, reactivated later

Plant viroids are infectious RNA molecules

Prions are protein molecules that may cause spongiform encephalopathies

Range in size from 20 to 300 nm in diameter

Naked capsid viruses have nucleic acid genome within capsid

Enveloped viruses have nucleocapsid packaged in lipoprotein envelope

Surface protrusions called spikes

Basic shapes: helical and icosahedral

Outer shell protective, aids in entry, packaging

Nucleic acid must be condensed during virion assembly

Genome RNA or DNA, not both

Genomes single- or double-stranded

RNA genomes (+) positive sense, negative (−) sense, or ambisense (+/−)

DNA viruses

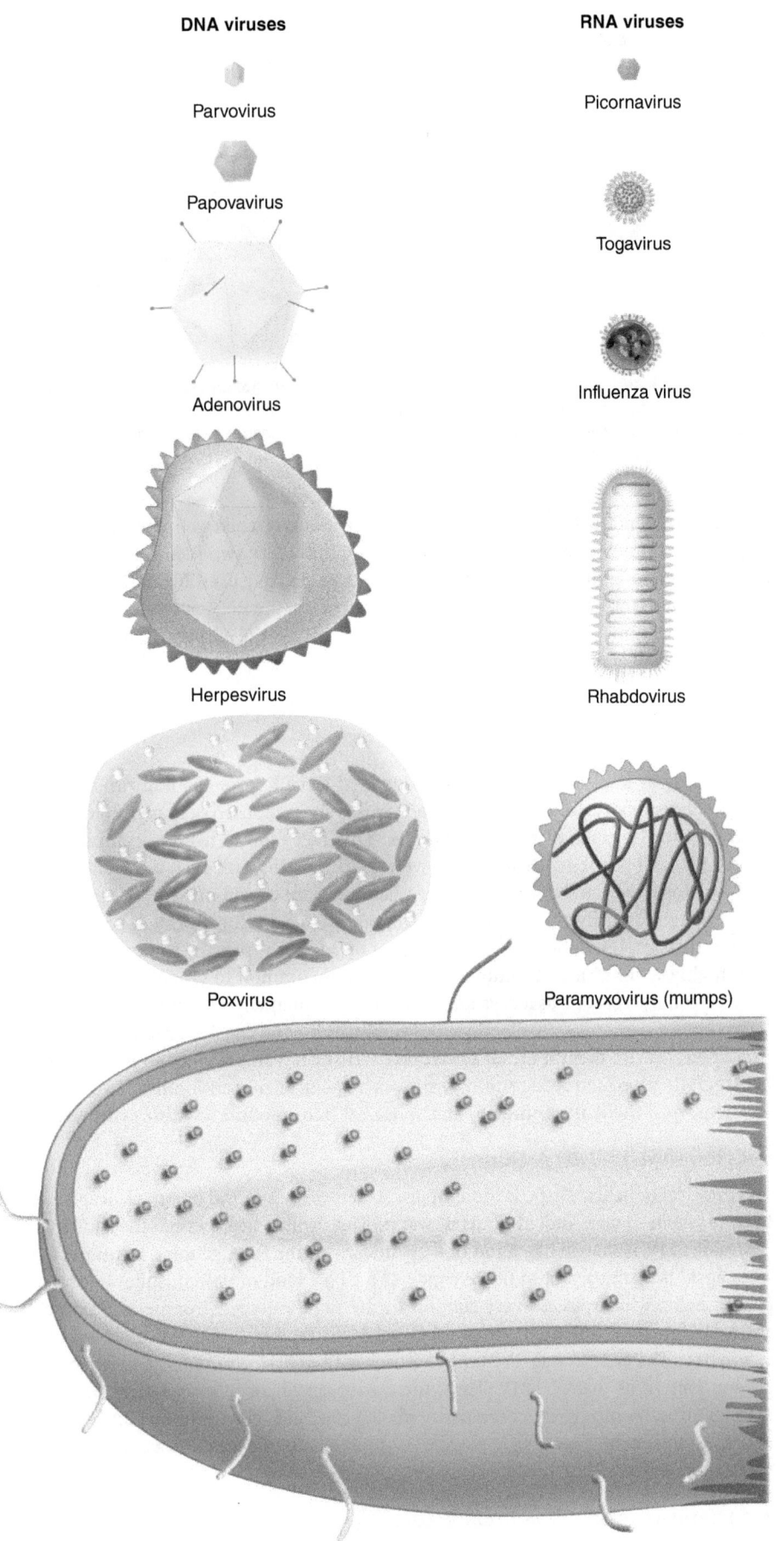

Parvovirus

Papovavirus

Adenovirus

Herpesvirus

Poxvirus

RNA viruses

Picornavirus

Togavirus

Influenza virus

Rhabdovirus

Paramyxovirus (mumps)

Escherichia coli

FIGURE 6–1. **Size comparison of viruses with other microbes.** (Adapted with permission from Willey JM: *Prescott, Harley, & Klein's Microbiology,* 7th ed. New York, NY: McGraw Hill; 2008.)

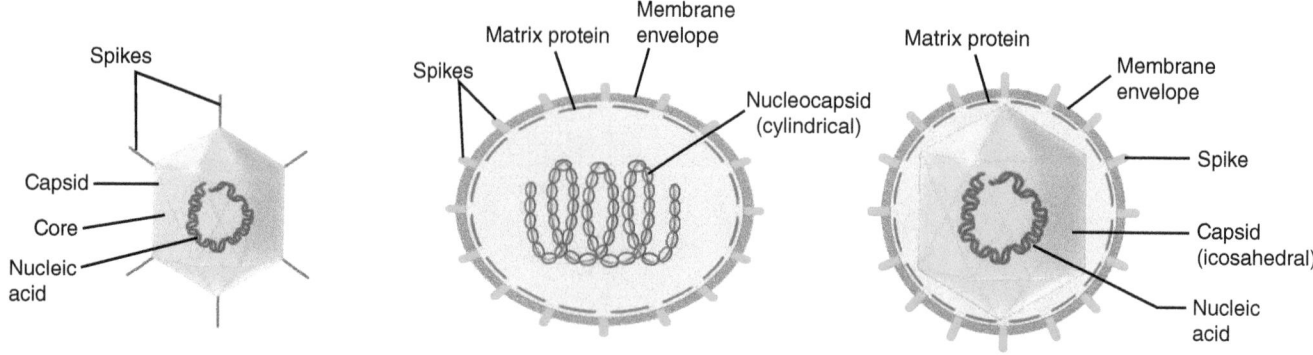

Naked capsid virus (icosahedral capsid)   Enveloped virus (helical nucleocapsid)   Enveloped virus (icosahedral capsid)

FIGURE 6–2. Schematic drawing of two basic types of virions, naked capsid virus and enveloped virus. In naked capsid virus, the genome is condensed with a defined external capsid (coat protein), whereas enveloped virus has a nucleocapsid or capsid wrapped in a lipid bilayer envelope. (Adapted with permission from Willey JM: *Prescott, Harley, & Klein's Microbiology*, 7th ed. New York, NY: McGraw Hill; 2008.)

The DNA genome of viruses can be both linear and circular genomes. Most viruses contain a single copy of their genome, except retroviruses that carry two identical copies of their genome and are, therefore, diploid. A few viral genomes (picornaviruses, hepatitis B virus, and adenoviruses) contain covalently attached protein on the ends of the RNA or DNA chains that are remnants of the replication process. Structural diversity among the viruses is most obvious when the makeup of viral genomes is considered.

Genomes linear or circular

Some genomes segmented

CAPSID STRUCTURE

■ Subunit Structure of Capsids

The capsids or nucleocapsids are virus-encoded specific proteins that protect the genome and confer shapes to viruses. The capsids of all viruses are composed of many copies of one or, at most, several different kinds of protein subunits. This fact follows from two fundamental considerations. First, all viruses code for their own capsid proteins, and even if the entire coding capacity of the genome were to be used to specify a single giant capsid protein, the protein would not be large enough to enclose the nucleic acid genome. Thus, multiple protein copies are needed, and, in fact, the simplest spherical virus contains 60 identical protein subunits. Second, viruses are such highly symmetrical structures that it is not uncommon to visualize naked capsid viruses in the electron microscope as a crystalline array (eg, simian virus 40 in Figure 6–3B).

Capsids and nucleocapsids composed of multiple copies of protein molecule(s)

The presence of many identical protein subunits in viral capsids or the existence of many identical spikes in the membrane of enveloped viruses has important implications for adsorption, hemagglutination, and recognition of viruses by neutralizing antibodies. Two main architectures are cylindrical (**helical symmetry**) and spherical (**icosahedral or cubic symmetry**).

■ Cylindrical (Helical) Architecture

A cylindrical or helical shape is the simplest structure for a capsid or a nucleocapsid. The first virus to be crystallized and studied in detail was a plant virus called tobacco mosaic virus (TMV). The capsid of TMV is shaped like a rod or a cylinder, with the RNA genome wound in a helix inside it. The capsid is composed of multiple copies of a single kind of protein subunit arranged in a close-packed helix, which places every subunit in the same microenvironment. Because of the helical arrangement of the subunits, viruses that have this type of design are often said to have **helical symmetry**. The architecture of human viruses with helical symmetry is likely to follow the same general pattern as that of TMV. Thus, the nucleocapsids of influenza virus, parainfluenza virus, measles virus, mumps virus, coronavirus, ebola virus, and rabies virus are likely constructed with a helical arrangement (Figure 6–2, middle) of protein subunits in close association with the nucleic acid genome.

Helical or cylindrical viruses have capsid protein molecules arranged in a helix

■ Spherical (Icosahedral) Architecture

The construction of a spherically (icosahedral) shaped virus similarly involves the packing together of many identical subunits, but, in this case, the subunits are placed on the surface of a

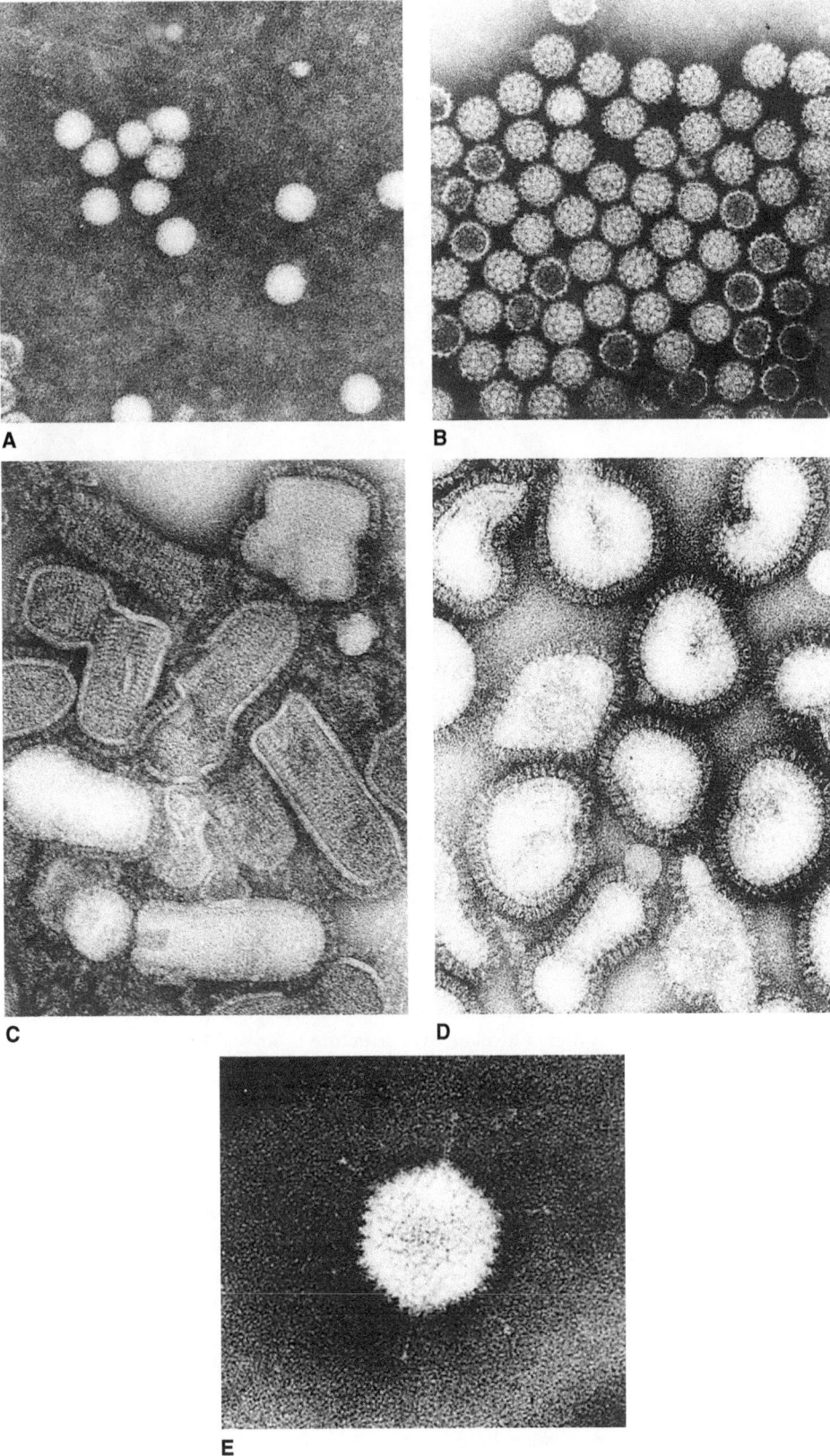

FIGURE   6–3. **Representative human/animal viruses. A.** Poliovirus. **B.** Simian virus 40. **C.** Vesicular stomatitis virus. **D.** Influenza virus. **E.** Adenovirus. (Used with permission from Dr. Robley C. Williams.)

geometric solid called an **icosahedron.** An icosahedron has 12 vertices, 30 sides, and 20 triangular faces (**Figure 6–4**). Because the icosahedron belongs to the symmetry group that crystallographers refer to as cubic (not the cube shape), spherically shaped viruses are said to have cubic symmetry, generally known as **icosahedral** capsid.

Spherical viruses exhibit icosahedral symmetry

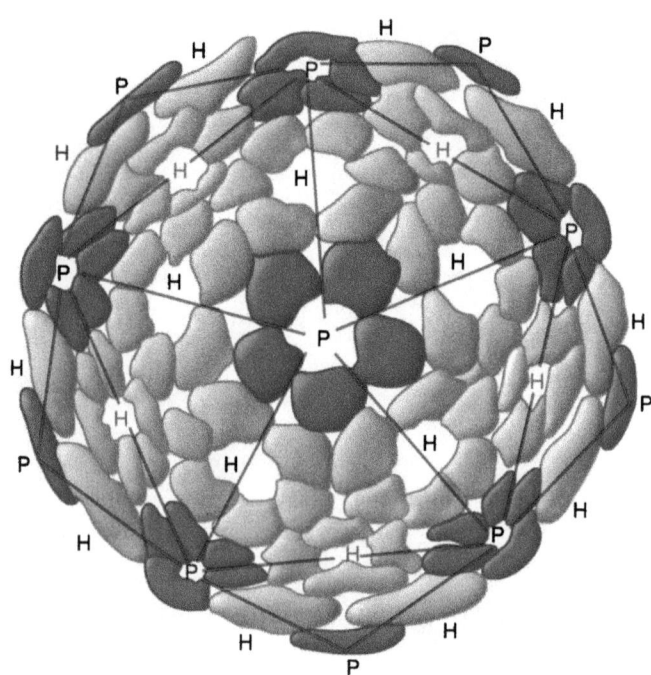

FIGURE 6–4. **Diagram of an icosahedron showing 12 vertices, 20 faces, and 30 sides.** The colored balls indicate the position of protomers forming a pentamer on the icosahedron. (Reproduced with permission from Willey JM: *Prescott, Harley, & Klein's Microbiology*, 7th ed. New York, NY: McGraw Hill; 2008.)

Capsomeres are surface structures composed of five or six protein molecules

When viewed in the electron microscope, many naked capsid viruses and some nucleocapsids appear as spherical particles with a surface topology that makes it appear that they are constructed of identical ball-shaped subunits (Figure 6–3B and E). These visible structures are referred to as **morphologic subunits** or **capsomeres.** A capsomere is generally composed of either five or six individual protein molecules, each one referred to as a **structural subunit** or **protomer.** In the simplest virus with cubic symmetry, five protomers are placed at each one of the 12 vertices of the icosahedron as shown in Figure 6–4 to form a capsomere called a **pentamer.** In this case, the capsid is composed of 12 pentamers, or a total of 60 protomers. Note that in the case of helical symmetry, this arrangement places every protomer in the same microenvironment as that of every other protomer.

To accommodate the larger cavity required by viruses with large genomes, the capsids contain many more protomers. These viruses are based on a variation of the basic icosahedron in which the construction involves a mixture of pentamers and hexamers rather than only pentamers. A detailed description of this higher level of virus structure is beyond the scope of this text. Examples of icosahedral capsids are shown in **Figure 6–5.**

■ Special Surface Structures

Surface structures are important in adsorption and penetration

Many viruses have structures that protrude from the surface of the virion generally known as spikes or peplomers. In virtually every case, these structures are important for the two earliest steps of infection—adsorption and penetration. The most dramatic example of such a structure is the tail of some bacteriophages which acts as a channel for the transfer of the genome into the bacterial cell. Other examples of surface structures include the spikes of adenovirus (Figure 6–3E) and the glycoprotein spikes found in the membrane of enveloped viruses (see influenza virus in Figure 6–3D). Even viruses without obvious surface extensions probably contain short projections which, like the more obvious spikes, are involved in the specific binding of the virus to the cell surface.

■ Envelope Structure

Viral envelopes are lipid bilayer membranes

Envelope glycoproteins called spikes or peplomers

Many human viruses have an outer lipid bilayer membrane that is derived from cellular membranes, mainly the plasma membrane, but also, in some cases, cytoplasmic or nuclear membranes. The viral envelope lipid layer membrane contains virus-encoded glycoproteins called **"spikes"** or **"peplomers"** or **"viral envelope proteins."** The envelope spikes bind to the receptor on the host cells, help the virus envelope membrane fuse with the cellular membrane of the host cells, and act as principal antigens against which the host mounts immune response for the recognition of the virus. Enveloped viruses have another protein, the matrix protein, which serves as a bridge between nucleocapsid and inner membrane of the envelope (Figure 6–2). Examples of enveloped

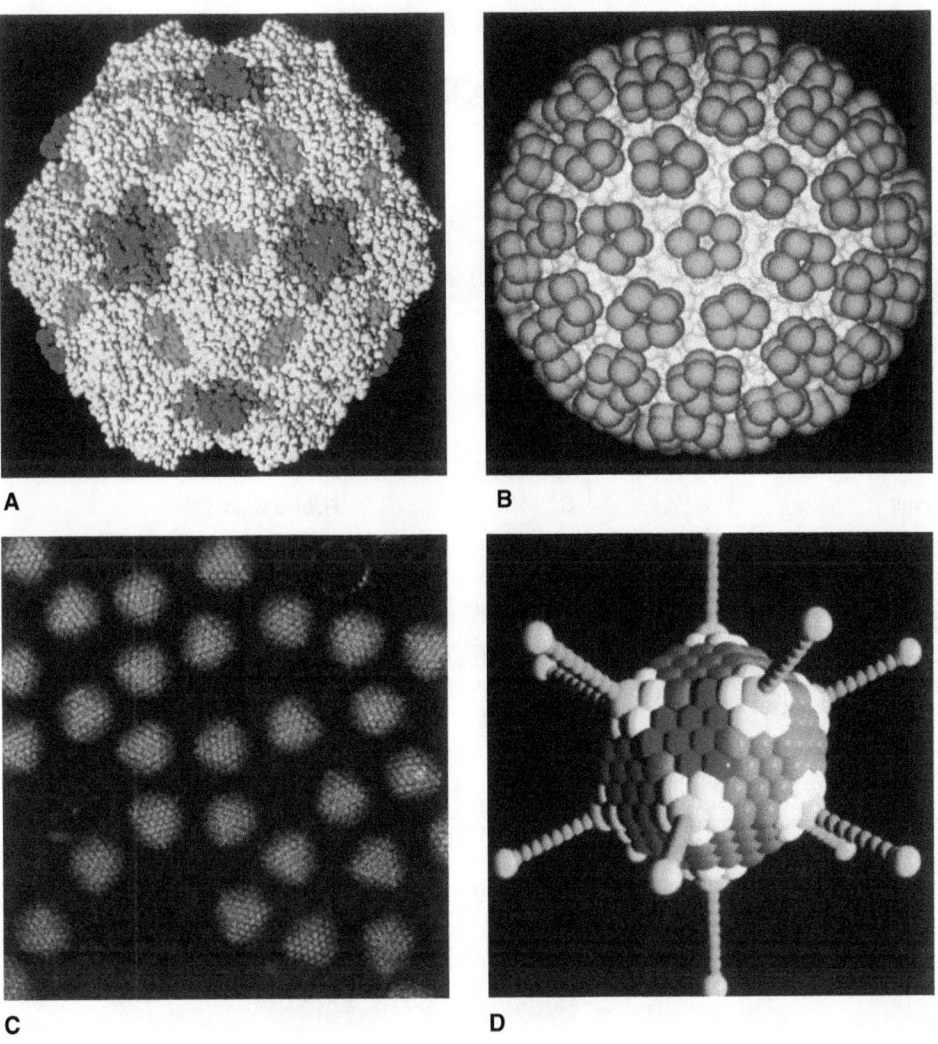

FIGURE 6–5. **Examples of icosahedral capsids.** (Reproduced with permission from Willey JM: *Prescott, Harley, & Klein's Microbiology*, 7th ed. New York, NY: McGraw Hill; 2008.)

A   B

C   D

viruses are shown in **Figure 6–6,** with both helical (Figure 6–6A and B) and icosahedral or cubic (Figure 6–6C and D) symmetry.

Enveloped viruses are more sensitive to detergents, solvents, ethanol, ether, and heat compared with nonenveloped (naked capsid) viruses whose outer coat is capsid protein. Both envelope glycoproteins and naked capsid viruses' spikes become antigens after infection and the host mounts both cell-mediated and humoral immune responses for the elimination of virus-infected cells and cell-free virus, respectively. These antigens determine the viral **serotypes** that are based on antigenic variation and are type-specific such as poliovirus serotypes 1, 2, and 3. Viral serotypes have cross-reactivity but, often, little cross-protection. Viral serotypes arise because of antigenic variations that allow viruses to escape preexisting immune response.

Envelope glycoproteins, like naked capsid viruses' spikes, bind to receptors on host cells for virus entry

Viral serotypes arise due to antigenic variation that have cross-reactivity but, often, little-cross protection

CLASSIFICATION OF VIRUSES

The classification of viruses has evolved at a slower pace than other microorganisms. The International Committee for Taxonomy of Viruses (ICTV) considered various properties, including virions, genome, proteins, envelope, replication, and physical and biologic properties. Based on these properties, virus families are designated with the suffix, -viridae (as in Herpesviridae), virus subfamilies with suffix -virinae (Herpesvirinae), virus genera with suffix -virus (Herpesvirus), and virus species designated by a virus type (herpes simplex virus 1). **Tables 6–1** and **6–2** present a classification scheme for human RNA and DNA viruses, respectively, which is based solely on their structure. The viruses are arranged in order of increasing virion size. It is important to bear in mind that phylogenetic relationships cannot be inferred from this taxonomic scheme. The tables should not be memorized but rather used as a reference guide to virus structure. In general, viruses with similar structures exhibit similar replication strategies, as discussed later.

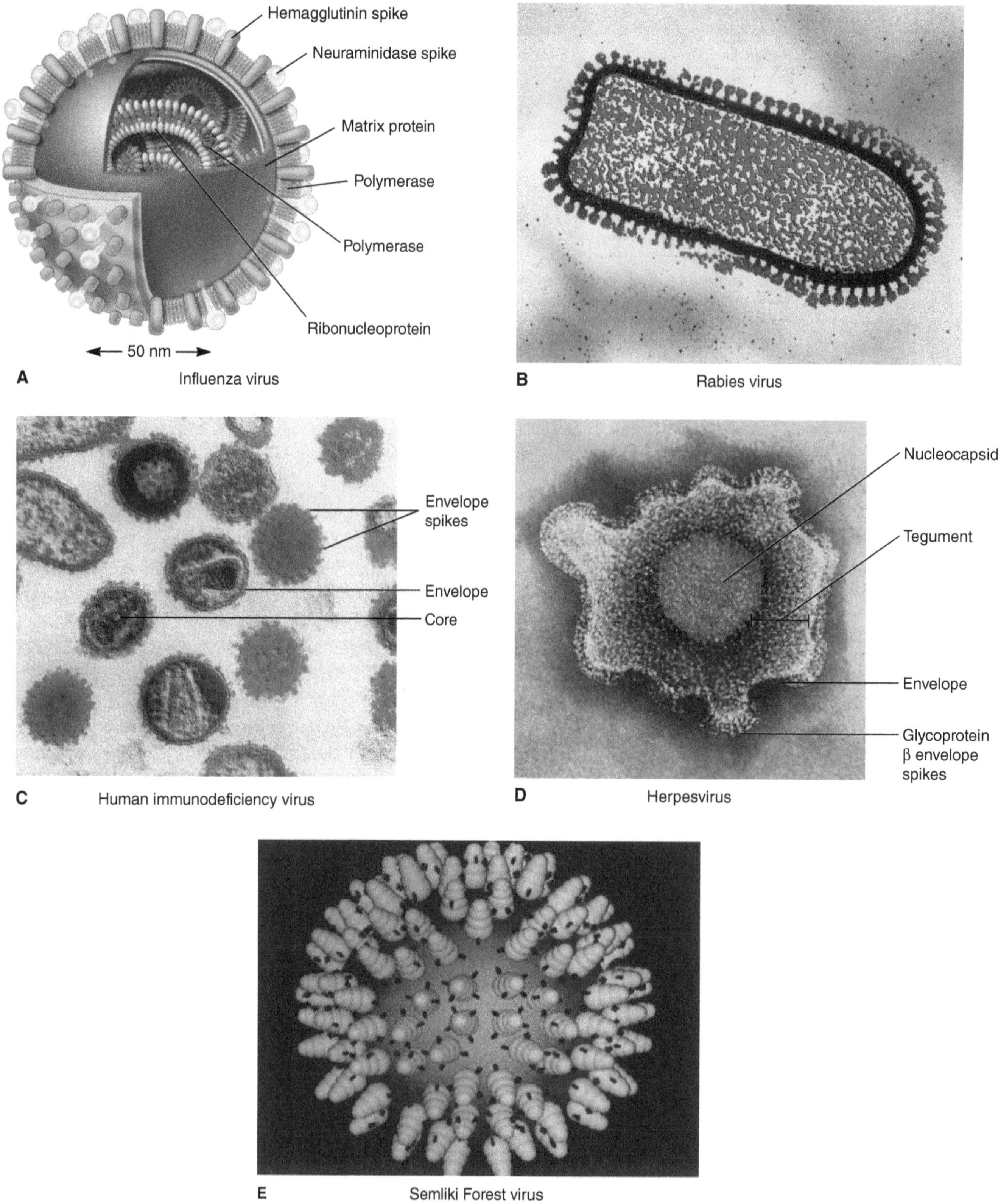

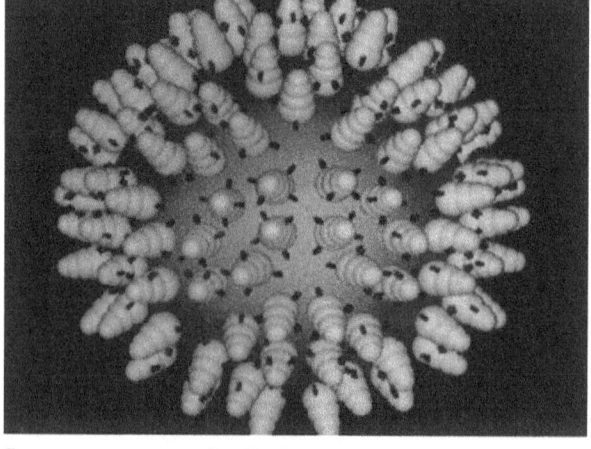

A Influenza virus

Hemagglutinin spike
Neuraminidase spike
Matrix protein
Polymerase
Polymerase
Ribonucleoprotein
← 50 nm →

B Rabies virus

C Human immunodeficiency virus

Envelope spikes
Envelope
Core

D Herpesvirus

Nucleocapsid
Tegument
Envelope
Glycoprotein β envelope spikes

E Semliki Forest virus

FIGURE 6–6. **Examples of enveloped viruses.** (Reproduced with permission from Willey JM: *Prescott, Harley, & Klein's Microbiology*, 7th ed. New York, NY: McGraw Hill; 2008.)

Representative and important bacteriophages are listed along with their properties in **Table 6–3.** In the chapters that follow, the properties of the well-studied temperate bacteriophage, λ, are described to illustrate the replicative strategies of the more medically important, but less well-studied, β phage of *Corynebacterium diphtheriae*.

TABLE 6–1	Classification of Human RNA Viruses		
FAMILY	VIRION STRUCTURE AND SIZE	GENOME STRUCTURE AND SIZE	REPRESENTATIVE MEMBERS INFECTING HUMANS
Picornaviridae (Picornaviruses)	Icosahedral, naked 22-30 nm	ss linear (+) (7.2-8.4 kb); protein attached	Human enteroviruses: poliovirus, coxsackieviruses, echoviruses, enteroviruses; hepatitis A virus (HAV); rhinoviruses
Caliciviridae (Caliciviruses)	Icosahedral, naked 27-38 nm	ss linear (+) (7.4-7.7 kb)	Norovirus; Norwalk virus; Sapovirus
Hepeviridae (Hepevirus)	Icosahedral, naked 27-34 nm	ss linear (+) (7.2 kb)	Hepatitis E virus (HEV)
Astroviridae	Icosahedral, naked 28-38 nm	ss linear (+) (7.2-7.9 kb)	Human astrovirus serotypes 1-8
Deltaviridae (Delta virus)	Icosahedral, enveloped 36-43 nm	ss circular (–) (1.7 kb)	Hepatitis D virus (HDV) or Hepatitis δ virus
Flaviviridae (Flaviviruses)	Icosahedral, enveloped 40-50 nm	ss linear (+) (9.5-10.7 kb)	Flaviviruses: Dengue virus, yellow fever virus, St. Louis encephalitis virus, West Nile virus, Zika virus, Japanese B encephalitis virus; Hepacivirus: Hepatitis C virus (HCV)
Togaviridae (Togaviruses)	Icosahedral, enveloped 70 nm	ss linear (+) (9.7-11.8 kb)	Alphaviruses: Western and Eastern equine encephalitis viruses, Venezuelan equine encephalitis virus, Chikungunya virus; Rubivirus: Rubella virus
Reoviridae (Reoviruses)	Icosahedral, naked 80 nm	10 ds linear segments (range 0.6-3.9 kb)	Human reoviruses; coltivirus; Colorado tick fever virus; rotavirus; human rotavirus
Rhabdoviridae (Rhabdoviruses)	Helical, enveloped 75-190 nm	ss linear (–) (13-16 kb)	Rabies virus; vesicular stomatitis virus
Orthomyxoviridae (Orthomyxoviruses)	Helical, enveloped 80-120 nm	8 ss linear segments (–) (range 0.2-2.3 kb, total 10-13.6 kb)	Type A, B, and C influenza viruses of humans, swine, horses, and avian
Coronaviridae (Coronaviruses)	Helical, enveloped 80-220 nm	ss linear (+) (20-30 kb)	Respiratory viruses of humans (Common cold causing coronaviruses), severe acute respiratory syndrome (SARS) coronavirus (SARS-CoV-1), Middle East Respiratory Syndrome Coronavirus (MERS-CoV), SARS-CoV-2 (COVID-19); Coronavirus-like diarrheal agent
Filoviridae (Filoviruses)	Helical, enveloped 80 nm diameter, 300-14,000 nm in length	ss linear (–) (19.1 kb)	Marburg and Ebola viruses
Bunyaviridae (Bunyaviruses)	Helical, enveloped 90-100 nm	3 ss linear segments (–) or (+/–) (11-21 kb)	Bunyavirus (bunyamwera virus, California virus), Phlebovirus (Rift Valley fever virus), Nairovirus and Hantavirus (Hantan virus, Sin Nombre virus)
Retroviridae (Retroviruses)	Icosahedral, enveloped 100 nm	ss linear (+), diploid (9.2 kb)	RNA tumor viruses of human; human T-lymphotropic virus (HTLV) type 1 and II (adult T cell leukemia and lymphoma and hairy T cell leukemia); lentiviruses; human immunodeficiency virus (HIV) type 1 and 2 (acquired immunodeficiency syndrome, AIDS)
Arenaviridae (Arenaviruses)	Helical, enveloped 110-130 nm	2 ss linear segments (+/–) (10-14 kb overall size)	Lassa virus (Africa); Junin virus, Machupo virus, Guanarito virus, Sabia virus (South America); Lymphocytic choriomeningitis virus (LCMV)
Paramyxoviridae (Paramyxoviruses)	Helical, enveloped 150-200 nm	ss linear (–) (16-20 kb)	Paramyxovirus (Mumps, parainfluenza viruses), Morbillivirus (measles virus); Pneumovirus (respiratory syncytial virus, RSV; human metapneumovirus); Henipavirus (Hendra and Nipah viruses)

ds, double-stranded; ss, single-stranded.

■ Virus Replication

Virus replication cycle typically consists of six discrete phases: (1) adsorption or attachment to the host cell, (2) penetration or entry, (3) uncoating to release the genome, (4) synthetic or virion component production, (5) assembly, and (6) release from the cell. These phases are shown in a general scheme of virus replication cycle in **Figure 6–7.**

TABLE 6–2 Classification of Human DNA Viruses

FAMILY	VIRION STRUCTURE AND SIZE	GENOME STRUCTURE AND SIZE	REPRESENTATIVE MEMBERS INFECTING HUMANS
Parvoviridae (Parvoviruses)	Icosahedral, naked 20 nm	ss linear (~5 kb)	Human parvovirus B-19; adeno-associated viruses; human bocavirus
Hepadnaviridae (Hepadnaviruses)	Icosahedral, enveloped 42 nm	ds circular (3.2 kb), gap in one strand; protein attached	Hepatitis B virus (HBV)
Polyomaviridae (Polyomaviruses)	Icosahedral, naked 45 nm	ds circular (5 kb)	JC virus, BK virus, KI virus, WU virus, Merkel cell virus, HPyV6, HPyV7 of humans
Papillomaviridae (Papillomaviruses)	Icosahedral, naked 55 nm	ds circular (8 kb)	Human papillomavirus (HPV), about 100 genotypes
Adenoviridae (Adenoviruses)	Icosahedral, naked 80-110 nm	ds linear (36-38 kb); protein attached	Human respiratory disease and gastroenteritis viruses
Herpesviridae (Herpesviruses)	Icosahedral, enveloped 180-200 nm	ds linear (124-235 kb)	Herpes simplex virus (HSV) types 1 and 2; varicella-zoster virus (VZV); cytomegalovirus (CMV); Epstein-Barr virus (EBV); human herpesviruses 6 and 7, human herpesvirus 8 (Kaposi sarcoma)
Poxviridae (Poxviruses)	brick-shaped or ovoid, enveloped 300 nm	ds linear (130-375 kb)	Smallpox; vaccinia; monkeypox virus; cowpox virus; orf; pseudocowpox virus; yabapox virus; tanapox virus; molluscum contagiosum

ds, double-stranded; ss, single-stranded.

TABLE 6–3 Some Important Bacteriophages

BACTERIOPHAGE	HOST	GENOME STRUCTURE AND SIZE	COMMENTS
MS2	*Escherichia coli*	ss linear RNA (3.5 kb)	Lytic
Filamentous (M13, fd)	*Escherichia coli*	ss linear RNA (7.6 kb)	No cell death
φX174	*Escherichia coli*	ss linear RNA (5.3 kb)	Lytic
β	*Corynebacterium diphtheriae*	ds linear DNA (42.9 kb)	Temperate, codes for diphtheria toxin
λ	*Escherichia coli*	ds linear DNA (48.5)	Temperate
T4	*Escherichia coli*	ds linear DNA (160-250 kb)	Lytic

ds, double-stranded; ss, single-stranded.

FIGURE 6–7. **Virus replication cycle.** A general scheme of the six discrete steps of virus replication cycle, including attachment, penetration, uncoating, synthetic phase (transcription, translation, and replication), assembly, and release.

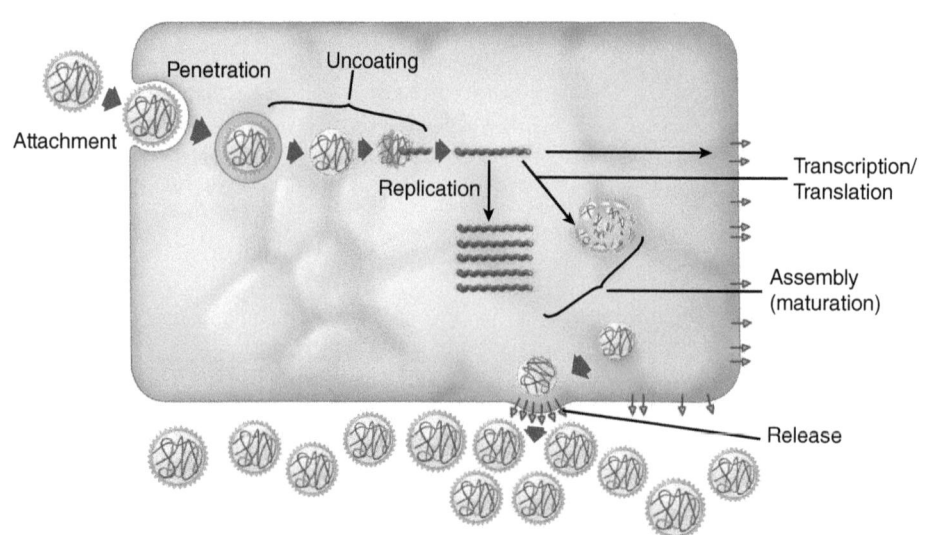

This series of events, sometimes with slight variations, describes what is called the **productive** or **lytic response;** however, this is not the only possible outcome of a virus infection. Some viruses can also enter into a very different kind of relationship with the host cell in which no new virus is produced, the cell survives and divides, and the viral genetic material persists indefinitely in a latent state. This outcome of an infection is referred to as the **nonproductive response.** The nonproductive response in the case of bacteriophages is called **lysogeny** and, in several human and animal viruses under some circumstances, may be associated with **oncogenic transformation.** (This use of the term transformation is to be distinguished from DNA transformation of bacteria discussed in Chapter 21.)

Some viruses can also cause a **chronic infection** where a low level of the virus is produced with little or no damage to the target tissue. Both latent infection and chronic infection are called **persistent infection.** Virus replication also depends on virus–host cell interaction such as the type of cells it infects—whether permissive or nonpermissive cells. **Permissive cells** are those that permit production of progeny virus particles and/or viral transformation. However, **nonpermissive cells** do not allow virus replication, but may allow virus transformation. Some viruses enter cells that do not support virus replication, but some early viral proteins cause cell death; this infection is termed **abortive infection.**

The outcome of an infection depends on the particular virus–host combination and on other factors such as the extracellular environment, multiplicity of infection, and physiology and developmental state of the cell. Viruses that can enter only into a productive relationship are called **lytic** or **virulent viruses.** Viruses that can establish either a productive or a nonproductive relationship with their host cells are referred to as **temperate viruses.** Some temperate viruses can be reactivated or "induced" to leave the latent state and enter into the productive response. Whether induction occurs depends on the particular virus–host combination, the physiology of the cell, and the presence of extracellular stimuli.

GROWTH AND ASSAY OF VIRUSES

Viruses are generally propagated in the laboratory by mixing the virus and susceptible cells together and incubating the infected cells until lysis occurs. After lysis, the cells and cell debris are removed by a brief centrifugation, and the resulting supernatant is called a **lysate.**

The growth of human viruses requires that the host cells be cultivated in the laboratory, mostly in human or animal cell lines (cell derived from tumors or cells transformed by viruses) and, in some cases, in primary cells derived from tissues. To prepare cells for growth *in vitro*, a tissue is removed from an animal, and the cells are disaggregated using the proteolytic enzyme trypsin. The cell suspension is seeded into a plastic Petri dish in a medium containing a complex mixture of amino acids, vitamins, minerals, and sugars. In addition to these nutritional factors, the growth of animal cells requires components present in animal serum. This method of growing cells is referred to as **tissue culture,** and the initial cell population is called a **primary culture.** The cells attach to the bottom of the plastic dish and remain attached as they divide and eventually cover the surface of the dish. When the culture becomes crowded, the cells generally cease dividing and enter a resting state. Propagation can be continued by removing the cells from the primary culture plate using trypsin and reseeding a new plate.

Cells taken from a normal (as opposed to cancerous) tissue cannot usually be propagated in this manner indefinitely. Eventually, most of the cells die; a few may survive, and these survivors often develop into a permanent **cell line.** Cell lines can also be generated directly from tumors or from virus transformed cells. Such cell lines are very useful as host cells for isolating and assaying viruses in the laboratory, but they rarely bear much resemblance to the tissue from which they originated. When cells are taken from a tumor and cultivated *in vitro*, they display a very different set of growth properties, including long-term survival, reflecting their tumor phenotype.

When a virus is propagated in tissue culture cells, the cellular changes induced by the virus, which usually culminate in cell death, are often characteristic of a particular virus and are referred to as the **cytopathic effect** of the virus.

Viruses are quantitated by a method called the plaque assay (see Plaque Assay under Quantitation of Viruses for a detailed description of the method). Briefly, viruses are mixed with cells on a Petri plate so that each infectious particle gives rise to a zone of lysed or dead cells called a **plaque.** From the number of plaques on the plate, the titer of infectious particles in the lysate is calculated. Virus titers are expressed as the number of plaque-forming units per milliliter (pfu/mL).

Viral infections may be productive or nonproductive

Some human viruses cause oncogenic transformation

Some cause persistent infection

Permissive cells allow replication and/or viral transformation

Nonpermissive cells do not permit virus replication, but may allow viral transformation

Temperate viruses can either replicate or enter a latent state

Viruses are cultivated in cell lines or cell cultures derived from animal tissues

Permanent cell lines are useful for growing viruses

Cytopathic effects are characteristic for individual viruses

Viruses are quantitated by a plaque assay

FIGURE 6–8. **One-step growth experiment.** The purpose of a one-step growth experiment is to understand the various phases of infection that occur following a viral infection. In the graph, red line measures virus in the culture medium (outside the cell) and blue line measures virus inside the cells. pfu, plaque-forming units.

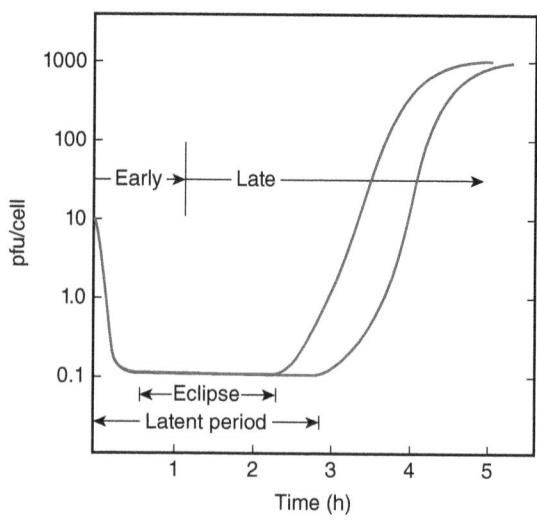

ONE-STEP GROWTH EXPERIMENT

The purpose of a one-step growth experiment is to understand various stages of viral infection. To describe an infection in temporal and quantitative terms, it is useful to perform a one-step growth experiment (**Figure 6–8**). The objective in such an experiment is to infect every cell in a culture so that the whole population proceeds through the infection process in a synchronous fashion. The ratio of infecting plaque-forming units to cells is called the multiplicity of infection (MOI). By infecting at a high MOI (eg, 10, as in Figure 6–8), one can be certain that every cell is infected.

One-step growth experiments are useful in the study of various stages of viral infection

The time course and efficiency of adsorption can be followed by the loss of infectious virus from the medium after removal of the cells (red line in Figure 6–8). In the example shown, adsorption takes approximately half an hour, and all but 1% of the virus is adsorbed. If samples of the culture containing the infected cells are treated so as to break open the cells before assaying for virus (blue line in Figure 6–8), it can be observed that infectious virus initially disappears, because no infectious particles are detectable above the background of unadsorbed virus. The period of infection in which no infectious viruses are found inside the cell is called the **eclipse phase** and emphasizes that the original virions lose their infectivity soon after entry. Infectivity is lost because, as is discussed later, the virus particles are dismantled as a prelude to their reproduction. Later, infectious virus particles rapidly reappear in increasing numbers and are detected inside the cell prior to their release into the environment (Figure 6–8). The length of time from the beginning of infection until progeny virions are found outside the cells is referred to as the **latent period.** Latent periods range from 20 minutes to hours for bacteriophages and from a few hours to many days for human viruses.

Shortly after infection, a virus loses its identity (eclipse phase)

Infectious virus reappears at the end of eclipse phase inside the cell

The time in the infection at which genome replication begins is typically used to divide the infection operationally into early and late phases. Early viral gene expression is largely restricted to the production of the proteins required for genome replication; later, the proteins synthesized are, primarily, those necessary for construction of the new virus particles.

Proteins for replication produced early, those for construction of virions late

The average number of plaque-forming units released per infected cell is called the burst size for the infection. In the example shown, the burst size is approximately 1000. Burst sizes range from less than 10 for some relatively inefficient infections to millions for some highly virulent viruses.

VIRUS REPLICATION CYCLE

■ Adsorption or Attachment

The first step in every viral infection is the attachment or adsorption of the infecting virus particle to the surface of the host cell. A prerequisite for this interaction is a collision between the virion and the cell. Viruses do not have any capacity for locomotion and, therefore, the collision event is simply a random process determined by diffusion. Therefore, similar to any bimolecular reaction, the rate of adsorption is determined by the concentrations of both the virions and the cells.

Only a small percentage of the collisions between a virus and its host cell lead to a successful infection because adsorption is a highly specific reaction that involves protein molecules on the surface of the virion called **virion attachment proteins** or **spikes** and certain molecules on the surface of the cell that are called **receptors.** Typically, 10^4 to 10^5 receptors are found on the cell surface. Receptors for some bacteriophages are found on pili of bacteria, although most adsorb to receptors found on the bacterial cell wall. Receptors for human viruses are usually glycoproteins located in the plasma membrane of the cell. **Table 6–4** lists some of the receptors that have been identified for medically important viruses. It appears that viruses have evolved to make use of a wide variety of surface molecules as receptors, which are normally signaling devices or immune system components. Any attempts to design antiviral agents that block viral infections by binding to the receptors for a long time must consider the possibility that the loss of the normal cellular function associated with the receptors would have serious consequences for the host organism.

For some viruses, two different surface molecules, called **coreceptors,** are involved in adsorption. Although CD4 was originally thought to be the sole receptor for human immunodeficiency virus type 1 (HIV-1), the discovery of a family of coreceptors that normally function as chemokine receptors (CCR5 and CXCR4) may explain why natural resistance against the virus is found in some individuals with variant forms (Δ32CCR5) of these signaling molecules (discussed in Chapter 18). Although receptors for some human viruses such as influenza viruses are present on lung cells, these receptors are also found on red blood cells of certain species that are responsible for the phenomena of hemagglutination and hemadsorption discussed later.

Virion attachment proteins are often associated with conspicuous features on the surface of the virion. For example, the virion attachment proteins for the bacteriophages with tails are located at the very end of the tails or the tail fibers. Similarly, the spikes found on adenoviruses (Figure 6–3E) and on virtually all the enveloped human viruses (Figure 6-3D) contain the virion attachment proteins.

In some cases, a region of the capsid protein serves the function of the attachment protein. For polioviruses, rhinoviruses, and probably other picornaviruses, the region on the capsid that binds to the receptor is found at the bottom of a cleft, trough, or canyon that is too narrow to allow access to antibodies. This particular arrangement is clearly advantageous to the virus because it precludes the production of antibodies that might directly block receptor recognition.

The repeating subunit structure of capsids and the multiplicity of spikes on enveloped viruses are probably important in determining the strength of the binding of the virus to the cell. The binding between a single virion attachment protein and a single receptor protein is relatively weak, but the combinations of many such interactions lead to a strong association between the virion and the cell. The fluid nature of the human cell membrane may facilitate the movement of receptor proteins to allow the clustering that is necessary for these multiple interactions.

A particular kind of virus is capable of infecting only a limited spectrum of cell types called its **host range.** Thus, although a few viruses can infect cells from different species, most viruses are limited to a single species. For example, dogs do not contract measles virus infection, and humans do not contract distemper, a viral disease of dogs. In many cases, human viruses infect only a particular subset of the cells found in their host organism. This kind of **tissue tropism** is clearly an important determinant of viral pathogenesis. In most cases studied, the specific host range of a virus and its associated tissue tropism are determined at the level of the binding between the cell receptors and virion attachment proteins. Thus, these two protein components must possess complementary surfaces that fit together in much the same way as a substrate fits into the active site of an enzyme. It follows that adsorption occurs only in that percentage of collisions that leads to successful binding between receptors and attachment proteins, and that the inability of a virus to infect a cell type is usually due to the absence of the appropriate receptors on the cell. A few cases are known in which the host range of a virus is determined at a step after adsorption and penetration, but these are the exceptions rather than the rule.

When a virus particle has penetrated to the inside of a cell, it is essentially hidden from the host immune system. Thus, if protection from a virus infection is to be accomplished at the level of antibody binding to the virions, it must occur before adsorption and prevent the virus from attaching to and penetrating the cell. It is, therefore, not surprising that most neutralizing antibodies—whether elicited as a result of natural infection or vaccination—are specific for virion attachment proteins.

Adsorption involves attachment of viral surface proteins or spikes to the cell surface receptor proteins

Viral spikes and phage tails carry attachment proteins

Adsorption is enhanced by presence of multiple attachment and receptor proteins

Differences in host range and tissue tropism are due to presence or absence of receptors

Neutralizing antibodies often specific for attachment proteins

TABLE 6–4	Examples of Cell Receptors for Human Viruses	
VIRUS	**RECEPTOR**	**CELLULAR FUNCTION**
Adenoviruses	Integrins	Cell surface receptors that interact with extracellular matrix
Arenaviruses	α-dystroglycan	Dystrophin-associated glycoproteins, transmembrane linkage
Cytomegalovirus	HSPGs, Integrins, EGFR, PDGFR, CD90, Nrp2, CD147, CD46	Glycoproteins, signaling, cell surface proteins, complement regulation and others
Coronavirus 229E	Aminopeptidase N	Protease
Coronavirus OC43, HKU1	Sialic acid	Glycoprotein
Coronavirus NL63, SARS-CoV-1, SARS-CoV-2 (COVID-19)	ACE-2	Angiotensin converting enzyme 2
MERS-CoV	Dipeptidyl peptidase 4	Serine exopeptidase
Dengue virus	Heparin sulfate	Glycoprotein
	Sulfated glycosaminoglycans	Polysaccharides
	Lectins	Glycoprotein
Epstein-Barr virus	CR2 (CD21)	Complement receptor
Filoviruses (Ebola and Marburg)	TIM-1	T-cell Ig and mucin domain 1
Hantavirus	Integerins	Cell surface proteins that interact with extracellular matrix
Hepatitis A virus	α_2-Macroglobulin	Plasma protein (inhibitor of coagulation, fibrinolysis)
Herpes simplex	Heparan sulfate	Glycoprotein
Human herpes 7	CD4	Immunoglobulin superfamily
HIV	CD4	Immunoglobulin superfamily
	CXCR4 and CCR5	Chemokine receptors
Influenza A	Sialic acid	Glycoprotein
Measles	CD46	Complement regulation
Papillomavirus	α-6 β-4 integrin	Cell surface proteins
Parvovirus B19	Erythrocyte P antigen	Erythroid precursors
Poliovirus	PVR	Immunoglobulin superfamily
Polyomavirus	Serotonin	G protein superfamily
Rabies	Acetylcholine receptor	Signaling
Reoviruses	Sialic acid	Glycoprotein
	EGFR	Signaling
Rhinoviruses	ICAM-1	Immunoglobulin superfamily
Rotavirus	$\alpha_2\beta_1$ and $\alpha_4\beta_1$, integrins	Cell surface receptors that interact with extracellular matrix
Vaccinia	EGF receptor	Signaling

COVID-19, coronavirus disease of 2019; EGF, endothelial growth factor receptor; HSPGs, heparin sulfate proteoglycans; HIV, human immunodeficiency virus; ICAM, intercellular adhesion molecule; MHC, major histocompatibility complex; Nrp2, neuropilin-2; PDGFR, platelet-derived growth factor receptor; PVR, poliovirus receptor; SARS, severe acute respiratory syndrome.

PENETRATION, ENTRY, AND UNCOATING

The disappearance of infectious virus during the eclipse phase is a direct consequence of the fact that viruses are dismantled before being replicated. As discussed later in the text, the uncoating step may be simultaneous with entry or may occur in a series of steps. Ultimately, the nucleocapsid or core structure must be transported to the site or compartment in the cell where transcription and replication will occur.

Viruses are dismantled before being replicated

■ The Bacteriophage Strategy

The processes of penetration and uncoating are simultaneous for all bacteriophages. Thus, the viral capsids are shed at the surface, and only the nucleic acid genome enters the cell. In some cases, a small number of virion proteins may accompany the genome into the cell, but these are probably tightly associated with the nucleic acid or are essential enzymes needed to initiate the infection.

Bacteriophages with tails are responsible for the attachment of the virion to the bacterial cell wall to facilitate the entry of the genome into the cell. The DNA of the bacteriophage is injected from the head directly into the cell through the hollow tail structure. The process has been likened to the action of a syringe.

Bacteriophage capsids are shed, only the genome enters host cell

Tailed bacteriophages attach by tail fibers, DNA injected through tail

■ Enveloped Human Viruses

There are two basic mechanisms for the entry of an enveloped human virus into the cell. Both mechanisms involve fusion of the viral envelope with a cellular membrane, and the end result in both cases is the release of the free nucleocapsid into the cytoplasm. What distinguishes the two mechanisms is the nature of the cellular membrane that fuses with the viral envelope.

Paramyxoviruses (eg, measles), some retroviruses (eg, HIV-1), and herpesviruses enter by a process called **direct fusion (Figure 6–9)**. The envelopes of these viruses contain protein spikes that promote fusion of the viral membrane with the plasma membrane of the cell, releasing the nucleocapsid directly into the cytoplasm. Because the viral envelope becomes incorporated into

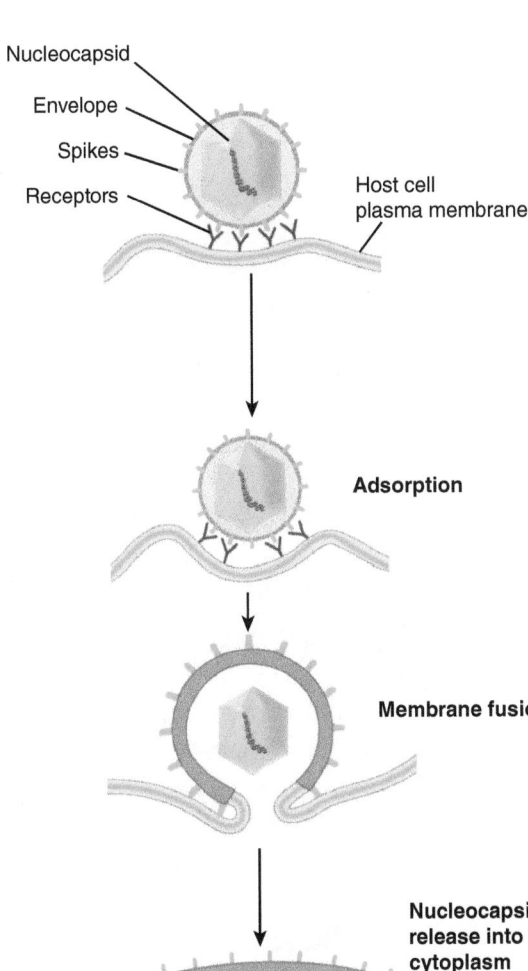

Nucleocapsid

Envelope

Spikes

Receptors

Host cell plasma membrane

Adsorption

Membrane fusion

Nucleocapsid release into cytoplasm

FIGURE 6–9. **Entry by direct fusion.** Some enveloped viruses enter cells by direct fusion mechanism. Viral envelope proteins (spikes) bind to the receptors on the host cell followed by fusion of the viral envelope with the plasma membrane of the host cells, which is promoted by one of the viral envelope spikes (F protein of RSV and Gp41 of HIV). After fusion, the nucleocapsid complex is released in the cytoplasm. This mode of virus entry is seen in enveloped viruses such as paramyxoviruses, herpesviruses, and some retroviruses (HIV).

Some enveloped viruses enter cells by direct fusion of plasma membrane and envelope

Other enveloped and naked viruses are taken in by receptor-mediated endocytosis (viropexis)

the plasma membrane of the infected cell and still possesses its fusion proteins, infected cells have a tendency to fuse with other uninfected cells. Cell-to-cell fusion is a hallmark of infections by paramyxoviruses and HIV-1, and can be important in the pathology of diseases such as measles, respiratory syncytial virus (RSV)-induced bronchiolitis, and acquired immunodeficiency syndrome (AIDS).

The mechanism for the entry of most of the remaining enveloped human viruses, such as orthomyxoviruses (eg, influenza viruses), togaviruses (eg, rubella virus), rhabdoviruses (eg, rabies), and coronaviruses, is shown in **Figure 6–10.** After adsorption, the virus particles are taken up by a cellular mechanism called **receptor-mediated endocytosis,** which is normally responsible for internalizing growth factors, hormones, and some nutrients. When it involves viruses, the process is referred to as **viropexis.**

In viropexis, the adsorbed virions become surrounded by the plasma membrane in a reaction that is probably facilitated by the multiplicity of virion attachment proteins on the surface of the particle. Pinching off of the cellular membrane by fusion encloses the virion in a cytoplasmic vesicle termed the **endosomal vesicle.** The nucleocapsid is now surrounded by two membranes: the original viral envelope and the newly acquired endosomal membrane. The surface receptors are subsequently recycled back to the plasma membrane, and the endosomal vesicle is acidified by a normal cellular process. The low pH of the endosome leads to a conformational change in a viral spike protein, which results in the fusion of the two membranes and release of the nucleocapsid into the cytoplasm. In some cases, the contents of the endosomal vesicle may be transferred to a lysosome before the fusion step that releases the nucleocapsid.

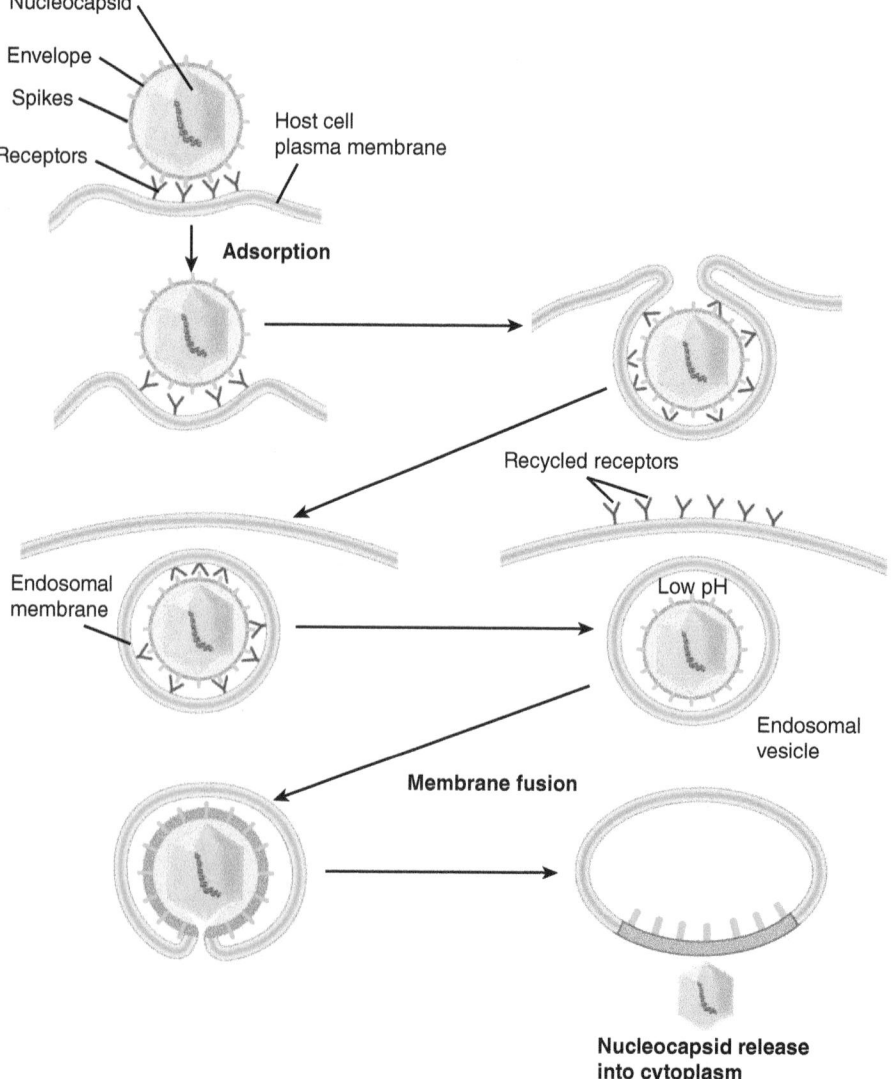

FIGURE 6–10. Viropexis. Several enveloped viruses and all naked capsid viruses enter cells by viropexis. In viropexis, viral spikes bind to the receptors on host cells followed by surrounding of the adsorbed virions by plasma membrane and formation of an endosomal vesicle. For enveloped viruses, low pH of the endosomes leads to a conformational change in a viral spike protein followed by fusion of the two membranes and release of the nucleocapsid into the cytoplasm. For naked capsid viruses, low pH of the endosomes expose hydrophobic domains resulting in binding of virions to the membrane or virions promoting lysis of the vesicle followed by release of viral genomes into the cytoplasm.

Nucleocapsid

Envelope

Spikes

Receptors

Host cell plasma membrane

Adsorption

Recycled receptors

Endosomal membrane

Low pH

Endosomal vesicle

Membrane fusion

Nucleocapsid release into cytoplasm

◼ Naked Capsid Human Viruses

Naked capsid human viruses, such as poliovirus, reovirus, and adenovirus, also appear to enter the cell by viropexis (Figure 6–10). However, in this case, the virus **cannot escape the endosomal vesicle by membrane fusion** as described earlier for some enveloped viruses. For poliovirus, it appears that the viral capsid proteins in the low-pH environment of the endosome expose hydrophobic domains. This process results in the binding of the virions to the membrane and release of the nucleic acid genome into the cytoplasm. In other cases, the virions may escape into the cytoplasm by simply promoting the lysis of the vesicle. This step is a potential target of antiviral chemotherapy, and some drugs have been developed that bind to the capsids of picornaviruses and prevent the release of the virus particles from the endosome.

Reovirus is unusual in that, before release into the cytoplasm, the contents of the endosome are transferred to a lysosome where the lysosomal proteases strip away part of the capsid proteins and activate virion-associated enzymes required for transcription.

Acidified endosome releases nucleocapsid to cytoplasm

Virions may escape endosome by dissolution of the vesicles

SYNTHETIC OR VIRION COMPONENT PRODUCTION

Synthetic or virion production is the most important step in the viral replication cycle because the virus must make mRNAs, proteins, and genomes for the assembly of progeny or daughter viruses. In the case of **bacteriophages**, there is evidence that the entering nucleic acid must be directed to a particular locus in the bacterial cell to initiate the infection process. **Pilot proteins** accompany the bacteriophage genome to a specific site into the bacterial cell where transcription and replication occur.

For **human viruses,** the ultimate fate of internalized virus particles depends on the particular virus and on the cellular compartment where replication occurs. Most RNA viruses replicate in the cytoplasm—the immediate site of entry with the exception of influenza viruses and the retroviruses that replicate in the nucleus. All DNA viruses must move from the cytoplasm to the nucleus to replicate, except the poxviruses that replicate in the cytoplasm. The larger DNA viruses, such as herpesviruses and adenoviruses, must uncoat to the level of cores before entry into the nucleus. The smaller DNA viruses, such as the parvoviruses and the papilloma/polyomaviruses, enter the nucleus intact through the nuclear pores and subsequently uncoat inside. The largest of the human viruses, the poxviruses, carry out their entire replicative cycle in the cytoplasm of the infected cell because they make both RNA and DNA polymerases.

Most RNA viruses replicate in the cytoplasm, except influenza viruses and retroviruses, which replicate in the nucleus

All DNA viruses replicate in the nucleus, except poxviruses, which replicate in the cytoplasm

TRANSCRIPTION

◼ From Genome to mRNA

An essential step in every virus infection is the production of virus-specific mRNAs that program the cellular ribosomes to synthesize viral proteins. Besides the structural proteins of the virion, viruses must direct the synthesis of enzymes and other specialized proteins required for genome replication, gene expression, and virus assembly and release. The production of the first viral mRNAs at the beginning of the infection is a crucial step in the takeover of the cell by the virus.

For some viruses, the presentation of mRNA to the cellular ribosomes poses no problems. Thus, the genomes of most DNA viruses are transcribed by the host DNA-dependent RNA polymerase (RNA polymerase II) in the nucleus to yield the viral mRNAs which are exported to the cytoplasm for translation. The (+) strand RNA viruses, such as the picornaviruses, the togaviruses, the flaviviruses, the coronaviruses, the caliciviruses, and the hepeviruses (hepatitis E virus) possess genomes that can be used directly as mRNAs and are translated (at least partially, as discussed later) immediately on entry into the cytoplasm of the cell. One of these viral proteins is **RNA-dependent RNA polymerase** (also known as viral RNA polymerase or RNA transcriptase) required to synthesize new mRNAs and genomic RNA.

However, for many viruses, the production of mRNA starting from the genome is not so straightforward. The fact that DNA virus such as poxvirus replicates in the cytoplasm means that the cellular RNA polymerase is not available to transcribe the viral DNA genome. Moreover, no cellular machinery exists in the cytoplasm that can use either single- or double-stranded RNA as a template to synthesize mRNA. Therefore, the poxviruses and viruses that use an RNA template, especially the (–) strand RNA viruses such as the rhabdoviruses, orthomyxoviruses,

Virus-specific mRNAs direct synthesis of viral proteins

DNA viruses synthesize mRNAs using host RNA polymerase

Positive-strand RNA virus genome serves as mRNA for early protein synthesis, and then uses viral RNA polymerase for transcription and replication

Negative-strand RNA viruses carry virion-associated RNA-dependent RNA polymerase to produce initial mRNAs

A variety of pathways exist for synthesis of mRNA by different virus groups

Retroviral RNA is copied to DNA by virion reverse transcriptase enzyme; host RNA polymerase transcribes viral DNA into viral mRNA and genomic RNA

paramyxoviruses, filoviruses, to make mRNAs must provide their own transcription machinery to produce the viral mRNAs at the beginning of the infection process. This feat is accomplished by synthesizing the polymerases or transcriptases in the later stages of viral development in the previous host cell and packaging the enzymes into the virions, where they remain associated with the genome as the virus enters the new cell and uncoats. In general, the presence of a polymerase or transcriptase in virions is indicative that the host cell is unable to use the viral genome as mRNA or as a template to synthesize mRNA. At later times in the infection, any special enzymatic machinery required by the virus and not initially present in the cell can be supplied among the proteins translated from the first mRNA molecules.

The pathways for the synthesis of mRNA by the major virus groups are summarized in **Figure 6–11** and related to the structure of viral genomes. The polarity of mRNA is designated as (+) and the polarity of antisense or complementary to mRNA as (–). The black arrows denote synthetic steps for which host cells provide the required enzymes, whereas the colored arrows indicate synthetic steps that must be carried out by virus-encoded enzymes. Several additional points should be emphasized. The parvoviruses and some bacteriophages have single-stranded DNA genomes. Although the RNA polymerase of the cell requires double-stranded DNA as a template, these viruses need not to carry special enzymes in their virions because host cell DNA polymerases can convert the single-stranded DNA genomes into double-stranded DNA. Note that the production of more mRNA by the picornaviruses and similar (+)-strand RNA viruses requires the synthesis of an intermediate (–)-strand RNA template. The enzyme required for this process is produced by translation of the genome RNA early in infection called RNA-dependent RNA polymerase.

The retroviruses are a special class of (+)-strand RNA viruses. Although their genomes are the same polarity as mRNA and could, in principle, serve as mRNAs early after infection, their replication scheme apparently precludes this. Instead, the RNA genomes of these viruses are copied into (–) DNA strands by an enzyme carried within the virion called **reverse transcriptase (RNA dependent DNA polymerase)**. The (–) DNA strands are subsequently converted by the same enzyme to double-stranded DNA in a reaction that requires the degradation of the original genomic RNA by the RNase H activity of the reverse transcriptase enzyme. The viral DNA product of reverse transcription is integrated into the host cell DNA and ultimately transcribed by the host RNA polymerase to complete the replication cycle as well as produce viral mRNA. The replication of the hepatitis B virus DNA genome is mechanistically similar to that of a retrovirus.

FIGURE 6–11. Pathways of mRNA synthesis for major virus groups.

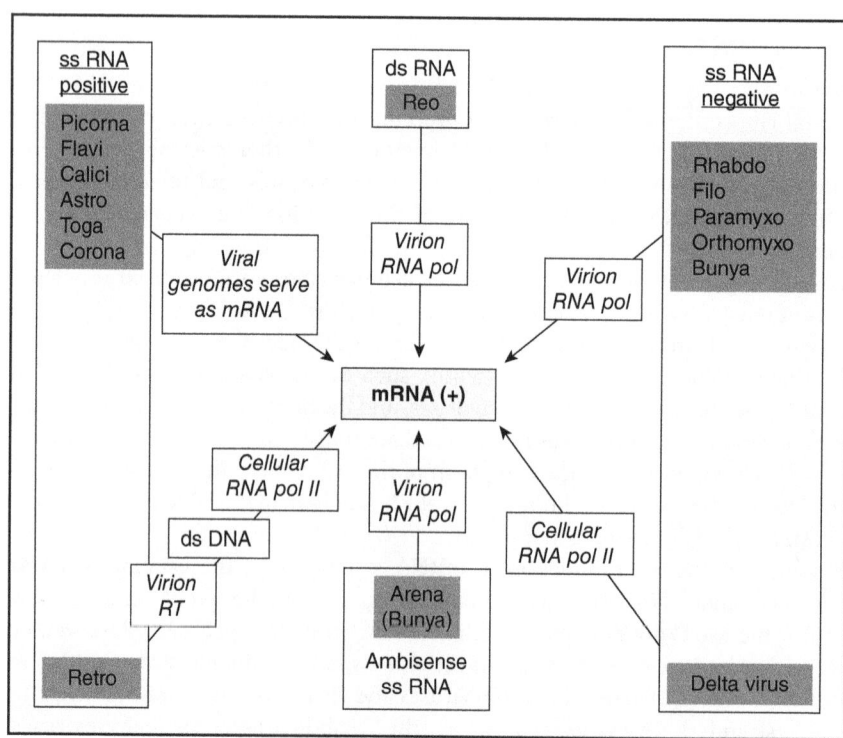

Thus, the hepatitis B viral DNA is transcribed to produce a single-stranded RNA by the host RNA polymerase, which in turn is reverse transcribed to produce the progeny viral DNA that is encapsidated into virions.

■ The Monocistronic mRNA Rule in Human Cells

The ribosome requires input of information in the form of mRNA. For a viral mRNA to be recognized by the ribosome, its production must conform to the rules of structure that govern the synthesis of the cellular mRNAs. Prokaryotic or bacterial mRNA is relatively simple and can be polycistronic, which means it can contain the information for several proteins. Each cistron or coding region is translated independently beginning from its own ribosome binding site.

> Prokaryotic (bacterial) mRNAs can be polycistronic

Eukaryotic mRNAs are structurally more complex, containing special 5'-cap and 3'-poly(A) attachments. In addition, their synthesis often involves removal of internal sequences (introns) and joining of coding sequences (exons) by a process called **splicing.** Most important, almost all eukaryotic mRNAs are monocistronic, which means one mRNA encodes one protein. Accordingly, eukaryotic translation is initiated by the binding of a ribosome to the 5'-cap, followed by movement of the ribosome along the RNA until the first AUG initiation codon is encountered. The outcome of this first AUG rule is that eukaryotic ribosomes, unlike prokaryotic ribosomes, generally cannot initiate translation at internal sites on an mRNA. To conform to the monocistronic mRNA, most human viruses produce mRNAs that are translated to yield only a single polypeptide chain (protein) following initiation near the 5' end of the mRNA.

> Human virus mRNAs are almost always monocistronic, one mRNA for one protein

Because most DNA human viruses replicate in the nucleus, they adhere to the monocistronic mRNA rule either by having a promoter precede each gene or by programming the transcription of precursor RNAs that are processed by nuclear splicing enzymes into monocistronic mRNAs (**Figure 6–12A**). The virion transcriptase or polymerase of the cytoplasmic poxviruses apparently must synthesize monocistronic mRNAs by initiation of transcription in front of each gene.

> Most DNA viruses generate monocistronic mRNA through splicing

RNA human viruses have evolved three strategies to circumvent or conform to the monocistronic mRNA rule. The simplest strategy involves having a segmented RNA genome (**Figure 6–12B**). For the most part, each genome segment of the orthomyxoviruses and the reoviruses corresponds to a single gene; therefore, the mRNA transcribed from a given segment constitutes a monocistronic mRNA. Unlike most RNA viruses, the orthomyxovirus virus (influenza virus) replicates in the nucleus, and some of its monocistronic mRNAs are produced by splicing of precursor RNAs by host cell enzymes. Moreover, orthomyxoviruses use small 5' RNA fragments derived from host cell pre-mRNAs, found in the nucleus, to prime the synthesis of their own mRNAs. However, the synthesis of mRNA and genomic RNA is completed by the viral RNA-dependent RNA polymerase.

> Some RNA viruses have segmented genomes to fulfill monocistronic mRNA rule

A second solution to the monocistronic mRNA rule is mainly seen in negative-strand RNA viruses that carry RNA-dependent RNA polymerase in their virus particle. The negative-strand RNA viruses, including paramyxoviruses, rhabdoviruses, filoviruses, bunyaviruses, and arenaviruses, and some positive-strand RNA viruses, such as togaviruses and coronaviruses, synthesize monocistronic mRNAs by initiating the synthesis of each mRNA at the beginning of a gene. In most cases, the RNA-dependent RNA polymerase terminates mRNA synthesis at the end of the gene such that each message corresponds to a single gene (**Figure 6–12C**). For coronaviruses and togaviruses, the positive-strand RNA is initially translated to synthesize RNA-dependent RNA polymerase, which transcribes positive-strand RNA into a negative-strand RNA intermediate that is used as a template for RNA synthesis. RNA synthesis is initiated on the negative-strand RNA intermediate template at the beginning of each gene and continues to the end of the genome so that a nested set of mRNAs is produced. However, each mRNA is functionally monocistronic and is translated to produce only the protein encoded near its 5' end.

> Negative-sense RNA viruses produce monocistronic RNAs by initiating synthesis at the start and pausing at the end of each gene

> Positive-sense RNA viruses make a polyprotein that is proteolytically cleaved later into individual proteins

The positive-strand RNA viruses such as picornaviruses and flaviviruses have evolved yet a third strategy to deal with the monocistronic mRNA requirement (**Figure 6–12D**). The (+)-strand genome contains just a single ribosome binding site near the 5' end. It is translated into one long polypeptide chain called a **polyprotein,** which is subsequently broken into the final set of protein products by a series of proteolytic cleavages. Most of the required protease activities reside within the polyprotein itself.

Several viruses use more than one of these strategies to conform to the monocistronic mRNA rule. For example, retroviruses, togaviruses, arenaviruses, and bunyaviruses synthesize multiple

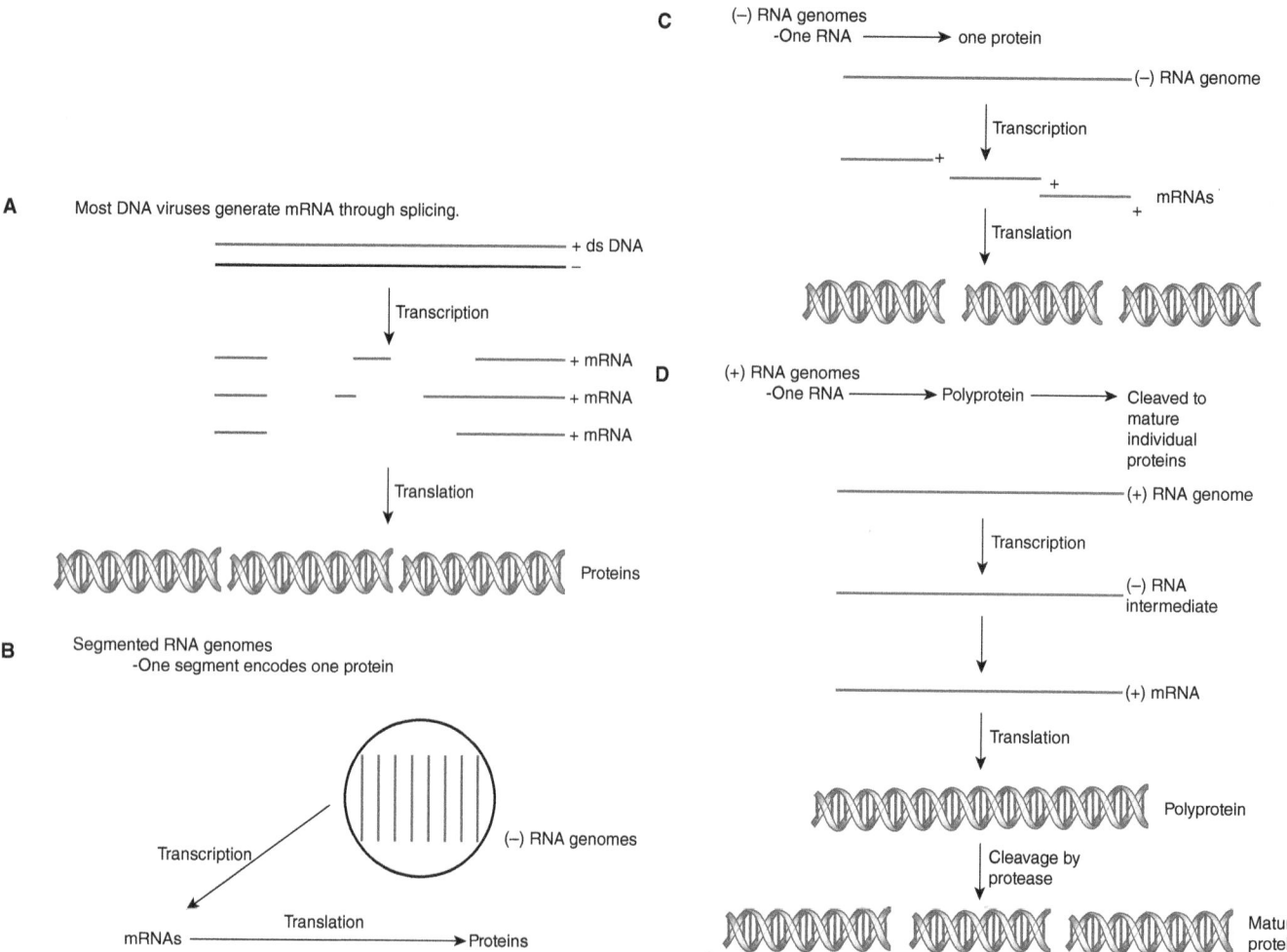

FIGURE 6–12. Monocistronic mRNA strategy for human viruses. Human viruses follow eukaryotic rule of mRNA synthesis, which means one mRNA encodes one protein. **A.** Most DNA viruses generate mRNA through splicing because they replicate inside the nucleus using host cell machinery. RNA viruses use three mechanisms to generate mRNA. **B.** Segmented genome, one segment encodes one protein. **C.** Viral RNA polymerase of negative-sense RNA viruses initiates transcription at the start of each gene and pauses at the end of the gene and continues to the end of the genome resulting in synthesis of a nested set of mRNAs. **D.** Positive sense RNA viruses' genome is translated into a polyprotein that is cleaved to mature proteins by protease enzyme.

HIV- and HCV-encoded proteases are targets for antiviral therapy (protease inhibitors)

mRNAs, each one coding for a polyprotein that is subsequently cleaved into the individual protein molecules. For some viruses such as retrovirus (HIV) and flavivirus (HCV), viral protease enzyme that cleaves polyprotein can be inhibited by potent antivirals (protease inhibitors) in infected patients.

GENOME REPLICATION

■ DNA Viruses

Host cells contain the enzymes and accessory proteins that are required for the replication of DNA. In bacteria, these proteins are present continuously, whereas in the eukaryotic cells they are present only during the S phase of the cell cycle and restricted to the nucleus. The extent to which viruses use the cell replication machinery depends on their protein-coding potential and, thus, on the size of their genome.

The smallest DNA viruses depend exclusively on host DNA replication machinery

The largest DNA viruses (poxviruses) encode for enzymes necessary for RNA transcription and DNA replication

The smallest of the DNA viruses, the parvoviruses, are so completely dependent on host machinery that they require the infected cells to be dividing to ensure that a normal S phase occurs and replicates the viral DNA together with the cellular DNA. At the other end of the spectrum are the large DNA viruses, which are relatively independent of cellular functions. The largest bacteriophages such as T4 degrade the host (bacterial) cell chromosome early in infection and replace all the host replication machinery with bacteriophage-specified proteins. The largest human viruses, the poxviruses, are similarly independent of the host. Because they replicate in the cytoplasm, they must code for almost all of the enzymes and other proteins required for replicating their DNA.

The remainder of the DNA viruses is only partially dependent on host machinery. For example, bacteriophages φX174 and λ code for proteins that direct the initiation of DNA synthesis to the viral origin. However, the actual synthesis of DNA occurs by the complex of cellular enzymes responsible for replication of the *Escherichia coli* DNA. Similarly, the small DNA human viruses, such as the polyomaviruses and papillomaviruses, code for a protein that is involved in the initiation of synthesis at the origin, but the remainder of the replication process is carried out by host machinery. The somewhat more complex adenoviruses and herpesviruses, in addition to providing origin-specific proteins, also encode for their own DNA polymerases and other accessory proteins required for DNA replication.

> Several complex DNA viruses such as adenoviruses and herpesviruses encode their own DNA polymerase

> Herpesvirus-encoded DNA polymerase is a target of antiviral therapy (eg, acyclovir)

The fact that the herpesviruses encode for their own DNA polymerase has important implications for the treatment of infections by these viruses and illustrates a central principle of antiviral chemotherapy. Certain antiviral drugs such as acyclovir (acycloguanosine) preferentially kill herpesvirus-infected cells because the viral thymidine kinase, unlike the cellular counterpart, phosphorylate the nucleoside analog, converting it to a form that inhibits further DNA synthesis when DNA polymerases incorporate it into DNA. The host cell enzyme is more discriminating and fails to phosphorylate the acyclovir analog and inhibit synthesis of cellular DNA; thus, this drug does not kill uninfected cells. Similar principle applies to the chain-terminating drugs such as zidovudine (ZDV or AZT) and dideoxyinosine (ddI) that are phosphorylated by cellular kinase and target not only the HIV-1 reverse transcriptase but also inhibit cellular DNA polymerase. In principle, any viral process that is distinct from a normal cellular process is a potential target for antiviral drugs such as HIV-1 protease and integrase inhibitors and HCV protease, polymerase (NS5B), and NS5A inhibitors. As more knowledge becomes available about the details of viral replication, more antiviral drugs will become available that are targeted to these unique viral processes.

> Viral processes that are distinct from normal cellular processes are potential targets for antiviral drugs

As noted earlier, with the exception of the poxviruses, all the DNA human viruses are at least partially dependent on host cell machinery for the replication of their genomes. However, unlike the parvoviruses, the other DNA viruses do not need to infect dividing cells for a productive infection to ensue. Instead, all these viruses code for a protein expressed early in infection that induces an unscheduled cycle of cellular DNA replication (S phase). In this way, these viruses ensure that the infected cell makes all the machinery required for the replication of their own DNA. It is noteworthy that all the DNA viruses except the parvoviruses are capable, in some circumstances, of transforming a normal cell into an abnormal or cancerous cell. This correlation suggests that the unlimited proliferative capacity of the cancer cells may be due to the continual synthesis of the viral protein(s) responsible for inducing the unscheduled S phase in a normal infection. The fact that these DNA viruses can induce oncogenic transformation of cell types that are nonpermissive for viral multiplication may simply be an accident related to the need to induce cellular enzymes required for DNA replication during the lytic infection.

> All DNA viruses except parvoviruses can transform host cells

All DNA polymerases, including those encoded by viruses, synthesize DNA chains by the successive addition of nucleotides onto the 3′ end of the new DNA strand. Moreover, all DNA polymerases require a primer terminus containing a free 3′-hydroxyl to initiate the synthesis of a DNA chain. In cellular replication, a temporary primer is provided in the form of a short RNA molecule. This primer (RNA) is synthesized by an RNA polymerase, and after elongation by the DNA polymerase, it is removed. With circular chromosomes, such as those found in bacteria and many viruses, the unidirectional chain growth and primer requirement of the DNA polymerase pose no structural problems for replication. However, as illustrated in **Figure 6–13,** when a replication fork encounters the end of a linear DNA molecule, one of the new chains (heavy lines) cannot be completed at its 5′ end, because there exists no means of starting the DNA portion of the chain exactly at the end of the template DNA. Thus, after the RNA primer is removed, the new chain is incomplete at its 5′ end. This constraint on the completion of DNA chains on a linear template is called the **end problem** in DNA replication. Some eukaryotic cells add short repetitive sequences to chromosome ends using an enzyme called telomerase to prevent the shortening of the DNA with each successive round of replication.

> Replication of linear viral DNAs must solve the end problem

Several viruses are faced with the end problem during replication of their linear genomes, but none uses the cellular telomerase to synthesize DNA ends. It is beyond the scope of this

FIGURE 6–13. **The end problem in DNA replication.** In linear DNA viruses, the replication fork encounters the end of a linear DNA molecule when one of the new chains (heavy lines) cannot be completed at its 5′ end after the removal of RNA primer.

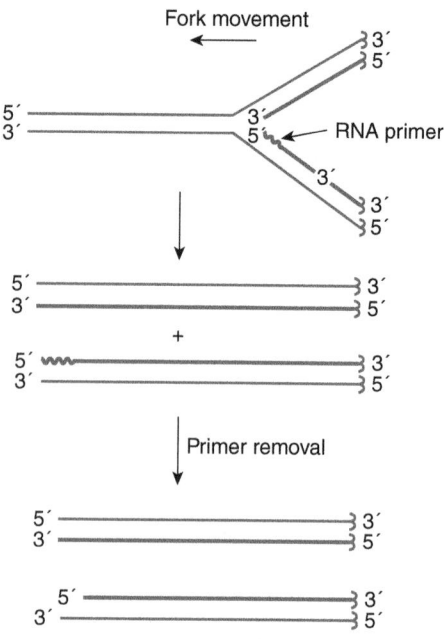

book to detail all of the strategies that viruses have evolved to deal with the end problem, but it is worth mentioning some of the structural features found in linear viral genomes whose presence is related to solutions of the end problem. These structures are diagrammed schematically in **Figure 6–14.** The linear double-stranded genome of bacteriophage λ possesses 12-bp single-stranded extensions that are complementary in sequence to each other and, thus, called **cohesive ends.** Very early after entry into the cell, the two ends pair up to convert the linear genome into a circular molecule to avoid the end problem in replication. The linear double-stranded adenovirus genome contains a protein molecule covalently attached to the 5′ end of both strands. These proteins provide the primers required to initiate the synthesis of the DNA chains during replication, circumventing the need for RNA primers and, thus, solving the end problem in replication. The single-stranded parvovirus genome contains a self-complementary sequence at the 3′ end, which causes the molecule to fold into a hairpin and make it self-priming for DNA replication. The poxviruses contain linear double-stranded genomes in which the ends are continuous. With the parvovirus and poxvirus genomes, the solutions to the end problem create additional problems that must be solved to produce replication products that are identical to the starting genomes.

■ RNA Viruses

Because nuclear functions are primarily designed for DNA metabolism, RNA viruses mostly replicate in the cytoplasm. Moreover, cells do not have RNA polymerases that can copy RNA templates (RNA-based RNA transcription or replication). Therefore, RNA viruses not only need to encode for transcriptases or polymerases (required for transcription), as discussed earlier, but

FIGURE 6–14. **Some solutions to the end problem.** Some of the structural features found in linear viral DNA genomes, including cohesive ends in bacteriophages, protein primers in adenoviruses, hairpin end in parvoviruses, and continuous ends in poxviruses are the solutions to the end problem in DNA replication.

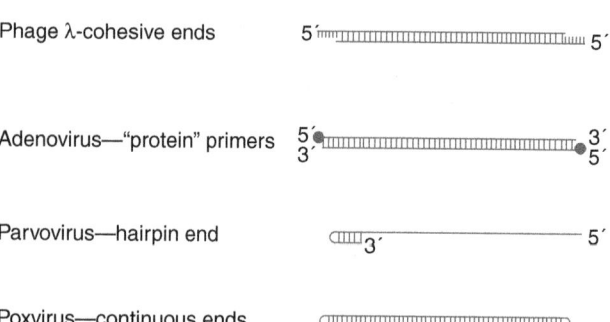

also must provide the replicases or polymerases required to duplicate the RNA genome into daughter RNA genomes. Furthermore, except in the cases of the picornaviruses, in which transcription and replication are synonymous, the RNA viruses must temporally and functionally separate transcription from replication. This requirement is especially apparent for the rhabdoviruses, paramyxoviruses, togaviruses, and coronaviruses, in which a complete genome, or complementary copy of the genome, is transcribed into a set of small monocistronic mRNAs early in infection. After replication begins, these same templates are used to synthesize full-length strands for replication.

RNA viruses must encode their own polymerases (transcriptase and replicase)

Two mechanisms exist to separate the process of transcription from replication. First, in some cases, transcription is restricted to subviral particles and involves a transcriptase transported into the cell within the virion. Second, in other cases, the replication process either involves a functionally distinct RNA polymerase or depends on the presence of some other viral-specific accessory protein that directs the synthesis of full-length copies of the template rather than the shorter monocistronic mRNAs. In reoviruses, the switch from transcription to replication appears to involve the synthesis of a replicase that converts the (+) mRNAs synthesized early in infection to the double-stranded genome segments.

Transcription and replication must be separated for most RNA viruses

Viral RNA polymerases, similar to DNA polymerases, synthesize chains in only one direction; however, in general, RNA polymerases can initiate the synthesis of new chains without primers. Thus, there is no obvious end problem in RNA replication. There is one exception to this general rule. The picornaviruses contain a protein that is covalently attached to the 5′ end of the genome, called **VPg.** This protein is present on the viral RNA because it is involved in the priming of new RNA viral genomes during the infection, similar to the process described earlier for adenoviruses.

Picornaviruses use a protein to prime RNA synthesis

ASSEMBLY OF NAKED CAPSID VIRUSES AND NUCLEOCAPSIDS

The process of enclosing the viral genome in a protein capsid is called assembly or **encapsidation.** Four general principles govern the construction of capsids and nucleocapsids. First, the process generally involves self-assembly of the component parts. Second, assembly is stepwise and ordered. Third, individual protein structural subunits or protomers are usually preformed into capsomeres in preparation for the final assembly process. Fourth, assembly often initiates at a particular locus on the genome called a **packaging site.**

Capsids and nucleocapsids self-assemble from preformed capsomeres

■ Viruses with Helical Symmetry

The assembly of the helical or cylindrically nucleocapsids has been extensively studied in the TMV. In helical symmetry, doughnut-shaped disks containing a number of individual structural subunits are preformed and added stepwise to the growing structure. Elongation occurs in both directions from a specific packaging site on the single-stranded viral RNA. The addition of each disk involves an interaction between the protein subunits of the disk and the genome RNA. The nature of this interaction is such that the assembly process ceases when the ends of the RNA are reached. The structural subunits as well as the RNA trace out a helical path in the final virus particle. The individual protein subunits are intimately associated with the RNA and that the nucleoprotein complexes are assembled by the stepwise addition of protein subunits or complexes of subunits.

Helical nucleocapsids are assembled by adding protein subunits to the RNA genome to form a helix

For influenza and other helical viruses with segmented genomes, the various genome segments are assembled into nucleocapsids independently and then brought together during virion assembly by a mechanism that is as yet poorly understood. It is notable that virtually all of the human RNA viruses with helical symmetry are enveloped.

■ Viruses with Icosahedral or Cubic Symmetry

For both human viruses and bacteriophages, icosahedral capsids are generally preassembled and the nucleic acid genomes, usually complexed with condensing proteins, are threaded into the empty structures. Construction of the hollow capsids appears to occur by a self-assembly process, sometimes aided by other proteins. The stepwise assembly of components involves the initial aggregation of structural subunits into pentamers and hexamers, followed by the condensation of these capsomeres to form the empty capsid. In some cases, it appears that a small complex of capsid proteins associates specifically with the viral genome and nucleates the assembly of the complete capsid around the genome.

Icosahedral capsids are preassembled and the genomes are complexed with condensing proteins

RELEASE OF VIRUS PARTICLES

■ Bacteriophages

Phages encode lysozyme or peptidases that lyse bacterial cell walls

Most bacteriophages escape from the infected bacterial cell by coding for one or more enzymes synthesized late in the latent phase, which causes the lysis of the cell. The enzymes are either lysozymes or peptidases that weaken the cell wall by cleaving specific bonds in the peptidoglycan layer. The damaged cells burst as a result of osmotic pressure.

● HUMAN VIRUSES

CELL DEATH

Naked capsid viruses are released with cell death

Some viruses block or delay apoptosis for virus replication cycle completion

Nearly all productively infected cells die (see further for exceptions), presumably because the viral genetic program is dominant and precludes the continuation of normal cell functions required for survival. In many cases, direct viral interference with normal cellular metabolic processes leads to cell death. For example, picornaviruses shut off host protein synthesis soon after infection, and many DNA human viruses interfere with normal cell-cycle controls. In many cases, the end result of such insults is a triggering of a cellular stress response called programmed cell death or **apoptosis.** Some viruses are known to code for proteins that block or delay apoptosis, probably to stave off cell death until the virus replication cycle has been completed. Ultimately, the cell lysis that accompanies cell death is responsible for the release of naked capsid viruses into the environment.

BUDDING

Most enveloped viruses acquire an envelope during release by budding

Poxviruses acquire membrane from the Golgi apparatus

Most enveloped human viruses acquire their membrane by budding either through the plasma membrane or, in the case of herpesviruses, through the nuclear membrane; however, in some other viruses such as coronaviruses and poxviruses, budding occurs through cytoplasmic membranes. Thus, for these viruses, release from the cell is coupled to the final stage of virion assembly. The herpesviruses ultimately escape from the cell when the membrane of the exocytic vesicle fuses with the plasma membrane. The poxviruses appear to program the formation of membrane structures and acquire membrane from Golgi apparatus that is lost upon the release of extracellular enveloped virions.

The membrane changes that accompany budding appear to be just the reverse of the entry process described before for those viruses that enter by direct fusion (compare Figure 6–9 and **Figure 6–15**). The region of the cellular membrane where budding is to occur acquires a cluster

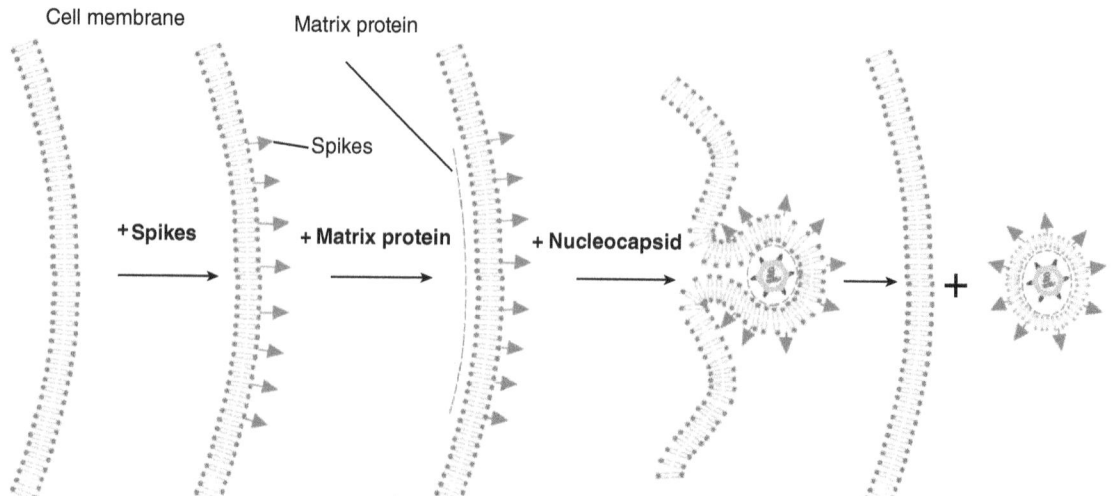

FIGURE 6–15. Viral release by budding. Human enveloped viruses acquire lipid bilayer membrane by budding generally from the plasma membrane. Viral spikes are expressed on the cell surface followed by synthesis of matrix protein that associates near the plasma membrane where viral spikes are present. The matrix protein attracts the assembled nucleocapsid (genome + nucleoprotein) near the plasma membrane expressing viral spikes followed by envelope membrane wrapping and release of the virus particle.

of viral glycoprotein spikes. These proteins are synthesized by the pathway that normally delivers cellular membrane proteins to the surface of the cell by way of the Golgi apparatus. At the site of the glycoprotein cluster, the inside of the membrane becomes coated with a virion structural protein called the **matrix** or **M protein.** The accumulation of the matrix protein at the proper location is probably facilitated by the presence of a binding site for the matrix protein on the cytoplasmic side of the transmembrane glycoprotein spike. The matrix protein attracts the completed nucleocapsid that triggers the envelopment process leading to the release of the completed particle to the outside (Figure 6–15).

> The membrane site for budding first acquires viral spikes and then matrix that attracts nucleocapsids

For viruses that bud, it is important to note that the plasma membrane of the infected cell contains virus-specific glycoproteins that represent foreign (viral) antigens. This means that infected cells become targets for the immune system. In fact, cytotoxic T lymphocytes that recognize these antigens can be a significant factor in combating a virus infection.

The process of initial viral budding usually does not lead directly to cell death because the plasma membrane can be repaired after budding. It is likely that cell death for most enveloped viruses, as for naked capsid viruses, is related to the loss of normal cellular functions required for survival or as a result of apoptosis. Unlike most retroviruses that do not kill the host cell, HIV-1 is cytopathic. Although the mechanism of HIV-1 cell killing is not entirely understood, factors such as the accumulation of viral DNA in the cytoplasm, the toxic effects of certain viral proteins, alterations in plasma membrane permeability, apoptosis, and cell–cell fusion are believed to contribute to the cytopathic potential of the virus.

> The initial budding rarely causes cell death but many daughter viruses released result in loss of cell membrane permeability
>
> Most retroviruses (except HIV) reproduce without cell death
>
> HIV causes cytopathic effects (cell death)

CELL SURVIVAL

For retroviruses (except HIV-1 and other lentiviruses) and the filamentous bacteriophages, virus reproduction and cell survival are compatible. Retroviruses convert their RNA genome into double-stranded DNA, which integrates into a host cell chromosome and is transcribed just like any other cellular gene (see Chapter 18). Thus, the impact on cellular metabolism is minimal. Moreover, these retroviruses bud through the plasma membrane without any permanent damage to the cell (except HIV). How the cell escapes permanent damage in this case is unknown. As with the retroviruses, the infected cell continues to produce virus indefinitely.

QUANTITATION OF VIRUSES

■ Hemagglutination Assay

For some human viruses such as influenza viruses, red blood cells from one or more human species contain receptors for the virion attachment proteins. Because the receptors and attachment proteins are present in multiple copies on the cells and virions, respectively, an excess of virus particles coats the cells and causes them to aggregate. This aggregation phenomenon was first discovered with influenza virus and is called **hemagglutination.** The virion attachment protein on the influenza virion is appropriately called the **hemagglutinin.** Furthermore, the presence of the hemagglutinin in the plasma membrane of the infected cell means that the cells as well as the virions bind the red blood cells. This reaction, called **hemadsorption,** is a useful indicator of infection by certain viruses.

> Virion and infected cell–attachment proteins also bind red blood cells

Hemagglutination can be used to estimate the titer of virus particles in a virus-containing sample. Serially diluted samples of the virus preparation are mixed with a constant amount of red blood cells, and the mixture is allowed to settle in a test tube. Agglutinated red blood cells settle to the bottom to form a thin, dispersed layer. If there is insufficient virus to agglutinate the red blood cells, they will settle to the bottom of the tube and form a tight pellet. The difference is easily scored visually, and the endpoint of the agglutination is used as a relative measure of the virus concentration in the sample. Furthermore, hemagglutination can be inhibited by virus attachment protein-specific antibodies known as hemagglutination inhibition (HI), which can be used to determine titer of the antibody.

■ Plaque Assay

The plaque assay is a method for determining the titer of infectious virions in a virus preparation or lysate. The sample is diluted serially, and an aliquot of each dilution is added to a vast excess of susceptible host cells. For a human virus, the host cells are usually attached to the bottom of a plastic Petri dish; for bacterial cells, adsorption is typically carried out in a cell suspension. In both

FIGURE 6–16. **Plaque assays.** **A.** Bacteriophage λ. **B.** Adenovirus. Plaque assays are used to determine the titer of infectious virus particles. Virus sample is diluted and mixed with appropriate cells and over-layered onto a soft agar plate. Virus release from the infected cells generates a clearing area called a plaque. The number of plaques is directly proportional to the amount of virus in the sample.

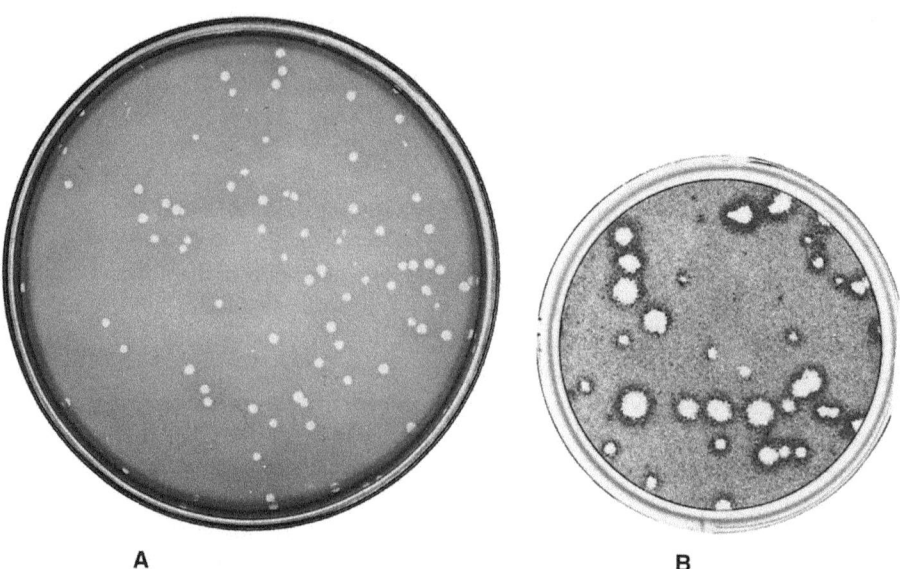

A   B

Plaque assay: Dilutions of virus are added to excess cells immobilized in agar

Replicated virus infects only neighboring cells, producing countable plaques

cases, the cells are then immersed in a semisolid medium such as agar, which prevents the released virions from spreading throughout the entire cell population. Thus, the virus released from the initial and subsequent rounds of infection can invade only the cells in the immediate vicinity of the initially infected cell on the plate. The end result is an easily visible clearing of dead cells at each of the sites on the plate where one of the originally infected cells was located. The clearing is called a **plaque** (**Figure 6–16**). Visualization in the case of human cells usually requires staining the cells. By counting the number of plaques and correcting for the dilution factor, the virus titer in the original sample can be calculated. The titer is usually expressed as the number of plaque-forming units per milliliter (pfu/mL).

■ Immunologic Assay

Using antigen–antibody specificity, viral antigens can be quantified by ELISA

EIA or ELISA can be used to detect antibodies produced during infection

Viral antigen can be quantified by using antigen–antibody specificity, as measured by enzyme immunoassay (EIA), enzyme-linked immunosorbent assay (ELISA), and immunofluorescence assay (IFA). Similar to other assays, in immunologic assays the antigen–antibody specificity and conditions should be worked out. For most viruses, commercial antibodies are available and can be used to detect or quantify the antigen of viruses in culture and body fluids, tissue biopsies, serum, plasma, and cerebrospinal fluid (CSF). The most common example is the detection and sometimes quantification of RSV by IFA in which RSV antigens can be measured in nasopharyngeal and throat washing, sputum, or bronchoalveolar lavage. In addition, viral antigens can be detected and quantified in blood (plasma or serum), which can then provide information on the amount of virus present in the blood. For example, HIV can be quantified by the levels of p24 (capsid) antigen in the culture fluid or blood. On the other hand, these immunoassays can also be used to detect antibodies produced during infection and are very powerful tools to diagnose infection. In this scenario, commercial antigens-coated plates are available that can be used to detect antibodies in patients' samples for diagnosis of infection and monitoring the effectiveness of vaccines.

■ Molecular Assay

DNA and RNA genomes of viruses can be quantified by PCR

Viral genomes, both RNA and DNA, can be quantified to determine the amount of virus (viral load) in blood (serum or plasma) or any given samples. The RNA genomes of the viruses are first reversely transcribed to cDNA by reverse transcriptase enzyme and then amplified by polymerase chain reaction (PCR) referred as RT-PCR. However, viral DNA genomes can be directly amplified by PCR to quantify the viral genomes. On the basis of the number of copies of the viral genomes, the amount of virus in any sample can be determined. This is the most sensitive and specific method to detect and quantify viral genomes. PCR is routinely used to determine viral load in HIV, hepatitis C virus, and other viral and microbial infections.

VIRAL GENETICS

Viruses generally use two mechanisms—mutation and recombination—by which viral genomes change during infection and there are virologic, immunologic, and clinical consequences of some of these changes. Typically, the majority of the virus particles derived from a cell infected with a human virus are noninfectious in other cells as determined by a plaque assay. Although some of this discrepancy may be attributable to inefficiencies in the assay procedures, it is clear that many defective particles are being produced. In part, this production of defective particles arises because the mutation rates for human viruses are unusually high and many infections occur at high multiplicities, where defective genomes are complemented by nondefective or normal (wild-type) viruses and therefore propagated.

Majority of the human virus particles from an infected cell are defective

■ Mutation

Many DNA viruses use the host DNA synthesis machinery for replicating their genomes. Therefore, they benefit from the built-in proofreading and other error-correcting mechanisms used by the host cell. However, the large human viruses (adenoviruses, herpesviruses, and poxviruses) code for their own DNA polymerases, and these enzymes are not as effective at proofreading as the cellular polymerases. The resulting higher error rates in DNA replication endow the viruses with the potential for a high rate of mutation, but they are also partially responsible for the high frequency of defective viral particles.

The replication of RNA viruses is characterized by even higher error rates of mutation because viral RNA polymerases do not possess any proofreading capabilities. The result is that error rates for RNA viruses commonly approach one mistake for every 2500 to 10,000 nucleotides polymerized. Such a high misincorporation rate means that, even for the smallest RNA viruses, virtually every round of replication introduces one or more nucleotide changes somewhere in the genome. If it is assumed that errors are introduced at random, most of the members of a clone (eg, in a plaque) are genetically different from all other members of the clone. The resulting mixture of different genome sequences for a particular RNA virus has been referred to as quasispecies to emphasize that the level of genetic variation is much greater than what normally exists in a species.

Because of the redundancy in the genetic code, some mutations are silent and are not reflected in changes at the protein level, but many occur in essential genes and contribute to the large number of defective particles found for RNA human viruses. The concept of genetic stability takes on a new meaning in view of these considerations, and the RNA virus population as a whole maintains some degree of homogeneity only because of the high degree of fitness exhibited by a subset of the possible genome sequences. Thus, strong selective forces continually operate on a population to eliminate most mutants that fail to compete with the few very successful members of the population. However, any time the environment changes (eg, with the appearance of neutralizing antibodies), a new subset of the population is selected and maintained as long as the selective forces remain constant.

High error rates for RNA viruses produce genetically heterogeneous populations

The high mutation rates found for RNA viruses endow them with a genetic plasticity that leads readily to the occurrence of genetic variants and permits rapid adaptation to new environmental conditions. The large number of serotypes of rhinoviruses causing the common cold, for instance, likely reflects the potential to vary by mutation. Although rapid genetic change occurs for most if not all viruses, no medically important RNA virus has exhibited this phenomenon as conspicuously as influenza virus. Point mutations accumulate in the influenza genes coding for the two envelope proteins (hemagglutinin and neuraminidase), resulting in changes in the antigenic structure of the virions. These changes lead to new variants not recognized by the immune system of previously infected individuals. This phenomenon is called **antigenic drift** (see Chapter 9). **Figure 6–17** shows the effect of mutations resulting in antigenic drift. Apparently, the domains of the two envelope proteins that are most important for immune recognition are not essential for virus entry and, as a result, can tolerate amino acid changes leading to antigenic variation. This feature may distinguish influenza from other human RNA viruses that possess the same high mutation rates, but do not exhibit such high rates of antigenic drift. Antigenic drift in epidemic influenza viruses from year to year requires continual updating of the strains used to produce annual influenza vaccines.

High mutation rates permit adaptation to changed conditions

Mutations or antigenic drift in influenza viruses allow escape from preexisting immunity

Antigenic drift requires updating or changing influenza strains for annual vaccination

The retroviruses likewise show high rates of variation because of error-prone reverse transcriptase enzyme that converts retroviral RNA into double-stranded DNA. For example, error

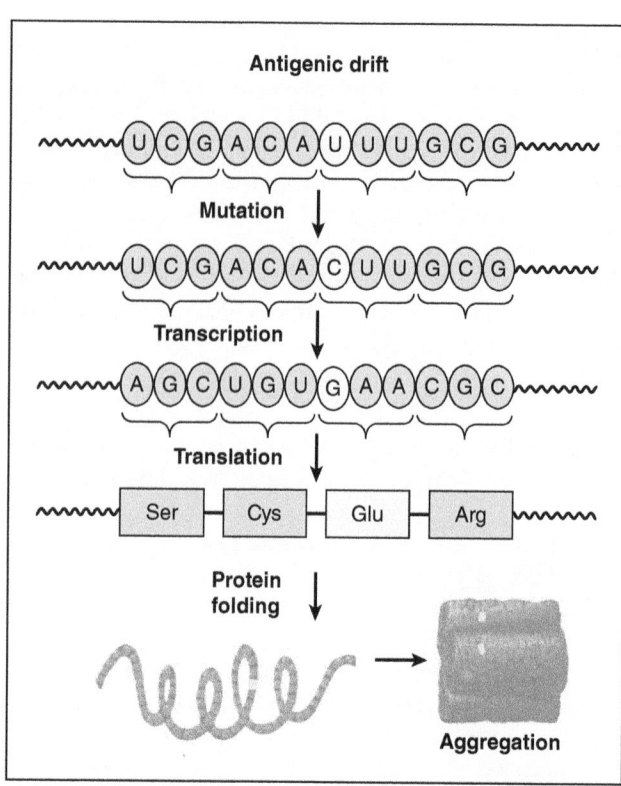

FIGURE 6–17. **Point mutation resulting in antigenic drift.** Point mutations occur in most RNA viruses and some DNA viruses because of errors caused by viral RNA or DNA polymerases due to lack of proofreading ability of the enzymes. Accumulation of point mutations in the viral genome may result in change of amino acids resulting in antigenic variation, which may allow the new viral variants to escape preexisting immunity.

High rates of mutation in retroviruses are due to error-prone reverse transcriptase

rate for HIV-1 reverse transcriptase is approximately four to five errors per reverse transcription of the genome. After the viral DNA has integrated into the chromosome of the host cell, the retroviral DNA is transcribed by the host RNA polymerase II, which is also capable of generating errors. Accordingly, HIV-1 exhibits a high rate of mutation, and this property gives HIV-1 the ability to evolve rapidly in response to changing conditions in the infected host. Genetic variation has resulted in several clades or subtypes of HIV-1 worldwide.

HIV-1 antigenic variation makes vaccine development difficult

Retroviruses that exhibit high rates of antigenic variation such as HIV-1 pose particularly difficult problems for the development of effective vaccines. Attempts are being made to identify conserved and, therefore, presumably essential domains of the envelope proteins for these viruses, which might be useful in developing a genetically engineered vaccine.

■ von Magnus Phenomenon and Defective Interfering Particles

In early studies with influenza virus, it was noted that serial passage of virus stocks at high multiplicities of infection led to a steady decline of infectious titer with each passage. At the same time, the titer of noninfectious particles increased. As discussed later, the noninfectious genomes interfere with the replication of the infectious virus and so are called **defective interfering (DI) particles.** Later, these observations were extended to include virtually all RNA and DNA human viruses. The phenomenon is now named after von Magnus, who described the initial observations with the influenza virus.

Defective interfering particles accumulate at high multiplicities of infection

A combination of two separate events leads to **von Magnus phenomenon.** First, deletion mutations occur at a significant frequency for all viruses. For DNA viruses, the mechanisms are not well understood, but deletions presumably occur as a result of mistakes in replication or by nonhomologous recombination. The basis for the occurrence of deletions in RNA viruses is better understood. All RNA polymerases (replicases) have a tendency to dissociate from the template RNA, but remain bound to the end of the growing RNA chain. By reassociating with the same or a different template at a different location, the replicase "finishes" replication, but, in the process, creates a shorter or longer RNA molecule. A subset of these variants possesses the proper signals for initiating RNA synthesis and continues replicating. Because the deletion variants in the population require less time to complete a replication cycle, they eventually predominate and constitute the DI particles.

Deletions result from mistakes in replication, recombination, or the dissociation–reassociation of polymerases

Second, as their name implies, the DI particles interfere with the replication of nondefective or normal (wild-type) particles. Interference occurs because the DI particles successfully compete with the nondefective genomes for a limited supply of replication enzymes. The virions released at the end of the infection are therefore enriched for the DI particles. With each successive infection, the DI particles can predominate over the normal particles as long as the multiplicity of infection is high enough that every cell is infected with at least one normal infectious particle. If this condition is satisfied, then the normal virus particle can complement any defects in the DI particles and provide all of the viral proteins required for the infection. This process is called **complementation.** Eventually, however, as serial passage is continued, the multiplicity of infectious particles drops below one, and the majority of the cells are infected only with DI particles. When this happens, the proportion of DI particles in the progeny virus decreases.

Defective interfering particles compete with infectious particles for replication enzymes

■ Recombination

Besides mutation, genetic recombination between related viruses is a major source of genomic variation. Bacterial cells as well as the nuclei of human cells contain the enzymes necessary for homologous recombination of DNA. Thus, it is not surprising that recombinants arise from mixed infections involving two different strains of the same type of DNA virus. The larger bacteriophages such as λ and T4 code for their own recombination enzymes, a fact that attests to the importance of recombination in the life cycles and possibly the evolution of these viruses. The fact that recombination has also been observed for cytoplasmic poxviruses suggests that they too code for their own recombination enzymes.

Homologous recombination is common in DNA viruses

As far as is known, cells do not possess the machinery to recombine RNA molecules. However, recombination among at least some RNA viruses has been observed by two different mechanisms. The first, which is unique to the viruses with segmented genomes (orthomyxoviruses and reoviruses), involves reassortment of segments during a mixed infection involving two different viral strains. Recombinant progeny viruses that differ from either parent can be accounted for by the formation of new combinations of the genomic segments that are free to mix with each other at some time during the infection. Reassortment of this type occurring during infections of the same cell by human and certain animal influenza viruses is believed to account for the occasional drastic change in the antigenicity of the human influenza A virus. These dramatic changes, called **antigenic shifts (Figure 6–18)**, produce strains to which much of the human population lacks immunity and, thus, can have enormous epidemiologic and clinical consequences (see Chapter 9).

Recombination for viruses with segmented RNA genomes involves reassortment of segments

Segment reassortment in mixed infections accounts for antigenic shifts in influenza virus

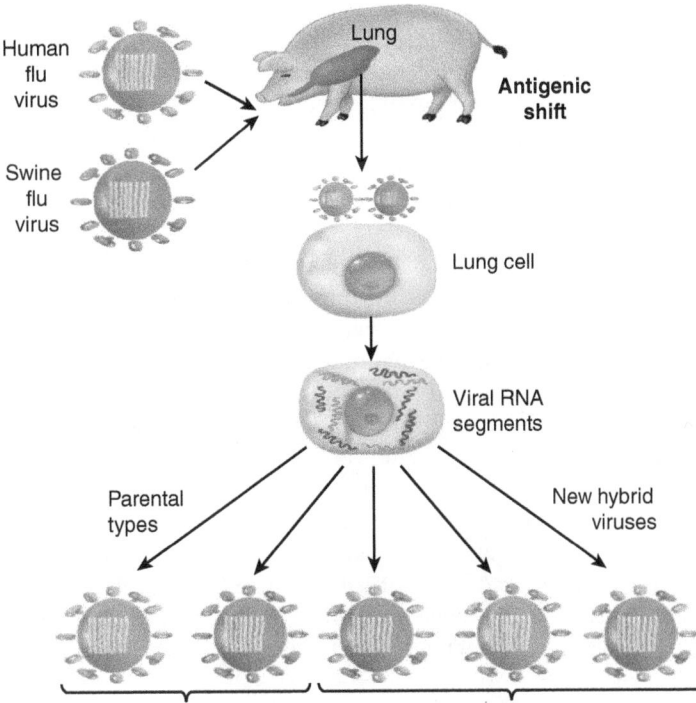

FIGURE 6–18. **Reassortment of influenza virus strains (antigenic shift) resulting in new strains.** Reassortment occurs when two closely related segmented viruses infect the same cell, resulting in drastic antigenic changes and formation of new viral strains. In this example, human influenza virus and swine influenza virus infect the lung cell of swine. Following replication of viral RNA segments of both viruses in the same cells, progeny viruses are assembled because of reassortment of newly synthesized RNA segments that may come from both viruses. Reassortment of newly synthesized RNA segments generates parental types, new hybrid viruses, and hundreds of other possible combinations. Some of these hybrid viruses could become new strains causing severe epidemics or pandemic influenza.

The second mechanism of RNA virus recombination is exemplified by the genetic recombination between different forms of poliovirus. Because the poliovirus RNA genome is not segmented, reassortment cannot be invoked as the basis for the observed recombinants. In this case, it appears that recombination occurs during replication by a "copy choice" type of mechanism. During RNA synthesis, the replicase (polymerase) dissociates from one template and resumes copying a second template at the exact place where it left off on the first. The end result is a progeny RNA genome containing information from two different input RNA molecules. Strand switching during replication, therefore, generates a recombinant virus. Although this is not frequently observed, it is likely that most of the RNA human viruses are capable of this type of recombination.

A "copy choice" mechanism has also been invoked to explain a high rate of recombination observed with retroviruses. Early after infection, the reverse transcriptase within the virion synthesizes a DNA copy of the RNA genome by a process called reverse transcription. In the course of reverse transcription, the enzyme is required to "jump" between two sites on the RNA genome (see Chapter 18). This propensity to switch templates apparently explains how the enzyme generates recombinant viruses. Because reverse transcription takes place in subviral particles, free mixing of RNA templates brought into the cell in different virus particles is not permitted. However, retroviruses are diploid, because each particle carries two copies of the genome. This arrangement appears to be a situation readymade for template switching during DNA synthesis, and most likely accounts for retroviral recombination.

Occasionally, animal retroviruses package a cellular mRNA into the virion rather than a second RNA genome. This arrangement can lead to copy choice recombination between the viral genome and a cellular mRNA. The end result is, sometimes, the incorporation of a cellular gene into the viral genome. This mechanism is believed to account for the production of highly oncogenic retroviruses containing modified cellular genes (see later).

■ Phenotype Mixing

Mixing of two closely related viruses, A and B, may result in generation of a hybrid virus with genome of virus A and outer surface protein of B. Upon infection of the new appropriate cells, the surface protein determines the tropism (means binds to the receptor on the host cells). However, the progeny viruses produced from this hybrid virus will be of type A virus because the genome in this hybrid virus belonged to type A virus.

THE LATENT STATE

Temperate viruses, which can establish both productive and nonproductive responses, can infect a cell and enter a latent state that is characterized by little or no virus production. The viral DNA genome is replicated and segregated along with the cellular DNA when the cell divides. There exist two possible states for the latent viral genome. It can exist extrachromosomally (herpesviruses) like a bacterial plasmid, or it can become integrated into the chromosome (retroviruses) like the bacterial F factor in the formation of a high-frequency recombination (HFR) strain (see Chapter 21). Because the latent genome is usually capable of reactivation and entry into the lytic cycle, it is called a **provirus** or, in the case of bacteriophages, a **prophage.** In many cases, viral latency goes undetected; however, limited expression of proviral genes can occasionally endow the cell with a new set of properties. For example, the latent herpes simplex virus infection is characterized by the presence of viral DNA (extrachromosomal) in the nerve ganglion without any production of infectious virus particles as well as no symptoms (clinical latency) in infected individuals. However, this latent state can be reactivated characterized by the presence of infectious virus particles and symptoms. For instance, lysogeny (latent state) can lead to the production of virulence-determining toxins in some bacteria (lysogenic conversion—details in Chapter 21) and latency by a human virus may produce oncogenic transformation.

The significance of lysogeny and lysogenic conversion is described in Chapter 21. Diphtheria, scarlet fever, and botulism all are caused by toxins produced by bacteria that have been "converted" by a temperate bacteriophage. In each case, the gene that codes for the toxin protein resides in the phage DNA and is expressed together with the repressor gene in the lysogenic state.

Poliovirus polymerase switches templates to generate recombinants

The diploid nature of retroviruses permits template switching and recombination during DNA synthesis

Occasional incorporation of host mRNA into retroviral particles may produce oncogenic variants

The latent state involves infection of a cell with little or no virus production

Latent virus may be silent, change cell phenotype, or be induced to enter the lytic cycle

Latent genomes can exist extrachromosomally or can be integrated

Lysogenic conversion results from expression of a prophage gene that alters cell phenotype

Several bacterial exotoxins are encoded in temperate bacteriophages

KEY CONCLUSIONS

- Viruses that have either RNA (RNA viruses) or DNA (DNA viruses) genomes covered with capsid protein are referred as naked capsid viruses.

- Some viruses have lipid bilayer membranes (envelope) external to the capsid protein. These viruses are called enveloped viruses.

- Viral RNA genomes are mainly single-stranded linear (+, –, or +/–), except reoviruses that have double-stranded RNA genomes. Some viruses have segmented RNA genomes. Viral DNA genomes are mainly double stranded, except parvoviruses that have single-stranded DNA genome.

- Viruses are considered intracellular microorganisms or parasites because they replicate inside the host cells using cellular structural components and metabolic functions.

- While many viruses cause acute infection that is cleared by the host immune system, some viruses cause persistent infection, latent or chronic. Latent viral infection can be reactivated periodically, whereas chronic viruses replicate at a low level without causing much damage to the target tissue.

- Capsid or envelop provides protection to viral genome. Nucleoprotein that binds to viral genome aids in condensation of the viral genome.

- Naked capsid viruses have icosahedral symmetry, whereas enveloped viruses have helical or icosahedral symmetry.

- Viral-encoded spikes (proteins or glycoproteins) are present on the outer capsid of naked capsid viruses and on the outer membrane of enveloped viruses that bind to the receptors on host cells for virus entry into the host cells.

- Some enveloped viral membranes fuse with the plasma membrane of the host cells, whereas other enveloped viruses and all naked capsid viruses enter cells via viropexis in which they form endosomal vesicles inside the cells.

- Positive sense RNA viruses immediately translate to produce RNA-dependent RNA polymerase and negative-sense RNA viruses bring viral RNA-dependent RNA polymerase for transcription in the cytoplasm. Exceptions are influenza viruses that replicate in the nucleus to prime the transcription but still use their own viral RNA polymerase and retroviruses following reverse transcription to DNA replicate in the nucleus.

- DNA viruses replicate in the nucleus by using host DNA-dependent RNA polymerase (host RNA polymerase) for transcription and either host (for parvovirus, papillomavirus, polyomavirus) or viral DNA-dependent DNA polymerase for replication. Exception is poxviruses that replicate in the cytoplasm by using their own viral RNA and DNA polymerases.

- Most enveloped viruses are assembled in the cytoplasm via matrix protein bringing the nucleocapsid complex near the plasma membrane and acquiring envelope membrane expressing viral spikes by budding.

- DNA naked capsid viruses are assembled in the nucleus and RNA naked capsid viruses in the cytoplasm and are released upon cell death.

- Infected cells may die because of cytopathic effects as too many daughter viruses are released from the cells.

- Viral-specific enzymes that are not present in the host cells are the ideal targets for antiviral drugs.

- Major genetic changes mechanisms include mutations and recombination or reassortment. Both mechanisms are responsible for allowing the virus to escape preexisting immunity requiring the need for updating strains for annual influenza vaccination and causing persistence viral infection such as HIV.

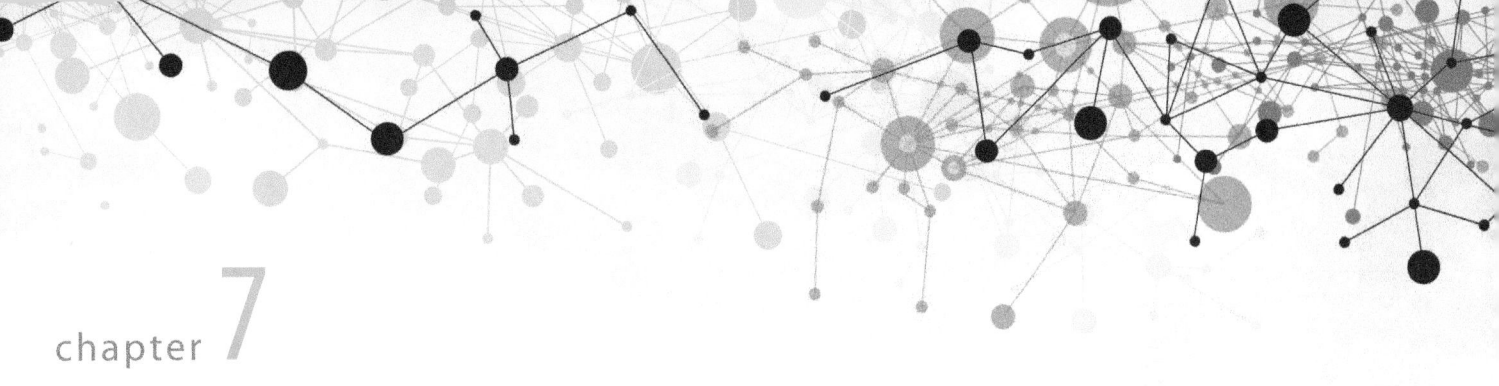

chapter 7

Pathogenesis of Viral Infection

OVERVIEW

Viral pathogenesis involves complex interactions between viruses and hosts comprising of transmission, replication, dissemination, immune response, and pathology to produce disease in humans. Viruses have found several routes to enter and spread in the host, and find a target cell/tissue where they can replicate efficiently, and cause cytopathic effects to damage the tissue. In some cases, the immune system is successful in eliminating the virus, whereas in other cases, viruses avoid elimination by the immune system and persist in the host. While in several cases, the disease is caused by direct viral lysis of the infected cells, in other cases, the disease is immune-mediated such as immune complexes, cytotoxic CD8 T cells, and cytokines. Many DNA viruses and some RNA viruses transform cells causing oncogenesis. Host factors and defenses play important roles in viral pathogenesis. It is interesting to note that the same virus may cause a mild disease in some hosts and a severe disease in other hosts. Innate and adaptive immune responses are critical to eliminate or control viral infections in hosts. Several viral infections cause immune suppression, including a risk of opportunistic and superinfections. Immunocompromised hosts are vulnerable to many viral diseases. Vaccination is the key to provide protection in the population.

Viral pathogenesis is the process by which viruses produce disease in the host. The factors that determine the viral transmission, multiplication, dissemination, and development of disease in the host involve complex and dynamic interactions between the virus and the susceptible host. Viruses cause disease when they breach the host's primary physical and natural protective barriers; evade local, tissue, and immune defenses; spread in the body; and destroy cells either directly or via bystander immune and inflammatory responses. Viral pathogenesis comprises of several stages, including (1) transmission and entry of the virus into the host, (2) spread in the host, (3) tropism, (4) virulence and cytopathogenicity, (5) patterns of viral infection and disease, (6) host factors, (7) host defense, and (8) virus-induced immunopathology. The stages of a typical viral infection and its pathogenesis (eg, poliovirus pathogenesis) are shown in **Figure 7–1.**

Process by which viruses cause disease in the host

Interactions between virus and host result in disease

TRANSMISSION AND ENTRY

Viruses are transmitted via horizontal (common route of transmission: person-to-person) and vertical (mother-to-child transmission) routes or vector transmission (from mosquitoes, animals; **Tables 7–1** and **7–2**). Human viruses cause either systemic or localized infections by entering the host through a variety of routes, including direct inoculation as well as respiratory, conjunctival, gastrointestinal, and genitourinary routes (**Figure 7–2**). In addition, viruses can enter the host through a break in the skin or via mucosal surfaces of various routes, such as respiratory, gastrointestinal, and genitourinary tracts. Mother-to-child transmission (vertical transmission) can occur in utero, during delivery (via birth canal), and through breastfeeding.

Zoonotic (animal-to-human) transmission of viral infections can occur from the bite of animals (eg, rabies) or insects (eg, dengue, yellow fever, West Nile) or from inhalation of animal excreta (eg, hantavirus, arenavirus; Table 7–2). In some cases, avian flu virus (bird flu) can be transmitted from birds or poultry to humans, and swine flu virus can also be transmitted to humans.

Viruses transmitted horizontally (common routes) and vertically (mother to child)

Some transmitted through sexual routes

Some transmitted through mosquito or animal bites

FIGURE 7–1. **Stages of poliovirus pathogenesis.** The diagram illustrates multiple steps of poliovirus pathogenesis, starting from virus entry through oropharynx (fecal–oral transmission), virus multiplication at the site of entry (gut), invasion of the virus to the regional lymph nodes, development of viremia, virus shed in feces, virus crossing the blood–brain barrier, virus replication in anterior horn cells, cell destruction, motor neurons are damaged, and development of paralysis.

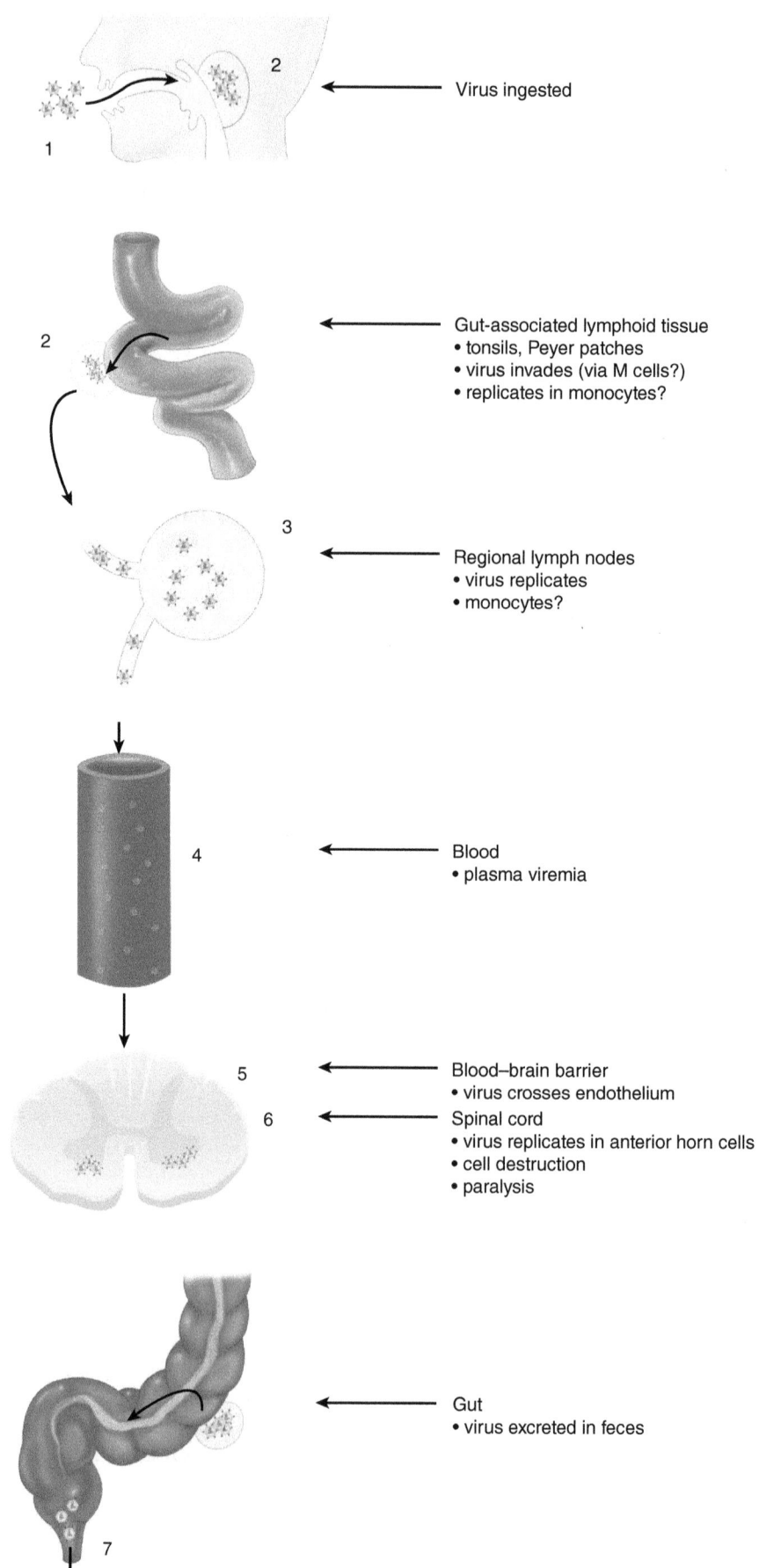

Virus ingested

Gut-associated lymphoid tissue
• tonsils, Peyer patches
• virus invades (via M cells?)
• replicates in monocytes?

Regional lymph nodes
• virus replicates
• monocytes?

Blood
• plasma viremia

Blood–brain barrier
• virus crosses endothelium

Spinal cord
• virus replicates in anterior horn cells
• cell destruction
• paralysis

Gut
• virus excreted in feces

TABLE 7–1   Common Routes of Transmission

ROUTE OF ENTRY	SOURCE/MODE OF TRANSMISSION	EXAMPLES/VIRUSES
Respiratory	Aerosol droplet inhalation	Influenza virus, parainfluenza virus, respiratory syncytial virus, coronavirus, measles, mumps, rubella, varicella-zoster virus, hantavirus
	Nose or mouth → hand or object → nose	Common cold (rhinovirus, coronavirus, adenovirus)
Salivary	Direct salivary transfer (eg, kissing)	Herpes simplex virus (oral-labial herpes), Epstein-Barr virus (infectious mononucleosis), cytomegalovirus
Gastrointestinal	Stool → hand → mouth and/or stool → object → mouth	Enteroviruses, hepatitis A virus, poliovirus, rotavirus
Skin	Skin discharge → air → respiratory tract	Varicella-zoster virus, smallpox virus
	Skin to skin	Human papillomavirus (warts)
	Animal bite to skin	Rabies virus
Blood	Blood products, transfusion, or needle prick	Hepatitis B virus, hepatitis C virus, hepatitis D virus, human immunodeficiency virus (HIV), human T lymphotropic virus, cytomegalovirus
	Insect bite	Arboviruses, dengue virus, yellow fever virus, West Nile virus, encephalitis causing arboviruses
Genital	Genital secretions	Hepatitis B virus, HIV, herpes simplex virus, cytomegalovirus
Urine	Urine	Polyomavirus (BK virus)
Eye	Conjunctival	Adenovirus, cytomegalovirus, herpes simplex virus 1
Zoonotic	Animal bite	Rabies
	Arthropod bite	Arboviruses
	Mammals excreta	Arenavirus, hantavirus, filovirus
	Chicken, wild birds—aerosol droplets	Avian influenza virus (bird flu, H5N1)
	Swine—aerosol droplets	Swine influenza virus (swine flu, H1N1)

After virus entry into the host, viruses have variable incubation periods. **Incubation period** is the time between exposure to the organism and appearance of the first symptoms of the disease. Viruses generally multiply at the site of entry to establish infection in the host. Some of the examples include respiratory viruses multiplying in the upper respiratory tract just after entry; rabies virus multiplying in the muscle cells after animal bite; and West Nile virus multiplying in Langerhans cells of skin after mosquito bite. Some viruses have short incubation periods (influenza—2-4 days), whereas others have long incubation periods (eg, hepatitis B virus—weeks to several months). Incubation periods of common viral infections are shown in

Incubation period is time between exposure and appearance of disease symptoms

Some (influenza, parainfluenza) have short incubation, others (hepatitis B, C) long

TABLE 7–2   Vertical Transmission of Viruses

SOURCE/MODE OF TRANSMISSION	EXAMPLES/VIRUSES
Prepartum or transplacental	Cytomegalovirus, parvovirus B19, rubella virus, HIV
Intrapartum or during delivery/birth	Hepatitis B virus, hepatitis C virus, herpes simplex virus, HIV, human papillomavirus
Postpartum or via breastfeeding	Cytomegalovirus, hepatitis B virus, human T lymphotropic virus, HIV

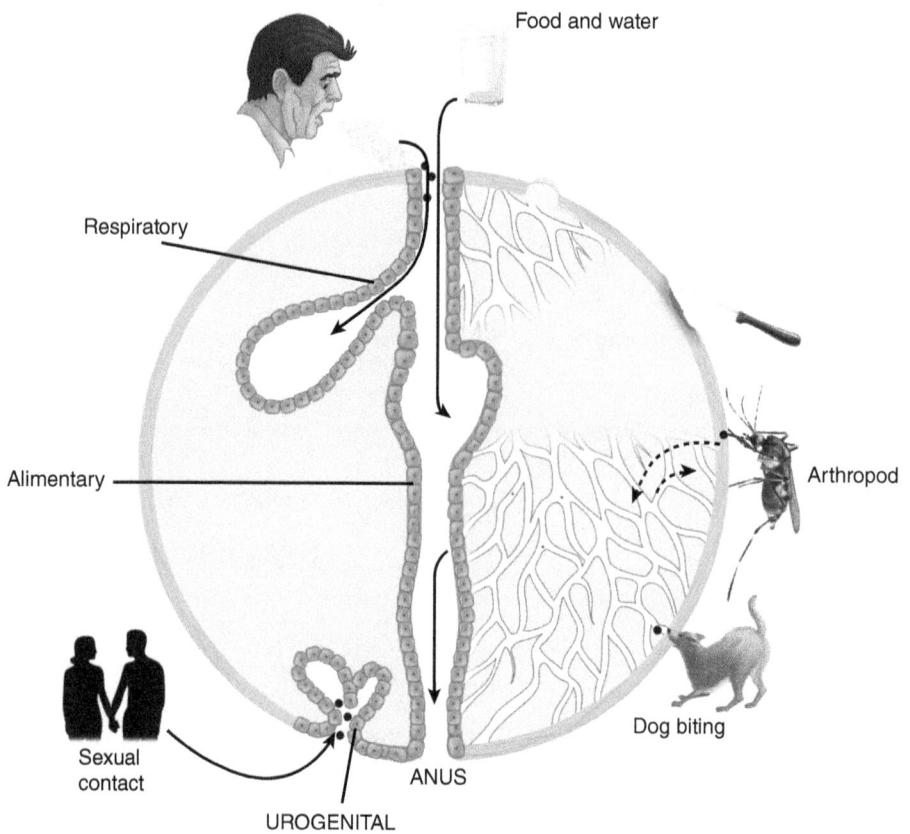

Food and water

Respiratory

Alimentary

Arthropod

Sexual contact

UROGENITAL

ANUS

Dog biting

Table 7-3. **Communicability** of a disease is the ability of the organism to shed in secretions, which may occur early in the incubation period. Some viruses can integrate into the host genome (HIV), survive by slow replication in the presence of an immune response (hepatitis B and C viruses [HBV, HCV]), or stay latent extrachromosomally (herpes simplex virus [HSV]). This dormancy or latency is dangerous because the virus may emerge long after the original infection has occurred and potentially infect others.

SPREAD IN THE HOST

Viral infections produce either **localized infection** at the site of entry or **disseminated infection** spread throughout the body. Localized infections include influenza, parainfluenza, common cold (rhinoviruses, coronaviruses, adenoviruses), gastrointestinal infections (rotaviruses, Norwalk viruses), and skin infections (papillomaviruses). In localized infections, the virus spreads mainly by infecting adjacent or neighboring cells.

Several viruses that cause systemic disease in the host spread from the site of entry to the target tissue, where they cause cell injury after multiplication. Viruses use two major routes to spread and cause systemic infection, that is, hematogenous (via the bloodstream) and neural (via neurons) spread. Some of the viruses that cause systemic or disseminated infection are poliovirus, flavivirus, rabies virus, HBV, HCV, HIV, measles, varicella-zoster virus (VZV), and others. Pathogenesis of poliovirus can be cited as an example of disseminated infection in which poliovirus is transmitted via the fecal–oral route, and the disease (paralytic poliomyelitis) is caused in the central nervous system (CNS; Figure 7–1). Poliovirus replicates at the sites of entry in the small intestine and spreads to the regional lymph nodes where it multiplies again and enters the bloodstream, resulting in **primary viremia.** The virus is spread via the bloodstream to other organs (liver, spleen), where it multiplies and enters the bloodstream causing **secondary viremia** followed by transmission to, and replication in, the CNS and resultant damage to motor neurons. The development of viremia allows the immune system to mount humoral and cell-mediated responses to control the poliovirus infection.

Some of the viruses that are spread by the neural route are HSV, poliovirus, rabies virus, and certain arboviruses, including West Nile virus and St. Louis encephalitis virus. HSV is transmitted

Communicability when infectious agents released in secretions, which may occur during incubation period

Viral infections cause either localized or systemic disease

Poliovirus enters by the fecal–oral route and multiplies in the small intestine, but causes major disease in the central nervous system

Viremia develops when the virus is detected in blood

TABLE 7–3	Incubation Periods of Human Pathogenic Viruses	
VIRUS	**INCUBATION PERIODS**	**DISEASE**
Respiratory viruses		
Influenza virus	~2 (1-4) days	Influenza (flu)
Parainfluenza virus	2-7 days	Laryngitis or croup
Respiratory syncytial virus (RSV)	4-6 days	Bronchiolitis mainly in infants
Rhinovirus	2-3 days	Common cold
Coronavirus 229E, NL63, OC43, HKU1	2-5 (mean 3) days	Common cold
SARS-CoV-1, MERS-CoV, SARS-CoV-2 (COVID-19)	2-14 (mean 5.5) days	SARS, MERS, COVID-19
Adenovirus	5-7 days	Pharyngitis, febrile illness
Childhood exanthems		
Mumps virus	12-29 days (average 16-18)	Parotitis (meningitis, orchitis)
Measles virus	7-18 days (average 9-11 days)	Measles
Rubella virus	14-21 days (average 16)	Rubella
Parvovirus B19	4-12 days	Erythema infectiosum (slapped face)
Poxviruses		
Smallpox virus	12-14 days	Smallpox (variola)
Enteroviruses		
Poliovirus	4-35 days (usually 7-14)	Poliomyelitis
Coxsackievirus	2-10 days	Herpangina, pleurodynia, myocarditis
Echovirus	2-14 days	Meningitis
Enterovirus	6-12 days	Rash, febrile illness
Hepatitis viruses		
Hepatitis A virus	15-45 (mean 25) days	Hepatitis A (acute, self-limiting)
Hepatitis B virus	60-150 (mean 90) days	Hepatitis B (acute, chronic)
Hepatitis C virus	14-182 (mean 14-84) days	Hepatitis C (chronic)
Hepatitis D virus	28-45 days	Delta hepatitis
Hepatitis E virus	15-60 (mean 40) days	Hepatitis E (acute, self-limiting)
Herpesviruses		
Herpes simplex virus 1	7-10 days	Gingivostomatitis
Herpes simplex virus 2, 1	2-12 (average 4) days	Genital herpes
Varicella-zoster virus	11-21 days	Chickenpox (primary), Shingles (reactivation)
Cytomegalovirus (CMV)	3-12 weeks	Heterophile-negative mononucleosis, congenital CMV
Epstein-Barr virus	30-50 days	Infectious mononucleosis (heterophile positive)
Viruses of diarrhea		
Rotavirus	1-3 days	Diarrhea
Calicivirus	0.5-2 days	Diarrhea
Astrovirus	1-2 days	Diarrhea

(continued)

TABLE 7–3	Incubation Periods of Human Pathogenic Viruses (continued)	
VIRUS	**INCUBATION PERIODS**	**DISEASE**
Adenovirus	8-10 days	Diarrhea
Zoonotic viruses		
Rabies virus	10 days to 1 year (average 20-90 days)	Encephalitis
Dengue virus	4-7 days	Hemorrhagic fever or febrile illness
St. Louis encephalitis virus	5-15 days	Encephalitis
Japanese B encephalitis virus	5-15 days	Encephalitis
Yellow Fever virus	3-6 days	Jaundice, shock, hemorrhage
California virus	5-15 days	Encephalitis
Chikungunya virus	2-12 days (average 3-7 days)	Fever, excruciating myalgia, polyarthritis
Hantavirus	7-39 days (average 18 days)	Fulminant respiratory disease, hantavirus pulmonary syndrome
Ebola virus	2-21 days (average 8-10 days)	Hemorrhagic fever
Marburg virus	2-21 days (average 5-10 days)	Hemorrhagic fever
West Nile virus	2-14 days (average 2-6 days)	Muscle weakness, flaccid paralysis, encephalitis, meningoencephalitis, poliomyelitis
Zika virus	3-14 days	Fever, rash, joint pain, muscle pain, headache, conjunctivitis, congenital (microcephaly)
Retroviruses		
HIV-1	2-4 weeks	Acute retroviral syndrome
HIV-1	2-10 years	Chronic, progressive AIDS
Human T-cell lymphotropic virus type I (HTLV-I)	15-20 years	Adult T-cell leukemia and lymphoma (ATLL)
HLTV-II	15-20 years	Hairy T-cell leukemia
Papillomaviruses		
Human papillomavirus (different genotypes)	50-150 days	Common and genital Warts
Polyomaviruses		
JC virus	Long, variable	Progressive multifocal leukoencephalopathy

Some viruses are spread via nerves to the target tissue

through vesicle fluids, saliva, and vaginal secretions and replicated in the mucoepithelial cells, causing primary infection and then traveling via sensory neurons to nerve bundles called ganglia where they establish latent infection. HSV can also travel into the CNS and infect the brain causing herpes encephalitis.

TROPISM

Tropism involves infection of a specific cell type within a tissue or organ

Tropism is governed by interaction of viral surface proteins with cellular receptors

Tropism is the capability of viruses to infect a discrete population of cells within an organ. Cellular or tissue tropism is most often determined by the specific interaction of viral surface proteins (spikes) and cellular receptors on the host cells. Some of the identified cellular receptors for viruses are shown in Table 6–5. However, it should be kept in mind that the presence of a receptor for a virus is not always sufficient for viral infection in the target cells. For example, the presence of CD4 (HIV receptor) alone on target cells does not allow virus entry into these cells, but it requires that target cells also express coreceptors, CXCR4 or CCR5 (chemokine receptors), for efficient viral attachment. Different viruses may use the same cellular molecule as receptors. Some examples are sialic acid residues functioning as important components of the receptor for influenza, corona, and reoviruses. Similarly, heparan sulfate is the receptor for HSV, cytomegalovirus (CMV), and adeno-associated virus (AAV). Conversely, angiotensin-converting enzyme-2 (ACE-2) receptor to which SARS-CoV-2 (COVID-19) binds is expressed on several tissues, including lungs, heart, blood vessels, kidneys, liver, and gastrointestinal tract.

Viruses such as HIV use a receptor (CD4) and coreceptor (CCR5 or CXCR4)

Different viruses may use the same receptor on host cells

Tropism can also be determined by intracellular factors, including host transcription factors and other factors necessary for viral replication. After attachment of viral surface proteins to the cellular receptor, the viral genome-protein complex is released in the cytoplasm followed by transcription, replication, and virus assembly. While enveloped viruses use two mechanisms for entry—fusion and receptor-mediated endocytosis (viropexis), naked capsid viruses use viropexis without membrane–membrane fusion. Influenza virus is tropic to cells that express sialic acid residues containing glycoproteins where the influenza virus attachment protein, hemagglutinin (HA), binds to the receptor, following which the virion is internalized into an endosomal vesicle and the viral envelope membrane fuses with the vesicle's membrane. For other enveloped viruses, such as HIV, viral envelope gp120 binds to the cellular receptor (CD4) and coreceptor (CXCR4 or CCR5) for attachment, and envelope gp41 fuses the viral envelope with the plasma membrane. Naked capsid viruses, such as poliovirus and hepatitis A virus, use outer capsid spikes to begin attachment to the cellular receptor; the virion is internalized and the viral genome is released in the cytoplasm without membrane–membrane fusion.

Enveloped viruses enter cells via viropexis and/or fusion

Naked capsid viruses enter cells via viropexis without fusion

Both RNA and DNA viruses undergo genetic changes, including mutation and recombination (see Chapter 6). Viral tropism can be altered in the case of some viruses because of genetic variation in the viral surface proteins. Avian influenza virus (H5N1) does not bind to the receptor of human influenza virus (H1N1), but mutation or reassortment in H5N1 may allow binding of H5N1 to H1N1 receptor (see Chapter 9). Similarly, genetic changes in the variable region 3 (V3 region) of HIV-1 Env gp120 during infection in patients switch the coreceptor requirement from CCR5 to CXCR4. CCR5 is predominantly expressed on macrophages, Langerhans cells, and mucosal T lymphocytes, whereas CXCR4 is mainly expressed on naïve T lymphocytes (see Chapter 18).

Genetic changes in viral surface proteins may alter viral tropism

Although interaction of the viral surface proteins with the receptors on the host cell plays a critical role in determining tropism, other factors such as viral gene expression, especially in the case of retroviruses, hepatitis B viruses, and papillomaviruses, contribute to tropism. For example, HBV replicates more efficiently in liver cells, and papillomavirus in skin cells, because of regulation of individual viral promoter transcription.

Viral gene expression also contributes to tropism

VIRULENCE AND CYTOPATHOGENICITY

The ability of a virus to cause disease in an infected host is called **pathogenicity.** Virulence is the relative ability of a virus to cause disease. Viral **virulence** is, basically, the degree of pathogenicity of a virus. A virus may be of high or low virulence for a particular host. Different strains of the same virus may differ in the degree of pathogenicity. The ability of a virus to cause degenerative changes in cells or cell death is called **cytopathogenicity.** Viral strains that kill target cells and cause disease are called **virulent viruses,** but other strains that have mutated and lost their ability to cause cytopathic effects (CPE) and disease are termed as **avirulent, nonvirulent,** or **attenuated** strains. Some attenuated strains can be used as live vaccines. Examples of live attenuated vaccines are MMRV (measles, mumps, rubella, varicella), rotavirus, poliovirus (not used in the United States), and yellow fever.

Pathogenicity is the ability of a virus to cause disease in a host

Virulence is the relative ability of a virus to cause disease

Virulence is the degree of pathogenicity between closely related viruses to cause disease

Three major outcomes can be attributed to a viral infection: (1) **abortive infection,** in which no progeny virus particles are produced, but the cell may die because early viral functions can occur; (2) **lytic infection,** in which active virus production is followed by cell death; and (3) **persistent infection,** in which small numbers of virus particles are produced with little or no CPE. Persistent infections include **latent infection,** in which viral genetic material remains in host cell without production of virus and may be activated at a later time to produce virus and/or transform the host cell; **chronic infection,** which involves a low level of virus production with little or no CPE; and **viral transformation,** in which viral infection or viral gene product induces unregulated cellular growth, and cells form tumors in the host. If two closely related viruses infect a host, then infection by the first virus can inhibit the function of the second virus; this is termed **interference.**

Cytopathogenicity is the ability of a virus to cause degenerative changes in cells or cell death

Viruses can cause abortive, lytic, or persistent infections

Persistent infections could be latent or chronic

CPE caused by a virus include morphologic changes of the cell followed by cell death

Virulence and cytopathogenicity depend on the nature of viruses and the characteristics of cells such as permissive and nonpermissive cells. A **permissive cell** permits production of progeny virus particles and/or viral transformation. A **nonpermissive cell** does not allow virus replication, but it may permit transformation of the cell. Replication of the virus results in alterations of cellular morphology and function as well as antigenicity of the virus. When a lytic virus infects a permissive cell, many daughter viruses are produced followed by lysis of the infected cells, called **cytopathic effects** (CPE) of the virus (Figure 4–9). The features of CPE are morphologic changes of the cell organelles, including nucleus (inclusion bodies, thickening of the nucleus, swelling, nucleolar changes, margination of chromatin), cytoplasm (inclusion bodies, vacuoles), and membranes (cells round up, loss of adherence, cell fusion [syncytia]), followed by cellular lysis (disintegration).

Molecular and genetic determinants of viral virulence are located throughout the viral genome

The molecular and genetic determinants of viral virulence are complex. Viral gene products influence pathogenesis and virulence. As previously described, viral surface proteins, both in enveloped and naked capsid viruses, determine tropism and spread, and alterations in these surface proteins may result in change in tropism, spread, and virulence. However, other regions of the viral genome contribute to pathogenicity and virulence. There is no single master gene or protein that determines virulence. For example, live attenuated vaccine of poliovirus, also called oral polio vaccine (OPV), contains all three serotypes of poliovirus that are attenuated and have markedly reduced neurovirulence compared with wild-type polioviruses. The neurovirulence determinants are located in the 5′ untranslated region of the genome involved in initiation of translation and an internal ribosomal entry site, structural capsid proteins (VP1-VP4), and nonstructural proteins, such as viral polymerase.

Viruses such as poxviruses and herpesviruses encode virokines and viroreceptors to help cells proliferate and avoid host defenses, respectively

Some viruses encode a new class of proteins called **virokines** and **viroreceptors,** which contribute to viral virulence by mimicking cellular proteins. It is believed that some large DNA viruses, such as poxviruses and herpesviruses, have acquired these genes by recombination from the cells in which they replicated. Virokines are secreted from infected cells and act as cytokines, helping the cells to proliferate and increase virus production. Viroreceptors resemble cytokine receptors and attract cellular cytokines. In addition, some viruses encode proteins that bind antibodies or components of complement pathways to avoid lysis of virus-infected cells. For example, a member of the poxvirus family, vaccinia virus (strain used in smallpox vaccine), encodes a vaccinia complement control protein (VCP) that abrogates the complement-mediated killing of virus-infected cells. Similarly, two glycoproteins of HSV act together as a receptor for the Fc domain of immunoglobulins to avoid antibody-directed cell-mediated cytotoxicity (ADCC).

PATTERNS OF VIRAL INFECTION AND DISEASE

Infections more common than disease

Infection involves multiplication in the host, disease represents clinical manifestations

Not every viral infection results in a disease. **Infection** involves multiplication of the virus in the host, whereas **disease** represents a clinically **apparent** response. Infections are much more common than disease; **unapparent** infections are termed **subclinical,** and the individual is referred to as a **carrier.** Although some primary infections are invariably accompanied by clinical manifestations of the disease (influenza, measles), other infections may propagate and spread for long periods before the extent of problem is recognized (HIV, HBV, and HCV).

The severity of the disease is influenced by both viral and host factors

Relative susceptibility of a host for a viral infection in terms of severity of the disease depends on several factors such as virulence, molecular and genetic determinants of the virus, and host factors (immune status of the host, age, health, and genetic background). After viral transmission, the virus multiplies in the host; this phase is referred to as the **incubation period,** which varies for different viruses (Table 7–3). Initial virus replication generally results in viremia, which allows the virus to travel to the target tissues and replicate further to cause cell damage and clinical symptoms. The host immune system plays a pivotal role in determining the course of infection and progression of disease.

Viral infections could be lytic, latent, or chronic

Viral infection results in either a lytic or persistent (latent or chronic) infection. **Lytic infections** are those in which productive virus replication results in cell death because viral replication is not compatible with essential cellular functions. Several viruses interfere with the synthesis of cellular macromolecules and other factors that prevent cellular growth, maintenance, and repair, thus leading to cell death. For example, poliovirus blocks the synthesis of cellular proteins by inhibiting the translation of cellular mRNA and competing for ribosomes. Accumulation of progeny viruses and viral proteins can destroy the structure and function, and enhance the process of apoptosis, resulting in cell death. In enveloped viruses, such as respiratory syncytial virus (RSV),

HIV, and HSV, replication of the virus and cell surface expression of the envelope glycoproteins (spikes) cause cell-to-cell spread and formation of multinucleated giant cells (**syncytia**) causing cell death (**cytopathic effect**).

Persistent viral infections are those in which the infected cells survive the effect of viral replication. Persistent infections are of two kinds: latent (viral genome without virus production) and chronic (low level of virus production without immune clearance). In addition, some persistent viruses cause oncogenic transformations. Several DNA viruses have the potential to cause oncogenic transformation; some viruses can cause tumors in their natural hosts (human papillomaviruses, HPV; HBV), whereas others can cause tumors in other species or only transform cells in vitro (human adenoviruses, human polyomaviruses). Some RNA viruses, such as retroviruses (human T lymphotropic virus, HTLV) and HCV, can cause oncogenic transformation in infected hosts. In these human oncogenic viruses, viral gene products transform the cells either by interfering with the tumor suppressor gene pathways (eg, HPV) or increasing the expression of protooncogenes (HTLV).

Based on patterns and levels of detectable infectious virus in the host and the role of immune response in clearing the virus, viral infections can be divided into five categories: (1) acute infection that is cleared by the immune response; (2) acute infection that becomes latent and periodically reactivated; (3) acute infection that becomes chronic; (4) acute infection followed by persistent infection (viral set point) established by immune response and followed by virus overproduction, immune dysfunction, and opportunistic infections; and (5) slow chronic infections. These patterns are shown in **Figure 7–3A-E**. In acute infection, the virus enters the host, then multiplies at the site of entry and in the target tissue, and this is followed by viremia and CPE. This type of infection is a lytic infection. The immune system mounts both cellular and humoral responses and successfully eliminates the virus from the host. Examples of acute viral infections followed by clearance of the virus from the host by immune responses are hepatitis A, influenza, parainfluenza, rhino, and coronaviruses. After causing acute or lytic infection, some viruses are not eliminated by the immune response but persist in the host either in a noninfectious latent form or an infectious chronic form. Most of the viruses opting to persist in the host have evolved various mechanisms for persistence, including restriction of viral CPE, infection of immunologically privileged sites, maintenance of viral genomes without full viral gene expression, antigenic variation, suppression of immune components, and transformation of host cells.

In some viral infections, acute infection may result in either asymptomatic or symptomatic disease followed by latent infection in which the viral genome persists without any infectious virus production. This latent virus could be periodically reactivated, with virus shedding at or near the primary infections along with some symptomatic disease, as seen in HSV infections. In this case, productive (lytic) infection takes place in permissive cells (mucoepithelial cells), whereas latent infection occurs in nonpermissive cells (neurons).

In some persistent infections, acute infection causes initial disease, which is followed by a chronic infection in which a low level of infectious virus is continuously produced with little or no damage to the target tissue. Initially, the immune system controls the infection by bringing the viral load lower than seen in acute infection; however, the immune system is unable to eliminate the infection during the acute phase. During chronicity, the virus is maintained via several mechanisms, such as infection of nonpermissive cells, spread to other cell types, antigenic variation, and inability of the immune response to completely eliminate the virus. Examples of viruses that cause this type of infection are HBV and HCV.

In other persistent infections such as HIV, the acute infection results in high viremia and mono-like illness known as "acute retroviral syndrome" followed by a persistent infection in which the immune responses bring down the high viral load to a "viral set point." The viral set point is maintained because of the robust immune response against the mutating virus for a long time in most infected patients. Because of impairment of the immune system and downregulation of immune components by HIV, the mutating and highly replicating HIV could not be contained by the immune system depletion of CD4+ T lymphocytes, which also offers an opportunity for other pathogens (opportunistic infections) to establish infection and cause full-blown AIDS. These processes and manifestations mainly occur in untreated HIV-infected patients.

Some unconventional infectious agents cause slow, chronic infection without acute infection, such as caused by prions. **Prions** are infectious protein molecules without any genes, causing slow, chronic infection in humans, such as Creutzfeldt-Jacob disease (CJD) and bovine spongiform encephalopathy (BSE, mad cow diseases) (see Chapter 20).

Persistent infection could be either latent or chronic

Some persistent viruses can cause oncogenic transformation

Most infections have acute phase followed by immune clearance or becoming latent or chronic

Acute viral infections that are cleared by the immune system are mainly RNA viruses such as picornaviruses, orthomyxo, and paramyxoviruses

Acute infection caused by herpes simplex virus is followed by a latent infection and periodic reactivation

Acute infection caused by HBV and HCV can be followed by a chronic infection and accumulation of the damage occurs over time

HIV acute infection is followed by a persistent infection leading to impairment of the immune system

Some unconventional infectious agents cause slow, chronic infection without acute symptoms

FIGURE 7-3. **Patterns of viral infection.** In these line diagrams, various patterns of viral infection are shown, including: **A.** Acute viral infection followed by viral clearance by the immune response (eg, Hepatitis A virus, influenza virus, parainfluenza virus, rhinovirus). **B.** Acute viral infection followed by viral latency and periodic reactivation (eg, herpes simplex viruses). **C.** Acute viral infection followed by chronic infection (eg, HBV and HCV). **D.** Acute viral infection followed by persistent infection (viral set point) and clinical latency followed by virus overproduction, immune dysfunction, and opportunistic infections (eg, HIV), and **E.** Slow chronic infections (eg, prions).

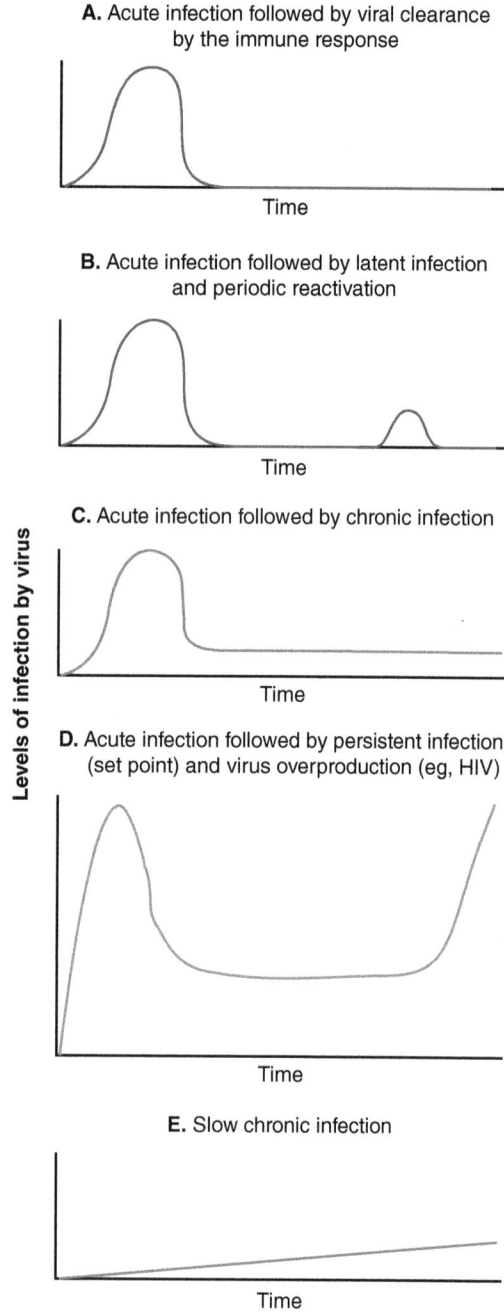

VIRAL TRANSFORMATION

Many DNA and some RNA viruses, especially the retroviruses and HCV, can transform normal cells into abnormal cells called tumors (benign or malignant). This process is called **viral transformation,** and these viruses are referred as **oncogenic viruses.** Viruses that can either cause tumors in their natural hosts or other species or can transform cells in vitro are considered to have oncogenic potential. Specifically, a tumor is an abnormal growth of cells and is classified as **benign or malignant**—depending on whether it remains localized or has a tendency to invade or spread by metastasis. Therefore, malignant cells have at least two defects. They fail to respond to controlling signals that normally limit the growth of nonmalignant cells, and they fail to recognize their neighbors and remain in their proper location.

When grown in tissue culture in the laboratory, these tumor cells exhibit a series of properties that correlate with the uncontrolled growth potential associated with the tumor in the organism. They have altered cell morphology and fail to grow in the organized patterns found for normal

Many DNA, and some RNA, viruses can transform normal cells into tumors cells. In addition, they grow to a much higher cell density than do normal cells under conditions of unlimited nutrients and can lose contact inhibition and the requirement for growth on a solid substrate; therefore, they appear unable to enter the resting G0 state. Furthermore, they have lower nutritional and serum requirements than normal cells and can grow indefinitely in cell culture. These transformed or tumor cells often are used as **cell lines** for the culture or propagation of viruses in the laboratory.

In addition to the listed properties, viral transformation usually, but not always, endows the cells with the capacity to form a tumor when introduced into the appropriate animal. Although the original use of the term **transformation** referred to the changes occurring in cells grown in the laboratory, current usage often includes the initial events in the animal that lead to the development of a tumor. In recent years, it has become increasingly clear that some, but not all, of these viruses cause cancers in the host species from which they were isolated.

> Malignant cells fail to respond to signals controlling the growth and location of normal cells

> Some DNA viruses and some retroviruses can accomplish malignant transformation of cells in culture

■ Transformation by DNA Human Viruses

The oncogenic potential of human DNA viruses is summarized in **Table 7–4.** With the exception of parvoviruses, most DNA virus families have some members capable of causing aberrant cell proliferation under some conditions. For some viruses, transformation or tumor formation has been observed only in species other than their natural host. Apparently, infections of cells from the natural host are so cytocidal that no survivor cells remain to be transformed. In addition, some viruses have been implicated in human tumors without any indication that they can transform cells in culture.

> Some oncogenic viruses cause tumors in species other than their natural hosts

In nearly all cases that have been characterized, viral transformation is the result of the continual expression of one or more viral genes that are directly responsible for the loss of cell growth control. Two targets have been identified that appear to be critical for the transforming potential of these viruses. Adenoviruses, papillomaviruses, and polyomaviruses (simian virus 40) all code for either one or two proteins that interact with the tumor suppressor proteins such as p53 and pRb (for retinoblastoma protein) to block their normal function, which is to exert a tight control over cell-cycle progression. The end result is endless cell cycling and uncontrolled cell growth.

> Many DNA viruses encode proteins that interfere with cell cycle causing uncontrolled growth and transformation

Some viruses integrate into the host chromosome at random sites (with a high efficiency for retroviruses and a very low efficiency for adeno-, polyo-, papillomaviruses), although the DNAs of papillomaviruses and herpesviruses are found in transformed cells as extrachromosomal DNA.

TABLE 7–4	Oncogenicity of DNA and RNA Human Viruses		
VIRUS OR VIRUS GROUP	TUMORS IN NATURAL HOST[a]	TUMORS IN OTHER SPECIES[b]	TRANSFORM CELLS IN TISSUE CULTURE
DNA viruses			
Parvoviruses	No	No	No
Polyomaviruses	No	Yes	Yes
Papillomaviruses	Yes, often benign	?	Yes
Human hepatitis B virus	Yes	?	No
Human adenoviruses	No	Yes	Yes
Human herpesviruses (EBV, HHV-8 or KSHV)	Yes	Yes	Yes
Poxviruses (Molluscum contagiosum)	Occasionally, usually benign	Yes	No
RNA viruses			
Retroviruses	Yes	Yes	Yes
Human T-lymphotropic viruses I and II (HTLV-I and II)			
Hepatitis C virus	Yes	Yes	Yes

[a]"Yes" means that at least one member of the group is oncogenic.
[b]Test usually done in newborns of immunosuppressed hosts.

Unlike retroviruses that code for the enzymes necessary for integration, papillomaviruses, polyomaviruses, and adenoviruses may integrate by nonhomologous recombination using enzymes present in the host cell. In summary, two events appear to be necessary for viral transformation: a persistent association of viral genes with the cell, and the expression of certain viral "transforming" proteins.

■ Transformation by Retroviruses

Two features of the replicative cycle of retroviruses are related to the oncogenic potential of this class of viruses known as oncoretroviruses. First, most retroviruses (exception human immunodeficiency virus, HIV) do not kill the host cell but rather set up a permanent infection with continual virus production. Second, a DNA copy of the RNA genome is maintained in cell via integration into the host cell DNA by a virally encoded integrase (IN).

Retroviruses are known to transform cells by **three** different mechanisms; the first and second mechanisms for animal retrovirus and the third mechanism for human retrovirus (HTLV). **First,** many animal retroviruses have acquired transforming genes called **oncogenes.** These retroviruses require a helper virus as the insertion of the oncogene replaces a viral gene. More than 30 such oncogenes have now been found since the original oncogene was identified in animal Rous sarcoma virus (called v-*src*, where v stands for viral). Because normal cells possess homologs of these genes called **proto-oncogenes** (eg, c-*src*, where c stands for cellular), it is generally thought that viral oncogenes originated from host DNA. It is possible they were picked up by "copy choice" recombination involving packaged cellular mRNAs, as previously described. Because these transforming viruses carry cellular genes, they are sometimes referred to as **transducing retroviruses.** Most of the viral oncogenes have undergone mutations that make them different from the cellular proto-oncogenes. These changes presumably alter the protein products such that they cause transformation. Although the mechanisms of oncogenesis are not completely understood, it appears that transformation results from inappropriate production of an abnormal protein that interferes with normal signaling processes within the cell, causing uncontrolled cell proliferation. Because tumor formation in vitro by retroviruses carrying an oncogene is efficient and rapid, these viruses are often referred to as **acute transforming viruses.** Although common in some animal species, this mechanism has not yet been recognized as a cause of any human cancers.

The second mechanism is called **insertional mutagenesis** and is not dependent on continued production of a viral gene product. Instead, the presence of the viral promoter or enhancer is sufficient to cause the inappropriate expression of a cellular gene residing in the immediate vicinity of the integrated provirus. This mechanism was first recognized in avian B-cell lymphomas caused by an avian leukosis virus, a disease characterized by a very long latent period in birds. Tumor cells from different hosts were found to have a copy of the provirus integrated at the same place in the cellular DNA. The site of the provirus insertion was found to be next to a cellular proto-oncogene called c-*myc*. The *myc* gene had previously been identified as a viral oncogene called v-*myc*. In this case, transformation occurs not because the c-*myc* gene is altered by mutation but because the viral promoter adjacent to the gene turns on its expression continuously and the gene product is overproduced. The disease has a long latent period because, although the birds are viremic from early life, the probability of an integration occurring next to the c-*myc* gene is very low. After such an integration event does occur, however, cell proliferation is rapid and a tumor develops. No human tumors are known to be caused from insertional mutagenesis caused by a retrovirus. However, some human cancers such as Burkitt lymphoma and chronic myelogenous leukemia (CML) are known to occur in which a chromosome translocation has placed an active cellular promoter next to a cellular proto-oncogene. In addition, a few retroviral gene therapy trials were stopped because of the induction of leukemia likely due to retroviral insertion near a proto-oncogene.

The **third** mechanism was revealed by the discovery of the first human retrovirus, human T lymphotropic virus type 1 (HTLV-1), the causative agent of adult T-cell leukemia and lymphoma (ATLL). HTLV-I sequences are found integrated in the DNA of the leukemic cells, and all tumor cells from a particular individual have the proviral DNA in the same location. This observation indicates that the tumor is a clone derived from a single cell; however, the sites of integration in tumors from different individuals are different. Thus, HTLV-I does not cause malignancy by promoter insertion near a particular cellular gene. Instead, HTLV has a regulatory gene called *tax* that encodes for Tax protein that transactivates or upregulate, not only the transcription of its own

Margin notes

In human viruses, viral transforming proteins (oncoproteins) and not integration events are responsible for transformation

Retroviruses produce virions without causing host cell death

DNA copy of retroviral genome integrated, but not at specific site

Animal retroviruses may carry transforming oncogenes

Oncogenes encode a protein that interferes with cell signaling causing transformation in some animal species

Insertional mutagenesis causes inappropriate expression of a proto-oncogene adjacent to integrated retroviral genome in animal retroviruses

Human T-cell leukemia is caused by transactivating factor (Tax) encoded in integrated HTLV

proviral DNA but also the transcription of many cellular genes, including proto-oncogenes. The resulting cellular proteins cooperate to cause uncontrolled cell proliferation. HTLV-I is commonly described as a **transactivating** retrovirus. The same mechanism is also observed in the second human retrovirus, HTLV-II that causes hairy T cell leukemia.

Tax turns on cellular proto-oncogenes, causing cell proliferation

■ Transformation by Other RNA Viruses

HCV causes chronic infection in more than 80% of infected people. The chronicity in HCV infection increases the risk of cirrhosis of liver and hepatocellular carcinoma (HCC). HCC occurs on average approximately 20 to 30 years after chronic infection but alcohol and drug abuse can accelerate this process. It is thought that the constant inflammation and regeneration of hepatocytes leads to the eventual induction of the tumor and is, therefore, considered indirect oncogenesis. However, several studies suggest that HCV nonstructural proteins, NS3 and NS5A, NS5B, and the HCV core protein may be involved in transformation. These HCV proteins interfere with cellular proteins that are responsible for the regulation of cell cycle control.

HOST FACTORS

Viral infection also depends on host factors. Several viral infections have repeatedly shown a variable range of outcomes from asymptomatic to symptomatic infections and even fatal disease in some cases. Furthermore, host factors probably play an important role in reversion of some of the live attenuated vaccines to a virulent state. Several of the host factors, including immune status, genetic background, age, and nutrition, play important roles in determining the outcome of viral infection. Several innate immune responses (interferons α and β, natural killer (NK) cells, mucociliary responses, and others) and adaptive immune responses (antibody and T-cell responses) influence the outcome of viral infections. Individuals with weak immune systems or those who are immunocompromised or immunosuppressed often have more severe outcomes. Details of immune responses to infection are described in Chapter 2.

Host immune status, genetics, age, and nutrition play important roles in viral infections outcome

Host genetics is one of the most important factors that influence the outcome of viral infections. Several host genes, in addition to viral factors, contribute to the variable outcome of HIV infection in infected individuals; some become rapid progressors. The majority are slow progressors. Elevated levels of β-chemokines such as MIP1-α, MIP1-β, RANTES, which are natural ligands of CCR5 (HIV coreceptor), have been found to be associated with decline in the rate of HIV disease progression. These chemokines are also called HIV-suppressive β-chemokines. Genetic resistance to HIV-1 infection was found in individuals expressing a truncated CCR5 coreceptor, CCR5Δ32. Individuals homozygous for the Δ32 allele seem to have normal life expectancy and are strongly protected (not completely) against HIV infection, whereas the heterozygous Δ32 allele slows the cell-to-cell spread of HIV in infected patients. The Δ32 homozygous allele is found in 1% of Caucasians, predominantly in Northern European populations. Furthermore, long-term progressors also have a high frequency of Δ32CCR5 deletion. Although Δ32CCR5 deletion or antagonists of CCR5 provide some protection against HIV infection, it may cause a higher risk of symptomatic West Nile virus infection and a lower likelihood of clearing HCV. In addition, the human leukocyte antigen (HLA) alleles have been associated with slow disease progression or protection against HIV infection.

Elevated levels of chemokines or a Δ32CCR5 allele slow down HIV disease progression

Homozygous Δ32CCR5 allele provides strong protection against HIV infection but increases West Nile virus infection severity and HCV chronicity

Age-related correlation between the host and several viral infections has been observed. Several viruses such as VZV, mumps, polio, and Epstein-Barr virus (EBV) cause less severe infection in infants as compared with teens or adults, whereas others (rotaviruses, RSV) result in severe disease in infants. Although the same strain of HIV infects both mothers (adults) and infants, infants develop symptomatic AIDS faster than adults because HIV replicates more efficiently in infant's mononuclear cells than in adult cells. It appears that age-related increased resistance to viral infections might reflect the maturity of the immune system and other defense mechanisms.

Age of the host plays an important role in the severity of some viral infections

Some cause severe diseases in infants; adults more vulnerable to others

Production of hormones may also influence the outcome of some viral infections. For example, polio, hepatitis A, B, and E, and poxviruses are more severe during pregnancy, suggesting that hormones may influence viral pathogenesis. Polyomaviruses can also be reactivated during pregnancy.

Hormones influence some infections

Nutritional state and personal habits of the hosts can also influence viral pathogenesis. Protein deficiency has been shown to be associated with severity of measles infection, most likely owing to weak cellular immunity. Some personal habits, such as smoking, increase the severity in influenza

Malnutrition, personal habits may increase severity

Fever and inflammation
combat infections

virus infection. In addition, host responses such as fever and inflammation have been suggested to have an important role in combating viral infections.

HOST DEFENSES

The two major types of host defenses are nonspecific (**innate**) and specific (**adaptive**) immune responses. The innate immune response includes interferons (α, β), NK cells, macrophages (phagocytosis), α-defensing, mucociliary clearance, apolipoprotein B RNA editing enzyme (APOBEC3G, an anti-HIV enzyme), and fever among many other factors, whereas the adaptive immune response involves humoral and cell-mediated immunity. Details of specific immune response to infection are described in Chapter 2.

■ Interferons

Interferons are cytokines
produced by virally infected
cells that inhibit virus
production in infected and
other cells

Interferons are not virus-
specific but act on all viruses

Interferons are host-encoded proteins that provide the first line of defense against viral infections. They belong to the class of molecules called **cytokines,** which are proteins or glycoproteins that are involved in cell-to-cell communication. There are three types of interferon, interferon-α (leukocyte), interferon-β (fibroblast), and interferon-γ (lymphocyte). Interferon-α/β are also called Interferon-I and interferon-γ is referred as Interferon-II. Virus infection of all types of cells stimulates the production and secretion of either interferon-α or interferon-β, which acts on other cells to induce what is called the **antiviral state.** Unlike specific immunity, the interferons are not specific to a particular kind of virus; however, interferons usually act only on cells of the same species. Other agents such as antigens and mitogens stimulate the production of interferon-γ by lymphoid cells. In this case, the interferon appears to play an important role in the immune system regardless of any role as an antiviral protein (see Chapter 2).

Interferons produced in
response to accumulation of
double-stranded viral RNA
during viral replication

A major signal that leads to the production of interferon by an infected cell appears to be double-stranded RNA (dsRNA). This conclusion is based on the observation that treatment of cells with purified dsRNA or synthetic double-stranded ribopolymers results in the secretion of interferon. Viral infections, in general, lead to the accumulation of significant levels of dsRNA in the cell. DsRNA is known to activate interferon through the activation of specific receptors called toll-like receptors (TLR) or intracellular receptors called retinoic acid-inducible gene 1 (RigI) like receptors (RLR) or melanoma differentiation-associated gene 5 (*MDA5*)/mitochondrial antiviral signaling protein (MAVS). These receptors via several signaling molecules activate transcription factors interferon regulatory factor 3 (IRF3) and NF-κB leading to interferon production.

Interferon is the first line of
defense against viral infection
by activating two pathways
that degrade mRNA and inhibit
protein synthesis

Changes in the synthesis of many cellular proteins are characteristic of the antiviral state induced by interferon. However, the cells exhibit only minimal changes in their metabolic or growth properties. The machinery to inhibit virus production is mobilized only on infection. Interferon has multiple effects on cells, and three systems have been extensively studied. The first system involves a protein called Mx, which is induced by interferon and specifically blocks influenza infections by interfering with viral transcription. The second system involves the upregulation of protein kinase R (PKR), which is dependent on dsRNA recognition by PKR, which phosphorylates and inactivates one of the subunits of an initiation factor (eIF-2) necessary for protein synthesis. In some cases, viruses have evolved specific mechanisms to block the action of this protein kinase. The third system involves the induction of an enzyme called 2′, 5′-oligoadenylate synthetase, which synthesizes chains of 2′, 5′-oligo (A) up to 10 residues in length. In turn, the 2′, 5′-oligo (A) activates a constitutive ribonuclease, called RNase L, which degrades mRNA. The activities of both protein kinase and 2′, 5′-oligo (A) synthetase require the presence of dsRNA, the intracellular signal that an infection is occurring. This requirement prevents interferons from having an adverse effect on protein synthesis in uninfected cells.

Interferons inhibit viral protein
synthesis by inducing cellular
enzymes that require dsRNA

Interferons inhibit protein
synthesis in infected cells

In the latter two cases, viral infection of a cell that has been exposed to interferon results in a general inhibition of protein synthesis, leading to cell death and no virus production. A cell that was destined to die anyway from a viral infection is sacrificed for the benefit of the entire organism. Virus-induced interferon pathways are shown in **Figure 7–4.** In addition, interferon prepares uninfected cells to fight viral infections. Presence of interferon induces oligosynthetase and protein kinase but does not activate because there is no viral dsRNA in uninfected cells. Thus, interferon kills only infected cells but not uninfected cells.

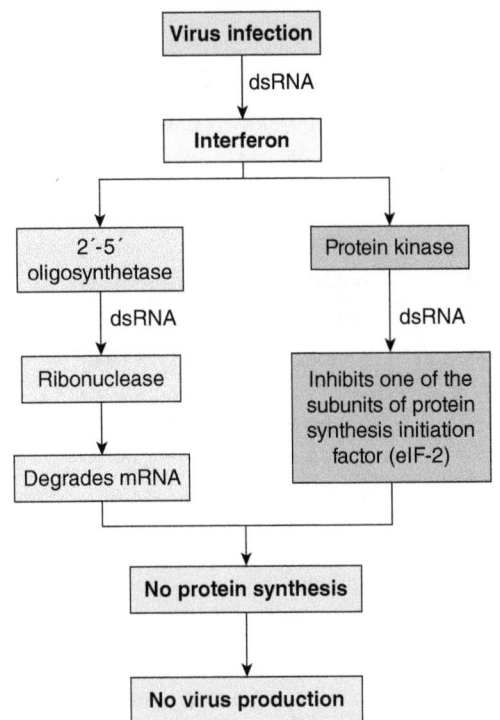

FIGURE 7-4. Virus-induced interferon pathways. Interferons are the first line of defense against viral infections. Interferons are induced after double-stranded viral RNAs are made after viral infection. Interferon activates two pathways; 2'-5' oligosynthetase (left panel) that, in the presence of dsRNA, induces ribonuclease, followed by degradation of RNA and no protein synthesis and virus production. The second pathway is protein kinase (right panel) that, in the presence of dsRNA, inhibits one of the subunits of protein synthesis initiation factor (eIF-2) resulting in no protein synthesis and virus production.

■ Other Host Defenses

NK cells, like interferons, are also not virus-specific but kill virus-infected cells by secreting perforins (pore-forming proteins) and granzymes (serine proteases), which cause apoptosis of infected cells. NK cell–induced killing of infected cells does not require immune components such as antigen, T-cell receptor, or major histocompatibility complex (MHC). NK cells recognize cells lacking class I MHC, which is downregulated by many viruses. Another important cell type that limits virus infection in a nonspecific manner via phagocytosis is the macrophage, especially alveolar macrophages and macrophages of the reticuloendothelial system. Macrophages also secrete interferon-γ upon activation, leading to further inhibition of virally infected cells. Furthermore, other factors show antiviral activity, especially against HIV infection, including α-defensins, APOBEC3G, and BST-2/CD317 (tetherin). α-Defensins are a class of peptides known to have antiviral activity against both enveloped (HSV) and nonenveloped viruses (adenovirus and papillomavirus), and have also been found to interfere with the interaction of HIV-1 Env gp120 with chemokine receptor CXCR4. On the other hand, APOBEC3G is an enzyme that hypermutates retroviral (HIV) DNA by deaminating cytosines in both viral DNA and mRNA, reducing viral infectivity. Bone marrow stromal antigen 2 (BST-2) is a type 2 integral membrane protein, which inhibits retroviruses, and other enveloped viruses infection by restricting the release of fully formed progeny virions from infected cells. However, HIV-1 Vif and Vpu proteins antagonize APOBEC3G and BST-2 activities, respectively.

Natural killer cells destroy virus-infected cells by secreting perforins and granzymes causing apoptosis

α–Defensins and APOBEC3G reduce HIV infectivity

ADAPTIVE IMMUNE RESPONSES

Adaptive immune responses involving humoral (antibody) and cell-mediated (cytotoxic T lymphocytes) immune responses are also described in Chapter 2. These are virus-specific immune responses directed against viral proteins (antigens). **Antibody** is effective in eliminating cell-free virus, and **cytotoxic T lymphocytes** (CTL) destroy virus-infected cells. The idea that adaptive or acquired immunity in patients is viral antigen-specific led the way in the development of vaccines against several viral infections. Immunity could be either **active,** in that it is elicited by exposure to a pathogen or vaccine, or **passive,** in which it is transferred by immune serum. After viral infection, the first specific immune response is T-cell mediated in which **CD8 T cells** recognize viral antigen presented by class I MHC and kill virus-infected cells by secreting perforins and granzymes and activating FAS proteins, causing apoptosis. It is important to differentiate that CD8 T-cell killing of virus-infected cells is viral antigen-specific, whereas NK cell killing

TABLE 7–5	Viral Vaccines Currently Used in Humans	
VIRUS	**VACCINE**	**IMMUNE RESPONSE**
SARS-CoV-2 (COVID-19)	mRNA-lipid nanoparticle	Antibody (IgG), T cells
Japanese encephalitis B virus	Inactivated or killed	Antibody (IgG)
Hepatitis A virus	Inactivated or killed	Antibody (IgG)
Hepatitis B virus	Subunit (HBsAg)	Antibody (IgG)
Human papillomavirus	Virus-like particles (VLPs)	Antibody (IgG) serum/mucosal
Influenza virus	Killed or inactivated	Antibody (IgG)
	Live attenuated (Nasal spray/ Flu mist)	Antibody (IgA, IgG), CD8 T cells
Measles virus	Live attenuated	Antibody (IgG), CD8 T cells
Mumps virus	Live attenuated	Antibody (IgG), CD8 T cells
Polio virus	Live attenuated (Sabin)	Antibody (IgA, IgG) serum/mucosal
	Killed (Salk)	Antibody (IgG)
Rabies virus	Killed	Antibody (IgG)
Rotavirus	Live attenuated	Antibody (IgA)
Rubella virus	Live attenuated	Antibody (IgG), CD8 T cells
Varicella-zoster virus (Chickenpox, shingles)	Live attenuated	Antibody (IgG), CD8 T cells
Yellow Fever virus	Live attenuated	Antibody (IgG), CD8 T cells

Adaptive immunity involves elimination of the virus by neutralizing antibodies and virus-infected cells by cytotoxic T lymphocytes

of infected cells is nonspecific. The second important control is **neutralization** of the virus in infected hosts by antigen–antibody interactions, preventing the virus from infecting target cells by blocking the virus-receptor interactions. Antibodies are generated against all viral antigens; however, antibody against surface antigens is most effective in eliminating the virus. Antibody in conjunction with complement can also kill virus-infected cells. The evidence that viral infection elicits antibody and CTL that help the clearance of viruses in many cases (acute infection) and control or suppress the viruses in certain cases (persistent infection) has allowed researchers to develop live attenuated vaccines. Live attenuated vaccines activate both arms of the immune system, are very effective in preventing infection, and are long lasting, but can carry a very small risk of reversion. On the other hand, killed or inactivated vaccines (pathogen-killed or inactivated) and subunit vaccines (one or few proteins of the virus) predominantly activate the humoral (antibody) response, may not confer long-lasting immunity, and are also needed in a larger quantity. Several of the live attenuated, killed, and subunit viral vaccines that are currently recommended for use in humans are listed in **Table 7–5**.

VIRUS-INDUCED IMMUNOPATHOLOGY

Immune responses may destroy target cells

Antigen–antibody complex, cytotoxic T lymphocytes, complement, cytokines mediate virus-induced immunopathology

Viral diseases are usually the result of virus-host cell interactions causing either a lytic infection and cell death or persistent infections and cell survival with some cellular dysfunction. However, sometimes both humoral and cellular immune responses against viral infections, especially those causing less cytopathic or persistent infections, mediate inflammation and disease. This could be true in viral infections in which a large number of cells are infected in an individual before the immune response is turned on and in which destruction of these infected cells by immune response may have severe or fatal pathologic outcomes. Specifically, proinflammatory cytokines, antigen–antibody complexes, complement activation pathways, CD4+ T–cell induced-delayed hypersensitivity, and CTL-mediated cell killing contribute to virus-induced immunopathology.

The most important mediators of virus-induced immunopathology are the CD4 T cells and CD8+ CTLs. They release several proinflammatory cytokines, including interferon-γ, tumor necrosis factor-alpha (TNF-α), several interleukins (ILs), and lytic granules, which play an important role in clinical manifestations of virus-induced immunopathology. Chronic HBV infection

TABLE 7–6	Selected Immune Mediated Viral Diseases of Humans	
VIRUS	VIRAL DISEASE	IMMUNE-MEDIATED MECHANISMS
Hepatitis B virus	Hepatitis B	CD8+ T cells, immune complexes
Hepatitis C virus	Hepatitis C	CD8 T cells
Flavivirus (dengue)	Hemorrhagic fever	Immune complexes T cells
Paramyxovirus (RSV)	Bronchiolitis	CD8+ T cells Antibody
Arenavirus	Choriomeningitis	CD8+ T cells
H5N1 (avian influenza)	Bird flu	Cytokine storm
H1N1 (swine influenza)	Swine flu	Cytokine storm

RSV, respiratory syncytial virus.

provided the first clue that the disease is caused by an indirect mechanism rather than the virus itself because a low level of virus can be present in chronically infected people without any damage to the target tissue (liver) for a long time. However, the circulating hepatitis B surface antigen (HBsAg) can form immune complexes that activate the complement system, causing inflammation and tissue damage. In addition, accumulation of these immune complexes in the kidney results in renal damage. In other viral infections, such as measles and mumps, many symptoms are caused by T cell–induced inflammatory responses as opposed to the direct CPE of the virus. Similar mechanisms of CD8 T cell–mediated cytotoxicity of the hepatocytes have been described for chronic HCV infection. Some selected examples of immune-mediated viral diseases are shown in **Table 7–6**. After viral infections, interferon-γ and other cytokines are secreted, which stimulate multiple organ systems to cause systemic infection (flu-like symptoms), and then other immune components such as antigen–antibody complex, complement, CTL and proinflammatory cytokines cause cell damage. This may be the case with several viral infections of the CNS and other tissues in which "cytokine storm" causes cell damage rather than direct viral replication (**Figure 7–5**), including H5N1 (avian influenza virus) and H1N1 (swine influenza of 2009). Recent emerging SASR-CoV-2 (COVID-19) pandemic causing multi-organ diseases involves viral load and excessive cytokine release induced damage.

An important example of acute antibody-mediated immunopathology is dengue hemorrhagic fever, in which a small percentage of infected patients develop dengue shock syndrome (DSS) with a mortality rate up to 10%. This syndrome mostly occurs in people who are either undergoing a second infection with a different serotype or in infants carrying maternal anti-dengue antibody and undergoing first infection. A nonneutralizing antibody (enhancing antibody) facilitates the adsorption of flaviviruses (dengue and yellow fever viruses) into macrophages through Fc receptors followed by replication, thereby changing the tropism of the virus. The infected macrophages secrete cytokines interferon-γ, TNF-α, and others. In addition, dengue-specific CD4+ and CD8+ T lymphocytes secrete similar types of cytokines, resulting in cytokine storm and causing hemorrhage and shock. The circulating immune complex activates the complement pathway, which also contributes to immunopathology.

Virus-initiated autoimmunity, in which a viral infection may induce an autoimmune response because the viral protein resembles a host cell protein, induces a phenomenon called **molecular mimicry.** Both viral epitope-specific antibody and T lymphocytes may react with cognate epitopes on the host proteins, which may elicit an autoimmune response. Viral proteins, such as the polymerase of hepatitis B, contain sequences similar to the encephalitogenic epitope of myelin basic protein (MBP), which is a major component of myelin sheath in the CNS. Immune responses against an epitope of hepatitis B polymerase induce an immune response against MBP, initiating an autoimmune disease process. Coxsackievirus infection has also been linked to autoimmune responses associated with type 1 diabetes as a result of molecular mimicry between a viral protein and a protein found in islet cells called glutamic acid decarboxylase (GAD).

Proinflammatory cytokines play roles in several viral diseases

CD8 CTL mediated chronic hepatitis B and C

Immune-mediated measles and mumps diseases

Viral and immune-mediated damage in COVID-19

Dengue hemorrhagic fever and shock syndrome is caused by antibody-mediated immunopathology

Some autoimmune diseases are initiated by viral infections because of molecular mimicry

FIGURE 7–5. **Cytokine storm.** In highly virulent viruses such as bird flu virus (H5N1) of 2006 or swine flu virus (H1N1) of 2009 and others, infected patients develop acute respiratory distress syndrome (ARDS) caused by a cytokine storm of a healthy, competent, and robust immune system. After viral infections, interferon-γ and other proinflammatory cytokines (mainly TNF-α, IL-1, and IL-6) are secreted that stimulate multiple organ systems. Cytokine storm is caused by rapidly proliferating and highly activated T cells or natural killer cells, which are activated by infected macrophages. Moreover, other immune components such as antigen–antibody complex, complement, CTLs, and proinflammatory cytokines cause cell damage.

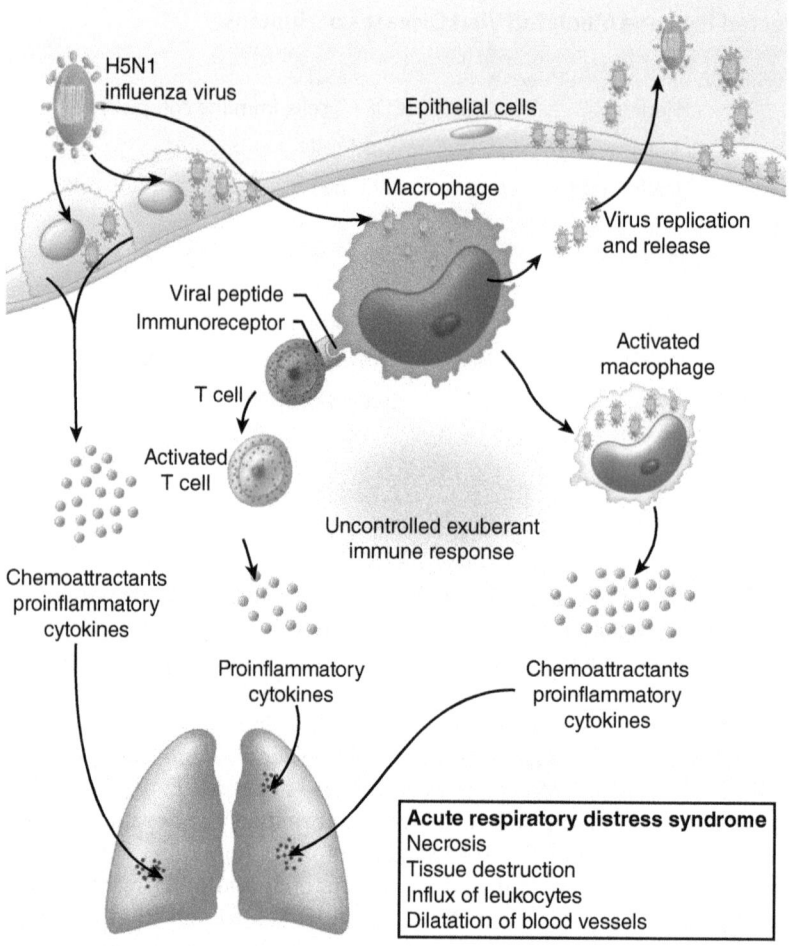

Viral infections can cause suppression of the immune response

Viruses infecting either CD4+ helper T cells or antigen-presenting cells cause immunosuppression

VIRUS-INDUCED IMMUNOSUPPRESSION

Viral infections, in several instances, can suppress the immune response. Immunosuppression can be achieved either by direct viral replication or by viral antigens. Some viruses specifically infect and kill immune cells. In some instances, immunosuppression is often associated with antenatal or perinatal infections. Historically, immunosuppression was first described approximately a century ago when patients lost their tuberculin sensitivity during, and weeks after, measles infection. In the last decade, immunosuppression has been the topic of discussion, concern, and treatment in the HIV/AIDS epidemic because HIV specifically infects and destroys the major type of immune cells, CD4+ T lymphocytes. **Table 7–7** shows the mechanisms of selected human viruses causing immune suppression. Several mechanisms have been proposed for virus-induced

TABLE 7–7	Immunosuppression by Some Human Viruses	
VIRUS	**DEGREE OF IMMUNOSUPPRESSION**	**MECHANISM OF IMMUNOSUPPRESSION**
HIV	High	CD4+ T-lymphocyte depletion Env gp120-induced syncytia formation and depletion of uninfected CD4+ T lymphocyte
Herpes simplex virus (HSV)	Low	HSV-encoded proteins that function as viroreceptors or virokines
Vaccinia	Low	Vaccina encodes viroreceptors and virokines
Measles	Moderate	Downregulation of IL-12, infection of monocytes/macrophages, T and B lymphocytes
Rubella	Moderate	Immune tolerance associated with fetal infection

immune suppression: (1) viral replication in a major immune cells (CD4+ helper T lymphocytes) or antigen-presenting cells (dendritic cells or macrophages) leading to apoptosis; (2) viral antigens stimulating proinflammatory cytokines causing cell death; (3) tolerance generated by clonal deletion of T lymphocytes by viral antigens, generally associated with perinatal infections; and (4) expression of viral proteins that destroy infected and uninfected cells such as HIV Env gp120 depleting uninfected and infected CD4+ T lymphocytes.

The extensively studied virus-induced immunosuppression problem is HIV/AIDS, which is a persistent infection. The primary target for HIV is CD4+ T lymphocytes and monocytes/macrophages. However, HIV is highly cytopathic to CD4+ T lymphocytes but not to monocytes/macrophages. Therefore, depletion of CD4+ T lymphocytes in HIV-infected patients results in immunosuppression. The mechanisms of depletion of CD4+ T lymphocytes include direct killing of CD4+ T lymphocytes as a result of HIV replication and also depletion of uninfected CD4+ T lymphocytes by HIV Env gp120-induced syncytia formation and apoptosis. Immunosuppression in HIV-infected patients causes opportunistic infection, whereas several other pathogens establish infection without immune challenge. However, antiretroviral therapy (ART) has significantly reduced the viral load, improved the CD4 T cell counts, and reduced the risk of opportunistic infections in infected patients.

Measles is an acute viral infection that produces immunosuppression, which appears during the incubation period and the clinical phase of the disease. Some results of measles-induced immunosuppression include increased susceptibility to other infections, possible aggravation of chronic latent infections such as tuberculosis, and remission of autoimmune diseases. The mechanisms of measles-induced immunosuppression involve infection of several cell types and pathways. However, during measles infection, the function of antigen-presenting cells such as monocytes/macrophages and CD4 and CD8 T lymphocytes is compromised, which may contribute to immunosuppression. An example of immunosuppression in utero or during infancy is rubella virus infection. Fetal infections that commonly produce congenital rubella (see Chapter 10) cause greatly reduced cellular immune responses to rubella virus antigens even several years after infection. In general, several factors or determinants could be responsible for virus-induced immunosuppression, such as the strain of the virus, dose, or amount of the virus entering the host, route of transmission or virus entry, age and immune status of the host, and other immunologic disorders in the host.

CONCLUSION

In the past decade, we have gained significant knowledge about how viruses interact with their hosts and cause disease as well as how the hosts, in turn, respond in ways that may be either beneficial or deleterious to their well-being. Our understanding of these processes is as yet incomplete, but the knowledge gained to date has enabled scientists to develop new strategies to deal with these issues. Two approaches that have already resulted in success are (1) prevention, including development of effective environmental controls, and vaccines for prevention and (2) development of specific antiviral agents that can cure, mitigate, or temporarily prevent infection. Better approaches to more advantageously manipulate specific and nonspecific host responses to such infections are expected as well. For now, all that can be stated with certainty is that exciting, meaningful progress will continue well into the future.

Viral gene products can cause immunosuppression by stimulating proinflammatory cytokines

Immunosuppression in HIV-infected individuals is due to direct and indirect depletion of CD4 T lymphocytes

In measles infection, the functions of CD4 and CD8 T lymphocytes are compromised

Immunosuppression in congenital rubella is due to reduced cellular immune response during fetal infection

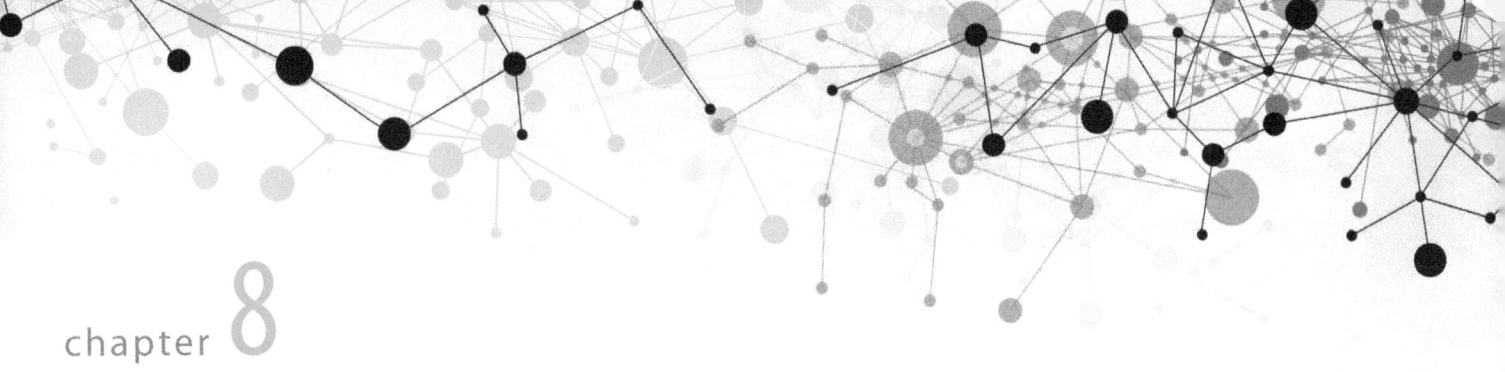

chapter 8

Antiviral Agents and Resistance

GENERAL CONSIDERATIONS

Viruses are composed of either DNA or RNA, a protein coat (capsid), and, in many, a lipid or lipoprotein envelope. The nucleic acid codes for enzymes involved in replication and for several structural proteins. Viruses use molecules (eg, amino acids, purines, pyrimidines) supplied by the cell and cellular structures (eg, ribosomes) for synthetic functions. Thus, one of the challenges in the development of antiviral agents is identification of the steps in viral replication that are unique to the virus and not used by the normal cell. Among the unique viral events are attachment, penetration, uncoating, RNA-directed DNA synthesis (reverse transcription) or RNA-directed RNA synthesis (RNA viruses), and assembly and release of the intact virion. Each of these steps may have complex elements with the potential for inhibition. For example, assembly of some virus particles requires a unique viral enzyme, protease, and this has led to the development of protease inhibitors (PIs). A general scheme for the points of action of antiviral agents is shown in **Figure 8–1.**

> Events in the cell unique to viral replication are the targets for antiviral therapy

In some cases, antiviral agents do not selectively inhibit a unique replicative event but inhibit viral polymerases. Inhibitors of these enzymes take advantage of the fact that the virus is synthesizing nucleic acids more rapidly than the cell; therefore, there is relatively greater inhibition of viral than cellular nucleic acids.

In many acute viral infections, especially respiratory ones, the bulk of viral replication has already occurred when symptoms are beginning to appear. Initiating antiviral therapy at this stage is unlikely to make a major impact on the illness. For these viruses, immuno- or chemoprophylaxis, rather than therapy, is a more logical approach. However, other viral infections are characterized by ongoing viral replication and do benefit from viral inhibition, such as human immunodeficiency virus (HIV) infection and chronic hepatitis B and C.

The principal antiviral agents in current use are discussed according to their modes of action. The first section deals with agents used for most of the non-HIV viruses; the later section reviews the therapeutic agents used for HIV and hepatitis infection. Their features are summarized in **Table 8–1.**

SELECTED ANTIVIRAL AGENTS

■ Inhibitors of Attachment

Attachment to a cell receptor is a unique virus-specific event. Antibodies can bind to the extracellular virus and prevent this attachment. However, although therapy with antibody is useful in prophylaxis, it has been minimally effective in treatment.

■ Inhibitors of Cell Penetration and Uncoating

Amantadine and rimantadine are symmetric amines, which are thought to inhibit viral uncoating as their primary antiviral effect.

They are extremely selective, with activity against only influenza A, where they act as inhibitors of the viral M2 protein. Unfortunately, since 2001, the rates of resistance to amantadine/rimantadine have increased so sharply (up to 100% for some strains) that they are no longer routinely recommended.

> Sharply rising resistance rates now preclude their routine use

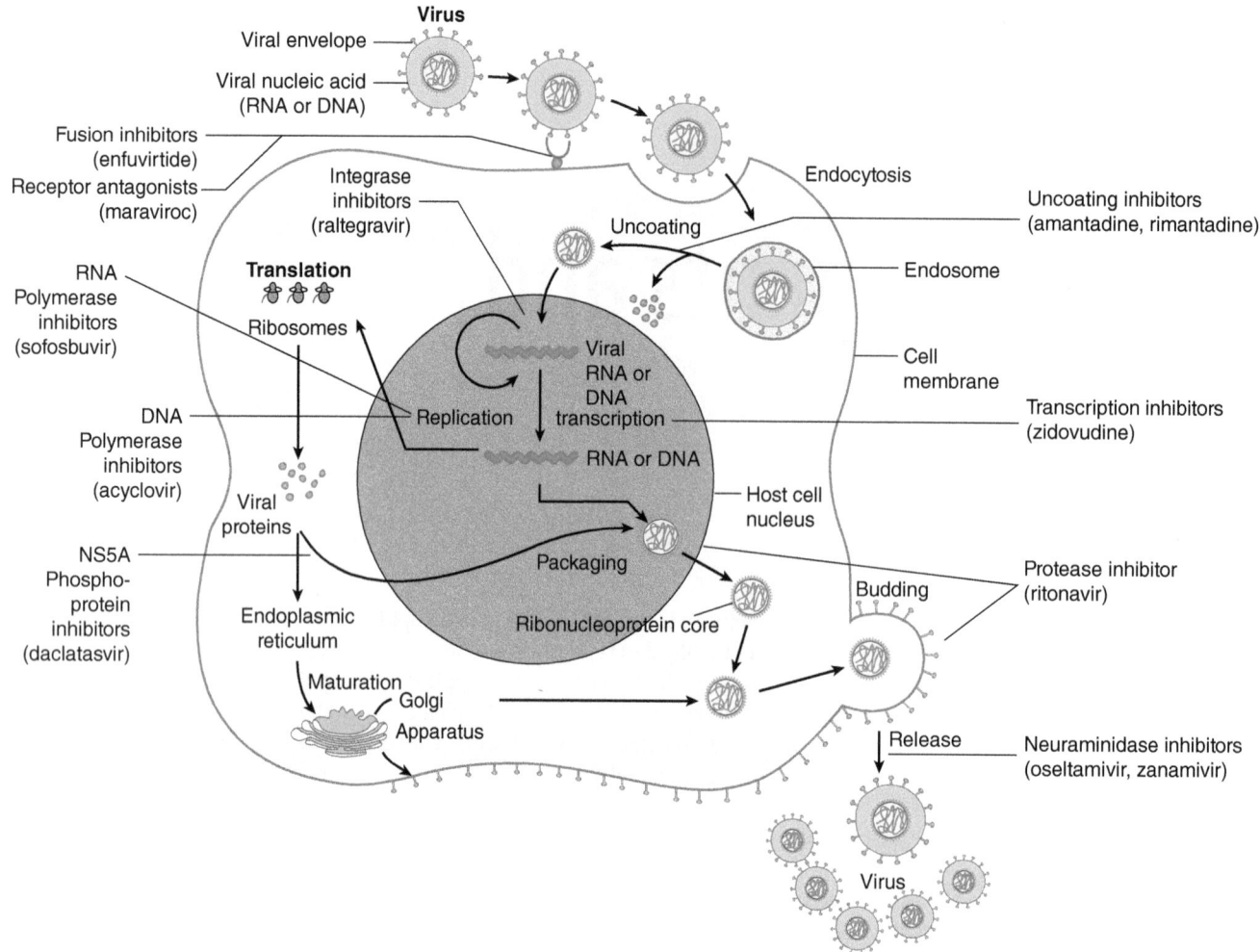

FIGURE 8–1. General scheme of antiviral action. The general sequence of viral replication, as in Figure 6–8, is shown with the points of action of selected antiviral agent.

■ Neuraminidase Inhibitors

Oseltamivir, zanamivir, and peramivir are antiviral agents that inhibit the neuraminidase of influenza A and B viruses. The neuraminidase cleaves terminal sialic acid from glycoconjugates and plays a role in the release of virus from infected cells. Due to limited bioavailability, zanamivir is given by inhalation using a specially designed device. Oseltamivir phosphate is the oral prodrug of oseltamivir, a drug comparable to zanamivir in antineuraminidase activity. Peramivir is only administered by intravenous infusion. Baloxavir, a newly approved anti-influenza drug, inhibits an enzyme within the viral RNA polymerase. It has similar efficacy as oseltamivir with only a single dose.

Treatment with either oseltamivir or zanamivir reduces influenza symptoms, shortens the course of illness by 0.5 to 1.5 days, and reduces the rate of complications. They are more effective if given prophylactically, that is, in nursing homes during an influenza outbreak.

Baloxavir, a prodrug, inhibits the function of the endonuclease within the influenza viral RNA polymerase. It was approved by the FDA for the treatment of uncomplicated influenza A or B in 2018 and more recently for patients at high risk for complications. As with the neurominidase inhibitors, that is, oseltamivir, it only reduces the illness by 24 hours and, for that, treatment should begin within 48 hours of illness onset. Also, like oseltamivir, baloxavir is more effective if given prophylactically to household contacts of patients with influenza.

A worldwide epidemic of COVID-19 the respiratory infection due to a coronavirus, SARS-CoV-2 began in late 2019. Globally it has caused over 2.8 million deaths as of early 2021. Remdesivir is the only antiviral agent approved for therapy. For the therapeutic use of convalescent plasma, corticosteroids, monoclonal antibodies and experimental drugs, see Chapter 9.

✳ Neuraminidase inhibitors are effective in treatment and prophylaxis of influenza A and B viruses

COVID-19 Epidemic

Immunotherapy

TABLE 8-1	Summary of Antiviral Agents	
VIRAL SPECTRUM	**ANTIVIRAL AGENT**	**MECHANISM OF ACTION**
Herpesvirus		
Cytomegalovirus	Ganciclovir, Foscarnet, Cidofovir	Inhibition of DNA polymerase
	Letermovir	Inhibition of viral terminase
	Maribavir	Inhibition of viral UL97 function
Herpes Simplex Virus	Acyclovir, Famciclovir, Valacyclovir, Docosanal (topical), Penciclovir (topical), Foscarnet (ACV resistant), Trifluridine (eye), Vidarabine (eye)	Inhibition of viral DNA polymerase
Varicella-Zoster	Acyclovir, Famciclovir, Valacyclovir	Inhibition of DNA polymerase
Hepatitis		
Hepatitis B	NRTIs	Inhibition of reverse transcriptase
	Interferon	Inhibitor of viral protein synthesis
Hepatitis C	Direct acting antivirals (DAA)	Protease, polymerase, NS5 inhibitors
	Ribavirin	Inhibitor of viral RNA synthesis
	Interferon a	Inhibitor of viral protein synthesis
Influenza		
Influenza A, B	Oseltamivir, Zanamivir	Neuraminidase inhibition
	Baloxavir	Inhibition of RNA polymerase
Human immunodeficiency virus		
HIV	Enfuvirtide	Inhibition of viral fusion
HIV	Maraviroc	Inhibition of viral entry
HIV	Zidovudine, Didoxinosine, Stavudine, Lamivudine, Abacavir, Emtricitabine, Tenofovir, Zalcitabine	NRTI[a]
HIV	Nevirapine, Delavirdine, Efavirenz, Etravirine, Rilpivirine, Doravirine	NNRTI[b]
HIV	Raltegravir, Elvitegravir, Dolutegravir, Bictegravir	Inhibition of viral integration
HIV	Saquinavir, Elvitegravir, Indinavir, Ritonavir, Nelfinavir, Lopinavir, Darunavir, Atazanavir, Fosamprenavir, Tipranavir, Amprenavir	Inhibition of viral protease
HIV	Ritonavir	Pharmacokinetic enhancer
Viral hemorrhagic fevers	Ribavirin	Inhibition of viral RNA synthesis
RSV	Ribavirin	Inhibition of viral RNA synthesis

[a]NRTI = nucleoside/nucleotide reverse transcriptase (RT) inhibitors.
[b]NNRTI = nonnucleoside RT inhibitors.

Recent investigation has revealed that certain viral infection may be complicated by "excessive" immune responses which may worsen the clinical course. This phenomenon, "cytokine storm" has been documented in severe influenza A and COVID-19. To address this plasma from convalescent patients has been tried with inconsistent effects. Monoclonal antibodies against one or more cytokines are being evaluated in COVID-19 patients. Dexamethasone has shown benefit in COVID-19 patients, possibly due to inhibition of the excessive immune response.

■ Inhibitors of Nucleic Acid Synthesis

At present, most antiviral agents are nucleoside analogs that are active against virus-specific nucleic acid polymerases or reverse transcriptases and have much less activity against analogous host enzymes. Some of these agents serve as nucleic acid chain terminators after incorporation into nucleic acids.

Idoxuridine and Trifluorothymidine

Idoxuridine (5-iodo-2′-deoxyuridine, IUdR) is a halogenated pyrimidine that blocks nucleic acid synthesis by being incorporated into DNA in place of thymidine and producing a nonfunctional molecule. It is phosphorylated by cellular thymidine kinase to the active compound, which inhibits both viral and cellular DNA polymerase. The resulting host toxicity precludes systemic administration in humans. Idoxuridine can be used topically as effective treatment of herpetic infection of the cornea (keratitis). Trifluorothymidine, a related pyrimidine analog, is effective in treating herpetic corneal infections, including those that fail to respond to IUdR. Trifluorothymidine has largely replaced IUdR.

Acyclovir

This antiviral agent differs from the nucleoside guanosine by having an acyclic (hydroxyethoxymethyl) side chain. The key to its benefit is that it must be phosphorylated by viral thymidine kinase to be active. Therefore, the compound is essentially nontoxic because it is not phosphorylated or activated in uninfected host cells. Viral thymidine kinase catalyzes the phosphorylation of acyclovir to a monophosphate. From this point, host cell enzymes complete the progression to the diphosphate and, finally, the triphosphate. Acyclovir triphosphate inhibits viral replication by competing with guanosine triphosphate and inhibiting the function of the virally encoded DNA polymerase. The selectivity and minimal toxicity of acyclovir is aided by its 100-fold or greater affinity for viral DNA polymerase than for cellular DNA polymerase. A second mechanism of viral inhibition results from incorporation of acyclovir triphosphate into the growing viral DNA chain. This causes termination of chain growth because there is no 3′-hydroxy group on the acyclovir molecule to provide attachment sites for additional nucleotides.

⁎ Acyclovir is effective against the herpesviruses, which induce thymidine kinase

Activity of acyclovir against herpesviruses directly correlates with the capacity of the virus to induce a thymidine kinase. Susceptible strains of herpes simplex virus types 1 and 2 (HSV-1 and -2) are the most active thymidine kinase inducers and are the most readily inhibited by acyclovir. Cytomegalovirus (CMV) induces little or no thymidine kinase and is not inhibited. Varicella-zoster and Epstein-Barr viruses are between these two extremes in terms of both thymidine kinase induction and acyclovir susceptibility.

Acyclovir inhibits viral DNA polymerase and terminates viral DNA chain growth

Resistant strains of HSV have been recovered from immunocompromised patients, including patients with acquired immunodeficiency syndrome (AIDS); in most instances, resistance results from mutations in the viral thymidine kinase gene, rendering it inactive in phosphorylation. Resistance may also result from mutations in the viral DNA polymerase. Remarkably, resistant virus has rarely been recovered from immunocompetent patients, even after years of drug exposure and frequent usage.

Pharmacology and Toxicity. Acyclovir is available in three forms: topical, oral, and parenteral. Topical acyclovir is rarely used. The oral form has low bioavailability (~10%), but achieves concentrations in blood that inhibit HSV and, to a lesser extent, varicella-zoster virus (VZV). Intravenous acyclovir is used for serious HSV infection (eg, congenital, encephalitis) as well as for VZV infection in immunocompromised patients. Because acyclovir is excreted by the kidney, the dosage must be reduced in patients with renal failure. Central nervous system toxicity and renal toxicity have been reported in patients treated with prolonged high intravenous doses. Despite its mechanism of action, acyclovir is remarkably free of bone marrow toxicity, even in patients with hematopoietic disorders—a feature attributable to the absence of its phosphorylation (ie, activation) in uninfected host cells.

Intravenous acyclovir used in serious HSV infections

Treatment and Prophylaxis. Acyclovir is most effective in the treatment of primary HSV mucocutaneous infections or for severe recurrences in immunocompromised patients. It can provide protection against recurrent genital infection when taken daily as well as reduced transmission to heterosexual partners. The agent is useful in neonatal herpes and encephalitis, infection in immunocompromised patients and for varicella in older children or adults. Acyclovir is beneficial against herpes zoster in elderly patients or any patient with eye involvement. Acyclovir is minimally effective in the treatment of recurrent genital or labial herpes in otherwise healthy individuals.

Valacyclovir, Famciclovir

Valacyclovir is an oral prodrug of acyclovir, that is, better absorbed and, therefore, is used in lower and less frequent dosage (bioavailability ~60%). When absorbed, it becomes acyclovir. It is currently approved for use in HSV and VZV infections. Dosage adjustment is necessary in patients with impaired renal function.

Famciclovir is similar to acyclovir in its structure and requirement for phosphorylation but differs slightly in its mode of action. After absorption, the agent is converted to penciclovir, the active moiety, which inhibits viral DNA polymerase. However, it does not irreversibly terminate DNA replication. Famciclovir is currently approved for the treatment of recurrent HSV and VZV infections. **Penciclovir** is approved for topical treatment of recurrent herpes labialis. **Docosanol**, known as Abreva, is the first FDA-approved over-the-counter antiviral and does not require a doctor's prescription. It is fatty alcohol which is only for oral–facial herpes simplex infection and not for genital herpes simplex infection. It can shorten healing time and the duration of symptoms, especially if given early in a symptomatic episode.

> Agents similar to or becoming acyclovir after absorption are available

Ganciclovir

Ganciclovir (DHPG), a nucleoside analog of guanosine, differs from acyclovir by a single carboxyl side chain. This structural change confers approximately 50 times more activity against CMV than acyclovir. Acyclovir has low activity against CMV because it is not well phosphorylated in CMV-infected cells due to the absence of the gene for thymidine kinase in CMV. However, ganciclovir is active against CMV because another viral-encoded phosphorylating enzyme (UL97) is present in CMV-infected cells that is, capable of phosphorylating ganciclovir and converting it to the monophosphate. Then, cellular enzymes convert it to the active compound, ganciclovir triphosphate, which inhibits the viral DNA polymerase (UL54). Since ganciclovir can be phosphorylated in normal, uninfected, host cells, toxicity, especially neutropenia, frequently limits therapy. Discontinuation of therapy is necessary in patients whose neutrophils do not increase during dosage reduction or in response to cytokines. Thrombocytopenia (platelet count less than $20,000/mm^3$) occurs in approximately 15% of patients. Ganciclovir is also active against herpes simplex, EB, and VZ viruses but is not the drug of choice for these viruses due to toxicity.

> ✳ Ganciclovir does not utilize viral thymidine kinase for phosphorylation

Oral ganciclovir is available but is inferior to the intravenous form. Oral valganciclovir, a prodrug of ganciclovir, has improved bioavailability and is equivalent to the intravenous form.

> Neutropenia and thrombocytopenia limit use

Clinical Use. Administration of ganciclovir or valganciclovir is indicated for the prevention or treatment of active CMV infection in immunocompromised patients. Because patients with AIDS with severe CMV infection frequently have concurrent illnesses caused by other herpesviruses, treatment with ganciclovir may benefit associated HSV and VZV infections.

Resistance. After several months of continuous ganciclovir therapy for treatment of CMV, between 5% and 10% of patients with AIDS excrete resistant strains of CMV. In almost all isolates, a mutation is found in the phosphorylating gene (*UL97*), and in a lesser number a mutation may also be found in the viral DNA polymerase (UL54). Most of these strains remain sensitive to foscarnet, which may be used as an alternate therapy. If only a *UL97* mutation is present, the strains remain susceptible to the nucleotide analog cidofovir (see later in the chapter); however, if the CMV strain has a ganciclovir-induced mutation in DNA polymerase (UL54), the virus is cross-resistant to cidofovir. Ganciclovir resistance has been noted in transplant recipients, in patients with lung or liver transplants, and those requiring prolonged prophylaxis or treatment.

> CMV resistance increases with continuous therapy

■ Ribavirin

Ribavirin is another analog of the nucleoside guanosine. Unlike acyclovir, which replaces the ribose moiety with a hydroxymethyl acyclic side chain, ribavirin differs from guanosine in that the base ring is incomplete and open. Similar to other nucleoside analogs, ribavirin must be phosphorylated to mono-, di-, and triphosphate forms, but cellular enzymes can carry out each of these, thus, heightening the risk of toxicity. Ribavirin is active against a broad range of viruses in vitro, but its in vivo activity is limited. The mechanism of the antiviral effect of ribavirin is not as clear as that of acyclovir. It is an inhibitor of RNA polymerase, and it also inhibits inosine monophosphate dehydrogenase—an enzyme important in the synthetic pathway of guanosine. Yet another mode of action is by decreasing synthesis of the mRNA 5′ cap because of interference with both guanylation and methylation of the nucleic acid base.

> Ribavirin has several modes of action

Aerosol administration enables ribavirin to reach concentrations in respiratory secretions up to 10 times greater than necessary to inhibit respiratory syncytial virus (RSV) replication and substantially higher than those achieved with oral administration. Problems encountered with aerosolized ribavirin include precipitation of the agent in tubing used for administration and exposure of healthcare personnel. Thus, its use for RSV infection is not generally recommended although when combined with monoclonal antibody, it may reduce mortality in highly immuno-compromised patients.

Oral and intravenous forms have been used for patients with Lassa fever and infections with other arenaviruses, with apparent benefit but the studies are uncontrolled. In a recent trial of hantavirus treatment, ribavirin was ineffective. A reversible anemia has been associated with oral administration of ribavirin and, in preclinical studies, it was teratogenic, mutagenic, and gonadotoxic.

■ Nonnucleoside Analogs—Letermovir

This new anti-CMV antiviral was approved by the FDA in 2017 for a very specific use: prevention of CMV infection and disease in adult allogenic stem cell transplant recipients. It is not approved for treatment of established CMV disease. Letermovir is a nonnucleoside that inhibits viral replication by targeting the viral terminase complex. Since this is a unique action, there is no cross resistance with CMV polymerase inhibitors, that is, ganciclovir. It is not active against other viruses but does not appear to be myelosuppressive, which makes its use in stem cell transplants appealing.

■ Nucleotide Analogs: Cidofovir

Cidofovir mimics a nucleotide, not nucleoside

The first example of the nucleotide analogs is **cidofovir.** This compound has a phosphonate group attached to the molecule and appears to the cell as a nucleoside monophosphate, in effect, a nucleotide. Cellular enzymes then add two phosphate groups to generate the active compound. In this form, the drug inhibits both viral and cellular nucleic acid polymerases, but selectivity is provided by its higher affinity for the viral enzyme.

Nucleotide analogs do not require phosphorylation, or activation, by a viral-encoded enzyme and remain active against viruses that are resistant due to mutations in codons for these enzymes, for example, a UL97 mutant CMV. Resistance to cidofovir can, of course, develop due to mutations in the viral DNA polymerase, UL54. An additional feature of cidofovir is a very prolonged half-life as a result of slow clearance by the kidneys.

Cidofovir is approved for intravenous therapy of CMV retinitis, and maintenance treatment may be given as infrequently as every 2 weeks. In addition, it is occasionally used to treat severe, disseminated adenovirus and BK virus infections although its efficacy/toxicity ratio for these is unfavorable. Nephrotoxicity is a serious complication of cidofovir treatment, and patients must be monitored carefully for evidence of renal impairment.

■ Inhibitors of Viral DNA Synthesis

Foscarnet

Foscarnet inhibits viral DNA polymerases

Effective against resistant CMV and HSV

Foscarnet, also known as phosphonoformate, is a pyrophosphate analog that inhibits viral DNA polymerase by blocking the pyrophosphate-binding site of the viral DNA polymerase and preventing cleavage of pyrophosphate from deoxyadenosine triphosphate. This action is relatively selective; CMV DNA polymerase is inhibited at concentrations less than 1% of that required to inhibit cellular DNA polymerase. Unlike such nucleosides as acyclovir and ganciclovir, foscarnet does not require phosphorylation to be an active inhibitor of viral DNA polymerases. This biochemical fact becomes especially important with regard to viral resistance, because the principal mode of viral resistance to nucleoside analogs is a mutation that eliminates phosphorylation of the drug in virus-infected cells. Thus, foscarnet can usually be used to treat patients with ganciclovir-resistant CMV and acyclovir-resistant HSV. Excretion is entirely renal without a hepatic component, and dosage must be decreased in patients with impaired renal function. Multiple metabolic abnormalities occur as evidence of toxicity.

Interferons

Recombinant DNA techniques allow large-scale production

Interferons are host cell-encoded proteins synthesized in response to double-stranded RNA (dsRNA) that circulate to protect uninfected cells by inhibiting viral protein synthesis. Ironically, interferons harvested in tissue culture were the first antiviral agents, but their clinical activity was disappointing. Recombinant DNA techniques now allow relatively inexpensive large-scale production of interferons by bacteria and yeasts.

Interferon α is beneficial in the treatment of chronic active hepatitis B and C infection, although its efficacy is often transient. Combinations of interferon-α with lamivudine, famciclovir, and certain nucleotides have been evaluated for treatment of hepatitis B but are being supplanted by newer drugs. Interferon combined with ribavirin is used for hepatitis C. Topical or intralesional interferon application is beneficial in the treatment of human papilloma virus infections. Parenteral use can cause symptomatic systemic toxicity (eg, fever, malaise), partly because of its effect on host cell protein synthesis.

Interferons inhibit viral protein synthesis

■ Maribavir

Maribavir is a benzimidazole riboside which inhibits viral DNA synthesis by a unique mechanism, inhibiting UL97 function. Initial evaluation, in vivo, indicated effective antiviral activity but a pivotal trial in hematopoietic transplant recipients failed to confirm efficacy. This result was at least partly due to inadequate dosage but the drug was shelved until more recent studies have proven benefit, especially in the treatment of patients whose CMV has become resistant to ganciclovir and other front line anti-CMV medications.

■ Inhibitors of HIV

There are now more than 30 antivirals for HIV in six different drug classes. Antiviral treatment is now recommended for everyone infected by HIV. This recommendation is a departure from the past when it was felt that treatment could wait while patients showed clinical or laboratory abnormalities attributed to HIV. For example, it was once felt that treatment could be withheld until the CD4 lymphocyte count was less than 200/mL. Treatment is beneficial at all stages of infection including primary, early infection, that is, within the first six months. In general, treatment consists of at least three different drug classes. These regimens are referred to as HAART (highly active antiretroviral treatment) or just ART. Treatment does not cure HIV infection or the disease, AIDS, but greatly prolongs life.

Treatment consists of at least three different drugs

1. **Fusion inhibitors.** Enfuvirtide is a synthetic peptide (36 amino acids) which inhibits the fusion of HIV-1 with CD4 cells. The latter is a complex process, including viral attachment and coreceptor binding and is necessary for subsequent viral entry into a cell. As with other HIV antagonists, it should only be used in combination with other classes of HIV inhibitors. There is no oral form, and it is usually reserved for patients failing other therapies.

2. **Receptor antagonists.** CCR5 is a molecule very similar to CD4 that acts as a viral receptor. Maraviroc blocks the predominant route of viral entry by interfering with the attachment of HIV gp 120 with the CCR5 receptor on the CD4 lymphocyte surface. Maraviroc is an oral drug which, like all anti-HIV agents, should not be used alone. Resistance may develop by the virus adapting to another receptor, CXCR4.

3. **Nucleoside reverse transcriptase inhibitors (NRTIs).** Zidovudine (AZT), the first true anti-HIV drug, a nucleoside analog of thymidine, inhibits the reverse transcriptase of HIV by terminating the developing DNA chain. As with other nucleosides, AZT must be phosphorylated; host cell enzymes carry out the process. The basis for the relatively selective therapeutic effect of AZT is that HIV reverse transcriptase is more than 100 times more sensitive to AZT than is host cell DNA polymerase. Nonetheless, toxicity frequently occurs.

   AZT was the first useful treatment for HIV infection, but as with virtually all HIV therapy is recommended for use only in combination with other inhibitors of HIV replication. Toxicity includes malaise, nausea, and bone marrow toxicity. All hematopoietic components may be depressed, but they usually reverse with discontinuation of the drug or dose reduction. Resistance is associated with one or more mutations in the HIV reverse transcriptase gene.

   A series of oral compounds similar to AZT have been developed and are used in combination with other HIV antivirals. Although they have similar mechanisms of action, their side effects may differ. These compounds include didanosine (ddI) and zalcitabine (ddC) which have serious adverse effects of treatment including peripheral neuropathy and pancreatitis; both conditions are dose related.

AZT is now used only in combination therapy

Stavudine (D4T) is another nucleoside analog that inhibits HIV replication by terminating the growth of the chain of viral nucleic acid. D4T is well absorbed and has a high bioavailability. Adverse effects include headache, nausea and vomiting, asthenia, confusion, and elevated serum transaminase and creatinine kinase. A painful sensory peripheral neuropathy that appears to be dose-related may occur. D4T should be used only in combination with other anti-HIV agents.

Lamivudine (3TC), another oral nucleoside reverse transcriptase inhibitor, is a comparatively safe and usually well-tolerated agent. It is used in combination with AZT or other nucleoside analogs.

Abacavir, tenofovir, and emtricitabine are newer oral NRTIs which, like those discussed earlier, should only be used in combination with other classes of HIV antivirals. They appear to be less toxic than older NRTIs especially for "mitochondrial toxicity" manifest as myopathy, neuropathy, hepatic failure, and lactic acidosis.

4. **Nonnucleoside reverse transcriptase inhibitors (NNRTIs).** Certain oral compounds that are not nucleoside analogs also inhibit HIV reverse transcriptase by binding to it and preventing conversion of HIV RNA, not HIV DNA. Several compounds, such as nevirapine, delavirdine, efavirenz, etravirine, rilpivirine, and doravirine have been evaluated alone or in combination with other nucleosides. They are collectively referred to as NNRTIs. These compounds are very active against HIV-1, do not require cellular enzymes to be phosphorylated, and bind to, essentially, the same site on reverse transcriptase. Cross-resistance does not occur between nucleoside RT inhibitors and NNRTIs, but does occur between one NNRTI and another. Unfortunately, drug resistance readily emerges with even a single passage of virus in the presence of drug in vitro and in vivo. Thus, NNRTIs should be used only in combination regimens with other drugs active against HIV.

5. **Protease inhibitors.** Additional oral agents that inhibit HIV are the PI. These agents block the action of the viral-encoded enzyme protease, which cleaves polyproteins to produce viral proteins. Inhibition of this enzyme leads to blockage of viral assembly and release. The PI are potent suppressors of HIV replication *in vitro* and *in vivo*, particularly when combined with other antiretroviral agents. These drugs do not require intracellular phosphorylation for activation.

In late 1995, **saquinavir** was the first PI to receive approval. **Ritonavir, indinavir, nelfinavir, darunavir, fosamprenavir, and tipranavir** and others are potent PI that have since been released. These drugs may cause hepatotoxicity as all agents inhibit P450, resulting in important drug interactions. They also appear to cause lipodystrophy. Because drug resistance to all PI develops, these agents should not be used alone without other anti-HIV drugs. Lopinavir is a PI which is marketed in combination with ritonavir. Atazanavir, another PI is usually prescribed with ritonavir to increase serum concentration of atazanavir. Ritonavir, itself, is a "booster," increasing the effectiveness of other PIs.

6. **Integrase inhibitors.** HIV integrase aids the insertion of viral DNA into host cell DNA. This occurs after the viral reverse transcriptase (RNA/DNA-dependent DNA polymerase) produces double-stranded viral DNA. This step is key to the cell becoming a permanent carrier. Four integrase inhibitors, raltegravir, elvitegravir, dolutegravir, and bictegravir are approved for use in the United States. They are oral and are used in combination with other classes of antiretrovirals.

ANTIVIRALS FOR HEPATITIS B

Acute hepatitis is not usually treated since most infections will resolve on their own. Treatment is reserved for patients with chronic active hepatitis B especially those with cirrhosis, liver inflammation, and high viral loads. The mainstays of treatment are: (1) interferons (interferon-α and Peg-IFN) or (2) inhibitors of hepatitis B DNA replication.

■ Interferon

In general, interferon slows the replication of the virus and/or enhances immune responses. Pegylated interferon can be given parenterally weekly, compared with thrice weekly for interferon-α and is the interferon of choice. Both products have a high incidence of side effects, with an "influenza-like" syndrome being very common. A 48-week course of pegylated interferon-based treatment is successful, that is, viral DNA and HBsAg clearance in approximately 30% of patients.

■ Nucleoside/Nucleotide (NUC) Analog Inhibitors

Lamivudine was the first inhibitor of hepatitis B DNA polymerase (reverse transcriptase [RT]) to be employed clinically. It has been followed—and supplanted—with similar molecules that are less prone to resistance development. Of these, entecavir and tenofovir have become the preferred agents for monotherapy due to their potency and very low rates of resistance development. The other polymerase inhibitors should not be used as monotherapy due to lesser efficacy and because of the ease with which resistance may develop.

✳ Treatment of hepatitis B may suppress but not eradicate virus

ANTIVIRALS FOR HEPATITIS C

There are at least 11 different FDA-approved antivirals for the treatment of hepatitis C. These include interferon and ribavirin as well as direct acting antivirals (DAA), which include protease polymerase and the NS5A phosphoprotein inhibitors. These are used in various combinations, but usually with at least two different drugs to enhance efficacy and/or reduce the development of resistance. Most of the studied combinations no longer require the use of ribavirin, thereby avoiding its associated anemia. The use of interferon is disappearing, a welcome development to eliminate unpleasant side effects and parenteral treatment. Recommended treatments vary with the genotype of the patient's virus. Genotype 1A, the cause of approximately 70% of cases in the United States is the most difficult to eradicate. The presence of cirrhosis also determines which combination regimen is recommended as does the subtype of genotype 1 (A vs B) and resistance due to prior treatment. Cures, defined as undetectable viral RNA for at least 12 weeks following the completion of treatment, may occur in over 90% of patients. This is referred to as a sustained viral response (SVR) and is 97% to 100% predictive of a cure.

✳ Hepatitis C is now considered curable

ANTIVIRAL RESISTANCE

Viral genomes and their replication, as well as the mechanisms of action of the available antiviral agents, have been intensively studied. Accordingly, an understanding of resistance to antiviral drugs has evolved; investigation of resistance mechanisms has shed light on the function of specific viral genes and the central role of gene mutations. For example, it has become clear that a common mechanism of resistance to nucleosides (eg, acyclovir and ganciclovir) by herpesviruses consists of mutations in the viral-induced enzyme responsible for phosphorylating the nucleoside. For HSV, this is thymidine kinase; for CMV, this gene is designated *UL97*.

✳ Herpesviruses develop resistance by mutations in phosphorylating genes

The likelihood of resistant mutants results from at least four factors:

1. **Rate of viral replication.** Herpesviruses, especially CMV and VZV, do not replicate as rapidly as HIV and hepatitis B and C viruses. Higher rates of replication are associated with higher rates of spontaneous mutations.

2. **Selective pressure of the drug.** The more effective an antiviral is in inhibiting susceptible viruses, the greater opportunity for resistant viruses to replicate.

3. **Rate of viral mutations.** In addition to viral replication, the rate of mutations differs among different viruses. In general, single-stranded RNA viruses (eg, HIV and influenza) have more rapid rates of mutation than double-stranded DNA viruses (eg, HSV).

4. **Rates of mutation in differing viral genes.** For example, within the herpesviruses, the genes for phosphorylating nucleosides (eg, *UL97*) are more susceptible to mutation than the viral DNA polymerase.

Resistance to antiviral agents may be detected in several ways:

• **Phenotypic.** This is the traditional method of growing virus in tissue culture in medium containing increasing concentrations of an antiviral agent. The concentration of the agent that reduces viral replication by 50% is the end point, and is referred to as the inhibitory concentration (IC_{50}). The IC_{50} of resistant virus is higher than that of susceptible virus. The degree of viral replication is obtained by counting viral plaques (ie, equivalent to bacterial "colonies") in the presence of drug versus controls. Other methods include measuring viral

Phenotypic resistance is detected by quantitative methods

✳ Genotypic = molecular
detection of resistance
mutation

**No reduction or increase in
patient's viral burden while
receiving an antiviral suggests
development of resistant
mutants**

antigen or nucleic acid concentration. Unfortunately, phenotypic assays are very time-consuming, requiring days to weeks for completion. IC_{50} values increase as the percentage of the viral population with the mutation increases.

- **Genotypic.** When the exact mutation or deletion responsible for antiviral resistance is known, it is possible to sequence the viral gene or detect it with restriction enzyme patterns. These tests are rapid but require knowledge of the expected mutation, and they do not provide quantitation of the percentage of the viral population harboring the mutation. If only 1% to 5% of the population has the mutation, this result may not be detected.

- **Viral quantitation in response to treatment.** Various methods of quantitating virus (eg, culture, polymerase chain reaction, antigen assay) provide a means of assessing the decline of viral titer in response to treatment with an antiviral agent. These assays are rapid and do not require knowledge of the expected mutation. If no decline occurs despite adequate dosage and compliance, viral resistance may be responsible. Likewise, if viral titer initially decreases but subsequently recurs and/or increases, then resistance may have developed.

KEY CONCLUSIONS

- Antiviral agents are ideally directed against replication events, unique to viruses, for example, attachment and penetration of cells as well as assembly or release of the final viral particle.
- Since only a few replicative events are unique to viruses, many antiviral agents are directed against metabolic events, shared by viruses and cells, for example, synthesis of DNA, RNA, and/or proteins.
- For inhibitors of viral DNA or RNA to be useful, they must be selective, for example, more inhibitory to viral DNA replication than against cellular DNA synthesis.
- Selectivity may be accomplished by using an antiviral which is activated intracellularly by a viral-induced enzyme but not in uninfected cells, for example, acyclovir.
- Selectivity can be obtained by inhibiting metabolic steps, unique to viruses, for example, synthesis of viral RNA via reverse transcription as exhibited by HIV.
- Other "viral unique" enzymes include proteases and integrases.
- Toxicities of antiviral drugs depend on their mechanism of action but are most notable for those which inhibit cellular as well as viral DNA synthesis, for example, ganciclovir.
- Inhibitors of DNA viruses, for example, the herpes viruses have DNA polymerase as their major target.
- RNA viruses are more mutable than DNA viruses, so antivirals for HIV and hepatitis C are usually combined (two or more) to reduce the development of resistance.
- Hepatitis C is considered curable, that is, viral eradication while hepatitis B replication can only be suppressed.
- Antiviral resistance is most readily assayed by genotyping for resistance mutations.

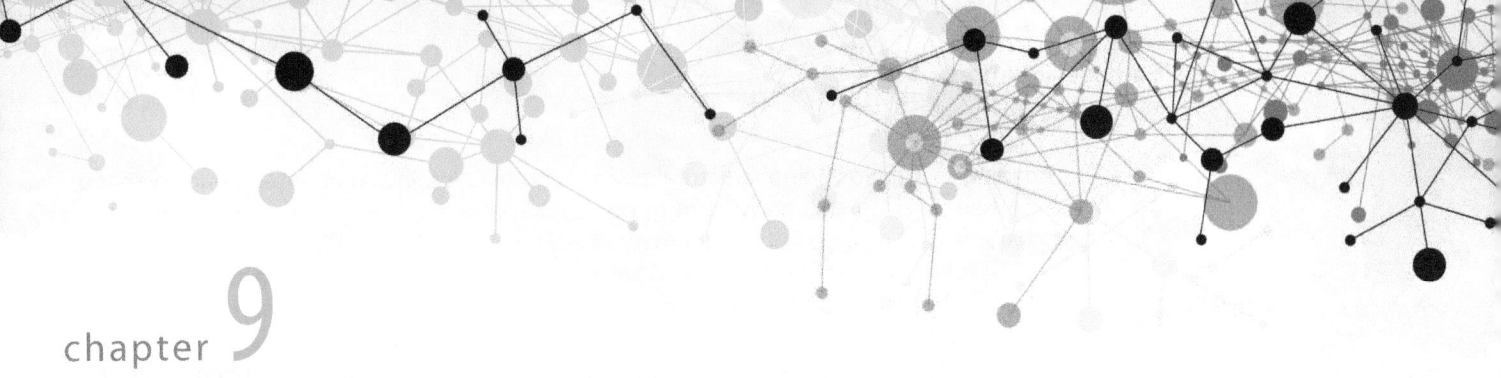

chapter 9

Respiratory Viruses

Influenza Virus · Parainfluenza Virus · Respiratory Syncytial Virus · Coronavirus · SARS-CoV-2 (COVID-19) ·

Human Metapneumovirus · Adenovirus · Rhinovirus · Bocavirus

> *Considering how common illness is, how tremendous the spiritual change that it brings, how astonishing, when the lights of health go down, the undiscovered countries that are then disclosed, what wastes and deserts of the soul a slight attack of influenza brings to view...*
>
> —Virginia Woolf, "On Being Ill"

Respiratory disease accounts for an estimated 75% to 80% of all acute morbidity in the United States, and most of these illnesses (approximately 80%) are viral infections. Although a majority of the episodes may not require medical attention, the overall average is three to four illnesses per year per person. Although the incidence varies inversely with age (ie, greater among younger children than healthy young adults), the morbidity is significantly higher in elderly population. Seasonality is also a feature; incidence is lowest in the summer months and highest in the winter.

The viruses that are major causes of acute respiratory disease (ARD) include influenza viruses, parainfluenza viruses, respiratory syncytial virus (RSV), coronaviruses (including COVID-19), adenoviruses, rhinoviruses, human metapneumovirus (hMPV), and bocaviruses (a member of parvovirus group). Reoviruses can also affect respiratory tract and are included in this chapter. Other viruses, such as enterovirus, measles virus, Epstein-Barr virus (EBV), cytomegalovirus (CMV), varicella-zoster VZV), herpes simplex virus (HSV), and hantavirus, can also cause respiratory symptoms but are discussed in other chapters of their principal diseases.

In addition to the ability to cause a variety of ARD syndromes, this group of viruses discussed in this chapter shares a relatively short incubation period, 1 to 4 days, but some up to 2 weeks and a person-to-person mode of spread. Transmission is direct, by infective droplet nuclei, or indirect, by hand transfer of contaminated secretions to nasal or conjunctival epithelium. These respiratory viral agents are associated with an increased risk of bacterial superinfection of the damaged tissue of the respiratory tract, and all have a worldwide distribution.

✳ Most of morbidity from respiratory diseases

✳ Viruses from different families

✳ Include influenza, parainfluenza, respiratory syncytial virus, human metapneumovirus, coronavirus, rhinovirus

✳ Transmission by droplet nuclei, transfer of secretions

✳ Incubation period 1 to 4 days, up to 14

INFLUENZA VIRUSES

Overview

Three types of influenza viruses (A, B, and C) infect humans. Influenza virus types A and B both cause more severe symptoms than does influenza virus type C. Influenza virus A, which has several subtypes based on hemagglutinin (H) and neuraminidase (N), undergo more genetic changes than types B and C. Influenza viruses are enveloped, helical, negative-sense segmented RNA virus that replicate in the nucleus of the infected cells by using its own viral RNA polymerase. Direct droplet spread is the most common mode of transmission and the incubation is period is about 2 days. The virus multiply in ciliated respiratory epithelial cells,

(Continued)

leading to functional and structural ciliary abnormalities, including interference with the mechanical clearance mechanism of the respiratory tract. The typical influenza illness is characterized by an abrupt onset (over several hours) of fever, diffuse muscle aches, and chills. This is followed within 12 to 36 hours by respiratory symptoms such as rhinitis, fever, myalgia, headache, cough, occasionally shaking chills, respiratory distress. The acute phase usually lasts 3 to 5 days, but a complete return to normal activities may take 2 to 6 weeks. Occasionally, patients develop a progressive viral infection causing viral pneumonia and some unusual manifestations such as CNS dysfunction, myositis, and myocarditis. The most common complication of influenza infection is bacterial superinfection usually resulting in bacterial pneumonia. Influenza virus infection can be prevented by annual vaccination, which is formulated every year because of antigenic drift that allows the virus to escape preexisting immunity from previous vaccination or infection.

 ## INFLUENZA VIRUS GROUP CHARACTERISTICS

* Influenza (orthomyxoviruses), types A, B, and C

* Influenza A has greatest virulence, epidemic predominance

A undergoes more genetic changes because of its existence in several species

* Enveloped, helical, negative segmented RNA viruses

Virus-specific hemagglutinin (H) and neuraminidase (N) spikes expressed on envelope

* Hemagglutinin binds to receptor (sialic acid glycoprotein) on host cell

Influenza viruses are members of the **orthomyxovirus** group or family, which are enveloped, pleomorphic, helical, single-stranded negative-sense segmented RNA viruses. They are classified into three major types, A, B, and C, based on antigenic differences in their ribonucleoprotein (NP) and matrix (M) protein antigens. Influenza A viruses are the most extensively studied because of their predominance in epidemics, and much of the following discussion is based on knowledge of influenza type A virus. They generally cause more severe disease and more extensive epidemics than the other types; naturally infect a wide variety of species, including mammals and birds; and have a great tendency to undergo significant antigenic changes (**Table 9–1**). Influenza B viruses are more antigenically stable, are known to infect humans and seals, and usually occur in more localized outbreaks. Influenza C viruses appear to be relatively minor causes of disease, affecting humans and pigs.

Influenza A and B viruses each consist of a nucleocapsid containing eight segments of negative-sense, **single-stranded RNA,** which is enveloped in a lipid bilayer membrane derived from the host cell plasma membrane. The inner side of the envelope contains a layer of virus-specified matrix protein (M1). Two virus-specified glycoproteins, **hemagglutinin (HA or H)** and **neuraminidase (NA or N),** are embedded in the outer surface of the lipid bilayer envelope and appear as "spikes" over the surface of the virion. The ratio of H to N is generally 4 or 5 to 1. There is another integral membrane protein in influenza A known as M2 ion channel protein. **Figure 9–1** illustrates the makeup of influenza A virus. Influenza B is somewhat similar but has a unique integral membrane protein, NB instead of M2, that is also believed to function as an ion channel. Influenza C differs from the others in that it possesses only seven RNA segments and only one spike protein, hemagglutinin-ester fusion (HEF) glycoprotein, and no neuraminidase and binds to a cell receptor different from that for types A and B.

The virus-specific glycoproteins are antigenic and have special functional importance in pathogenesis and immunity. **Hemagglutinin** has the ability to agglutinate red blood cells from certain species (eg, chickens and guinea pigs) *in vitro*. Its major biologic function is to attach

TABLE 9–1	Differences Among Influenza Viruses		
FEATURE	**INFLUENZA A**	**INFLUENZA B**	**INFLUENZA C**
Gene segments	8	8	7
Unique proteins	M2	NB	HEF
Host range	Humans, swine, avians, equines, marine mammals, bats	Humans, seals	Humans, swine
Disease severity	Often severe	Occasionally severe	Usually mild
Epidemic potential	Extensive; epidemics and pandemics (antigenic drift and shift)	Outbreaks; occasional epidemics (antigenic drift only)	Limited outbreaks (antigenic drift only)

HEF, hemagglutinin esterase fusion; M2, ion channel protein; NB, ion channel protein.

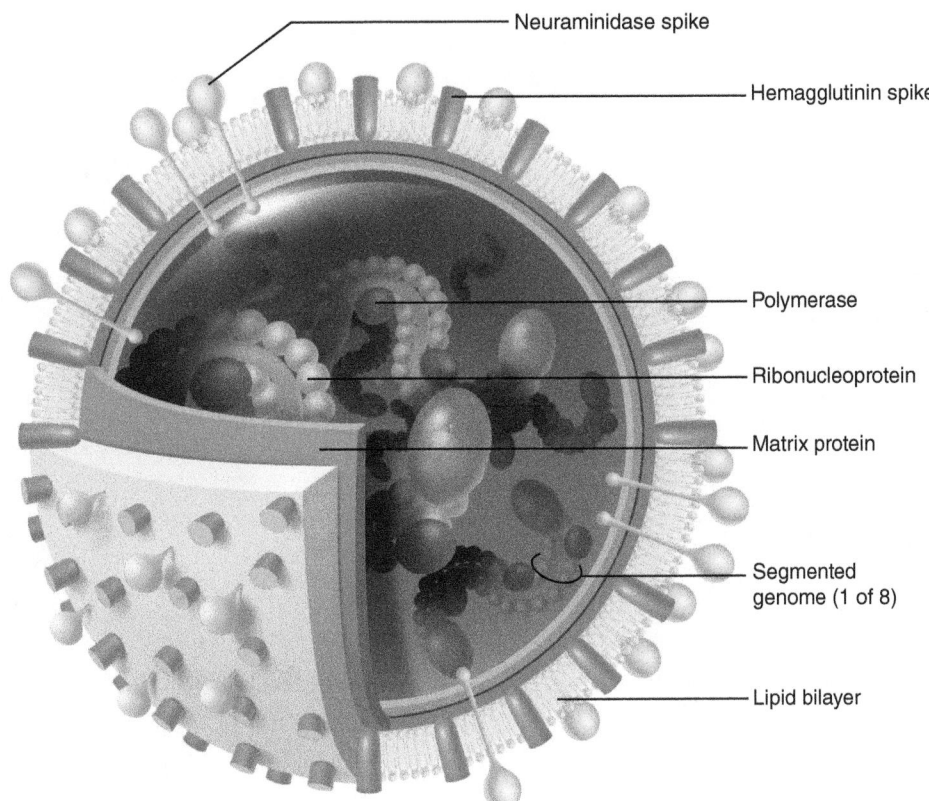

Neuraminidase spike

Hemagglutinin spike

Polymerase

Ribonucleoprotein

Matrix protein

Segmented genome (1 of 8)

Lipid bilayer

FIGURE 9–1. Diagrammatic view of influenza A virus. Three types of membrane proteins are inserted in the lipid bilayer: hemagglutinin (as trimer), neuraminidase (as tetramer), and M2 ion channel protein. The eight ribonucleoproteins segments each contain viral RNA surrounded by nucleoprotein and associated with RNA transcriptase. (Reproduced with permission from Willey JM: *Prescott, Harley, & Klein's Microbiology,* 7th ed. New York, NY: McGraw Hill; 2008.)

to *N*-acetylneuraminic (sialic) acid-only containing glycoprotein or glycolipid receptor sites on human respiratory cell surfaces, which is a critical first step in initiating infection of the cell.

Neuraminidase is an antigenic hydrolytic enzyme that acts on the hemagglutinin receptors by splitting off their terminal neuraminic (sialic) acid. The result is destruction of receptor activity, which may help in preventing superinfection or aggregation of virus particle in the infected cell. Neuraminidase serves several functions. It may inactivate a free mucoprotein receptor substance in respiratory secretions that could otherwise bind to viral hemagglutinin and prevent access of the virus to the cell surface. More importantly, neuraminidase aids in the release of newly formed virus particles from infected cells. The newly formed virus particles aggregate on the cell surface by attaching to sialic acid through their hemagglutinins, but neuraminidase removes the sialic acid from the cell surface receptor allowing the virus to be released and infect other cells. Type-specific antibodies to neuraminidase appear to inhibit the spread of virus in the infected host and to limit the amount of virus released from host cells.

Figure 9–2 illustrates the replication cycle of influenza virus. After viral entry in the cytoplasm of the host cells, nucleocapsids (viral RNA-protein complex) with viral RNA-dependent RNA polymerase complex (PB2, PB1, PA—see **Table 9–2**) move into the nucleus for transcription and replication (unique to RNA viruses). The priming of viral mRNA transcription is done by using host capped RNA primers, whereas viral RNA synthesis is performed by viral RNA-dependent RNA polymerase. Viral mRNAs are transported in the cytoplasm for protein synthesis followed by proteins translocation at various sites such as H and N on cell surface and nucleocapsid in the nucleus. Viral genomic (–) RNAs replication is carried out by viral RNA polymerase via positive-sense RNA intermediates followed by nucleocapsids assembly.

Nucleocapsids assembly takes place in the cell nucleus, but final virus assembly takes place at the plasma membrane. The ribonucleoproteins are enveloped by the plasma membrane, which by then contains hemagglutinin and neuraminidase. Virus "buds" are formed, and intact virions are released from the cell surface (Figure 9–2).

Influenza A viruses were initially isolated in 1933 by intranasal inoculation of ferrets, which developed febrile respiratory illnesses. The viruses replicate in the amniotic sac of embryonated hen's eggs, where their presence can be detected by the hemagglutination test. Most strains can

✳ Neuraminidase promotes passage by inactivating mucoprotein receptors in respiratory secretions

✳ Neuraminidase has major role in viral release from infected cells

Neuraminidase destroys viral receptor, preventing aggregation, superinfection

✳ Viral mRNA transcription and genomic RNA replication occur in the nucleus by using viral RNA polymerase and host cell RNA primers

✳ Nucleocapsids assemble in the nucleus and virus assembly occurs in the cytoplasm through budding from the plasma membrane

Viral propagation and isolation in eggs and mammalian cell cultures

1 The endonuclease activity of the PB1 protein cleaves the cap and about 10 nucleotides from the 5′ end of host mRNA (cap snatching). The fragment is used to prime viral mRNA synthesis by the RNA-dependent RNA polymerase activity of the PB1 protein.

2 Viral mRNA is translated. Early products include more NP and PB1 proteins.

3 RNA polymerase activity of the PB1 protein synthesizes +ssRNA from genomic −ssRNA molecules.

4 RNA polymerase activity of the PB1 protein synthesizes new copies of the genome using +ssRNA made in step 3 as templates. Some of these new genome segments serve as templates for the synthesis of more viral mRNA. Later in the infection, they will become progeny genomes.

5 Viral mRNA molecules transcribed from other genome segments encode structural proteins such as hemagglutinin (HA) and neuraminidase (NA). These messages are translated by ER-associated ribosomes and delivered to the cell membrane.

6 Viral genome segments are packaged as progeny virions bud from the host cell.

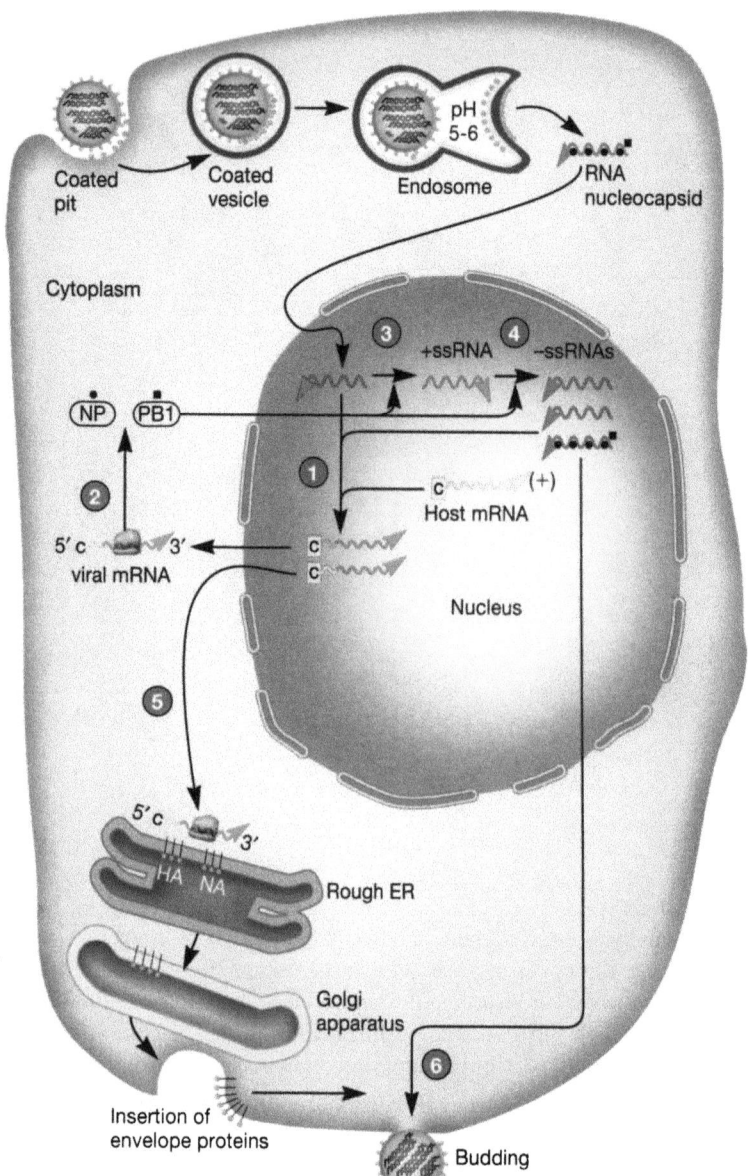

FIGURE 9–2. Diagrammatic view of influenza virus life cycle. (Reproduced with permission from Willey JM: *Prescott, Harley, & Klein's Microbiology*, 7th ed. New York, NY: McGraw Hill; 2008.)

TABLE 9–2	Virus-Coded Proteins of Influenza A	
RNA SEGMENT	**PROTEINS**	**FUNCTION**
1	PB2—Polymerase component	RNA synthesis, virulence
2	PB1—Polymerase component	RNA synthesis
3	PA—Polymerase component	RNA synthesis
4	HA—Hemagglutinin	Viral attachment
5	NP—Nucleocapsid	RNA synthesis, binds to RNA
6	NA—Neuraminidase	Virus release from infected cells
7	M1, M2—Matrix protein	Matrix, ion channel
8	NS1, NS2—Nonstructural proteins	NS1 is interferon antagonist

also be readily isolated in cell culture systems, such as primary monkey kidney cells. Some cause cytopathic effects in culture.

The most efficient method of detection is demonstration of hemadsorption by adherence of erythrocytes to infected cells expressing hemagglutinin or by agglutination of erythrocytes by virus already released into the extracellular fluid. The virus can then be identified specifically by inhibition of these properties by addition of antibody directed specifically against hemagglutinin. This method is called **hemadsorption inhibition** or **hemagglutination inhibition (HI)**, depending on whether the test is conducted on infected cells or on extracellular viruses, respectively. Because the hemagglutinin is antigenic, HI tests can also be used to detect antibodies in infected subjects. Research has shown that antibody directed against specific hemagglutinin is highly effective in neutralizing the infectivity of the virus.

Hemadsorption and hemagglutination inhibition used to detect virus

Antibodies to hemagglutinin detectable in patients' serum

Hemagglutination inhibition used to detect antibodies

■ Influenza A

Influenza A is considered in detail because of its great clinical and epidemiologic importance.

The influenza A virion contains eight segments of negative-sense, single-stranded RNA with defined genetic responsibilities. These functions include coding for virus-specified proteins (Figure 9–1; Table 9–2). A unique aspect of influenza A viruses is their ability to develop a wide variety of subtypes through the processes of **mutation** and whole-gene "swapping" between strains, called **reassortment.** Recombination, which occurs when new genes are assembled from sections of other genes, is thought to occur rarely, if at all. These processes result in antigenic changes called **drifts** (mutation) and **shifts** (reassortment or recombination), which are discussed shortly.

The 18 recognized subtypes of hemagglutinin (H) and 11 neuraminidase (N) subtypes known to exist among influenza A viruses that circulate in birds and mammals represent a reservoir of viral genes that can undergo reassortment or "mixing" with human strains. All subtypes of H and N have been found among aquatic birds, except H17N10 and H18N11 that have been identified only in bats. In other animals, pigs are generally infected with two major hemagglutinins (H1 and H3) and two neuraminidases (N1 and N2) and horses with two H (H3 and H7) and two N (N7 and N8), although H2, H4, H5, and H10 have been identified in pigs. Three hemagglutinins (**H1, H2, and H3**) and two neuraminidases (**N1 and N2**) appear to be of greatest importance in **human infections,** although other subtypes have also been identified such as H5-H7, H9-H10, and N6-N9. These major subtypes H1-H3 and N1-N2 are designated according to the H and N antigens on their surface (eg, H1N1, H3N2). There may also be more subtle, but sometimes important, antigenic differences (drifts) within each subtype. These differences are designated according to the major representative virus to which they are most closely related antigenically, using the place of initial isolation, number of the isolate, and year of detection. For example, two H3N2 strains that differ antigenically only slightly are A/Texas/1/77(H3N2) and A/Bangkok/1/79(H3N2).

Antigenic drifts within major subtypes can involve either H or N antigens, as well as the genes encoding other structural and nonstructural proteins, and may result from as little as a single or several mutations in the viral RNA. These mutations are caused by viral RNA polymerase enzyme because it lacks proofreading ability. The mutant may come to predominate under selective immunologic pressures in the host population (**Figure 9–3**). Such drifts are common among influenza A viruses, occurring every year to every few years and sometimes more even during a single epidemic. In addition, drifts can develop in influenza B viruses but considerably less frequently.

In contrast to the frequently occurring mutations that cause antigenic drift among influenza A strains, major changes (>50%) in the nucleotide sequences of the H or N genes can occur suddenly and unpredictably. These are referred to as antigenic shifts. Figure 9–3 illustrates the difference between antigenic drifts and shifts. When "new" epidemic strains emerge, they most likely have circulated into animal or avian reservoirs, where they have undergone genetic reassortment (and also mutations) and then are readapted and spread to human hosts when a sufficient proportion of the population has little or no immunity to the "new" subtypes. An example was the appearance of avian influenza A (H5N1) virus in Hong Kong in 1997 that caused infection in humans. The majority of human infections occurred in people below 40 years of age and the highest mortality was in young adults. The global spread of avian influenza (H5N1 and others) continued through 1997 and onward with several more cases every year. Studies indicated that all RNA segments were derived from an avian influenza A virus, but a single insert coding for several additional amino acids in the hemagglutinin protein facilitated cleavage by human cellular

✳ Virus has 8 negative-sense RNA segments each encoding at least one protein

✳ Mutation (antigenic drift) and reassortment (antigenic shift) produce antigenic changes

A virus subtypes based on 18 subtypes of H and 11 N in various species

✳ Three subtypes of H (H1-H3), two subtypes of N (N1-N2) in humans

✳ Subtle changes during antigenic drift (mutation) occurs in all strains

✳ Drastic changes antigenic shift (reassortment) occurs when closely related strains infect the same cell

✳ Antigenic drift occurs every year to few years with influenza A

✳ Antigenic shift occurs abruptly and unpredictably

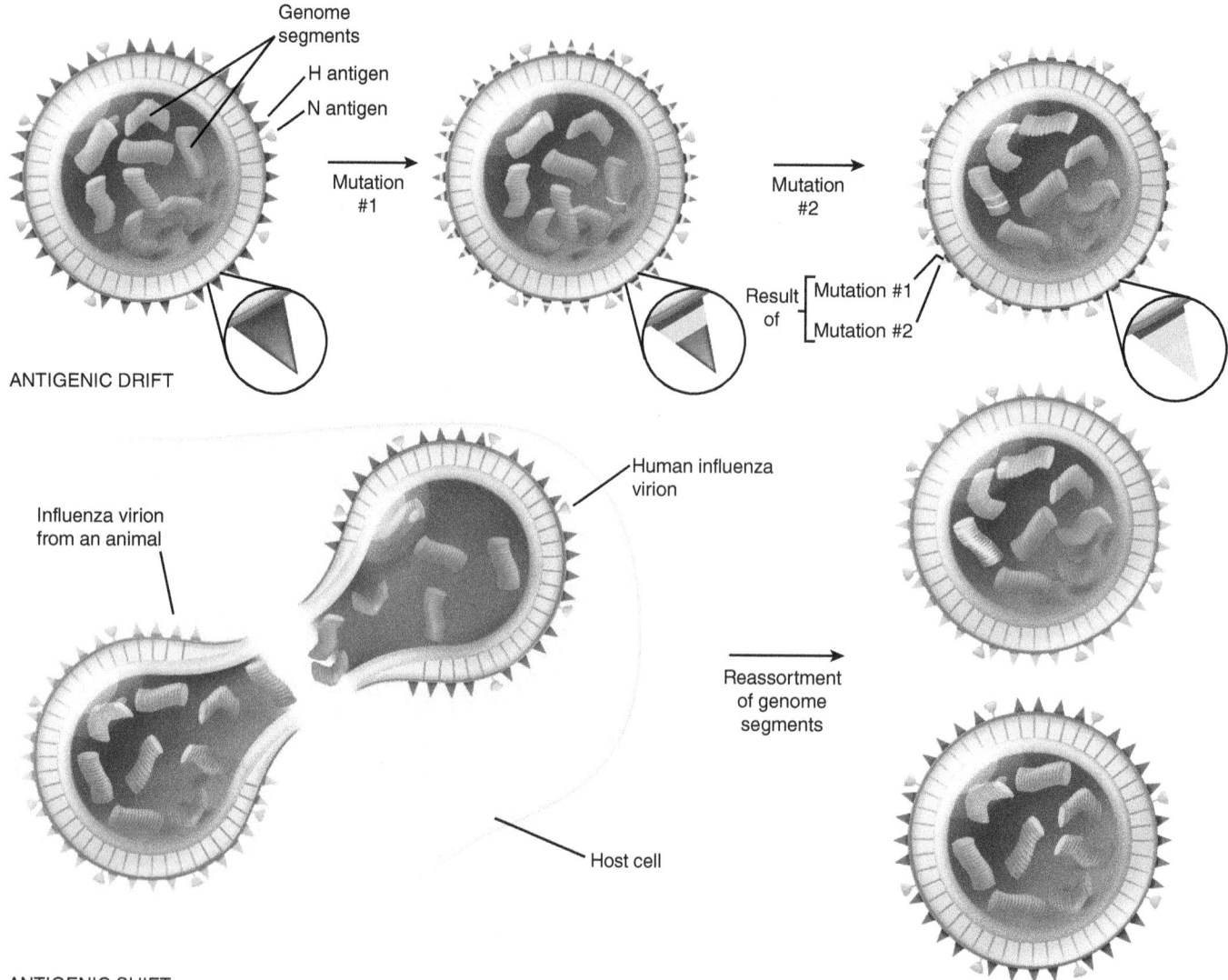

Genome
segments

H antigen

N antigen

Mutation
#1

Mutation
#2

Result
of
Mutation #1
Mutation #2

ANTIGENIC DRIFT

Influenza virion
from an animal

Human influenza
virion

Reassortment
of genome
segments

Host cell

ANTIGENIC SHIFT

FIGURE 9–3. Influenza virus: antigenic drift and antigenic shift. With drift, repeated mutations cause a gradual change in the antigens composing hemagglutinin, such that antibody against the original virus becomes progressively less effective. With shift, there is an abrupt, major change in the hemagglutinin antigens because the virus acquires a new genome segment, which in this case codes for hemagglutinin. Changes in neuraminidase could occur by the same mechanism. (Reproduced with permission from Nester EW, Anderson DG, Roberts CE Jr, et al: *Microbiology: A Human Perspective*, 6th ed. New York, NY: McGraw Hill; 2008.)

Newly generated subtypes of influenza virus also develop mutations

H5N1 infected fewer people but the fatality was 60%

enzymes. In addition, a single amino acid substitution in the PB2 polymerase protein occurred. These two mutations together made the virus more virulent for humans; fortunately, human-to-human transmission was poor as discussed further. In 2006, the WHO reported a highly mutating and pathogenic new strain of H5N1 in several bird species in Asia, Africa, and Europe. H5N1 infected humans who were in close contacts with poultry and birds with several cases with high fatality in many countries. In the past several years, 700 cases of H5N1 in humans with 60% fatality have been reported worldwide, including a case in Canada in 2014 in a traveler returning from China. A recent example is the emergence of swine influenza virus (H1N1) in Mexico and the southwestern United States in 2009 that contained segments from avian, human, and swine influenza A viruses (named as H1N1pdm09 virus), and was easily transmitted to humans and caused a severe disease, mainly in young immune-competent adults, including deaths. From April 2009 to April 2010, Centers for Disease Control and Prevention (CDC) estimated 60.8 million cases of (H1N1)pdm09, 274,304 hospitalizations, and 12,469 deaths mostly in young adults in the United States. Globally, the number of estimated cases were between 700 million and 1.4 billion and deaths were estimated between 151,700 and 575,400. Since then, (H1N1)pdm09 has been circulating every year and has been included in annual influenza vaccination starting from 2010 onwards. In 2013, a new strain of avian flu (H7N9) infected humans in eastern China resulting in severe illness, including deaths. H7N9 has been found in chickens, ducks, and pigeons in live poultry markets in eastern China. H7N9 continues to cause infections and deaths in humans in China even in 2017. There is no solid evidence of human-to-human transmission because most of the infected people had contacts with sick poultry. Based on genetic analysis, H7N9 is responsive to neuraminidase inhibitors and that the virus has acquired some mutations that may allow it to infect mammals and humans. A group of H1N1 swine viruses with features of being adapted to humans have been circulating in pigs in China since 2016 and has the pandemic potential.

Additional molecular barriers limit human-to-human transmission of avian influenza virus (H5N1). One of the most important barriers is that avian and human influenza viruses target different regions of the human respiratory tract. Although the receptor for influenza viruses is sialic acid (SA) glycoprotein, there is a major difference in the sialic acid sugar positions with SA α 2,6 galactose for human influenza virus and SA α 2,3 galactose for avian influenza virus H5N1. Human influenza virus receptor, SA α 2,6 galactose, is dominant on epithelial cells of nasal mucosa, paranasal sinuses, pharynx, trachea, and bronchi, whereas the H5N1 receptor SA α 2,3 galactose is mainly found on nonciliated bronchiolar cells at the junction between respiratory bronchioles and alveolus. It is interesting that A/Hong Kong/213/03 (H5N1) isolated from a patient recognized both SA α 2,6 galactose and SA α 2,3 galactose are bound extensively to both bronchial and alveolar cells. More importantly, H1N1 swine influenza of 2009 was transmitted from human-to-human easily because it binds to the receptor SA α 2,6 galactose found in the upper respiratory tract, and caused greater severity because it infected the lower portion of the lungs by interacting with the receptor SA α 2,3 galactose.

Major antigenic shifts, which occurred approximately every 8 to 10 years in the 20th century, often resulted in serious epidemics or pandemics among populations with little or no preexisting antibody to the new subtypes. Examples include the appearance of an H1N1 subtype in 1947, followed by an abrupt shift to an H2N2 strain in 1957, which caused the pandemic of Asian flu. A subsequent major shift in 1968 to an H3N2 subtype (the Hong Kong flu) led to another, but somewhat less severe, epidemic. The Russian flu, which appeared in late 1977, was caused by an H1N1 subtype very similar to that which dominated between 1947 and 1957 (**Table 9–3**). The swine flu that appeared in April 2009, in Mexico and southwestern United States was a previously unrecognized H1N1 strain, which caused a severe acute respiratory distress syndrome, including deaths, especially in young, healthy immune-competent adults. Further analysis revealed that H1N1 swine influenza virus of 2009 was a reassortant that contained genetic components from four different flu viruses—North American swine influenza, North American avian influenza, human influenza, and swine influenza virus of Eurasian origin. Over the subsequent 3 months, this strain, designated H1N1 swine-origin 2009 A (H1N1)pdm09 rapidly spread globally. Fortunately, the pandemic tapered down in the following seasons. So, the key requirements for a pandemic influenza strain are: (1) generation of a new influenza A subtype, (2) causing a serious illness, and (3) easily transmitted from human to human. Although two of these three requirements were met in 2006 by H5N1, all these three prerequisites were fulfilled in 2009 by H1N1 swine. Each new human infection is an opportunity for the virus to change.

H1N1 swine of 2009 caused pandemic, 60 million cases, 12,000 deaths in the United States

H1N1 and H5N1 target regions of respiratory tract

H1N1 receptors dominant in upper respiratory tract

H5N1 receptors in lower respiratory tract

H1N1 (swine) interacts with receptors in upper and lower tract

✳ Major antigenic shifts correlate with serious epidemics or pandemics

TABLE 9–3	Major Antigenic Shifts Associated With Influenza A Pandemics, 1947-2009	
YEAR	SUBTYPE	PROTOTYPE STRAIN
1918	H1N1	A (contained avian influenza genes)
1947	H1N1	A/FM1/47
1957	H2N2	A/Singapore/57
1968	H3N2	A/Hong Kong/68
1977	H1N1	A/USSR/77
1987	H3N2	No pandemic occurred; various strains of H1N1 and H3N2 continue circulating worldwide through 2008
2009	H1N1	A new pandemic swine-origin H1N1 originated from Mexico followed by spread to southwestern United States

The concepts of antigenic shift and drift in human influenza A virus infections can be approximately summarized as follows. Periodic shifts in the major antigenic components appear, usually resulting in major epidemics in populations with little or no immunologic experience with the subtype. As the population of susceptible individuals is exhausted (ie, subtype-specific immunity is acquired by increasing numbers of people), the subtype continues to circulate for a time, undergoing mutations with subtle antigenic drifts from season to season. This allows some degree of virus transmission to continue. Infectivity persists because subtype-specific immunity is not entirely protective against drifting strains; for example, an individual may have antibodies reasonably protective against influenza A/Texas/77(H3N2), yet be susceptible in succeeding years to reinfection by influenza A/Bangkok/79(H3N2). Eventually, however, the overall immunity of the population becomes sufficient to minimize the epidemic potential of the major subtype and its drifting strains. Unfortunately, the battle is never entirely won; the scene is set for the sudden and usually unpredictable appearance of an entirely new subtype that may not have circulated among humans for 20 years or more. One example we saw in 2009 was when an H1N1 swine influenza virus appeared that had not been seen previously, and the existing population had no immunity to its components.

Minor antigenic drifts allow influenza virus maintenance in population

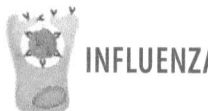

INFLUENZA

EPIDEMIOLOGY

Humans are the major hosts of the influenza viruses, and severe respiratory disease is the primary manifestation of infection. However, influenza A viruses closely related to those prevalent in humans circulate among many mammalian and avian species. As noted previously, some of these may undergo antigenic mutation or genetic recombination (reassortment) and emerge as new human epidemic strains.

✳ **Human, animal, and avian strains similar but may have differences in receptor specificities**

 Why does influenza virus A possess the ability to generate new strains?

Characteristic influenza outbreaks have been described since the early 16th century, and outbreaks of varying severity have occurred nearly every year. Severe pandemics occurred in 1743, 1889-1890, 1918-1919 (the Spanish flu), 1957-1958 (the Asian flu), 1968-1969 (Hong Kong flu), 1977-1978 (Russian flu), and 2009-2010 (Swine flu). Several of these episodes were associated with particularly high mortality rates; the Spanish flu was thought to have caused at least 30 to 50 million deaths, and some historians estimate the worldwide toll was closer to 100 million deaths. Usually, the elderly and persons of any age group with cardiac or pulmonary disease have the highest death rate. However, the severity in the 2009 swine flu pandemic was mainly seen among the young, healthy adult population, although the fatality rate was low.

Pandemic influenza generally has high mortality

Globally, the WHO estimates 1 billion cases, 3 to 5 million severe cases, and 290,000 to 650,000 influenza-related deaths every year. In the United States, the burden of influenza diseases has varied widely due to several factors, including the virulence of influenza strains, the number of people vaccinated and the efficacy of influenza vaccine. The CDC estimates 9 to 45 million influenza cases, 140,000 to 810,000 hospitalizations, and 12,000 to 61,000 influenza-related deaths annually in the United States since 2010. The 2011-2012 influenza season reported 9.3 million cases and 12,000 deaths, whereas 2017-2018 season reported 45 million cases and 61,000 deaths. The 2019-2020 season estimated 38 million cases and 22,000 deaths in the United States.

Globally, 1 billion cases and 290,000-650,000 deaths annually

In the United States, 36 to 45 million cases and 22,000-61,000 deaths annually

 Think ▸▸ Apply 9-1: Because influenza A virus exists in multiple subtypes such as H1N1, H3N2, etc. in several species. Two subtypes may infect the same cell of a host such as pig or humans followed by replication and reassortment (antigenic shift) to generate more than 250 combinations. Antigenic drift may also occur in these new subtypes.

Direct droplet spread is the most common mode of transmission. Influenza infections in temperate climates tend to occur most frequently during midwinter months. Major epidemics of influenza A usually occur at 2- to 3-year intervals, and influenza B epidemics occur irregularly, usually every 4 to 5 years. The typical epidemic develops over a period of 3 to 6 weeks, and can involve 10% of the population. Illness rates may exceed 30% among school-aged children, residents of closed institutions, and industrial groups. One major indicator of influenza virus activity is an abrupt rise in school or industrial absenteeism. In severe influenza A epidemics, the number of deaths reported in a given area of the country often exceeds the number expected for that period. This significant increase, referred to as **excess mortality,** is another indicator of severe, widespread illness. Influenza B rarely causes such severe epidemics. In general, human influenza viruses are not stable in the environment and are sensitive to heat, acid pH, and solvents. In contrast, avian influenza viruses (H5N1 and others) retain infectivity for several weeks outside the host. The avian virus is shed in respiratory secretions and feces, and the virus survives in the feces for a long time.

> Winter months allow influenza virus to survive longer in the environment
>
> Epidemic intervals usually a few years
>
> Excess mortality or increased absenteeism indicators of epidemics

PATHOGENESIS

Influenza viruses are transmitted by direct infective droplet spread and have a predilection for the respiratory tract because of the presence of their receptors. They multiply in ciliated respiratory epithelial cells, leading to functional and structural ciliary abnormalities and viremia is rarely detected. This is accompanied by a switch-off of protein and nucleic acid synthesis in the affected cells, the release of lysosomal hydrolytic enzymes, and desquamation of both ciliated and mucus-producing epithelial cells. Thus, there is substantial interference with the mechanical clearance mechanism of the respiratory tract. The process of programmed cell death (apoptosis) results in the cleavage of complement components, leading to localized inflammation. Early in infection, the primary chemotactic stimulus is directed toward mononuclear leukocytes, which constitute the major cellular inflammatory component. The respiratory epithelium may not be restored to normal for 2 to 10 weeks after the initial insult.

> ✳ Virus multiplies in upper respiratory tract ciliated epithelial cells
>
> ✳ Inhibition of host cell syntheses and release of lysosomal enzymes
>
> ✳ Desquamation of ciliated and mucous producing cells
>
> ✳ Clearance mechanisms of respiratory tract compromised

The virus particles are also toxic to tissues. This toxicity can be demonstrated by inoculating high concentrations of inactivated virions into mice, which produces acute inflammatory changes in the absence of viral penetration or replication within cells. Other host cell functions are also severely impaired, particularly during the acute phase of infection. These functions include chemotactic, phagocytic, and intracellular killing functions of polymorphonuclear leukocytes and, perhaps, of alveolar macrophage activity.

> Viral toxicity causes inflammation
>
> Phagocytic host defenses compromised

The net result of these effects is that, on entry into the respiratory tract, the viruses cause cell damage, especially in the respiratory epithelium, which elicits an acute inflammatory response and impairs mechanical and cellular host responses. This damage renders the host highly susceptible to invasive bacterial **superinfection.** *In vitro* studies also suggest that bacterial pathogens such as staphylococci can more readily adhere to the surfaces of influenza virus-infected cells. Recovery from infection begins with interferon (α/β) production, which limits further virus replication, and with rapid generation of natural killer cells. Shortly thereafter, class I major histocompatibility complex (MHC)-restricted cytotoxic T cells appear in large numbers to participate in the lysis of virus-infected cells and, thus, in initial control of the infection. This is followed by the appearance of local and humoral antibody together with an evolving, more durable cellular immunity. Finally, there is repair of tissue damage.

> Tissue damage creates susceptibility to bacterial invasion
>
> Interferon and cytotoxic T-cell responses associated with recovery

 Why is clearance mechanism of respiratory tract compromised in influenza virus infection?

IMMUNITY

Although cell-mediated immune responses are undoubtedly important in influenza virus infections, humoral immunity has been investigated more extensively. Typically, patients respond to infection within a few days by producing antibodies directed toward the group ribonucleoprotein antigen, the hemagglutinin, and the neuraminidase. Peak antibody titer levels are usually reached within 2 weeks of onset and then gradually wane over the following months to varying low levels. Antibody to the ribonucleoprotein appears to confer little or no protection against reinfection because it is an internal protein of the virus particle that cannot be recognized by the circulating antibody. Antibody to hemagglutinin (H) is considered the most protective; it has the ability to neutralize the virus on reexposure because it is a surface protein of the virus and easily recognized by the antibody. However, such immunity is relative, and quantitative differences in responsiveness exist among individuals. Furthermore, antigenic shifts and drifts often allow the virus to subvert the antibody response on subsequent exposures. Antibody to neuraminidase antigen is not as protective as antibody to hemagglutinin, but plays a role in limiting virus spread within the host.

* Antibody to hemagglutinin has protective effect

Antibody to neuraminidase may limit viral spread

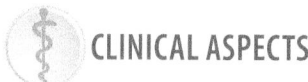 **CLINICAL ASPECTS**

MANIFESTATIONS

Influenza A and B viruses tend to cause the most severe illnesses, whereas influenza C seems to occur infrequently and generally causes milder disease. The typical acute influenza syndrome is described here.

The incubation period is brief, lasting an average of 2 (1-4) days. Onset is usually abrupt, with symptoms developing over a few hours. These include fever, myalgia, headache, and occasionally shaking chills. Within 6 to 12 hours, the illness reaches its maximum severity, and a dry, nonproductive cough develops. The acute findings persist, sometimes with worsening cough, for 3 to 5 days, followed by gradual improvement. By about 1 week after onset, patients feel significantly better. However, fatigue, nonspecific weakness, and cough can remain frustrating lingering problems for an additional 2 to 6 weeks.

Occasionally, patients develop a progressive infection that involves the tracheobronchial tree and lungs. In these situations, pneumonia, which can be lethal, is the result. Other unusual acute manifestations of influenza include central nervous system dysfunction, myositis, and myocarditis. In infants and children, a serious complication known as Reye syndrome may develop 2 to 12 days after onset of the infection. It is characterized by severe fatty infiltration of the liver and by cerebral edema. This syndrome is associated not only with influenza viruses but with a wide variety of systemic viral illnesses. The risk is greatly enhanced by exposure to salicylates, such as aspirin.

The most common and important complication of influenza virus infection is **bacterial super-infection**. Such infections usually involve the lung, but bacteremia with secondary seeding of distant sites can also occur. The superinfection, which can develop at any time in the acute or convalescent phase of the disease, is often heralded by an abrupt worsening of the patient's condition after initial stabilization. The bacteria most commonly involved include *Streptococcus pneumoniae*, *Haemophilus influenzae*, and *Staphylococcus aureus*.

In summation, there are essentially three ways in which influenza may cause death:

* Short incubation period

Symptoms include fever, myalgia, headache, dry cough

* Gradual improvement in 1 week, residual, lingering problems 2-6 weeks

* Progressive infection may lead to lethal pneumonia

* Reye syndrome, a serious complication, may develop 2 to 12 days after infection

* Sudden worsening of symptoms suggests bacterial superinfection

* Bacterial superinfection includes *S pneumoniae*, *H influenzae*, *S aureus*

Underlying disease with decompensation. Individuals with limited cardiovascular or pulmonary reserves can be further compromised by any respiratory infection. Thus, the elderly and those of any age with underlying chronic cardiac or pulmonary disease are at particular risk.

Superinfection. Superinfection can lead to bacterial pneumonia and, occasionally, disseminated bacterial infection.

Direct rapid progression. Less commonly, progression of the viral infection can lead to overwhelming viral pneumonia with asphyxia with seasonal influenza virus. However, this phenomenon has been seen most commonly in severe pandemics; for example, the Spanish flu in 1918-1919 often produced fulminant death in healthy young soldiers and H5N1 in 2006, and H1N1 swine flu pandemic in 2009 also caused a severe disease (viral pneumonia due to cytokine storm) and fatality in young immunocompetent people.

 Think ▸▸ Apply 9-2: **Because the ciliated epithelial cells are damaged leading to loss of the functions of cilia.**

Clinical manifestations of avian flu (H5N1) and swine flu (H1N1) varied with high fever, respiratory symptoms, neurologic symptoms, lymphopenia, and diarrhea. The virus replicated in the lower portion of the lung via interacting with the SA α 2,3 galactose receptor resulting in primary viral pneumonia in the absence of any secondary bacterial infection, including deaths, especially in healthy young adults. The cause of death was believed to be related to systemic dissemination, alveolar flooding, Na+ channel blockage, and **cytokine storm** (see Figure 7–5).

 Why is H5N1, avian flu virus, not easily transmitted to humans?

DIAGNOSIS

During the acute phase of illness, influenza viruses can be readily detected or isolated from respiratory tract specimens, such as nasopharyngeal, nasal, and throat swabs. However, nasopharyngeal specimens typically have higher yield of virus than nasal or throat swabs. Various diagnostic tests, including virus culture, serology, rapid antigen and molecular (viral nucleic acid) assays, immunofluorescence, and reverse transcription polymerase chain reaction (RT-PCR) are available. However, the widely and most often used diagnostic tests are **molecular assays** (rapid viral RNA assay, RT-PCR, and other nucleic acid amplification tests) and **antigen detection tests** (rapid viral antigen test by immunoassay and immunofluorescence assay). The rapid antigen and RNA assays take about 15 to 20 minutes, rapid immunofluorescence (antigen) assay 1 to 4 hours, real-time RT-PCR takes 1 to 8 hours, and virus culture takes 3 to 10 days. These tests detect both influenza A and B viruses. To detect a specific influenza A virus subtype such as (H1N1)pdm09 or H3N2, specific RT-PCR tests are performed. Nucleic acid–based BioFire test for 14 to 19 respiratory pathogens include influenza A and B viruses. Virus culture is done in cell lines because most strains grow in primary monkey kidney cell cultures, and they can be detected by hemadsorption or hemagglutination. Serologic diagnosis (antibody test) is of considerable help epidemiologically and is usually made by demonstrating a fourfold or greater increase in HI antibody titers in acute and convalescent specimens collected 10 to 14 days apart. For details about the HI assay, see Chapter 4.

* Rapid viral antigen detection by immunoassay and RNA by RT-PCR often used

* Virus can be cultured in cell lines

Antibody diagnosis useful epidemiologically

TREATMENT

The two basic approaches to management of influenza disease are symptomatic care and anticipation of potential complications, particularly bacterial superinfection. After the diagnosis has been made, rest, adequate fluid intake, conservative use of analgesics for myalgia and headache, and antitussives for severe cough are commonly prescribed. It must be emphasized that nonprescription drugs must be used with caution. This applies particularly to drugs containing salicylates (aspirin) given to children, because the risk of Reye syndrome must be considered.

Supportive therapy indicated

Bacterial superinfection is often suggested by a rapid worsening of clinical symptoms after patients have initially stabilized. Antibiotic prophylaxis has not been shown to enhance or diminish the likelihood of superinfection, but can increase the risk of acquisition of more resistant bacterial flora in the respiratory tract and make the superinfection more difficult to treat. Ideally, physicians should instruct patients regarding the natural history of the influenza virus infection and be prepared to respond quickly to bacterial complications, if they occur, with specific diagnosis and therapy.

Antibiotic prophylaxis does not prevent bacterial superinfection

Four antiviral agents, including three neuraminidase inhibitors and one cap-dependent endonuclease inhibitor, are approved by FDA for use against influenza viruses' infection (**Table 9–4**). The neuraminidase inhibitors are oseltamivir (Tamiflu), zanamivir (Relenza), and peramivir (Rapivab) and cap-dependent endonuclease inhibitor is baloxavir marboxil (Xofluza). These neuraminidase inhibitors block the function of neuraminidase enzyme of both influenza A and B viruses, which is required for viral release, spread, and infectivity. The mechanism of action of these neuraminidase inhibitors is to competitively inhibit the function of the viral neuraminidase

 Think ▸▸ Apply 9-3: H5N1 is not easily transmitted to humans because its receptor (SA α 2, 3 galactose) is not expressed on cells of upper respiratory tract but found in cells of lower respiratory tract.

TABLE 9–4   Comparison of Antiviral Drugs for Influenza

FEATURE	AMANTADINE* RIMANTADINE*	OSELTAMIVIR	ZANAMIVIR	PERAMIVIR	BALOXAVIR
Susceptible viruses	Influenza A only	Influenza A and B	Influenza A and B	Influenza A and B	Influenza A and B
Administration	Oral	Oral	Inhalation	Intravenous	Oral
Treatment age group	≥ 1 year	≥ 2 weeks	≥ 7 years	≥ 2 years	≥ 12 years
Chemoprophylaxis age group	≥ 1 year	≥ 3 months	≥ 5 years	Not recommended	≥12 years
Mechanism	M2 inhibitor	N inhibitor	N inhibitor	N inhibitor	Endo inhibitor
Emergent resistant strains	Yes (++++)	Yes (+)	Yes (+)	?	?

*Amantadine and *Rimantadine not recommended for use due to resistance. N, Neuraminidase; Endo, Endonuclease cap-dependent; + indicates the severity of resistance.

enzyme. As neuraminidase removes sialic acid from the glycoprotein receptors, the inhibitors do not cleave sialic acid residues on the surfaces of host cells and influenza viral envelopes. Therefore, viral hemagglutinin (H) binds to the uncleaved sialic acid residues, resulting in viral aggregation at the surface of the host cell and inhibition of virus release and reinfection of uninfected cells. These drugs are effective in reducing the severity of influenza virus if taken within 48 hours of the onset of illness. Oseltamivir is taken orally and recommended for treatment in subjects 2 weeks and older, and chemoprophylaxis in 1 year and older. Zanamivir is recommended for treatment in subjects 7 years and older, and chemoprophylaxis in 5 years and older. Zanamivir that is administered as oral inhalation is not recommended for people with underlying respiratory disease. Peramivir is an injectable antiviral recommended for treatment in subjects 2 years and older, but not approved for prophylaxis. Baloxavir is an oral antiviral drug recommended for treatment in people 5 years and older and approved for postexposure prophylaxis at 12 years and older. Baloxavir is a cap-dependent endonuclease inhibitor that interferes with viral RNA transcription and blocks viral replication. Viral resistance has now been demonstrated for some strains of influenza A and is currently low, but this might change in the future.

Historically, antivirals amantadine and rimantadine (the two symmetric amines) that were considered for influenza A treatment and prophylaxis but not for influenza B virus are not currently recommended because resistance has developed against influenza A virus. The mechanism of action of both amantadine and rimantadine was to block the ion channel of the viral M2 protein, resulting in interference with the key role of M2 protein in early virus uncoating.

PREVENTION

The best available method of controlling influenza infection is to annually vaccinate all people aged 6 months and older. Although everybody older than age 6 months should be vaccinated, it is important that vaccination be directed primarily toward the elderly, individuals of all ages who are at high risk (eg, those with chronic lung or heart disease), and their close contacts, including medical personnel and household members and pregnant women.

There are three types of influenza vaccines—**inactivated influenza vaccine (IIV), recombinant influenza vaccine (RIV),** and **live attenuated influenza vaccine (LAIV).** The IIV and RIV are given as intramuscular injection known as flu shots and the LAIV is administered as nasal spray known as FluMist. These **viral vaccines** are reformulated each year to most closely match the influenza A and B antigenic subtypes [two influenza A viruses and one B virus (**trivalent**) or two influenza A and two influenza B viruses (**quadrivalent**)] currently causing infections. There are three different technologies approved by the FDA to produce influenza vaccines in the United States: (1) egg-based flu vaccine, (2) cell-based flu vaccine, and (3) recombinant flu vaccine. Egg-based flu vaccine is the most common and oldest technology used to produce both inactivated and live attenuated vaccines. The candidate vaccine viruses are grown in chicken eggs, harvested, and either inactivated (flu shot) or weakened for live attenuated vaccine (nasal spray). In the cell-based vaccine, the candidate vaccine viruses are grown in mammalian cell cultures followed by harvesting and preparing of the vaccines. This method requires less time than egg-based vaccine and prevents allergic reaction with eggs to some people. The recombinant flu vaccine utilizes expression of hemagglutinin (HA), the major antigen of influenza that produces protective immune response in people, in insect cells followed by purification of the antigen. This is the fastest technology to produce influenza vaccine, free of egg allergies. Some of these vaccines also include adjuvants.

There are different types of flu shots made available recently: (1) a trivalent flu shot with adjuvant to create a stronger immune response for people 65 years and older, (2) a standard dose quadrivalent influenza shot grown in eggs (Afluria, Fluarix, FluLaval, Fluzone) for people aged 6 months and older. The quadrivalent Afluria has two options for delivery; either with a needle or with a jet injector for people aged 18 years to 64 years, (3) a quadrivalent cell-based influenza shot (Flucelvax) grown in cell culture (egg-free) for people 4 years and older, (4) recombinant quadrivalent influenza shot (Flublok), also egg-free, for people 18 years and older, (5) a quadrivalent flu shot with adjuvant for people 65 years and older, (6) a quadrivalent high dose influenza shot for people 65 years and older, (7) a quadrivalent live attenuated influenza vaccine (FluMist) given as intranasally to people 2 years through 49 years of age (not recommended for pregnant women and immunocompromised people). The flu shots are commonly used in two doses given 1 month apart to immunize children (aged 6 months to 8 years) who may not have been immunized previously. Among older children and adults, single annual doses are recommended just before influenza season. Vaccine efficacy is variable, and annual revaccination is necessary to ensure maximal protection. Recent studies show that vaccination reduces the risk of fluillness by 40% to 60%. Two weeks after vaccination, protective antibodies against influenza viruses are formed in the body that provide variable protection.

A problem unique to influenza vaccinology is the inherent, often unexpected variation in antigenic drift from year to year. This often requires annual reformulation of vaccines that are hoped to provide the best protection before the onset of the next influenza season. Prediction of which strains should be used for vaccine production is based on international surveillance—always a difficult task indeed. After the emergence of the swine-origin 2009 A (H1N1) virus, this virus was added to annual influenza vaccine strains starting 2010. The dilemma to vaccine composition will continue as new strains abruptly develop.

> **Why does the influenza vaccine have to be reformulated every year?**

A major factor contributing to this dilemma is related to difficulties in timely production of a vaccine. Up until very recently, all available vaccines had to be prepared in embryonated hen's eggs—a cumbersome process that required at least 22 weeks of preparation. There are new methods whereby new strains can be identified quickly and mass-produced in mammalian cell culture (as described earlier) instead of eggs, thus reducing the production time by as much as 50%, with far higher vaccine quantities. In addition, the cell-based vaccine could be given to people with egg allergies. Newer platforms such as mRNA, viral-vector based and nanoparticles-based vaccines are under development that may reduce some of these issues and increase the efficacy and protection.

● PARAINFLUENZA VIRUSES

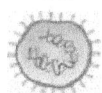 ## VIROLOGY

Parainfluenza viruses belong to the paramyxovirus genus and paramyxoviridae family. There are four serotypes of parainfluenza viruses: parainfluenza 1, 2, 3, and 4. These enveloped viruses contain linear (nonsegmented), negative-sense, single-stranded RNA genome. Similar to influenza viruses, parainfluenza viruses possess a hemagglutinin and neuraminidase, but on the same spike. The structure of paramyxovirus is shown in **Figure 9–4.** The single-stranded,

Sidebar notes:

Flu vaccine recommended for ages 6 months and older and high-risk individuals

A high-dose vaccine available for ages 65 years and older

✳ Annual revaccination against most current strains necessary to achieve protection

Two weeks after vaccination, protective antibodies formed

When antigenic drift occurs unexpectedly, vaccine efficacy in the subsequent year may fall to unacceptable levels

 Think ▸▸ Apply 9-4: The preexisting immunity from previous infection or vaccination does not prevent the new infecting virus from subsequent years because the virus has changed mainly due to antigenic drift (mutation). Antigenic shift (reassortment) may abruptly occur for which there may not be preexisting immunity in the population.

FIGURE 9–4. **Schematic diagram of a paramyxovirus PIV, parainfluenza virus; RSV, respiratory syncytial virus.** The virion contains a negative sense, single-stranded, linear RNA genome bound to a nucleoprotein forming the nucleocapsid that is surrounded by a membrane associated matrix (M) protein, which is then packaged into a lipid bilayer envelope. The envelope contains surface attachment protein (H and N on the same spike) and the fusion protein (F) for PIV and attachment protein (G) and fusionprotein (F) for RSV. Inside the virion, there is RNA-dependent RNA polymerase comprising of large polymerase complex and phosphoprotein.

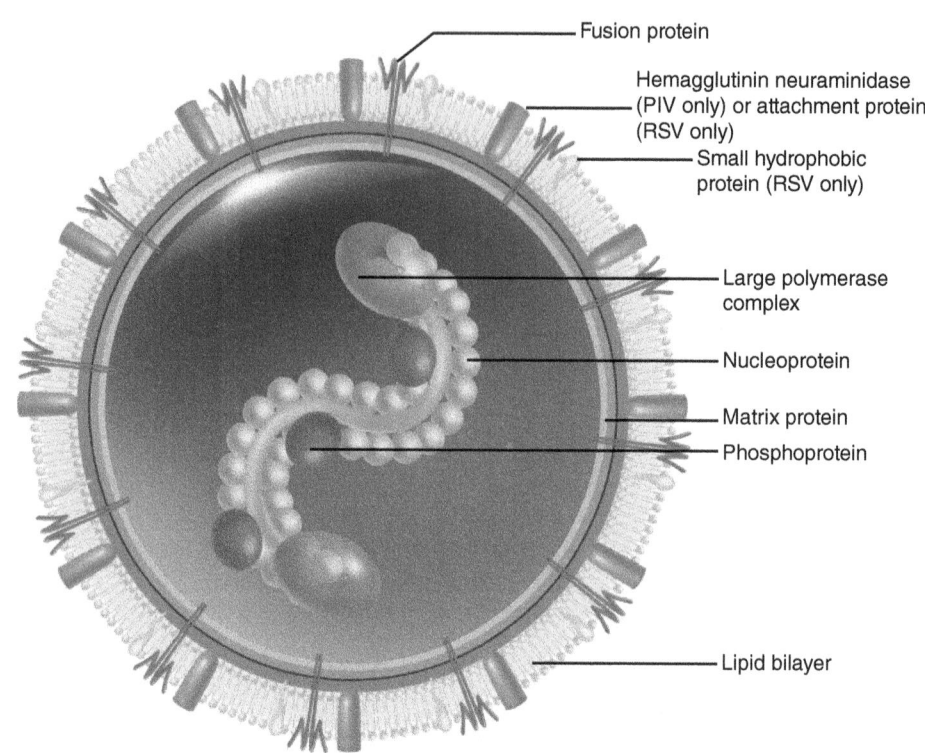

Fusion protein
Hemagglutinin neuraminidase (PIV only) or attachment protein (RSV only)
Small hydrophobic protein (RSV only)
Large polymerase complex
Nucleoprotein
Matrix protein
Phosphoprotein
Lipid bilayer

＊ Negative-sense linear RNA, helical, enveloped with H and N on the same spike

Four serotypes of parainfluenza viruses, antigenically stable

Immunity to reinfection transient

Humoral immunity important in infection control

Cell-mediated immunity prevents severe disease

negative-sense linear RNA genome is bound to a nucleoprotein (helical nucleocapsid), and the matrix protein surrounds the nucleoprotein complex, which is packaged into a lipid bilayer envelope containing attachment protein (H and N on the same spike) and the fusion protein (F). Their mode of spread and pathogenesis are similar to those of the influenza viruses. They differ from the influenza viruses in that RNA synthesis of parainfluenza virus, like most RNA viruses, occurs in the cytoplasm rather than in the nucleus. All events related to parainfluenza virus replication occur in the cytoplasm, similar to any other negative-sense RNA viruses (see Chapter 6 for details about replication of negative-sense RNA viruses). The virus buds out through plasma membranes. In addition, the antigenic makeup of the four serotypes is relatively stable, and significant antigenic shift or drift does not occur. Each serotype is considered separately.

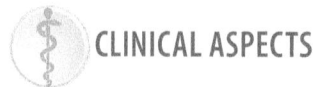 **PARAINFLUENZA DISEASE**

The parainfluenza viruses are important because of the serious diseases they can cause in infants, young children, older adults, and people with weakened immune system, but anyone can be infected. Parainfluenza 1 and 3 are particularly common in this regard. Overall, the group is thought to be responsible for 15% to 20% of all nonbacterial respiratory diseases requiring hospitalization in infancy and childhood. Immunity to reinfection is transient. Although repeated infections can occur in older children and adults, they are usually milder than the illnesses of infancy and early childhood. Humoral immunity plays an important role in controlling parainfluenza virus infection. Antibodies against surface protein, HN, and F are detected in infected patients. Cell-mediated immunity might play an important role in preventing infected people from getting severe diseases.

CLINICAL ASPECTS

MANIFESTATIONS

Parainfluenza virus is transmitted through infectious droplets or airborne spread through sneezing and coughing. The virus infects the upper respiratory tract and the incubation period is 2 to 7 days. The onset of illness from parainfluenza virus may be abrupt, as in acute spasmodic croup, but usually begins as a mild upper respiratory infection (URI) with variable progression over 1 to 3 days to involvement of the middle or lower respiratory tract. Symptoms may include fever, runny nose, sneezing, sore throat, barking cough, hoarse voice, ear pain and in some cases wheezing, croup, bronchitis, bronchiolitis, and pneumonia. Duration of acute illness can vary from 4 to 21 days but is usually 7 to 10 days. Some of the symptoms and diseases associated with each serotype are described below.

■ Parainfluenza 1

Parainfluenza 1 is the major cause of acute croup (laryngotracheitis) in infants and young children, but it also causes less severe diseases such as mild URI, pharyngitis, and tracheobronchitis in individuals of all ages. Outbreaks of infection tend to occur most frequently during the fall months.

✳ Severe croup and tracheobronchitis in infants and young children

Mild URI, pharyngitis and tracheobronchitis at all ages

■ Parainfluenza 2

Parainfluenza 2 is of slightly less significance than parainfluenza 1 or 3. It has been associated with croup, primarily in children, with mild URI, and occasionally with acute lower respiratory disease. As with parainfluenza 1, outbreaks usually occur during the fall months.

Croup is primary disease in children

■ Parainfluenza 3

Parainfluenza 3 is a major cause of severe lower respiratory disease in infants and young children. It often causes bronchitis, pneumonia, and croup in children younger than 1 year of age. In older children and adults, it may cause URI or tracheobronchitis. Infections are common and can occur in any season; it is estimated that nearly 50% of all children have been exposed to this virus by 1 year of age.

✳ Causes severe lower respiratory disease in infants; croup, bronchitis, pneumonia

■ Parainfluenza 4

Parainfluenza 4 is the least common of the group. It is generally associated with mild upper respiratory illness only.

Causes upper respiratory tract infections

DIAGNOSIS, TREATMENT, AND PREVENTION

Specific diagnosis is based on RT-PCR, rapid antigen assay (by enzyme-immunoassay or immunofluorescence), virus isolation, usually in monkey kidney cell cultures, or serology using HI, enzyme immunoassay (EIA), or neutralization assays on paired sera to detect a rising antibody titer. Nucleic acid–based BioFire test for 14 to 19 respiratory pathogens include all four parainfluenza viruses. Currently, there is no method of control or specific therapy for these infections. However, symptoms could be relieved by using some over-the-counter medication to relieve pain and fever. Rest and drinking plenty of fluids are recommended.

Laboratory diagnosis by RT-PCR, antigen assay, or virus isolation

No specific therapy for croup and URI

RESPIRATORY SYNCYTIAL VIRUS

Overview

Respiratory syncytial virus (RSV) belongs to *Pneumovirus* genus of the Paramyxoviridae family. It is an enveloped, helical, negative-sense linear RNA virus that primarily infects the bronchi, bronchioles, and alveoli of the lung. RSV is transmitted by the respiratory route through infective secretions and the incubation period is 4 to 6 days. The illnesses clinically categorized as croup, bronchitis, bronchiolitis, or pneumonia are extremely common in infants. The duration of acute illness is 10 to 14 days. The acute phase of cough, wheezing, and respiratory distress lasts 1 to 3 weeks. Clinical findings include hyperexpansion of the lungs, hypoxemia, and hypercapnia. Interstitial infiltrates, often with areas of pulmonary collapse, may be seen on chest radiography. The severity of respiratory involvement and high prevalence during outbreaks require many hospitalizations each year for infants. Elderly or immunocompromised patients are also frequently susceptible and can be severely affected. RSV envelope fusions (F) protein plays an important role in pathogenesis by forming syncytia and multinucleated giant cells causing cell death. Th2 cytokines and immune complex formation makes the disease worse. Immunity is incomplete as infants get multiple bouts of reinfection in the same season. Supportive therapy is recommended. In some circumstances, aerosol ribavirin can be given. Currently, there is no vaccine available but palivizumab (a monoclonal antibody against viral F protein) can be used for prophylaxis in high-risk infants such as those born prematurely or with chronic lung disease.

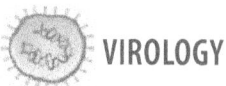

VIROLOGY

Respiratory syncytial virus (RSV) is classified as a *Pneumovirus* within the paramyxoviridae family. Its name is derived from its ability to produce cell fusion in tissue culture (syncytium formation). Unlike influenza or parainfluenza viruses, RSV possesses no hemagglutinin or neuraminidase. The virion structure is similar to parainfluenza virus except that the envelope glycoproteins are an attachment (G) protein and a fusion (F) protein. The RNA genome is linear (nonsegmented), negative-sense, and single stranded and codes for at least 10 different proteins. Among these are a nucleoprotein bound to genomic RNA (helical nucleocapsid), a phosphoprotein, and two matrix (M) proteins in the viral envelope. One forms the inner lining of the viral envelope; the function of the other is uncertain. The virion also contains the viral RNA polymerase enzyme (RNA-dependent RNA polymerase). RSV, similar to other paramyxoviruses, replicates in the cytoplasm and buds out from the plasma membrane.

The antigens on the surface spikes of the viral envelope include the G glycoprotein, which mediates virus attachment to host cell receptors, and the fusion (F) glycoprotein, which induces fusion of the viral envelope with the host cell surface to facilitate entry. F glycoprotein is also responsible for fusion of infected cells in cell cultures, leading to the appearance of multinucleated giant cells (syncytium formation). Antibodies directed at the F glycoprotein are more efficient than G glycoprotein antibodies in neutralizing the virus *in vitro*.

At least two antigenic subgroups (A and B) of RSV are known to exist. This dimorphism is due primarily to differences in the G glycoprotein. The epidemiologic and biologic significance of these variants is not yet certain; however, epidemiologic studies have suggested that group A infections tend to be more severe. RSV is the single most important etiologic agent in respiratory diseases of infancy, and it is the major cause of bronchiolitis and pneumonia among infants under 1 year of age. In addition, older adults aged 65 years and older, adults with heart or lung disease, and people with weakened immune system develop severe RSV disease.

RESPIRATORY SYNCYTIAL VIRUS DISEASE

EPIDEMIOLOGY

Community outbreaks of RSV infection occur annually, commencing at any time from late fall to early spring. The usual outbreak lasts 8 to 12 weeks and can involve nearly 50% of all families with children. In the family setting, it appears that older siblings often introduce the virus into the home, and secondary infection rates can be almost 50%. The usual duration of virus shedding is 5 to 7 days; young infants, however, may shed virus for 9 to 20 days or longer.

Spread of RSV in the hospital setting is also a major problem. Control is difficult including careful attention to handwashing between contacts with patients, isolation, and exclusion of personnel and visitors who have any form of respiratory illness. Masks are not effective in controlling nosocomial spread.

In the United States, 2.1 million RSV-infected outpatient visits and 58,000 hospitalizations among children younger than 5 years old, and 100 to 500 deaths occur annually. The number of RSV-related deaths in infants and children have significantly dropped in the United States in the past few decades due to medical care provided during hospitalization and intensive care units, and availability of monoclonal antibody against RSV (palivizumab) for prophylaxis for high-risk infants. On the contrary, 177,000 people older than 65 years are hospitalized for RSV-related disease, including 14,000 deaths annually in the United States.

PATHOGENESIS

RSV is spread to the upper respiratory tract by contact with infective secretions. Infection appears to be confined primarily to the respiratory epithelium, with progressive involvement of the middle and lower airways. Viremia occurs rarely. Viral surface F protein plays an important role in pathogenesis by forming syncytia and multinucleated giant cells leading to cell death. The direct effect of virus on respiratory tract epithelial cells is similar to that previously described for influenza viruses, and cytotoxic T cells appear to play a similar role in early control of the acute infection.

Sidebar notes (left margin):

✳ RSV, an enveloped, helical (-) RNA virus, forms syncytia in culture

Two envelope glycoproteins (spikes), G and F, mediate attachment and syncytium formation

RSV most important respiratory virus causing severe infection in infants

✳ Major cause of bronchiolitis, pneumonia in infants under 1 year

✳ RSV F protein important in pathogenesis, causing syncytia formation and cell death

High attack rate, introduced by older siblings

Nosocomial infection reduced by careful handwashing

58 thousand hospitalizations and 100-500 deaths among children < 5 years annually

177 thousand hospitalizations and 14 thousand deaths among adults > 65 years annually

Confined to respiratory epithelium

The apparent enhanced severity of RSV, particularly in very young infants, is not yet clearly understood but may have an immunologic basis. Factors that have been proposed to play a role include: (1) qualitative or quantitative deficits in humoral or secretory antibody responses to critical virus-specified proteins; (2) formation of antigen–antibody complexes within the respiratory tract resulting in complement activation; and (3) excessive damage from inflammatory cytokines. Experimental evidence suggests that patients who respond to RSV infections with CD4+ T cells that are predominantly of the T_H type 2 have more severe disease than those with predominant T_H type 1 responses. This is thought to be due to the inflammatory cytokines produced by T_H type 2 cells, including interleukin (IL)-4, IL-5, IL-6, IL-10, and IL-13. Several of these cytokines are involved in promoting increased infiltrations of eosinophils and neutrophils into the lung tissues. In addition, this allergic-like response diminishes the activation and effector functions of cytotoxic CD8+T cells followed by a delay in RSV clearance, induction of lung damage, and dissemination of the virus.

✳ Enhanced disease in infants may have immunologic basis

✳ T_H2-stimulated cytokines cause injury and make the disease worse

 What is the mechanism of RSV-induced bronchiolitis?

The major pathologic findings of RSV are in the bronchi, bronchioles, and alveoli. These include necrosis of epithelial cells; interstitial mononuclear cell inflammatory infiltrates, which sometimes also involve the alveoli and alveolar ducts; and plugging of smaller airways with material containing mucus, necrotic cells, and fibrin (**Figure 9–5**). Multinucleated syncytial cells with intracytoplasmic inclusions are occasionally seen in the affected tracheobronchial epithelium.

Necrosis and inflammation plug bronchioles and alveoli

IMMUNITY

Infection with RSV results in IgG and IgA humoral and secretory antibody responses. However, immunity to reinfection is tenuous, as shown by patients who have recovered from a primary acute episode and have become reinfected with disease of similar severity in the same or succeeding year. Illness severity appears to diminish with increasing age and successive reinfection. Cell-mediated immunity is dampened due to activation of the Th2 response.

Immunity to reinfection is brief

✳ Multiple bouts of infection in the same season

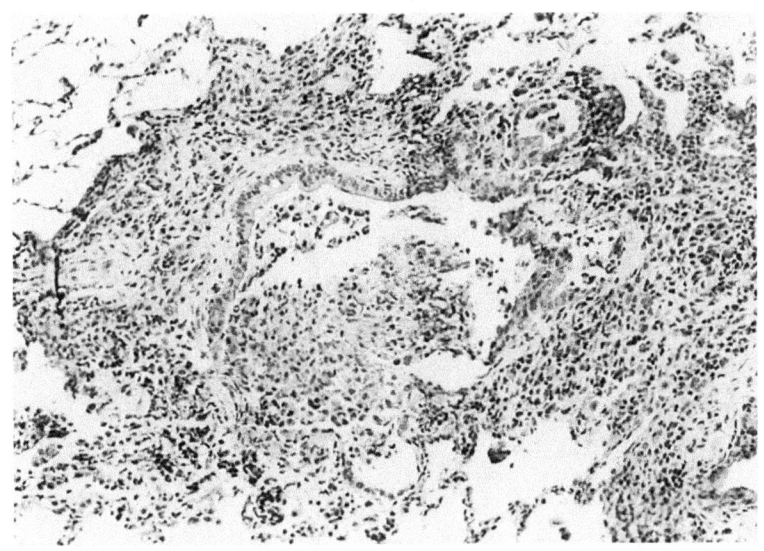

FIGURE 9–5. Photomicrograph illustrates the bronchiolar and surrounding interstitial inflammation in respiratory syncytial virus infection. (Original magnification ×100.)

 Think ▸▸ Apply 9-5: **The F protein of RSV causes syncytia and multinucleated giant cells followed by cell death. In addition, immune complex formation and proinflammatory cytokine production cause damage.**

Why are the same infants reinfected with RSV in the same or succeeding season?

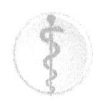 **CLINICAL ASPECTS**

MANIFESTATIONS

✳ RSV single most important agent of bronchiolitis and pneumonia in infants younger than 1 year

Infant bronchiolitis and pneumonitis lasts up to 2 weeks

Mortality is highest with underlying diseases

Children and adults have milder illness

Can trigger wheezing in asthmatics

Older people > 65 years develop severe disease and death

The usual incubation period for RSV is 4 to 6 days, followed by the onset of rhinitis; severity of illness progresses to a peak within 1 to 3 days. In infants, this peak usually takes the form of bronchiolitis and pneumonitis, with cough, wheezing, and respiratory distress. Clinical findings include **hyperexpansion** of the lungs, **hypoxemia** (low oxygenation of blood), and **hypercapnia** (CO_2 retention). Interstitial infiltrates, often with areas of pulmonary collapse, may be seen on chest radiography (**Figure 9–6**). Fever is variable. The duration of acute illness is often 10 to 14 days.

The fatality rate among hospitalized infected infants is estimated to be between 0.5% and 1%; however, this rises higher in children receiving cancer chemotherapy, infants with congenital heart disease, and those with severe immunodeficiency. Infants with underlying chronic lung disease are also at high risk. Causes of death include respiratory failure, right-sided heart failure (corpulmonale), and bacterial superinfection. Death has sometimes resulted from unnecessary procedures in patients in whom RSV infection was not considered. Bronchoscopy, lung biopsy, or overly aggressive therapy with corticosteroids and bronchodilators for presumed asthma all can pose a danger to such patients.

Older infants, children, and adults are also readily infected. The clinical illnesses in these groups are usually milder and include croup, tracheobronchitis, and URI; however, elderly persons can experience severe morbidity. In addition, RSV can cause acute flare-ups of chronic bronchitis and trigger acute wheezing episodes in asthmatic children. However, older adults above 65 years of age, adults with lung or heat disease, and adults with compromised immune system are at a higher risk of developing severe RSV disease, including hospitalizations and deaths.

FIGURE 9–6. Chest radiograph of an infant with a severe case of respiratory syncytial virus pneumonia and bronchiolitis. Bilateral interstitial infiltrates, hyperexpansion of the lung, and right upper lobe atelectasis (*arrow*) are present.

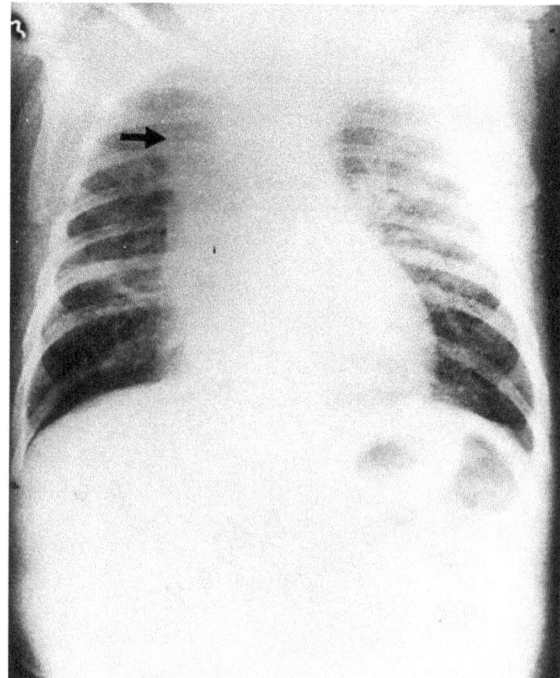

 Think ▸▸ Apply 9-6: **Because immunity to both RSV subtypes is incomplete or ineffective to provide protection to subsequent infections.**

DIAGNOSIS

Rapid diagnosis of RSV infection can be made by detection of viral genome by RT-PCR, and/or viral antigen by immunofluorescence or EIA from respiratory tract specimens. The nucleic acid–based BioFire test for 14 to 19 respiratory pathogens includes RSV. The virus can also be isolated from the respiratory tract by prompt inoculation of specimens into cell cultures. Syncytial cytopathic effects develop over 2 to 7 days. Serodiagnosis may also be used but requires acute and convalescent sera and is less sensitive than antigen-detection methods, PCR, or culture.

TREATMENT AND PREVENTION

Treatment for RSV is directed primarily at the underlying pathophysiology and includes adequate oxygenation, ventilatory support when necessary, and close observation for complications such as bacterial superinfection and right-sided heart failure. Some studies suggest that ribavirin aerosol treatment may be effective in selected circumstances.

No vaccine is currently available for RSV. RSV vaccines and immune globulins containing high antibody titers to RSV are also under active investigation. However, a high-titered monoclonal antibody against F protein called palivizumab has been used for prophylaxis in high-risk infants (those born prematurely or with chronic lung disease). This method requires monthly injections during the RSV season (usually 5 months). This monoclonal antibody can prevent development of severe RSV disease, but cannot cure or treat infants already infected with RSV.

Supportive treatment indicated

Aerosol ribavirin may be effective

✳ No RSV vaccine available

✳ Monoclonal antibody to F protein (Palivizumab) for prophylaxis in high-risk infants

● HUMAN METAPNEUMOVIRUS

Human metapneumovirus (HMPV), a *Pneumovirus* of paramyxoviridae family, was discovered in 2001 and can cause upper and lower respiratory tract infection in people of all age groups. HMPV has subsequently been found to be a significant cause of ARD in infants and young children. It may account for approximately 10% of the respiratory tract infections for which there are no previously identified causative agents. It is second only to RSV as a cause of bronchiolitis during the winter-spring seasons, and it produces illnesses that are comparable in their severity and symptoms to those of RSV. Infection with HMPV generally occurs in slightly older children compared with RSV, which infects younger children. The incubation period is approximately 3 to 6 days. Symptoms include fever, nasal congestion, cough, and shortness of breath, which may progress to bronchiolitis or pneumonia. Both viruses, HMPV and RSV, can coinfect the same child, and this is generally associated with worse disease. Two genotypes are known to exist, but it is not known whether either produces more severe disease or protective immunity. The usual diagnostic methods of choice are viral genome amplification by RT-PCR or viral antigen detection by enzyme immunoassay or immunofluorescence. The BioFire test for 14 to 19 respiratory pathogens includes human metapneumovirus. Virus culture is rarely done. No specific treatment is available. Preventive measures such as handwashing, avoiding sharing drinks and kissing, and covering coughs and sneezes may prevent the spread to others.

✳ HMPV causes bronchiolitis and pneumonia, second to RSV, in infants and children

HMPV is a paramyxovirus, enveloped and negative-sense RNA

Clinical, epidemiologic behaviors like RSV

CORONAVIRUSES

Overview

Coronaviruses are the largest RNA viruses comprised of a positive-sense RNA genome, a helical nucleocapsid and a lipid bilayer envelope containing viral Spike (S) glycoprotein, membrane glycoprotein, and small envelope glycoprotein. The virus replicates in the cytoplasm by using its newly synthesized viral RNA-dependent RNA polymerase and assembles in the cytoplasm acquiring an envelope from ER-Golgi membranes. Four common human coronaviruses (Hu-CoV) -229E, -NL63, -OC43, and -HKU1 have been contributing to 5% to -10% common cold every year for decades. In addition, three novel human coronaviruses have been identified causing severe acute respiratory syndrome, SARS-CoV-1, MERS-CoV, and SARS-CoV-2 in 2019 (COVID-19). While SARS and MERS were highly fatal they were limited in spread and number of cases. COVID-19 has become a pandemic infection involving most countries and causing 178 million cases and 3.86 million deaths globally. The United States has the greatest number of cases, and deaths of any country. SARS-CoV-2 is transmitted through respiratory droplets and its Spike glycoprotein interacts with ACE2 receptor in the upper and lower respiratory tract, and also utilizes TMPRSS2 host transmembrane

(Continued)

protein for virus entry followed by viral replication, increasing viral copies number, upregulation of proinflammatory cytokines and chemokines and recruitment of T lymphocytes, monocytes, and neutrophils. In the late stage, pulmonary edema can fill the alveolar spaces with hyaline membrane formation, consistent with early-phase acute respiratory distress syndrome. About 80% of infected people develop mild to moderate flu-like symptoms, ~15% develop severe disease such as viral pneumonia, and ~5% have critical illness such as acute hypoxemic respiratory failure, shock, or multiorgan dysfunction. Older people above 65 years of age develop more severe COVID-19 than younger people and the majority of deaths have occurred in this group, especially above 85 years. Molecular (RT-PCR) and antigen tests are available to detect SARS-CoV-2. Treatment includes antiviral remdesivir and dexamethasone. Combination monoclonal antibodies against SASR-CoV-2 Spike glycoprotein are available to prevent severe disease progression. Two mRNA vaccines (Pfizer and Moderna) given in two doses and a one-dose adenovirus-virus vector encoding Spike glycoprotein have been authorized for emergency use in the United States, and are highly effective in preventing moderate to severe COVID-19.

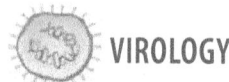

VIROLOGY

Coronaviruses are large family of RNA viruses and named for the crown-like or petal or club-shaped spikes on the surface of the virus giving crown of thorns or solar corona. There are four subgroups of coronaviruses infecting humans and animals, including alpha-, beta-, gamma-, and delta-coronaviruses. The first human coronavirus was identified in the mid-1960s. There are four **common or routine human coronaviruses** (Hu-CoV) that cause the common cold, including Hu-CoV-229E, Hu-CoV-NL63, Hu-CoV-OC43, and Hu-CoV-HKU1. In addition, three **novel human coronaviruses** causing severe acute respiratory syndromes (SARS) have been identified, including SARS-CoV-1 and SARS-CoV-2 (COVID-19) and the Middle-East respiratory syndrome (MERS) causing coronavirus, MERS-CoV. These novel coronaviruses have probably jumped from animals and evolved to infect humans causing severe acute respiratory diseases such as SARS, MERS and COVID-19, involving multi-organs diseases and deaths.

Coronaviruses are the largest RNA viruses that contain a positive-sense single-stranded linear RNA genome, which is bound to a helical nucleocapsid (N) protein surrounded by a lipid bilayer envelope containing virus-encoded spike (S) proteins. In addition, the envelope has several other proteins, including membrane (M) glycoprotein, small envelope (E) glycoprotein, and hemagglutinin-acetyl esterase (HE) protein (only in β−coronaviruses). The lipid bilayer is derived from intracellular rough endoplasmic reticulum and Golgi membranes of infected cells. The S glycoprotein (spikes or peplomers) plays an important role in binding to the host cell receptor and inducing neutralizing antibodies and cellular immune responses. The structure of coronavirus is shown in **Figure 9–7.** The S protein is made up of two units, S1 and S2. S1 forms the head of the spike (S) protein and contains the receptor binding domain (RBD) which interacts with the receptor on host cells such as ACE2 for SARS-CoV-2. S2 makes the stem of the S protein and anchors with the viral envelope and mediates fusion of viral and host cell membranes for viral entry.

Coronaviruses replicate in the cytoplasm, generally like other positive-sense RNA viruses (see Chapter 6), but acquire an envelope from the endoplasmic reticulum and/or the Golgi apparatus. Brief replication of SARS-CoV-2 (COVID-19) is discussed later.

Enveloped, helical, positive-sense RNA viruses

Replicate in the cytoplasm using viral RNA polymerase

EPIDEMIOLOGY, PATHOGENESIS, AND DISEASE

■ Common Cold Human Coronaviruses

Like the rhinoviruses, the **four common human coronaviruses** (Hu-CoV -229E, -NL63, -OC43, and -HKU1) are distributed worldwide and considered primary causes of the **common cold**. Based on serologic studies, it is estimated that they may cause up to 5% to 10% of common colds in adults, and a similar proportion of lower respiratory illnesses in children. Some of these common human coronaviruses have been studied to some extent; they can cause outbreaks like those

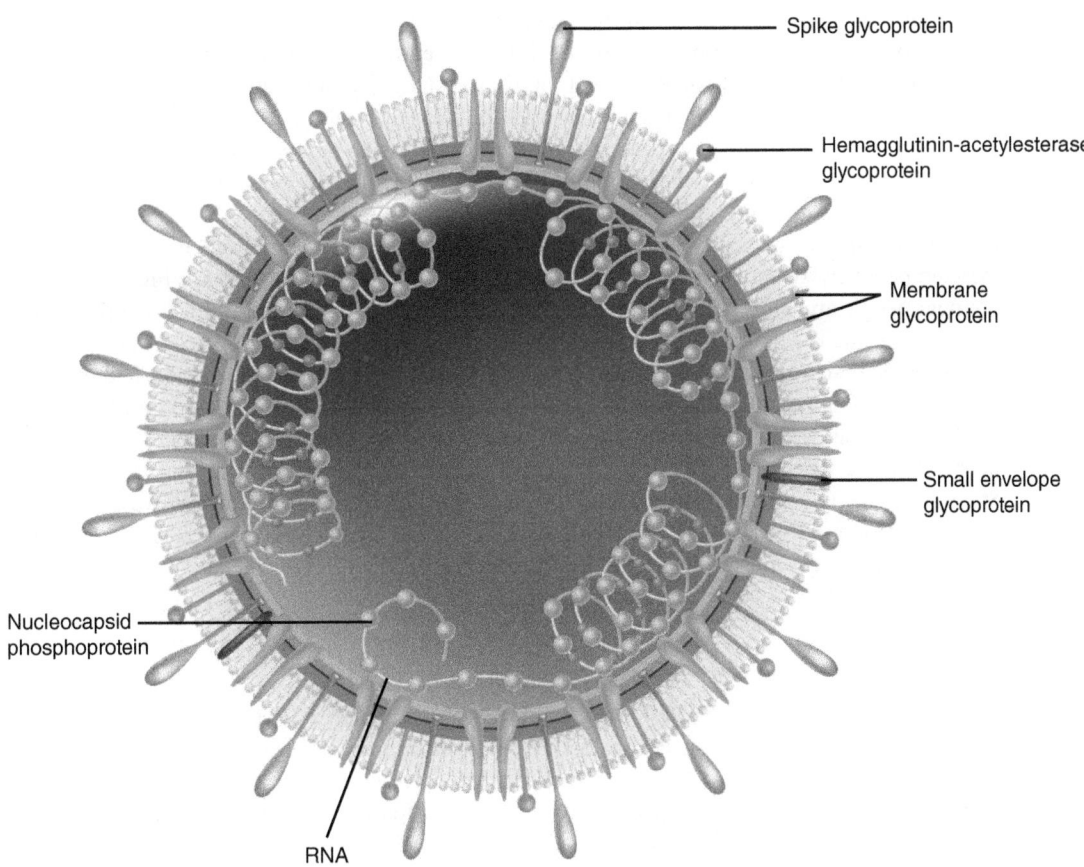

Spike glycoprotein

Hemagglutinin-acetylesterase
glycoprotein

Membrane
glycoprotein

Small envelope
glycoprotein

Nucleocapsid
phosphoprotein

RNA

FIGURE 9–7. Virion structure of a coronavirus. Coronavirus particle is shown to contain a single-stranded, positive-sense RNA genome bound to a nucleoprotein (helical nucleocapsid) surrounded by a lipid bilayer envelope. Petal- or club-shaped spikes (Spike glycoprotein) project from the surface of the envelope giving the appearance of a crown of thorns or a solar corona. There are several other surface proteins, including hemagglutinin-acetylesterase glycoprotein, membrane glycoprotein, and small envelope glycoprotein.

of rhinoviruses, and reinfection with the same serotype can occur. The HuCoV-229E was discovered in 1966 and binds to cellular receptor aminopeptidase N (CD13), OC43 in 1967 and receptor is 9-*O*-Acetylated sialic acid, NL63 in 2004 and receptor is ACE2 (same as COVID-19), and HKU1 in 2005 and receptor is 9-*O*-Acetylated sialic acid. All these four common coronaviruses produce similar syndromes ranging from upper to lower respiratory illness. Transmission occurs through respiratory droplets, through air by coughing and sneezing, close contact and hand-to-face transfer from touching contaminated surfaces. The incubation period is generally 2 to 5 days followed by symptoms, including runny nose, sore throat, low-grade fever, cough, headache. In some people who have cardiopulmonary disease, weakened immune system, infants, and elderly, common coronaviruses can cause lower respiratory tract infection, including pneumonia. There is no antiviral or vaccine to prevent common cold coronavirus infections.

Four common human coronaviruses causing common cold

Contribute to 5% to 10% of common colds

No specific treatment or vaccine

■ Severe Acute Respiratory Syndrome (SARS)—SARS-COV-1

In late 2002, an illness called severe acute respiratory syndrome (SARS) appeared in Guangdong Province, China, spread throughout Asia in early 2003, and to several countries in Europe, North America, and South America. The etiology was identified as another previously undescribed coronavirus named SARS-CoV-1, with unusually high virulence for humans. The genome of the SARS-causing coronavirus has been sequenced, and the virus has some ability to mutate like other RNA viruses, but not like influenza viruses. The immediate origin of SARS-CoV-1 wes likely the exotic animals such as palm civets and raccoon dogs which harbored very similar coronaviruses. SARS-CoV-like viruses have been isolated from several bat species, especially horseshoe bats and the lack of overt disease in the bats make them reservoirs for the virus. The route of transmission is similar to that of other common cold viruses such as direct contact, via the eyes, nose, and mouth with infectious droplets and through aerosolized inhalation. The incubation period is 2 to

7 days (as long as 10 days and in some cases up to 14 days). The risk of transmitting the infection to a person is greatest around day 10 of the illness, when the maximum amount of virus is shed from the respiratory tract. SARS-CoV-1 binds to ACE2 (angiotensin-converting enzyme 2) receptor to enter the cells of the respiratory tract followed by viral replication and assembly in the cytoplasm leading to various respiratory symptoms and disease. Symptoms start with a high fever with chills, headache, body aches, and mild respiratory symptoms, including diarrhea in some patients. After 2 to 7 days, SARS patients may develop nonproductive cough leading to hypoxia, and 10% to 20% of the cases require intubation and mechanical ventilation. While most of the infected people were between 25 and 70 years old, the older population was at a higher risk than younger people and children. SARS can be diagnosed by RT-PCR of viral RNA. An antibody test can be performed to detect past exposure. There is no specific treatment or vaccine approved for SARS, other than supportive treatment based on patient's symptoms. Prevention included frequent washing of hands with soap and water or wiping hands with alcohol-based sanitizers. During the outbreak, people used face covering and masks for protection. In this outbreak, 8098 people became sick with SARS and 774 people died (9.6% fatality) worldwide. In the United States, eight people were infected with SARS with a travel history where SARS was spreading. Control to contain the outbreak included measures such as testing, surveillance, isolation of suspected cases, tracing, quarantine for 10 days, screening travelers and disinfecting the aircrafts, etc. Fortunately, SARS-CoV-1 spread was contained.

■ Middle East Respiratory Syndrome (MERS)—MERS-COV

In 2012, an illness called Middle East respiratory syndrome (MERS) appeared in Saudi Arabia that caused a fatal ARD leading to renal failure and was caused by new novel coronavirus known as MERS coronavirus (MERS-CoV). Three to four people out of every 10 with MERS have died (30%-40% fatality) with a total of 858 deaths worldwide. Most of the MERS cases have been linked with travel or living in the Arabian Peninsula. MERS affects people of all age groups. The largest group of MERS cases outside the Arabian Peninsula occurred in South Korea linked to a traveler from that region. MERS-CoV is a zoonotic virus transmitted from infected dromedary camels to humans and has been identified in dromedaries in several countries in the Middle East, Africa, and South Asia. This virus is similar to SARS, but still different than SARS and other human coronaviruses. While the origin of MERS-CoV is not fully understood, several studies suggest, based on viral genome sequencing and analysis, that the virus may have originated from bats and later transmitted to camels. Although the exact mechanisms of transmission to humans are not known, it most likely occurs through close contact with sick people or caring or living with an infected people and in healthcare setting and hospitals. The incubation period is from 2 to 14 days (average 5-6 days). Most people infected people have symptoms of severe acute respiratory syndrome, including fever, cough, and shortness of breath. While some patients experience nausea, vomiting, and diarrhea, many patients develop severe complications such as pneumonia and renal failure. The fatality rate with MERS is about 30% to 40%. People with other underlying conditions such as diabetes, cancer, chronic lung, heart and kidney diseases, and weakened immune system develop severe disease. Diagnostic tests include RT-PCR of viral RNA and an antibody test is available for surveillance programs. There is no specific treatment or vaccine approved. However, several vaccines are under development against MERS. Supportive care is recommended, including support of vital organs functions. Preventive measures to protect respiratory infection such as in SARS are recommended.

■ Coronavirus Diease-2019 (COVID-19)—SARS-COV-2

Epidemiology. In December 2019, a cluster of cases of viral pneumonia were reported in Wuhan, Hubei province, China and the etiologic agent identified was a novel coronavirus related to SARS coronavirus, and therefore named SARS-CoV-2 and the disease as Coronavirus Disease-2019 (COVID-19). By January 2020, it was confirmed that this novel coronavirus is easily transmitted from human to human through respiratory droplets and spreading in China's neighboring countries. On January 21, 2020, the United States confirmed its first case of SARS-CoV2 in Washington State in a man who had travelled to the Wuhan area. On January 11-12, 2020, the genomic sequence of SARS-CoV-2 was published by Chinese scientists and on January 24, 2020 by French scientists. SARS-CoV-2 is a β-coronavirus like SARS-CoV-1 and MERS-CoV and shares ~80% and ~50% of genome identity, respectively. By February 2020, the virus had spread in several

---

Margin notes:

✳ SARS caused by a novel coronavirus, SARS-CoV-1 with ~10% fatality

Risk of transmission of SARS greatest around day 10 of illness

Supportive treatment, no specific treatment or vaccine

Middle east respiratory syndrome (MERS) caused by novel coronavirus

✳ MERS-CoV causes acute respiratory syndrome leading to pneumonia, renal failure

Fatality rate 30% - 40%

countries in Asia, North America, South America, Europe, the Middle-East, Australia, and Africa. On March 11, 2020, the WHO declared the SARS-CoV2 (COVID-19) outbreak a pandemic, which led to travel restrictions, lockdowns, closures of schools and businesses. As of June 20, 2021, 178 million cases of COVID-19 and 3.86 million deaths have occurred worldwide involving 219 countries and territories. In the United States, 33.5 million cases and 0.6 million deaths have occurred, with 80% of those in people 65 years and older and 38% in people 85 years and older. While the origin of this virus is not established, it is presumed that it either emerged from its likely animal reservoir, horseshoe bats, and possibly adapted to an intermediate host and then became easily transmitted from person to person.

Transmission. SARS-CoV-2 is transmitted from person to person through respiratory droplets when an infected person coughs or sneezes and the respiratory droplets land on another's face, nose, and eyes. In addition, hand-to-face, -nose, or -eyes transfer following touching surfaces contaminated with infected respiratory droplets. The virus transmission has also been shown to be transmitted through aerosol inhalation with some fine respiratory droplets. One unique feature of this virus is that many asymptomatic infected individuals transmit the virus to others. The virus is highly transmissible and contagious, and the stability of the virus may also influence these processes. SARS-CoV-2 has been found to be stable for about 2 to 4 hours in aerosolized form, 72 hours on plastic, 48 hours on steel, 24 hours on cardboard, and 8 hours on copper surfaces.

Pathogenesis and disease progression. SARS-CoV-2 enters via the respiratory tract and nasopharyngeal and/or oropharyngeal cells are the initial targets for viral entry and replication. This is followed by reproduction in airways, bronchial epithelium, alveolar epithelial cells, vascular endothelial cells, and alveolar macrophages. Viral Spike (S) glycoprotein's RBD (receptor binding domains) binds to ACE2 followed by cleavage of S1/S2 by cellular cathepsin L and the transmembrane protease serine 2 (TMPRSS2), which mediates the viral entry at the plasma membrane and forming an endosomal vesicle. S2 helps the viral envelope to fuse with cellular membranes. Following viral entry, the viral genome is released in the cytoplasm and the genomic RNA is translated in a polyprotein which is cleaved by the host and viral proteases into several individual proteins such as RNA-dependent RNA polymerase (RdRp) and other nonstructural proteins, including an exonuclease activity with proofreading function protein (ExoN), which probably controls mutations. The RdRp directs the synthesis of genomic and subgenomic RNAs and the subgenomic RNAs are translated into structural proteins such as envelope and nucleocapsid. The virus is assembled in the cytoplasm and acquires its envelope from the ER-Golgi membranes that have already envelope proteins expressed, including the Spike glycoprotein, and released from infected cells. The binding affinity of SARS-CoV-2 with ACE2 may also influence the viral infectivity and possibly transmission efficiency. One of the variants in Spike RBD, D614G, binds ACE2 with higher affinity and increases viral infectivity and load in the upper respiratory tract which increases human-to-human transmission. While the ExoN probably limits mutations to some extent in coronaviruses, SARS-CoV-2 has mutated, but not like other RNA viruses including influenza viruses that lack proof reading ability. Several variants have been generated worldwide and associated with transmission, pathogenesis, and immunity, noticeably, B.1.1.7 (emerged in UK—alpha variant), B. 1.351 (emerged in South Africa—beta variant), P.1 (emerged in Brazil—gamma variant), and B. 1.617.1 and B. 1.617.2 (emerged in India—delta variant). These variants are circulating in many countries, including the United States and are known to spread easily and faster, because of their higher binding affinity with ACE2, and are more pathogenic and likely to cause more cases of increased morbidity and mortality.

Damage caused in COVID-19 includes both viral and immune-mediated, mainly proinflammatory cytokines, pathologic changes in the lung. In the lower respiratory tract, the virus infects and replicates in alveolar airway epithelial cells, vascular endothelial cells, and alveolar macrophages increasing the viral load or copy numbers and release of inflammatory signaling molecules leading to recruitment of T lymphocytes, monocytes, and neutrophils leading to cell death by apoptosis. SARS-CoV-2 interaction with the innate immune cells and its strategy of innate immune evasion is important for the progression of infection. While the innate immune pathways, especially antiviral molecules IFN-I (α and β) and cytokines are activated in response to viral RNA, some of the SARS-CoV-2 nonstructural proteins antagonize IFN genes. In patients with severe COVID-19, very little IFN-1 is seen in serum, although higher levels of proinflammatory cytokines are found. In the late stage, pulmonary edema can fill the alveolar spaces with hyaline membrane formation, compatible with early-phase acute respiratory distress syndrome. ACE2 is also expressed at higher levels in many extrapulmonary cells, including enterocytes,

* Novel coronavirus SARS-CoV-2 cause of COVID-19 pandemic

178 million cases and 3.86 million deaths worldwide

33.5 million cases and 0.6 million deaths in the United States

* Transmission through respiratory droplets direct or indirect and aerosol

Virus stable in air and on several surfaces for several hours

Virus utilizes ACE2 receptor expressed in lungs, heart, kidneys

Mutations in RBD increase affinity to ACE2 and infectivity and transmissibility efficiency

Recruitment of lymphocytes, monocytes, neutrophils

cholangiocytes, myocardial cells, kidney cells, and bladder urothelial cells making these cells vulnerable to SARS-CoV-2 assault.

Cell damage is viral and immune mediated

Older individuals suffer from severe COVID-19 manifestations more than younger people most likely due to higher levels of lymphocytopenia and neutrophilia and elevated inflammation and coagulation markers which are consistently seen in older patients compared with younger adults. In addition, higher levels of proinflammatory cytokines (IL-1β, IL-6, IL-8, TNF-α, and others) and chemokines (CCL2, MIP1-α, and others) result in a cytokine storm (see Chapter 7, Figure 7-5) in severe COVID-19 patients more than nonsevere patients. Moreover, the recruitment of activated neutrophils and monocytes may be driven by pulmonary endothelial cell impairment through vascular leakage, tissue edema, and possibly disseminated intravascular coagulation (DIC) pathways. It has been found that these inflammatory mononuclear cells are accumulated in multiple organs such as lung, heart, kidney, liver etc. with elevated D-dimer and longer prothrombin time.

Proinflammatory cytokines cause damage in severe disease

Older people develop more severe disease than younger

Immunity. Both cell-mediated and humoral immunity play important roles in acute SARS-CoV-2 infection. Recent studies suggest that T cell responses may be important in controlling infection, whereas antibodies may provide longer protection. Furthermore, T cell responses were higher in mild COVID-19 patients compared with moderate to severe patients. On the contrary, COVID-19 patients with moderate to severe disease had more robust antibody responses than patients with mild disease. More research is needed to determine the duration of immunity and long-term protection by cellular and humoral immune responses in recovered COVID-19 patients or vaccinated individuals.

Cell-mediated immunity controls infection, reduces disease severity

Antibodies provide longer protection but do not reduce disease severity

Manifestations. Following respiratory route transmission and an incubation period of 2 to 14 (median 5-6) days, 80% of the people who develop symptoms will have mild to moderate findings. Symptoms develop within 11.5 days and in some cases 5 to 6 days. These may include (several of these but not all) fever or chills, cough, shortness of breath, fatigue, muscle or body aches, headache, new loss of taste or smell, sore throat, congestion or runny nose, nausea or vomiting, diarrhea. Severe symptoms include shortness of breath or trouble in breathing, persistent pain or pressure in the chest, new confusion, inability to wake or stay a wake, bluish lips on face, and many more. Impairment of olfactory function (anosmia) may be present in ~10% of cases. Dermatologic findings are nonspecific, consisting of maculopapular or urticarial lesions. Some people (~15%) develop severe diseases such as viral pneumonia and ~5% have critical illnesses such as acute hypoxemic respiratory failure, shock, or multiorgan dysfunction. There are reports that suggest an increased risk of thrombosis of large and small vessels and of neurologic complications of COVID-19, including stroke. There are several risk factors for severe illness. While people of any age can be infected, middle aged are most commonly affected, and older individuals are most likely to develop severe disease. Several other conditions associated with severe illness are immunocompromise, severe obesity, cardiovascular disease, diabetes, hypertension, chronic lung disease, cancer, and chronic kidney disease. Postinfectious complications of COVID-19 have been reported, including bacterial superinfections and Guillain-Barré syndrome (acute flaccid myelitis). In children, a multisystem inflammatory syndrome known as MIS-C that may manifest with myocarditis, shock, or features similar to those of Kawasaki disease that includes the development of coronary artery aneurysms. Some patients experience lingering symptoms following COVID-19 such as fatigue, body aches, shortness of breath, difficulty concentrating, inability to exercise, headache, and difficulty sleeping also referred as "long haulers" or as named by the NIH "post-acute sequelae of SARS-CoV-2 infection" (PASC). While most people recover from COVID-19 within weeks or months, some will likely suffer from chronic damage to their lungs, heart, kidneys or brain.

Majority of infected people have mild flu-like symptoms

Severe symptoms; shortness of breath, chest pain, confusion, bluish lips

Critical illness; pneumonia, respiratory failure, shock, or multiorgan dysfunction

Diagnosis. Two types of diagnostic tests, molecular (viral RNA by RT-PCR) nucleic acid test (NAT) and antigen (viral antigen mainly nucleocapsid, N) using nasal swab specimen are approved and manufactured by several companies. Antigen tests may require confirmation by RT-PCR. In addition, a nucleic acid–based BioFire Respiratory panel 2.1 (RP2-1) is available for emergency use (EU) to detect 15 viral and four bacterial respiratory pathogens, including common cold coronaviruses and SARS-CoV-2. An antibody test is also approved to detect past infection but not recommended to diagnose current infection.

Viral RNA by RT-PCR and viral antigen tests for diagnosis

Antibody test for past exposure

BioFire detects nucleic acids of SARS-CoV-2

Treatment. Treatment includes the antiviral remdesivir and dexamethasone. Monoclonal antibodies cocktail against SARS-CoV-2 Spike glycoprotein, bamlanivimab, and casirivimab plus imdevimab are available under FDA emergency authorization for patients at high risk of disease

Remdesivir and dexamethasone for treatment

progression and severe illness. Severe COVID-19 patients require ICU care, including intubation and mechanical ventilation. Current guidelines for COVID-19 treatment can be seen at www.cdc.gov or www.covid19treatmentguidelines.nih.gov.

Prevention. Preventive measures include COVID-19 vaccination, wearing mask and/or face shield, social distancing (staying 6 feet from others), avoiding crowded and poorly ventilated places, frequent washing hands with soap and water or using a hand sanitizer with at least 60% alcohol (ethanol), covering your cough or sneeze, and disinfecting frequently touched spaces.

Three vaccines, including two mRNA vaccines encoding SARS-CoV-2 Spike glycoprotein (manufactured by Pfizer and Moderna) and one replication-incompetent human adenovirus vector (Ad26) encoding SARS-CoV-2 Spike glycoprotein (made by Johnson & Johnson) were authorized by the FDA in the United States. Pfizer and Moderna mRNA vaccines are given in two doses 3 and 4 weeks apart, respectively, while Johnson & Johnson vaccine is administered as a single dose. All these vaccines are recommended for people 12 to 18 years of age and older. These vaccines mount neutralizing antibodies and T cell responses and provide a very high efficacy of preventing moderate to severe disease. Recent studies suggest a high level of protection by these vaccines against SARS-CoV-2 infection. There are several other vaccines made and authorized for emergency in other countries. COVID-19 vaccines are being distributed to many developing countries through WHO program known as COVAX.

● ADENOVIRUSES

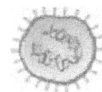 ### VIROLOGY

Adenoviruses are naked capsid, icosahedral, and double-stranded DNA viruses. There are 68 different adenovirus serotypes that infect humans, which are classified into one of seven subgroups (A-G) based on multiple biologic properties of the virus. The virion size is in the range of 90 to 100 nm and it contains a linear double-stranded DNA genome covered with an icosahedral capsid (**Figure 9–8**). The capsid is composed of 252 subunits (capsomeres), including 240 hexons and 12 pentons and fibers. The penton on the surface of the capsid contains a base and a projecting fiber that varies in length based on the serotypes. The fiber is modified by addition of glucosamine. The fiber is like a spike that interacts with the receptor on host cells. The variability in the fiber determines cellular tropism for the virus. The hexon and the fiber contain most of the neutralizing antibodies' epitopes, although some epitopes on penton base have been recognized. Adenoviruses enter cells via viropexis and replication occurs in the nucleus by using host RNA polymerase for transcription and viral DNA–dependent DNA polymerase (viral DNA polymerase) for replication of DNA genomes. The assembly of the virus occurs in the nucleus, and virions are released by cell destruction (see Chapter 6 for DNA virus replication). All adenoviruses share a common group-specific, complement-fixing antigen associated with the hexon component of the viral capsid. Adenoviruses are characterized by their ubiquity and persistence in host tissues for periods ranging from a few days to several years. Their ability to produce infection without disease

Monoclonal antibodies cocktail for high risk

Social distancing, wearing mask, frequent handwashing

Hand sanitizer with 60% alcohol

✳ Two mRNA vaccines and one adenovirus-vector vaccine authorized for emergency use

Vaccines highly efficacious in preventing moderate to severe disease

✳ Multiple serotypes of naked capsid, double-stranded DNA virus

✳ Replication in nucleus, transcription by host RNA polymerase genome synthesis by DNA polymerase

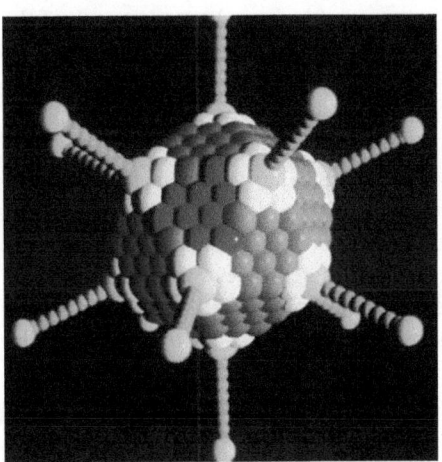

FIGURE 9–8. **Virion structure of an adenovirus.** The double-stranded DNA genome is covered with an icosahedral capsid composed of 252 subunits (capsomeres), including 240 hexons and 12 pentons and fibers. The penton on the surface of the capsid contains a base and a projecting fiber that varies in length among serotypes. The fiber is modified by addition of glucosamine and interacts with the receptor on host cells.

is illustrated by the frequent recovery of virus from tonsils or adenoids removed from healthy children (the group name is derived from its discovery in 1953 as a latent agent in many adenoid tissue specimens) and by prolonged intermittent shedding of virus from the pharynx and intestinal tract after initial infection. Adenoviruses most commonly cause respiratory infection but depending on the serotypes, they can also cause gastroenteritis, conjunctivitis, cystitis, hepatitis, myocarditis, and less commonly, neurologic diseases. In addition, people with weakened immune system are at high of developing severe illness.

EPIDEMIOLOGY

Potential for prolonged infection without disease

Types 1, 2, and 3 adenoviruses are highly endemic; type 5 is the next most common. Most primary infections with these viruses occur early in life and are spread by the respiratory route, fecal–oral route, and by contact with contaminated fomites. Neonates can acquire infection from exposure to cervical secretions at birth. Adenoviruses can survive for a long period on surfaces and are relatively resistant to disinfectants but inactivated by heat, formaldehyde, or bleach. Overall, only about 45% of adenovirus infections result in disease. Their most significant contribution to acute illness is in children, particularly those younger than 2 years of age (~10% of acute febrile illness). Adenoviruses are also major causes of ARD in military recruits, usually by types 4 (prevalence > 90%), 14, 7, 3, and 21.

Disease in children, military recruits is spread by respiratory or fecal–oral route

✳ Naked capsid virus relatively resistant to disinfectants than enveloped respiratory viruses

Infections caused by serotypes 1, 2, and 5 are generally most common during the first few years of life. All serotypes can occur during any season of the year but are encountered most frequently during late winter or early spring. Sharp outbreaks of disease caused by serotypes 3 and 7 have been traced to inadequately chlorinated swimming pools. Conjunctivitis is the illness most commonly associated with these episodes. Other outbreaks of conjunctivitis have been traced to physicians' offices and appear to have been spread by contaminated ophthalmic medications or diagnostic equipment.

Swimming pool and medication-associated conjunctivitis occur in outbreaks

PATHOGENESIS

The adenoviruses usually enter the host by inhalation of droplet nuclei or by the oral route. Direct inoculation onto nasal or conjunctival mucosa by hands, contaminated towels, or ophthalmic medications may also occur. The incubation period in most infected people is 5 to 7 days. The virus replicates in epithelial cells, producing cell necrosis and inflammation. Viremia sometimes occurs and can result in spread to distant sites, such as the kidney, bladder, liver, lymphoid tissue (including mesenteric nodes), and, occasionally, the central nervous system. In the acute phase of infection, the distant sites may also show inflammation; for example, abdominal pain is occasionally seen with severe illnesses and is believed to result from mesenteric lymphadenitis caused by the viruses.

Infects by droplet, oral route, or direct inoculation

Epithelial cell replication may follow viremic spread and remote disease

After the acute phase of illness, the viruses may remain in tissues, particularly lymphoid structures such as tonsils, adenoids, and intestinal Peyer patches, and may become reactivated and shed without producing illness for 6 to 18 months thereafter. This reactivation is enhanced by stressful events (stress reactivation), such as infection by other agents.

Viral DNA can persist and reactivate

Like the viruses described previously, adenoviruses have a primary pathology involving epithelial cell necrosis with a predominantly mononuclear inflammatory response. In some instances, smudgy intranuclear inclusions may be seen in infected cells (**Figure 9–9**). A potentially important pathogenic feature of the virion is the presence of pentons, which are located at each of the 12 corners of the icosahedron. These fiber-like projections with knob-like terminal structures are believed to bind to a cellular receptor that is similar or identical to the one for group B coxsackieviruses. Moreover, the pentons appear to be responsible for a toxic effect on cells, which manifests as clumping and detachment *in vitro*.

Penton projections are toxic to cells

In addition, adenoviruses have developed other novel strategies to survive in the host, yet produce deleterious effects. These include encoding a protein in its early E3 genomic region that binds class I MHC antigens in the endoplasmic reticulum, thus restricting their expression on the surface of infected cells and interfering with recognition and attack by cytotoxic T cells. This ability to evade immunosurveillance may be vital to establishment of latency. Another early protein (E1A) has been associated with increased susceptibility of epithelial cells to destruction by tumor necrosis factor and other cytokines. Other adenoviral proteins have been described that have a variety of effects on cell function and susceptibility to cytolysis. One of these, called the **adenovirus death protein,** is considered important for efficient lysis of infected cells and release of newly formed virions.

Proteins restrict cytotoxic T cells and enhance cytokine susceptibility

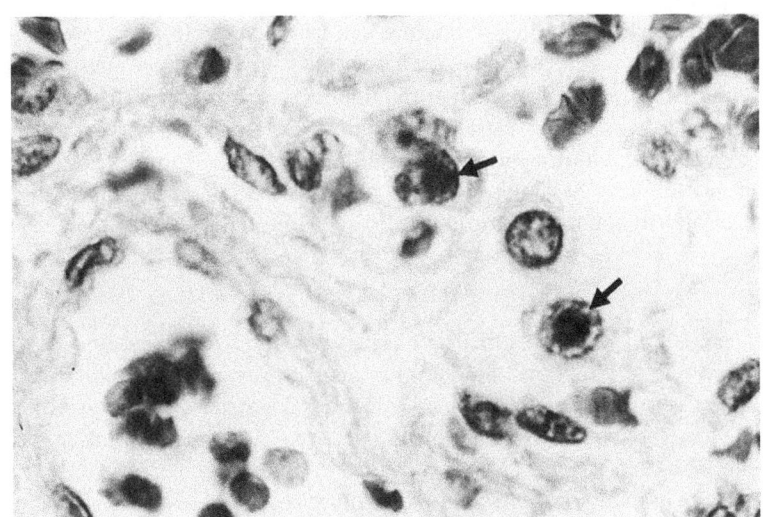

FIGURE 9-9. **Lung tissue from a fatal case of adenovirus type 7 pneumonia.** Large, smudgy intranuclear inclusions in alveolar epithelial cells (*arrows*), which are sometimes seen in adenovirus infections, are present. (Original magnification ×100.)

IMMUNITY

Immunity to adenoviruses after infection is serotype-specific and usually long lasting. In addition to type-specific immunity, group-specific complement-fixing antibodies appear in response to infection. These antibodies are useful indicators of infection, but do not specify the infecting serotype.

Immunity is serotype-specific

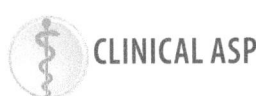 CLINICAL ASPECTS

MANIFESTATIONS

The diversity of major syndromes and serotypes commonly associated with adenoviruses are summarized in **Table 9-5.** The acute respiratory syndromes vary in both clinical manifestations and severity. Symptoms include fever, rhinitis, pharyngitis, cough, and conjunctivitis. Adenoviruses are also common causes of nonstreptococcal exudative pharyngitis, particularly among children younger than 3 years of age. Acute and, occasionally, chronic conjunctivitis and keratoconjunctivitis have been associated with several serotypes. More severe diseases, such as laryngitis, croup, bronchiolitis, and pneumonia, may also occur. A syndrome of pharyngitis and conjunctivitis (pharyngoconjunctival fever) is classically associated with adenovirus infection. Adenoviruses can also cause acute hemorrhagic cystitis, in which hematuria and dysuria are prominent findings. Some serotypes are significant causes of gastroenteritis (see Chapter 15).

Multiple upper respiratory syndromes, conjunctivitis, and pharyngitis are common

＊ More severe diseases include croup, bronchiolitis, and pneumonia

＊ Pharyngoconjunctival fever is a classical manifestation

DIAGNOSIS

Adenovirus infection can be diagnosed by genome amplification by PCR, antigen detection by enzyme immunoassay, virus isolation, and serology. The nucleic acid–based BioFire test for 14 to 19 respiratory pathogens includes adenovirus. Many serotypes of adenoviruses, other than those

TABLE 9-5	Clinical Syndromes Associated With Adenovirus Infection
SYNDROME	**COMMON SEROTYPES**[a]
Childhood febrile illness; pharyngoconjunctival fever	1, 2, **3**, 5, 7, **7a**, 21
Pneumonia and other acute respiratory illnesses	1, 2, **3**, 5, 7, **7a, 7b, 14a,** 21 (4 in military recruits)
Pertussis-like illness	1, 2, **3**, 5, **19**, 21
Conjunctivitis	2, 5, 7, 8, 19, 21
Keratoconjunctivitis	**3**, 8, 9, **19**, 37
Acute hemorrhagic cystitis, interstitial nephritis	11, 34, 35
Acute gastroenteritis	40, 41

[a]Serotypes in **boldface** are commonly associated with outbreaks.

associated with acute gastroenteritis, can be readily isolated in heteroploid cell cultures. There is little difficulty in relating the virus detected to the illness in question when the isolate has been obtained from a site other than the upper respiratory or gastrointestinal tract (eg, lung biopsy, conjunctival swabs, urine). However, because of the known tendency for intermittent asymptomatic shedding into the oropharynx and feces, isolates from these latter sites must be interpreted more cautiously. Serologic testing of acute and convalescent sera may be necessary to confirm the relation between the virus and the illness in question.

Diagnosis by PCR, antigen detection, virus isolation, or serology

Viral isolation from oropharynx or feces may not mean disease

TREATMENT AND PREVENTION

There is no specific treatment for adenovirus infection. Most infections are treated or managed based on the symptoms. Some *in vitro* and *in vivo* data combined with clinical observations in patients with severe disseminated infections suggest that cidofovir (nucleotide analog) might be effective for adenovirus infection. A live virus vaccine containing serotypes 4 and 7, enclosed in enteric-coated capsules and administered orally, has been used in military recruits. The viruses are released into the small intestine, where they produce an asymptomatic, nontransmissible infection. This vaccine has been found effective but is neither available nor recommended for civilian groups.

Cidofovir (antiviral) in severe adenovirus infections

Live enteric vaccine used in military

 Why are some respiratory viruses such as adenovirus and rhinovirus relatively resistant to disinfectants compared with respiratory viruses like influenza virus, parainfluenza virus, RSV, and coronavirus?

● RHINOVIRUSES

The rhinovirus group comprises of more than 100 serotypes as well as more that are not yet classified, all of which are members of the picornavirus family. They are small (20-30 nm), naked capsid virus particles containing single-stranded, positive-sense RNA genomes. They are distinguished from other picornaviruses, namely enteroviruses by their acid lability and an optimum temperature of 33°C for *in vitro* replication. This temperature approximates that of the nasopharynx in the human host and may be a factor in the localization of pathologic findings at that site. Rhinoviruses are most consistently isolated in cultures of human diploid fibroblasts. The receptor for most rhinoviruses (and some coxsackieviruses) is glycoprotein intercellular adhesion molecule 1 (ICAM-1), a member of the immunoglobulin supergene family. ICAM-1 is best known for its role in immunologic cell adhesion; its ligand is the lymphocyte function-associated antigen-1.

⁎ **Small, naked capsid, positive-sense RNA viruses include multiple serotypes**

Optimum growth temperature is 33°C

Virus binds to ICAM intercellular adhesion molecule receptor

Rhinoviruses are known as the common cold viruses. They represent the major causes of mild URI syndromes in all age groups, especially older children and adults. Lower respiratory tract disease caused by rhinoviruses is uncommon. The usual incubation period is 2 to 3 days, and acute symptoms commonly last 3 to 7 days. It is interesting to note that mucosal cell damage is minimal during the illness. Data suggest that activation and an increase in kinins, particularly bradykinin, may have a major role in the pathogenesis of increased secretions, vasodilation, and sore throat. Rhinovirus infections may be seen at any time of the year. Epidemic peaks tend to occur in the early fall or spring months.

⁎ **Rhinoviruses (common cold viruses) cause mild URI**

Minimal cell injury produced

DIAGNOSIS, TREATMENT, AND PREVENTION

Rhinoviruses can be diagnosed by viral genome amplification by RT-PCR in nasopharyngeal specimens. At present, there is no specific therapy and no method of prevention with vaccines. Prospects for the development of an appropriate vaccine appear less promising. The multiplicity of serotypes and their tendency to be type-specific in the production of antibodies seem to demand the development of a multivalent vaccine, which would be extremely difficult to

Diagnosis by RT-PCR

Multiple serotypes make vaccine difficult

 Think ▸▸ Apply 9-7: While influenza virus, parainfluenza virus, RSV, and coronavirus are enveloped with lipid membranes that are lysed in disinfectants, adenovirus and rhinovirus are naked capsids and relatively resistant to lipid-based disinfectants.

accomplish. However, recent studies have suggested that a monoclonal antibody directed at the virus receptor or the use of a recombinant soluble receptor (ICAM-1) might block attachment of rhinoviruses. It remains to be seen whether these observations can be translated into effective preventive or therapeutic applications. At present, the attitude toward these viruses is best summed up by Sir Christopher Andrewes, who suggested that we should accept these infections as "one of the stimulating risks of being mortal."

Monoclonal antibody block attachment to ICAM

BOCAVIRUS

Human bocavirus was first discovered in 2005 by using molecular screening methods. It is a novel parvovirus which is a small (20 nm) naked capsid, single-stranded DNA virus. Unlike another human parvovirus, parvovirus B19 that causes erythema infectiosum (slapped face—see Chapter 10 detailed virology of parvovirus), it has been primarily implicated as a cause of wheezing and other respiratory illnesses in children. In addition, bocavirus has also been isolated from feces of infants with gastroenteritis symptoms. Three strains of human bocavirus (HBoV), HBoV-1, 2, and 3 have been identified. Symptoms include cough, fever, and wheezing. Diagnosis requires PCR methods. Further studies are ongoing to determine its epidemiologic behavior and relative contribution to respiratory morbidity.

✳ **Bocavirus associated with wheezing and respiratory illness in infants and children**

REOVIRUSES

Reoviruses have been associated with upper respiratory tract infection, fever, gastroenteritis, febrile illness, and childhood exanthem. The reoviruses (also known as respiratory enteric orphans for "reo") are naked capsid virions that contain segmented, double-stranded RNA genomes and an outer and inner (double) protein shell. In addition, the virions contain RNA-dependent RNA polymerase. These double-stranded viruses transcribe and replicate in the cytoplasm by using their own RNA polymerase. The progeny viruses are assembled in the cytoplasm of infected cells and released by cell lysis. They are ubiquitous and have been found in humans, simians, rodents, cattle, and a variety of other hosts. They have been studied in detail as experimental models, revealing much basic knowledge about viral genetics and pathogenesis at the molecular level. Three serotypes are known to infect humans and associated with several conditions; however, their role and mechanisms in human disease remain to be understood. Reoviruses causing diarrheal disease are discussed in Chapter 15 and arboviral diseases are discussed in Chapter 16.

Reoviruses associated with respiratory, enteric, and febrile illness

Role and mechanisms in human respiratory disease are unclear

KEY CONCLUISONS

- Major influenza epidemics are caused by influenza A virus and also B virus but not C virus. Influenza A has eight segments of negative-sense RNA, enveloped virus containing H and N spikes. H binds to the receptor on host cells and N is involved in smooth passage of the virus in the respiratory tract and virus release.

- Three types of H (H1, H2, and H3) and two types of N (N1 and N2) dominate in human influenza A virus infection.

- Influenza virus replicates in the nucleus of the infected cells by using host cell RNA primers and its own viral RNA polymerase for transcription and replication.

- Influenza A virus undergoes antigenic drift more frequently than B and C viruses. Antigenic shift only takes place in influenza A virus.

- Clinical disease involves abrupt onset of respiratory symptoms for 1 to 4 days after exposure which include fever, myalgia, and cough lasting for 3 to 5 days. Nonspecific weakness and coughing may continue for 2 to 6 weeks. Some patients may develop progressive infection resulting in viral pneumonia.

- The most common and important complication is bacterial superinfection leading to bacterial pneumonia, occasionally disseminated bacterial infection. People with underlying cardiovascular and pulmonary conditions develop complications, including death.

- Pathogenic mechanisms of influenza involve damage to structural and functional ability of ciliated epithelial cells followed by host cell synthesis shut off, release of lysosomal enzymes, and desquamation of ciliated and mucus producing epithelial cells. This causes a significant interference in the clearance mechanism of the respiratory tract.

- Humans can also be infected with influenza viruses from other species such as avian (H5N1) and swine (H1N1). Both avian and swine influenza viruses cause more severe diseases, especially viral pneumonia with high fatality in younger adults.

- H5N1 is not easily transmitted to humans because it does not bind to human influenza virus receptor SA α 2,6 galactose located in the cells of upper respiratory tract; however, it binds to its receptor SA α 2,3 galactose located in the cells of lower respiratory tract. H1N1 swine binds to both receptors, SA α 2,6 galactose and SA α 2,3 galactose. Both H5N1 and H1N1 swine cause viral pneumonia because they can infect and replicate in lower respiratory tract cells and cause cytokine storm.

- Parainfluenza virus is a paramyxovirus with a negative-sense RNA genome and lipid bilayer envelope containing spikes HN and F. They cause upper respiratory tract infections in all age groups, especially croup and bronchitis in infants.

- RSV is a *Pneumovirus* (paramyxovirus) with a negative-sense RNA genome and a lipid bilayer envelope with spikes G and F. G binds to a receptor and F protein causes syncytia formation leading to cell death.

- RSV is the single most important agent to cause acute bronchiolitis and pneumonia in infants under 1 year of age. Symptoms include cough, wheezing, and respiratory distress.

- Clinical findings include hyperexpansion of the lungs, hypoxemia, and hypercapnia. Interstitial infiltrates with areas of pulmonary collapse may be seen on chest X-ray.

- Th2 cytokines and immune complex formation make the RSV-induced bronchiolitis worse.

- Human metapneumovirus (paramyxovirus) and bocavirus (parvovirus) cause bronchiolitis and pneumonia in infants.

- Coronaviruses (positive-sense RNA, helical, enveloped) cause common cold like rhinovirus. However, three novel coronaviruses have emerged that cause severe respiratory infections; they are SARS, MERS, and COVID-19.

- Of the three novel coronaviruses, SARS-CoV-2 emerged in 2019 in China and spread worldwide causing a pandemic by infecting 178 million and killing 3.86 million people, including 33.5 million cases and 0.6 million deaths in the United States.

- SARS-CoV-2 is transmitted through the respiratory route and causes flu-like illness in the majority of infected people; however, 15% of infected people develop severe COVID-19 including pneumonia and 5% of patients develop critical illness such as acute hypoxemic respiratory failure, shock, or multiorgan dysfunction.

- Three highly efficacious vaccines for COVID-19, including two mRNA (Pfizer, Moderna) and one adenovirus vector–based expressing Spike glycoprotein have been authorized for emergency use in the United States.

- Adenoviruses are naked capsid double-stranded DNA viruses mainly causing respiratory infections. However, depending on the serotypes, they can also cause gastroenteritis, conjunctivitis, cystitis, hepatitis, myocarditis, and, unusually, neurologic diseases.

- Severe form of adenoviral disease includes croup, bronchiolitis, and pneumonia, whereas pharyngoconjunctival fever is a classical manifestation.

- Rhinoviruses (picornavirus, naked capsid, positive-sense RNA virus) cause common cold, like common coronavirus.

- Bocavirus, a single-stranded DNA, naked capsid parvovirus is associated with coughing and wheezing in infants and children.

CASE STUDY

An Infant with Respiratory Distress

This 9-month-old boy was born prematurely, requiring treatment in a neonatal intensive care unit for the first month of life. After discharge, he remained well until 3 days ago, when symptoms of a common cold progressed to cough, rapid and labored respiration, lethargy, and refusal to eat. On examination, his temperature was 38.5°C, respiratory rate 60/min, and pulse 140/min. Auscultation of the chest revealed coarse crackles and occasional wheezes. Abnormal laboratory findings included hypoxemia and hypercapnia. A chest radiograph showed hyperinflation, interstitial perihilar infiltrates, and right upper lobe atelectasis.

QUESTIONS

1. Which of these viruses is the least likely cause of this baby's illness?
   A. Influenza
   B. Parainfluenza
   C. Reovirus
   D. Respiratory syncytial virus
   E. Adenovirus

2. The mechanism of "antigenic drift" in influenza viruses includes all of the following, *except*:
   A. Can involve either H or N antigens
   B. Mutations caused by viral RNA polymerase
   C. Can predominate under host selective immune pressures
   D. Reassortment between human and animal or avian reservoirs
   E. Can involve genes encoding structural or nonstructural proteins

3. Which of the following is involved in pathogenesis of RSV-induced bronchiolitis?
   A. G protein
   B. F protein
   C. Neuraminidase
   D. Hemagglutinin
   E. M protein

4. Which of the following can be used to prevent RSV pneumonia?
   A. Vaccine
   B. Oseltamivir
   C. Zanamivir
   D. Palivizumab (Monoclonal antibody against F)
   E. Monoclonal antibody against G

ANSWERS

1. **(C)**

2. **(D)**

3. **(B)**

4. **(D)**

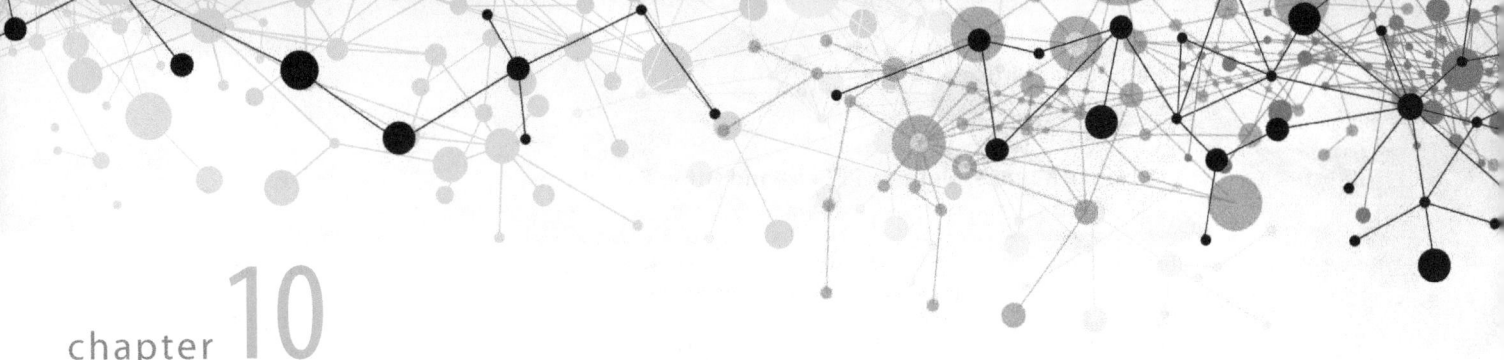

chapter 10

Viruses of Mumps, Measles, Rubella, and Other Childhood Exanthems

Mumps Virus · Measles Virus · Rubella Virus · Parvovirus B19

> They wondered
>
> If wheezeles
>
> Could turn
>
> Into measles,
>
> If sneazles
>
> Would turn
>
> Into mumps
>
> —A.A. Milne, *Now We Are Six*

The major viruses described in this chapter are mumps, measles, rubella, and the human parvovirus B19, which are from different virus families and genetically unrelated, but share several common epidemiologic and clinical characteristics, including (1) worldwide distribution, with a high incidence of infection in nonimmune individuals; (2) humans as sole reservoir of infection; and (3) person-to-person spread primarily by the respiratory (aerosol) route.

The other diseases discussed in this chapter are roseola infantum and rubella-like rashes caused by many different viruses that are mainly common illnesses occurring in early life. Key characteristics of these major viruses are summarized in **Table 10–1**.

TABLE 10–1   Comparison of Mumps, Measles, Rubella and Other Exanthems

FEATURE	MUMPS	MEASLES	RUBELLA	PARVOVIRUS B19	ROSEOLA
Virus type	Paramyxoviridae (Paramyxovirus) enveloped, helical, single-stranded (-) RNA	Paramyxovirus (Morbillivirus) enveloped, helical, single-stranded (-) RNA	Togavirus (Rubivirus) enveloped, icosahedral, single-stranded (+) RNA	Parvovirus, naked capsid, icosahedral, single-stranded DNA	Human herpesviruses 6 or 7, enveloped, icosahedral, double-stranded DNA
Transmission	Respiratory	Respiratory	Respiratory	Respiratory	Oral secretions
Incubation period (days)	12-29 (average 16-18)	7-18 (average 9-11)	14-21 (average 16)	4-12	Unknown
Symptoms	Fever, parotitis	Fever, cough, conjunctivitis, Koplik spots	Fever (low grade), upper respiratory symptoms	Mild fever, malaise, headache, myalgia, itching	High fever, occasional late sudden rash
Characteristic rash	None	Widespread, maculopapular	Faint, macular	Macular, reticular, often faint	Transient, faint macular
Duration of illness	7-10 days	3-5 days	1-3 days	1-2 weeks	3-5 days
Severity and/or complications	Meningitis, encephalitis, pancreatitis, orchitis, oophoritis	Bacterial superinfection, encephalitis, keratitis, reactivation of tuberculosis, subacute sclerosing panencephalitis (rare)	Overt arthritis, congenital infection	Aplastic crisis (in chronic[a] hemolytic diseases), arthritis, arthralgias	
Fetal infection	No[a]	No[a]	Yes—multiple defects	Yes—stillbirth, fetal hydrops	No[a]
Vaccine	Live attenuated	Live attenuated	Live attenuated	No	No

[a]Fetal infection may rarely occur, but with no apparent consequences.

MUMPS

Overview

Mumps virus, a member of paramyxoviridae family and paramyxovirus genus, is a negative-sense single-stranded RNA, helical, enveloped virus with glycoprotein spikes, HN, and F that replicates in the cytoplasm by using viral RNA polymerase. Mumps is transmitted through respiratory tract and replicate in the respiratory tract epithelium and local lymph nodes followed by fever and swelling of parotid glands (parotitis) unilateral or bilateral. The incubation period is 12 to 29 days and the symptoms persist for 7 to 10 days. The development of viremia allows the virus to travel to all body organs, including salivary glands and central nervous system. The complications of mumps include aseptic meningitis, encephalitis, pancreatitis, orchitis, and oophoritis. Pathogenesis involves cell necrosis and inflammation with predominant infiltration of mononuclear cells. Humoral and cell-mediated immunity are involved in containing the infection; however, IgG persists for lifelong. An effective live, attenuated mumps vaccine (part of MMR or MMRV vaccine) is recommended at 12 to 15 months of age and a second dose at 4 to 6 years. In recent years, there has been a resurgence of outbreaks of mumps in the United States and elsewhere, underscoring the ongoing necessity to ensure adequate surveillance and immunization efforts.

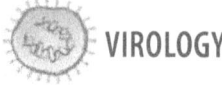 VIROLOGY

✳ Enveloped, helical, single-stranded (-) RNA virus with hemagglutinin and neuraminidase activity (HN) and fusion protein F spikes

Mumps virus is a paramyxovirus, and only one major antigenic type is known. Like fellow members of its genus, it contains a single-stranded, negative-sense RNA genome, and a helical nucleocapsid that is surrounded by a matrix protein followed by a lipid bilayer envelope (see Figure 9–4). Two glycoproteins are expressed on the surface of the envelope; one mediates hemagglutination and neuraminidase (HN) activity and the other is responsible for viral lipid membrane fusion (F) to the host cell. Similar to other paramyxoviruses, mumps virus initiates infection by attachment of the HN spike to sialic acid on the cell surface, and F protein promotes fusion with the plasma membrane. It replicates in the cytoplasm by using its own RNA-dependent RNA polymerase, and the progeny viruses are released by budding from the plasma membranes. Details about the structure of the virus are described in Chapter 9 and replication of negative-sense RNA viruses (paramyxoviruses) are in Chapter 6.

⁕ Viral replication in cytoplasm using viral RNA polymerase

⁕ High frequency of mumps at 5 to 15 years

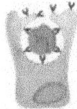 ## MUMPS INFECTION

EPIDEMIOLOGY

Mumps infection is observed to occur most frequently in the 5- to 15-year age group. Infection is rarely seen in the first year of life. Mumps is transmitted from person to person through the respiratory route (aerosol), such as in respiratory viruses. Although approximately 85% of susceptible household contacts acquire infection, approximately 30% to 40% of these contacts do not develop clinical disease. The disease is communicable from approximately 7 days before until 9 days after the onset of illness; however, virus has been recovered in urine for up to 14 days after onset. The highest incidence of infection is usually during the late winter and spring months, but it can occur during any season. In the United States, mumps cases range from couple hundred to couple thousand every year. For example, from 2011 to 2015, mumps cases ranged from 229 to 1329. However, mumps cases saw an increase in recent years, including 6366 cases in 2016, 6109 in 2017, 2251 in 2018, and 3474 in 2019. The increase in recent mumps cases is attributed to lack of vaccination, incomplete doses of vaccines, living in crowded environments such as community gatherings, schools and universities, and sports team.

Person-to-person transmission via respiratory route

High infectivity 7 days before and 9 days after onset

⁕ Few hundred to few thousand cases in the United States

⁕ Replicates in the upper respiratory tract epithelium, local lymph nodes

Viremia allows virus dissemination

PATHOGENESIS

After initial entry into the respiratory tract, the virus replicates locally in the respiratory tract epithelium and local lymph nodes. Replication is followed by viremic dissemination to target tissues such as the salivary glands (parotid glands) and central nervous system (CNS). It is also possible that, before the development of immune responses, a secondary phase of viremia may result from virus replication in target tissues (eg, initial parotid glands involvement with later spread to other organs). There is painful swelling of one or both parotid glands. Viruria is common, probably as a result of direct spread from the blood into the urine, in addition to active viral replication in the kidney. The tissue response is that of cell necrosis and inflammation, with predominantly mononuclear cell infiltration. In the salivary glands, swelling and desquamation of necrotic epithelial lining cells, accompanied by interstitial inflammation and edema, may be seen within dilated ducts. The pathogenesis, clinical disease, and immune response are summarized in **Figure 10–1.**

⁕ Viral replication in salivary glands with painful swelling of parotid glands

Viruria common due to direct spread from blood to urine, replication in kidney

Necrosis, inflammation, infiltration of mononuclear cells in tissues

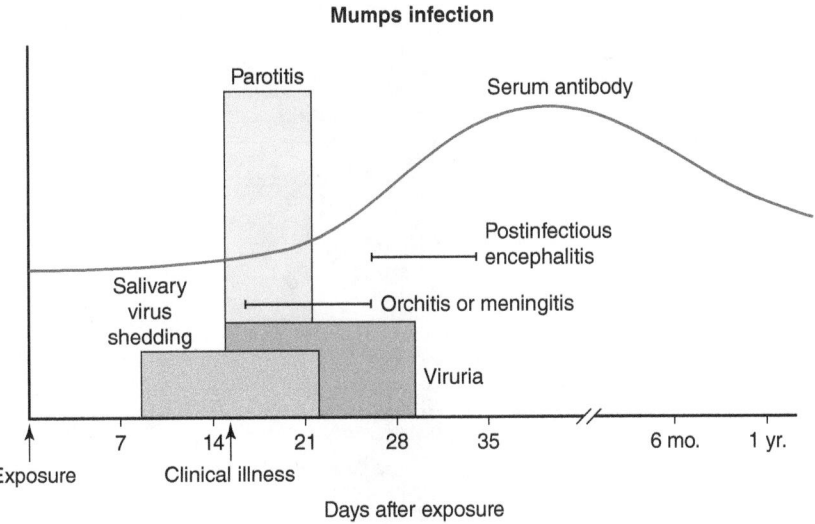

FIGURE 10–1. Pathogenesis of mumps virus infection. After exposure, the virus multiplies in the respiratory tract epithelium (incubation period of 16-18 days on average) and spreads to local lymph nodes followed by viremia, which spreads throughout the body. The virus is also shed in salivary glands and urine. Fever follows painful swelling of one or both parotid glands (parotitis). The symptoms last 7 to 10 days. Humoral and cellular immune responses eliminate the virus from the infected hosts. IgM appears early in infection followed by IgG that persists for life. Some of the common complications of the mumps include meningitis, encephalitis, orchitis, oophoritis, pancreatitis, and myocarditis.

IMMUNITY

＊IgM suggests recent infection

As in most viral infections, the early antibody response in mumps is predominantly with immunoglobulin M (IgM), which is switched gradually over several weeks to a specific IgG antibody. The latter persists for a lifetime, but can often be detected only by specific neutralization assays. Immunity is associated with the presence of neutralizing antibody. The role of cellular immune responses has also been investigated and is found to contribute both to the pathogenesis of the acute disease and to recovery from infection. After primary infection, immunity to reinfection is, virtually, always permanent.

IgG persists lifelong

Neutralizing antibody (IgG) protective

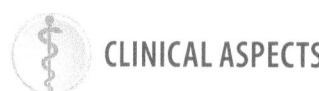 **CLINICAL ASPECTS**

MANIFESTATIONS

Incubation period 12 to 29 days

＊Parotitis, unilateral or bilateral, may last 7 to 10 days

After an incubation period of 12 to 29 days (average, 16-18 days), the typical case of mumps is characterized by fever and swelling with tenderness of the salivary glands, especially the parotid glands (**Figure 10–2**). Swelling may be unilateral or bilateral and persists for 7 to 10 days. Several complications can occur, usually within 1 to 3 weeks of onset of illness. All appear to be a direct result of virus spread to other sites and illustrate the extensive tissue tropism of mumps.

The common complications of mumps infection, which can occur without parotitis, include the following:

＊Complications include meningitis, encephalitis, pancreatitis, orchitis, oophoritis

Meningitis: Approximately 10% of all infected patients develop meningitis. It is usually mild, but can be confused with bacterial meningitis. In approximately one-third of these cases, associated or preceding evidence of parotitis is absent.

Encephalitis: Encephalitis is occasionally severe.

Spinal cord and peripheral nerves are involved, causing transverse myelitis and polyneuritis in rare cases.

Pancreatitis: Pancreatitis is suggested by upper abdominal pain, nausea, and vomiting.

＊Orchitis in 10% to 20% of men, unilateral or bilateral; sterility rare

Orchitis: Orchitis (inflammation of the testes) is estimated to occur in 10% to 20% of infected men, which could be unilateral or bilateral in postpubertal men. Although subsequent sterility is a concern, it appears that this outcome is rare.

Oophoritis: Oophoritis (inflammation of ovaries) is an unusual, usually benign, inflammation of the ovarian glands.

FIGURE 10–2. **Mumps parotitis.** The swelling just below the earlobe is due to enlargement of the parotid gland. (Reproduced with permission from Nester EW, Anderson DG, Roberts CE Jr, et al *Microbiology: A Human Perspective*, 6th ed. New York, NY: McGraw Hill; 2008.)

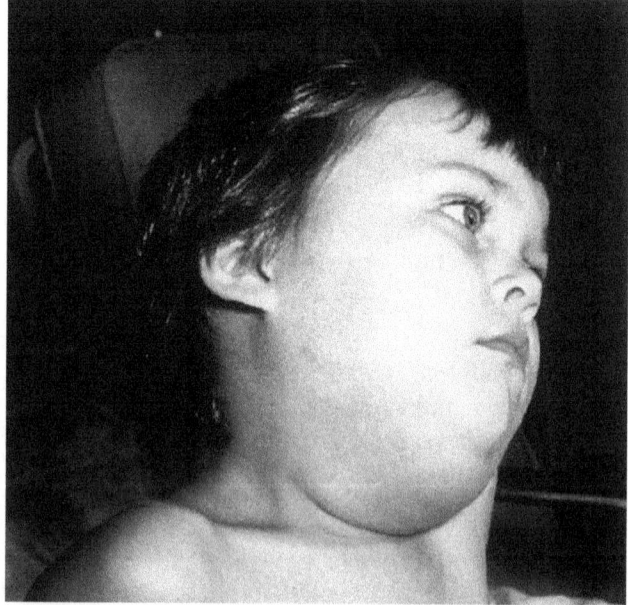

Other rare and transient complications include myocarditis, nephritis, arthritis, thyroiditis, thrombocytopenic purpura, mastitis, and pneumonia. Most complications resolve without sequelae within 2 to 3 weeks. However, occasional permanent effects have been noted, particularly in severe CNS infection, in which sensorineural hearing loss and other impairment can occur.

 While the mumps virus enters through and replicates in respiratory tract cells and causes parotitis, how does it cause other diseases such as meningitis, pancreatitis, and orchitis?

DIAGNOSIS

Mumps virus can be readily detected or isolated early in the illness from the saliva, pharynx, and other affected sites, such as the cerebrospinal fluid (CSF). In addition, urine is an excellent source for virus isolation. Rapid diagnosis can be made by direct detection of viral nucleic acid by reverse transcription-polymerase chain reaction (RT-PCR). Mumps virus grows well in primary monolayer cell cultures derived from monkey kidney, producing syncytial giant cells and viral hemagglutinin. Virus culture is gold standard.

The usual serologic tests are enzyme-linked immunoassay (EIA) or enzyme-linked immunosorbent assay (ELISA) and indirect immunofluorescence (IF) to detect IgM- and IgG-specific antibody responses. Other serologic tests are also available, such as complement fixation, hemagglutination inhibition, and neutralization. Of these, the neutralization test is the most sensitive for detection of immunity to infection.

Rapid detection by RT-PCR

Culture in cell lines from saliva, throat, CSF, urine

ELISA, EIA, IF detect IgM IgG

IgM early provides diagnosis

PREVENTION

There is no specific treatment available for mumps. Since 1967, a live attenuated vaccine that is safe and highly effective has been available. As a result of its routine use, infections in the United States before 2005 were exceedingly rare; however, in the late 2005 and into 2006, a large outbreak (greater than 6000 proved or probable cases) developed in Iowa and eight neighboring midwestern states. Most occurred in persons 18 to 25 years of age, many of whom had been previously vaccinated at least once. The mumps strain identified was genotype G, a common strain similar to the one that involved more than 70,000 cases in the United Kingdom from 2004 to 2006. Thus, it has been reemphasized that a two-dose vaccine regimen is essential to ensure adequate immunity. The vaccine is produced by serial propagation of virus in chick embryo cell cultures. Mumps is commonly combined with measles and rubella (MMR) vaccine or measles, rubella, and varicella (chickenpox virus) vaccine (MMRV), and given as a single injection to a child at 12 to 15 months of age. A second dose of MMR or MMRV is recommended at 4 to 6 years of age; those who have missed the second dose should receive it no later than 11 to 12 years of age. A single dose causes seroconversion in approximately 80% of recipients, and it increases only to about 90% after two doses. The vaccine must be given at least 2 to 4 weeks before exposure to be at all effective in postexposure prophylaxis. In approximately 10% of the people who have received the two doses of the vaccine and, probably, partially seroconverted could still be infected with the mumps virus because of living in close contacts, such as at schools and colleges. In 2009-2010, a mumps outbreak occurred in the northeastern United States, spreading in a camp, followed by spread in schools and household. This infection most likely came through a boy who traveled to the United Kingdom and later joined the camp. In 2010, more than 2000 cases and in 2016, more than 5000 cases of mumps were reported in the United States. In 2015-2016, several outbreaks were reported from many university campuses, including the largest outbreaks from Iowa and Illinois campuses that held MMR vaccination campaigns.

Furthermore, cases of mumps have increased in recent years, including 6366 cases in 2016, 6109 in 2017, 2251 in 2018, and 3474 in 2019. In 2017, Advisory Committee on Immunization Practices (ACIP) recommended a third dose of MMR vaccine to improve protection in people living in crowded settings.

✳ Live attenuated vaccine (MMR or MMRV) ideally given at 12 to 15 months of age, repeated at 4 to 6 years

 Think ▸▸ Apply 10-1: Viremia develops due to viral replication in the respiratory tract, regional lymph nodes, and parotid glands probably before the development of immune response. The virus travels to various body organs such as CNS, pancreas, testis, and others causing damage and inflammation.

Overview

Measles virus, a member of paramyxoviridae family and *Morbillivirus* genus, is a negative-sense RNA, helical, enveloped virus with H and F spikes, which replicates in the cytoplasm by using viral RNA polymerase. Measles (also known as rubeola or 5-day measles) is transmitted through respiratory inhalation (incubation period 7-18 days) and replicates in respiratory mucosal epithelium infections followed by spread to regional lymph nodes and development of viremia and transportation of virus to all body organs. Measles often produce severe illness in children, associated with fever, cough, coryza, widespread rash, and transient immunosuppression. One to 2 days before the development of rash, Koplik spots (small bluish-yellow spots) appear on the buccal mucosa opposite the molar teeth. Severity of measles includes high fever, delirium, conjunctivitis and photophobia. The virus is one of the most contagious agents among humans. Serious complications include encephalitis, pneumonia, otitis media, mastoiditis, sinusitis and bleeding disorders. Pathogenesis involves infection of immune cells, downregulation of IL-12 and depressed cell-mediated immunity. Skin lesions show vasculitis and presence of viral components in rash. Immune-mediated postinfectious encephalitis may occur in some patients through CD8 T cells infiltration in the CNS. Long-term sequelae, such as blindness, may occur, and, rarely, a few patients develop a slowly fatal condition called subacute sclerosing panencephalitis (SSPE) with onset years after the initial infection. Immunity to reinfection is lifelong associated with the presence of neutralizing antibodies. However, patients with defects in cell-mediated immunity and malnutrition have a prolonged infection with severe complication. An effective live attenuated vaccine is recommended (as part of MMR or MMRV) in the first year of life and a booster between 4 and 6 years of age. In the past several years, cases and outbreaks of measles have been reported in the United States and elsewhere underscoring the importance of surveillance and immunization.

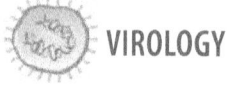

VIROLOGY

The measles virus is classified in the paramyxoviridae family, genus *Morbillivirus*. It contains a linear, negative-sense, single-stranded RNA genome surrounded by a helical nucleocapsid protein and a lipid bilayer envelope containing two glycoprotein spikes (peplomers), namely hemagglutinin (H), that mediates virus adsorption to the cell surfaces, and fusion (F) protein that mediates cell fusion, hemolysis, and viral entry into the cell. On the inside of the envelope surface, there is a matrix (M) protein that plays a key role in viral assembly. The virions also contain the viral RNA polymerase (RNA-dependent RNA polymerase) required for viral RNA transcription and replication. Unlike the mumps virus, the measles virus lacks neuraminidase (N) activity. The receptor for measles virus is CD46 (membrane cofactor protein), a regulator of complement activation. Replication of measles virus is similar to other paramyxoviruses, which is described in Chapter 6 for negative-sense RNA viruses. Only a single serotype restricted to human infection is recognized; however, subtle antigenic and genetic variations among wild-type measles strains do occur. These variations can be determined by sequencing analyses, enabling more precise epidemiologic tracking of outbreaks and their origins. Such ongoing molecular surveillance is also extremely important in determining whether significant antigenic drifts evolve over time.

✳ Enveloped, helical, negative-sense, single-stranded RNA virus has hemagglutinin, fusion glycoproteins

CD46 a cell receptor

✳ Replicates in cytoplasm using viral RNA polymerase

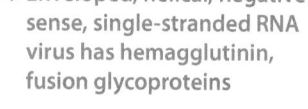

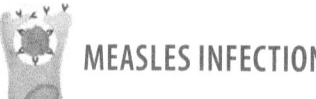

MEASLES INFECTION

EPIDEMIOLOGY

The highest attack rates of measles have been in children, usually sparing infants less than 6 months of age because of passively acquired antibody. However, a shift in age-specific attack rates to greater involvement of adolescents and young adults was observed in the United States in the 1980s. A marked decline in measles in the United States during the early 1990s may reflect decreased transmission as increased immunization coverage takes effect. However, in developing countries, an estimated one million children still die from this disease each year. Furthermore, measles remains endemic in most countries in the world, including parts of Europe. In 2007 to 2008, large outbreaks of measles were occurring in Switzerland and Israel, resulting in imported cases leading to localized spread within the United States. In the United States, approximately 60 people are reported to have measles each year. In 2011, 222 people were infected with measles, including 40% imported from Europe and Asia involving more than a dozen outbreaks in various communities in the United States. In 2013 and 2014, the United States reported 11 outbreaks (3 outbreaks have more than 20 cases and 1 with 58 cases) and 23 outbreaks (1 outbreak with 383 cases in unvaccinated Amish community in Ohio and many cases brought from the Philippines—a total of 667 cases), respectively. In 2015, the United States experienced a large, multistate measles outbreak (188 cases) linked to an amusement park in California, likely from a traveler. Several states in the United States reported a total of 86 cases in 2016, 120 cases in 2017, 375 cases in 2018, and 1282 cases in 2019, although 2019 saw higher number of cases than previous years. It is believed that many measles cases are seen in unvaccinated people and travelers becoming infected abroad and bringing into the United States. Thus, continued vigilance is required for all who care for patients and live in crowded environment.

> Although a childhood disease, infections in young adults are also seen
>
> Dramatic decrease in the United States, but importation of infections is still a problem
>
> ✳ Many recent outbreaks in the United States

Epidemics tend to occur during the winter and spring and, increasingly, are limited to one-dose vaccine failures or groups who do not accept immunizations. The infection rate among exposed susceptible subjects in a classroom or household setting is estimated at 85%, and more than 95% of those infected become ill. The period of communicability is estimated to be 3 to 5 days before appearance of the rash to 4 days afterward.

> Epidemics occur in unimmunized or partially immunized groups

PATHOGENESIS

Measles is transmitted through respiratory inhalation and, after implantation of the virus in the upper respiratory tract, viral replication proceeds in the respiratory mucosal epithelium. The effect within individual respiratory cells is profound. Although measles does not directly restrict host cell metabolism, susceptible cells are damaged or destroyed by virtue of the intense viral replicative activity and the promotion of cell fusion with formation of syncytia. This results in disruption of the cellular cytoskeleton, chromosomal disorganization, and the appearance of inclusion bodies within the nucleus and cytoplasm. Replication is followed by viremic and lymphatic dissemination throughout the host to distant sites, including lymphoid tissues, bone marrow, abdominal viscera, and skin. The virus can be demonstrated in the blood during the first week after illness onset, and viruria persists for up to 4 days after the appearance of rash. Viremia also allows the infection of conjunctiva, urinary tract, small blood vessels, and the CNS. **Figure 10–3** summarizes the pathogenesis, clinical disease, and immunity in measles virus infection.

> Respiratory cell multiplication disrupts cytoskeleton
>
> Viremia disseminates to multiple sites

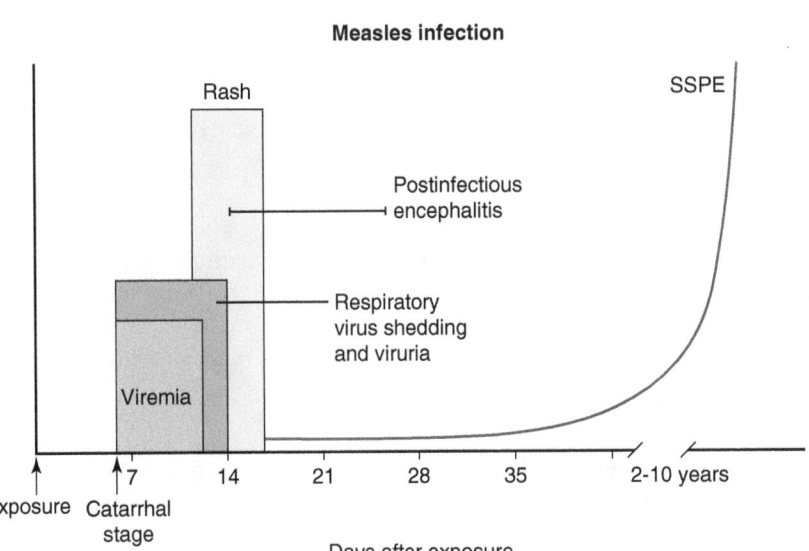

Measles infection

FIGURE 10–3. Pathogenesis of measles virus infection. After exposure, the virus multiplies in the respiratory tract epithelium (incubation period of 9-11 days, on average) and spreads to regional lymph nodes followed by viremia, which helps the virus to be transported throughout the body. Moreover, the virus is also shed in saliva and excreted in the urine. Koplik spots appear on the tongue before appearance of rash on head, then trunk and other extremities. Humoral immune response plays an important role in clearing the virus from the hosts, with IgM appearing early in infection followed by IgG that persists for a long time. Cell-mediated immunity plays a role in disease progression. Postinfectious encephalitis and bacterial superinfections are major complications of measles virus infection. In some patients, there is a rare persistent infection of the CNS known as subacute sclerosing panencephalitis (SSPE).

T and B lymphocytes, monocytes infected

Leukocyte function impaired

✴ IL-12 downregulation leads to depressed cell-mediated immunity, disease severity

Susceptibility to bacterial superinfections enhanced

Vasculitis, giant cells, and inclusions are seen

Encephalitis lesions are due to cytotoxic T-cell (CD8 T cells) activity

During the viremic phase, measles virus infects T and B lymphocytes, circulating monocytes, and polymorphonuclear leukocytes without producing cytolysis. Profound depression of cell-mediated immunity occurs during the acute phase of illness and persists for several weeks thereafter. This is believed to be a result of virus-induced downregulation of interleukin-12 (IL-12) production by monocytes and macrophages. The effect on B lymphocytes has been shown to suppress immunoglobulin synthesis; in addition, generation of natural killer cell activity appears to be impaired. Moreover, there is evidence that the capability of polymorphonuclear leukocytes to generate oxygen radicals is diminished, perhaps directly by the virus or by activated regulatory T cells. This may further explain the enhanced susceptibility to bacterial superinfections. Virion components can be detected in biopsy specimens of Koplik spots and vascular endothelial cells in the areas of skin rash.

In addition to necrosis and inflammatory changes in the respiratory tract epithelium, several other features of measles virus infection are noteworthy. The skin lesions show vasculitis characterized by vascular dilation, edema, and perivascular mononuclear cell infiltrates. The lymphoid tissues show hyperplastic changes, and large multinucleated reticuloendothelial giant cells are often observed (Warthin-Finkeldey cells). Some of the giant cells contain intracytoplasmic and intranuclear inclusions. Similarly involved giant epithelial cells can be found in a variety of mucosal sites, the respiratory tract, skin, and urinary sediment.

In some patients with measles, an immune-mediated postinfectious encephalitis occurs after the rash. The major findings in measles encephalitis include areas of edema, scattered petechial hemorrhages, perivascular mononuclear cell infiltrates, and necrosis of neurons. In most cases, perivenous demyelination in the CNS is also observed. The pathogenesis is thought to be related to infiltration by cytotoxic (CD8+) T cells, which react with myelin-forming or virus-infected brain cells.

 Why does IL-12 downregulation result in severity of measles?

IMMUNITY

Lifelong immunity associated with neutralizing antibody

✴ Cell-mediated immunity defects, protein-calorie malnutrition lead to measles complications, including viral pneumonia

✴ Vitamin A may benefit

Cell-mediated immune responses to other antigens may be acutely depressed during measles infection and persist for several months. There is evidence that measles virus-specific cell-mediated immunity developing early in infection plays a role in mediating some of the features of disease, such as the rash, and is necessary to promote recovery from the illness. Antibodies to the virus appear in the first few days of illness, peak in 2 to 3 weeks, and then persist at low levels. Immunity to reinfection is lifelong and is associated with the presence of neutralizing antibody. In patients with defects in cell-mediated immunity, including those with severe protein-calorie malnutrition, infection is prolonged, tissue involvement is more severe, and complications such as progressive viral pneumonia are common. In addition, use of vitamin A may have some benefits in reducing the severity and complications of measles, especially in malnourished children.

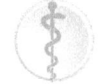 **CLINICAL ASPECTS**

MANIFESTATIONS

✴ Incubation period 7 to 18 days

✴ Onset with cough, coryza, conjunctivitis, fever

✴ Koplik spots on buccal mucous membranes before rash

Common synonyms for measles include **rubeola,** 5-day measles, and hard measles. The incubation period ranges from 7 to 18 days. A typical illness usually begins 9 to 11 days after exposure, with cough, coryza, conjunctivitis, and fever. One to three days after onset, pinpoint gray-white spots surrounded by erythema (grains-of-salt appearance) appear on mucous membranes. This

 Think ▸▸ Apply 10-2: **Downregulation of IL-12 results in suppression of Th1 cells response and release of antiviral cytokines causing reduced CD8 T cells response to control the infection.**

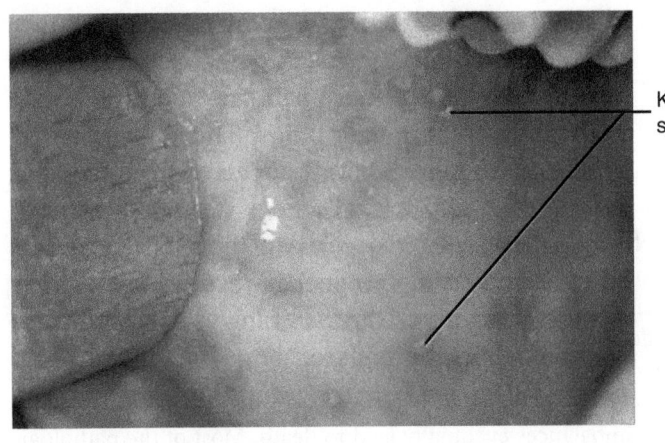

Koplik
spots

FIGURE 10-4. **Oral Koplik spots on day 3 of measles.** (Reproduced with permission from Nester EW, Anderson DG, Roberts CE Jr, et al: *Microbiology: A Human Perspective*, 6th ed. New York, NY: McGraw Hill; 2008.)

sign, called **Koplik spots,** is usually most noticeable over the buccal mucosa opposite the molar teeth and persists for 1 to 2 days (**Figure 10-4**). Within a day of the appearance of Koplik spots, the typical measles rash begins—first on the head, then on the trunk and extremities. The rash is maculopapular and semiconfluent; it persists for 3 to 5 days before fading (**Figure 10-5**). Fever and severe systemic symptoms gradually diminish as the rash progresses to the extremities. Lymphadenopathy is also common, with particularly noticeable involvement of the cervical nodes.

Measles can be very severe, especially in immunocompromised or malnourished patients. Death can result from overwhelming viral infection of the host, with extensive involvement of the respiratory tract and other viscera. In some developing countries, mortality rates of 15% to 25% have been recorded.

✳ Rash first on head then trunk, extremities

✳ Maculopapular, semiconfluent rash for 3 to 5 days

■ Complications

Bacterial superinfection, the most common complication, occurs in 5% to 15% of all cases. Such infections include acute otitis media, mastoiditis, sinusitis, pneumonia, and sepsis. Clinical signs of encephalitis develop in 1 per 500 to 1000 cases. This condition usually occurs 3 to 14 days after onset of illness and can be extremely severe. The mortality in measles encephalitis is approximately 15%, and permanent neurologic damage among survivors is estimated at 25%. Acute thrombocytopenic purpura may also develop during the acute phase of measles, leading to

✳ Bacterial superinfection is a common complication

✳ Encephalitis can be severe with 15% mortality and permanent neurologic damage in 25% survivors

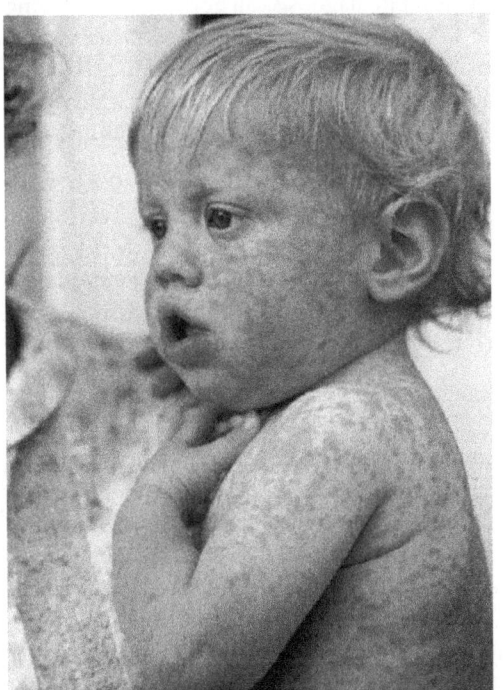

FIGURE 10-5. **Measles rash on day 4 of illness.** (Reproduced with permission from Nester EW, Anderson DG, Roberts CE Jr, et al: *Microbiology: A Human Perspective*, 6th ed. New York, NY: McGraw Hill; 2008.)

Thrombocytopenic purpura and bleeding occur in acute phase

bleeding episodes. Abdominal pain and acute appendicitis can occur secondary to inflammation and swelling of lymphoid tissue.

■ Subacute Sclerosing Panencephalitis (SSPE)

SSPE a rare, progressive neurologic disease 2 to 10 years after measles

Neurologic deterioration progressive in children

Inclusions in neuronal cells

SSPE patients have higher oligoclonal IgG

Subacute sclerosing panencephalitis (SSPE) is a rare, progressive neurologic disease of children, which usually begins 2 to 10 years after a measles infection. In rare instances, measles virus persists in the CNS and the disease is a result of chronic measles virus infection of the CNS. It is characterized by insidious onset of personality change, poor school performance, progressive intellectual deterioration, development of myoclonic jerks (periodic muscle spasms), and motor dysfunctions, such as spasticity, tremors, loss of coordination, and ocular abnormalities, including blindness. Neurologic and intellectual deterioration generally progresses over 6 to 12 months, with children eventually becoming bedridden and stuporous. Dysfunctions of the autonomic nervous system, such as difficulty with temperature regulation, may develop. Progressive inanition, superinfection, and metabolic imbalances eventually lead to death. Most of the pathologic features of the disease are localized to the CNS and retina. Both the gray matter and the white matter of the brain are involved, the most noteworthy feature being the presence of intranuclear and intracytoplasmic inclusions in oligodendroglial and neuronal cells. Cerebral spinal fluid (CSF) findings generally include no significant pleocytosis, normal glucose, and protein, but significantly higher levels of oligoclonal IgG.

Chronic measles infection causes SSPE

Incomplete virus present in brain tissue

The disease is a result of chronic wild-type measles virus infection of the CNS. Studies have shown that patients have a variety of patterns of missing measles virus structural proteins in brain tissue. Thus, any of several defects in viral gene expression may prevent normal viral assembly, allowing persistence of defective virus at an intracellular site with failure of immune eradication.

Rarely, a similar progressive, degenerative neurologic disorder may be related to persistent rubella virus infection of the CNS. This condition is seen most often in adolescents who have had congenital rubella syndrome. Rubella virus has been isolated from brain tissue in these patients, again using cocultivation techniques.

SSPE declined after introduction of measles vaccine

The incidence of SSPE is approximately 1 per 100,000 measles cases. Its occurrence in the United States has decreased markedly over the last 25 years with the widespread use of live measles vaccine. At present, there is no accepted effective therapy for SSPE.

DIAGNOSIS

RT-PCR in respiratory specimens

IgM suggests current or recent infection

The typical measles infection can often be diagnosed on the basis of clinical findings, but laboratory confirmation is necessary. Detection of measles in throat, nasal or nasopharyngeal specimens can be performed by RT-PCR or virus isolation. A rapid diagnosis can be done by employing real-time RT-PCR to detect measles viral genome in respiratory specimens and urinary sediments. Virus isolation from the respiratory specimens or urine is usually most productive in the first 5 days of illness. Measles grows on a variety of cell cultures, producing multinucleated giant cells similar to those observed in infected host tissues. Serologic diagnosis, IgM and IgG may involve HI, ELISA, or indirect fluorescent antibody methods.

TREATMENT

No specific therapy is available other than supportive measures and close observation for the development of complications such as bacterial superinfection. Intravenous ribavirin has been suggested for patients with severe measles pneumonia, but no controlled studies have been performed.

PREVENTION

Live attenuated vaccine highly immunogenic, in the first year of life with booster at 4 to 6 years

Vaccination contraindicated in pregnant, immunocompromised

Passive protection for immunocompromised

Highly immunogenic live attenuated measles vaccine is available and is most commonly administered as MMR or MMRV. To ensure effective immunization, the vaccine should be administered to infants at 12 to 15 months of age with a second dose at 4 to 6 or 11 to 12 years of age. Immunity induced by the vaccine may be lifelong. Because the vaccine consists of live virus, it should not be administered to immunocompromised patients and is not recommended for pregnant women. Exceptions to these guidelines include susceptible human immunodeficiency virus (HIV)-infected persons. Exposed susceptible patients who are immunologically compromised (including small infants) may be given immune serum globulin intramuscularly. This treatment can modify or prevent disease if given within 6 days of exposure, but protection is transient.

While measles virus entry and replication in respiratory tract mucosa result in a significant IgA response, why does the live, attenuated measles (MMR) vaccine predominantly generate IgG response?

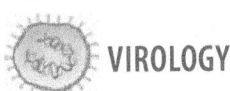

Overview

Rubella virus, a member of Togaviridae (Togavirus) family and *Rubivirus* genus, is a positive-sense single-stranded RNA, icosahedral, enveloped virus containing two glycoprotein spikes, E1 and E2 that replicates in the cytoplasm by using viral RNA polymerase. In primary rubella infection, the virus enters through inhalation (incubation period 14-21 days), replicates in the upper respiratory tract and spreads via bloodstream to lymphoid tissues, skin, and other organs. Rubella, also known as German or 3-day measles, is often mild, or even asymptomatic. However, when symptomatic, it is often manifested as fever, malaise, faint rash (on head, neck, and trunk), and arthralgia. The symptoms persist for 1 to 3 days. Immunity to reinfection is generally lifelong. The major concerns are the profound effects of congenital (maternal) infection during the first trimester of pregnancy, which can affect developing fetuses, resulting in multiple congenital malformations, such as cardiac and ocular defects, deafness, hepatosplenomegaly, thrombocytopenia, microcephaly, and failure to thrive. An effective live attenuated vaccine (part of MMR or MMRV) is recommended in the first year of life and a second dose between 4 and 6 years of age that provides protection via antibody response.

Rubella, commonly known as **German measles** or 3-day measles, was considered a mild, benign exanthem of childhood until 1941, when the Australian ophthalmologist Sir Norman Gregg described the profound defects that could be induced in the fetus as a result of maternal infection. Since 1962, when the virus was first isolated, knowledge regarding its extreme medical importance and biologic characteristics has increased rapidly.

VIROLOGY

Rubella virus is classified as a member of the Togaviridae family, *Rubivirus* genus. It is a simple, icosahedral, enveloped virus, and contains a single-stranded, positive-sense RNA genome. There is a single species of capsid protein, and the lipid bilayer envelope contains two glycoproteins—E1 and E2. E1 interacts with the receptor on the host cell and comprises the principal antigenic determinants or epitopes involved in virus neutralization and hemagglutination. E2 interacts with capsid and E1 to reach the Golgi apparatus for viral assembly. There is only one serotype of rubella; however, some strain variation in virulence and antigenicity has been reported. In addition, there are no extrahuman or animal reservoirs for rubella virus as well as any related animal viruses. There is no serologic cross-reactivity between rubella virus and other members of the togavirus family such as alphaviruses (transmitted via arthropods). The details of viral structure of the togavirus are described in Chapter 16. The virus can agglutinate some types of red blood cells, such as those obtained from 1-day-old chicks and trypsin-treated human type O cells.

Rubella virus enters target cells via receptor-mediated endocytosis. Viral positive-sense RNA is translated to produce viral proteins, including RNA-dependent RNA polymerase. These proteins are required for the synthesis of replicative intermediates, full-length genomic RNA, and subgenomic RNA. The subgenomic RNA encodes the structural proteins of the virus, including capsid and envelope proteins. The full-length genomic RNA encodes for nonstructural proteins and RNA polymerase and also serves as genomic RNA for progeny viruses. Virus assembly takes place in either the Golgi complex or cytoplasmic membranes.

✳ Enveloped, icosahedral Togavirus (Rubivirus) positive sense, single-stranded RNA

✳ Viral spikes E1 and E2; E1 binds to receptor and involved in virus neutralization

✳ Replicates in the cytoplasm using viral RNA polymerase

Genomic RNA encodes for nonstructural proteins and subgenomic RNA for structural proteins

 Think ▸▸ Apply 10-3: **Because the live attenuated MMR or MMRV vaccine is given as intramuscular injection shot, the immune response is to the isotype found in serum (IgG).**

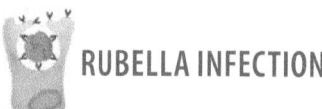 RUBELLA INFECTION

EPIDEMIOLOGY

While endemic rubella has been eliminated in the United States due to vaccination, it is a serious concern in various parts of the world, including Africa, Asia, and elsewhere. In the United States, most of the rubella cases are imported. Rubella infections are usually observed during the winter and spring months. In contrast to measles, which has a high clinical attack rate among exposed susceptible individuals, only 30% to 60% of rubella-infected susceptible persons develop clinically apparent disease. A major focus of concern is susceptible women of childbearing age, who carry a risk of exposure during pregnancy and transmitting the virus to their babies (congenital infection). Patients with primary acquired rubella infections are contagious from 7 days before to 7 days after the onset of rash; congenitally infected infants may spread the virus to others for 6 months or longer after birth. In the United States, less than a dozen cases of congenital rubella are seen. However, more than 100,000 babies are born with congenital rubella syndrome (CRS) every year worldwide. CRS is the highest in Africa and Southeast Asia where the vaccination is the lowest. The disease is preventable by vaccination.

PATHOGENESIS

In acquired infection, the virus enters the host through the upper respiratory tract, replicates, and then spreads by the bloodstream to distant sites, including lymphoid tissues, skin, and organs. Viremia in these infections has been detected for as long as 8 days before and 2 days after the onset of the rash, and virus shedding from the oropharynx can be detected up to 8 days after onset (**Figure 10–6**). Cellular immune responses and circulating virus–antibody immune complexes are thought to play a role in mediating the inflammatory responses to infection, such as rash and arthritis.

Congenital infection occurs as a result of maternal viremia that leads to placental infection and then transplacental spread to the fetus. The risk of congenital infection correlates with the timing of transmission of the virus to the fetus. If the virus is transmitted to the fetus early in gestation, then the risk of development of CRS is very high. After fetal infection occurs, it persists chronically. Such persistence is probably related to an inability to eliminate the virus by immune or interferon-mediated mechanisms. There is too little inflammatory change in the fetal tissues to explain the pathogenesis of the congenital defects. The possibilities include placental and fetal vasculitis with compromise of fetal oxygenation, chronic viral infection of cells leading to impaired mitosis, cellular necrosis, and induction of chromosomal breakage. Any or all of these factors may operate at a critical stage of organogenesis to induce permanent defects. Viral persistence with circulating virus–antibody immune complexes may evoke inflammatory changes postnatally and produce continuing tissue damage.

Rubella virus has high infectivity but low virulence

✴ Childbearing women major concern for congenital rubella

✴ Fewer cases of congenital rubella in the United States; higher in other parts of the world

✴ Cellular immune responses and antigen–antibody complexes mediate arthritis and rash

✴ Transplacental transmission of rubella to fetus

✴ Risk of developing congenital rubella syndrome high during the early weeks of gestation

Fetal infection becomes chronic

FIGURE 10–6. Antibody response and viral isolation in a typical case of acquired rubella.

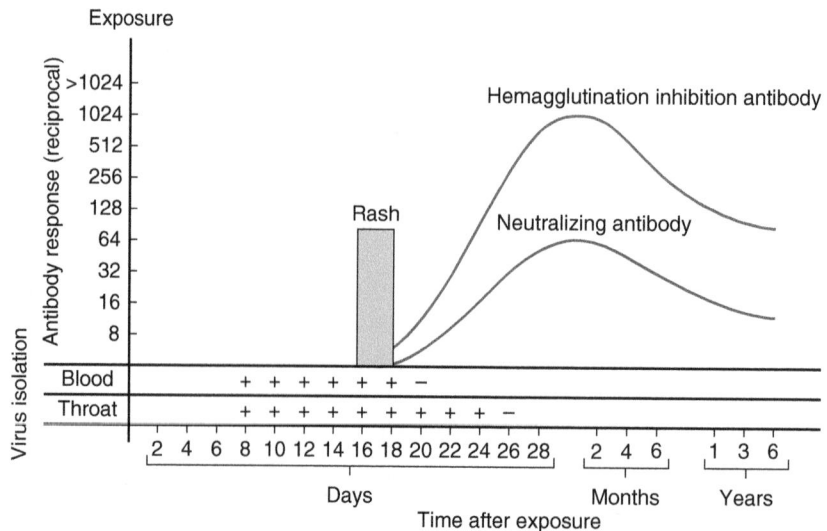

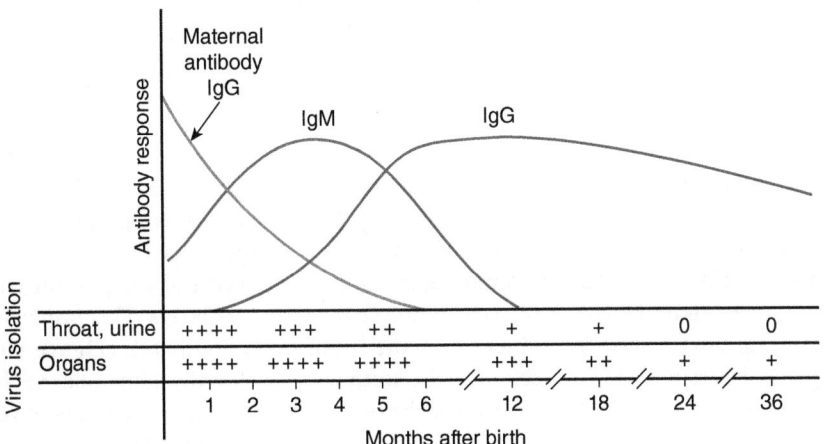

 Why does congenital rubella infection result in major organ defects?

After birth, infants affected with rubella continue to excrete the virus in the throat, urine, and intestinal tract (**Figure 10–7**). Virus may be isolated from virtually all tissues in the first few weeks of life. Shedding of virus in the throat and urine, which persists for at least 6 months in most cases, has been known to continue for 30 months. Rubella virus has also been isolated from lens tissue removed 3 to 4 years later. These observations underscore the fact that such infants are important reservoirs in perpetuating virus transmission. The prolonged virus shedding is somewhat puzzling; it does not represent a typical example of immunologic tolerance. The affected infants are usually able to produce circulating IgM and IgG antibodies to the virus (Figure 10–7), although antibodies may decrease to undetectable levels after 3 to 4 years. Many infants have evidence of depressed rubella virus-specific cell-mediated immunity during the first year of life.

Infection and virus shedding continue long after birth

Virus persists despite antibody

PATHOLOGY

Because postnatally acquired disease is usually mild, little is known about the pathology of rubella. Mononuclear cell inflammatory changes can be observed in tissues, and viral antigen can be detected in the same sites (eg, skin and synovial fluid). Congenital infections are characterized primarily by the various malformations. Necrosis of tissues such as myocardium and vascular endothelium may also be seen, and quantitative studies suggest a decrease in cell quantity in affected organs. In severe cases, normal calcium deposition in the metaphyses of long bones is delayed, sometimes referred to as a "celery stalk" appearance on a radiograph.

Fetal disease includes multiple malformations

IMMUNITY

After infection with rubella, the serum antibody titer rises, reaching a peak within 2 to 3 weeks of onset (Figure 10–7). Natural infection also results in the production of specific secretory IgA antibodies in the respiratory tract. Immunity to disease is nearly always lifelong; however, reexposure can lead to transient respiratory tract infection, with an anamnestic rise in IgG and secretory IgA antibodies, but without resultant viremia or illness.

Lasting immunity is associated with IgG and IgA

 Think ▶▶ Apply 10-4: Transmission of rubella early in gestation causes chronic infection and deformities of the fetal organs. The virus interferes with the organogenesis processes causing damage to various organs. In addition, lack of immunity makes it difficult to control virus replication.

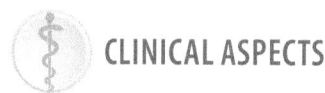

CLINICAL ASPECTS

MANIFESTATIONS

Mild illness with lymphadenopathy, macular rash for 1 to 3 days

※ Arthralgia or arthritis is common, more frequently in women

Rubella is commonly known as **German measles** or 3-day measles. The incubation period for acquired infection is 14 to 21 days (average, 16 days). Illness is generally very mild, consisting primarily of low-grade fever, sore throat and other upper respiratory symptoms, and lymphadenopathy, which is most prominent in the posterior cervical and postauricular areas. A macular rash often follows within a day of onset and lasts 1 to 3 days. This rash, which is often quite faint, is usually most prominent over the head, neck, and trunk (**Figure 10–8**). In addition, petechial lesions may be seen over the soft palate during the acute phase. The most common complication is arthralgia or overt arthritis, which may affect the joints of the fingers, wrists, elbows, knees, and ankles. The joint problems, which occur most frequently in women, rarely last longer than a few days to 3 weeks. Other, rarer complications include thrombocytopenic purpura and encephalitis.

The major significance of rubella is not the acute illness but the risk of fetal damage in pregnant women, particularly when they contract either symptomatic or subclinical primary infection during the first trimester. The risk of fetal malformation and chronic fetal infection, which is estimated to be as high as 80% if infection occurs in the first 2 weeks of gestation, decreases to 6% to 10% by the 14th week. The overall risk during the first trimester is estimated at 20% to 30%.

※ High risk for fetal damage with infection in first trimester

※ Congenital rubella syndrome includes cardiovascular stenosis, eye defects, hearing loss, hepatosplenomegaly, thrombocytopenia, microcephaly.

※ Rash appears as blueberry muffin due to extramedullary hematopoiesis

※ Part of TORCHS for congenital infections screening and evaluation

Clinical manifestations of congenital rubella syndrome vary, but may include any combination of the following major findings: cardiac defects, commonly patent ductus arteriosus and pulmonary valvular stenosis; eye defects such as cataracts, chorioretinitis, glaucoma, coloboma, cloudy cornea, and microphthalmia; sensorineural deafness; enlargement of liver and spleen; thrombocytopenia; and intrauterine growth restriction. There is also appearance of purpura more often on head, neck, and trunk due to extramedullary hematopoiesis, also referred as blueberry muffin. Other findings include CNS defects such as microcephaly, mental retardation, and encephalitis; anemia; transient immunodeficiency; interstitial pneumonia; intravascular coagulation; hepatitis; rash; and other congenital malformations. Late complications of congenital rubella syndrome have also been described, including an increased risk of diabetes mellitus, chronic thyroiditis, and, occasionally, the development of a progressive subacute panencephalitis in the second decade of life. Some congenitally infected infants may appear entirely normal at birth, and sequelae such as hearing or learning deficits may not become apparent until months later. The spectrum of defects, thus, varies from subtle to severe. Congenital rubella is considered as part of TORCHS (toxoplasma, others, rubella, CMV, herpes, syphilis) in clinical evaluation and screening of congenital infections.

FIGURE 10–8. **Rubella rash.** Diffuse, macular in appearance, usually beginning on the face and spreading to the trunk. (Reproduced with permission from Nester EW, Anderson DG, Roberts CE Jr, et al: *Microbiology: A Human Perspective,* 6th ed. New York, NY: McGraw Hill; 2008..)

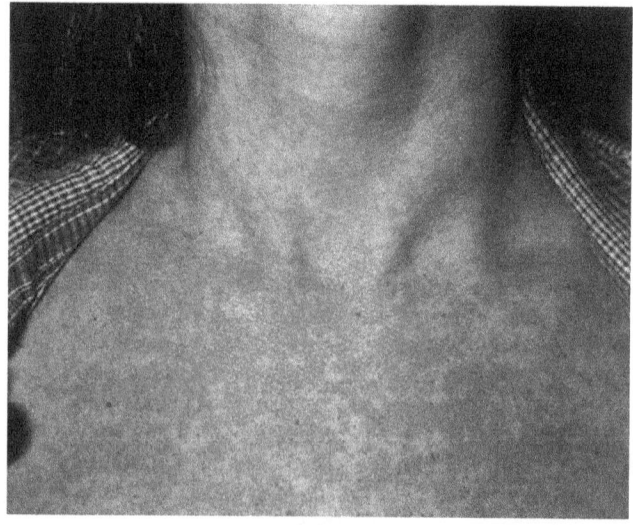

DIAGNOSIS

Because of the rather nonspecific nature of the illness, a diagnosis of rubella cannot be made on clinical grounds alone. More than 30 other viral agents, which are discussed later in this chapter, can produce a similar illness. Confirmation of the diagnosis requires laboratory studies. The virus may be detected by RT-PCR or isolated from respiratory secretions in the acute phase (and from urine, tissues, and feces in congenitally infected infants) by inoculation into a variety of cell cultures. Serologic diagnosis is most commonly used in acquired infections; paired acute and convalescent samples collected 10 to 21 days apart are used. Hemagglutination inhibition, IF, EIA, and other tests are available.

Determination of IgM-specific antibody is, sometimes, useful to ascertain whether an infection occurred in the last several months; it has also been used in the diagnosis of congenital infections. Unfortunately, there are certain pitfalls in interpreting this test. Some individuals (less than 5%) with acquired infections may have persistent elevations of IgM-specific antibodies for 200 days or more afterward, and some congenitally infected infants do not produce detectable IgM-specific antibodies. However, RT-PCR can be used to detect congenital rubella infection in infants.

Detected by RT-PCR or virus culture from respiratory secretions

Acquired infections diagnosed serologically

IgM and RT-PCR tests can help detect congenital infections

TREATMENT AND PREVENTION

Other than supportive measures, there is no specific therapy for either the acquired or the congenital rubella infection.

Since 1969, a live attenuated rubella vaccine has been available for routine immunization either as MMR or MMRV. As a result of the widespread use of the vaccine in the United States, the number of cases of rubella has declined dramatically. From 1990 through 1999, the median number of cases reported annually was only 232. The current vaccine virus—grown in human diploid fibroblast cell cultures (RA 27/3)—has been shown to be highly effective. It causes seroconversion in approximately 95% of recipients. Routine immunization is now recommended for infants after the first year of life and for other individuals with no history of immunization and lack of immunity by serologic testing. Target groups include female adolescents and hospital personnel in high-risk settings. The vaccine is contraindicated in many immunocompromised patients and in pregnancy. To date, more than 200 instances of accidental vaccination of susceptible pregnant women have been reported, with no clinically apparent adverse effects on the fetus. However, it is strongly recommended that immunization be avoided in this setting, and that nonpregnant women avoid conception for at least 3 months after receiving the vaccine.

✳ *MMR or MMRV given at 1 year of age and a second dose at 4 to 6 years*

Vaccine also indicated for hospital workers

Vaccine does not produce defects in fetus

Vaccine-induced immunity may be lifelong

PARVOVIRUS B19 INFECTIONS

Parvoviruses are very small (18-26 nm), naked icosahedral capsid virions that contain a linear single-stranded DNA genome. Parvovirus B19 causes disease in humans (children) known as erythema infectiosum, slapped face, or fifth disease. The other parvovirus that infects humans is human bocavirus, believed to cause wheezing and respiratory infections in children. Parvovirus also causes disease in animals, including canine parvovirus and feline panleukopenia virus, which produce severe infections among puppies and kittens, respectively. These do not appear to cross species barriers such as infecting humans. The other parvovirus that is of some interest is adenoassociated virus (AAV) because of its potential in gene therapy. The human parvovirus B19 has been well described, but its origin is not yet known.

Parvovirus B19 encodes three capsid proteins (VP1, VP2, and VP3) that encapsidate a single-stranded DNA molecule into an icosahedral symmetry. VP2 is the major capsid protein that comprises almost 90% of the virion capsid. The virus can be grown in primary cultures of human bone marrow cells, fetal liver cells, hematopoietic progenitor cells generated from peripheral blood, and a megakaryocytic leukemia cell line. The major cellular receptor for the virus is globoside (also known as blood group P antigen, which is commonly found on erythroid progenitors, erythroblasts, megakaryocytes, and endothelial cells). All represent potential targets for disease production. A primary site of replication appears to be the nucleus of an immature cell in the erythrocyte lineage that is mitotically active. Such infected cells then cease to proliferate, resulting in an impairment of normal erythrocyte development. Parvovirus enters the cells after binding to P antigen (globoside) followed by internalization, uncoating, and delivery of single-stranded DNA to the nucleus. The single-stranded DNA genome is converted to

Small naked, icosahedral, single-stranded DNA viruses

✳ *Replicates in erythroid precursor nuclei*

Globoside is virus receptor

* Endothelial cells and megakaryocytes can also be affected

double-stranded DNA by host DNA polymerase, which is transcribed by host RNA polymerase to produce viral mRNAs, followed by synthesis of viral proteins. After synthesis of single-stranded DNA genomes by host DNA polymerase, progeny viruses are assembled in the nucleus and released upon cell lysis.

The clinical consequences of this effect on erythrocytes are generally trivial, unless patients are already compromised by a chronic hemolytic process, such as sickle cell disease or thalassemia, in which maximal erythropoiesis is continually needed to counterbalance increased destruction of circulating erythrocytes. Primary infection by parvovirus B19 in such individuals often produces an acute, severe, and sometimes fatal anemia manifested as a rapid fall in red blood cell count and hemoglobin. These patients may present initially with no clinical symptoms other than fever; this is commonly referred to as **aplastic crisis.** Immunocompromised patients such as those with acquired immunodeficiency syndrome (AIDS), sometimes, have difficulty clearing the virus and develop persistent anemia with reticulocytopenia. Parvovirus B19 has also been occasionally implicated as a cause of persistent bone marrow failure and an acute hemophagocytic syndrome. In addition, it is now recognized as sometimes causing severe, protracted anemia in many settings of immune compromise, including in patients with AIDS, organ transplant recipients, and leukemic patients undergoing chemotherapy. Parvovirus B19 has also been implicated in triggering various forms of autoimmune diseases affecting joints, connective tissues, and small and large vessels both in children and adults. Furthermore, autoimmune neutropenia, thrombocytopenia, and hemolytic anemia are known sequelae of parvovirus B19 infection.

* Aplastic crisis develops in patients with chronic hemolytic anemias

* Parvovirus B19 implicated with autoimmune diseases causing symptoms like rheumatoid arthritis

 What are the causes of arthritis-like symptoms in parvovirus B19 and rubella infections?

■ Erythema Infectiosum

Erythema infectiosum (also referred to as fifth disease or academy rash) is a more common disease that is clearly attributable to parvovirus B19. The virus is primarily transmitted by the respiratory route. In addition, it can be transmitted through blood or blood products as well as from mother to child. After an incubation period of 4 to 12 days, a mild illness appears, characterized by fever, malaise, headache, myalgia, and itching in varying degrees. A confluent, indurated rash appears on the face, giving a "slapped-cheek" appearance. The rash spreads in 1 or 2 days to other areas, particularly exposed surfaces such as the arms and legs, where it is usually macular and reticular (lace-like). During the acute phase, generalized lymphadenopathy or splenomegaly may be seen, together with a mild leukopenia and anemia.

The illness of erythema infectiosum lasts 1 to 2 weeks, but rash may recur for periods of 2 to 4 weeks thereafter, exacerbated by heat, sunlight, exercise, and emotional stress. Arthralgia sometimes persists or recurs for weeks to months, particularly in adolescent or adult females. Overt arthritis or vasculitis have also been reported in some individuals. Serious complications such as hepatitis, thrombocytopenia, nephritis, or encephalitis are rare. However, like rubella, active transplacental transmission of parvovirus B19 can occur during primary infections in the first 20 weeks of pregnancy, sometimes resulting in stillbirth of fetuses that are profoundly anemic. The progress can be so severe that hypoxic damage to the heart, liver, and other tissues leads to extensive edema (hydrops fetalis). The frequency of such adverse outcomes is as yet undetermined.

It is important to be aware that erythema infectiosum is extremely variable in its clinical manifestations; even the "classic" presentation can be mimicked by other agents, such as rubella and echoviruses. Before a firm diagnosis is made on clinical grounds, especially during outbreaks, it is wise to exclude the possibility of atypical rubella infection.

Epidemiologic evidence suggests that spread of the virus is primarily by the respiratory route, and high transmission rates occur in households. Outbreaks tend to be small and localized, particularly during the spring months, with the highest rates among children and young adults.

* Erythema infectiosum (fifth disease) is usually a mild "slapped cheek" rash

Fetal infection is occasionally severe

* Fetal anemia leads to hydrops fetalis (excessive edema)

Detection requires DNA probe or PCR

 Think ▸▸ Apply 10-5: **Because of autoimmune-like conditions such as formation of immune complexes cause arthritis-like joint pains.**

Seroepidemiologic studies have demonstrated evidence of past infection in 30% to 60% of adults. Viremia usually lasts 7 to 12 days but can persist for months in some individuals. It can be detected by a specific DNA probe or PCR methods. Alternatively, the presence of IgM-specific antibody late in the acute phase or during convalescence strongly supports the diagnosis.

There is currently no definitive treatment for erythema infectiosum. Commercial immune globulins with antibodies to parvovirus B19 have been used with salutary effects and reduction of serum viral DNA in some patients with refractory infection in a setting of immunodeficiency.

A recombinant parvovirus B19 virus-like particle vaccine (VLP) has been developed, but not approved by the FDA. This vaccine could potentially benefit groups especially at risk because of chronic hemolytic disease, immunodeficiency, or seronegative pregnancies (to prevent hydrops fetalis), and perhaps even benefit children with acute anemia due to malaria, in whom the hematologic effects may be more profound, if there is parvovirus B19 coinfection.

IgM-specific antibody supports diagnosis

Immunoglobulin treatment may be useful in selected cases

ROSEOLA INFANTUM (EXANTHEM SUBITUM)

Roseola infantum is a common illness observed in infants and children 6 months to 4 years of age. Its alternative name, exanthem subitum, means "sudden" rash. Roseola has more than one cause: the most common is human herpesvirus type 6 (HHV-6) and, less frequently, human herpesvirus type 7 (HHV-7). HHV-6 and HHV-7 are members of the *Roseolovirus* genus of herpesvirus family (see Chapter 14). HHV-6 is classified into two groups; HHV-6A and HHV-6B. HHV-6B is a major cause of roseola infantum, whereas HHV-6A is not clearly associated with any disease. Several other agents, including adenoviruses, coxsackieviruses, and echoviruses, have occasionally been noted to cause similar manifestations. The illness is characterized by abrupt onset of high fever, sometimes accompanied by brief, generalized convulsions (seizures) and leukopenia. After 3 to 5 days, the fever diminishes rapidly, followed in a few hours by a faint, transient, macular rash.

Associated generally with human herpesvirus type 6 and to lesser extent with type 7

✳ Abrupt onset of high fever, sometimes seizures, and macular rash

OTHER CAUSES OF RUBELLA-LIKE RASHES

In addition to erythema infectiosum, diseases caused by numerous other agents can mimic rubella. These include at least 17 echoviruses, nine coxsackieviruses, several adenoviral serotypes, arboviruses (such as dengue, West Nile virus, Zika virus), Epstein-Barr virus, Cytomegalovirus, scarlet fever (caused by Group A Streptococcus discussed in Chapter 25), and toxic drug eruptions. Because of the wide variety of diagnostic possibilities, it is not possible to diagnose or rule out rubella confidently on clinical grounds alone. Therefore, a specific diagnosis requires specific laboratory studies. Because rubella is an infection with such significant impact on the fetus, serologic study to rule out the possibility is mandatory if the diagnosis is suspected during early pregnancy—both in the woman and potentially infective contacts.

KEY CONCLUSIONS

- Mumps, measles, and rubella (MMR) cause childhood exanthems. Immunity to these viral infections is lifelong. An effective live, attenuated vaccine, MMR or MMRV that produces an IgG response is recommended.

- Mumps is a paramyxovirus comprising of a negative-sense single-stranded linear RNA, a helical nucleocapsid and a lipid bilayer envelope with HN and F spikes. The virus replicates in the cytoplasm by using viral RNA polymerase for both transcription and replication.

- Mumps enters via respiratory tract, multiplies in respiratory tract epithelium and regional lymph nodes followed by viremia and dissemination to target tissues such as salivary glands and the CNS.

- Mumps infection (incubation period 16-18 days average) is characterized by fever and swelling of one or both parotid gland (parotitis) that persists for 7 to 10 days. Complications include meningitis, encephalitis, pancreatitis, orchitis, and oophoritis.

- Measles is a *Morbillivirus* of paramyxovirus family comprising of a negative-sense single-stranded linear RNA, a helical nucleocapsid and a lipid bilayer envelope with H and F spikes. Unlike mumps, it lacks N activity. Like mumps, it replicates in the cytoplasm by using viral RNA polymerase for both transcription and replication.

- Measles enters through respiratory tract, replicates in respiratory mucosal epithelium leading to disintegration of cellular cytoskeleton and viremic and lymphatic dissemination to all body organs. The virus also infects immune cells such as T and B lymphocytes and antigen-presenting cells leading to downregulation of IL-12 and lack of control of viral infection.

- In measles infection, the skin lesions show vasculitis with vascular dilation and edema. The lymphoid tissue shows large multinucleated reticuloendothelial giant cells known as Warthin-Finkeldy cells.

- Clinical manifestation of measles includes fever, cough, coryza, conjunctivitis, and Koplik spots on buccal mucosa (1-3 days after the onset) and within 1 day, a maculopapular and semiconfluent rash that persists for 3 to 5 days. Complications of measles are bacterial superinfection, pneumonia, and encephalitis.

- Measles virus can persist in the CNS and cause a rare, progressive neurologic diseases, subacute sclerosing panencephalitis (SSPE) 2 to 10 years after the primary infection.

- Rubella virus (Rubivirus genus of Togavirus family) is a positive-sense linear RNA, icosahedral capsid and enveloped with E1 and E2 glycoproteins and replicate in the cytoplasm by using viral RNA polymerase both for transcription and replication.

- Rubella virus enters and replicates in the respiratory tract and spreads through bloodstream to various tissues such as lymphoid tissues, skin, and others. Cellular immune response and antigen–antibody immune complex mediate rash and arthritis.

- Symptoms of primary rubella (German or 3-day measles) include low-grade fever, upper respiratory symptoms, lymphadenopathy, and a macular rash lasting for 1 to 3 days. The most common complication is arthralgia and arthritis, more frequent in women, lasting few days to 3 weeks.

- Congenital rubella is a serious concern because the virus can be transmitted from mother to child transplacentally causing congenital rubella syndrome (CRS) with severe deformities of various organs, if the transmission occurs early in gestation. CRS manifestations include cardiac and ocular defects, microcephaly, deafness, thrombocytopenia, failure to thrive, and other developmental defects.

- Parvovirus B19 is a single-stranded linear DNA, icosahedral naked capsid virus that replicates in the nucleus of erythroid precursor by using host RNA polymerase for transcription and host DNA polymerase for replication.

- Parvovirus B19 causes erythema infectiosum (aka fifth disease) characterized by fever, headache, myalgia and a confluent, indurated rash on the face with a slapped-face appearance.

- Overt arthritis or vasculitis is seen in some patients, in addition to some rare complications such as hepatitis, thrombocytopenia, nephritis, or encephalitis.

- Parvovirus B19 can also be transmitted transplacentally and causes hydrops fetalis.

- HHV-6 or 7, a member of herpesvirus family, causes roseola infantum (sudden rose-like rash) of the face. Other viruses that can cause similar type of rashes are adenoviruses, coxsackieviruses, and echoviruses.

- Rashes may be seen in several other viral infections such as echoviruses, coxsackieviruses, adenoviral serotypes, arboviruses (dengue, West Nile virus, Zika virus), Epstein-Barr virus, cytomegalovirus, and others.

CASE STUDY

A Preventable Illness?

A 12-year-old boy returned to the United States 2 days ago, after 3 weeks of travel with his family throughout southern Europe and northern Africa.

Yesterday, he developed a fever, dry cough, runny nose, and bilateral conjunctivitis. Twenty-four hours later, the fever has reached 39.1°C, and the other symptoms have worsened somewhat.

Physical examination reveals pharyngeal and conjunctival inflammation, and swollen, nontender anterior cervical lymph nodes. A rash is seen on the head and trunk.

He received all routinely recommended childhood immunizations by 5 years of age, but none since.

QUESTIONS

1. Which of the following viruses do you consider to be the most likely cause of the symptoms in this patient?
    A. Measles
    B. Mumps
    C. Rubella
    D. Human herpesvirus 6
    E. Parvovirus B19

2. Which of the following tests would you perform to obtain a diagnosis?
    A. Obtain a complete blood count
    B. Obtain a microscopic exam
    C. IgM-specific antibody or RT-PCR
    D. Obtain a blood culture
    E. Obtain a radiologic test

3. The pathogenesis of infection includes a significant tropism for vascular endothelial cells in all the following viruses *except*:
    A. Mumps
    B. Measles
    C. Rubella
    D. Human herpesvirus 6
    E. Parvovirus B19

4. Which of the following is mechanism of pathogenesis of this disease?
    A. Toxicity of CD4 T cells mediated by immune complex
    B. IL-12 downregulation
    C. Replication of the virus in the nucleus
    D. Upregulation of TNF-alpha
    E. Cell lysis by viral neuraminidase

ANSWERS

1. **(A)**

2. **(C)**

3. **(A)**

4. **(B)**

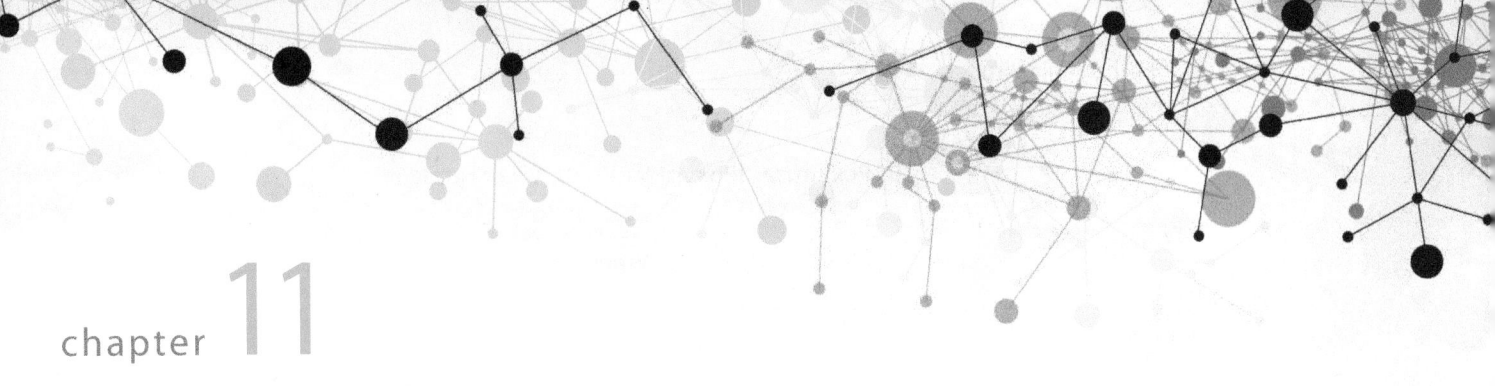

chapter 11

Poxviruses

Variola Virus · Vaccinia Virus · Monkeypox · Cowpox · Parapoxvirus · Molluscum Contagiosum

You have erased from the calendar of human afflictions one of its greatest. Yours is the comfortable reflection that mankind can never forget that you have lived. Future nations will know by history only that the loathsome small-pox has existed.

—Thomas Jefferson, Letter to Edward Jenner, 1806

Poxviruses belong to Poxviridae family that are the largest and most complex viruses infecting humans, other mammals, birds, and even insects. Poxviruses that infect vertebrates are classified into eight genera, and four of these genera cause disease in humans, including *Orthopoxvirus, Parapoxvirus, Yantapoxvirus*, and *Molluscipoxvirus*. *Orthopoxvirus* genus members that cause disease in humans include variola (smallpox), cowpox, vaccinia (strain used for smallpox vaccination), and monkeypox viruses. *Parapoxvirus* genus members cause disease mainly in animals but sometimes also in humans, including orf and pseudocowpox viruses. *Molluscipoxvirus* causes molluscum contagiosum (pearl-like lesions) in humans and *Yantapoxvirus* comprises tanapox and yabapox viruses that mainly infect animals but may also cause mild disease in humans. The most important agents in human disease are variola (smallpox), vaccinia, monkeypox, molluscum contagiosum, orf, cowpox, and pseudocowpox (**Table 11–1**). Although smallpox has been eliminated, it has the potential to be used in germ warfare or in bioterrorism. In addition, monkeypox causes similar disease in humans like smallpox but usually milder. Therefore, knowledge and understanding of smallpox pathogenesis and disease are important for any future control of outbreaks of poxviral diseases.

POXVIRUSES: GROUP CHARACTERISTICS

Poxviruses are large, brick-shaped or ovoid, linear double-stranded DNA (130-300 kbp) containing core within a double membrane and a lipoprotein envelope carrying virions measuring approximately 350 × 270 nm (vaccinia virus) (**Figures 11–1 and 11–2**). The core is flanked by two lateral bodies containing several viral enzymes and proteins, including DNA-dependent RNA polymerase and transcription factors required for viral replication. The poxvirus genome encodes all essential enzymes, proteins, and factors needed for viral replication in the cytoplasm of infected cells, including transcription, DNA synthesis, and virus assembly. The envelope is acquired in the cytoplasm either from the Golgi apparatus or other cellular organelles, but not by budding from the plasma membrane and may not be essential for viral infectivity.

Poxvirus replication is unique among DNA viruses in that the viral replication cycle takes place in the cytoplasm of the infected cell (**Figure 11–3**). The viral replication cycle starts with attachment, rapid adsorption to receptors followed by viral entry, and release of cores in the cytoplasm. Viral DNA-dependent RNA polymerase in the cores initiates early transcription to synthesize several proteins, including DNA and RNA polymerases, transcription factors, growth factors, and immune defense molecules. The uncoating of the cores uses viral DNA to synthesize concatemeric DNA molecules, which are eventually resolved into viral DNA genomes for progeny viruses. The late mRNAs synthesize viral structural proteins required for virus assembly and early transcription factors for packaging in the virions. Assembly of the progeny viruses begins with the

Largest, most complex enveloped, double-stranded DNA virus

✳ Only DNA viruses that completely replicate in the cytoplasm

TABLE 11–1	Poxviruses (Poxviridae) That Affect Humans
GENERA	**MEMBERS THAT CAUSE DISEASE**
Orthopoxvirus	Variola (smallpox) Vaccinia (strain used for smallpox vaccination) Cowpox[a] Monkeypox[a]
Parapoxvirus	Bovine papular stomatitis[a] Orf[a] Pseudocowpox[a]
Molluscipoxvirus	Molluscum contagiosum
Yatapoxvirus	Tanapox[a] Yabapox[a]

[a]Viruses that have nonhuman reservoirs but can cause disease in humans (usually mild and localized).

FIGURE 11–1. **Schematic diagram of the structure of poxvirus virion.** Viral DNA and several viral proteins within the core form the nucleosome (N). The core is covered with a 9 nm thick core membrane (CM) and assumes a dumbbell shape because of two lateral bodies (LB), which is eventually enclosed within a protein shell of 12 nm thickness (outer membrane) containing irregular surface tubules (T). The virion is enclosed in a lipid bilayer envelope containing virus-specific proteins. (Reproduced with permission from Willey JM: *Prescott, Harley, & Klein's Microbiology*, 7th ed. New York, NY: McGraw Hill; 2008.)

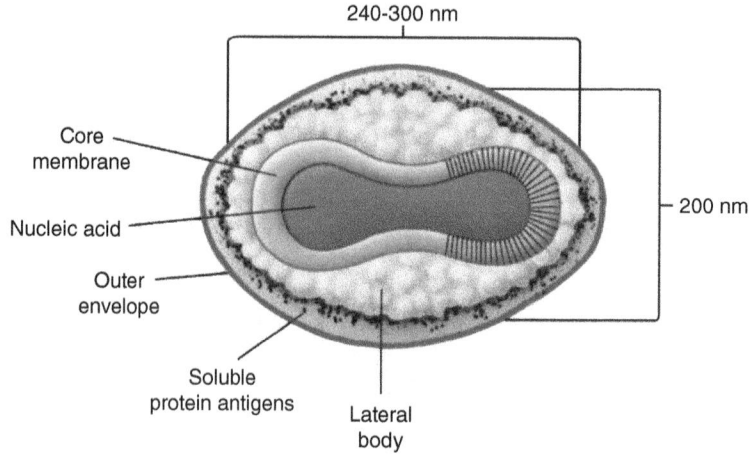

FIGURE 11–2. **Electron microscopic appearance of a poxvirus (vaccinia).** (Negative stain; original magnification ×60000.) (Used with permission from Dr Claire M. Payne.)

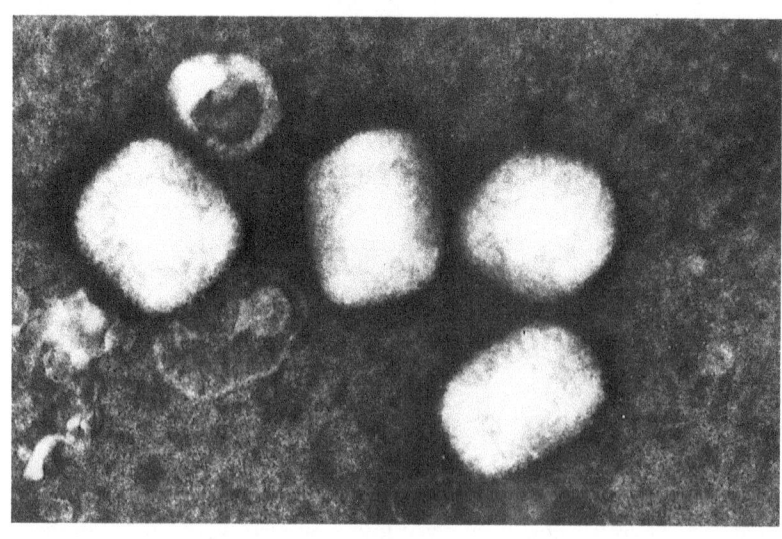

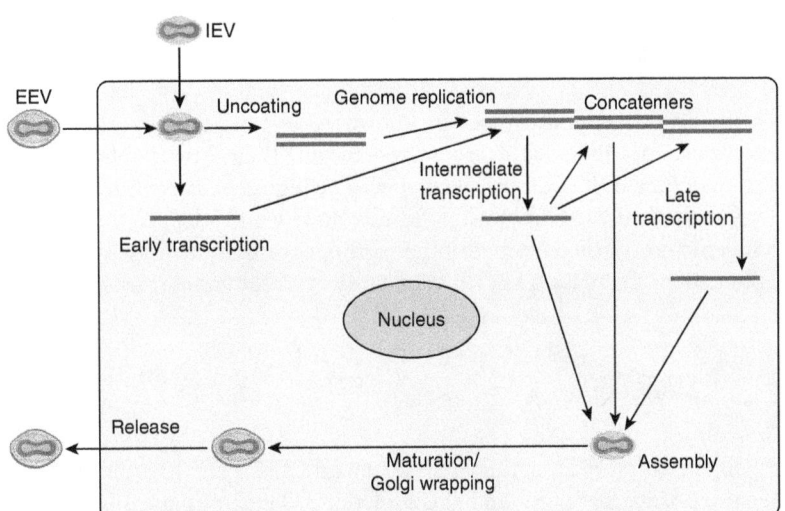

FIGURE 11–3. **Replication cycle of poxviruses.** All the events in sequence are listed in the diagram, including: (1) attachment, (2) entry, (3) early mRNA synthesis, (4) uncoating, (5) genome replication, (6) intermediate mRNA synthesis, (7) late mRNA synthesis, (8) assembly, (9) DNA genome packaging, (10) maturation, (11) envelope wrapping from Golgi, and (12) exit or virus release. EEV, extracellular enveloped virus; IEV, intracellular enveloped mature virus.

formation of membrane structures followed by maturation of intracellular mature virions (IMV). The virions are further wrapped by membranes from the Golgi apparatus that are lost upon the release of extracellular enveloped virions (EEV).

 Unlike other DNA viruses that replicate in the nucleus, why does poxvirus replicate in the cytoplasm?

VARIOLA (SMALLPOX)

Overview

Although smallpox virus has been eliminated from the world, it caused an acute infection with a high fatality rate. Smallpox or variola virus is a poxvirus with a double-stranded linear DNA genome and a lipoprotein envelope that replicates in the cytoplasm by using its own viral RNA and DNA polymerases. Smallpox virus enters through inhalation and replicates in the upper respiratory tract epithelium, spreads to the regional lymph nodes, infects phagocytic cells followed by development of viremia and dissemination to various organs such as liver, spleen, and skin. Eosinophilic inclusions called Guarnieri bodies can be seen in the cytoplasm. Viral proteins such as complement regulatory and immunomodulatory proteins interfere with activities of Th1 response, cellular cytokines, chemokines, and other immune mediators. Enormous inflammatory responses were also accountable for main characteristics of illness. The incubation period is 12 to 14 days (occasional fulminant case; 4-5 days). Clinical manifestations are fever, chills, and malaise preceding lesions after 4 to 5 days. A dominant feature is a uniform papulovesicular rash that evolves to pustules over 1 to 2 weeks. Vesicles appear on face, arms, and lower extremities (all at the same time). Some cases are fulminant with a hemorrhagic rash. Complications include keratitis, encephalitis, pneumonia, and bacterial superinfections. Intensive worldwide epidemiologic control measures, including vaccination (live vaccinia virus vaccine), are currently thought to have achieved global eradication of the disease; nevertheless, it is imperative to continue careful surveillance in case the virus may unexpectedly reemerge. Other poxviruses such as monkeypox and others are occasionally transmitted from animals to humans, and can sometimes mimic smallpox in a much milder form.

 Think ▸▸ Apply 11-1: **Poxviruses replicate in the cytoplasm because they can make their own RNA and DNA polymerases and other enzymes and proteins required for transcription of mRNA and replication of genomes.**

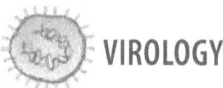

VIROLOGY

Generally, two types of viruses are known: variola major and variola minor (alastrim). Although the viruses are indistinguishable antigenically, their fatality rates differ considerably (>1% for variola minor, 3-40% for variola major). The high replicative fidelity of variola DNA polymerase enzyme limited its ability to significantly mutate and adapt to the humans, which preserved the antigenic cross-reactivity with other orthopoxviruses such as vaccinia virus that was used for vaccination. There is no known animal reservoir for variola virus.

✳ Smallpox was caused by variola major (3-40% fatality) and variola minor (>1% fatality)

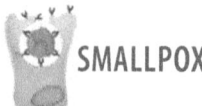

SMALLPOX

Smallpox has played a significant role in world history with respect to both the serious epidemics recorded since antiquity and the sometimes dangerous measures taken to prevent infection. Smallpox virus is highly contagious and can survive well in the extracellular environment. Acquisition of infection by infected saliva droplets or by exposure to skin lesions, contaminated articles, and fomites has been well documented. Variola caused a severe systemic illness when inhaled but a milder disease when inoculated into the skin.

In 1967, the World Health Organization (WHO) launched an ambitious program aimed at eradication of smallpox. This goal was considered realistic for two major reasons: (1) no extra-human reservoir of the virus was known to exist, and (2) asymptomatic carriage apparently did not occur. The basic approach included intensive surveillance for clinical cases of smallpox, prompt quarantine of such patients and their contacts, and immunization of contacts with vaccinia virus (vaccination) to prevent further spread. A tremendous amount of effort was involved, but the results were astonishing: The last recorded case of naturally acquired smallpox occurred in Somalia in 1977. Global eradication of smallpox was confirmed in 1979 and accepted by WHO in May 1980. Since then, the virus has been solely secured in two WHO-restricted laboratories: One at the United States Centers for Disease Control and Prevention (CDC) in Atlanta, Georgia, and the other at a similar facility in Moscow, Russia.

High communicability by respiratory droplets, fomites

✳ Highly contagious, survival in environment, threat to bioterrorism

WHO eradication campaign based on lack of nonhuman reservoir and asymptomatic cases

Immunization and case tracing led to success in 1980

 Why does poxvirus pose threat to potential bioterrorism?

Unfortunately, the dramatic world events that occurred in 2001 have raised the chilling possibility that clandestine virus stocks of smallpox may exist elsewhere and could be effectively used for major bioterrorist attacks. Reasons for such concern include: (1) smallpox is one of the most stable viruses; (2) it can remain stable for a long time, if freeze-dried; (3) it is unaffected by environmental conditions; (4) scab forms are stable for 1 year at room temperature and in one case, it was found stable for 13 years in a laboratory; (5) it has high infectivity among humans; (6) it is associated with high susceptibility among populations (routine vaccination against smallpox ended in 1972, and current vaccine supplies are limited); (7) there is a risk that healthcare providers may not promptly recognize and respond to early cases; and (8) there is no specific antiviral treatment.

A response plan and guidelines for such threats are posted on CDC website (www.cdc.gov/smallpox) and are updated at regular intervals.

Continuing surveillance also includes studies of poxviruses of animals (eg, buffalopox, monkeypox), which are antigenically somewhat similar to smallpox. Some virologists remain legitimately concerned that an animal poxvirus, such as monkeypox, could mutate to become highly virulent to humans—a further reminder that complacency could be dangerous.

✳ Potential for bioterrorism germ warfare

✳ One of the most stable viruses unaffected by environmental conditions

Freeze-dried form of smallpox virus and scab form very stable for a long time

No proven antiviral treatment

Animal poxviruses could be a future threat

 Think ▸▸ Apply 11-2: **Smallpox virus poses threat to human welfare because it can be used as a weapon in bioterrorism. Poxviruses are stable in the environment and stay intact in a lyophilized powder.**

PATHOGENESIS

The virus enters the mucous membranes of the upper respiratory tract through inhalation followed by viral replication at the site of entry and infection of mononuclear phagocytic cells in the regional lymph nodes. Viremia allows the virus to be transported to liver, spleen, and other tissues. At the end of the incubation period, inflammatory mediators are released causing fever and other symptoms. In variola, a secondary viremic phase has been demonstrated. The virus spreads through the capillaries to the skin followed by viral replication and evolution of rash. The virus further spreads cell-to-cell or through the mid and basal layers of skin causing necrosis and vesicles. The orthopoxviruses as a group cause a dramatic effect on host cell macromolecular function, leading to a switch from cellular to viral protein synthesis, changes in cell membrane permeability, and cytolysis. Eosinophilic inclusions, called **Guarnieri bodies,** can be seen in the cytoplasm. Multiple viral proteins, such as complement regulatory and immunomodulatory proteins are encoded by the virus that can interfere with induction or activities of multiple host mononuclear cell cytokines, chemokines, and other immune mediators. This serves to impair the host innate defenses that are important in the early control of infection. Some immunomodulatory proteins interfere with the T_H1 response, causing depressed cell-mediated immunity in controlling primary infection. Enormous inflammatory responses were also accountable for main characteristics of illness. In some patients, high levels of circulating virus caused hemorrhagic disease that resembled septic shock. Although variola was found in several tissues of infected patients, the lesions are limited to skin and oropharyngeal mucosa because the virus produces a homolog of epidermal growth factor that proliferates keratinocytes, followed by virus replication and spread.

✳ Replicates in upper respiratory tract followed by viremia, dissemination

Profound effect on host cell protein synthesis

✳ Viral proteins interfere with host defenses causing depressed cell-mediated immunity

✳ Eosinophilic inclusions, Guarnieri bodies, in cytoplasm

Enormous inflammatory responses were also accountable for main characteristics of illness

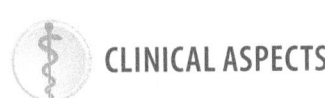

CLINICAL ASPECTS

MANIFESTATIONS AND DIAGNOSIS

The incubation period of smallpox is usually 12 to 14 days, although in occasional fulminating cases it can be as short as 4 to 5 days. The typical onset is abrupt, with fever, chills, and myalgia, followed by a rash 3 to 4 days later. The rash evolves to firm papulovesicles that become pustular over 10 to 12 days, then crust and slowly heal. Only a single crop of lesions (all in the same stage of evolution) develop; these lesions are most prominent over the head and extremities (**Figure 11–4**). Some cases are fulminant, with a hemorrhagic rash ("sledgehammer" smallpox). Death can result from the overwhelming primary viral infection or from bacterial superinfection. Diagnostic methods

✳ Fever, chills, myalgia, and single-stage rash become pustules over 10 to 12 days

Vesicular scrapings used for diagnosis

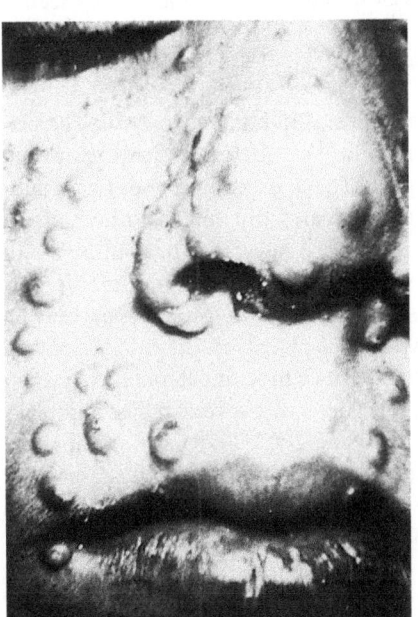

FIGURE 11–4. **Close-up of facial lesions of smallpox during the first week of the illness.**

use vesicular scrapings and include culture, electron microscopy, gel diffusion, and polymerase chain reaction.

PREVENTION

Jenner vaccinated with cowpox

The first major step toward modern prevention and subsequent eradication of smallpox can be credited to Edward Jenner, who noted that milkmaids who develop mild cowpox lesions on their hands appeared immune to smallpox. In 1798, he published evidence indicating that purposeful inoculation of individuals with cowpox material could protect them against subsequent infection by smallpox. The concept of vaccination gradually evolved, with the modern use of live vaccinia virus, a poxvirus of uncertain origin to be discussed later, which produced specific immunity.

● VACCINIA

Origin unclear, likely hybrid of smallpox and cowpox

✳ Live vaccinia virus vaccine used in humans

✳ Vaccination produces strong local reactions

Severe reactions seen in immunocompromised patients

Immunity was believed to wane after 3 to 5 years

Studies suggest vaccination immunity persisted for decades

Vaccinia virus is serologically related to smallpox, although its exact origin is unclear. Some virologists believe it is a recombinant virus derived from smallpox and cowpox, and others suggest it originated from a poxvirus of horses. The virus is usually propagated by dermal inoculation of calves, and the resultant vesicle fluid ("lymph") is lyophilized and used as a live virus vaccine in humans. The vaccine is inoculated into the epidermis and produces a localized lesion, which indicates successful immunization. The lesion becomes vesicular, then pustular, followed by crusting and healing over 10 to 14 days. The local reaction is sometimes severe and accompanied by systemic symptoms such as fever, rash, and lymphadenopathy. Patients who are immunocompromised may experience severe reactions, such as progressive vaccinia. Vaccinia-produced immunity to smallpox was believed to wane rapidly after 3 to 5 years, and the duration of long-term immunity beyond that time was uncertain. However, several studies, including the Baltimore Longitudinal Study of Aging, suggested that the immunity (IgG neutralizing antibody) to smallpox vaccine (vaccinia) persisted for decades.

Vaccinia and canarypox as vectors for delivery of vaccines and gene therapy

There has been a resurgence of scientific interest in vaccinia as a possible vector for active immunization against other diseases, such as hepatitis B, herpes simplex, and human immunodeficiency virus. It has been shown that gene sequences coding for specific immunogenic proteins of other viruses can be inserted into the vaccinia virus genome, with subsequent expression as the virus replicates. For example, a recombinant vaccinia strain carrying the gene sequence for hepatitis B surface antigen (HBsAg) can infect cells, lead to production of HBsAg, and stimulate an antibody response to it. Theoretically, gene sequences coding for a variety of antigens could be packaged in a single viable vaccinia virus, thus allowing simultaneous active immunization against multiple agents. It has been suggested that use of other poxviruses of animal or avian origin, such as canarypox, may be even safer, yet effective vectors for use in humans. These vectors are being used to develop gene therapy approaches and vaccines for HIV and other infections. Whether such approaches become routinely applicable to clinical medicine remains to be seen.

● MONKEYPOX

✳ Monkeypox, other animal poxviruses can be transmitted to humans by close animal contact

Monkeypox was first reported in laboratory monkeys in 1958 and in humans in 1970. The primary reservoir for monkeypox is not monkeys but Central and West African rodents. However, two other African viruses classified in the *Yatapoxvirus* genus (tanapox and yabapox) have subhuman primates as their primary reservoirs. All these three viruses can spread to humans by direct contact producing generally mild illness that, in more severe cases, may be confused with smallpox. While the symptoms of monkeypox in humans are milder than smallpox, another difference is that there is swelling of lymph nodes in monkeypox infection. Monkeypox causing infection in humans is also referred to as human monkeypox.

The first case of human monkeypox was first identified in 1970 Democratic Republic of Congo (DRC) followed by majority of cases occurring in this region. There were several major outbreaks reported in the same region of Central Africa. Between 1970 and 2007, 1378 cases of monkeypox in humans were reported in DRC, including 830 cases in 2005-2007. Sporadic cases have been reported in West African countries. Two strains of monkeypox virus, the Central African strain and West African strain, have been found. In 2003, at least 47 cases of human monkeypox occurred in the Midwestern United States. There were no fatalities. The contact sources were ill pet prairie dogs that had been housed with various exotic rodents imported from Ghana. In 2005, 19 cases of human monkeypox were reported in Sudan. In total, 88 cases were reported in

Republic of Congo (2017), 115 cases in Nigeria (2017-2019), 45 cases in Central African Republic (2015-2018), 3 cases in the United Kingdom (2018), and 1 case in Israel (2018). Continued surveillance is needed for this emerging infection.

Direct transmission to humans occurred by close contact with the ill animals, including direct contact with blood, bodily fluids, or rashes of infected animals. Secondary, human-to-human transmission occurs from close contact to respiratory secretions, lesions, or droplet nuclei of infected people. However, the transmission efficiency is far less than smallpox virus. Monkeypox could be transmitted through the placental route.

After transmission, there is an incubation period of 6 to 16 days, in which the virus replicates in the lymphatic system followed by viremia and transportation of the virus to all body organs, including multiplication within the epithelial cells of the skin. Human monkeypox infection can be divided into two phases, the invasion phase and the skin eruption phase. In the invasion phase that lasts from 0 to 5 days after incubation period, fever, severe headache, lymphadenopathy (swelling of the lymph nodes), back pain, myalgia, and an extreme asthenia (lack of energy) are noted. The skin eruption phase is characterized by the appearance of maculopapular rash on the face in about 95% of the cases, on the palms of the hands and soles of the feet in 75% of the cases, and on the body concurrently. The maculopapular rash develops into vesicles, pustules, followed by crusts in about 10 days, which is generally eliminated in about 3 weeks. The symptoms of human monkeypox last about 12 to 14 days. One of the characteristics of monkeypox is that there may be severe lymphadenopathy in some patients before the development of rash, unlike smallpox or chickenpox. The fatality is less than 10%.

The clinical diagnosis may be confusing because of similarities with smallpox, chickenpox, measles, and other rash-like diseases. Therefore, laboratory diagnosis by ELISA (antibody), antigen detection, PCR (genome amplification), or virus isolation by cell culture must be performed.

No specific treatment is available for monkeypox. However, smallpox vaccine (vaccinia virus) provides more than 85% protection.

● MOLLUSCUM CONTAGIOSUM

Molluscum contagiosum is a benign, cutaneous poxvirus disease of humans, spread by direct contact with infected cells. It is usually acquired by inoculation into minute skin abrasions; events that commonly lead to transmission include "roughhousing" in shower rooms and swimming pools, sharing of towels, bathing sponges, pool equipment, toys, and sexual contact. Most infection occurs in children over 1 year of age. Patients with AIDS are especially prone to develop widespread lesions. Some of the other risk factors include atopic dermatitis because of broken skin and immune dysfunction.

After an incubation period between 2 weeks and 6 months, nodular, pale, firm (pearl-like) lesions or papules known as Mollusca that are usually 2 to 5 mm in diameter develop in the epidermis. These lesions are painless, flesh-colored papules, and umbilicated in appearance (**Figure 11–5**). They may become itchy, red, sore, and swollen. A cheesy material may be expressed from the pore at the center of each lesion. Local trauma may cause a spread of lesions in the involved skin area. Since the virus is localized in the epidermis, there is no viremia and no spread to other body organs. The lesions are not associated with systemic symptoms, and they disappear in 6 to

Marginal notes

* Monkeypox illness can mimic smallpox

* Human-to-human, secondary transmission occurs at a low efficiency

Incubation period 6 to 16 days

Vesicles and pustules on face, palms, hands, feet, other body areas

Symptoms last 12 to 14 days

Severe lymphadenopathy in some

Smallpox (vaccinia) vaccine provides protection

Transmission direct skin-to-skin

* Painless pearl-like lesions express cheesy material

* Lesions flesh colored and umbilicated

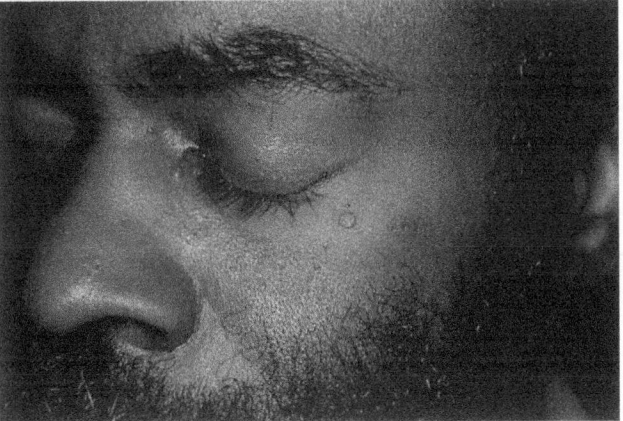

FIGURE 11–5. **Several papular lesions of molluscum contagiosum on the face of a patient with AIDS.** The larger lesion (near the eye) is raised, fleshy, and slightly umbilicated. (Reproduced with permission from Connor DH, Chandler FW, Schwartz DQ, et al: *Pathology of Infectious Diseases.* Stamford CT: Appleton & Lange; 1997.)

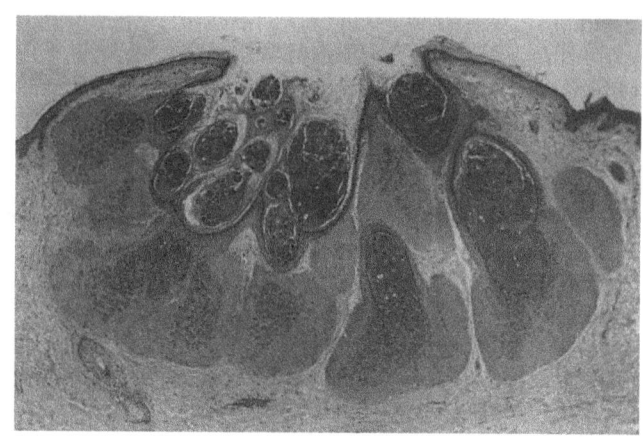

FIGURE 11–6. **Molluscum contagiosum of skin.** The epithelium has a crater-form indentation with inverted lobules of keratinocytes containing eosinophilic inclusion. The epithelium over the edge of the lesion is raised (hematoxylin-eosin × 40). (Reproduced with permission from Connor DH, Chandler FW, Schwartz DQ, et al: *Pathology of Infectious Diseases.* Stamford CT: Appleton & Lange; 1997.)

✳ Virus confined to epidermis

✳ Molluscum bodies in cytoplasm are diagnostic

Smallpox (vaccinia) vaccine does not provide protection

12 months without treatment but may take as long as 4 years. The lesions are classified into three categories, including the common skin lesions generally seen on faces, trunks, and limbs of children, sexually transmitted lesions seen on genitals, groin area, inner thighs, and lower abdomen, and the diffuse lesions seen in AIDS, immunocompromised, or immunosuppressed patients. Specific treatment, if desired, is usually by curettage or careful removal of the central core by expression with forceps. Some oral (cimetidine for pediatric cases) and topical (podophyllotoxin) agents are also available. HIV/AIDS and other immunocompromised patients may develop lesions more than 15 mm in diameter that do not respond to therapy.

Pathologic findings, which are limited to the epidermis, include hyperplasia, ballooning degeneration, and acanthosis. The diagnosis, made on clinical grounds, can be confirmed by demonstration of large, eosinophilic cytoplasmic inclusions (molluscum bodies) in the affected superficial epithelial cells (**Figure 11–6**).

People who recover from molluscum infection are not protected against new infections. The virus does not persist indefinitely. The smallpox (vaccinia) vaccine does not provide any protection either.

● ORF

Orf is an old Saxon term for a human infection caused by a parapoxvirus of sheep and goats. Synonyms for the infection in animals include contagious pustular dermatitis, ecthyma contagiosum, pustular ecthyma, and "scabby mouth." Humans usually acquire the infection by close contact with infected animals and accidental inoculation through cuts or abrasions on the hands or wrists. The typical skin lesion is solitary; it begins as a vesicle and evolves into a nodular mass that later develops central necrosis (**Figure 11–7**). Regional lymphadenopathy sometimes develops. Dissemination is rare. The average duration of the lesion is 35 days, followed by complete resolution. The diagnosis is usually made on the basis of clinical appearance and occupational history. Serologic confirmation or electron microscopy of the lesion can be performed but is rarely necessary.

Vesicular skin lesions seen in sheep- or goat-herders

FIGURE 11–7. A boggy indurated plaque on the dorsal surface of the hand characteristic of orf, a parapoxvirus infection transmitted by sheep and goats. (Reproduced with permission from Connor DH, Chandler FW, Schwartz DQ, et al: *Pathology of Infectious Diseases.* Stamford CT: Appleton & Lange; 1997.)

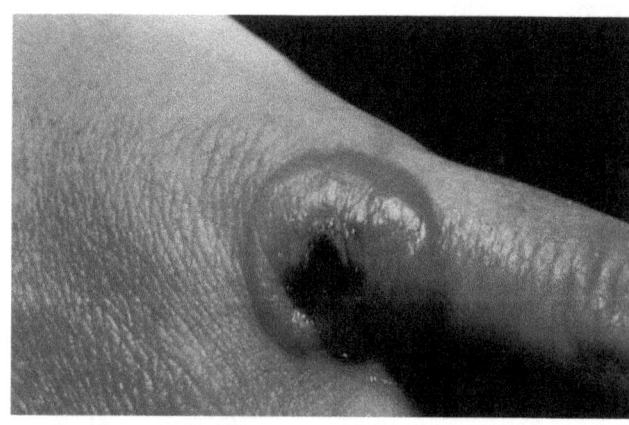

MILKER'S NODULES AND COWPOX

Milker's nodules (pseudocowpox) constitute a cutaneous parapoxvirus disease of cattle, distinct from cowpox, which can cause local skin infections similar to those of orf in exposed humans. Healing of the skin lesions may take 4 to 8 weeks. There is no cross-immunity to cowpox. Cowpox is now very rare in the United States. It produces a vesicular eruption on the udders of cows and similar, usually localized, vesicular skin lesions in humans (referred as cowmaid blisters) who are accidentally exposed.

Localized infection acquired by direct contact with bovines

KEY CONCLUSIONS

- Poxviruses are the largest, most complex, enveloped, double-stranded DNA viruses with lateral bodies in their core.
- Poxviruses replicate in the cytoplasm, unlike all other DNA viruses that replicate in the nucleus. Poxviruses synthesize RNA and DNA polymerases and other necessary enzymes and proteins required for transcription and replication. Poxvirus particles bring their own RNA polymerase that transcribes mRNAs in the cytoplasm which are translated into many proteins, including DNA polymerase, that are used for replication of the DNA genomes. Viral assembly takes place in the cytoplasm by wrapping envelope from the Golgi bodies.
- Smallpox virus enters through inhalation and multiplies in upper respiratory tract epithelium and phagocytic cells. Viremia develops that allows the virus to travel in the body organs such as skin and eosinophilic inclusions, called **Guarnieri bodies** that can be seen in the cytoplasm. Viral proteins interfere with host defenses causing depressed cell-mediated immunity. More importantly, massive inflammatory responses are responsible for the illness.
- Smallpox symptoms are fever, chills, and malaise preceding lesions starting with a dominant and uniform papulovesicular rash that evolves to pustules over 1 to 2 weeks. Vesicles appear on face, arms, and lower extremities (all at the same time).
- Several complications of smallpox such as keratitis, encephalitis, pneumonia, bacterial superinfections have been found.
- Vaccinia virus (a likely hybrid of cowpox and smallpox virus) was used as a live vaccine that allowed eradication of the smallpox globally. However, the vaccine can cause several adverse reactions such as generalized vaccinia and others, especially in immunocompromised people.
- Monkeypox and other animal poxviruses can be transmitted to humans and cause similar diseases that mimic smallpox but at a milder level.
- Molluscum contagiosum is transmitted through contact and causes pearl-like lesions that are flesh colored and umbilicated and express cheesy material.
- Poxvirus vectors have potential to be used in gene therapy and vaccination.

CASE STUDY

An Aftermath of War

A 22-year-old soldier has returned home after a 6-month tour of duty along the northeastern border of Afghanistan. The area consisted of scattered, small villages, where the main activities included raising goats and sheep, along with cultivation of poppies.

On arrival, the man was found to have a fever of 38.4°C and headache. The symptoms persisted, and by the third day of illness, papulopustular skin lesions began to appear over his face and upper chest.

Laboratory studies included a mild leukocytosis (11,000/mm³) but no other abnormalities.

QUESTIONS

1. Which of the following is the least likely cause of the man's condition?

   A. Vaccinia
   B. Variola minor
   C. Cowpox
   D. Monkeypox
   E. Variola major

2. Which is currently the most important aspect of smallpox transmission?
   A. Animal-to-human
   B. Human-to-human
   C. Asymptomatic human carriage
   D. Evolution of mutant virus
   E. Rodent contact

3. Which of the following is true about smallpox vaccine that could provide protection against cowpox?
   A. It is a live, vaccinia virus vaccine.
   B. It is a live, attenuated smallpox virus vaccine.
   C. It only induces cellular immunity and no humoral immunity.
   D. It has rarely any adverse reactions in immunocompromised people.
   E. It is a killed, smallpox virus vaccine.

ANSWERS

1. (C)

2. (B)

3. (A)

chapter 12

Enteroviruses

Poliovirus · Coxsackievirus · Echovirus · Paraechovirus · Other Enteroviruses

Ann Arbor. *The world learned today that its hopes for finding an effective weapon against paralytic polio had been realized.*
—*The New York Times*, April 12, 1955

OVERVIEW

Enteroviruses constitute a major subgroup of small, icosahedral, naked capsid, positive-sense RNA viruses belonging to the family Picornaviridae (picornaviruses). Their name is derived from their ability to infect intestinal tract epithelial and lymphoid tissues and shed into the feces, but they do not commonly cause gastrointestinal diseases. They are transmitted by the fecal–oral route and readily infect the intestinal tract and further spread to cause paralytic disease, mild aseptic meningitis, exanthems, myocarditis, pericarditis, and nonspecific febrile illness. These viruses include the polioviruses, coxsackieviruses, echoviruses, parechoviruses, and other agents that are simply designated as enteroviruses. There is another member of the picornavirus family called rhinoviruses that are not enteroviruses, because they are transmitted through respiratory route and cause common colds. Enterovirus infections can produce a great diversity of clinical disease. Some cause paralytic disease that may persist permanently (a typical feature of polioviruses), acute inflammation of the meninges with or without involvement of cerebral or spinal tissues, or sepsis-like illnesses in newborn infants. Inflammatory effects at other sites, such as the lungs, pleura, heart, and skin have also been observed, often without concomitant or preceding central nervous system (CNS) involvement. Occasionally, infections may result in chronic, active disease processes. For poliovirus, two types of vaccines, inactivated polio vaccine (IPV) and live attenuated oral polio vaccine (OPV), have been in use in preventing polio worldwide. Moreover, IPV is recommended for use in the United States.

● ENTEROVIRUSES: GROUP CHARACTERISTICS

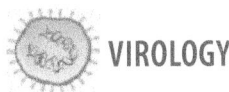 **VIROLOGY**

MORPHOLOGY AND BIOLOGIC FEATURES

Enteroviruses constitute polioviruses (3 serotypes), coxsackieviruses (Group A, 23 serotypes and Group B, 6 serotypes), echoviruses (32 serotypes), parechoviruses (8 serotypes), and other enteroviruses (4 serotypes). As a group, the enteroviruses are picornaviruses that are extremely small (22-30 nm in diameter), naked capsid virions with icosahedral symmetry. Enteroviruses possess a single-stranded, positive-sense RNA with a covalently bound small virus-encoded protein (VPg) and a capsid formed from 60 copies of four nonglycosylated proteins (VP1, VP2, VP3, and VP4). The basic building block of the capsid is the protomer containing one copy each of VP1, VP2, VP3, and VP4. Five protomers (pentamers) are placed at each of the 12 vertices of the icosahedron to form a capsomere of 60 protomers. The shell is composed of VP1, VP2, and VP3, whereas VP4 is attached on the inner surface. On the surface of the virus, there is a deep depression or canyon around each pentameric vertex. The receptor-binding site is located at the floor of

* Small, naked capsid, icosahedral, single-stranded (+) RNA viruses

* Replicate in the cytoplasm using viral RNA polymerase

the canyon. The virion structure of a picornavirus member is shown in Chapter 13 (Figure 13–1). Replication and assembly occur exclusively in the cellular cytoplasm; one infectious cycle can occur within 6 to 7 hours. This results in cessation of host cell protein synthesis and cell lysis with release of new infectious progeny. The replication cycle is shown in **Figure 12–1.** Picornaviruses enter the host cell via receptor-mediated endocytosis (viropexis) following interaction of a viral surface protein with a specific receptor on the host cell. Picornaviruses use a wide variety of host cell receptors, including PVR or CD155 (poliovirus), CD55 (coxsackieviruses, echoviruses, enterovirus 70), and ICM1 (some coxsackieviruses A). After the removal of capsid protein, uncoating takes place followed by removal of VPg, and the positive-sense RNA viral genome is released into the cytoplasm, which acts as an mRNA. This genomic viral mRNA is translated in a cap-independent manner using internal ribosomal entry site (IRES) into a polyprotein, which is processed into mature proteins, including an RNA-dependent RNA polymerase. RNA-dependent RNA polymerase directs both transcription of mRNA and synthesis of genomic RNA via negative-sense RNA intermediates. After the synthesis of viral proteins, the genomic RNA (+) is packaged into progeny virions that are assembled in the cytoplasm and released upon cell death.

Unlike rhinoviruses, which are also members of the picornavirus family, enteroviruses are resistant to an acidic pH (as low as 3.0). This feature undoubtedly helps ensure their survival during passage through the stomach to the intestines. Enteroviruses are also resistant to many common disinfectants such as 70% alcohol, substituted phenolics, ether, and various detergents that readily inactivate most enveloped viruses. Chemical agents, such as 0.3% formaldehyde or free residual chlorine at 0.3 to 0.5 ppm, are effective. However, if sufficient extraneous organic debris is present, the virus can be protected and survive long periods. Glutaraldehyde (2%, pH 7.4, temperature 25°C) can reduce the infectivity of the virus by $2\log_{10}$ in less than 1 minute and was not negatively affected by the presence of high concentration of organic matters.

✳ (+) RNA IRES allows ribosome to translate in a cap-independent manner

✳ (+) RNA is translated into a polypeptide which is cleaved into individual proteins

✳ Enteroviruses resistant to acid, detergents, and many disinfectants

✳ Formaldehyde, hypochlorite active against enteroviruses

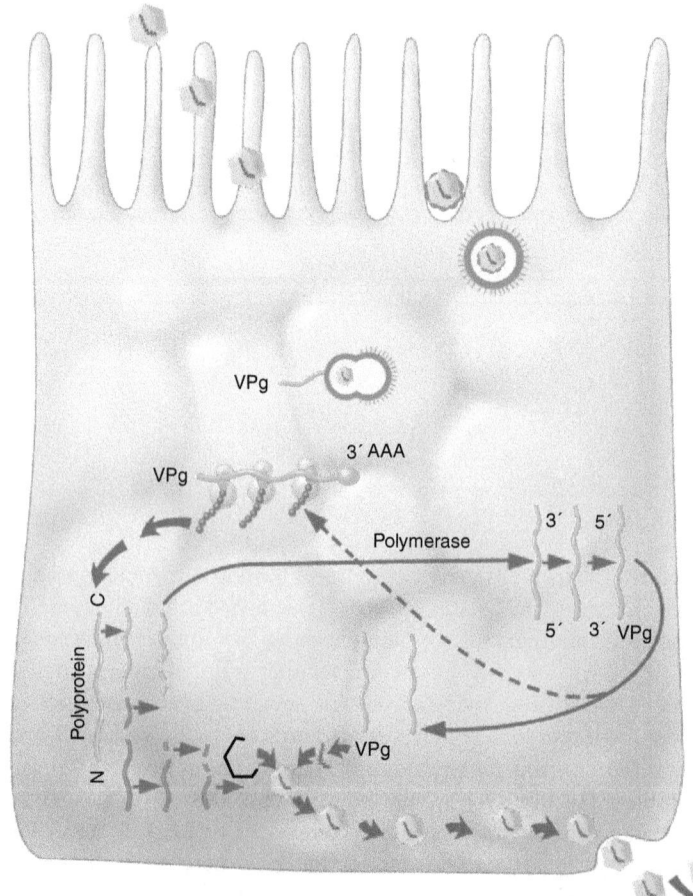

FIGURE 12–1. Replication cycle of picornaviruses. Picornaviruses interact with a specific receptor on the host cell for entry via receptor-mediated endocytosis (viropexis). Following uncoating, VPg (viral protein genome) is removed and the positive-sense genomic RNA is released in the cytoplasm. The genomic RNA (+) is translated in a cap into a polyprotein, which is processed into mature proteins, including an RNA-dependent RNA polymerase. RNA-dependent RNA polymerase directs both transcription of mRNA and synthesis of genomic RNA via negative-sense RNA intermediates. After the synthesis of viral proteins, the genomic RNA (+) is packaged into progeny virions that are assembled in the cytoplasm and released upon cell death.

TABLE 12–1	Human Enteroviruses
CLASS	**NUMBER OF SEROTYPES**[a]
Poliovirus	3
Coxsackievirus	
Group A	23
Group B	6
Echovirus	32
Parechovirus	8
Enterovirus	4

[a]More recently discovered enteroviruses, which have overlapping biologic characteristics, are identified numerically (types 68-71). Four of the original 30 numbered echovirus serotypes have been reclassified; however, the remaining retain their original serotype number (eg, echovirus 30).

 Why are enteroviruses resistant to detergents and disinfectants despite being simple, naked capsid viruses?

Some of the enterovirus serotypes share common antigens, but there are no significant serologic relationships between the currently recognized major classes listed in **Table 12–1.** Genetic variation within specific strains occurs, and mutants that exhibit antigenic drift and altered tropism for specific cell types are now recognized. Polioviruses, which have been most extensively studied as enterovirus prototypes, are known to have epitopes on three surface structural proteins (VP1, VP2, and VP3) that induce type-specific neutralizing antibodies. This appears to be generally the case for all enteroviruses; definitive identification of isolates usually requires neutralization or molecular analysis tests.

Antigenic mutations, drifts occur

✴ Antibody to surface proteins neutralize infectivity

✴ Type-specific neutralizing antibodies

GROWTH IN THE LABORATORY

Most enteroviruses can be propagated and isolated in primate (human or simian) cell cultures and show characteristic cytopathic effects. Some strains, particularly several coxsackievirus A serotypes, are more readily detected by inoculation of newborn mice. In fact, the newborn mouse is one basis for originally classifying group A and B coxsackieviruses. Group A coxsackieviruses primarily cause a widespread, inflammatory, necrotic effect on skeletal muscle, leading to flaccid paralysis and death. Similar inoculation of group B coxsackieviruses causes encephalitis, resulting in spasticity and occasionally convulsions. Other enteroviruses rarely have an adverse effect on mice unless special adaptation procedures are first used. The higher-numbered enteroviruses (types 68-71), which have overlapping variable growth and host characteristics, have been classified separately.

Growth of some in primate cell cultures

Coxsackie A and B viruses have different effects on newborn mice

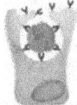 ## ENTEROVIRUS DISEASE

EPIDEMIOLOGY

Humans are the major natural host for the polioviruses, coxsackieviruses, and echoviruses. There are enteroviruses of other animals with limited host ranges that do not appear to extend to humans. Conversely, viruses thought to be identical or related to human enteroviruses have been

Worldwide distribution

 Think ▸▸ Apply 12-1: Unlike enveloped viruses' lipid membranes easily inactivated by solvent-based disinfectants, enteroviruses, outer capsid proteins are not easily inactivated by these disinfectants. However, formaldehyde and hypochlorite are active against enteroviruses.

Animals are not involved in human disease

Proportion of asymptomatic infections varies with strain

Dominant epidemic strains come and go

Greater prevalence during summer and fall in temperate climates

✳ **Person-to-person fecal–oral transmission correlates with predominance in children**

✳ **Virus in respiratory secretions, saliva, sputum, blister fluids, stool**

Incubation periods typically short

Initial attachment of viral surface protein to cell surface receptors immunoglobulin or integrin families

Initial replication in epithelial and lymphoid cells followed by viremic spread

isolated from dogs and cats. Whether these agents cause disease in such animals is debatable, and there is no evidence of disease spreading from animals to humans.

The enteroviruses have a worldwide distribution, and asymptomatic infection is common. The proportion of infected persons who develop illness varies from 2% to 100%, depending on the serotype or strain involved and the age of the patient. Secondary infections in households are common and range as high as 40% to 70%, depending on factors such as family size, crowding, and sanitary conditions.

In some years, certain serotypes emerge as dominant epidemic strains; they then may wane, only to reappear in epidemic fashion years later. From 2009 to 2013, coxsackievirus A6 were the most common infections reported in the United States. Coxsackievirus A16 is the most common cause of hand-foot-and-mouth disease (HFMD) in the United States and coxsackievirus A24 and echovirus 70 have been associated with conjunctivitis. Coxsackievirus B1 was common in 1963; echovirus 9 in 1962, 1965, 1968, and 1969; echovirus 13 and 18 in 2001; echovirus 16 in 1951 and 1974; and echovirus 30 in 1968, 1969, between 1989 and 1992, and in 2003. Echoviruses 13, 18, and 30 have caused viral meningitis in the United States. Enterovirus 71 has caused HFMD and encephalitis in Asia and have also been associated with neurologic disease in the United States. Enterovirus D68 has caused a widespread outbreak of severe respiratory disease in 2014, 2016, and 2018 in the United States. Recently, ED68 has been shown to be associated with acute flaccid myelitis in young children. The emergence of dominant serotypes is unpredictable from year to year. All enteroviruses show a seasonal predilection in temperate climates; epidemics are usually observed during the summer and fall months. In subtropical and tropical climates, the transmission may occur year-round.

Direct or indirect fecal–oral transmission is considered the most common mode of spread. After infection, the virus persists in the oropharynx for 1 to 4 weeks, and it can be shed in the feces for 1 to 18 weeks. The virus is present in respiratory secretions, including saliva, sputum, nasal mucous, and blister fluids as well as stool of infected people. Thus, sewage-contaminated water, fecally contaminated foods, or passive transmission by insect vectors (flies, cockroaches) may occasionally be the source of infection. More commonly, however, the spread is directly from person to person. This mode of transmission is suggested by the high infection rates seen among young children, whose hygienic practices tend to be less than optimal, and in crowded households. Approximately two-thirds of all isolates are from children 9 years of age or younger. The risk of transmission is higher in those who do not have antibodies from previous infections, including during pregnancy. Mothers infected around the time of delivery can pass the virus to the infants.

Incubation periods vary (Table 7–3), but relatively short intervals (2-10 days) are common. Often, illness is seen concurrently in more than one family member, and the clinical features vary within the household.

PATHOGENESIS

Initial binding of an enterovirus to the cell surface is commonly between an attachment protein in a "canyon" configuration on the virion surface and cell receptors belonging to the immunoglobulin gene superfamily. These receptors map to chromosome 19. A different receptor, belonging to the integrin group of adhesion molecules, has been identified for at least one echovirus serotype. After attachment, the virion is endocytosed by the cell membrane, and its (+) RNA is released into the cellular cytoplasm, where it binds to ribosomes and commences protein synthesis. Newly synthesized virions are released by lysis to spread to the other cells. Enteroviruses shut off host cell synthesis by destroying the cellular mRNA cap-binding complex (CBC) required for cellular protein synthesis (translation) and still favor their own protein synthesis by allowing ribosomes to bind onto IRES on viral RNA.

 How do enteroviruses inhibit host protein synthesis but not their own?

After primary replication in epithelial cells and lymphoid tissues in the upper respiratory and gastrointestinal tracts, viremic spread to other sites can occur. Potential target organs vary according to the virus strain and its tropism, but may include the CNS, heart, vascular endothelium, liver, pancreas, lungs, gonads, skeletal muscles, synovial tissues, skin, and mucous membranes. Histopathologic findings include cell necrosis and mononuclear cell inflammatory infiltrates; in the CNS, the inflammatory cells are localized most prominently in perivascular sites. The initial tissue damage is thought to result from the lytic cycle of virus replication; secondary spread to other sites may ensue. Viremia is usually undetectable by the time symptoms appear, and termination of virus replication appears to correlate with the appearance of circulating neutralizing antibody, interferon, and mononuclear cell infiltration of infected tissue. The early dominant antibody response is with immunoglobulin M (IgM), which usually wanes 6 to 12 weeks after onset to be replaced progressively by increased IgG-specific antibodies. The important role of antibodies in termination of infection, demonstrated in mouse models of group B coxsackievirus infections, is supported by the observation of persistent echovirus and poliovirus replication in patients with antibody deficiency diseases.

Injury by cell lysis localized in perivascular sites

Antibody response terminates replication

Although initial acute tissue damage may be caused by the lytic effects of the virus on the cell, the secondary sequelae may be immunologically mediated. Enterovirus-caused poliomyelitis, disseminated disease of the newborn, aseptic meningitis, encephalitis, and acute respiratory illnesses, thought to represent primary lytic infections, can usually be identified through routine methods of virus isolation and determination of specific antibody titer changes. On the other hand, syndromes such as myopericarditis, nephritis, and myositis have been associated with enteroviruses primarily because of serologic and epidemiologic evidence. In many of these cases, viral isolation is the exception rather than the rule. The pathogenesis of these latter infections is not clear; however, observations suggest that the acute infectious phase of the virus may be mild or subclinical and often subsides by the time clinical illness becomes evident. Illness may represent a host immunologic response to tissue injury by the virus or to viral or virus-induced antigens that persist in the affected tissues.

In experimental group B coxsackievirus myocarditis, mononuclear inflammatory cells (monocytes, natural killer lymphocytes) seem to play a greater role than antibody in termination of infection, and the persistence of inflammation after disappearance of detectable infectious virus or viral antigen appears to be mediated by cytotoxic T lymphocytes. Experimental findings have led to another hypothesis regarding pathogenic mechanisms, called **molecular mimicry.** This is best conceptualized as a form of virus-induced autoimmune response. It is known that small peptide sequences on viral epitopes can sometimes be shared by host tissues. Thus, an immune response produced by the virus may also generate antibodies or cytotoxic cross-reactive effector T lymphocytes that recognize shared determinants located on host cells. For example, a monoclonal antibody directed against a neutralizing site of a group B coxsackievirus has also been shown to react strongly with normal myocardial cells.

In addition to lytic effects of virus, there are probable immunopathologic manifestations

Disease may follow the acute infection

Coxsackie B myocarditis may involve virus-induced cross-reacting antibody

IMMUNITY

Infection by a specific serotype in an immunologically normal host is followed by a humoral antibody response, which can often be detected by neutralization methods for many years thereafter (**Figure 12–2**). There is relative immunity to reinfection by the same serotype; however, reinfection has been reported, usually resulting in subclinical infection or mild illness.

Immunity is serotype specific

CLINICAL ASPECTS

DIAGNOSIS

Currently, the polymerase chain reaction (PCR) with reverse transcription and complementary DNA amplification (RT-PCR) is being increasingly used to detect enteroviral RNA sequences in tissue and body fluids, thus greatly enhancing diagnostic sensitivity and speed. Alternatively, classical virus isolation methods can be used. The disadvantages of the latter approach are longer time to detection (3-10 days versus several hours for RT-PCR) and lower sensitivity; one advantage is that virus isolates can be more readily further characterized antigenically and genetically.

RT-PCR enhances diagnostic speed and sensitivity

Think ▶▶ Apply 12-2: **Enteroviruses destroy the cellular mRNA cap-binding complex that is required for initiation of protein synthesis but allow ribosomes to bind onto IRES of its RNA for protein synthesis.**

FIGURE 12–2. **Antibody response and viral isolation from various sites in a typical case of enteroviral infection.**

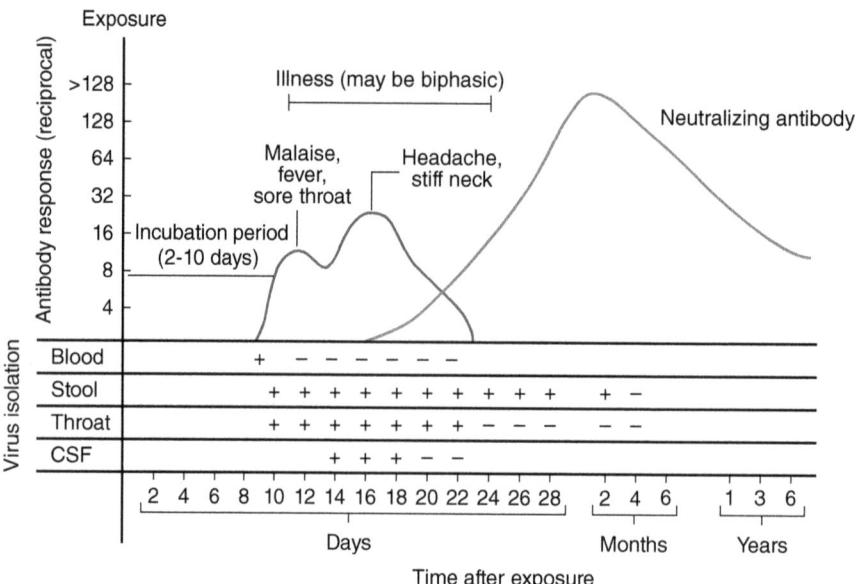

In acute enterovirus-caused syndromes, diagnosis is most readily established by virus detection in throat swabs, stool or rectal swabs, body fluids, and occasionally tissues. Viremia may be undetectable by the time symptoms appear. When there is a CNS involvement, cerebrospinal fluid (CSF) specimens taken during the acute phase of the disease may be positive in 10% to 85% of cases, depending on the stage of illness and the viral serotype involved. Direct detection of virus from affected tissues or body fluids in enclosed spaces (eg, pleural, joint, pericardial, or CSF) usually confirms the diagnosis. Detection of an enterovirus from the throat is highly suggestive of an etiologic association; the virus is usually present at this site for only 2 days to 2 weeks after infection. Detection of virus from fecal specimens only must be interpreted more cautiously; asymptomatic shedding from the bowel may persist for as long as 4 months (Figure 12–2).

The diagnosis may be further supported by fourfold or greater neutralizing antibody titer changes between paired acute and convalescent serum samples. However, this method is often expensive and cumbersome, requiring careful selection of serotypes for use in antigens. Quantitative interpretations of antibody titers on single serum samples are rarely helpful, because of the wide range of titers to different serotypes that can be found among healthy individuals.

Viral isolation from pharynx or closed space is significant

Prolonged shedding in stool

Serodiagnosis cumbersome due to many serotypes

TREATMENT AND PREVENTION

None of the currently available, approved antiviral agents has been shown to be effective in treatment or prophylaxis of enterovirus infections. Treatment is symptomatic and supportive. Vaccines for the prevention of poliovirus infections are available and discussed later in this chapter. Vaccines of other nonpolio enteroviruses are not available. Although proper disposal of feces and careful personal hygiene are recommended, the usual quarantine or isolation measures are relatively ineffective in controlling the spread of enteroviruses in the family or community.

✳ **Poliovirus vaccines available**

Nonpolio enteroviruses have no vaccines

Hygienic factors make prevention difficult

● ENTEROVIRUSES: SPECIFIC GROUPS

POLIOVIRUSES

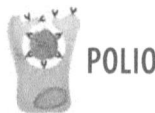 POLIO

EPIDEMIOLOGY

Worldwide, the most important enteroviruses are the three poliovirus serotypes (types 1, 2, and 3). They first emerged as important causes of disease in developed temperate zone countries during the latter part of the 19th century, and they have become increasingly important elsewhere as living conditions improve in developing countries. This somewhat paradoxical situation is related to the fact that the risk of paralytic disease resulting from infection increases with age. Improvement of sanitary conditions tends to impede the spread of the viruses; thus, individuals may become infected not in early infancy but later in life, when paralysis is more likely to occur. Polio affects mainly children below 5 years of age. More importantly, polio cases have decreased by more than 99% since 1988. In 1988, there were 350 000 polio cases in 125 endemic countries, whereas only 223 cases in 3 endemic countries were reported in 2012, 74 cases in 2015, and 37 cases in 2016 in two endemic countries (Afghanistan and Pakistan). However, the number of cases in these two endemic countries during 2017-2020 has increased, including 21 cases in 2018, 29 in 2019, and 41 in 2020. In 2016, type 2 containing oral poliovirus vaccine (OPV) was withdrawn globally due to higher incidence of reversion, the number of circulating vaccine-derived poliovirus type 2 (cVDP2) outbreaks have increased, and 547 cVDP2 cases have been reported in 21 countries between 2018 and 2020. It has been suggested that 10 million cases of polio-induced paralysis and 0.5 million deaths have been prevented since 1988 due to polio vaccination. It seems that polio eradication is within reach, provided vaccination is continued in endemic countries. However, complete eradication has been hampered by political strife, severe poverty, wars, and myths in many underdeveloped nations in Africa, Asia, and the Middle East. In addition, the coronavirus (COVID-19) pandemic and mitigation have resulted in suspension of polio immunization and surveillance activities. In the United States, the last case of endogenous polio was seen in 1979 after the implementation of IPV in 1955 and live OPV in 1961. However, only IPV is now used in the United States.

* Polio cases reduced by more than 99% since 1988 due to vaccination

* Risk of paralytic disease increases with age

* Polio affects mainly children below 5 years of age

PATHOGENESIS

The schematic diagram of the pathogenesis of poliovirus is shown in Chapter 7 (Figure 7–1). Poliovirus is spread by fecal–oral route. Virus enters oropharynx and multiplies in the mucosa, shed in oral secretions and swallowed, and then multiplies in the intestine. The virus enters the cells by binding to poliovirus receptor (PVR) or CD155 (an immunoglobulin-like receptor). The virus takes over the host cell synthesis by shutting it down and favoring its own replication. After primary replication in epithelial cells and lymphoid tissues in the upper respiratory and gastrointestinal tracts, including the M cells of Peyer patches, viremia spreads to other sites. The specific tropism of polioviruses for the CNS, which they usually reach by passage across the blood–CNS barrier, is perhaps favored by reflex dilatation of capillaries supplying the affected motor centers of the anterior horn of the brainstem or spinal cord. An alternate pathway is via the axons or perineural sheaths of peripheral nerves. The virus replicates in the CNS and motor neurons are particularly vulnerable to infection and variable degrees of neuronal destruction. The histopathologic findings in the brainstem and spinal cord include necrosis of neuronal cells and perivascular "cuffing" by infiltration with mononuclear cells, primarily lymphocytes (**Figure 12–3**).

* CNS tropism by blood or peripheral nerves

* Motor neuron cells destroyed

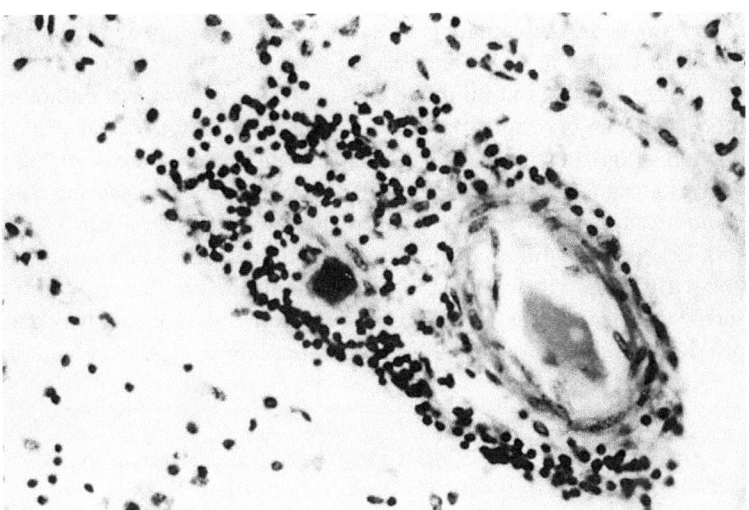

FIGURE 12–3. **Section of spinal cord from a fatal case of poliomyelitis, demonstrating perivenous mononuclear cell inflammatory reaction.** (Used with permission from Dr Peter C. Johnson.)

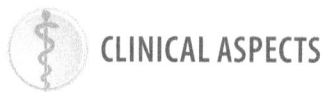 **CLINICAL ASPECTS**

MANIFESTATIONS

Most infections (perhaps 80-90%) are either completely subclinical or so mild that they do not gather attention. One out of four people may experience flu-like symptoms such as sore throat, fever, tiredness, nausea, headache, and stomach pain for few days. The incubation period ranges from 4 to 35 days but is usually between 7 and 14 days. Three types of disease can be observed. **Abortive poliomyelitis** is a nonspecific febrile illness of 2 to 3 days duration with no signs of CNS localization. **Aseptic meningitis** (nonparalytic poliomyelitis) is characterized by signs of meningeal irritation (stiff neck, pain, and stiffness in the back) in addition to the signs of abortive poliomyelitis; recovery is rapid and complete, usually within a few days. **Paralytic poliomyelitis** occurs in less than 2% of infections. It is the major possible outcome of infection and is often preceded by a period of minor illness, sometimes with two or three intervening symptom-free days. There are signs of meningeal irritation, but the hallmark of paralytic poliomyelitis is asymmetric flaccid paralysis, with no significant sensory loss. The extent of involvement varies greatly from case to case; however, in its most serious forms, all four limbs may be completely paralyzed or the brainstem may be attacked, with paralysis of the cranial nerves and muscles of respiration (bulbar polio). The maximum extent of involvement is evident within a few days of first paralysis. Thereafter, as temporarily damaged neurons regain their function, recovery begins and may continue for as long as 6 months; paralysis persisting after this time is permanent.

Subclinical, abortive poliomyelitis common

Aseptic meningitis recovers rapidly

✳ *Paralytic poliomyelitis manifests flaccid paralysis without sensory loss*

Recovery of function up to 6 months, after which it becomes permanent

 How does poliovirus cause flaccid paralysis?

PREVENTION

Two types of poliovirus vaccines are currently available: Inactivated or killed polio vaccine (IPV) and live, attenuated virus, oral polio vaccine (OPV). Each contains all three poliovirus serotypes 1, 2, and 3. IPV is currently used in the United States.

Inactivated or killed polio vaccine (IPV) was developed by Jonas Salk and introduced in 1955; its use was associated with a dramatic decline in paralytic cases (**Figure 12–4**). Vaccination is by subcutaneous injection. Primary vaccination with four doses of the present enhanced-potency IPV at ages 2, 4, 6 through 18 months, and 4 through 6 years of age produces antibody responses in more than 98% of recipients. IPV stimulates the production of IgG antibodies that eliminate the virus during viremia. The current product is considered safe, with no significant deleterious side effects. Inactivated (Salk) vaccine is used in many developed countries, including the United States, and will be replacing OPV, which is used in several developing countries.

✳ *Four doses of IPV at ages 2, 4, 6-18 months, and 4-6 years recommended in the United States*

✳ *IPV predominantly elicits IgG antibody*

OPV is composed of live, attenuated viruses that have undergone serial passage in cell cultures from humans and subhuman primates. OPV was developed by Albert Sabin and first licensed in the United States in 1963. The vaccine is given orally as a primary series of four doses 2, 4, 6 through 18 months, and 4 through 6 years of age and produces antibodies to all three serotypes in more than 95% of recipients; these antibodies persist for several years. OPV stimulates the production of IgA that eliminates the virus in the mucosal areas, including gastrointestinal tract. OPV is given at a lower dose than IPV because OPV replicates in the intestinal epithelial cells without causing pathogenicity and the titer of antibodies is much higher in OPV than IPV. As with IPV, recall boosters are recommended to maintain adequate antibody levels. Like wild-type poliovirus, OPV viruses infect and replicate in the oropharynx and intestinal tract and can be spread to other persons. The WHO also recommends that countries that are using only OPV add one dose of IPV (3 doses of OPV plus 1 dose of IPV).

✳ *Live (Sabin) vaccine is given orally (OPV), requires low dose, mounts IgA response*

Vaccine virus replicates and can spread

 Think ▶▶ Apply 12-3: Poliovirus damages motor neurons leading to loss of muscle function causing flaccid paralysis.

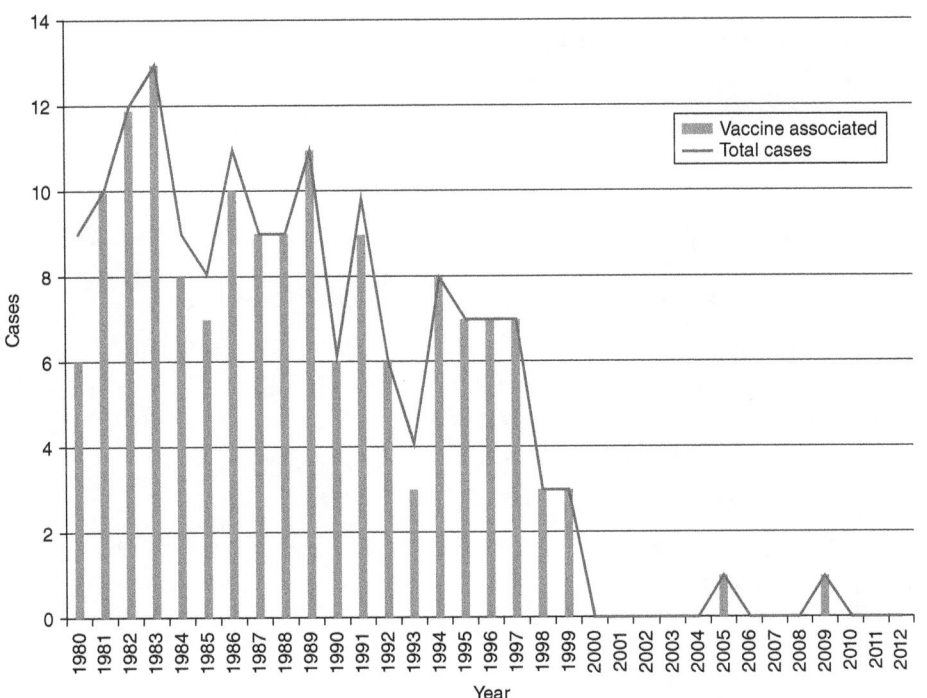

FIGURE 12–4. **Total number of reported paralytic poliomyelitis cases (including imported cases) and number of reported vaccine-associated cases—United States, 1980-2012.** (Reproduced with permission from Centers for Disease Control and Prevention.)

One disadvantage of OPV is the remote risk of vaccine-associated paralytic disease in some recipients or their household contacts, including immunocompromised persons. The incidence of vaccine-associated paralytic poliomyelitis is estimated at approximately 1 per 2.4 million doses distributed. In September 2015, poliovirus type 2 was officially eradicated, therefore, bivalent OPV (poliovirus type 1 and 3) was recommended for use in April 2016 to avoid reversion of poliovirus type 2 vaccine virus. However, the number of circulating vaccine-derived poliovirus type 2 (cVDP2) outbreaks have increased and 547 cVDP2 cases have been reported in 21 countries between 2018 and 2020. It is also being hoped that eventually there will be a withdrawal of OPV once poliovirus transmission has been interrupted and replaced by IPV. In the United States, exclusive use of IPV has been recommended for all routine immunizations since the end of 1999.

＊ Vaccine-associated poliomyelitis is a remote risk with OPV

＊ IPV is currently preferred in the United States

No cases of paralytic poliomyelitis attributed to indigenously acquired wild poliovirus have occurred in the United States since 1979. Nevertheless, it must be kept in mind that importation of these strains can readily occur from endemic areas in developing nations. Once introduced into a community, the virus can spread rapidly among susceptible individuals. Thus, continuing immunization programs are of utmost importance in preventing spread of this disease. Even an immunized adult traveling to polio-endemic areas should be vaccinated with IPV.

Coxsackieviruses, Echoviruses, and Enteroviruses

 Why is OPV a better vaccine than IPV despite a risk of reversion?

EPIDEMIOLOGY

The coxsackieviruses, echoviruses, and other enteroviruses are widespread throughout the world. Their epidemiology and pathogenesis are much the same as those of the polioviruses. Unlike polioviruses, they have a greater tendency to affect the meninges and occasionally the cerebrum,

Millions of infections and thousands of hospitalizations every year in the United States

 Think ►► Apply 12-4: OPV is a live, attenuated vaccine, which when given to people orally, replicates in the intestine and elicits both cell-mediated (CD8 T cells and CD4 T cells) and humoral (B cells, predominantly IgA) responses that are stronger, robust and long-lasting than IPV that mainly mounts humoral response with the help of CD4 T cells.

TABLE 12–2   Clinical Syndromes and Commonly Associated Enterovirus Serotypes[a]

	COXSACKIEVIRUS		
SYNDROME	**GROUP A**	**GROUP B**	**ECHOVIRUS, PARECHOVIRUS (PEV), AND ENTEROVIRUS (E)**
Aseptic meningitis, encephalitis	2, 4, 7, **9**, 10	1, **2, 3, 4, 5**	**4, 6, 9, 11, 13, 16, 18, 30**, E70, E71
Muscle weakness and paralysis (poliomyelitis-like disease)	7, **9**	2, 3, 4, 5	2, 4, 6, 9, 11, 18, 30, **E71**, ED68
Cerebellar ataxia	2, 4, **9**	3, 4	4, 6, 9
Exanthems and enanthems, HFMD	**4, 5, 6, 9, 10, 16**	2, 3, 4, 5	**2, 4, 5, 6, 9, 11, 16, 18, 25, E71**
Pericarditis, myocarditis	4, 16	**2, 3, 4, 5**	1, 6, 8, 9, 19
Epidemic myalgia (pleurodynia), orchitis	9	1, **2, 3, 4, 5**	1, 6, 9
Respiratory	9, 16, **21**, 24	1, 3, 4, 5	**4, 9, 11**, 20, 25, **ED68**
Conjunctivitis	**24**	1, 5	7, **E70**
Generalized disease (viral sepsis in neonates)	–	1, **2, 3, 4, 5**	3, 6, 9, 11, 14, 17, 19, PEV3

[a]Serotypes most commonly associated with the syndrome are in **boldface.**

Often do not affect motor neurons

Most infections are subclinical

Wide range of clinical manifestations

but only a few such as enterovirus 71 affect anterior horn cells. These group of viruses are also referred as nonpolio enteroviruses. These viruses cause 10 to 15 million infections with tens of thousands of hospitalizations every year in the United States.

The consequences of infection with these agents are highly variable and related only in part to virus subgroup and serotype. Most infections are subclinical or cause mild common cold-like illness. Infants and children and people with weakened immune system experience severe disease, whereas infected adults get mild form. The main interest in these agents stems from their ability to cause more serious illness, which becomes most evident during epidemics of infection with a particular agent. Unapparent infection is common. Illness manifestations vary from mild to lethal. **Table 12–2** lists the major syndromes and serotypes commonly associated with each. However, considerable overlap occurs, and one should not be surprised if an enteroviral serotype found in connection with a specific syndrome differs from that most often encountered.

MANIFESTATIONS

Respiratory symptoms, fever, skin rash, mouth blisters, and muscle ache seen

Conjunctivitis, meningitis, HFMD, myocarditis, and pericarditis are the severe forms

✱ **Major cause of viral (nonbacterial) CNS infections in infants and children**

✱ **Aseptic meningitis is the most common syndrome**

Myocarditis is often associated with group B coxsackieviruses

Following fecal–oral transmission, and from eyes, nose, and mouth secretions, blister fluids close contact with infected people and an incubation period of 2 to 10 days (see Table 7–3 for different enterovirus groups). Some people may get symptoms such as fever, runny nose, sneezing, cough, skin rash, mouth blisters, and body and muscle pain. Some infections, especially in infants and immunocompromised, may result in conjunctivitis, meningitis, encephalitis, HFMD, myocarditis, pericarditis, acute flaccid paralysis, and inflammatory muscle disease. In addition, newborns may develop viral sepsis that in some instances causes organ damage and failure, including death. It can also be transmitted perinatally.

Nonpolio enteroviruses are the major cause of CNS infections (nonbacterial) in the United States during summer and fall months, especially in infants and young children. Aseptic meningitis is the most frequently recognized clinical illness associated with enterovirus infections. This syndrome can be mild and self-limiting, lasting 5 to 14 days. However, it is sometimes accompanied by encephalitis, which can lead to permanent neurologic sequelae.

Acute inflammation of the heart muscle (myocarditis), its covering membranes (pericarditis), or both can be caused by a variety of viral agents. Group B coxsackieviruses are the most commonly implicated enteroviruses. Such infections are usually self-limiting but may be fatal in the acute phase (arrhythmia or heart failure) or progress to chronic dilated myocardiopathy.

In 2014, Enterovirus D68 (EV-D68) caused a severe respiratory illness in the United States. Although EV-D68 was discovered in 1962 in California, small number of cases have been reported

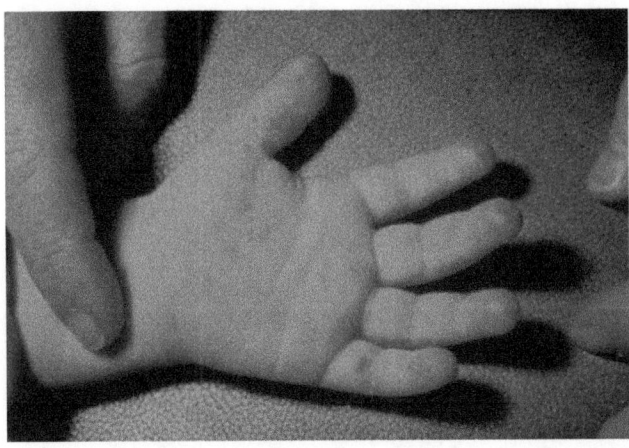

FIGURE 12–5. **Vesicular lesions of hand-foot-and-mouth disease (HFMC).**

since 1987. However, several outbreaks have occurred, in addition to 2014, in 2016 and 2018 during the months of August and November. It is transmitted through respiratory secretions either directly or indirectly, including saliva, nasal mucus, and sputum with mild symptoms such as fever, runny nose, sneezing, cough, and body and muscle aches. However, the severe symptoms include wheezing and difficulty breathing. Other symptoms may include arm or leg weakness, pain in the neck, arms, back or legs, difficulty in swallowing, slurred speech, or facial droop. An uncommon but serious neurological condition, acute flaccid myelitis (AFM), has been reported mostly in young children, which affects the gray matter area of spinal cord causing muscle weakness.

The exanthems are often not associated with CNS inflammation. They can resemble rubella, roseola infantum, or adenoviral macular or maculopapular exanthems, but may also appear as vesicular or hemangioma-like lesions. One interesting syndrome is **HFMD,** which usually affects children younger than 5 years of age and is characterized by fever, blister-like sores in the mouth (herpangina), and a skin rash (**Figure 12–5**). Coxsackievirus A16 is most commonly implicated, but others, such as enterovirus 71, can cause a similar illness. When associated with enterovirus 71 infection, the illness can be especially severe, with encephalitis, permanent polio-like limb weakness, and often fatal cardiorespiratory failure. Herpangina is an enanthematous (mucous membrane-affecting) febrile disease in which small vesicles or white papules (lymphonodules) surrounded by a red halo are seen over the posterior palate, pharynx, and tonsillar areas (**Figure 12–6**). This mild, self-limiting (1- to 2-week) illness has usually been associated with infection by several different group A coxsackievirus serotypes.

Epidemic myalgia (pleurodynia or Bornholm disease) is characterized by fever and sudden onset of intense upper abdominal or thoracic pain. The pain may be aggravated by movement, such as breathing or coughing, and can persist for as long as 14 days. Group B coxsackieviruses are often implicated.

Generalized disease of the newborn is a disseminated, sometimes lethal, enteroviral infection due to viral sepsis characterized by pathologic changes in the heart, brain, liver, and other organs.

✳ Enterovirus D68 associated with respiratory illness, including coughing and wheezing

Exanthems can mimic other diseases

Herpangina is an infection of palate and tonsils

Coxsakievirus A 16 and enterovirus 71 cause HFMD

Epidemic myalgia, with pleuritic pain

✳ Viral sepsis may cause organ damage and failure and death in newborns

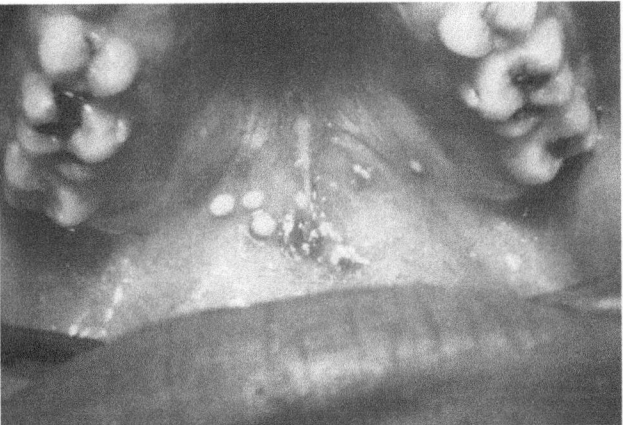

FIGURE 12–6. **Herpangina.** Localized lymphonodules and vesicles (mostly ruptured) in the posterior oropharynx.

Enterovirus 70 associated with conjunctivitis and enterovirus 71 with paralytic disease

Coxsackievirus type B liked to pathogenesis of type 1 diabetes, arthritis, polymyositis, and nephritis

It is apparent from Table 12–2 that the spectrum of disease produced by these viruses is enormous and that many other illnesses may also result from infections by this subgroup. Epidemics of acute hemorrhagic keratoconjunctivitis associated with enterovirus 70 and localized outbreaks of disease resembling paralytic poliomyelitis caused by enterovirus 71 infection have been described. In addition, there is evidence that certain enteroviruses, particularly group B coxsackievirus serotypes, may sometimes participate in the pathogenesis of type 1 diabetes, acute arthritis, polymyositis, and idiopathic acute nephritis via molecular mimicry mechanisms. Further investigations are required to establish whether such associations are significant.

KEY CONCLUSIONS

- Enteroviruses are picornaviruses which are simple, icosahedral naked capsid, positive-sense RNA and replicate in the cytoplasm by using viral RNA polymerase for transcription and replication.
- Enteroviruses are transmitted fecal–oral and from respiratory secretions, multiply in gastrointestinal tract but cause diseases such as paralytic disease, mild aseptic meningitis, exanthems, myocarditis, pericarditis, and nonspecific febrile illness.
- Enteroviruses (Picornaviruses) shut off host cell protein synthesis by destroying the cellular initiation factor complex but allow ribosomes to bind onto IRES on viral RNA for protein synthesis.
- Polioviruses cause abortive poliomyelitis (no sign of CNS involvement), aseptic meningitis (rapid recovery), and paralytic poliomyelitis (less than 2% of infections).
- Poliovirus damages motor neurons with variable degree of destruction from meningeal irritation and asymmetric flaccid paralysis to most serious form involving paralysis of all four limbs, cranial nerves, and muscles of respiration (bulbar polio).
- Two vaccines, inactivate polio vaccine (IPV) and live-attenuated oral polio vaccine (OPV) are available for polio prevention. IPV is given in four doses as intramuscular infection and mounts mainly IgG response, whereas OPV is given orally and mounts IgA and cell-mediated immune response. IPV is recommended for use in the United States, whereas OPV is used in developing countries.
- In general, infection with nonpolio enteroviruses (coxsackieviruses, echoviruses, and other enteroviruses) are subclinical. While some people get mild symptoms of fever, respiratory symptoms, skin rash, mouth blisters, and muscle ache, others have severity such as conjunctivitis, meningitis, HFMD, myocarditis, and pericarditis are the severe forms.
- Nonpolio enteroviruses are the major cause of viral (nonbacterial) CNS infections in the United States, especially in infants and young children.
- Enterovirus D68 (EV D68) has been found to cause severe respiratory illness, including coughing and wheezing in children.

CASE STUDY

A Severe Headache

A 2-year-old girl is on a summer visit to her grandparents in the midwestern United States, when she develops irritability, vomiting, low-grade fever, and frontal headache over 2 days.

Physical examination reveals only a stiff neck, wherein the patient resists attempts to flex it.

A lumbar puncture is done to quickly rule out bacterial meningitis. The CSF results are 90 cells/mm³, 70% mononuclear, glucose 60 mg/dL, and protein 45 mg/dL. Gram stain is negative for bacteria.

QUESTIONS

1. Which of the following tests would be most sensitive and specific at this stage of illness?
   A. IgM-specific serology on CSF
   B. Viral culture of CSF
   C. RT-PCR on CSF
   D. RT-PCR on rectal swab specimen
   E. IgM-specific serology on serum

2. All of the below are common characteristics of enteroviruses in humans, *except*:
    A. Seasonal peaks in temperate climates
    B. Fecal–oral transmission
    C. Resistance to 70% alcohol
    D. Replication in cell cytoplasm
    E. Animal reservoirs.

3. Live, attenuated, oral polio vaccine (OPV) and inactivated polio vaccine (IPV) are both available. In which one of the following situations is the use of OPV preferred?
    A. Routine infant vaccination
    B. Mass immunization programs in areas of high poliomyelitis endemicity
    C. Adult immunization
    D. Patients who are receiving immunosuppressive therapy
    E. Family contacts of immunocompromised patients

ANSWERS

1. (C)

2. (E)

3. (B)

chapter 13

Hepatitis Viruses

Hepatitis A · Hepatitis B · Hepatitis C · Hepatitis D · Hepatitis E · Hepatitis G

Jaundice is the disease that your friends diagnose.

—Sir William Osler

The causes of hepatitis (inflammation of the liver) are varied and include viruses, bacteria, and protozoa, as well as drugs and toxins (eg, isoniazid, carbon tetrachloride, and ethanol). The clinical symptoms and course of acute viral hepatitis can be similar, regardless of etiology, and determination of a specific cause depends primarily on the use of laboratory tests. Hepatitis may be caused by at least five viruses, including hepatitis A virus (HAV), hepatitis B virus (HBV), hepatitis C virus (HCV), hepatitis D virus (HDV), and hepatitis E virus (HEV) belonging to different virus families, whose major characteristics are summarized in **Table 13–1. Non-A, non-B hepatitis** is a term previously used to identify cases of hepatitis not due to HAV or HBV. With the discovery of HCV and HEV, virtually all the viral etiologies of non-A, non-B hepatitis can be specifically identified. One additional hepatitis virus, hepatitis G virus (HGV) or GB virus C (GBV-C), has been identified that is not associated with any clinical disease so far, but found in some blood donors as well as some patients who are either infected with HCV or human immunodeficiency virus (HIV). Other viruses, such as Epstein-Barr virus and cytomegalovirus, can cause inflammation of the liver, but hepatitis is not the primary disease caused by them. Yellow fever virus is also associated with hepatitis, but is described in Chapter 16.

HEPATITIS A

Overview

Hepatitis A virus (HAV) is a positive-sense RNA, icosahedral naked capsid virus belonging to Picornavirus family, which replicates in the cytoplasm by using viral RNA-dependent RNA polymerase for transcription and replication. It is the cause of what was formerly termed as infectious hepatitis or short-incubation hepatitis. This virus is spread by the fecal–oral route, and outbreaks may be associated with contaminated food or water. HAV replicates in the intestinal mucosa (incubation period 15-45 days) followed by viremia and spread to the liver where the replication causes lymphoid cell infiltration, necrosis of liver parenchymal cells, and proliferation of Kupffer cells. The illness is subclinical in up to 50% of infected adults. When symptomatic, there is usually fever, anorexia, nausea, right upper quadrant abdominal pain, and jaundice. Before the development of jaundice, dark urine and clay-colored stool may be noticed. Diagnosis is done by detecting IgM against HAV. Serum aminotransferases such as ALT and AST as well as bilirubin levels are elevated. Recovery occurs in weeks as it follows self-limiting rule. In rare cases, fulminant fatal hepatitis with extensive liver necrosis may occur. There is no specific treatment for HAV. However, an effective inactivated HAV vaccine given in two doses 6-12 months apart is recommended for use in children at age 1 year and in adults in the United States that also provides protection if given shortly after exposure.

TABLE 13–1	Comparison of Hepatitis A, B, D (Delta), C, and E				
FEATURE	**A**	**B**	**D**	**C**[a]	**E**
Virus type	Single-stranded RNA (+)	Double-stranded DNA	Single-stranded RNA (−)	Single-stranded RNA (+)	Single-stranded RNA (+)
Incubation period (weeks)	15-45 (mean, 25)	60-150 (mean 90)	21-49	14-182 (mean 14-84)	15-60 (mean, 40)
Onset	Usually sudden	Usually slow	Variable	Insidious	?
Age preference	Older children, young adults	All ages	All ages	All ages	Young adult
Transmission					
Fecal–oral	+++	±	±	−	+++
Sexual	+	++	++	+	+?
Parenteral	−	+++	++	+++	
Chronicity (%)	None	10	50-80	85	Rare
Carrier state	None	Yes	Yes	Yes	No
Immune serum globulin protective	Yes	Yes[b]	Yes[c]	No	No
Vaccine	Yes	Yes	Yes[c]	No	No

Plus and minus signs indicate relative frequencies.
[a]Many individuals with hepatitis C virus are also infected with hepatitis G virus, which is similar to hepatitis C virus.
[b]Hyperimmune globulin is more protective.
[c]Prevention of hepatitis B prevents hepatitis D.

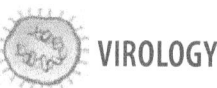 ## VIROLOGY

HAV is a picornavirus with only one serotype

Hepatitis A virus (HAV) belongs to the Picornaviridae (picornaviruses) family and *Hepatovirus* genus. It is a naked capsid (unenveloped), linear single-stranded, positive-sense RNA virus with a cubic (icosahedral) symmetry and a diameter of 27 nm (**Figure 13–1**). The genome of HAV is a 7.4 kb positive-sense, single-stranded RNA bound to a protein called VPg, and each capsid unit comprises four proteins, VP1, 2, 3, and 4, which cover the genome and form a naked capsid icosahedral virion. VP1 is the spike of HAV that binds to the receptor on the host cells. On the surface of the virus, there is a deep depression or canyon around each pentameric vertex. The receptor-binding site is located at the floor of the canyon. There is only one serotype and multiple genotypes of HAV. This virus possesses several characteristics of enteroviruses; for example, it resists inactivation and is stable at −20°C with low pH. The virus has been successfully cultivated in primary marmoset liver cell cultures and in fetal rhesus monkey kidney cell cultures.

* **Naked capsid, icosahedral, positive-sense RNA virus**

Replicates in the cytoplasm by using viral RNA polymerase

HAV replicates in the cytoplasm, like other positive-sense RNA viruses (Figure 12–1). HAV interacts with the receptor (α_2-macroglobulin) on the target cells (liver cells and few other cell types) and enters via receptor-mediated endocytosis (viropexis). The positive-sense RNA is translated into a polyprotein in a cap-independent manner by allowing ribosomes to bind onto internal ribosomal entry site (IRES), which is cleaved into various mature proteins, including RNA-dependent RNA polymerase. RNA-dependent RNA polymerase directs transcription of mRNAs to produce viral proteins as well as replication to make full-length viral RNA genomes. The assembly of the progeny viruses takes place in the cytoplasm after the packaging of viral genomes into HAV capsid proteins. Virions are released upon cell lysis.

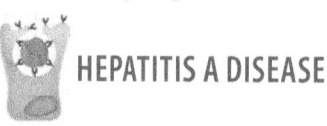 ## HEPATITIS A DISEASE

EPIDEMIOLOGY

HAV is endemic in several parts of the world, including Asia, Africa, the Middle East, Central and South America, and Western Pacific. Humans appear to be the major natural hosts of HAV. Several other primates (including chimpanzees and marmosets) are susceptible to experimental infection, and natural infections of these animals may occur. The major mode of transmission of

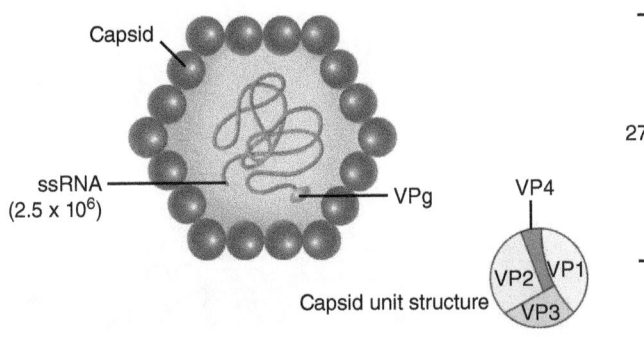

FIGURE 13-1. Diagram of the proposed structure of the hepatitis A virus. The protein capsid is made up of four viral polypeptides (VP1-VP4). Inside the capsid is a single-stranded (ss) molecule of RNA (molecular weight 2.5 × 10⁶), which has a genomic viral protein (VPg) on the 5' end.

HAV is through ingestion of contaminated food or water or through direct contact with an infected individual, person-to-person by fecal–oral exposure. Transmission through blood transfusion, though possible, is not an important means of spread, but persons with hemophilia who are given plasma products are at risk. High risk of infection is also observed in men who have sex with men, oral sex, in illicit drug users, and in travelers from the developed countries visiting developing areas of the world. While most HAV-infected people recover from the infection, a small number of infected people die due to the development of fulminant hepatitis. The WHO estimates that in 2016, 7134 died due to HAV infection worldwide, accounting for 0.5% of the mortality due to viral hepatitis.

In the United States, most cases of hepatitis A are not linked to a single contaminated source and occur sporadically, but several outbreaks have been described. The disease is common under conditions of crowding, and it occurs very frequently in nursing home settings and day care centers. A chronic carrier state has not been observed with hepatitis A; perpetuation of the virus in nature presumably depends on sporadic subclinical infections and person-to-person transmission. Outbreaks of hepatitis A have been linked to the ingestion of undercooked seafood, usually shellfish from waters contaminated with human feces. Common-source outbreaks related to other foods, including vegetables and fruits as well as contaminated drinking water, have also been reported. In 2013, 165 people became sick, including hospitalizations, with HAV in 10 states in the United States that was linked to contaminated pomegranate seeds imported from Turkey. In 2016, 143 people came down with hepatitis A in nine states in the United States from frozen strawberries imported from Egypt. There has been an estimated 2000 to 3000 HAV cases, including deaths in the United States between 2011 and 2014. Since 2016, HAV cases have increased considerably due to large person-to-person outbreaks in the United States. As of February 5, 2021, 37,691 cases, 23,053 hospitalizations, and 345 deaths have been reported from 35 states of the United States. These outbreaks underscore the importance of surveillance and vaccination of hepatitis A in the United States.

Less than 35% of the general population of the United States had serologic evidence of HAV infection between 1988 and 1994, and rates have been decreasing apparently because of better sanitation, less crowding, and the introduction of hepatitis A vaccination since 1995. In contrast, more than 90% of the adult population in many developing countries shows evidence of previous hepatitis A infection. The risk of clinically evident disease is much higher in infected adults than in children. Patients are most contagious in the 1 to 2 weeks before the onset of clinical disease.

PATHOGENESIS

HAV is believed to replicate initially in the enteric mucosa. The incubation period is 15 to 45 days (mean 25 days). It can be demonstrated in feces by electron microscopy for 10 to 14 days before the onset of disease. In most patients with symptoms of the disease, virus is no longer found in fecal specimens. Multiplication in the intestines is followed by a period of viremia with spread to the liver. The response to replication in the liver consists of lymphoid cell infiltration, necrosis of liver parenchymal cells, and proliferation of Kupffer cells (**Figure 13–2**). A variable degree of biliary stasis may be present. It is also believed that cytotoxic T lymphocytes (CTLs) damage the hepatocytes. Except in the rare instance of acute hepatic necrosis, the infection is cleared, liver damage is reversed, and HAV does not establish a chronic infection. Initial immune response is

---

Fecal–oral transmission

Contaminated food or water, person-to-person

✳ Early outbreaks linked to uncooked seafood, contaminated food, produce, water

✳ Recent outbreaks due to person-to-person spread in the United States

No chronic carriage

90% of adults seropositive in developing countries

Subclinical infection common in children

✳ Replicates in intestinal mucosa, incubation 15 to 45 days

Contagion greatest 10 to 14 days before symptoms

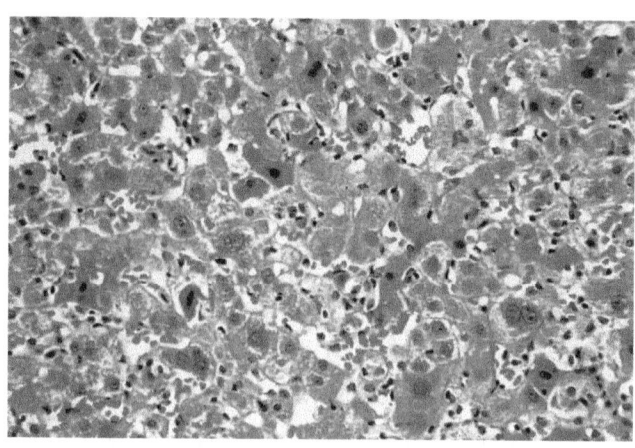

FIGURE 13–2. **Acute viral hepatitis, moderately severe.** There is a lobular disarray with degeneration, apoptosis, and necrosis of liver cells. Disruption of liver cell plates, hypertrophy of Kupffer cells, a predominantly lymphocytic inflammatory infiltrate, and regeneration of surviving liver cells also are seen. (Reproduced with permission from Connor DH, Chandler FW, Schwartz DQ, et al: *Pathology of Infectious Diseases.* Stamford CT: Appleton & Lange; 1997.)

✳ IgG-specific antibody protective

the development of HAV-specific IgM antibody followed by appearance of IgG after a few weeks. Detectable levels of IgG antibody to HAV persist indefinitely in serum, and patients with anti-HAV antibodies are immune to reinfection. Although virus-specific IgA has been demonstrated in stool, secretory immunity has not been shown to be important for hepatitis A. The immunopathogenic events associated with HAV infection are shown in **Figure 13–3.**

FIGURE 13–3. **Sequence of appearance of viremia, virus in feces, alanine aminotransferase (ALT), symptoms, jaundice, and IgM and IgG antibodies in hepatitis A virus (HAV) infection.**

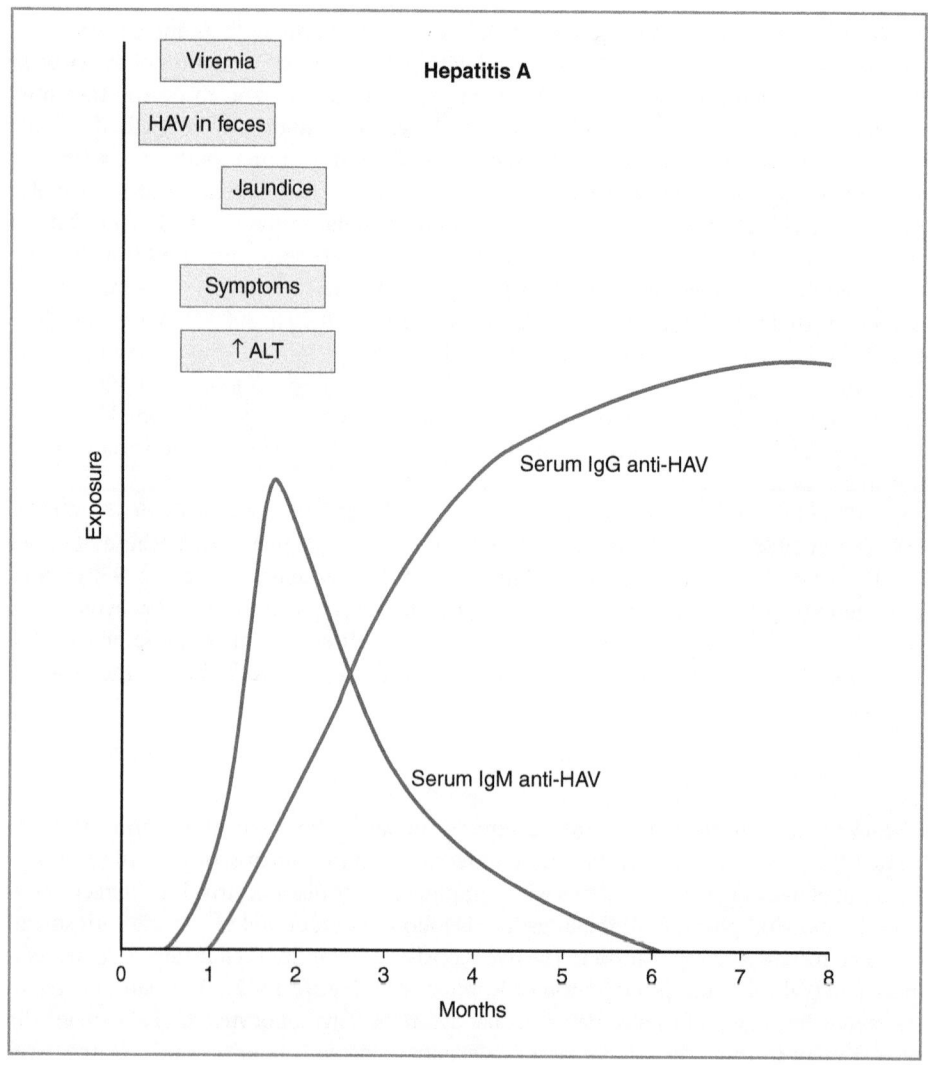

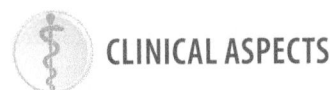 **CLINICAL ASPECTS**

MANIFESTATIONS

In HAV infection, an incubation period of 15 to 45 days (mean 25 days) is usually followed by fever; anorexia (poor appetite); nausea; pain in the right upper abdominal quadrant; and, within several days, jaundice. Dark urine and clay-colored stools may be noticed by the patient 1 to 5 days before the onset of clinical jaundice. The liver is enlarged and tender, and serum aminotransferase and bilirubin levels are elevated as a result of hepatic inflammation and damage. Recovery occurs in days to weeks.

* Fever, anorexia, jaundice common

* Dark urine, clay-colored stool, elevated ALT, and bilirubin

 Why do acute hepatitis patients have dark-colored urine and clay-colored stool?

Many persons who have serologic evidence of acute HAV infection are asymptomatic or only mildly ill, without jaundice (anicteric hepatitis A). The infection-to-disease ratio is dependent on age; it may be as high as 20:1 in children and approximately 1:1 in older adults. Almost all cases (99%) of HAV are self-limiting. Chronic hepatitis such as that seen with hepatitis B is very rare. In rare cases, fulminant fatal hepatitis associated with extensive liver necrosis may occur (~0.1%).

Chronic infection does not occur

DIAGNOSIS

Antibody to HAV can be detected during early illness, and most patients with symptoms or signs of acute HAV already have detectable antibody in serum. Early antibody responses are predominantly IgM, which can be detected for several weeks and up to several months (Figure 13–3). During convalescence, antibody of the IgG class predominates. The best method for documentation of acute HAV infection is the demonstration of high titers of virus-specific IgM antibody in serum drawn during the acute phase of illness. Because IgG antibody persists indefinitely, its demonstration in a single serum sample is not indicative of recent infection; a rise in titer between acute and convalescent sera must be documented. Reverse transcriptase polymerase chain reaction (RT-PCR) can also be used to detect HAV. Immunoelectron microscopic identification of the virus in fecal specimens and isolation of the virus in cell cultures remain research tools.

* IgM-specific antibody denotes acute infection

TREATMENT AND PREVENTION

There is no specific treatment for patients with acute hepatitis A. Supportive measures include adequate nutrition and rest. Avoidance of exposure to contaminated food or water or infected persons are important measures to reduce the risk of hepatitis A infection. More importantly, hepatitis A virus vaccination is the most effective way to attain protection in the population.

Inactivated hepatitis A virus (HAV), which is grown in human cell culture, is used as a vaccine that induces antibody titers similar to those of wild-type virus infection, is almost 100% protective, and is now recommended for all children at age 1 year and for adults with a high risk of infection. Two doses are given 6 to 12 months apart to achieve long-term protection (at least 25 years in adults and 14-20 years in children). In the United States, two inactivated HAV vaccines, HAVRIX (GlaxoSmithKline) and VAQTA (Merck & Co) are currently licensed. In addition, a combination vaccine, TWINRIX (GlaxoSmithKline) that contains both HAV and HBV antigens given in three or four doses to adults of age 18 years and above, is also available.

Immune serum globulin (ISG), manufactured from pools of plasma from large segments of the general population that has HAV antibodies, is protective if given before or during the incubation

* Inactivated hepatitis A virus vaccine confers long-term protection

 Think ▶▶ Apply 13-1: Dark-colored urine is due to excessive bilirubin in urine and clay-colored stool is due to lack of drainage of bile salts in the stool through the biliary system due to liver infection.

ISG provides temporary
protection

period of the disease. It has been shown to be about 80% to 90% effective in preventing clinically apparent type A hepatitis. In some cases, infection occurs but disease is ameliorated; that is, patients develop anicteric, usually asymptomatic, hepatitis A. ISG could be administered to household and intimate contacts of hepatitis A patients and those known to have eaten uncooked foods prepared or handled by an infected person. When clinical symptoms have appeared, the patient is already producing antibody, and administration of ISG is not indicated.

✳ Hepatitis A vaccine prevents
postexposure infection

Based on scientific evidence that active immunization (HAV vaccine) is as effective as ISG if given shortly after exposure, the guidelines were revised in 2007 in the United States to give hepatitis A vaccine after exposure to prevent infection in healthy individuals of 1 to 40 years of age. More importantly, the rates of HAV infection have declined by 92% in the United States since the vaccine was made available in 1995.

KEY CONCLUSIONS

- HAV is a picornavirus comprising of icosahedral naked capsid, positive-sense RNA, which replicates in the cytoplasm by using viral RNA polymerase.

- HAV is transmitted through fecal–oral route and replicates in the intestinal mucosa (incubation period 15-45 days) followed by viremia and spread to the liver and cause lymphoid cell infiltration, necrosis of liver parenchymal cells, and proliferation of Kupffer cells.

- Symptoms of acute HAV include fever, poor appetite, nausea, headache, malaise, vomiting, abdominal pain, and jaundice (ALT and bilirubin levels are elevated). Recovery occurs within weeks. IgM is diagnostic. No chronic infection.

- Inactivated HAV vaccine is recommended for use at age 1 year and adults at risk as well as for postexposure (should be given shortly after exposure).

HEPATITIS B

Overview

Hepatitis B virus (HBV) virion, also known as Dane particle, contains an incomplete double-stranded DNA genome, a core protein (HBcAg), viral DNA polymerase (reverse transcriptase), and surface protein (HBsAg). There is also another viral protein, hepatitis B e antigen (HBeAg) which is secreted during infection. HBV replication is unique in the sense that it utilizes reverse transcriptase enzyme to convert its pregenomic full-length RNA into genomic partially double-stranded DNA. HBV is the cause of what was formerly known as "serum hepatitis" just to distinguish it from "infectious hepatitis" (HAV). HBV is transmitted through sexual contact, sharing needles and syringes, injecting drugs, blood and blood-derived products, and mother-to-child. The virus replicates (incubation period range 60-150, average 90 days) in the liver. However, the pathogenesis is mainly immune mediated, including serum sickness like rash, arthritis, and development of jaundice (symptoms like acute hepatitis A) due to circulating immune complexes that activate complement and cytotoxic CD8 T cells causing liver damage. In addition, accumulation of immune complexes in the kidney results in renal damage. Antibody to HBsAg is protective and associated with resolution of the disease. About 90% of the patients resolve the infection after acute disease that may be asymptomatic; however, 10% of the patients develop chronic infection, probably due to insufficient cellular immunity. The chronicity is more than 90% if the virus is transmitted from mother to child. Chronicity may lead to cirrhosis of the liver with an increased risk of hepatocellular carcinoma (HCC). Acute diagnosis is made by the presence of HBsAg and IgM to HBcAg and chronic by HBsAg (for more than 6 months) and IgG to HBcAg. Treatment for chronic infection includes alpha interferon and reverse transcriptase inhibitors. An effective subunit vaccine, HBsAg, is recommended for use in infants starting at age 0 to 2 months and in adults given in three doses at 0, 1, and 6 months, which provides long-term protection.

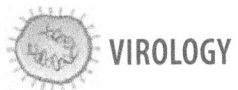 VIROLOGY

STRUCTURE

Hepatitis B virus (HBV) is an enveloped DNA virus belonging to the family Hepadnaviridae (hepadnaviruses). It is unrelated to any other human virus; however, related hepatotropic agents have been identified in woodchucks, ground squirrels, and kangaroos. A schematic of the HBV is illustrated in **Figure 13–4.** The complete virion is a 42 nm spherical particle that consists of an envelope around a 27 nm core. The core comprises a nucleocapsid that contains the DNA genome.

The viral genome consists of partially double-stranded DNA with a short, single-stranded piece. It comprises 3200 nucleotides, making it the smallest known DNA virus with respect to genome size but capable of encoding surface (envelope) protein (hepatitis B surface antigen [HBsAg]), core (nucleocapsid) protein (hepatitis B core antigen [HBcAg]), DNA polymerase (reverse transcriptase), and HBx protein (a transcriptional activator). Closely associated with the viral DNA is a viral DNA polymerase (reverse transcriptase), which has RNA-dependent DNA polymerase, DNA-dependent DNA polymerase, and RNase H activities. Another component of the core is hepatitis B e antigen (HBeAg), which is a low–molecular-weight glycoprotein secreted from the infected cells. The virion has a lipid bilayer envelope containing the HBsAg, which is composed of one major and two other proteins. The complete virus particle is called a **Dane particle.**

Smallest known human DNA virus genome

✳ Enveloped DNA virus with viral DNA polymerase (reverse transcriptase) activity

 Being a DNA virus, why does HBV need a reverse transcriptase enzyme?

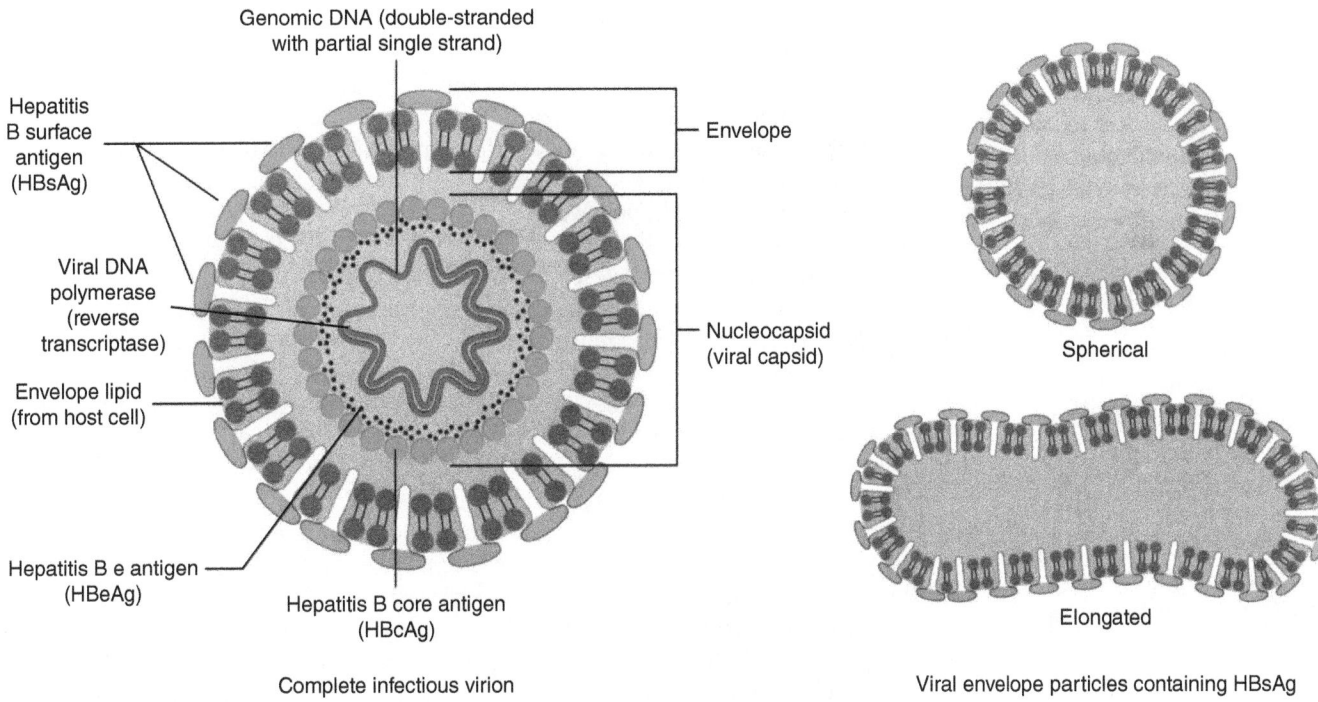

FIGURE 13–4. **Schematic diagram of hepatitis B virion. A.** The 42 nm particle is the "Dane particle" or the hepatitis B virus. **B.** The 22-nm particles are the filamentous and circular forms of hepatitis B surface antigen (HbsAg) or protein coat. (Reproduced with permission from Nester EW, Anderson DG, Roberts CE Jr, et al: *Microbiology: A Human Perspective*, 6th ed. New York, NY: McGraw Hill; 2008.)

 Think ▸▸ Apply 13-2: Due to lack of accurate DNA synthesis from the HDV DNA template, it utilizes the pregenomic RNA as a template to synthesize its genomic DNA through the action of reverse transcriptase enzyme that makes both strands of DNA, although one strand is incomplete.

✳ HBsAg produced in great abundance, presence indicates active infection

HBsAg in cytoplasm of hepatocytes

Four HBsAg serotypes

Ten genotypes vary with geographic distribution

Partially incomplete ds DNA becomes complete double-stranded, covalently closed circular DNA (cccDNA) before transcription

✳ Host RNA polymerase directs viral mRNA synthesis

✳ Unique replication using a reverse transcriptase step

✳ Pregenomic RNA converted to incomplete ds DNA by viral DNA polymerase

HBsAg acquired from endoplasmic reticulum or Golgi

Viral DNA integration in some with HCC but not essential

Humans are major hosts

Aggregates of HBsAg are often found in great abundance in serum during infection. They may assume spherical or filamentous shapes with a mean diameter of 22 nm (Figure 13–4). HBV DNA can also be detected in serum and is an indication that infectious virions are present. In infected liver tissue, evidence of HBcAg, HBeAg, and hepatitis B DNA is found in the nuclei of infected hepatocytes, whereas HBsAg is found in cytoplasm. There are four major serotypes of HBV (*adr, adw, ayr, ayw*) based on HBsAg antigenic epitopes. HBV also encodes a small protein, HBX, which may play a multifactorial role in viral transcription and replication and cellular transformation.

Furthermore, there are 10 hepatitis B genotypes (A-J) based on nucleotide sequence variation of HBV genome, which may be associated with different clinical outcomes. These genotypes vary in geographic distribution with genotype A primarily found in North America, Northern Europe, India, and Africa; genotypes B and C in Asia; genotype D in Southern Europe, Middle East, and India; genotype E in West and South Africa; genotype F in South and Central America; genotype G in the United States and Europe, and genotype H in Central America and California. Genotype I was recently identified and reported in Vietnam and Laos genotype J in Ryukyu Islands, Japan.

REPLICATION CYCLE

The replication of HBV involves a reverse transcription step, and, as such, is unique among DNA viruses (**Figure 13–5**). HBV has a specific tropism for the liver. HBV infection to hepatocytes (liver cells) is initiated by the interaction of the viral envelope protein or surface antigen (HBsAg) with heparan sulfate proteoglycan, followed by specific attachment to a receptor, sodium taurocholate cotransporting polypeptide (NTCP), and virus internalization mediated by epidermal growth factor receptor (EGFR). After viral entry, uncoating occurs allowing the release of nucleocapsid in the cytoplasm and the partially double-stranded DNA (incomplete) is transported to the nucleus. The double-stranded DNA is organized as two strands. One, a short strand, is associated with the viral DNA polymerase and is of positive polarity, and the complete or long strand is complementary and thus is of negative polarity.

The partially incomplete strand is formed into a complete double-stranded, covalently closed circular DNA (cccDNA), which serves as a template for transcription. Host RNA polymerase directs the transcription of viral mRNAs to encode early proteins, including HBcAg, HBeAg, and viral DNA polymerase as well as full-length RNA (pregenomic RNA). HBsAg is encoded later and associates with the membranes of endoplasmic reticulum or Golgi apparatus. HBcAg forms the core by enclosing the full-length, positive-sense viral pregenomic RNA along with viral DNA polymerase (reverse transcriptase) into maturing core particles late in the replication cycle. These full-length RNA strands form a template for a reverse transcription step in which negative-stranded DNA is synthesized by the RNA-dependent DNA polymerase activity of reverse transcriptase activity. The RNA template strands are then degraded by ribonuclease H activity of the reverse transcriptase. A positive-stranded DNA is then synthesized by the DNA-dependent DNA polymerase activity of reverse transcriptase, although this is not completed before virus maturation in which HBsAg-containing membranes of the endoplasmic reticulum or Golgi apparatus are wrapped over the nucleocapsid core, resulting in the variable-length, short, positive DNA strands found in the virions. The virions are released by exocytosis.

HBV DNA has also been found to integrate into the host chromosomes, especially in HBV-infected patients with hepatocellular carcinoma (HCC). However, the significance of integrated HBV DNA in viral replication is not known. While past extensive attempts to propagate HBV in cell culture in the laboratory were not successful, recent advances in developing various cell lines, including hepatocytes cell lines to culture HBV have been performed. These cell culture systems have aided in the screening of antivirals. Humans appear to be the major host; however, as with hepatitis A, infection of subhuman primates has been accomplished experimentally.

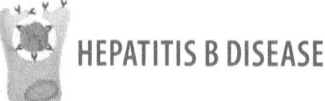 **HEPATITIS B DISEASE**

EPIDEMIOLOGY

Hepatitis B infection is found worldwide. The WHO estimates that 257 million people are living chronically infected with hepatitis B virus and an estimated 887,000 deaths occurred mostly from cirrhosis of liver and HCC in 2015 worldwide. The prevalence rates varying markedly among

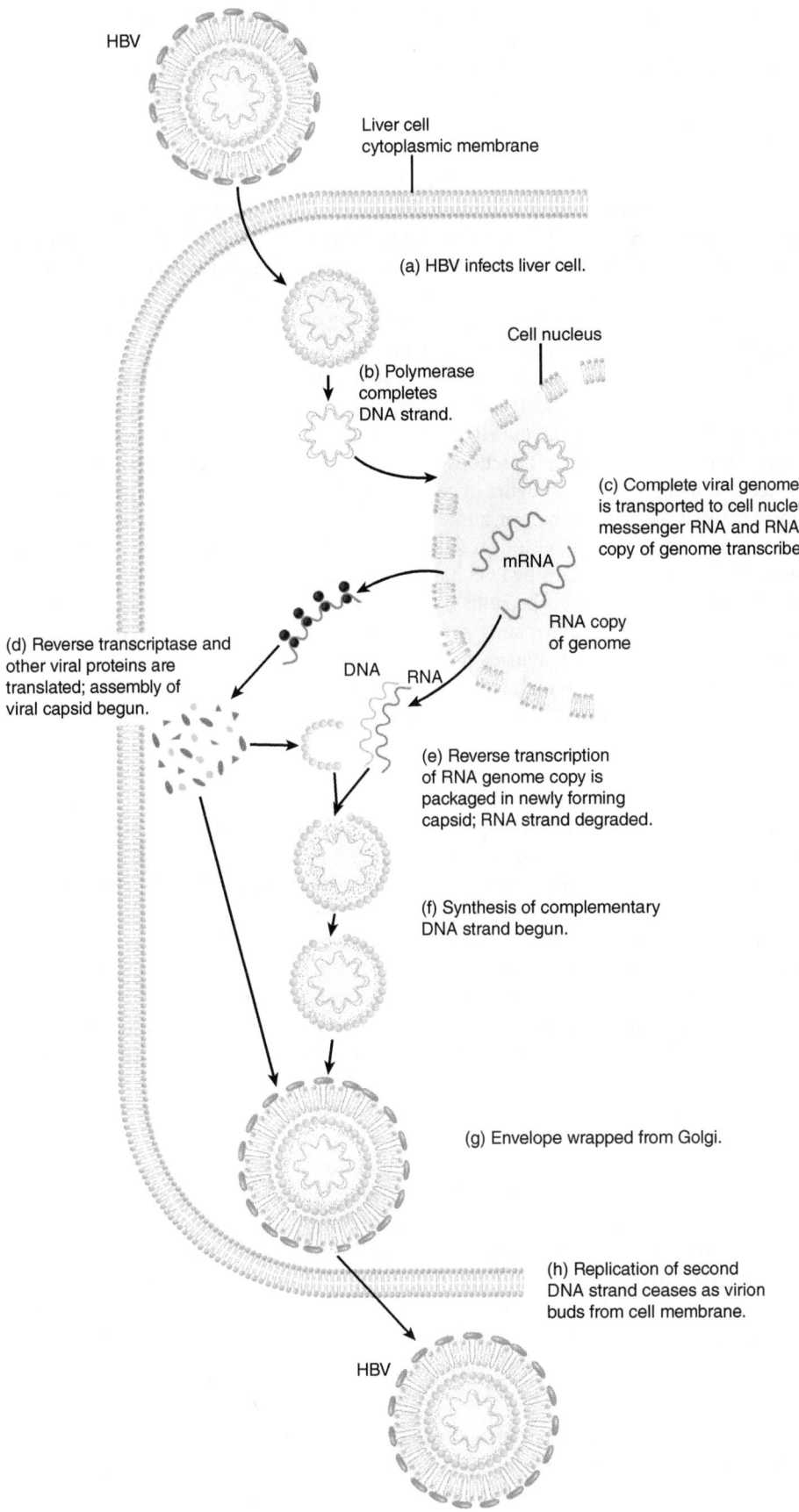

HBV

Liver cell
cytoplasmic membrane

(a) HBV infects liver cell.

Cell nucleus

(b) Polymerase
completes
DNA strand.

(c) Complete viral genome
is transported to cell nucleus,
messenger RNA and RNA
copy of genome transcribed.

mRNA

RNA copy
of genome

(d) Reverse transcriptase and
other viral proteins are
translated; assembly of
viral capsid begun.

DNA   RNA

(e) Reverse transcription
of RNA genome copy is
packaged in newly forming
capsid; RNA strand degraded.

(f) Synthesis of complementary
DNA strand begun.

(g) Envelope wrapped from Golgi.

(h) Replication of second
DNA strand ceases as virion
buds from cell membrane.

HBV

FIGURE 13–5. **Replication cycle of hepatitis B virus (HBV).** HBV replication requires reverse transcription step, unique among DNA viruses. (Reproduced with permission from Nester EW, Anderson DG, Roberts CE Jr, et al: *Microbiology: A Human Perspective*, 6th ed. New York, NY: McGraw Hill; 2008.)

Highest rates in regions of
Western Pacific, Africa

Lower rates in the Americas

countries with highest in WHO Western Pacific Region and WHO African region, where 6.2% and 6.1% of the adult population is chronically infected, respectively. In addition, WHO Eastern Mediterranean region, South-east Asia region, and European region, have the population infected at an estimated rate of 3.3%, 2.0%, and 1.6%, respectively. However, the WHO Region of the Americas has 0.7% of the population chronically infected. About 7.4% of HIV-infected individuals are chronic carriers of HBV.

In the United States, CDC reports that an estimated 862,000 people (actual number may be as high as 2.2 million) were living chronically infected with hepatitis B in 2016. In 2018, 14,207 new cases of chronic hepatitis B were reported in the United States. The rates of HBV infection have declined since 1990 due to HBV vaccination and have remained stable over the past decade, with a slight increase in 2017. In 2017 and 2018, 3409 and 3322 new acute HBV cases were reported, respectively, which are estimated to be 6.5 times higher (22,200 and 21,600) than the reported cases. About 200 to 300 of these patients die of acute fulminant hepatitis, and 10% of infected patients become chronic HBV carriers. The number of reported deaths have declined from 1837 in 2014 to 1649 in 2018 (0.47 to 0.43 per 100,000 population) in the United States, and most deaths are due to hepatitis B-related cirrhosis and HCC. The virus is spread vertically, parenterally, and by sexual contact. Approximately 50% of infections in the United States are sexually transmitted, and the prevalence of HBsAg in serum is higher in certain populations, such as among men who have sex with men, patients on hemodialysis or immunosuppressive therapy, patients with Down syndrome, and injection drug users. Routine screening of blood donors for HBsAg and antibody to HBcAg (anti-HBcAg) and HBV DNA by PCR has markedly decreased the incidence of postblood transfusion and postplasma products hepatitis B transmission. Multiple-pool blood products still cause occasional cases. Exposure to hepatitis viruses from direct contact with blood or other body fluids, probably through needlestick injuries, has resulted in a risk of hepatitis B infection in medical personnel. Attack rates are also high in the sexual partners of infected patients.

✳ About 50% of the US
infections is sexually
transmitted

**Needlestick transmission is a
risk for healthcare workers**

Hepatitis B infection of infants does not appear to be transplacentally transmitted to the fetus in utero but is acquired during the birth process due to newborn contact with mother's infected secretion or blood, through abrasions, or probably swallowing of infected blood or fluids. The rate of virus acquisition is very high (70-90%) in infants born to mothers who have acute hepatitis B infection and are positive to both HBsAg and HBeAg, and low (10-40%) in mothers who are positive for HBsAg and negative for HBeAg. Some of the risk factors associated with a higher rate of vertical transmission include high maternal viral load (higher HBV DNA copies), HBeAg positivity, young age of infected mother, coinfection with HIV. Most infected infants do not develop clinical disease during the neonatal period or early in infancy. However, infection in the neonatal period or during the first year of life is associated with more than 80% to 90% chronicity in these infected neonates/infants, most likely due to failure of humoral and cell-mediated immune responses because of an immature immune system of the neonates. Moreover, 30% to 50% chronicity rate is seen in children infected between the ages of 1 and 6 years, and about 10% chronicity in children infected above the age of 6 years as well as in adults. The prevention of neonatal HBV infection includes treatment of exposed newborns with hepatitis B immune globulin (HBIG) and HBV vaccine that has significantly reduced vertical transmission.

**Vertical transmission usually
occurs during birth process**

✳ Chronicity extremely high in
vertically infected infants

HCC has been strongly associated with persistent carriage of HBV by serologic tests and by detection of HBV DNA integrated in tumor cell genomes. In many parts of Africa and Asia, primary liver cancer accounts for 20% to 30% of all types of malignancies, but in North and South America and in Europe, it is only 1% to 2%. The estimated risk of developing the malignancy for persons with chronic HBV is increased to between 10-fold and more than 300-fold in different populations. The risk of HCC further increases in patients with chronic hepatitis B infection and high viral loads.

✳ Strong association between
HBV chronic infection and
HCC

PATHOGENESIS

In the past, hepatitis B was known as posttransfusion hepatitis or as hepatitis associated with the use of illicit parenteral drugs (serum hepatitis). However, over the last few years, it has become clear that the major mode of acquisition is through close personal contact with body fluids of infected individuals through sexual transmission. HBsAg has been found in most body fluids, including saliva, semen, and cervical secretions. Under experimental conditions, as little as 0.0001 mL of infectious blood has produced infection. Transmission is therefore possible by vehicles such as inadequately sterilized hypodermic needles and instruments used in tattooing and ear piercing.

**Virus found in blood, saliva,
and semen**

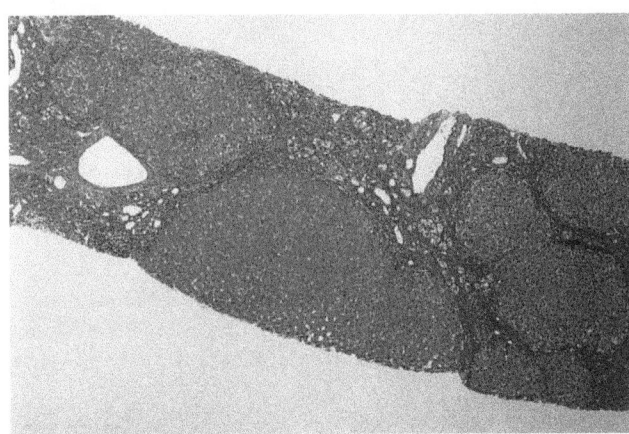

FIGURE 13–6. **Cirrhosis of liver in chronic hepatitis B infection (HBV).** This is a needle biopsy of Masson trichrome stain that shows cirrhotic nodules and portion of nodules separated by fibrous scars. (Reproduced with permission from Connor DH, Chandler FW, Schwartz DQ, et al: *Pathology of Infectious Diseases.* Stamford CT: Appleton & Lange; 1997.)

The factors determining the clinical manifestations of acute hepatitis B are not fully known; however, the pathogenesis appears to be immune-mediated. The serum sickness-like rash and arthritis that may precede the development of symptoms and jaundice appear to be related to circulating immune complexes that activate the complement system. In addition, accumulation of these immune complexes in the kidney results in renal damage. Antibody to HBsAg is protective and associated with resolution of the disease. Cellular immunity such as cytotoxic CD8 T lymphocytes (CTLs) is also important in the host response to contain the infection because patients with insufficient T-lymphocyte function have a high incidence of chronic infection with HBV. However, HBV-specific CTLs destroying infected cells cause damage to liver and is a major pathogenic mechanism of the disease. Antibody to HBcAg, which appears during infection, is present in chronic carriers with persistent hepatitis B virion production and does not appear to be protective.

The morphologic lesions of acute hepatitis B resemble those of other hepatitis viruses. In chronic active hepatitis B, the continued presence of inflammatory foci of infection results in necrosis of hepatocytes, collapse of the reticular framework of the liver, and progressive fibrosis. The increasing fibrosis can result in the syndrome of postnecrotic hepatic cirrhosis (**Figure 13–6**).

* Immunologic factors contribute, including cytotoxic T lymphocyte
* Serum sickness-like rash, arthritis precede symptoms
* Antibody to HBsAg protective
* Cellular immunity important
* Defects in cellular immunity in chronic infection
* Chronic infection leads to fibrosis, cirrhosis

 Why is HBV pathogenesis more immune-mediated than viral-mediated?

Integrated hepatitis B viral DNA can be found in nearly all HCCs. The virus has not been shown to possess a transforming gene but may well activate a cellular oncogene. It is also possible that the virus does not play a direct molecular role in oncogenicity, because the natural history of chronic hepatitis B infection involves cycles of damage or death of liver cells interspersed with periods of intense regenerative hyperplasia. This significantly increases the opportunity for spontaneous mutational changes that may activate cellular oncogenes. HBV transcriptional transactivator protein, HBx, is known to activate the Src kinase, which may influence HBV-induced carcinogenesis. HBx protein has been shown to interact with tumor suppressor gene, p53, which may result in the development of oncogenesis and HCC. Whatever the mechanisms may be, the association between chronic hepatitis B infection and HCC is clear, and liver cancer is a major cause of disease and death in countries in which chronic hepatitis B infection is common. The proven success of combined active and passive immunization in aborting hepatitis B infection in infancy and childhood makes HCC a potentially preventable disease.

Mechanism of HCC development is not clearly known

* Strong association between chronic viral infection and HCC

 Think ▸▸ Apply13-3: Since HBV replication in hepatocytes is noncytopathic, the damage to liver starts with the cytotoxic T cells killing infected cells followed by recruitment of mononuclear cells and production of proinflammatory cytokines causing further liver damage. Formation of immune complexes also causes liver and extrahepatic damage such as kidneys.

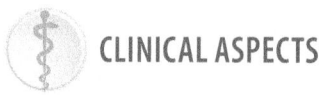

CLINICAL ASPECTS

MANIFESTATIONS

The clinical picture of hepatitis B is highly variable. The incubation period may be as brief as 60 days or as long as 150 days (mean approximately 90 days). Acute hepatitis B is usually manifested by the gradual onset of fatigue, loss of appetite, nausea and pain, and fullness in the right upper abdominal quadrant. Early in the course of disease, pain and swelling of the joints and occasional frank arthritis may occur. Some patients develop a rash. With increasing involvement of the liver, there is increasing cholestasis, and hence clay-colored stools, darkening of the urine, and jaundice. Symptoms may persist for several months before finally resolving.

In general, the symptoms associated with acute hepatitis B are more severe and more prolonged than those of hepatitis A; however, anicteric disease and asymptomatic infection occur. The infection-to-disease ratio, which varies according to patient age and method of acquisition, has been estimated to be approximately 3:1. Fulminant hepatitis, leading to extensive liver necrosis and death, develops in less than 1% of the cases. One important difference between hepatitis A and hepatitis B is the development of chronic hepatitis, which occurs in approximately 10% of all patients with hepatitis B infection, with a much higher risk for newborns (~90%), children (~50%), and the immunocompromised. In immunocompetent adults, the strong cellular immune response results in acute hepatitis and only rarely (~1%) in chronic hepatitis. Chronic infection is associated with ongoing replication of virus in the liver and usually with the presence of HBsAg in serum. Chronic hepatitis may lead to cirrhosis, liver failure, or HCC in up to 30% of the patients.

 Why does HBV cause higher chronicity in infected neonates/infants than adults?

DIAGNOSIS

The nomenclature of hepatitis B antigens and antibodies is shown in **Table 13–2** and the sequence of their appearance is shown in **Figure 13–7.** During the acute episode of disease, when there is active viral replication, large amounts of HBsAg and HBV DNA can be detected in

TABLE 13–2	Nomenclature for Hepatitis B Virus Antigens and Antibodies
ABBREVIATION	**DESCRIPTION**
HBV	Hepatitis B virus; 42 nm, double-stranded DNA virus; Dane particle
HBsAg	Hepatitis B surface antigen; found on surface of virus; formed in excess and seen in serum as 22 nm spherical and tubular particles; four subdeterminants (*adw, ayw, adr,* and *ayr*) identified
HBcAg	Core antigen (nucleocapsid core); found in nucleus of infected hepatocytes by immunofluorescence
HBeAg	Glycoprotein; associated with the core antigen; used epidemiologically as marker of potential infectivity; seen only when HBsAg is also present
Anti-HBs	Antibody to HBsAg; correlated with protection against and/or resolution of disease; used as a marker of past infection or vaccination
Anti-HBc	Antibody to HBcAg; seen in acute infection and chronic carriers; anti-HBc IgM used as indicator of acute infection; anti-HBc IgG used as a marker of past or chronic infection; apparently not important in disease resolution; does not develop in response to vaccine
Anti-HBe	Antibody to HBeAg

 Think ▸▸ Apply 13-4: **The higher rate of chronicity in neonates/infants than adults is most likely due to relative immaturity of the immune system of the neonates/infants, which is unable to contain HBV replication.**

Average incubation 90 days; range 60 to 150

✳ Chronic hepatitis is most common with infection in early infancy or childhood

✳ Acute HBV infection demonstrates HBsAg and IgM anti-HBc in serum

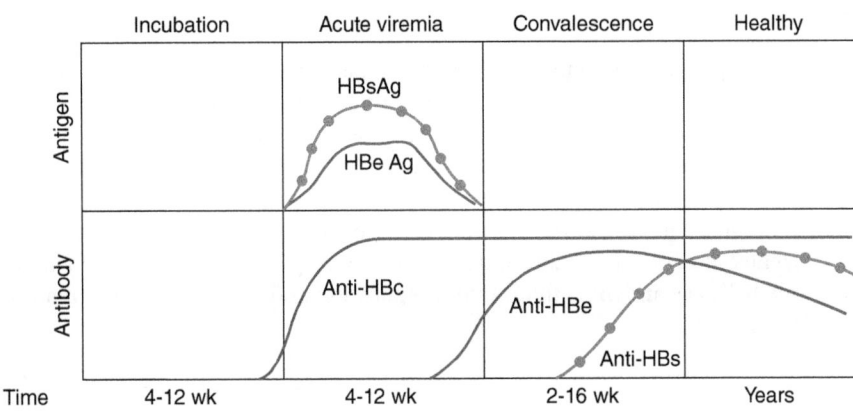

FIGURE 13–7. **Sequence of appearance of viral antigens and antibodies in acute self-limiting cases of hepatitis B.** Anti-HBc, antibody to hepatitis B core antigen; anti-HBe, antibody to HBeAg; anti-HBs, antibody to HBsAg; HBeAg, hepatitis B e antigen; HBsAg, hepatitis B surface antigen.

the serum, as can fully developed virions and high levels of DNA polymerase and HBeAg. Although HBcAg is also present, but antibody against it (anti-HBc) invariably occurs and prevents HBcAg detection. Upon resolution of acute hepatitis B, HBsAg and HBeAg disappear from serum with the development of antibodies (anti-HBs and anti-HBe) against them. There is small period "window period" or equivalence zone characterized by the disappearance of HBsAg and before the appearance of anti-HBs. During this window period, HBsAg and anti-HBs are absent but anti-HBc (IgM) is present (anti-Hbe may also be present). The development of anti-HBs is associated with elimination of infection and protection against reinfection. Anti-HBc is detected early in the course of disease and persists in serum for years. It is an excellent epidemiologic marker of infection, but is not protective. The laboratory diagnosis of acute hepatitis B infection is best made by demonstrating the presence of HBsAg and IgM anti-HBc in serum, since this antibody disappears within 6 months of the acute infection. Almost all patients who develop jaundice are anti-HBc IgM-positive at the time of clinical presentation. Past infection with hepatitis B is best determined by detecting IgG antibody to HBcAg, HBsAg, or both, whereas vaccine induces only antibody to HBsAg. While the HBV antigens and antibodies are demonstrated by enzyme immune assay, HBV DNA is detected by PCR.

* Appearance of anti-HBs signals elimination

* Window period shows anti-HBc and may be anti-HBe, but neither HBsAg nor anti-HBs

In patients with chronic hepatitis B, evidence of viral persistence can be found in serum (**Figure 13–8**). HBsAg can be detected throughout the active disease process, and anti-HBs do not develop, which probably accounts for the chronicity of the disease. However, anti-HBc (IgG) is detected. Two types of chronic hepatitis can be distinguished. In one, HBsAg is detected, but not HBeAg; these patients usually show progressive liver dysfunction. In the other, both antigens are found; development of antibody to HBeAg is associated with clinical improvement. Chronic infection with hepatitis B is best detected by persistence of HBsAg in blood for more than 6 to 12 months and IgG anti-HBc. Progression of liver disease is associated with more than 1000 IU/mL (5600 copies/mL) of HBV DNA. Persons with levels lower than 1000 IU/mL and normal liver function have a low risk of progression. HBV DNA is monitored to determine the efficacy of antiviral treatment. Moreover, a new test has been recently approved that would quantify the levels of HBsAg in HBV infected patients, which could be used as a predictive marker for antiviral efficacy, disease progression, risks of liver damage, and sign of recovery.

* Chronic infection demonstrates persistence of HBsAg for >6 months and IgG anti-HBc

HBV DNA determines antiviral efficacy

Quantitative HBsAg for prognosis, antiviral efficacy

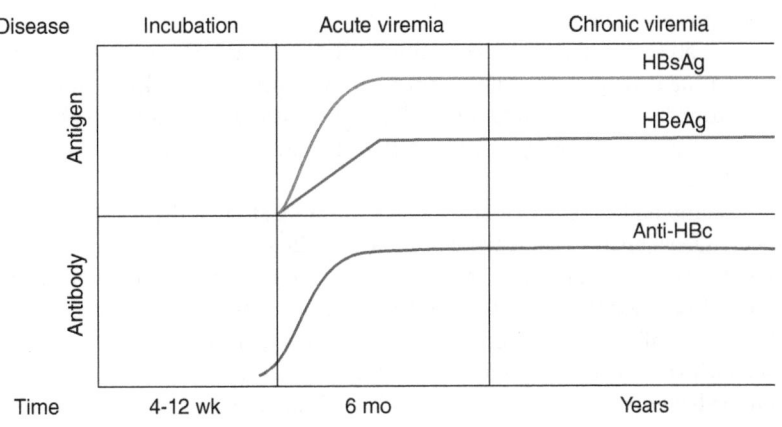

FIGURE 13–8. **Sequence of appearance of viral antigens and antibodies in chronic active hepatitis B.** Antibodies to HBsAg and HBeAg are not detected. Anti-HBc, antibody to hepatitis B core antigen; HBeAg, hepatitis B e antigen; HBsAg, hepatitis B surface antigen.

TREATMENT

No treatment for acute infection

Interferon and nucleoside and nucleotide reverse transcriptase inhibitors of benefit in chronic infection

There is no specific treatment recommended for acute hepatitis B. A proper nutrition with plenty of fluid and rest is recommended and drugs that are toxic to the liver should be avoided. Treatment should be considered for patients with rapid deterioration of liver function, cirrhosis, or complications such as ascites, hepatic encephalopathy, or hemorrhage as well as those who are immunosuppressed. For chronic hepatitis B diseases, pegylated or regular interferon-α provides benefit in some patients. Antiviral such as nucleoside reverse transcriptase inhibitors, lamivudine (3TC), entecavir and telbivudine and nucleotide analogs, adefovir and tenofovir are active against hepatitis B. These antivirals inhibit viral replication and may reduce viral load but do not cure HBV infection.

PREVENTION

Postexposure treatment with HBIG temporarily reduces risk

Screening of blood and plasma product donors for HBsAg, anti-HBcAg, and HBV DNA has greatly reduced the incidence of hepatitis B in recipients. Similarly, screening pregnant women and treatment of exposed newborns with hepatitis B immune globulin (HBIG) and HBV vaccine have significantly reduced vertical transmission. Safe sexual practices and avoidance of needle-stick injuries or injection drug use are approaches to diminishing the risk of hepatitis B infection. Both active prophylaxis and passive prophylaxis against hepatitis B infection can be accomplished. Most preparations of immune serum globulin (ISG) contain only moderate levels of anti-HBs; however, specific HBIG with high titers of hepatitis B antibody is now available. HBIG is prepared from sera of subjects who have high titers of antibody to HBsAg but are free of the antigen itself. Administration of HBIG soon after exposure to the virus greatly reduces the development of symptomatic disease. Postexposure prophylaxis with HBIG should be followed by active immunization with vaccine.

The vaccine for HBV infection is the surface protein of the virus, HBsAg. Initially, purified inactivated HBsAg protein (HBsAg subunit vaccine) from chronic carriers was used for vaccination, but it is no longer in use. The current vaccine candidate, HBsAg (ENGERIX-B, RECOMBIVAX-HB, HEPLISAV-B) is a recombinant product expressed in yeast. This recombinant vaccine mounts a strong humoral immune response (IgG) and provides more than 90% protection. Excellent protection has been shown in studies of men who have sex with men and in medical personnel. These groups and others, such as laboratory workers, injection drug users, travelers to endemic areas, persons at risk for sexually transmitted diseases, and those in contact with patients who have chronic hepatitis B, should receive hepatitis B vaccine as the preferred method of preexposure prophylaxis. Recently, immunization of newborns, all children, and adolescents has been recommended. Three intramuscular doses (at 0, 1, and 6 months) are given to achieve maximum titer. Protection is long term (approximately 20 years) but may not be lifelong. Neonates receive the first dose soon after birth and before leaving the hospital.

Recombinant (HBsAg) vaccine recommended for all children and high-risk persons

Protection is long term, probably not lifelong

Some people do not respond to HBV vaccine. Several factors could be attributed to this nonresponse such as dose, schedule, injection site, age (older adults), obesity and chronic illness. People who fail to seroconvert with the first series of HBV vaccine should be vaccinated for a second three-dose series in the deltoid muscle. Failure to respond after six doses of HBV vaccine may be because of persistent HBV infection, which should be evaluated. In addition, people who do not respond to vaccine should be given HBIG for prophylaxis and/or for other known risks.

Combination vaccines available with age restrictions for delivery

Several combination vaccines are also available. These include COMVAX (hepatitis B-*Haemophilus influenzae* conjugate vaccine, cannot be given before 6 weeks or after 71 months), PEDIARIX (hepatitis B, diphtheria, tetanus, acellular pertussis, and inactivated polio, cannot be given before 6 weeks or after 7 years), and TWINRIX (hepatitis A and hepatitis B is recommended at the age of 18 years or above).

Combination of HBIG and vaccine reduces vertical transmission

A combination of active and passive immunization is the most effective approach to prevent neonatal acquisition and chronic carriage in the neonate. Routine screening of pregnant women for the presence of HBsAg is recommended. Infants born to those who are positive should receive HBIG in the delivery room followed by three doses of hepatitis B vaccine beginning 24 hours after birth. A similar combination of passive and active immunization is used for unimmunized persons who have been exposed to a needlestick or similar injuries. The procedure varies depending on the hepatitis B status of the "donor" case linked to the injury.

KEY CONCLUSIONS

- Hepatitis B virus (HBV) is a hepadnavirus comprising of a partially double-stranded DNA genome surrounded by HBcAg and carrying viral DNA polymerase (reverse transcriptase) and wrapped in a lipid bilayer membrane containing HBsAg. HBeAg is made during infection.

- HBV transcribes in the nucleus using host RNA polymerase followed by viral protein synthesis. HBcAg packages the pregenomic RNA, viral DNA polymerase, and dNTP pool and then reverse transcriptase synthesizes double-stranded DNA (incomplete) followed by wrapping of envelope from Golgi body or endoplasmic reticulum with HBsAg on its surface.

- HBV is transmitted through blood and blood-derived products and sexual route causing acute hepatitis followed by clearance by the immune response (in 90% of the cases) and in 10% of the cases establishes chronic infection.

- Pathogenesis involves immune-mediated serum sickness-like rash and arthritis leading to acute hepatitis symptoms and jaundice. The major pathogenic mechanism is the liver damage caused by cytotoxic CD8 T lymphocytes (CTL). Immune complexes activate complement causing liver damage and deposition in kidney resulting in liver damage.

- Appearance of antibody to HBsAg resolves the infection, whereas lack of antibody to HBsAg response and defects in cellular immunity result in chronic infection.

- Presence of HBsAg and antibody to HBcAg (IgM) confirms acute hepatitis B infection, whereas presence of HBsAg for more than 6 months and antibody to HBcAg (IgG) suggest chronic infection.

- Treatment for chronic HBV includes interferon-α and reverse transcriptase inhibitors.

- HBsAg, a subunit vaccine, given in three doses (0, 1, and 6 months) to provide long-term protection by producing IgG.

- Combination of HBIG and HBV vaccine is used to prevent vertical transmission. Vertically infected infants develop chronicity in more than 90% cases. HBV vaccination in mothers has significantly reduced vertical transmission in the United States.

HEPATITIS D (DELTA HEPATITIS)

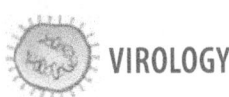 VIROLOGY

Delta hepatitis is caused by the hepatitis D virus (HDV) belonging to Deltaviridae. This small, single-stranded circular (–) RNA virus has an icosahedral naked capsid, HDV or delta capsid antigen, and a lipid bilayer envelope containing hepatitis B surface antigen (HBsAg). This means that HDV requires the presence of HBsAg for its transmission, and is thus found only in persons with acute or chronic HBV infection. Strategies directed at preventing HBV are also effective in preventing HDV. Associated with the circular RNA, which forms a rod because of extensive base pairing, are proteins of 27 and 29 kDa, which constitute the delta capsid antigen (HDV capsid antigen). This protein–RNA complex is surrounded by HBsAg (**Figure 13–9**). Thus, although the delta virus produces its own capsid antigens, it co-opts the HBsAg in assembling its coat or envelope. Unlike other RNA viruses, HDV genome is not capable of encoding its own RNA polymerase.

✳ Hepatitis D is found only in HBV-infected persons

Small, icosahedral, single-stranded (–) circular RNA virus

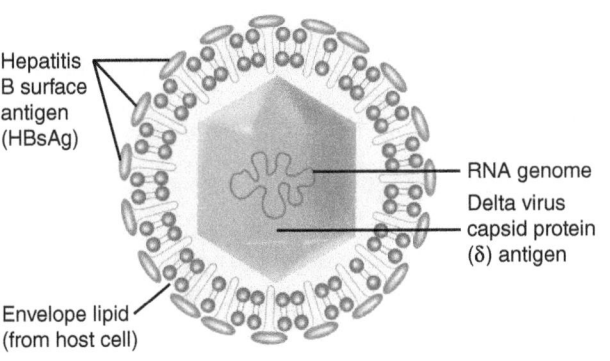

Hepatitis B surface antigen (HBsAg)

RNA genome

Delta virus capsid protein (δ) antigen

Envelope lipid (from host cell)

FIGURE 13–9. Schematic of hepatitis D (delta) virus (HDV). A single-stranded, circular RNA forms an icosahedral capsid with HDV-encoded capsid protein, which is wrapped by a lipid bilayer membrane containing hepatitis B virus surface antigen (HBsAg). HDV is only assembled when there is HBsAg present in the same infected cell.

Virus uses HBsAg for
transmission and assembly

Replication of HDV complex,
unique

Transcription and replication
in nucleus using host RNA
polymerase

HBV (HBsAg) required for HDV
assembly

The replication of HDV involves virus entry in hepatocytes (liver cells) just like HBV by using NTCP, because HDV contains HBsAg on its surface. Because HDV lacks an RNA polymerase required for transcription and replication, it uses host cell RNA polymerase to synthesize mRNA and RNA genome in the nucleus. This is unique for an RNA virus to replicate in the nucleus without encoding its own RNA polymerase. The extensive base pairing in some regions of the HDV genome allows the cellular RNA polymerase to bind the base-paired RNA sequences, as RNA polymerase binds to DNA sequences, and to transcribe HDV mRNA. The RNA genome further forms a ribozyme structure that allows self-cleaving of the RNA genome to generate mRNA. The delta capsid antigens are synthesized and associate with HDV circular RNA genomes followed by acquiring an envelope from the endoplasmic reticulum or Golgi apparatus containing HBsAg. Thus, the presence of HBsAg is essential for assembly of HDV virions.

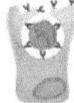 DELTA HEPATITIS DISEASE

Greatest risk is among injection
drug abusers

Delta hepatitis affects 5% of people worldwide who are chronically infected with hepatitis B and currently is most prevalent in countries such as Mongolia, Republic of Moldova, and in Western and Middle Africa. Injection drug users are those at greatest risk in the western parts of the world, and up to 50% of such individuals may have IgG antibody to the delta virus antigen. Other risks include sexual transmission and dialysis. Vertical transmission can also occur. Interestingly, overall number of hepatitis D infection has decreased in the past few decades due to successful hepatitis B vaccination program.

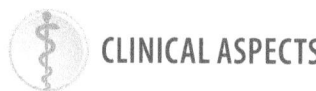 CLINICAL ASPECTS

MANIFESTATIONS

✳ Simultaneous hepatitis B and
D infections cause severe
disease

✳ Delta superinfection with
chronic hepatitis B causes a
severe hepatitis with risk of
chronic cirrhosis

Two major types of delta infection have been noted: Simultaneous hepatitis D or delta and hepatitis B infections or delta superinfection in those with chronic hepatitis B infection. Simultaneous infection with both delta and hepatitis B may result in clinical hepatitis that is indistinguishable from acute hepatitis A or B, but it may manifest as a second rise in liver enzymes (ALT, AST). Persons with chronic hepatitis B who acquire superimposed infection with hepatitis D suffer relapses of jaundice and have a high likelihood of developing chronic cirrhosis. Epidemics of delta infection have occurred in populations with a high incidence of chronic hepatitis B and have resulted in rapidly progressive liver disease, and HCC causing death in up to 20% of infected persons.

DIAGNOSIS

✳ Diagnosis is by detection of
antibodies to delta antigen

Diagnosis of delta infection is made most commonly by demonstrating IgM or IgG antibodies, or both, to the delta (HDV) capsid antigen in serum and/or by detection of HDV RNA by RT-PCR. The IgM antibodies appear within 3 weeks of infection and persist for several weeks, whereas IgG antibodies persist for years. In coinfection, the patient has both anti-HBc and anti-D antibodies, whereas in superinfection, the anti-HBc is already present and anti-D capsid antibodies appear later. In chronic HBV infection, superinfection with HDV will demonstrate HBsAg and antibody to delta capsid antigen.

TREATMENT AND PREVENTION

✳ Major strategies for
prevention of hepatitis B also
prevent hepatitis D

Interferon-α has shown some efficacy but the viral clearance is low. Other anti-HBV therapies (nucleosides, nucleotide analogs) have not shown any benefits against HDV. Response to treatment in patients with delta hepatitis (and hepatitis B) is less than in those with hepatitis B alone. Because the surface of HDV is HBsAg, measures aimed at limiting the transmission of hepatitis B (eg, vaccination, blood screening) prevent the transmission of delta hepatitis. People vaccinated with HBV vaccine (HBsAg) are protected against HDV. Persons infected with hepatitis B or D virus should not donate blood, organ, tissues, or semen. Safe sex should be practiced unless there is only a single sex partner who is already infected. Methods of reducing transmission include decreased use of contaminated needles and syringes by injection drug users and use of needle safety devices by healthcare workers.

Overview

Hepatitis C virus (HCV), a flavivirus, has a positive-sense single-stranded RNA genome, icosahedral capsid (core protein), and lipid bilayer envelope with E1 and E2 proteins. The virus replicates in the cytoplasm by using viral RNA-dependent RNA polymerase for transcription and replication and viral protease for processing of viral structural proteins. HCV is transmitted parenterally, including blood and blood-derived products, injection drug use, needle stick injuries, and organ transplantation. It can also be transmitted through sex and from mother to child. The virus initially replicates in the mononuclear cells and at a higher level in the liver, since about 10% of the hepatocytes are infected. However, pathogenesis is mainly mediated by immune-mediated cytotoxic T cells and proinflammatory cytokines that cause damage to the liver. Following an average incubation period of 2 to 12 weeks, about 75% of the infected people are asymptomatic, whereas about 25% develop symptoms such as fever, fatigue, abdominal pain, poor appetite, joint pain, and jaundice. Cell-mediated and humoral immune responses control acute infection. However, about 80% to 85% of infected people become chronic/carrier that develop chronic hepatitis over a period of 10 to 18 years. Chronic hepatitis tends to wax and wane, is often asymptomatic, and may be associated with either elevated or normal ALT values in serum. These chronically infected patients may develop cirrhosis of liver with increased risk of HCC. Additionally, the pathogenesis involves immune complexes formation due to HCV antibodies and deposition in other tissues and causes some of the other extrahepatic problems, including vasculitis, arthritis, glomerulonephritis, and others. HCV diagnosis is done by detecting HCV antibodies and/or HCV RNA by RT-PCR. Current potent treatment includes interferon-α and ribavirin and direct-acting antivirals (DDAs) such HCV (NS3/4A) protease, HCV (NS5B) RNA polymerase, and HCV (NS5A) phosphoprotein inhibitors, which can functionally cure most HCV-infected people in 8 to 12 weeks. There is no vaccine for HCV but screening of blood and blood products reduces the risk of transmission.

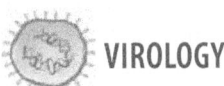 **VIROLOGY**

HCV is an RNA-enveloped virus in the Flaviviridae family and *Hepacivirus* genus that is transmitted through blood and blood-derived products. Several other important members of Flaviviridae that cause disease in humans belong to *Flavivirus* genus, including yellow fever virus, dengue virus, West Nile virus that are arboviruses and transmitted through bite of arthropods (discussed in Chapter 16). HCV has a positive-sense, single-stranded RNA genome, consisting of just three structural (C, core; E1 and E2, envelope) and six nonstructural (NS2, NS3, NS4A, NS4B, NS5A, and NS5B) genes. Several of these nonstructural proteins are enzymes that are essential for HCV replication and have potent antivirals against them, including NS2-3 HCV protease, NS3 HCV serine protease and RNA helicase, NS5A (HCV phosphoprotein required for replication and assembly, interferon resisting protein), and NS5B (HCV RNA-dependent RNA polymerase). The HCV virion of 50 nm in diameter contains an RNA genome of 9.5 kb, which is enclosed in an icosahedral capsid or core (C) protein and a lipid-bilayer envelope containing two virus-specific glycoproteins E1 (gp31) and E2 (gp70) (**Figure 13–10**). The RNA genome is encoded into a polyprotein, which is processed into individual proteins by viral and host proteases. The envelope glycoproteins interact with receptor and coreceptor on the host cell for virus entry into target cells. In addition, antibodies against these envelope glycoproteins are involved in virus neutralization.

HCV is highly heterogeneous because the genome of HCV is highly mutable, because its RNA-dependent RNA polymerase lacks proofreading ability. Mutations give rise to HCV quasispecies (variants) and antigenic variation, most noticeably in the E2 glycoprotein hypervariable regions (HVR1 and HVR2), which may allow the virus to escape immune response and cause chronic or persistent infection in infected persons. The hypervariable region in E2 contains the epitope for neutralization, and mutations allow the newly generated HCV variants to escape preexisting immune response.

Enveloped RNA virus of Flaviviridae family, *Hepacivirus* genus

(+) RNA genome encodes three structural, six nonstructural proteins

Two envelope glycoproteins, E1 and E2 and a core or capsid protein, C

✳ NS2-NS3, NS5A, and NS5B encode HCV protease, phosphoprotein, and polymerase; antivirals available against these targets

Highly heterogeneous virus, hypervariable regions (HVR1 and HVR2) in E2 envelope glycoprotein

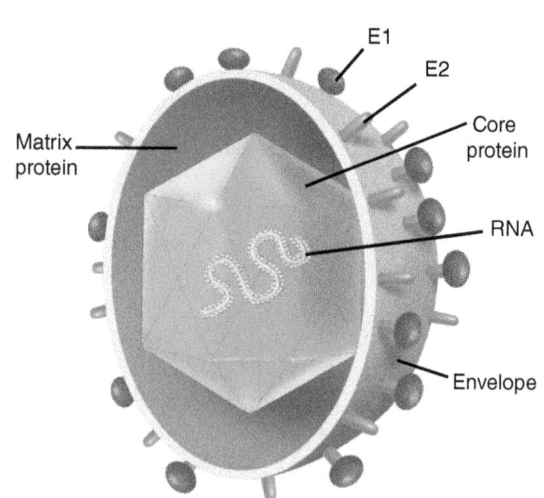

FIGURE 13–10. **Structure of hepatitis C virion.** Inside the icosahedral core is a single-stranded, positive-sense RNA enclosed in a lipid bilayer membrane containing viral specific glycoproteins, E1 and E2. E2 glycoprotein interacts with the receptor on the host cells.

* Six genotypes have different distribution, treatment sensitivity

* Genotype 1 (1a) in North America

Genotypes important for predicting therapy response

There are at least six genotypes with multiple subtypes. The genotypes have different geographic distributions and may be associated with differing severity of disease as well as response to therapy. Genotypes 1-3 have worldwide distribution, with genotype 1 predominating in the world, including North America; genotype 3 in South Asia; genotype 4 in central Africa to the Middle East; genotype 5 in southern Africa; and genotype 6 in East and Southeast Asia. In the United States, 1 is the major genotype followed by 1b, 2, 3, and 4.

The HCV genome also encodes a nonstructural protein that is involved in sensitivity to interferon. HCV heterogeneity and generation of multiple HCV genotypes, like HIV, hinder the development of an HCV vaccine.

Similar to other positive-sense RNA viruses, HCV also replicates in the cytoplasm of the infected cell. Because of lack of a tissue culture system for HCV propagation, the replication cycle of HCV is not fully understood. In infected people, the virions of HCV are firmly associated with lipoproteins to form a complex particle called lipoviroparticle (LVP). These LVPs attach to heparan sulfate proteoglycans on the hepatocytes. HCV-LVPs may then interact with low-density lipoprotein receptor (LDLR) leading to a nonproductive infection. However, in the productive infection, HCV enveloped glycoprotein (E2) interacts with scavenger receptor class B type I (SCARB1), the tetraspanin CD81 (a member of the transmembrane 4 superfamily), and claudin-1 followed by virus entry into target cells probably via receptor-mediated endocytosis. After virus entry, uncoating takes place followed by translation of a full-length genomic, positive-sense RNA via binding of ribosome to the internal ribosome entry site (IRES) located on viral RNA into a polyprotein, which is cleaved into viral structural proteins (C, and E1 and E2) and nonstructural proteins (NS2, NS3, NS4A, NS4B, NS5A, and NS5B) by viral (NS3/NS4A) and host proteases in the cytoplasm. One of these proteins, NS5B, is an RNA-dependent RNA polymerase that directs transcription and replication via negative-sense RNA intermediates. Another viral phosphoprotein (NS5A) helps NS5B in viral replication and assembly. Virus assembly takes place in the cytoplasm by the formation of vesicles that fuses with the plasma membranes for virus release.

HCV uses a series of cellular receptors, such as SCARB1 and CD81

* HCV replicates in the cytoplasm via negative-sense RNA intermediates

* HCV RNA is translated into a polyprotein, which is cleaved into mature proteins by viral and host proteases

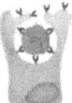 ## HEPATITIS C DISEASE

EPIDEMIOLOGY

Similar to HBV, HCV is spread parenterally. The transmission of HCV by blood was well documented. Indeed, until screening blood for transfusions was introduced, it caused most cases of posttransfusion hepatitis. Screening of donor blood for antibody has reduced posttransfusion hepatitis by 80% to 90%. HCV may be sexually transmitted but to a much lesser degree than HBV. Needle sharing accounts for up to 40% of the cases. Worldwide, about 71 million are chronically infected with HCV and approximately 2 million people are infected every year as well as about 399,000 people died in 2016 mostly from cirrhosis and HCC. The highest prevalence of HCV in the WHO Eastern Mediterranean Region is about 2.5% that includes countries in the Middle East and North Africa, especially in Egypt and 1.5% in WHO European Region. In the

* Transmission from blood, blood products, is now from "needle sharing"

United States, an estimated 2.4 million people are living chronically infected with HCV and a total of 3621 acute new cases were reported, but an estimated 50,300 new cases occurred in 2018, including 143,286 confirmed cases of chronic HCV and 15,713 deaths. It is important to note that new cases of HCV have been increasing every year for the past several years. Since the 1980s, outbreaks of hepatitis C have been associated with intravenous immune globulin (IVIG). To reduce this risk, all US-licensed IVIG products now have additional viral inactivation steps included in the manufacturing process. Furthermore, all immunoglobulin products (including intramuscular immunoglobulin products that have not been associated with hepatitis C) that lack viral inactivation steps are now excluded if HCV is detected by polymerase chain reaction (PCR). Other individuals considered at risk for hepatitis C are healthcare workers because of needlesticks and chronic hemodialysis patients and their spouses. Vertical transmission also occurs during deliveries.

PATHOGENESIS

HCV is transmitted via blood and blood-derived products and invades and infects the peripheral blood B and T lymphocytes and monocytes and moves to the main site of infection—the liver. The rate of HCV replication in hepatocytes is very high (~1×10^{12} virions per day), as 10% of the hepatic cells are infected. The high rate of viral replication results in an increased level of viral heterogeneity, which allows the virus to evade the host immune response. Although little evidence exists regarding a direct effect of HCV-induced cytopathic effects on the hepatocytes (liver cells), hepatocytes are likely killed by immune-mediated cytotoxic CD8 T cells (CTLs). Several recent studies suggest that HCV replication can cause cytopathic lesions in the liver, such as histologic lesions with scant inflammatory infiltrate, and fulminant hepatitis C after chemotherapy in liver transplant recipients. The innate immune response results in the activation of cytokines and interferon, which initially control viral replication in some cases. However, HCV-encoded proteins help the virus to evade innate immune response, including interaction of HCV core with tumor necrosis factor (TNF) receptor, which decreases cytolytic T-cell activity and interference of an HCV nonstructural protein(s) with interferon pathways. In addition, the natural killer (NK) cells respond to HCV infection by releasing perforins, which fragment nuclei of infected cells and induce apoptosis. HCV infection is inhibited by the release of interferon-γ, which recruits intrahepatic inflammatory cells, stimulates helper T1 (T_H1) response, and induces necrosis or apoptosis of HCV-infected cells.

Adaptive immune responses, including cell-mediated and humoral responses are elicited after expression of HCV proteins, especially the envelope glycoproteins E1 and E2. HCV antibodies appear several weeks after infection, and because of selective pressure from the host, mutations take place in the E2/E1 proteins, allowing the virus to evade the humoral immune response and establish persistent infection. More importantly, HCV antibodies have been implicated in tissue damage because of immune complex formation. Examples of such tissue damage are antinuclear antibodies, autoantibodies that act against cytochrome P450, and antibodies that work against the liver and kidney.

The immune complexes are also deposited in other tissues and cause some of the other extrahepatic problems, including vasculitis, arthritis, glomerulonephritis, and others. In the absence of strong humoral immune response against HCV infection, CTLs or CD8 T cells are critical to the elimination of HCV infection, and any impairment in cell-mediated immunity could be a major factor for a high level of chronicity in infected patients. The CD8 T cells eliminate HCV by apoptosis of infected hepatocytes and interferon-γ-induced inhibition of viral replication. The CTL response is less effective in chronically HCV-infected patients compared with that in acutely infected patients. Also, CD4 T cells play an important role in HCV pathogenesis by secreting several proinflammatory cytokines related to hepatocyte death. During acute infection, the rise in serum transaminases corresponds with cell damage, and the hepatic lesion is immune mediated by CTLs. The chronic infection probably progresses as a result of imbalance between T_H1 and T_H2 cytokines. T_H1 cytokines such as interleukin 2 (IL-2) and TNF-α are associated with aggressive hepatic disease, whereas T_H2 cytokines (IL-10) are related to the milder presentation. Expression of TNF-α causes hepatic injury and triggers "cytokine storm" to cause liver damage in chronically infected patients (**Figure 13–11**). Chronic HCV infection promotes insulin resistance in hepatocytes by increasing the inflammatory response due to increased expression of TNF-α and IL-6 and oxidative stress. Insulin resistance may lead to the progression of fibrosis and hepatocarcinogenesis.

Sexual transmission likely but to lower than HBV

❋ Needle sharing accounts for more than 40% of cases

71 million chronically infected, highest in the Middle East, Egypt

2.4 million chronic cases in the United States; numbers on rise for years

Cellular receptors, host factors contribute to liver tropism

Mutations allow evasion of host immune response

❋ Disease immune mediated by cytotoxic CD8 T cells

❋ Cytokines cause inflammation in HCV infection

❋ Antibody immune complexes cause liver damage, vasculitis, arthritis, glomerulonephritis

HCV infection causes imbalance between T_H1 and T_H2 cytokines

Cytokine expression triggers cytokine storm, liver damage

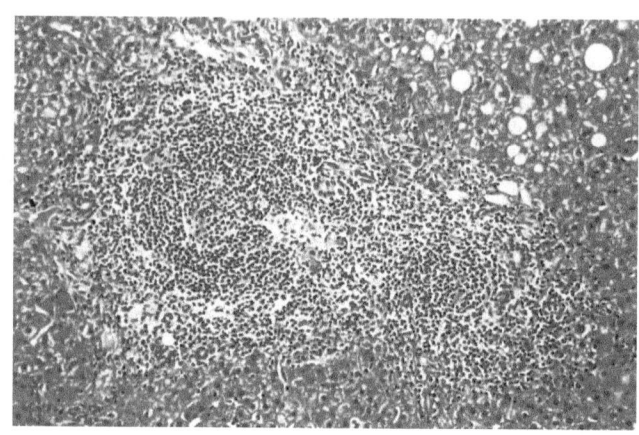

FIGURE 13–11. **Inflammation in chronic hepatitis C virus (HCV) infection.** Chronic inflammation of the portal area with a lymphoid aggregate in the center can be seen. At the edges of the portal area, the interface between the parenchyma and portal connective tissue, inflammation spreads outward, destroying hepatocytes and expanding the portal tract by piecemeal necrosis. (Reproduced with permission from Connor DH, Chandler FW, Schwartz DQ, et al: *Pathology of Infectious Diseases.* Stamford CT: Appleton & Lange; 1997.)

Host factors important in disease progression

Alcohol abuse, smoking influence severity

In addition to immune status of the host, genetic host factors play an important role in HCV pathogenesis. One such factor is major histocompatibility complex (MHC) class II DR5 allele, which has been shown to be associated with a lower incidence of cirrhosis in HCV-infected individuals. One study identified CTLs restricted by HLA A2 in 97% of chronic hepatitis C patients. Several extrinsic factors, such as alcohol abuse and smoking, are related to progression of chronic hepatitis C. The influence of age, gender, and race due to genetic factor variation has been implicated with progression of hepatitis C. Coinfection with other viruses such as HIV, HBV, HAV, and human T-lymphotropic virus influence the outcome of HCV disease.

❋ **Increased risk of HCC with chronic hepatitis C**

HCV core and NS3 and NS5A implicated with oncogenesis

HCV-infected patients may develop cirrhosis of liver with an increased risk of HCC. It has also been suggested that alcoholism increases the rate of HCC in HCV-infected patients. It is also believed that HCC is probably caused by long-term damage followed by rapid growth rate of hepatocytes during regeneration of liver, which may be mediated by some cytokines. Recent studies suggest that various HCV protein–host-cell interactions may play a role in the development of HCC, including disturbance in the cell cycle, upregulation of oncogenes, and loss of tumor suppressor gene functions. HCV core protein has been shown to perturb and modify the growth of the cell cycle. HCV core interacts directly or indirectly with components or pathways that lead to oncogeneses such as tumor suppressor genes (p53, p73, pRb), protein kinase, cell cycle, and cell proliferation and differentiation. In addition, HCV nonstructural proteins, NS3 and NS5A, play a role in cell transformation, differentiation, and oncogenesis.

 Despite a high rate of HCV replication, why is the disease immune mediated?

 ## CLINICAL ASPECTS

MANIFESTATIONS

Acute illness mild or asymptomatic

The incubation period of hepatitis C averages 2 to 12 weeks (range 2-26 weeks). The infection is usually asymptomatic in 75% of the infected people, whereas about 25% develop mild symptoms such as fever, fatigue, abdominal pain, poor appetite, joint pain, and jaundice. While some of these acutely infected people may clear the infection within 6 months, about 85% of the cases results in chronic carrier state in adult patients. Fulminant hepatitis due to hepatitis C is very rare in the United States. The average duration of time from infection to the development of chronic

 Think ▸▸ Apply 13-5: While there may be some direct effect of HCV on liver pathology, the major pathogenic mechanisms, although not well understood, are mediated by cytokines, oxidative stress, immune complex, and steatosis induction.

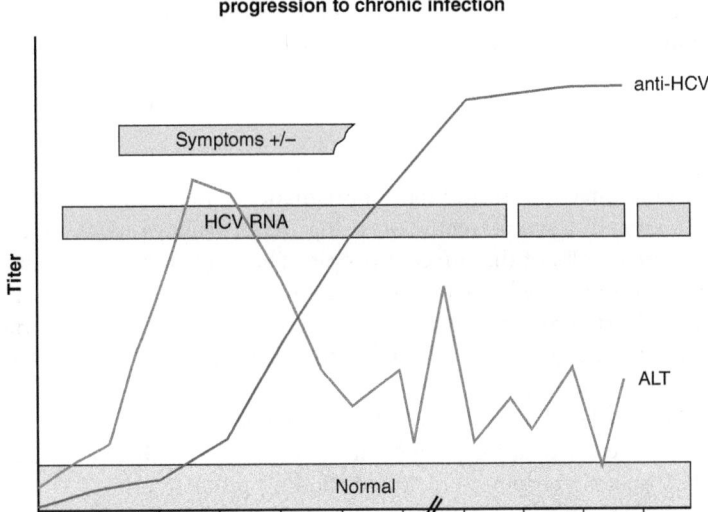

Serologic pattern of acute HCV infection with progression to chronic infection

FIGURE 13–12. **Sequence of appearance of viremia, alanine aminotransferase (ALT), symptoms, antibodies in acute hepatitis C virus (HCV) infection, and progression to chronic infection.**

hepatitis C is 10 to 18 years. Cirrhosis and HCC are late sequelae of chronic hepatitis. Chronic hepatitis C tends to wax and wane, is often asymptomatic, and maybe associated with either elevated or normal ALT values in serum (**Figure 13–12**). Chronic hepatitis C has been the leading infectious cause of chronic liver disease and liver transplantation in the United States. New treatments may reduce the severity of HCV-related liver diseases.

Chronic infection in 85%

Chronic hepatitis tends to wax and wane; asymptomatic, elevated, or normal ALT

 Despite being an RNA virus, how does HCV cause chronicity in 85% of the infected patients?

DIAGNOSIS

Two types of diagnostic tests are available to detect HCV infection: HCV antibodies and HCV RNA. However, the antibody response in acute disease may be detectable between 6 to 12 weeks after infection, about 50% to 70% of infected patients may have detectable levels at the onset of symptoms, whereas after 3 to 6 months about 90% of the infected patients may have HCV antibodies. On the other hand, HCV RNA can be detected in most infected people 2 to 3 weeks after infection, even before the elevation of ALT levels (**Figure 13–12**). Therefore, the current recommendations are to combine HCV antibodies and HCV RNA for the diagnosis of HCV infection. To detect HCV antibodies, enzyme-linked immunosorbent assay (ELISA) and enhanced chemiluminescence immunoassay (CIA) employing multiple HCV antigens (core, NS3, and NS5) are used. For positive HCV antibody results, confirmation is made by detecting HCV RNA by RT-PCR. People who test positive for both HCV antibodies and HCV RNA, HCV treatment is recommended. For those who are suspected of recent exposure or from high-risk groups and test negative for HCV antibodies such as immunocompromised or receiving chronic hemodialysis, HCV RNA test is performed. People who test positive for HCV antibodies and negative for HCV RNA, a follow-up HCV RNA test should be performed. CDC recommends one-time HCV testing of all adults of the age of 18 years and older and all pregnant women during pregnancy and regular testing of people who inject drugs. Quantitative assays of HCV RNA by RT-PCR are used for predicting the responsiveness and monitoring the efficacy of antiviral therapy, but there is not a very good correlation between viral load and histology. Usually, genotyping may not be needed

Antibody responses usually delayed

✳ ELISA to detect HCV antibody; RT-PCR to detect HCV RNA for confirmation

HCV RNA quantitated by PCR to monitor antiviral efficacy

One-time testing recommended at 18+ years

 Think ▸▸ Apply 13-6: **While most RNA genomes are unable to persist in infected cells, HCV RNA probably persists by a folding or conformation change mechanism, and HCV proteins suppress components of innate and adaptive immunity.**

✳ HCV genotypes important for cirrhosis, treatment failures

for starting of therapy because the new line of drugs works on many genotypes. However, pre-treatment genotyping continues to be recommended for patients with cirrhosis, past treatment failures, and drug resistance in order to develop treatment strategies for better outcomes.

TREATMENT AND PREVENTION

Treatment for HCV infection is recommended for all HCV-infected people with acute or chronic infection, including nonpregnant women and children aged more than 3 years and adolescents. Current treatments using DDAs usually involve oral pills for 8 to 12 weeks results in cure of 90% of the infected people. The guidelines and recommendations for HCV treatment are provided at www.hcvguidelines.org. While earlier combination treatment therapy with interferon-α (in the form of injection) and ribavirin (as oral pill) was used for patients with chronic hepatitis C, this treatment is not commonly used due to the availability of potent and safer DDAs.

Since 2011, FDA has approved several potent DDAs that target specific HCV enzymes/proteins which are essential for HCV replication. Currently, there are four classes of DDAs that target HCV-specific enzymes/proteins, including protease (NS3/4A) inhibitors, polymerase (NS5B) inhibitors (nucleotide), polymerase (NS5B) inhibitors (nonnucleoside), and phosphoprotein (NS5A) inhibitors. Several of these DDAs are available in fixed doses pills and recommended for use in many genotypes. However, pretreatment genotyping is recommended for patients with cirrhosis and past unsuccessful HCV treatment, including some drug combination and resistance.

- **HCV protease (NS3/4A) inhibitors:** (1) The first-generation HCV protease inhibitors were boceprevir and telaprevir that are used in combination of interferon-α and ribavirin in patients infected with HCV genotype 1. Side effects of telaprevir included anemia, rash, nausea, diarrhea, headache, and rectal irritation and pain. These drugs are not commonly used because of the development of second generation of protease inhibitors. (2) The second generation of protease inhibitors includes simeprevir, paritaprevir, grazoprevir, and glecaprevir. Side effects with simeprevir include photosensitivity and rash.
- **HCV RNA polymerase (NS5B) inhibitor:** The nucleotide HCV RNA polymerase inhibitor includes sofosbuvir (Sovaldi) that terminates the RNA synthesis of HCV. Side effects include fatigue, headache, and nausea. The nonnucleoside HCV polymerase inhibitor includes dasabuvir that inhibits HCV RNA polymerase. Side effects are nausea, itching, and insomnia.
- **HCV NS5A (phosphoprotein) inhibitors:** The inhibitors of HCV NS5A phosphoprotein, which are critical for HCV replication, include daclatasvir, elbasvir, ledipasvir, ombitasvir, pibrentasvir, and velpatasvir. Common side effects include headache, feeling tired, and nausea.

✳ New direct-acting antivirals (DDAs) target HCV protease, HCV polymerase, HCV NS5A phosphoprotein

✳ Combination therapy uses HCV protease/NS5A or HCV polymerase/NS5A inhibitors for 8 to 12 months

- **Treatment combinations:** The recommendations, including pretreatment assessment such as blood work, hepatic panel, HCV viral load, HBsAg test, HIV antigen/antibody test, cirrhosis, drug interactions, genotyping, and others have been developed by American Association for the Study of Liver Diseases (AASLD) and Infectious Diseases Society of America (IDSA) are provided at **www.hcvguidelines.org.** Initial treatment of adults is separated into two categories. (1) Simplified pangenotypic HCV treatment for treatment-naïve adults without cirrhosis includes glecaprevir (protease NS3/4A inhibitor)/pibrentasvir (NS5A inhibitor) for 8 weeks or Sofosbuvir (polymerase NS5B inhibitor)/velpatasvir (NS5A inhibitor) for 12 weeks, (2) Simplified pangenotypic HCV treatment algorithm for treatment-naïve adults with compensated cirrhosis includes: for Genotype 1-6 glecaprevir (protease NS3/4A inhibitor)/pibrentasvir (NS5A inhibitor) for 8 weeks or for genotype 1, 2, 4, 5, or 6 Sofosbuvir (polymerase NS5B inhibitor)/velpatasvir (NS5A inhibitor) for 12 weeks. Follow-up is recommended for 12 weeks or later after completion of the therapy by assessing HCV viral load and hepatic panel to confirm virologic cure (HCV RNA undetectable) and normal levels of transaminases. Patients who have treatment failures will be evaluated for retreatment based on AASLD/IDSA guidelines.

Immune globulin may not be protective; no vaccine

Corticosteroids are not beneficial. Avoidance of injection drug use and screening of blood products are important preventive measures. Prophylactic ISG does not protect against hepatitis C. There is no vaccine for HCV.

KEY CONCLUSIONS

- HCV, a Flavivirus, virion contains an icosahedral core (C) and a lipid bilayer envelope with two glycoproteins, E1 and E2. E2 binds to receptor and has hypervariable regions that allow the virus to escape immune responses. There are six nonstructural proteins made by HCV such as NS2, NS3/4A (protease), NS4B (interferon resistance), NS5A (phosphoprotein), and NS5B (RNA polymerase).

- HCV replicates in the cytoplasm by translating its positive-sense RNA into a polyprotein that is cleaved into mature proteins by protease, including RNA-dependent RNA polymerase that is used for transcription and replication. Assembly and release takes place in and from the cytoplasm.

- HCV pathogenesis (average incubation period 2-12 weeks) is mainly immune mediated where liver damage is caused by cytotoxic CD8 T cells and proinflammatory cytokines. In addition, immune complexes are formed that cause liver damage and extrahepatic problems such as vasculitis, arthritis, glomerulonephritis.

- HCV acute infection is usually asymptomatic in 75% of infected people and 25% may get mild symptoms of acute hepatitis. About 85% of the infected people develop chronic hepatitis that leads to cirrhosis of liver in 10 to 18 years with increased risk of HCC.

- Humoral and cell-mediated immune responses are responsible in controlling the infection but also exacerbating the disease. Moreover, depressed cell-mediated immunity is seen in chronic infection.

- During HCV infection, HCV RNA appears before (2-3 weeks after exposure) the elevation of ALT and HCV antibodies (6-12 weeks after exposure).

- HCV diagnosis is done by detecting HCV antibodies (ELISA) and confirming by HCV RNA (RT-PCR).

- Successful HCV treatment involves combination therapy, including HCV protease (NS3/4A), HCV polymerase (NS5B), and HCV phosphoprotein (NS5A) inhibitors leading to a functional cure.

- There is no vaccine available.

● HEPATITIS E

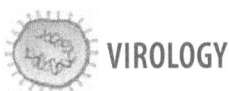 ### VIROLOGY

Hepatitis E virus (HEV), a member of Hepeviridae (hepevirus), is the cause of another form of hepatitis that is spread by the fecal–oral route, and therefore resembles hepatitis A disease. It used to be referred as enterically transmitted (ET) non-A, non-B hepatitis. HEV is a positive-sense, single-stranded RNA virus that is similar to, but distinct from, caliciviruses. The viral particles in stool are naked capsid, 27 to 34 nm in diameter with icosahedral symmetry, and they exhibit spikes on their surface. The genome of HEV is 7.2 kb in size and contains three open reading frames (ORFs). ORF-1 encodes the nonstructural proteins, including methyltransferase, protease, helicase, and RNA-dependent RNA polymerase. ORF-2 encodes capsid protein and ORF-3 a multifunctional small protein.

Like other positive-sense RNA viruses, HEV replicates in the cytoplasm. HEV enters host cells via an unidentified receptor. After uncoating, the positive-sense RNA genome is released in the cytoplasm that acts as an mRNA for synthesis of ORF-1 (nonstructural proteins). The viral RNA-dependent RNA polymerase transcribes a replicative intermediate negative-sense RNA that serves template for a subgenomic RNA and full-length genomic RNA. The subgenomic RNA synthesizes ORF-2 (capsid) and ORF-3. Virus assembly takes place in the cytoplasm and ORF-3 helps virus release from the infected cells.

Spreads in similar manner to hepatitis A

Naked capsid, icosahedral, positive-sense RNA virus

Genome encodes ORF-1, 2, and 3

Replication in cytoplasm

Nonstructural proteins encoded by full-length genomic RNA

Subgenomic RNA encodes capsid protein

EPIDEMIOLOGY

Worldwide, an estimated 20 million HEV infections occur every year, including 3.3 million symptomatic acute cases and approximately 44,000 deaths in 2015. Most cases of hepatitis E infection have been identified in developing countries with poor sanitation including Asia (mainly East and South Asia), Africa, Central America, Mexico, and the Indian subcontinent, and recurrent epidemics have been described in these areas. Cases have been recently recognized in developed countries such as the United States; most have been in visitors or immigrants from endemic areas. There are four genotypes of HEV, including genotype 1 in Asia and Africa, genotype 2 in Mexico and West Africa, genotype 3 in developed countries (isolated cases in the United States) and genotype 4 in China, Taiwan, and Japan. Genotypes 1 and 2 are commonly found in contaminated water, whereas genotypes 3 and 4 in uncooked/undercooked pork, boar or deer meat. Shellfish are also a risk factor for HEV infection.

Most cases in East Asia, Africa, Mexico, and the Indian subcontinent

CLINICAL ASPECTS

HEV is transmitted fecally–orally, mainly from contaminated drinking water. Several other transmission routes have been documented, including foodborne transmission from ingestion of infected animal products, zoonotic transmission from animals to humans, transfusion of infected blood products, and vertical transmission. Whereas major outbreaks are caused by contaminated water or food supplies, sporadic outbreaks occur from ingesting raw or uncooked shellfish. Similar to hepatitis A, infection with HEV is frequently subclinical. The incubation period for hepatitis E ranges from 15 to 60 days (average 40 days). In endemic, developing areas, hepatitis E has the highest attack rate in young adults aged 15 to 44 years. Symptoms of HEV include jaundice, loss of appetite, enlarged liver, nausea and vomiting, fever, itching, skin rash, or joint pain that typically last between 1 and 6 weeks. There is also dark urine and clay-colored stool. The virus is excreted in feces 1 week before and 4 weeks after the onset of jaundice. While most people recover from HEV infection, the overall case fatality rate is about 1% during outbreaks. In rare cases, acute HEV can result in fulminant hepatitis (acute liver failure), including deaths. Pregnant women infected with HEV during pregnancy, especially in second or third trimester, develop fulminant hepatitis more frequently with an increased risk of acute liver failure, fetal loss, and mortality. The fatality is reported between 10% and 30%.

Fecal–oral transmission from contaminated water, food

Frequently subclinical, like hepatitis A

Indistinguishable from other acute hepatitis

Highest attack in young adults

✳ **Fulminant hepatitis in pregnant women**

 Why does HEV cause fulminant hepatitis in pregnant women?

DIAGNOSIS

Because HEV is clinically indistinguishable from other acute hepatitis, the diagnosis is confirmed by demonstrating the presence of specific IgM antibody to HEV. HEV RNA may be detected by RT-PCR in blood and/or stool, especially in those areas where HEV is seen infrequently.

Demonstrate IgM to hepatitis E for diagnosis

✳ **RT-PCR detects HEV RNA**

TREATMENT AND PREVENTION

There is no specific treatment available other than supportive measures and proper nutrition. ISG does not appear to provide protection. The risk of transmission can be reduced by upholding safe hygienic practices, drinking safe and boiled water, and avoiding eating raw and uncooked seafood, pork, deer and boar meat, vegetables, and fruits in endemic areas. In seriously ill patients with liver failure, liver transplantation may be the only recourse. A recombinant subunit HEV vaccine was approved in China in 2012 but not approved in other countries, including the United States.

No specific treatment

ISG does not protect

Hygienic measures reduce transmission risk

HEPATITIS G

In 1995, hepatitis G virus (HGV), or GB virus C (GBV-C), was discovered in sera from two patients. HGV and GBV-C are two isolates of the same virus. Hepatitis G is a (+) sense RNA virus of 9.3 kb, similar to that of hepatitis C and members of the Flaviviridae family but has not been associated with any clinical disease. The virion structure of hepatitis G is similar to that of HCV. The genome encodes two structural envelope proteins (E1 and E2) and five nonstructural proteins (NS2, NS3, NS4b, NS5a, and NS4b). The other structural protein, core or capsid, has not

 Think ▸▸ Apply 13-7: Probably due to several maternal factors (eg, malnutrition), pregnancy factors (hormonal changes), Th1 to Th2 switch, and viral factors (viral load, genotypes) contribute to fulminant hepatitis in pregnant women.

been characterized. The virus encodes its own RNA-dependent RNA polymerase. HGV has been found to replicate in lymphocytes rather than in hepatocytes. HGV is mainly transmitted parenterally, including blood and blood-derived products. There may be a sexual component of transmission as seen in HBV and HCV. HGV infection is widely distributed worldwide with a high prevalence in blood donors in the United States. Approximately 10% to 30% of the blood donors have antibody against HGV. An antibody assay can detect past, but not present, infection, and detection of acute infection with hepatitis G requires a PCR assay for viral RNA in serum. Up to 5% of volunteer blood donors and 35% of HIV-infected patients are positive for hepatitis G RNA. In addition to being closely related to hepatitis C, data suggest that 10% to 20% of patients infected with hepatitis C are also infected with hepatitis G. Given this association, it has been difficult to ascertain the contribution of hepatitis G to clinical disease. Patients infected with both viruses (HCV and HGV) do not appear to have a worse disease than those infected by HCV only. Currently, there is no useful serologic test and no therapy is established for patients with HGV.

Recent studies suggest that persistent coinfection of HGV and HIV is associated with lower viral (HIV) load, higher CD4$^+$ T-cell count, and prolonged survival of HIV-infected individuals. Some studies suggest that HGV E2 protein inhibits processing of HIV Gag precursor protein resulting in inhibition of virus assembly and release. Other studies suggest that HGV stimulates cytokine production that inhibits HIV replication, decreases T-cell activation and proliferation, and downregulates chemokine receptors, CCR5 and CXCR4 (HIV coreceptors). However, more research is needed before any of these findings are translated into therapeutic advances.

Enveloped RNA (+) virus similar to hepatitis C

Transmission parenteral

High prevalence in blood donors

Uncertain Role in human disease

HGV and HCV coinfection does not worsen HCV disease

HGV and HIV coinfection may prolong AIDS survival

HGV may inhibit HIV replication

CASE STUDY
A Laboratory Discovery

A 45-year-old man has a routine physical in connection with a request for life insurance. All physical and laboratory examinations are normal except for a bilirubin of 2.6 mg/mL. The patient visited Nepal 1 year ago and acknowledged sharing intravenous drugs as a collegian. He has never had an acute hepatitis illness.

QUESTIONS

1. What was the most likely cause of the man's elevated bilirubin?
   A. Hepatitis A
   B. Hepatitis B
   C. Hepatitis C
   D. Hepatitis D
   E. Hepatitis E

2. Which laboratory test would be most likely to indicate the diagnosis?
   A. Specific IgM antibody and Western blot assay
   B. Specific IgG antibody and RT-PCR assay
   C. Quantitative viral DNA assay
   D. Viral genotypic assay
   E. Serum alanine aminotransferase

3. What would be an effective treatment?
   A. Interferon and Ribavirin
   B. Polymerase and NS5A inhibitor
   C. Protease and polymerase inhibitor
   D. Ribavirin and NS5A inhibitor
   E. Quantitative enzyme immunoassay

ANSWERS

1. (C)

2. (B)

3. (B)

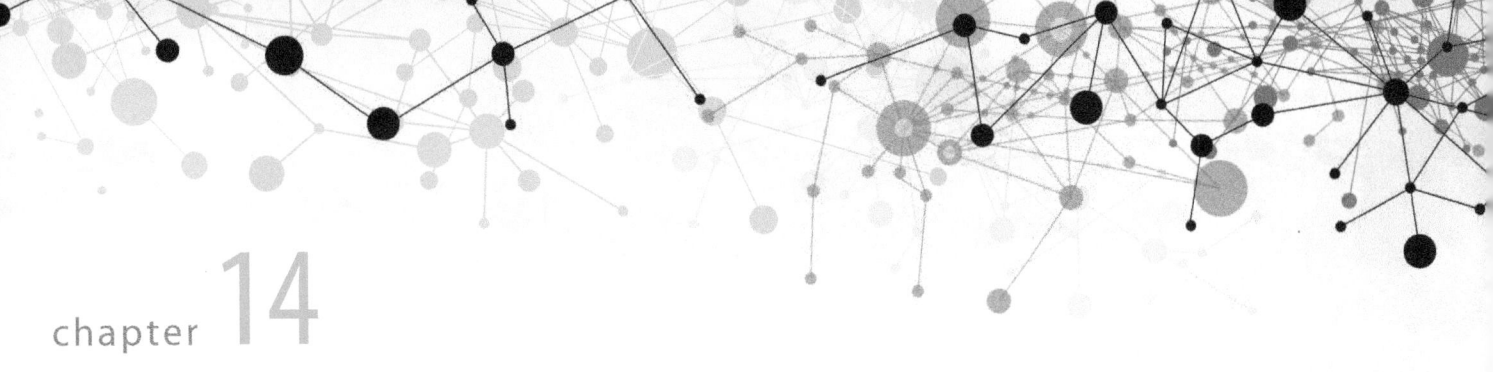

chapter 14

Herpesviruses

Herpes Simplex 1 and 2 • Varicella-Zoster Virus • Epstein-Barr Virus • Cytomegalovirus • Human Herpesvirus 6 and 7

Kaposi's Sarcoma Herpesvirus 8

I'm kinda like herpes, I just keep coming back.

—George Carlin

The Herpesviridae family is composed of large, enveloped, icosahedral, double-stranded DNA viruses. There are eight known human herpesviruses (HHVs) and a very large number of animal herpesviruses. The HHVs causing diseases include herpes simplex virus-1 (HSV-1) and HSV-2, which cause orofacial and genital lesions; varicella-zoster virus (VZV), which causes primary chickenpox and reactivated shingles; Epstein-Barr virus (EBV), an infectious cause of mononucleosis, Burkitt lymphoma (BL), and other B-cell lymphomas; cytomegalovirus (CMV) cause mononucleosis symptoms in adults and pneumonia, diarrhea, and retinitis in immunocompromised, and the most common congenital infection; HHV types 6 and 7 (HHV-6 and HHV-7), which cause roseola in infants; and HHV-8 also known as Kaposi Sarcoma (KS)-associated herpesvirus (KSHV), which causes KS and some B-cell lymphoma (**Table 14–1**). In addition, the simian herpesvirus, herpes B virus, has occasionally caused lethal human disease in primate center workers. All herpesviruses establish lifelong latent infections in their hosts with periodic reactivation events.

* Large, enveloped, icosahedral, double-stranded DNA viruses

Eight HHVs cause a range of diseases

● HERPESVIRUSES: GROUP CHARACTERISTICS

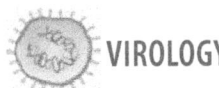 ### VIROLOGY

All herpesviruses are morphologically similar, with an overall size of 180 to 200 nm. An example of an HSV virion is shown in **Figure 14–1** as a representative virion structure for herpesviruses. The linear, double-stranded DNA genome and core proteins are encapsidated by an icosahedral capsid forming a diameter of 75 nm. The capsid is surrounded by the tegument, a relatively amorphous protein-filled region unique to herpesviruses. The **tegument** contains viral proteins and enzymes that play a structural role and many are required immediately for viral replication upon initial infection. Surrounding the tegument is a lipoprotein envelope originally derived from the nuclear membrane of the infected host cell forming the complete virus particle or virion of 180 to 200 nm. The envelope contains multiple viral glycoproteins such as gB to gE and gH to gM that in various combination in different members act as viral binding, fusion, and entry proteins.

Icosahedral capsid surrounded by a tegument and a lipid envelope from nuclear membrane

Herpesvirus genomes range from 125 kbp (VZV) to 240 kbp (CMV) of DNA, and code from around 75 viral proteins to over 200. However, it is now clear from next-generation RNA sequencing and proteomics that the coding capacity is much more complex than originally thought and many more genes may be expressed in the infected cell. Herpesviruses express the enzymes

TABLE 14-1   Human Herpesviruses

NAME	COMMON NAME	TRANSMISSION	INCUBATION PERIOD	PRIMARY INFECTION SITE	DISEASE	LATENT INFECTION SITE
HHV-1	Herpes simplex virus 1 (HSV-1)	Close contact	7-10 days	Mucoepithelial cells	Oral (fever blisters), ocular lesions; encephalitis	Nerve ganglia
HHV-2	Herpes simplex virus 2 (HSV-2)	Close contact Sexual transmission	2-12 days	Mucoepithelial cells	Genital, anal lesions; severe neonatal infections; meningitis	Nerve ganglia
HHV-3	Varicella-zoster virus (VZV)	Respiratory route Inhalation Close contact	11-21 days	Mucoepithelial cells	Chickenpox (primary infection); shingles (reactivation)	Nerve ganglia
HHV-4	Epstein-Barr virus (EBV)	Saliva Kissing	30-50 days	B cell, oral epithelium	Infectious mononucleosis (primary infection); tumors, including B-cell tumors (Burkitt lymphoma, immunoblastic lymphomas of the immunosuppressed); nasopharyngeal carcinoma, some T-cell tumors	B lymphocytes
HHV-5	Cytomegalovirus (CMV)	Close contact, sexual transmission Congenital Blood-to-blood Transplant	21-84 days	Leukocytes (T and B) Lymphocytes Monocytes	Mononucleosis; severe congenital infection; infections in immunocompromised (gastroenteritis, retinitis, pneumonia)	Monocytes, neutrophils, vascular endothelial cells
HHV-6	Human herpesvirus 6	Close contact Respiratory route	7-14 days	T lymphocytes	Roseola in infants (primary infection); infections in allograft recipients (pneumonia, marrow failure)	T lymphocytes monocytes, macrophages
HHV-7	Human herpesvirus 7	Saliva Close contact		T lymphocytes	Some cases of roseola (primary infection)	CD4+ T cells
HHV-8	Kaposi sarcoma-associated herpesvirus (KSHV), human herpesvirus 8	Saliva, blood?		B lymphocytes Peripheral blood mononuclear cell Oral epithelium	Tumors, including Kaposi sarcoma; some B-cell lymphomas	B-lymphocytes Virus-infected tumors

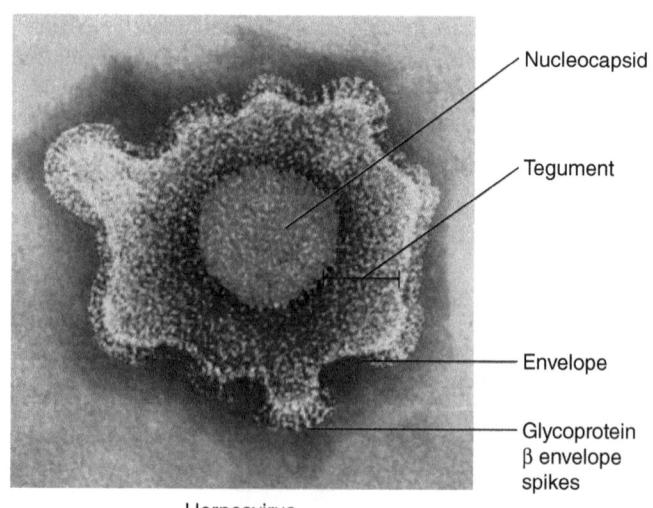

FIGURE 14-1. Virion structure of herpes simplex virus. (Reproduced with permission from Willey JM: *Prescott, Harley, & Klein's Microbiology*, 7th ed. New York, NY: McGraw Hill; 2008.)

Nucleocapsid

Tegument

Envelope

Glycoprotein β envelope spikes

Herpesvirus

necessary for viral DNA synthesis allowing herpesviruses to infect both dividing and quiescent cells. The HHVs have six blocks of orthologous genes with interspersed species-specific viral genes. There are substantial differences in their genomic sequences particularly in the unique coding regions of each herpesvirus. Antigenic analysis of both conserved and nonconserved genes is an important means for differentiation among herpesviruses despite some cross-reactions (eg, between HSV-1 and HSV-2).

Based on certain virologic similarities, the herpesviruses may be divided into three subfamilies α, β, and γ herpesviruses. HSV-1 and HSV-2, as well as VZV, are in the α subfamily, characterized by relatively rapid replication time and neuronal latency; CMV, HHV-6, and HHV-7 are in the β subfamily, characterized by slow replication rates and extremely limited host range; EBV and KSHV (HHV-8) are in the γ subfamily characterized by relatively rapid replication, replication in lymphocytes, and restricted host range. These characterizations are now made on the basis of genomic sequences but the original classifications have held up in the genomic era.

Cell tropism for the individual viruses varies significantly. HSV has the widest range; it can infect many different animal hosts and replicates in numerous animal and human host cells, although in nature it is only found in humans. VZV infects only humans and is best grown in cells of human origin, although some laboratory-adapted strains can grow in primate cell lines. Human CMV replicates well only in limited human cell lines including human foreskin fibroblasts. HHV-6 and HHV-7 preferentially grow in T-lymphocyte cell cultures. EBV does not replicate in most commonly used cell culture systems, but can be grown in continuous human or primate lymphoblastoid cell cultures where it is present in the latent state. KSHV infects many cell types but generally establishes latency in cultured cells, where only a low percentage of the cells support active replication.

■ Replication

The replication of HSV has been comprehensively studied and is representative of all herpesviruses, as shown in **Figure 14–2**. HSV generally causes lytic infection in epithelial cells and subsequently establishes latency in neuronal cells. The glycoproteins in the HSV envelope interact with cellular receptors, including initial binding to heparan sulfate and subsequent interaction with higher affinity receptors, leading to fusion with the cell membrane. For most herpesviruses, fusion occurs at the cytoplasmic membrane but for some viruses or in specific cell types, the virus is first endocytosed and fusion occurs in the endosome. Fusion delivers tegument proteins into the cytoplasm as well as the capsid containing viral DNA. The capsid migrates to the nucleus where the genome is then extruded into the nucleus. In the nucleus, the viral DNA genome circularizes and viral gene expression can be initiated. Transcription by host RNA polymerase of the large, complex genome is sequentially regulated in three distinct classes of mRNAs: (1) immediate early (IE) mRNAs, encoded by α genes, are synthesized 2 to 4 hours after infection. IE genes do not require de novo viral protein synthesis prior to expression and generally encode for proteins involved in regulation of viral gene expression and host defense; (2) early (E) mRNAs encoded by β genes require prior protein synthesis of IE genes and generally encode proteins involved in viral replication (DNA binding proteins, DNA polymerase, thymidine kinase, etc), and (3) late (L) mRNAs encoded by γ genes require viral genome replication for full expression and encode major structural proteins: capsid subunits, tegument proteins, and envelope glycoproteins. The early (E) proteins thymidine kinase and DNA polymerase are distinct from host cell enzymes and are, therefore, important targets of antiviral chemotherapy as discussed later. Synthesis of IE genes is required for E genes, and E genes shut off the IE genes. The E genes are required for viral genomic replication, which in turn is required for optimal synthesis of most L genes. However, some of the late structural proteins are produced to lower levels independently of genome replication. Viral DNA replication occurs in a rolling circle fashion producing high–molecular-weight DNA concatemers. Genomic concatemers are cleaved and packaged into pre-assembled capsids in the nucleus.

Herpesviruses assemble in the nuclei and a proteolytic cleavage event is necessary for the maturation of the capsid. A viral protease is responsible for the maturation. The envelope is acquired from the inner lamella of the nuclear membrane. Budding occurs at the nuclear membranes, and virions are then transported through the ER and Golgi. Re-envelopment and de-envelopment through the ER and Golgi and ultimately the cytoplasmic membrane is thought to occur. Host cell protein synthesis shut-off occurs for both α- and γ-herpesviruses and is thought to occur by

Herpesviruses encode a large number of proteins

Three subfamilies of herpesvirus, α, β, and γ

Herpes simplex has widest range of cell tropism

Three classes of mRNAs produced by α (immediate early), β (early), and γ (late) genes

Coordinated, sequential gene expression of the three classes

Host RNA polymerase directs transcription, viral DNA polymerase genome replication

Herpesvirus capsids assemble in the nucleus, envelope acquired from nuclear membrane

1 Circularization of genome and
transcription of immediate early
genes

2 α-Proteins, products of immediate early
genes, stimulate transcription of early
genes.

3 β-Proteins, products of early genes,
function in DNA replication, yielding
concatemeric DNA. Late genes are
transcribed.

4 γ-Proteins, products of late genes,
participate in virion assembly.

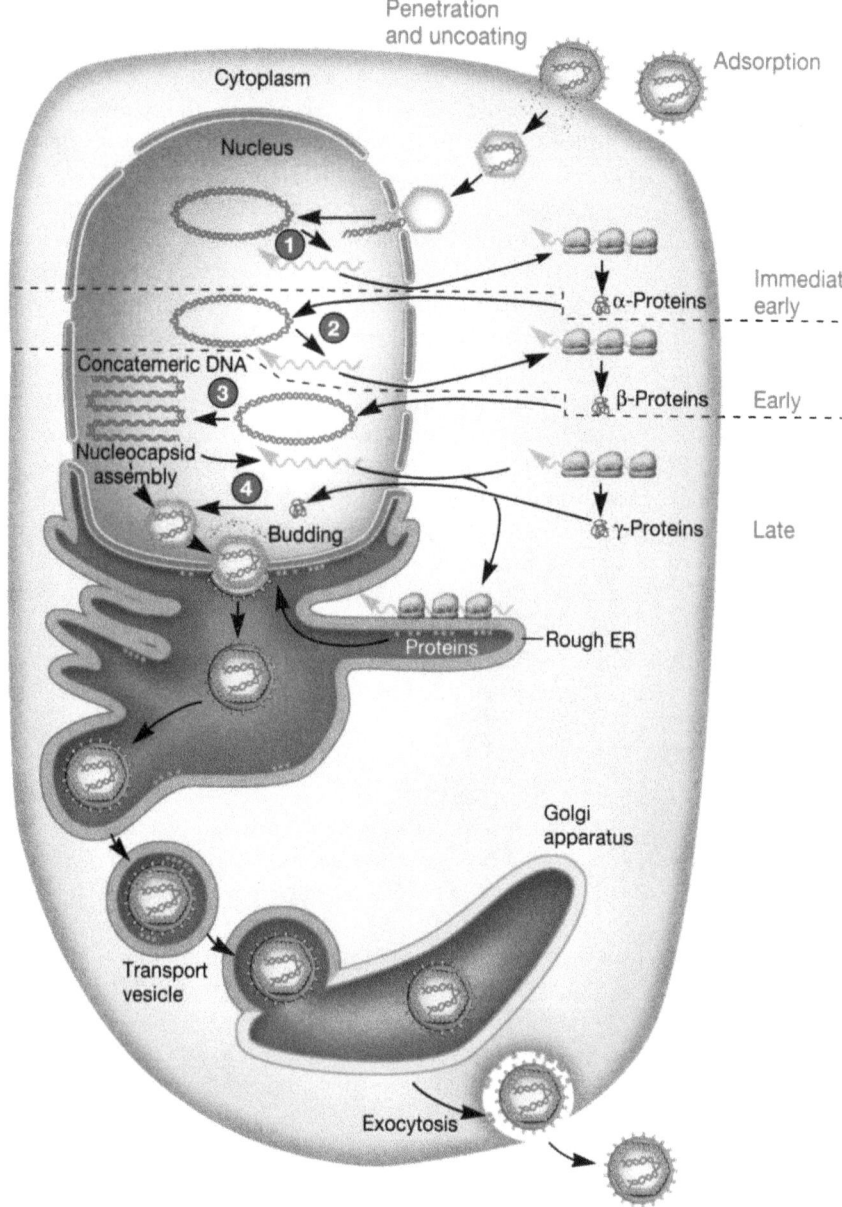

FIGURE 14–2. Replication cycle of herpes simplex virus 1. (Reproduced with permission from Willey JM: *Prescott, Harley, & Klein's Microbiology*, 7th ed. New York, NY: McGraw Hill; 2008.)

α- and γ-Herpesviruses shut-off host cell protein synthesis

cleavage of mRNAs by viral protein complexes. Ultimately, viral replication and host cell shut-off lead to death of the infected cell. Due to their long replication cycle, β-herpesviruses do not exhibit host cell shut-off.

■ Latency

In vivo, herpesviruses generally produce an initial lytic infection which is eventually controlled by the host immune system. However, during the initial infection, latent infection is also established. Latent infection allows all herpesvirus infection to be maintained for the life of the host. During latency, the genome of the virus is present in cells, but infectious virus is not recovered. The viral DNA is maintained as an episome in the nucleus. Latent infection is different from chronic infection in that the viral genome is not rapidly replicated and virions are not produced. During latency, there is minimal viral gene expression with only 1 to 10 latent genes being regularly expressed, depending on the virus. Latent genes encode functions for maintenance of the viral episome, preventing host cell death and inhibiting the host immune response. Many herpesviruses also express microRNAs during latency. MicroRNAs are small regulatory RNAs that control gene expression without producing a peptide product. This allows the virus to alter host and viral gene expression without producing antigens that could be recognized by the host immune system. HSV-1 expresses only microRNAs during latent infection and no proteins, minimizing the ability of the immune system to recognize the latently infected cells. Periodic reactivation provides a constant source of new infections in the population. There is a range of reactivation rates depending on the virus and the host. In immunosuppressed patients, reactivation is more common and severe, indicating that the immune system must play a role in the suppression of reactivation.

✱ Viral latency and
typical for all herp   ⌐ses

✱ Viral genome maintained as episomes

● HERPES SIMPLEX VIRUS

OVERVIEW

Herpes simplex virus (HSV), HSV-1 and HSV-2 are double-stranded DNA, icosahedral, enveloped viruses that have 50% homology and replicate in the nucleus by using host RNA polymerase for transcription and viral DNA polymerase for genome replication and acquire envelope from the nuclear membrane. HSV is transmitted through direct contact with lesions and infected secretions. Both HSV-1 and HSV-2 initially infect and replicate in the muco-epithelial cells and initiate viral-mediated multinucleated giant cells and cellular death leading to lytic or productive infection at the site of contact with associated inflammatory response followed by establishing latent infection in the nerve ganglion. HSV-1 usually causes orofacial infections involving skin, mouth, conjunctiva, and the nervous system. Genital infections are predominantly caused by HSV-2, but HSV-1 can also cause genital infection, and some of these individuals may develop aseptic meningitis. Both HSV-1 and HSV-2 cause latency and the site of latency is determined by the location of primary infection with orofacial infection (by HSV-1) residing as extrachromosomal episomal DNA in trigeminal ganglion and genital infection (HSV-2 ~70%, HSV-1~30%) in dorsal ganglion in the sacral region. Neonates can also acquire HSV during birth with a high mortality and neurologic sequalae in survivors. Both humoral and cell mediated immunity play an important role in controlling the virus, but CD8 T cells destroy virus-infected cells. Latent HSVs are reactivated periodically by factors such as sunlight, ultraviolet light, fever, excitement, emotional stress, and trauma. Acyclovir, a nucleoside analog, that is monophosphorylated by HSV thymidine kinase and inhibits viral DNA synthesis, is used for acute treatment and prevents frequent reactivation. There is no vaccine approved against HSV infection.

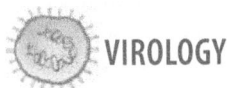 VIROLOGY

The genomes of herpes simplex 1 and 2 (HSV-1 and HSV-2, respectively) are both approximately 150 kbp of DNA. Although they are distinct epidemiologic and antigenic viruses, their genomes contain approximately 50% homology, making them the most closely related HHVs. Nearly all of the genes of HSV-1 have colinear homologs in HSV-2. HSV-1 and HSV-2 share many glycoprotein and structural antigens, but differences in glycoprotein B, among other glycoproteins, enable them to be distinguished antigenically. The viruses can also be distinguished by PCR assays.

HSV-1 and HSV-2 closely related

HSV-1 and HSV-2 distinguished epidemiologically, antigenically, and by DNA homology

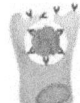 HERPES SIMPLEX DISEASE

EPIDEMIOLOGY ✦

Herpes simplex viruses are distributed worldwide, with an estimated 3.7 billion people under age 50 (67%) have HSV-1 and 491 million people aged 15 to 49 (13%) have HSV-2 infection globally. There are no known animal vectors, and humans appear to be the only natural reservoir. Direct contact with infected secretions is the principal mode of transmission or spread. HSV-1 is more often associated with disease "above the waist" or orofacial herpes, whereas HSV-2 is most often associated with genital infections or "below the waist" infections. However, an increasing number of genital infections are caused by HSV-1, with an estimated 122 to 192 million aged 15 to 49 years worldwide mostly in the Americas, Europe, and Western Pacific. HSV-1 is most often spread by direct contact of mucosal tissue, especially the lip area. Both HSV-1 and HSV-2 are prevalent worldwide. Seroepidemiologic studies indicate that the prevalence of HSV antibody varies by age and socioeconomic status of the population studied. In most developing countries, up to 90% of the population has HSV-1 antibody by the age of 30 years. In the United States, HSV-1 antibody is found in 18% to 35% of children by the age of 5 years with the percentages varying according to the population studied. In the United States, the seroprevalence rises to approximately 60% to 70% by the age of 30 years for middle-class populations; among lower socioeconomic groups, however, the percentage is higher. Detection of HSV-2 antibody before puberty is less common. Direct sexual transmission is the major mode of spread. Approximately 15% to 30% of sexually active adults in Western industrialized countries have HSV-2 antibody and seropositive rates are positively correlated with the number of sexual partners. The virus can be isolated from the cervix and urethra of approximately 5% to 12% of adults attending sexually transmitted disease clinics; many of these patients are asymptomatic or have small, unnoticed lesions on penile or vulvar skin. Asymptomatic shedding accounts for transmission from a partner who has no active genital lesions and often no history of genital herpes. There are 18.6 million people infected with HSV-2 and 572,000 infected annually in the United States. Genital herpes, which includes both HSV-2 and HSV-1, is not a reportable disease in the United States, but it is estimated that one out of every six people aged 14 to 49 years have genital herpes and more than 750,000 new cases occur per year. Infection with genital herpes increases the risk of other sexually transmitted infections, including HIV.

PATHOGENESIS

■ Acute Infections

Transmission occurs by direct contact with infection secretions. Both HSV-1 and HSV-2 initially infect and replicate in the mucoepithelial cells with an incubation period of 7 to 10 days and 2 to 12 days, respectively, and initiate viral-mediated cellular death leading to lytic or productive infection at the site of contact with associated inflammatory response. Pathologic changes during acute infections consist of ballooning degeneration of epithelial cells with condensed chromatin within the nuclei of cells, nuclear degeneration, and cells lose intact plasma membranes and form multinucleated giant cells (**Figure 14–3**). There is focal necrosis, eosinophilic intranuclear inclusion bodies, and an inflammatory response characterized by an initial polymorphonuclear neutrophil (PMN) infiltrate and a subsequent mononuclear cell infiltrate. Upon cell lysis, a clear fluid-containing virus is found between the epidermis and dermis layer and the fluid becomes pustular with healing upon the recruitment of inflammatory cells. The virus spreads to local sensory neurons and travels in retrograde fashion to the sensory ganglia that innervate the site of infection. In the case of facial herpes, the virus infects neurons in the trigeminal ganglia and in the case of genital herpes, the dorsal root or sacral ganglia. Latency is established in the ganglionic neurons. A round of replication may occur in the ganglia, but is not necessary for the establishment of latency.

■ Latent Infection

In humans, latent infection by HSV-1 initially causing orofacial acute infection has been demonstrated in trigeminal, superior cervical, and vagal nerve ganglia, and occasionally in the S2-S3

Sidebar notes:

＊ HSV-1 highly prevalent in the population

＊ HSV-2 more associated with sexual activity

＊ Genital herpes includes HSV-2 and HSV-1

＊ Contact with secretions mode of transmission, spread

No known animal vectors for HSV-1 or HSV-2

Lytic replication at the site of infection produces inflammation and giant cells

Virus can infect and spread to neurons and establishes latency in sensory ganglia

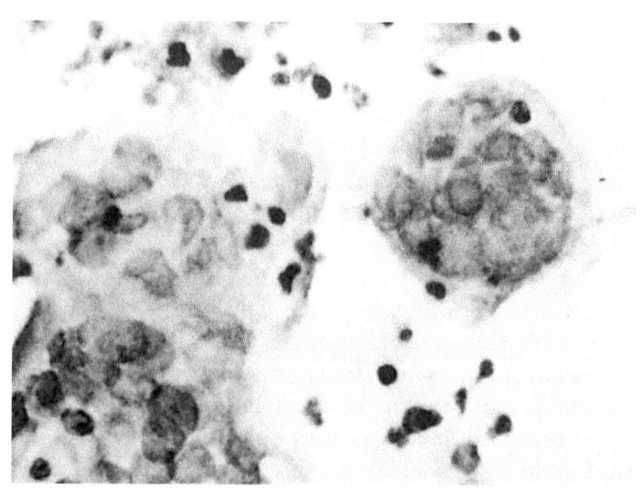

FIGURE 14–3. Multinucleated giant cells from herpes simplex virus lesion.

dorsal sensory nerve root ganglia when the acute infection initiates in the genital areas. Latent HSV-2 infection causing acute genital infection has been demonstrated in the sacral (S2-S3) region in the dorsal sensory root ganglia. Therefore, the site of latency is determined by the location of the primary acute infection and not the type of HSV. Latent infection of neurons by HSV does not result in the death of the cell. Multiple viral genomes exist in a circular extrachromosomal (episome) form in the nucleus, and transcription of only a small portion of the viral genome occurs, limited to a single viral transcript, the latency-associated transcript (LAT). The LAT encodes a number of miRNAs that serve as regulatory RNAs that can alter host cell gene expression without expressing foreign proteins. Some of the microRNAs of LAT are antisense to ICP0 or α-0 mRNA that encodes an immediate early protein necessary for lytic viral replication. Because latency is established in nondividing neurons, HSV does not encode direct functions to maintain the viral episome. Latent infection does not require synthesis of early or late viral polypeptides and, therefore, antiviral drugs directed at the thymidine kinase enzymes or viral DNA polymerase do not eradicate the virus in its latent state.

✳ HSV genomes exist as episomes during latency, no viral protein synthesis

✳ Orofacial HSV infection latency in trigeminal and genital HSV latency in sacral region/dorsal ganglia

No drugs treat latent HSV infections

■ Reactivation

A subset of patients exhibit overt clinical disease from reactivation of the virus. This can occur over the entire life of the host. However, people without obvious clinical disease can also reactivate and spread the virus through subclinical shedding. The mechanisms by which latent infection is reactivated are unknown. Precipitating factors that are known to initiate reactivation of HSV and subsequent clinical disease include exposure to ultraviolet light, sunlight, fever, excitement, emotional stress, and trauma (eg, oral intubation). However, it is clear that reactivation and viral shedding between overt disease episodes is common, and may account for some of the spread of the virus. Upon reactivation, the virus initiates lytic replication and virus particles travel down the neuronal axons (anterograde transport), most often to the site of or near the site of initial infection. The virus replicates in the epithelium, which is subsequently infected, produces vesicles and leads to localized spread and ulceration in a subset of reactivations. While immunocompetent hosts generally contain the viral infection, the virus may spread to proximate skin surfaces.

✳ Reactivation induced by sun exposure, fever, trauma, stress

Only subset of infected patients exhibit clinical disease

Two theories were proposed on how latent herpes reaches the peripheral sites, including ganglionic and skin trigger theories. In ganglionic theory, metabolic changes switch on the virus replication cycle, and the virus travels down the peripheral nerves to the skin, where it replicates in the epidermal cells and produces lesions. The skin trigger theory proposes that because of chronic multiplication of the virus in the ganglion, there is intermittent shedding of the virus through the nerve axon to the skin.

IMMUNITY

Host factors have a major effect on clinical manifestations of HSV infection. Many episodes of HSV infection are either asymptomatic or mildly symptomatic. Initial symptomatic clinical episodes of the disease are often more severe than recurrent episodes, likely due to the presence of anti-HSV antibodies and immune lymphocytes in persons with recurrent infections. Prior infection with HSV-1 may provide some level of protection against or shorten the duration of symptoms and lesions from subsequent infection with HSV-2 as a result of some degree of cross-protection, though dual infections certainly occur.

Both cellular and humoral immune responses are important in immunity to HSV. Neutralizing antibodies directed against HSV envelope glycoproteins appear to be important in preventing exogenous reinfection. Antibody-dependent cellular cytotoxicity (ADCC) may be important in limiting the early spread of HSV. By the second week after infection, cytotoxic T lymphocytes can be detected, which have the ability to destroy HSV-infected cells before completion of the replication cycle. Conversely, in immunosuppressed patients, especially those with depressed cell-mediated immunity, reactivation of HSV may be associated with prolonged viral excretion and persistence of lesions as well as more disseminated lesions. During latency, the HSV-1 and HSV-2 do not express viral proteins and are thus effectively hidden from the immune system. However, the immune system plays a role in keeping latency in check as immunosuppression leads to more common reactivation. It is possible that the virus may initiate reactivation more often than previously thought and that the adaptive immune system shuts down those cells once they reactivate.

✳ ADCC may limit early spread of HSV; cytotoxic T lymphocytes destroy HSV-infected cells

Reactivation controlled by adaptive immune system

HSVs express a number of genes that have evolved to inhibit innate and adaptive immunity. There are a number of genes capable of inhibiting interferon pathways at different stages. HSV-1

HSV encodes inhibitors of innate and adaptive immunity

also encodes an IE protein that blocks peptide loading onto MHC-I and prevents the complex from reaching the cell surface. Additionally, HSV inhibits apoptosis during both latent and lytic phases.

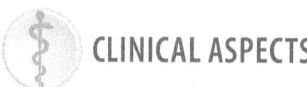

CLINICAL ASPECTS

MANIFESTATIONS

■ Herpes Simplex Type 1

Infection with HSV-1 is more often associated with orofacial disease though it causes an increasing number of genital infections. It consists characteristically of grouped or single vesicular lesions that become pustular and coalesce to form single or multiple ulcers. On dry surfaces, these ulcers scab before healing; on mucosal surfaces, they re-epithelialize directly. HSV can be isolated from almost all ulcerative lesions, but the titer of virus decreases as the lesions evolve. Infections generally involve ectoderm (skin, mouth, conjunctiva, and the nervous system).

❋ Vesicular lesions become pustular and then ulcerate

Primary infection with HSV-1 is most often asymptomatic. When symptomatic, typically in children (1-6 years of age), it appears most frequently as **gingivostomatitis,** with fever and ulcerative lesions involving the buccal mucosa, tongue, gums, and pharynx. The lesions are painful, and the acute illness usually lasts 5 to 12 days. During this initial infection, HSV spreads to the sensory neurons and becomes latent within neurons of the trigeminal ganglia, the ganglia that innervated the oral and nasal area.

Primary infections are often asymptomatic

Gingivostomatitis most commonly in children

Lesions usually recur on a specific area of the lip and the immediate adjacent skin; these lesions are referred to as mucocutaneous and are commonly called "cold sores" or "fever blisters" known as labialis (**Figure 14–4**). Lesions are typically unilateral. Their recurrence may be signaled by premonitory tingling or burning in the area. Systemic complaints are unusual, and the episode generally lasts approximately 7 days. It should be noted that HSV may be reactivated and excreted into the saliva with no apparent mucosal lesions present. HSV has been isolated from saliva in 5% to 8% of children and 1% to 2% of adults who were asymptomatic at the time.

❋ Recurrent cold sores or labialis are usually unilateral

Virus in saliva with asymptomatic reactivation

HSV sometimes infects the finger or nail area. This infection, termed **herpetic whitlow,** usually results from the inoculation of infected secretions through a small cut in the skin or from needle sticks. Painful vesicular lesions of the finger develop and pustulate; they are often mistaken for bacterial infection and mistreated accordingly.

Herpetic whitlow mimics bacterial paronychia

HSV infection of the eye is one of the most common causes of corneal damage and blindness in the developed world. Infections usually involve the conjunctiva and cornea, and characteristic dendritic ulcerations are produced. With recurrence of disease, there may be deeper involvement with corneal scarring. Occasionally, there may be an extension into deeper structures of the eye, especially when topical steroids are used.

❋ Herpetic corneal and conjunctival infection can cause blindness

In rare cases, encephalitis may result from HSV-1 infection. Most cases occur in adults with high levels of anti-HSV-1 antibody, suggesting reactivation of latent virus in the trigeminal nerve root ganglion and extension of productive (lytic) infection into the temporoparietal area of the brain. Primary HSV infection with neurotropic spread of the virus from peripheral sites up the

FIGURE 14–4. Coalesced, localized lesions characteristic of reactivated herpes simplex virus type 1 (HSV-1) infection.

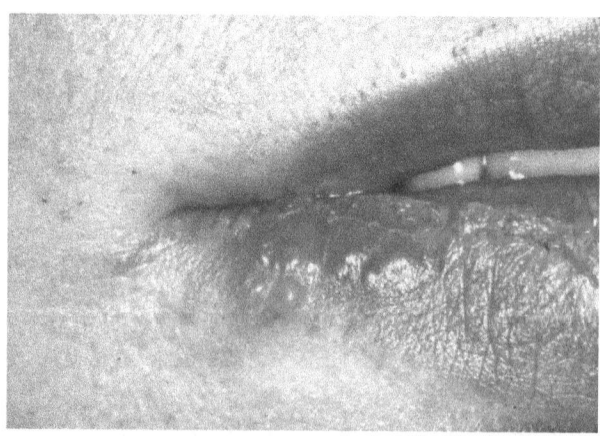

olfactory bulb into the brain may also result in parenchymal brain infection. Classically, HSV encephalitis affects one temporal lobe, leading to focal neurologic signs and cerebral edema. If untreated, mortality rate is approximately 70%. Clinically, the disease can resemble brain abscess, tumor, or intracerebral hemorrhage. Rapid diagnosis by polymerase chain reaction (PCR) of cerebrospinal fluid (CSF) has replaced brain biopsy as the diagnostic test. Intravenous acyclovir reduces the morbidity and mortality of the disease, especially if treatment is initiated early. There are small number of familiar genetic mutations leading to increased herpes encephalitis. These mutations appear to be in genes involved in specific innate immune responses.

* HSV encephalitis typically localized to temporal lobe and has high mortality without treatment

Rapid PCR diagnosis of CSF allows antiviral therapy

■ Herpes Simplex Type 2

Genital herpes is a significant sexually transmitted disease. Both HSV-1 and HSV-2 can cause genital disease, and the symptoms and signs of acute infection are similar for both viruses. Seventy percent of the first episodes of genital HSV infection in the United States are caused by HSV-2, and genital HSV-2 disease is also more likely to recur than genital HSV-1 infection. Ninety percent of the HSV-2 antibody-positive patients have never had a clinically evident genital HSV episode. In many instances, the first clinical episode is years after primary infection.

* HSV-2 associated with genital infections

HSV-2 patients may not exhibit overt disease

Primary Genital Herpes Infection

For individuals who develop clinically evident primary genital HSV disease, the mean incubation period from sexual contact to onset of lesions is 4 days. Lesions begin as small erythematous papules, which soon form vesicles and then pustules (**Figure 14–5**). Within 3 to 5 days, the vesiculopustular lesions break to form painful coalesced ulcers that subsequently dry; some form crusts and heal without scarring. With primary disease, the genital lesions are usually multiple (mean number 20), bilateral, and extensive. The urethra and cervix are also infected frequently, with discrete or coalesced ulcers on the exocervix. Bilateral, enlarged, tender inguinal lymph nodes are usually present and may persist for weeks to months. About one-third of patients show systemic symptoms such as fever, malaise, and myalgia, and approximately 1% develop aseptic meningitis with neck rigidity and severe headache. First episodes of disease last an average of 12 days.

* Multiple painful vesiculopustular lesions

Systemic symptoms and adenopathy can occur

Recurrent Genital Herpes Infection

In contrast to primary infection, recurrent genital herpes is a disease of shorter duration, usually localized in the genital region and without systemic symptoms. A common symptom is prodromal paresthesias in the perineum, genitalia, or buttocks that occur 12 to 24 hours before the

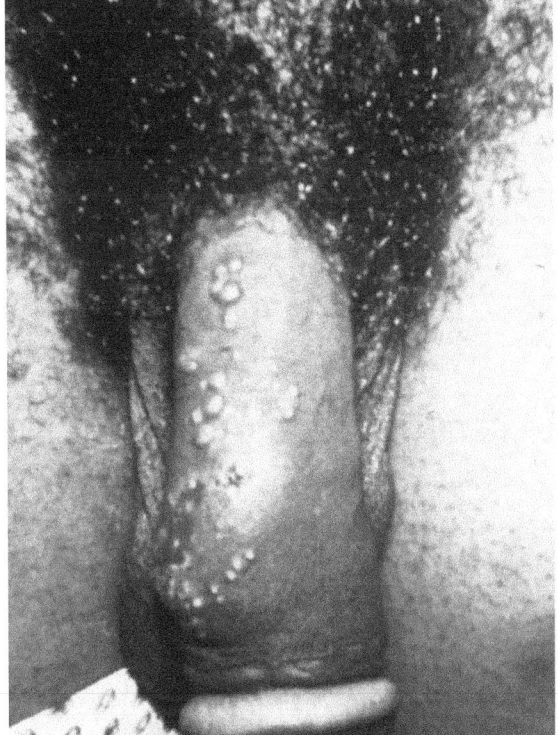

FIGURE 14–5. Multiple grouped vesicles of primary genital herpes.

appearance of lesions. Recurrent genital herpes usually presents with grouped vesicular lesions in the external genital region. Local symptoms such as pain and itching are mild, lasting 4 to 5 days, and lesions usually last 2 to 5 days.

At least 80% of patients with primary, symptomatic, genital HSV-2 infection develop recurrent episodes of genital herpes within 12 months. In patients whose lesions recur, the median number of recurrences is four or five per year. They are not evenly spaced, and some patients experience a succession of monthly attacks followed by a period of quiescence. Over time, the number of recurrences decreases by a median of one-half to one recurrence per year. Recurrences result from reactivation of virus from dorsal root ganglia. Recurrent infections due to reinfection with a different strain of HSV-2 are extremely rare. Recurrent viral shedding from the genital tract often occurs without clinically evident disease.

■ Neonatal Herpes

Neonatal herpes usually results from transmission of virus during delivery through infected genital secretions from the mother. In utero infection, though possible, is uncommon. In most cases, severe neonatal herpes is associated with primary infection of a seronegative woman near the time of delivery. This results in an intense viral exposure of a seronegative infant as it passes through the birth canal. The risk of transmission is 25% to 50% with primary HSV infection during pregnancy, whereas the risk is less than 2% with reactivation at delivery. The incidence of symptomatic neonatal herpes simplex infection varies greatly among populations, but it is estimated at between 1 per 6000 and 1 per 20,000 live births in the United States. Because a normal immune response is absent in the neonate born to a mother with recent primary infection, neonatal HSV infection is an extremely severe disease with an overall mortality rate of approximately 60%, and neurologic sequelae are high in those who survive. Manifestations vary. Some infants show disseminated vesicular lesions with widespread internal organ involvement and necrosis of the liver and adrenal glands; others have involvement of the central nervous system only, with listlessness and seizures. Intervention of transmission includes clinical exam, PCR test, C-section, and antiviral therapy. Neonatal care includes clinical exam, PCR test, and initiation of antiviral therapy (intravenous acyclovir) in suspected cases while PCR results are awaited.

DIAGNOSIS

Several diagnostic tests are available for the detection of herpes simplex virus infection, including viral culture, antigen detection, viral DNA by PCR, and antibody test.

Viral culture: HSV can be cultured in cell lines inoculated with infected secretions or lesions. The cytopathic effects of HSV can usually be demonstrated 24 to 48 hours after inoculation of the culture. Isolates of HSV-1 and HSV-2 can be differentiated by staining virus-infected cells with type-specific monoclonal antibodies. Culture can also be performed from throat, urine, and CSF samples.

Tzanck test: A direct smear prepared from the base of a suspected lesion and stained by either Giemsa or Papanicolaou method may show intranuclear inclusions or multinucleated giant cells typical of herpes (Tzanck test), but this is less sensitive than viral culture and not specific. Similar changes can be seen in cells infected with VZV.

Antigen test: Enzyme immunoassays and immunofluorescence are rapid and relatively sensitive assays for direct detection of herpes antigen in lesions. Although early versions of these noncultural tests lacked sensitivity, more recent procedures have correlations with culture that approach 90%.

HSV DNA by polymerase chain reaction (PCR): A PCR test can be performed to detect HSV genomic DNA in samples such as lesions, cells, secretions, blood, and CSF. CSF and blood is the best test to diagnose HSV encephalitis.

Antibody test: Serology should not be used to diagnose active HSV infections, such as those affecting the genital or central nervous systems; frequently, there is no change in antibody titer when reactivation occurs. Serology can be useful in detecting those with asymptomatic HSV-2 infection.

TREATMENT

Several antiviral drugs that inhibit HSV have been developed. The most commonly used is the nucleoside analog acyclovir, which is converted by a viral enzyme (thymidine kinase) to a monophosphate form and then by cellular enzymes to the triphosphate form. The triphosphate form is

Prodromal paresthesias and shorter duration

Recurrent episodes common; may involve shedding without lesions

Primary infection of mother late during pregnancy is the most common cause

✳ Usually transmitted during birth and leads to high mortality if disseminated

✳ Virus can be isolated from lesions and grown in cell culture

HSV-1 and HSV-2 distinguished by type-specific monoclonal antibodies

✳ PCR of CSF used for diagnosis of herpes encephalitis

then incorporated by the viral polymerase into the ongoing replicating viral genome leading to chain termination due to the lack of a hydroxyl group to build upon. Acyclovir significantly decreases the duration of primary infection and has a lesser but definite effect on recurrent mucocutaneous HSV infections. If taken daily, it has been shown to suppress recurrences of genital and oral–labial HSV. In its intravenous form, it is effective in reducing mortality of HSV encephalitis and neonatal herpes. Acyclovir-resistant HSV has been recovered from immunocompromised patients with persistent lesions, especially those with acquired immunodeficiency syndrome (AIDS). Foscarnet is active against acyclovir-resistant HSV.

The US Food and Drug Administration has approved both valacyclovir and famciclovir for the treatment of recurrent genital HSV. Valacyclovir is an oral prodrug of acyclovir with better bioavailability than acyclovir (54% compared with 15-20%). It is rapidly converted to acyclovir and, in every characteristic except absorption, it is identical with the parent compound. Valacyclovir is not more effective than acyclovir, but can be given in lower doses and less frequently (500 mg twice daily). Famciclovir is the prodrug of another guanosine nucleoside analog, penciclovir. The bioavailability of famciclovir is also high (77%). After conversion, penciclovir must be phosphorylated, similarly to acyclovir. Penciclovir has a longer tissue half-life than acyclovir and can be given as 125 mg twice daily for treatment of recurrent genital HSV. Valacyclovir and famciclovir are now also approved for chronic suppression of recurrent genital HSV. Valacyclovir taken daily was shown to decrease spread between discordant partners in a long-term study.

> Intravenous acyclovir effective in HSV encephalitis and neonatal disease

> ✳ Acyclovir or prodrugs can decrease duration of acute and recurrent disease

> Daily valacyclovir can decrease the spread of HSV-2 between partners

PREVENTION

Avoiding contact with individuals with lesions reduces the risk of spread; however, virus may be shed asymptomatically and transmitted from the saliva, urethra, and cervix by individuals with no evident lesions. Safe sexual practices, including condom usage reduce the risk of transmission, but the areas not covered by condom are not protected. Acyclovir has been shown to reduce asymptomatic shedding and transmission of genital herpes, especially from males to females. Because of the high morbidity and mortality rates of neonatal infection, special attention must be paid to preventing transmission during delivery. Where active HSV lesions are present on maternal tissues, Cesarean section delivery may be used to minimize contact of the infant with infected maternal genital secretions, but Cesarean delivery may not be effective if rupture of the membranes precedes delivery by more than several hours. Avoiding the birth canal is particularly important if the mother has a primary HSV infection late during pregnancy. Intravenous acyclovir is used to treat suspected cases of neonatal HSV infection. There is no current HSV vaccine available though a number have been under study for years.

> Cesarean section may be performed to reduce neonatal infection

> Intravenous acyclovir treatment for suspected neonatal infection

KEY CONCLUSIONS

- Two types of herpes simplex viruses (HSV) 1 and 2 that are enveloped, icosahedral, double-stranded DNA, and replicate in the nucleus.
- HSV is transmitted by direct contact from oral and genital lesions, saliva, and infected and genital secretions resulting in primary acute infection mainly asymptomatic followed by latency in the ganglion and periodic reactivation.
- HSV-1 causes orofacial infection such as gingivostomatitis but may also cause keratoconjunctivitis, encephalitis, eczema, and herpetic whitlow followed by latency in trigeminal root ganglion and periodic reactivation.
- HSV-2 mainly, but also HSV-1, causes genital infections in female and male, vulvovaginitis and progenitalis, respectively, followed by latency in dorsal root ganglion (sacral region) followed by periodic reactivation.
- Pathologic changes include ballooning degeneration of epithelial cells, nuclear degeneration, and formation of multinucleated giant cells.
- HSV genome is maintained as extrachromosomal DNA as episomes. Reactivation factors include sunlight, UV light, stress, trauma, etc.
- Neonates are infected during birth. Suspected cases treated with intravenous acyclovir.
- Acyclovir is monophosphorylated by HSV thymidine kinase to terminate viral DNA synthesis and used for treatment of acute and frequent recurrent infections.
- No preventive vaccine approved.

While HSV-1 causes latency in trigeminal and HSV-2 in dorsal/sacral ganglion, how does genital infection of HSV-1 latently reside in dorsal/sacral ganglion?

● VARICELLA-ZOSTER VIRUS

OVERVIEW

Varicella-zoster virus (VZV) is a member of Herpesviridae family with same morphologic and genomic features as other herpes viruses, transmitted through respiratory route and causes primary infection (chickenpox) in children and recurrent infection (shingles) mainly in older adults. Pathogenesis includes viral replication in respiratory epithelium and spread to lymph nodes followed by viremia and dissemination to various organs, including reticuloendothelial system and skin leading to formation of pustular vesicles. Symptoms include fever and lesions generally appear on the back of the head and ears, and then spread centrifugally to the face, neck, trunk, and proximal extremities. Both humoral and cell-mediated immunity play important roles, but cell-mediated immunity control infection and dissemination. Immunocompromised hosts develop viral pneumonia, encephalitis, hepatitis, etc. VZV establishes latency in sensory root ganglion like HSV. Reactivation occurs with increasing age (50% in >50 years of age) causing shingles, although it can occur at any age. Acyclovir provides some benefits in extreme cases. A two-dose live attenuated varicella virus vaccine, Vairvax or ProQuad (MMRV) is recommended for use in children (at age 1 and 4 years) and a two-dose recombinant protein subunit shingles vaccine, Shingrix, ≥age 50 years 2 to 6 months apart.

 VIROLOGY

VZV has the same general structural and morphologic features of herpes simplex and other HHVs such as enveloped, icosahedral, double-stranded DNA virion, but it contains distinct gly-coproteins and is antigenically different. The genome of VZV is approximately 125 kbp, which is the smallest genome of the HHVs. Similar to HSV, VZV encodes a thymidine kinase and is responsive to acyclovir. Cellular features of infected cells such as multinucleated giant cells and intranuclear eosinophilic inclusion bodies are similar to those of HSV. VZV is more difficult to isolate in cell culture than HSV. The virus often remains attached to the membrane of the host cell with less release of virions into fluids and thus does not spread well in culture. However, this is not the case *in vivo*, where it is the most infectious HHV.

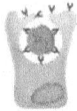 **VARICELLA-ZOSTER DISEASE**

EPIDEMIOLOGY

VZV infection occurs worldwide. In the prevaccine era, 4 million people used to get chickenpox, 10,000 to 13,000 hospitalization, and 100 to 150 deaths occurred annually in the United States. In temperate climates, greater than 90% of people contract varicella (chickenpox) by the time they reach adulthood, and most cases occur before the age of 10 years. In contrast, the mean age of infection in tropical countries is over 20 years, and the seroprevalence at the age of 70 years may be only 50%. Since the implementation of chickenpox vaccination program in 1996, the incidence of chickenpox declined 97% by 2014 from the prevaccine years in the United States. The virus is highly contagious, with attack rates among susceptible contacts of 75% making it the most infectious of the HHVs. Varicella occurs most frequently during the winter and spring months. The incubation period is 11 to 21 days. The major mode of transmission is the respiratory route, although direct contact with vesicular or pustular lesions may result in transmission. Communicability is greatest 24 to 48 hours before the onset of rash and lasts 3 to 4 days into the rash phase. Virus is difficult to isolate from patients once lesions have crusted over.

✳ VZV is acquired by respiratory route, usually before adulthood

Communicability greatest 1 to 2 days before rash onset

Think ▸▸ Apply 14-1: Orofacial infection caused by HSV-1 becomes latent, whereas genital infection by HSV-2 resides in dorsal/sacral ganglion because of the close proximity of the ganglia. Therefore, HSV-1 causing genital infection becomes latent in dorsal/sacral ganglion, because it's the location of the primary infection that determines the site of latency, not the HSV type.

Shingles or zoster results from a reactivation of VZV and occurs in approximately 20% of the population. Shingles occurrences depend on the severity of the initial infection. Shingles can occur at any age but uncommon in children. After the age of 50 years the incidence of shingles increases dramatically. Shingles provides a constant source of VZV for spread. Initial infection with VZV or spread from shingles/zoster will result in varicella or chickenpox.

PATHOGENESIS

Spread of virus by the respiratory route leads to infection of the patient's upper respiratory tract followed by replication in regional lymph nodes and primary viremia. The latter results in infection of the reticuloendothelial system and a subsequent secondary viremia associated with T lymphocytes. After secondary viremia, there is infection of the skin and ultimately, a host immune response. Latency is established in the same sensory ganglia as HSV-1 and HSV-2.

The relation between zoster and varicella was first described by Von Bokay in 1892, when he observed several instances of varicella in households after the introduction of a case of zoster. On the basis of these epidemiologic observations, he proposed that zoster and varicella were different clinical manifestations of a single agent. The cultivation of VZV *in vitro* by Weller in 1954 confirmed Von Bokay hypothesis that the viruses isolated from chickenpox and from zoster (or shingles) are identical. Latency of VZV occurs in sensory ganglia, in the dorsal root ganglia, and trigeminal ganglia. VZV latency-associated transcript (VLT) has been found to be expressed in ganglion where VZV DNA resides, suggest a role for VLT in VZV latency.

Herpes zoster (shingles) occurs when latent VZV reactivates and multiplies within a sensory ganglion and then travels back down the sensory nerve to the skin. In immunocompetent patients, the rash of herpes zoster is generally confined to the area of the skin (ie, dermatome) innervated by the sensory ganglion in which reactivation occurs. The factors that may reactivate VZV to cause shingles include advancing age, decreasing VZV-specific T cells, immunosuppression, and conditions that cause decreased immunity, etc.

IMMUNITY

Both humoral immunity and cell-mediated immunity are important factors in the VZV immune response. Cell-mediated immunity is thought to be important for cessation of spread of VZV in the body as most spread is cell associated. Reinfection with VZV is rare and is prevented by circulating antibody, whereas reactivation of VZV is apparently controlled by cell-mediated immunity.

The increase in the incidence and severity of herpes zoster observed with increasing age in immunocompetent individuals is correlated with an age-related decrease in VZV-specific cellular immunity. Beginning in the fifth decade of life, there is a marked decline in cellular immunity to VZV, which can be measured by delayed cutaneous hypersensitivity as well as by a variety of *in vitro* assays. This occurs many years before any generalized decline in cellular immunity. In patients with depressed cell-mediated immune responses, especially those with bone marrow transplants, Hodgkin disease, AIDS, lymphoproliferative disorders, and immune cancers as well as other conditions such as diabetes, reactivation often occurs, and is more frequent and severe.

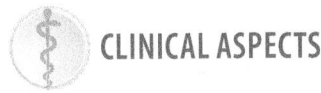

CLINICAL ASPECTS

MANIFESTATIONS

■ Varicella (Chickenpox)

VZV produces a primary infection in normal children characterized by a generalized vesicular rash termed **chickenpox** or **varicella.** After clinical infection resolves, the virus persists for decades with no clinical manifestation. Chickenpox lesions generally appear on the back of the head and ears, and then spread centrifugally to the face, neck, trunk, and proximal extremities. Involvement of mucous membranes is common, and fever may occur early in the course of disease. Lesions appear in stages of spread during the course of disease (**Figure 14–6**); this characteristic was one of the major features used to differentiate varicella from smallpox, in which lesions are concentrated on the extremities and all have a similar appearance. Skin lesions form rapidly as fluid-filled vesicles that become turbid after 1 to 2 days and then crust over. Varicella lesions are pruritic (itchy), and the number of lesions may vary from 10 to several hundred.

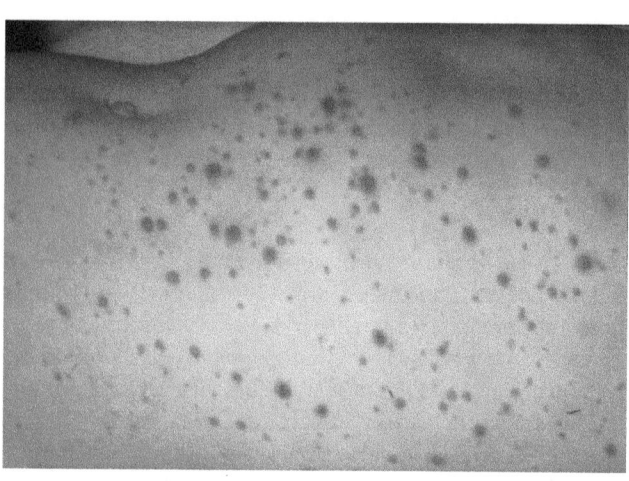

FIGURE 14–6. **Primary varicella.** Shows multiple stages of vesicles, papules, and crusted lesions on the abdomen.

Immunocompromised children may develop progressive varicella, which is associated with prolonged viremia and visceral dissemination as well as pneumonia, encephalitis, hepatitis, and nephritis. Progressive varicella has an estimated mortality rate of 20%. In thrombocytopenic patients, the lesions may be hemorrhagic. Susceptible adults upon primary infection have a higher risk (15 times) for VZV pneumonia during chickenpox. Mortality in children aged 1 to 14 years is less than 1 in 100,000 patients. However, mortality increases in primary infection of adult populations to 25 per 100,000 patients between 30 and 49 years of age.

Mortality is rare but increases with age of primary infection

Severe disease in immunocompromised patients

■ **Herpes Zoster (Shingles)**

Reactivation of VZV is associated with the disease herpes zoster. Although shingles can be found in patients of all ages, the frequency of patients developing shingles greatly increases with advancing age. Clinically, pain in a sensory nerve distribution may herald the onset of the eruption, which occurs several days to 1 or 2 weeks later. The vesicular eruption is usually unilateral, involving one to three dermatomes (**Figure 14–7**). New lesions may appear over the first 5 to 7 days. Multiple attacks of VZV reactivation and disease are uncommon; if recurrent attacks of a vesicular eruption occur in one area of the body, HSV infection should be considered. Shingles is 20% as infectious as varicella (primary infection) and contact with shingles rash causes varicella, not shingles.

Reactivation to shingles most common in elderly

✳ **Follows sensory nerve distribution**

The complications of VZV infection are varied and depend on age and host immune factors. Postherpetic neuralgia (PHN) is a common complication of herpes zoster in elderly adults. It is characterized by persistence of pain in the dermatome for months to years after resolution of the lesions of zoster and appears to result from damage to the involved nerve root. Immunosuppressed patients may develop localized shingles followed by dissemination of virus with visceral infection, which resembles progressive varicella. Bacterial superinfection is also possible. Maternal varicella infection during early pregnancy can result in fetal embryopathy with skin scarring, limb hypoplasia, microcephaly, cataracts, chorioretinitis, and microphthalmia. Severe varicella can also occur in seronegative neonates, with a mortality rate as high as 30%.

✳ **Postherpetic neuralgia can occur after zoster**

Dissemination with visceral infection in immunocompromised persons

DIAGNOSIS

Varicella or herpes zoster lesions can be diagnosed clinically as the rash is quite characteristic, and therefore laboratory diagnosis is not generally necessary. However, the lesions are occasionally difficult to distinguish from those caused by HSV. Scrapings of lesions may reveal multinucleated

FIGURE 14–7. **Herpes zoster lesion of the thorax.** Note dermatomal distribution and presence of vesicles, pustules, and ulcerated and crusted lesions.

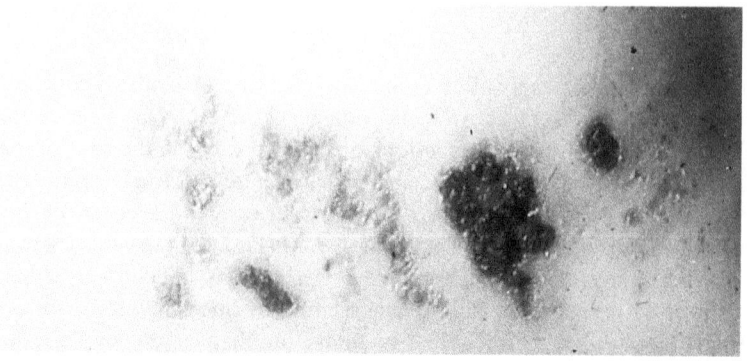

giant cells characteristic of herpesviruses, but cytologic examination does not distinguish HSV lesions from those due to VZV. For rapid viral diagnosis, varicella-zoster antigen can be identified in cells from lesions by immunofluorescent antibody staining. VZV can be isolated from vesicular fluid or cells inoculated onto human diploid fibroblasts. However, the virus is difficult to grow from zoster lesions older than 5 days, and cytopathic effects are usually not seen for 5 to 9 days, therefore PCR detection is more commonly done. PCR of CSF may be useful in the diagnosis of VZV encephalitis; culture is rarely positive.

Diagnosis usually on clinical symptoms

Rapid confirmation by antigen test or viral DNA by PCR

TREATMENT

Antiviral therapy is not recommended for healthy children with chickenpox. Acyclovir therapy can be considered for patients of >12 years of age who are at increased risk for moderate to severe disease, which has been shown to reduce fever and skin lesions in patients with varicella. In immunocompromised patients, intravenous acyclovir has been effective in reducing dissemination, and the use of this agent is indicated. In addition, controlled trials of acyclovir have demonstrated effectiveness in the treatment of herpes zoster in immunocompromised patients. Acyclovir may be used to treat herpes zoster in immunocompetent adults, but it appears to have only a moderate impact on the development of PHN, an important complication of zoster. Treatment should be started within 3 days of the onset of shingles. VZV is less susceptible than HSV to acyclovir, so the dosage for treatment is substantially higher. Famciclovir or valacyclovir is more convenient and may be more effective.

✳ Acyclovir recommended for immunocompromised patients

PREVENTION

A live, attenuated varicella virus vaccine (Varivax) derived from Oka strain given in two doses, which is 98% effective in preventing varicella and 100% effective against severe varicella disease, has been in use since 1995 in the United States. Another vaccine, ProQuad is a combination of measles, mumps, rubella, and varicella (MMRV) is also available for use in the United States. Routine immunization with Varivax or MMRV at 12 to 15 months for the first dose and 4 to 6 years of age for the second dose is recommended. For children 12 months to 12 years, two doses should be separated by 3 months and 13 years and older seronegative people, two doses 4 to 8 weeks apart is recommended. The vaccine is used routinely in immunocompetent seronegative adults, especially those with occupational risk, such as healthcare workers. The vaccine can be helpful when given to a seronegative, immunocompetent adult shortly after exposure. For the use of varicella vaccine in HIV infected patients and people with various degree of immunodeficiencies, recommendation can be found on CDC website.

✳ Live, attenuated varicella vaccine is effective and safe

Vaccination for shingles, Zostavax (a single high dose, live attenuated virus vaccine) was recommended for all people over the age of 60 years by CDC in 2006 in the United States. The vaccine stimulates the waning cellular immunity, and thereby decreases reactivation. This vaccine has been shown to be approximately 51% effective in preventing shingles and 67% effective in reducing PHN. Chronic conditions such as renal failure, heart disease, or diabetes are not contraindications, but this vaccine is not recommended for immunosuppressed patients. Varicella is a highly contagious disease and rigid isolation precautions must be instituted in all hospitalized cases. Zostavax is no longer available since November 18, 2020 for use in the United States.

A new recombinant protein (glycoprotein E antigen) with adjuvant, Shingrix, was approved on October 20, 2017 for use in the United States. Shingrix is recommended as two doses separated by 2 to 6 months for immunocompetent adults aged 50 years and older, including those who had received the older shingles vaccine (Zostavax) and whether they had or not had previous episode of shingles. This vaccine (Shingrix) has been found to be more than 90% effective in preventing shingles and PHN. Currently, it is not recommended to immunocompromised, pregnant and breastfeeding women, patients with active shingles disease, varicella seronegative individuals or with allergic reactions with any component of the vaccine.

✳ Recombinant shingles vaccine recommended for 50 years and older

Postexposure prophylaxis

High-titer immune globulin (VariZIG) administered as soon as possible and as late as 10 days after exposure is useful in preventing infection in people with lack of VZV immunity or ameliorating disease in patients at risk for severe primary infection (eg, immunosuppressed children with contact of patients with varicella or shingles). Once skin lesions have occurred, however, high-titer immune globulin has not proved useful in ameliorating disease or preventing dissemination. Immune globulin is not indicated for the treatment or prevention of reactivation (ie, zoster or shingles). In nonimmunosuppressed children, varicella is a relatively mild disease, and passive immunization is not indicated.

Varicella vaccine is recommended for postexposure prophylaxis in unvaccinated healthy people as soon as possible within 5 days after exposure. In children, the protective efficacy was reported to be >90% if given within 3 days after exposure. These people should be given the second dose of the vaccine to complete the two doses of the vaccine.

 Can an elderly person directly contract shingles from another person? Is it possible for a person to contract chickenpox from someone with shingles?

KEY CONCLUSIONS

- VZV is a member of Herpesviridae family with an enveloped, icosahedral, double-stranded DNA virus that replicates in the nucleus by using host RNA polymerase for transcription and viral DNA polymerase for genome replication.
- VZV is transmitted through inhalation and causes chickenpox (primary infection) mainly in children, and symptoms include fever and vesicular rash on head and ears, and then spread to the face, neck, trunk, and proximal extremities, and recovery in 2 weeks.
- Immunocompromised children may develop progressive varicella, including pneumonia, encephalitis, hepatitis, and nephritis.
- Viral latency in dorsal and trigeminal ganglion and reactivation mainly in older adults with increasing age and waning immunity resulting in herpes zoster or shingles, usually vesicular rash unilateral. One of the complications of shingles is PHN.
- Acyclovir can be used in extreme cases of chickenpox and shingles.
- Line attenuated varicella vaccine (Varivax) or MMRV (ProQuad) is recommended in children (first dose at age 12-15 months and second dose at 4-6 years) and recombinant shingles vaccine (Shingrix) in adults aged 50 years and older.

● EPSTEIN-BARR VIRUS

OVERVIEW

EBV, a member of Herpesviridae with similar morphological, structural, and genomic features, is the etiologic agent of infectious mononucleosis (IM) and associated with several malignancies such as African Burkitt lymphoma (BL), nasopharyngeal carcinoma (NPC), Hodgkin lymphoma, etc. Epidemiology of EBV includes 90% seroprevalence worldwide by age 2 years in developing countries and in late childhood and adolescence in developed countries. EBV is transmitted via infected secretions (saliva) and replicates in epithelial cells and B lymphocytes and later becomes latent in B lymphocytes. Most primary infections are asymptomatic, but infection in adolescence age results in clinical IM and symptoms include fever, malaise, pharyngitis, tender lymphadenitis, and splenomegaly. Complications of IM may include laryngeal obstruction, meningitis, encephalitis, hemolytic anemia, thrombocytopenia, or splenic rupture. Diagnosis is generally done by presence of a nonspecific heterophile antibodies (monospot test). CBC demonstrates 10% atypical lymphocytosis (Downey cells). EBV specific antibody panel for acute infection includes high titer anti-VCA and no titer to anti-EBNA. Treatment is supportive for IM and in some extreme cases acyclovir can be used. There is no preventive vaccine available.

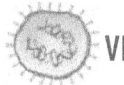 **VIROLOGY**

EBV is the main etiologic agent of IM and associated with African BL, NPC, Hodgkin lymphoma, and a number of other B-cell lymphomas. EBV is a γ-herpesvirus and the morphological and structural features are similar to members of Herpesviridae family such as enveloped,

 Think ▸▸ Apply 14-2: An elderly person cannot contract shingles because it can only be caused by neuronal reactivation from an earlier chickenpox infection. However, a person can contract chickenpox from a person with shingles (though shingles is much less infectious than chickenpox itself). Chickenpox is a primary infection and shingles is reactivation.

icosahedral, double-stranded DNA virus particle. The viral DNA genome is 172 kbp in length and contains about 100 open reading frames. The virion has glycoprotein (GP) spikes and viral capsid antigen (VCA) and teguments proteins. In lytic phase, immediate early genes include transactivators and enhancers; early genes also known as early antigens (EA) include enzymes for replication, metabolism, and immune blockage; and late genes include viral capsid proteins, VCA, and glycoproteins, Gps. *In vivo*, EBV has tropism for both human B lymphocytes and epithelial cells. *In vitro*, EBV can be cultured only in human or some primate B cells as well as limited epithelial cultures. In cultured B lymphocytes, the virus establishes a latent infection. Therefore, the virus does not produce cytopathic effects or the characteristic intranuclear inclusions of other herpesvirus infections. A low percentage of cultured primary human B cells infected with EBV grow out to form immortal lymphoblastoid cell lines (LCLs) that can grow permanently in culture and maintain EBV infection. The viral DNA in LCLs remains in a circular extrachromosomal, nonintegrated form, and is only very rarely found in the integrated state. Lytic replication can be found in LCLs induced to reactivate by cross-linking the B-cell receptor or other chemical means and follows similar gene regulation cascades as the other herpesviruses.

* Etiologic agent of infectious mononucleosis and certain lymphomas

EBV-infected cultured B cells can form immortal LCLs

■ EBV Latency

A number of different forms of latency have been described for EBV, each with a different viral gene profile. Three main types of latent infection have been characterized, though slightly different gene expression has been described in specific settings. LCLs support type III latency which is characterized by the expression of four EBV nuclear antigens (EBNAs), including EBNA-1 that is necessary to maintain the episome, and two integral membrane proteins, LMP-1 and LMP-2. A number of small RNAs are also expressed including the abundant EBERs and the BARTs that encode a number of regulatory miRNAs. Type II latency, found in NPC cells, does not express the full range of EBNA proteins but expresses many of the other viral genes found in type III latency. Type I latency is found in most BL cells and has more limited gene expression with only EBNA-1 and small regulatory RNAs expressed.

EPSTEIN-BARR VIRUS DISEASE

EPIDEMIOLOGY

Over 90% of the population is seropositive for EBV worldwide. In developing countries, most children are infected by the age of 2 years, whereas in the developed world, EBV infection occurs more often in late childhood or adolescence. When primary infection with EBV is delayed until the second decade of life or later, it is accompanied by symptoms of IM in about 50% of the cases. There are two main strains of EBV (types 1 and 2) that both circulate widely, and can coinfect a single individual. EBV is spread by direct contact of oropharyngeal secretions. The virus can be routinely cultured from saliva in 10% to 20% of healthy adults and is intermittently recovered from most seropositive individuals. It is of low contagiousness, and most cases of IM are contracted after repeated contact between susceptible persons and those asymptomatically shedding the virus. Secondary attack rates of IM are low (<10%) because most family or household contacts already have antibody to the agent. IM has also been transmitted by blood transfusions; most transfusion-associated mononucleosis syndromes, however, are attributable to CMV.

Widespread asymptomatic infection especially in children

* Mononucleosis most common in primary infection of young adults

PATHOGENESIS

Although EBV initially infects epithelial cells in the oral environment, the hallmark of EBV disease involves subsequent infection of B lymphocytes and polyclonal B-lymphocyte activation with benign proliferation. The virus enters B lymphocytes by means of envelope glycoprotein (Gp) binding to a surface receptor (CR2 or CD21), which is the receptor for the C3d component of complement system; 18 to 24 hours later, EBNAs are detectable within the nucleus of infected cells. Infection is associated with immortalization and proliferation of the B cell. The EBV-infected B lymphocytes are polyclonally activated to produce immunoglobulin and express a lymphocyte-encoded membrane antigen that is the target of host cellular immune responses to EBV-infected B lymphocytes. During the acute phase of IM, up to 20% of circulating B lymphocytes demonstrate EBV antigens. After infection subsides, EBV can be isolated from only about 1% of such cells.

* Infects oral epithelium and B cells

EBV has been associated with several lymphoproliferative diseases, including African BL and posttransplant lymphomas in immunocompromised patients. EBV is also associated with an epithelial tumor, NPC. The factors that render the EBV infections oncogenic in these cases are not clear, but a few of the type III latency genes are necessary for immortalization of B cells, in particular latent membrane protein-1. The distribution of EBV infections in Africa has suggested an infectious cofactor, such as malaria, which may lead to further activation of infected B cells and enable BL formation. *In vivo,* EBV-associated lymphomas have been shown to be of both monoclonal and polyclonal origin. In BL, translocations, involving the *c-myc* oncogene and immunoglobulin heavy or light loci, are almost invariable. These translocations lead to increased *c-myc* expression and subsequent expression of oncogenic pathways that may contribute to B-cell activation and ultimately to malignancy. EBV is present in many forms of NPC and is thought to play an etiologic role. However, environmental carcinogens and genetic factors may also be operative. Some breakdowns in immune surveillance also appear to play a role in the development of malignancy, because immunosuppressed patients are more prone to develop EBV-associated B-cell lymphomas. Furthermore, studies suggest an association of EBV with Hodgkin lymphoma in young adults, although the risk is low with 1 in 1000. The role of EBV is not clear but parts of EBV genome have been found in Reed Sternberg (RS) cells in 1 out of 4 people with classical Hodgkin lymphoma. While some studies suggest the presence of EBV early RNA (EBER1 and EBER2) in RS cells, others EBNA1, LMP1, LMP2, and Bam HIA transcripts.

EBV-associated lymphomas can develop in immunocompromised patients

EBV association with Hodgkin lymphoma

IMMUNITY

Virus-induced IM is associated with circulating antibodies against specific viral antigens, as well as against unrelated antigens found in sheep, horse, and some bovine red blood cells. The latter, referred to as **heterophile antibodies**, are a heterogeneous group of predominant IgM antibodies long known to correlate with episodes of IM, and are commonly used as diagnostic tests (monospot test) for the disease. They do not cross-react with antibodies specific to EBV, and there is no good correlation between the heterophile antibody titer and the severity of illness. Cutaneous anergy and decreased cellular immune responses to mitogens and antigens are seen early in the course of mononucleosis. The "atypical" lymphocytosis associated with IM is caused by an increase in the number of circulating T cells, which appear to be activated cells developed in response to the virus-infected B lymphocytes. With recovery from illness, the atypical lymphocytosis gradually resolves, and cell-mediated immune functions return to preinfection levels, although memory T cells maintain the capacity to limit proliferation of EBV-infected B cells. In rare cases, the initial EBV-induced proliferation of B cells is not contained, and EBV lymphoproliferative disease ensues. This syndrome is most often seen in immunocompromised organ transplant recipients.

✳ Suppressed cell-mediated immune responses in acute infection

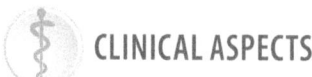 **CLINICAL ASPECTS**

MANIFESTATIONS

■ Infectious Mononucleosis

Most primary EBV infections are asymptomatic. However, infections in the second decade of life often lead to clinically apparent IM. IM is characterized by fever, malaise, pharyngitis, tender lymphadenitis, and splenomegaly. These symptoms persist for days to weeks; they slowly resolve. Complications such as laryngeal obstruction, meningitis, encephalitis, hemolytic anemia, thrombocytopenia, or splenic rupture may occur in 1% to 5% of patients. Many of these IM patients are heterophile antibody positive.

Primary infection asymptomatic or infectious mononucleosis heterophile-positive

Splenomegaly can occur

■ Lymphoproliferative Syndrome

Patients with primary or secondary immunodeficiency are susceptible to EBV-induced lymphoproliferative disease. The incidence of these lymphomas is 1% to 2% after renal transplantations and 5% to 9% after heart–lung transplantations. The risk is greatest in patients experiencing primary EBV infection rather than reactivation. The most characteristic symptoms are persistent fever, lymphadenopathy, and hepatosplenomegaly.

Lymphoproliferative disease occurs, especially in immunocompromised

■ Burkitt Lymphoma

In sub-Saharan Africa, endemic BL is the most common malignancy in young children, with an incidence of 8 to 10 cases per 100,000 people per year. Endemic BL is almost always associated with EBV. The risk is greatest in equatorial Africa, where there is a high incidence of malaria. Endemic BL commonly occurs along the jawline or orbit of the eye in children. Endemic BL is thought to result from an early EBV infection that produces a large pool of infected B lymphocytes. Malarial infection may further increase the size of this pool and provide a constant antigenic challenge. Such stimuli can increase the chances of c-*myc* chromosomal translocations, which are pathognomonic for this lymphoma. Serologic screening for increased IgA antibody levels to both VCA and early EBV antigens (EA) can be used for early diagnostic purposes. In the United States and other countries where BL is not endemic, EBV is associated with 15% to 30% of sporadic BL while c-*myc* translocations are still invariable in all forms.

＊ African endemic BL is strongly associated with EBV

c-*myc* translocations occur in EBV-associated and unassociated BL

■ Other EBV-associated lymphomas

Hodgkin lymphoma: There are four histologic subtypes of Hodgkin lymphoma (HL) with a broad range of EBV association. Overall, approximately 30% of HL are associated with EBV in the United States and other developed countries. A much higher percentage of HL is associated with EBV in developing countries. In 1 out of 4 HL cases, EBV is present in Reed-Sternberg cells, large often multinucleated cells of B-cell origin.

Non-Hodgkin lymphoma: Additionally, EBV is associated with a lower percentage of other B-cell lymphoma including diffuse large B-cell lymphoma (DBCL). EBV is also associated with some T-cell lymphomas as well.

■ Nasopharyngeal Carcinoma

NPC, an epithelial-derived tumor, is endemic in southern China, where it is responsible for approximately 25% of the mortality from cancer. The high incidence of NPC among the southern Chinese people suggests that in addition to EBV, genetic or environmental factors may also be important in the pathogenesis of the disease.

EBV-associated endemic NPC in southern China

■ AIDS Patients

In patients with AIDS, several distinct additional EBV-associated diseases may occur, including hairy leukoplakia of the tongue, interstitial lymphocytic pneumonia (especially in infants), and increased incidence of lymphoma described earlier. EBV is also associated with posttransplant lymphoproliferative disorders (PTLD).

DIAGNOSIS

Laboratory analysis of EBV IM is usually documented by the demonstration of atypical lymphocytes and heterophile antibodies or positive EBV-specific serologic findings. Hematologic examination reveals a markedly raised lymphocyte and monocyte count with more than 10% atypical lymphocytes, called **Downey cells** (**Figure 14–8**). Atypical lymphocytes, which are probably both EBV-specific and nonspecific, are present with the onset of symptoms and disappear with resolution of disease. Alterations in liver function tests may also occur, and enlargement of the liver and spleen is a common finding.

＊ Atypical lymphocytosis common in acute infection

Though not specific for EBV, tests for heterophile antibodies generally known as monospot test are used most commonly for diagnosis of IM. In commercial kits, animal erythrocytes are used in simple slide agglutination methods, which incorporate absorptions to remove cross-reacting antibodies that may develop in other illnesses, such as serum sickness. The IM heterophile antibody is absorbed by sheep erythrocytes but not by guinea pig kidney cells. Heterophile antibodies can usually be demonstrated by the end of the first week of illness, but are occasionally delayed until the third or fourth week. They may persist for many months. Approximately 5% to 15% of EBV-induced cases of IM in adults and a much greater proportion in young children and infants fail to induce detectable levels of heterophile antibodies.

＊ Non-specific heterophile antibodies (monospot test) detected in EBV IM

EBV-specific serologic tests are available as summarized in **Table 14–2** and may be used to establish the diagnosis of EBV infection. The panel includes antibodies to VCA, which rise quickly (IgM) and disappears with 4 to 6 weeks followed by the appearance of IgG that persists for life (IgG). Antibodies to EBV nuclear antigens (EBNAs) rise later in disease (after about 2 months)

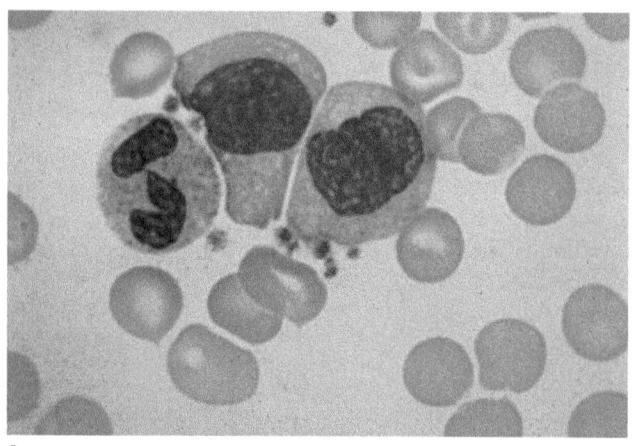

A

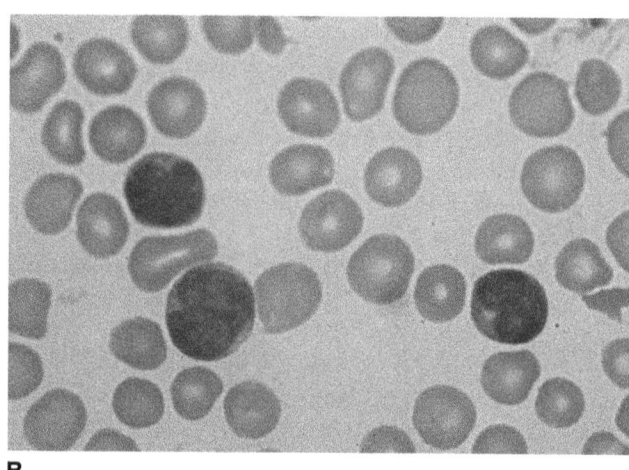

B

FIGURE 14–8. **A.** Atypical lymphocytes (Downey cells) in blood smear from a patient with infectious mononucleosis. Note indented cell membranes. Polymorphonuclear leukocyte is adjacent to the two affected cells. **B.** Normal lymphocytes contrast sharply with those in A.

and also persist at low titers for life. Thus, a high titer to VCA and no titer to EBNA antibodies suggest recent EBV infection, whereas antibody titers to both antigens are indicative of past infection. The presence of IgM antibody to VCA is theoretically diagnostic of acute, primary EBV infection, but low levels may occur during reactivation of EBV, and cross-reactions with antigens of other herpesviruses occur. Antibodies to EBV early antigens (EA-D or EA-R) appears in acute infection and becomes undetectable, however; persistence of EA antibodies indicates ongoing infection and may correlated with severe diseases such as NPC, NPC (anti-EA-D), or African BL (anti-EA-R), but are not useful in diagnosing IM. Isolation of EBV from clinical specimens is not practical, because it requires fresh human B cells or fetal lymphocytes obtained from cord blood.

* IgM or high IgG anti-VCA with negative anti-EBNA suggest primary infection

Virus isolation is impractical for routine diagnosis

TREATMENT AND PREVENTION

Treatment of IM is largely supportive. More than 95% of patients recover uneventfully. In a small percentage of patients, splenic rupture may occur; restriction of contact sports or heavy lifting during acute illness is recommended. Lytic replication of EBV has been shown to be sensitive to acyclovir, and acyclovir can decrease the amount of replication of EBV in tissue culture and

TABLE 14–2	Epstein-Barr Virus—Specific Antibodies		
ANTIBODY SPECIFICITY	TIME OF APPEARANCE	DURATION	COMMENTS
Viral capsid antigen (VCA)			
IgM	Early in illness	1-2 months	Indicator of primary infection
IgG	Early in illness	Lifelong	Standard Epstein-Barr virus (EBV) titer reported by most commercial and state laboratories; major usefulness is as marker for prior infection in epidemiologic studies; if present without EBNA (Epstein-Barr nuclear antigen) antibody, indicates current infection
EBNA IgG	3-6 weeks after onset	Lifelong	Late appearance of anti-EBNA IgG antibodies in infectious mononucleosis (IM) makes absence or seroconversion a useful marker for primary infection; persists for life
Early antigen (EA) diffuse protein (EA-D)	Peaks 3-4 weeks after onset	3-6 months	Present in IM patients; IgA antibodies useful for prediction of nasopharyngeal carcinoma in high-risk populations
EA restricted (EA-R)	Several weeks after onset	Months to years	Present in higher titer in African Burkitt lymphoma; may be useful as indicator of reactivation of EBV

in vivo. Despite this antiviral activity, systemic acyclovir makes little or no impact on the clinical illness. Laryngeal obstruction should be treated with corticosteroids. Hairy leukoplakia in patients with AIDS does respond to acyclovir treatment. There is currently no approved vaccine for EBV and few preventative measures other than limiting saliva transmission.

IM treatment is supportive

Immunization of humans not available

KEY CONCLUSIONS

- EBV is a member of γ-herpesvirus and some of the viral components that are important for diagnosis and pathogenesis include viral EA, VCA, glycoprotein (Gp), EBV nuclear antigens (EBNAs), and LMPs.

- Pathogenesis includes transmission though infected secretions such as saliva and infection of epithelial cells in the oral environment and subsequent infection of B lymphocytes by viral Gp binding to a surface receptor CR2 or CD21. Infection is associated with immortalization and proliferation of the B cell and EBNAs are detected in the nucleus of these cells.

- Acute infection causes IM (heterophile antibody positive) in which 20% of B lymphocytes demonstrate EBV antigens. There are also activated T cells with 10% atypical lymphocytes known as Downey cells.

- There are nonspecific heterophile antibodies seen during EBV infection in majority of the patients which could be used for diagnosis by monospot test.

- EBV-specific tests for acute infection included IgM or high titer IgM anti-VCA and no titer to anti-EBNAs.

- No specific treatment or preventive vaccine.

- EBV is associated with lymphoproliferative disease in immunocompromised people.

- Several other diseases associated with EBV include NPC (endemic in southern China), BL (endemic in sub-Saharan Africa), Hodgkin lymphoma, and hairy leukoplakia (in AIDS patients).

CYTOMEGALOVIRUS

OVERVIEW

Cytomegalovirus (CMV) is a β-herpesvirus with similar morphological, structural, and genomic features as other herpesviruses. It produces cytopathic effects in cell culture with nuclear inclusion which looks like owl's eyes and cytoplasmic inclusion and enlargement (cytomegaly). In developed countries, 50% to 75% of people and more than 90% in developing countries are infected with CMV. CMV is found in all bodily fluids and transmitted through close contact and infects mucosal epithelial cells, vascular endothelial cells, leukocytes, monocytes, and CD34+ pluripotent stem cells that can differentiate into monocytes maintain latency for CMV. Most people are asymptomatic, some people have mild symptoms such as fever, sore throat, swollen lymph nodes, and some have mononucleosis (heterophile-negative) or hepatitis. In immunosuppressed and immunocompromised patients, interstitial pneumonia, chorioretinitis, gastroenteritis, and neurologic disorders have been described. Pathogenesis include disease caused by viral-mediated direct tissue damage and immunologic damage. Congenital CMV infection occurs in 1% of the infants worldwide. Most infants appear normal at birth, but may develop hearing loss or some mental retardation often later. Infants with symptomatic illness at birth demonstrate hepatosplenomegaly, jaundice, anemia, low weight, microcephaly, rash, thrombocytopenia, chorioretinitis. Diagnosis is generally done by PCR or antigen test. Ganciclovir can be used for treatment. There is no vaccine available but several candidates are under development.

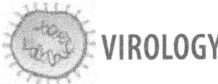 VIROLOGY

Human cytomegalovirus (CMV) is a β-herpesvirus named for the cytopathic effect it produces in cell culture. In addition to nuclear inclusions ("owl's eye cells"), CMV produces perinuclear cytoplasmic inclusions and enlargement of the cell (cytomegaly) (**Figure 14–9**). CMV possesses the largest genome of the HHVs (approximately 240 kbp). Similar to the α-herpesviruses, CMV gene expression is highly regulated with the sequential appearance of IE, E, and L gene products, though the replication cycle is much slower. The viral DNA is transcribed to mRNA by host RNA polymerase and the viral genome is replicated by viral DNA polymerase. CMV also encodes a viral kinase encoded by UL97 gene, which is utilized to efficiently monophosphate antiviral, ganciclovir, that terminates the elongating viral DNA synthesis. Based on genomic and phenotypic

✳ Nuclear and perinuclear cytoplasmic inclusions and cell enlargement

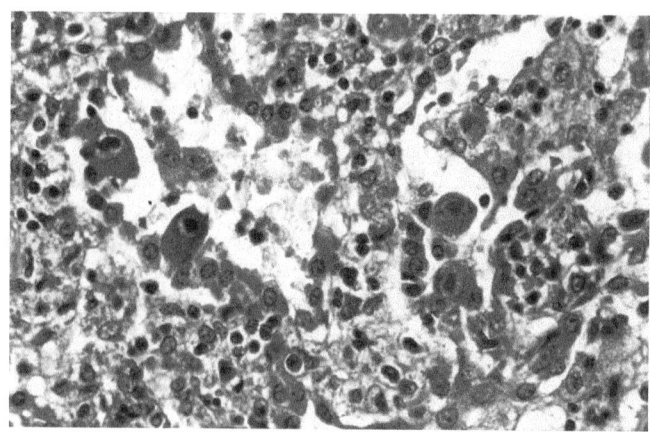

FIGURE 14–9. **Cytomegalovirus-infected cells showing "owl's eye" appearance of intranuclear inclusions.** (Reproduced with permission from Nester EW, Anderson DG, Roberts CE Jr, et al: *Microbiology: A Human Perspective*, 6th ed. New York, NY: McGraw Hill; 2008.)

heterogeneity, innumerable strains of CMV exist. Antigenic variations have been observed but are not of clinical importance. Laboratory-adapted strains grown in cell culture rapidly lose a 10 to 15 kbp region of CMV genomic DNA that limits tropism in culture.

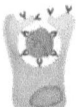

CYTOMEGALOVIRUS DISEASE

EPIDEMIOLOGY

CMV infection is distributed worldwide. In developed countries approximately 50% to 75% of adults have developed antibody with even higher percentages (more than 90%) in lower socioeconomic strata and in the developing world. Age-specific prevalence rates show that approximately 10% to 15% of children are infected by CMV during the first 5 years of life, after which the rate of new infections levels off. The rate subsequently increases by 1% to 2% per year during adulthood. Infection probably occurs through close personal contact, including sexual contact with a virus-excreting person. CMV has been isolated from saliva, cervical secretions, semen, urine, and white blood cells for months to years after infection. Excretion of CMV is especially prolonged after congenital and perinatal infections, with 35% of infected infants excreting virus for as long as 5 years after birth. Transmission of infection in day care centers has been shown to occur from asymptomatic excreters to other children and, in turn, to seronegative parents. By 18 months, up to 80% of infants in day care centers are infected and actively excreting virus in saliva and urine. Seroconversion rates in seronegative parents who have children attending day care centers are approximately 20% per year, as parents are infected by the children. In contrast to day care centers, there is no substantial evidence for the spread of CMV infection to healthcare workers in hospitals.

Latent infection occurs in leukocytes and their precursors and accounts for transfusion transmission, but this route is relatively infrequent—only 1% to 2% of blood units are believed to be infectious. Organ donation may also transmit latent virus, which causes primary infection in CMV-seronegative recipients and reinfection in seropositive patients.

PATHOGENESIS

CMV infects mucosal epithelial cells, vascular endothelial cells, and leukocytes and produces characteristic inclusions in the vascular endothelial cells. *In vitro*, CMV DNA can be demonstrated in monocytes showing no cytopathology, indicating a restricted growth potential in these cells. It is conjectured that these as well as the CD34+ pluripotent stem cells that can differentiate into monocytes maintain latency for CMV.

CMV can cause disease by a variety of mechanisms, including direct tissue damage and immunologic damage. Although direct infection and damage of mucosal epithelial cells in the lung is a potential mechanism for pneumonia, animal models have suggested that immunologic destruction of the lung by the host immune response to CMV infection may be the major mechanism of viral disease in this tissue. This hypothesis is supported by the observation that the degree of viral infection in lung tissue cannot account for the severity of CMV pneumonia; likewise, the disease does not respond well to antiviral therapy. Although cytolytic T-lymphocyte activity may contribute to lung pathology, cytokines released by these cells have also been implicated.

* High infection rates in early childhood and early adulthood

Present in urine, saliva, semen, and cervical secretions

Viral latency in leukocytes

CMV DNA in monocytes

Immune-mediated tissue damage in lungs

IMMUNITY

Both humoral and cellular immune responses are important in CMV infections. In immunocompetent persons, clinical disease, if it occurs at all, results from primary infection. Reactivation and viral excretion in cervical excretions or semen are invariably subclinical. In immunocompromised patients, both primary infection and reactivation are much more likely to be symptomatic. Furthermore, CMV infection of monocytes results in dysfunction of these phagocytes in immunocompromised patients, which may increase predisposition to fungal and bacterial superinfection. When latently infected monocytes are in contact with activated T lymphocytes, the former are activated to differentiate into macrophages that produce infectious virus. These monocyte–T cell interactions may occur after transfusion or transplantation and may explain not only the transmission of CMV but also activation of latent virus in the allograft recipient.

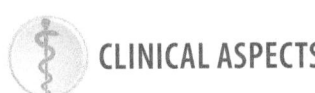

CLINICAL ASPECTS

MANIFESTATIONS

CMV infection in healthy people is usually asymptomatic. In some cases, there can be mild illness with symptoms, including fever, sore throat, fatigue, and swollen glands. However, in some healthy young adults, CMV may cause a mononucleosis-like syndrome (heterophile antibody negative) or hepatitis. In immunosuppressed patients, both primary infection and reactivation may be severe. For example, in patients receiving bone marrow transplants, interstitial pneumonia caused by CMV is a leading cause of death (50-90% mortality rate), and in patients with AIDS, CMV often disseminates to visceral organs, causing chorioretinitis, gastroenteritis, and neurologic disorders. CMV retinitis is the main cause of blindness in patients with AIDS. More importantly, antiretroviral therapy in HIV-infected patients, which has reduced the viral load and improved CD4 T cell counts, has resulted in a significant reduction of these opportunistic infections.

> CMV infection usually asymptomatic in healthy adults
>
> Some have mononucleosis-like syndrome, heterophile-negative
>
> CMV lung, visceral, eye infections in immunocompromised

Congenital infection in CMV is a huge concern because CMV can be transmitted vertically to the fetus in utero leading to deafness or other congenital defects. Worldwide, 1% of infants excrete CMV in urine or nasopharynx at delivery as a result of infection in utero. On physical examination, 90% of these infants appear normal or asymptomatic; however, long-term follow-up has indicated that 10% to 20% go on to develop sensory nerve hearing loss, psychomotor mental retardation, or both. Infants with symptomatic illness (about 0.1% of all births) have a variety of congenital defects or other disorders, such as hepatosplenomegaly, jaundice, anemia, thrombocytopenia, low birth weight, microcephaly, and chorioretinitis. Almost all infants with clinically evident congenital CMV infection are born to mothers who experienced primary CMV infection during pregnancy. The apparent explanation is that the fetus is exposed to virus in the absence of maternal antibody. It is estimated that one-third of maternal primary infections are transmitted to the fetus and that fetal damage is most likely to occur in the first trimester. Congenital infection frequently also results from reactivation in the mother with spread to the fetus, but such infection rarely leads to congenital abnormalities because the mother also transmits antibody to the fetus. It is more common for second children to have congenital CMV infection. This is thought to be due to the first child obtaining CMV in day care, a common place for spread, and infecting the naïve pregnant mother.

> * Serious disease of fetus with primary maternal infection
>
> Most infants asymptomatic at birth
>
> Some have symptoms at birth and defects; hepatosplenomegaly, jaundice, anemia, thrombocytopenia, microcephaly, chorioretinitis
>
> Congenital infection a leading cause of deafness

In contrast to the devastating findings with some congenital infections, neonatal infection acquired during or shortly after birth is rarely associated with adverse outcomes. Most population-based studies have indicated that 10% to 15% of all mothers are excreting CMV from the cervix at delivery. Approximately one-third to one-half of all infants born to these mothers acquire infection. Illness is rare in perinatally infected infants unless the infant is premature or immunocompromised. CMV can also be efficiently transmitted from mother to child by breast milk, but these postpartum infections are also usually benign. As with intrapartum acquisition of infection, most CMV infections during childhood are asymptomatic.

DIAGNOSIS

Laboratory diagnosis of CMV infection depends on (1) detecting CMV cytopathology, antigen, or DNA in infected tissues; (2) detecting viral DNA or antigen in body fluids; (3) isolating the virus from tissue or secretions; or (4) demonstrating seroconversion. CMV can be grown in serially propagated diploid fibroblast cell lines. Demonstration of viral growth generally requires 1 to

14 days, depending on the concentration of virus in the specimen and whether fluorescence immuno-staining is used to speed detection. The presence of large inclusion-bearing cells in urine sediment may be detected in widespread CMV infection. This technique is insensitive, however, and provides positive results only when large quantities of virus are present in the urine. Culture of blood to detect viremia is now superseded by detection and quantitation of CMV antigen in peripheral blood leukocytes or detection of CMV DNA in plasma or leukocytes by PCR. These procedures are significantly more sensitive than culture.

Because of the high prevalence of asymptomatic carriers and the known tendency of CMV to persist for weeks or months in infected individuals, it is frequently difficult to associate a specific disease entity with the isolation of the virus from a peripheral site. Thus, the isolation of CMV from the urine of immunosuppressed patients with interstitial pneumonia does not constitute evidence of CMV as the cause of that illness. CMV pneumonia or gastrointestinal disease is best diagnosed by demonstrating CMV inclusions in biopsy tissue.

The procedures listed below are recommended to facilitate the diagnosis of CMV infection in specific clinical settings:

1. *Congenital infection*—Virus culture or viral DNA assay positive at birth or within 1 to 2 weeks (to distinguish from natally or perinatally infected infants, who will not begin to excrete virus until 3-4 weeks after delivery).

2. *Perinatal infection*—Culture-negative specimens at birth but positive specimens at 4 weeks or more after birth suggest natal or early postnatal acquisition. Seronegative infants may acquire CMV from exogenous sources, such as from blood transfusion.

3. *CMV mononucleosis in nonimmunocompromised patients*—Seroconversion and presence of IgM antibody specific for CMV are best indicators of primary infection. Urine culture positivity supports the diagnosis of CMV infection, but may reflect remote infection because positivity may continue for months to years. A positive blood assay for CMV antigen or DNA, however, is diagnostic in this patient population.

4. *Immunocompromised patients*—Demonstration of virus by viral antigen or DNA in blood documents viremia. Demonstration of inclusions or viral antigen in diseased tissue (eg, lungs, esophagus, or colon) establishes the presence of CMV infection, but does not provide proof that CMV is the cause of disease unless other pathogens are excluded. Seroconversion is diagnostic but rarely occurs, especially in patients with AIDS, because more than 95% of these patients are seropositive for CMV before infection with human immunodeficiency virus (HIV). CMV-specific IgM antibody may not be present in immunocompromised transplant patients, especially during reactivation of virus. Conversely, in patients with AIDS, this antibody frequently is present even when clinically important infection is absent.

TREATMENT

Ganciclovir, a nucleoside analog of guanosine structurally similar to acyclovir, has been shown to inhibit CMV replication, prevent CMV disease in patients with AIDS and transplant recipients, and reduce the severity of some CMV syndromes such as retinitis and gastrointestinal disease. Combining immune globulin with ganciclovir appears to reduce the very high mortality from CMV pneumonia in bone marrow transplant recipients more than that achieved with ganciclovir alone. However, unlike acyclovir, ganciclovir has some toxicity. Foscarnet, a second approved drug for therapy of CMV disease, is also efficacious. Its toxic effects are primarily renal, whereas ganciclovir is most apt to inhibit bone marrow function. Ganciclovir is phosphorylated by the viral kinase, UL97 and acts as a chain terminator when incorporated by the CMV DNA polymerase. Valganciclovir, also approved for use as a CMV therapeutic, is a prodrug of ganciclovir and provides increased bioavailability. Foscarnet inhibits the CMV polymerase and is used as a second-line drug for CMV. A third drug, cidofovir, a nucleotide analog, is approved for therapy of retinitis, but its use is limited to ganciclovir-resistant infections in immunosuppressed patients because of nephrotoxicity.

PREVENTION

The use of blood from CMV-seronegative donors or blood that is treated to remove white blood cells decreases transfusion-associated CMV. Similarly, the disease can be avoided in seronegative transplant recipients by using organs from CMV-seronegative donors. Washing hands, avoiding

* DNA detection by PCR or antigen detection is useful to identify viremia

Histologic detection of inclusions in lung, gastrointestinal tissues is useful

CMV-seronegative donors for seronegative recipients decrease risk of posttransplant complications

contact with tears, saliva, and sharing food and drinks, and safe sexual practices including condom usage may reduce transmission. There is currently no vaccine available. However, several vaccines are under development, including an mRNA-style vaccine.

 Why is HSV-2 primary infection of a pregnant mother of more concern late during pregnancy, while CMV infection is of more concern early in pregnancy?

KEY CONCLUSIONS

- CMV is an enveloped, icosahedral, double-stranded DNA virus that replicates in the nucleus by using host RNA polymerase for RNA synthesis and viral DNA polymerase for genomic DNA synthesis.
- CMV is transmitted through saliva and other bodily secretions, infects mucosal epithelial cells, vascular endothelial cells, and leukocytes, and produces characteristic inclusions in the vascular endothelial cells.
- While most people are asymptomatic, some get mild illness and mononucleosis or hepatitis. The diseases take a severe form in immunocompromised patients, including lungs, eye, visceral organs, and neurological disorders.
- Congenital infection is a major concern which may cause hepatosplenomegaly, jaundice, anemia, thrombocytopenia, low birth weight, microcephaly, chorioretinitis, and hearing loss.
- Some conditions are treated by ganciclovir or foscarnet for ganciclovir resistance.
- Currently no vaccine is available, but several are under development.

● HUMAN HERPESVIRUS 6

In 1986, a herpesvirus, now called human herpesvirus type 6 (HHV-6), was identified in cultures of peripheral blood lymphocytes from patients with lymphoproliferative diseases. HHV-6 is β-herpesvirus subfamily. The virus is morphologically similar to other herpesviruses with similar replication patterns of other herpesviruses. HHV-6 replicates in lymphoid tissue, especially CD4+ T lymphocytes, and has two distinct variants, A and B, that are genetically disparate enough that some consider them different species.

✴ Replicates in CD4+ T lymphocytes

EPIDEMIOLOGY

Of the herpesviruses, HHV-6 is the most rapidly spread and is shed in the throats of 10% of infants by age 5 months, 70% by 12 months, and 30% of adults. Greater than 90% of the population has antibody to this virus by the age of 5 years.

Infection common in infancy

MANIFESTATIONS

HHV-6 type B is the main etiologic agent of exanthem subitum (roseola), and both types A and B can cause acute febrile illnesses with or without seizures or rashes. Exanthem subitum generally occurs in infants aged 6 months to 1 year. In the first 6 months, infants are generally protected by the mother's IgG. Exanthem subitum is characterized by fever (usually about 39°C) for 3 days, followed by a faint maculopapular rash spreading from the trunk to the extremities, which begins during defervescence. Exanthem subitum is one of the six classic childhood exanthems. Some of the other symptoms may include otitis, gastrointestinal or respiratory distress, and seizures. The manifestation of seizures indicates neurotropism for HHV-6.

✴ Associated with roseola in infants

HHV-6 also appears to reactivate in transplant recipients. It may contribute to graft rejection and clinical illnesses such as meningoencephalitis, pneumonia, and bone marrow suppression after bone marrow transplantation. The virus reactivates in other immunocompromised patients

 Think ▸▸ Apply 14-2: HSV-2 is most often vertically transmitted during the birth process. So infection late in pregnancy leads to neonatal herpes since the newborn has not received antibodies from the mother. CMV crosses the placental barrier leading to birth defects that are more severe during early fetal development.

including those with AIDS, lymphoma, and leukemia, but its clinical significance is not fully understood. Attempts have been made to associate HHV-6 persistence with many other disease states including multiple sclerosis, chronic fatigue syndrome, and Alzheimer's disease. However, due to the ubiquitous nature of the virus, disease association is difficult to assess.

HHV-6 infects mainly T lymphocytes and establishes a latent infection in T cells but maybe activated to a productive lytic infection by mitogenic stimulation. Resting lymphocytes and lymphocytes from normal immune individuals are resistant to HHV-6 infection. *In vivo*, HHV-6 replication is controlled by cell-mediated factors.

DIAGNOSIS

Primary virus infection can be documented by seroconversion. Active virus infection can be documented by culture, antigenemia, or DNA detection in the blood (by PCR). Because asymptomatic viremic reactivation is common, it is very difficult to use these tools to identify HHV-6 as the cause of febrile or other miscellaneous syndromes.

TREATMENT

Definitive therapy has not been established, but like the better characterized β-herpesvirus, CMV, HHV-6 appears to be susceptible *in vitro* to ganciclovir and foscarnet. It is less susceptible to acyclovir because the virus has no thymidine kinase.

● HUMAN HERPESVIRUS 7

Isolation of human herpesvirus 7 (HHV-7) was first reported in 1990. The virus was isolated from activated CD4+ T lymphocytes of a healthy individual. The CD4 molecule appears to be a receptor for virus attachment. HHV-7 is closely related to HHV-6 and is in the β-herpesvirus genus. Seroepidemiologic studies indicate that this virus usually does not infect children until after infancy, but that nearly 90% of children are antibody positive by 3 years of age. As with HHV-6, this virus is frequently isolated from saliva, and close personal contact is the probable means of transmission. HHV-7 DNA has been detected in skin, lungs, tonsils, liver, and kidneys. There is little disease associated with HHV-7; however, it may also be a cause of exanthem subitem and some other erythemato-papular rash, but the association has only been found in rare cases. The diagnosis of acute infection can be made by the demonstration of seroconversion. No treatment has been identified.

● HUMAN HERPESVIRUS 8

During the AIDS epidemic in the 1980 in the United States, Kaposi Sarcoma (KS) occurred in 20% to 30% of men who have sex with men (MSM) or bisexual males with AIDS but in only around 1% of hemophiliacs with AIDS. This led to the proposal that there was another infectious agent associated with KS. In 1994, unique viral DNA sequences were identified in KS tumors using subtractive hybridization analysis. The sequences bore homology to γ-herpesviruses and were used to clone the entire 165 kbp genome of the eighth HHV, commonly known as KS-associated herpesvirus (KSHV) or HHV-8. KSHV is found in 100% of KS tumors.

EPIDEMIOLOGY

KSHV is the least widespread HHV. In the United States, 5% or less of healthy blood donors are seropositive. Worldwide the seroprevalence varies dramatically. In central Africa, where KS is endemic, KSHV seroprevalence can reach 50%. Classic KS is more common in Southern Italy where seroprevalence approaches 25%, whereas in Northern Italy where KS is less common, where the seroprevalence is closer to 10%. As noted earlier, in the United States, KS was common in the gay and bisexual AIDS community where the seroprevalence rates perfectly match the KS rates at around 25%, whereas in hemophiliacs with AIDS, the seroprevalence rates were similar to healthy blood donors. The relationship of seroprevalence rates and KS probability were critical for collaring KSHV as the etiologic agent of KS. KSHV is also associated with two rare lymphoproliferative diseases, primary effusion lymphoma, where KSHV is nearly 100% associated, and multicentric Castleman disease (MCD), where it is associated with 50% of AIDS-related cases.

KSHV seropositive rates correlate with numbers of sexual partners and was originally thought to be transmitted sexually. However, the virus is not found in sexual secretions but is shed in saliva. Because the virus is not ubiquitous like the other saliva-transmitted herpesvirus, it is not likely to be easily transmitted by kissing and may require more prolonged intimate contact.

KSHV can be shed in saliva but is not easily transmitted

PATHOGENESIS

KSHV infects the oral epithelium and can be shed into saliva for transmission. KSHV is also found in the B-cell fraction of peripheral blood mononucleocytes. In B cells, KSHV is predominantly in the latent state although lytic antigens can be found in a low percentage of the cells. In KS tumors, KSHV is found in the main tumor cell, the spindle cell, a cell of endothelial origin. KSHV is found in all spindle cells in later-stage tumors. Again, the virus is found predominantly in the latent state, though 1% to 5% of the spindle cells support lytic antigens and likely replication and virus production. In culture, KSHV can infect many cell types where it establishes latency in most of the cells. Similar to the KS tumor, a low percentage of endothelial cells infected in culture also express lytic antigens.

CLINICAL MANIFESTATIONS

■ KS—Four Forms of Disease

There are four main forms of KS: classic, endemic, iatrogenic, and epidemic or AIDS-associated. The forms vary in the degree of severity but are indistinguishable at the pathologic level. KSHV is associated with all four forms.

1. *Classic KS*—Originally described in the 1800s by Moriz Kaposi, it is a rare, fairly indolent tumor mainly found on the lower extremities. It is mostly seen in elderly men of Mediterranean origin and was also described in Ashkenazi jews.
2. *Endemic KS*—In the middle of the 20th century, KS became common in central Africa, where in countries like Uganda, it is the most common tumor reported in hospitals. It is more aggressive than classic KS and tumors can be seen higher on the extremities and in the oral cavity and the torso.
3. *Iatrogenic KS*—KS also arises in posttransplant patients but generally regresses upon the removal of immunosuppression.
4. *Epidemic or AIDS-associated KS*—This is the most aggressive form of KS, with the tumors often appearing first in the mouth, on the torso, and face, and can also be found on internal organs. Without treatment for HIV, it can lead to death.

Primary effusion lymphoma (PEL): PELs have high mortality and KSHV is associated with nearly 100% of this pleural cavity B-cell lymphoproliferative disease. EBV is also present in 50% to 70% of PELs and may play a contributing role in these cases. Unlike BL, there are no known obvious genetic abnormalities in PELs.

Multicentric Castleman disease (MCD): MCD is a B-cell lymphoproliferative disease of the lymph nodes and 50% of AIDS-associated MCD is associated with KSHV. The infected cells in MCD have a much higher percentage of cells expressing lytic antigen than other KSHV-associated tumors.

DIAGNOSIS

Diagnosis for KSHV infection is currently imperfect. Immunofluorescence with sera from infected patients is a standard technique but has a sensitivity of only 70% to 90%. PCR from peripheral blood mononucleocytes of patients with KS is possible, but in seropositive patients without KS, KSHV DNA is difficult to detect.

TREATMENT AND PREVENTION

A number of antiherpesviral drugs inhibit lytic replication of KSHV with foscarnet being the most active followed by ganciclovir. There is evidence that treatment with ganciclovir is positively indicated for MCD because it is a more lytic disease. No treatment for latently infected cells or vaccine is available.

Can EBV- or KSHV-related cancers be treated with herpesvirus antivirals?

CASE STUDY

A "Kissing" Disease

A 17-year-old girl was healthy before entering college as a freshman. Two months later, she noted an illness that progressed over a few days, beginning with fatigue and difficulty concentrating. Other symptoms followed, including fever, sore throat, headache, and "fullness" in the neck.

The physical examination revealed conjunctival and pharyngeal inflammation and enlarged, slightly tender lymph nodes in the anterior and posterior cervical triangles.

QUESTIONS

1. Which one of the following agents most likely caused the infection in this patient?
    A. HSV-1
    B. HSV-2
    C. VZV
    D. EBV
    E. CMV

2. If this patient has acute, primary Epstein-Barr virus infection, which of the following would be the most sensitive and specific confirmatory test?
    A. IgG-specific anti-VCA antibody and undetectable anti-EBNA antibody
    B. IgG-specific anti-EBNA antibody
    C. Heterophile antibodies
    D. Circulating atypical lymphocytosis of 20% or greater
    E. PCR of serum

3. The major sites of herpesvirus latency are listed in the right-hand column. Match these with the viruses in the left-hand column.
    a. HSV-1 _____
    b. HSV-2 _____   A. Nerve ganglia
    c. CMV _____   B. Monocytes
    d. VZV _____   C. B lymphocytes
    e. EBV _____

4. Which one of the following infections/diseases can be prevented by vaccination?
    A. HSV-1 primary infection
    B. Varicella-zoster reactivation
    C. HSV-2 reactivation
    D. CMV primary infection
    E. EBV reactivation

ANSWERS

1. **(D)**

2. **(A)**

3. a(A), b(A), c(B), d(A), e(C)

4. **(B)**

 Think ▸▸ Apply 14-3: Both EBV- and KSHV-related cancers are primarily associated with latent infection. All herpesvirus antivirals solely target lytic infection and so have less effect. However, MCD has a large lytic gene component so there is some benefit to antiviral treatment.

Viruses of Diarrhea

OVERVIEW

Viral gastroenteritis (inflammation of stomach, small, and large intestine) is caused by rotaviruses, caliciviruses, astroviruses, and some adenoviruses serotypes (enteric), which results in vomiting and/or diarrhea. In addition to the bacterial and protozoal agents responsible for approximately 20% to 25% of these cases, these viruses are a significant cause of the balance. Acute diarrheal disease is an illness, usually of rapid evolution (within several hours), that lasts less than 3 weeks. Worldwide, diarrhea caused by rotavirus resulted in an estimated 528,000 infants' death in 2000, which has dropped to an estimated 128,500 in 2016 due to rotavirus vaccination. The vaccine has averted 28,000 deaths in 2016. In the United States, the total annual deaths before the vaccine era used to be less than 60, but these viruses were still the major causes of severe illness and hospitalization in early life. Since the introduction of rotavirus vaccine in the United States in 2006, rotaviruses-related illness, and hospitalizations have significantly dropped, and deaths are rare. Symptoms of the rotavirus disease like vomiting, abdominal cramps, and low-grade fever followed by watery stools that usually do not contain mucus, blood, or pus, are all characteristics of the acute phase of illness and can also be seen with infections due to caliciviruses, astroviruses, and adenoviruses. Following successful rotavirus vaccination, caliciviruses have become the leading cause of viral diarrhea in the United States.

GENERAL FEATURES

Until the 1970s, proof of viral causation of acute diarrhea was usually based on exclusion of known bacterial or protozoan pathogens and supported by feeding cell-free filtrates of diarrheal stools to volunteers to reproduce the disease. As might be expected, the results of such experiments were variable, and the methods were impractical for routine laboratory diagnosis. One aspect of such infections that proved to be of great help was the frequent association with abundant excretion of virus particles during the acute phase of illness. Virion numbers greater than 10^8 per gram of diarrheal stool are relatively common, allowing ready visualization with an electron microscope **(Figure 15–1)**. Direct electron microscopy and immunoelectron microscopy were used to detect and identify the presumed causative viruses; the latter method was also used to detect humoral antibody responses to infection. More recently, polymerase chain reactions (PCRs) and enzyme immunoassays (EIAs) are employed in diagnosis.

A diagnosis of exclusion

Viral particles in stool by electron microscopy

Confirmation by PCR or EIA

Several criteria were used to establish the role of viruses in diarrheal diseases, including detecting viruses in symptomatically ill patients more frequently than in asymptomatic individuals, demonstrating significant antibody response in patients shedding the virus, reproducing the disease by experimental inoculation of nonimmune human or animal hosts, and excluding other known causes of diarrhea such as bacteria, bacterial toxins, and protozoa.

Multiple criteria for establishing etiologic relationship

Using the above criteria, four groups of viruses have been clearly established as important causes of gastrointestinal disease: rotaviruses, caliciviruses, astroviruses, and some adenovirus serotypes ("enteric" adenoviruses). Other viruses have also been implicated, but many of the preceding criteria have not been fulfilled; therefore, they are currently regarded as "candidate" causes of gastrointestinal disease.

✳ Rotaviruses, caliciviruses, astroviruses, adenoviruses serotypes established causes

The currently established viruses are listed in **Table 15–1,** and all have several features in common, including a tendency toward brief incubation periods; fecal–oral spread by direct or indirect routes; and production of vomiting, which generally precedes or accompanies diarrhea.

"Candidate" viruses meet some criteria

FIGURE 15–1. **Viruses of diarrhea.** All are photographed at the same magnification to illustrate the size and morphologic differences. **A.** *Rotavirus.* **B.** Calicivirus. **C.** Astrovirus. (Used with permission from Claire M. Payne.)

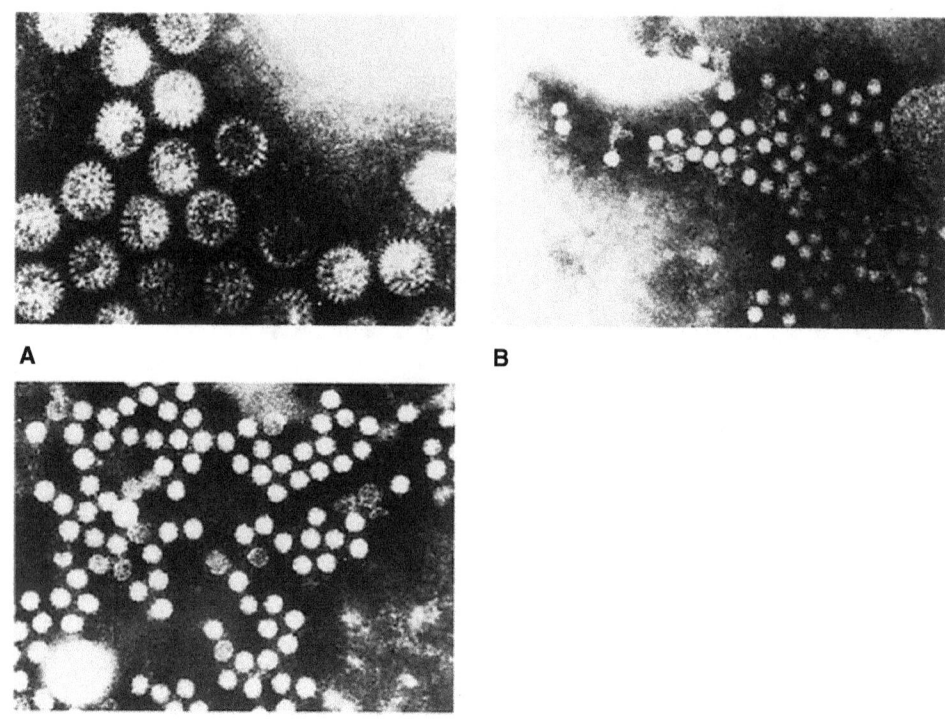

A

B

C

TABLE 15–1	Biologic and Epidemiologic Characteristics of Viruses That Cause Diarrhea			
SPECIAL FEATURES	**ROTAVIRUS**	**CALICIVIRUS**	**ASTROVIRUS**	**ADENOVIRUS**
Biologic				
Nucleic acid	Double-stranded RNA	Single-stranded (+) RNA	Single-stranded (+) RNA	Double-stranded DNA
Diameter, shape	65-75 nm, naked, icosahedral, double-shelled capsid	27-38 nm, naked, icosahedral, round	28-38 nm, naked, star-shaped	70-90 nm, naked, icosahedral
Replication in cell culture	Yes	Yes	Yes	Yes
Number of serotypes	5 important to humans	More than 4	8, perhaps more	2, perhaps 7
Pathogenic				
Site of infection	Duodenum, jejunum	Jejunum	Small intestine	Small intestine
Mechanism of immunity	Local intestinal IgA	Unknown	Unknown	Unknown
Epidemiologic				
Epidemicity	Epidemic or sporadic	Family and community outbreaks	Sporadic	Sporadic
Seasonality	Usually winter	None known	None known	None known
Ages primarily affected	Infants, children aged <2 years	Older adults, adults, children, infants	Infants, children	Infants, children
Method of transmission	Fecal–oral	Fecal–oral; contaminated water and shellfish	Fecal–oral	Fecal–oral
Incubation period (days)	1-3	0.5-2	1-2	8-10
Major diagnostic tests	PCR, EIA, EM	PCR, EM, IEM	PCR, EM	PCR, EIA, EM

EIA, enzyme immunoassay; EM, electron microscopy; IEM, immunoelectron microscopy; PCR, polymerase chain reaction.

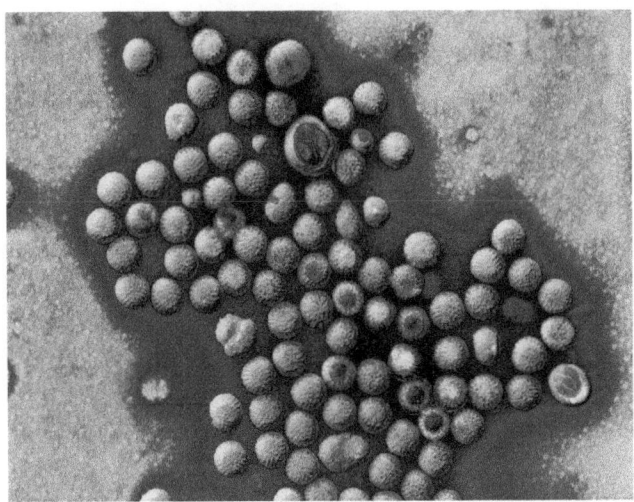

FIGURE 15-2. *Rotavirus* struc-ture. (Reproduced with permission from Willey JM: *Prescott, Harley, & Klein's Microbiology*, 7th ed. New York, NY: McGraw Hill; 2008.)

The last feature has influenced physicians to use the term **acute viral gastroenteritis** to describe the syndrome associated with these agents.

Vomiting, short incubation period

Just general knowledge.

● ROTAVIRUSES

The human intestinal rotaviruses were first found in 1973 by electron microscopic examination of duodenal biopsy specimens from infants with diarrhea (**Figure 15–2**). Since then, they have been found worldwide and are believed to account for 40% to 60% of cases of acute gastroenteritis occurring during the cooler months in infants and in children less than 5 years of age, with most serious disease in 3 to 35 months of age. Worldwide, more than 528,000 deaths in children younger than 5 years of age in 2000 were attributed to rotavirus infections mainly in Sub-Saharan Africa, South Asia, and Southeast Asia, which has dropped to 128,000 in 2016 due to rotavirus vaccination. Four countries, including India, Nigeria, Pakistan, and Democratic Republic of Congo accounted for 49% of rotavirus-related deaths under 5 years of age in 2013, with 22% alone in India. In the United States, more than 400,000 doctor visits, 200,000 emergency room visits, 50,000 to 70,000 hospitalizations, and 20 to 60 deaths were reported before the rotavirus vaccine was introduced in 2006. Now such deaths in the United States are rather infrequent; the annual morbidity rate has significantly dropped. Before the introduction of rotavirus vaccines in 2006, almost all children were infected in the United States before their fifth birthday. The routine use of rotavirus vaccine in infants has significantly reduced rotavirus infection in the United States. These viruses have been detected in intestinal contents and in tissues from the upper gastrointestinal tract.

✴ Most common cause of winter gastroenteritis and serious diarrheal disease in unvaccinated children

VIROLOGY

The rotaviruses belong to the family Reoviridae. The genome of rotaviruses is unique in the sense that they have 11 segments of double-stranded RNA. The 11 segments of the genome encode six structural (VP1–VP4 and VP6–VP7) and six nonstructural (NSP1–NSP6) proteins (**Figure 15–3A**). There are three types of virus particles, including triple layered (previously called double shelled), double layered (previously called single shelled), and single layered (empty capsids, usually lacking genomes) (Figures 15–1A, 15–2). The complete virus particle of rotavirus is a wheel-shaped virus and the name is derived from the Latin *rota* ("wheel") because of the outer capsid, which resembles a wheel attached by short spokes to the inner capsid and core (Figures 15–1, 15–2, 15–3A). Eleven segments of double-stranded RNA genome are packaged into an icosahedral capsid making the spherical particles of 65 to 75 nm in diameter in size (smaller forms have also been described) (**Figure 15–3B-D**). The virus particle has a virion-associated RNA-dependent RNA polymerase and a double-shelled outer capsid; two segments encode proteins of the outer capsid (VP4 or P and VP7 or G), which are targets for neutralizing antibodies. The major outer capsid proteins are VP4 and VP7. VP4 performs several functions, including viral attachment protein, whereas VP7 is a type-specific antigen and facilitates viral attachment and entry.

Wheel-shaped naked capsid spherical viruses

✴ Eleven segments of double-stranded RNA genome replicates in the cytoplasm

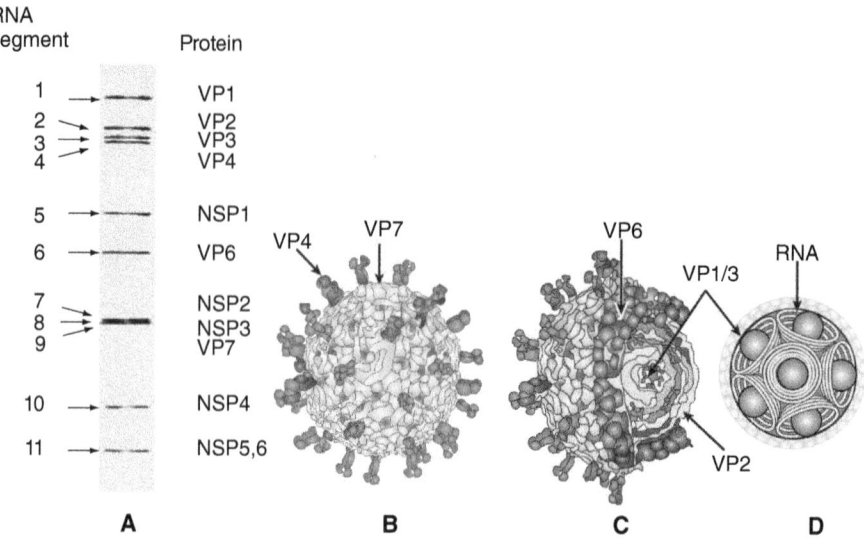

FIGURE 15–3. **Structure of Rotavirus. A.** Eleven segments of rotavirus are shown on a gel, each segment encoding corresponding structural (VP1–VP7) or nonstructural (NSP1–NSP6) proteins are shown. **B.** Structure of rotavirus showing outer layer capsid proteins, including VP4 (spikes) and VP7 (outer capsid layer). **C.** A cutaway view of rotavirus showing the inner VP6 (blue) and VP2 (green layers). **D.** Rotavirus ds RNA genome segments represented as inverted conical spirals. (Used with permission from BVV Prasad.)

✳ Double-shelled (triple-layered) outer capsid

Group A rotaviruses infect humans

Five antigenic types based on capsid proteins VP4, VP7

Rotaviruses are classified into seven groups, A to G, based on the internal capsid protein, VP6. Human infections are predominantly caused by group A and less commonly by group B or C. Based on VP4 and VP7 type-specific antigens on the outer capsid, G (VP7 is a glycoprotein) and P (VP4 is protease-sensitive) serotypes have been designated. Five serotypes (G1, G2, G3, G4, and G9) are of major epidemiologic importance because they represent more than 90% of all serotypes detected worldwide. G1 serotype represents more than 75% of the isolates. The outer capsid is proteolytically cleaved in the gastrointestinal tract to generate intermediate infectious subviral particle (ISVP), which activates the virus for infection. Rotaviruses can replicate in the cytoplasm of infected cell cultures in the laboratory and successful propagation of human strains *in vitro* has been achieved in cell lines.

Rotavirus replication is depicted in **Figure 15–4.** Rotavirus is transmitted by fecal–oral route, and the virus particle is partially digested in the gastrointestinal tract and activated by protease

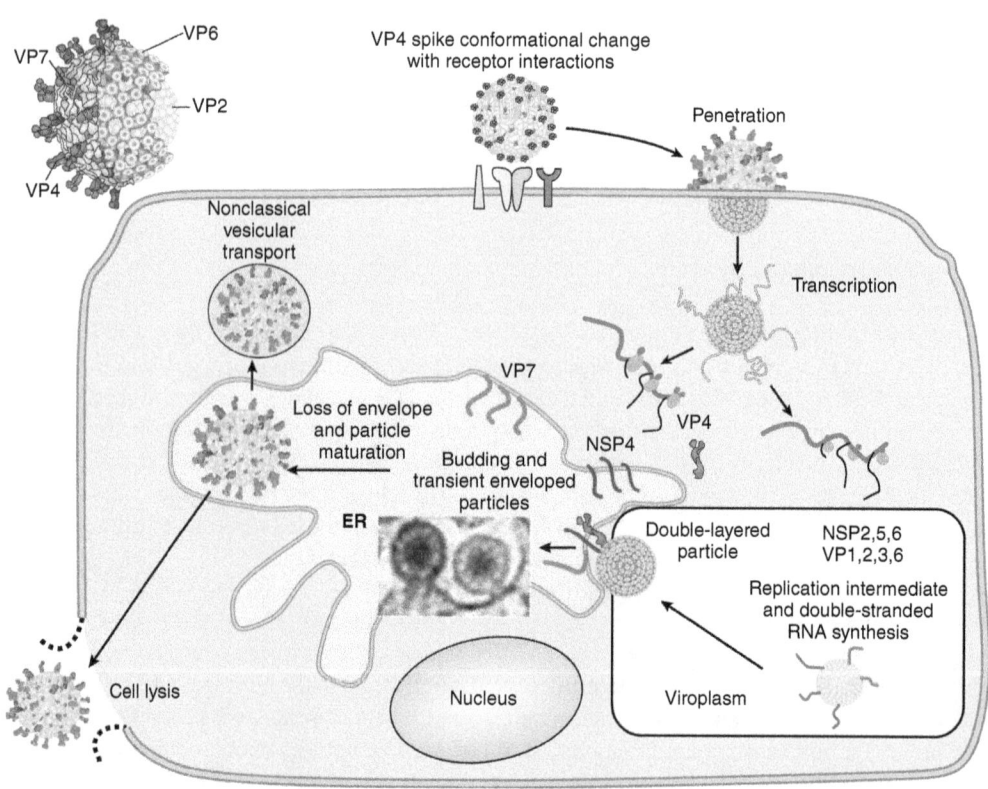

FIGURE 15–4. **Schematic diagram of Rotavirus replication.** Rotavirus outer capsid spike (VP4) binds to the receptor (sialic acid-containing glycoprotein) followed by a conformational change, removal of outer layer, and penetration of the virus in the target cells. Following partial uncoating, viral RNA-dependent RNA polymerase directs the transcription of viral mRNAs followed synthesis of viral proteins, by genome replication by using the negative-strand RNA of the double-stranded RNA genome. Rotavirus assembles by associating its core with a nonstructural protein (NSP4) and acquiring VP7 and a membrane budding from the ER. The virus eventually loses the membrane in the ER and is released upon cell lysis. (Used with permission from MK Estes.)

cleavage resulting in the loss of VP7 and cleavage of VP4 to generate ISVP. The VP4 binds to sialic acid-containing glycoproteins on epithelial cells, and the ISVP penetrates the target cells. The generation of ISVP is necessary for rotavirus infection because the double-shelled virus particle, after entering the cells via receptor-mediated endocytosis, is unable to establish infection owing to a dead-end pathway. After entry of the ISVP, the core containing double-stranded RNA genomes and the RNA-dependent RNA polymerase is partially released into the cytoplasm. Rotaviruses use negative-sense RNA strategy for transcription and replication. RNA-dependent RNA polymerase directs the synthesis of early and late mRNAs followed by genome replication by using the negative-strand RNA of the double-stranded RNA genome. Early proteins are produced that are required for virus replication, whereas late proteins are mainly the structural proteins. Rotavirus assembles by associating its core with a nonstructural protein (NS28, a product of NSP4) and by acquiring VP7 and a membrane budding into the endoplasmic reticulum (ER). The virus eventually loses the membrane in the ER and is released upon cell lysis.

Fecal–oral trans

ISVP infectious, virion

VP4 binds to sialic acid-glycoprotein

＊ Viral RNA polymerase directs the synthesis of mRNA and genomic RNA using negative-strand RNA of ds RNA genome

Assembly takes place at the ER

Release on cell lysis after losing membrane

 Why does rotavirus contain 11 segments of RNA?

Rotaviruses of animal origin are also highly prevalent and produce acute gastrointestinal disease in a variety of species. Very young animals, such as calves, suckling mice, piglets, and foals, are particularly susceptible. The animal rotaviruses can often replicate in cell cultures, and infection across species has been accomplished experimentally; however, there is no evidence that such interspecies spread occurs in nature (eg, animal rotaviruses are not known to affect humans and vice versa).

One unique feature of rotaviruses is the ease with which the 11 RNA segments can undergo reassortment. This has enabled the development of live vaccines that combine genes from readily cultivated animal rotaviruses with human rotavirus genes that encode serotype-specific capsid proteins.

Animal rotaviruses produce diarrhea, but not humans

Reassortment of the 11 RNA segments occurs

Live, attenuated vaccines incorporate genes from animal viruses

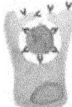 HUMAN *ROTAVIRUS* INFECTIONS

EPIDEMIOLOGY

Outbreaks of rotavirus infection were common in the prevaccine era, particularly during the cooler months, among infants and children of less than 5 years of age, but the incidence of clinical illness was highest among 3 to 35 months of age. Older children and adults can also be affected, but attack rates are usually much lower, and the disease is milder. Outbreaks among elderly, institutionalized patients have also been recognized.

Although newborn infants can be readily infected with the virus, such infections often result in little or no clinical illness. This finding is illustrated by reported infection rates of 32% to 49% in some neonatal nurseries, but mild illness in only 8% to 28% of the infants. It is unclear whether this transient resistance to disease is a result of host maturation factors or transplacentally conferred immunity. Seroepidemiologic studies have been useful in demonstrating the ubiquity of these viruses and may help to explain the age-specific attack rates. By the age of 5 years, almost all individuals have humoral antibodies, suggesting a high rate of virus infection early in life.

＊ Primarily affects infants and children in colder months

Most of the older children and adults are immune

PATHOGENESIS

Rotaviruses appear to localize primarily in the duodenum and proximal jejunum, causing destruction of villous epithelial cells with blunting (shortening) of villi and variable, usually mild, infiltrates of mononuclear and a few polymorphonuclear inflammatory cells within the villi. The gastric and colonic mucosa is unaffected; however, for unknown reasons, gastric emptying time is markedly delayed. The primary pathophysiologic effects are a decrease in absorptive surface in the small intestine and decreased production of brush border enzymes, such as the disaccharidases. The net result is a transient malabsorptive state, with defective handling of fats and

Think ▸▸ Apply 15-1: **Rotavirus has 11 segments of RNA so it can follow the monocistronic rule of one RNA one protein.**

sugars. It may take as long as 3 to 8 weeks to restore the normal histologic and functional integrity of the damaged mucosa. Although the specific gene product associated with virulence is not yet known, some evidence suggests that one nonstructural protein, NSP4, may behave as an enterotoxin in a manner similar to that of the heat-labile enterotoxin (LT) of *Escherichia coli* and cholera toxin. This may further explain the excess fluid and electrolyte secretion in the acute phase of illness. Viral excretion usually lasts 2 to 12 days but can be greatly prolonged in malnourished or immunodeficient patients with persistent symptoms.

* Destroys villous cells of jejunum and duodenum

Absorptive surface is decreased

* Enterotoxin-like effects are also present

 Why does rotavirus infection cause malabsorption in infected children?

IMMUNITY

* Long-term immunity after subsequent infections

Type-specific humoral, secretory IgA antibodies protective

IgA, mucin glycoproteins confer protective role of breastfeeding

Rotavirus infection responds with production of type-specific humoral antibodies that probably do not last for a lifetime after the first infection. Recovery from the first infection provides 38% protection against infection, 77% protection against diarrhea, and 87% protection against severe diarrhea. Subsequent infections provide long-term immunity. In addition, type-specific secretory IgA antibodies are produced in the intestinal tract, and their presence seems to correlate best with immunity to reinfection. Breastfeeding also seems to play a protective role against rotavirus disease in young infants. Secretory IgA antibodies to rotaviruses appear in colostrum and continue to be secreted in breast milk for several months postpartum. Human breast milk mucin glycoproteins have also been shown to bind to rotaviruses, inhibiting their replication *in vitro* and *in vivo*.

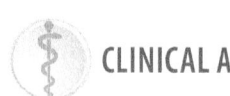 **CLINICAL ASPECTS**

MANIFESTATIONS

* Severe dehydration can lead to death

* Short incubation, vomiting, watery diarrhea lead to dehydration

After an incubation period of 1 to 3 days, there is usually an abrupt onset of vomiting, followed within hours by frequent, copious, watery, brown stools. In severe cases, the stools may become clear; the Japanese refer to the disease as **hakuri**, the "white stool diarrhea." Fever, usually low grade, is often present. Vomiting may persist for 1 to 3 days, and diarrhea for 4 to 8 days. The major complications result from severe dehydration, occasionally associated with hypernatremia.

DIAGNOSIS

Viral RNA by RT-PCR or antigen by EIA in stool specimen detects virus

Diagnosis of acute rotavirus infection is usually by detection of virus particles, antigen, or virion RNA in the stools during the acute phase of illness. This can be accomplished by immunologic detection of antigen with EIA methods or virion RNA by RT-PCR. Direct examination of the specimen by electron microscopy can also be done primarily in research setting. However, RT-PCR of the viral RNA is widely used for diagnosis.

TREATMENT AND PREVENTION

No specific treatment

* Vigorous fluid, electrolyte replacement

There is no specific treatment for rotavirus infection. Vigorous replacement of fluids and electrolytes is required in severe cases and can be lifesaving. The rotaviruses are highly infectious and can spread quickly in family and institutional settings. Control consists of rigorous hygienic measures, including careful handwashing and adequate disposal of enteric excretions.

Previously developed live attenuated or reassortant rhesus-based rotavirus vaccine was developed and licensed in the United States in 1998 but withdrawn because of some side effects (intussusception). In 2006, a live, attenuated, oral bovine/human reassortant vaccine that contains five reassortant rotaviruses (RV5) developed from human and bovine strains (RotaTeq developed by Merck) was licensed for routine use in the United States. It is a three-dose series at 2, 4, and 6 months of age. A second live, attenuated oral vaccine, RV1 (Rotarix) that contains one live,

 Think ▸▸ Apply 15-2: **Rotavirus damages villous cells that reduce the absorptive space in the intestine causing transient malabsorption.**

attenuated human strain (developed by GlaxoSmithKline) was licensed in 2008 for a two-dose series, administered at 2 and 4 months. The minimum age for the first dose administration is 6 weeks and maximum age is 14 weeks and 6 days. The minimum interval between doses is 4 weeks and all doses should be completed by 8 months of age. To date, its efficacy after a three-dose series has been excellent, and no safety concerns have arisen. The efficacy of the vaccine in preventing infection is between 85% and 98%. However, rotavirus vaccine should not be given to infants aged 15 months and above due to lack of availability of safety data. While the vaccine is safe, mild problems such as temporary diarrhea or vomiting may occur. In addition, 1 in 20,000 to 1 in 100,000 infants may have intussusception (a bowel blockage) with rotavirus vaccination.

Rigorous hygienic measures to prevent the spread

✳ Live, attenuated oral rotavirus vaccines are available and recommended for infants

Vaccine dose administration important

● CALICIVIRUSES

Although the caliciviruses were the first to be clearly associated with outbreaks of gastroenteritis, considerably less is known about their biology than about that of the rotaviruses. Caliciviruses belong to Caliciviridae family. Two genera, *Norovirus* and *Sapovirus*, infect humans. Caliciviruses were first associated with an outbreak in Norwalk, Ohio, in 1968, and their role was confirmed by production of disease in volunteers fed fecal filtrates. The original virus was thus called the **Norwalk agent,** and similar viruses have been given names such as Hawaii agent, Montgomery County agent, Ditchling agent, and so on. Following rotavirus vaccination, norovirus has become the leading cause of viral gastroenteritis in infants and children in the United States.

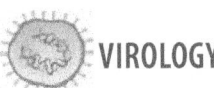 ## VIROLOGY

Caliciviruses are small, naked capsid, icosahedral symmetry, positive-sense RNA-containing particles 27 to 38 nm in diameter; their appearance is similar to that of parvoviruses and hepatitis A virus (Figure 15–1B). The viral capsid is made up of two proteins, VP1 and VP2. The nonstructural proteins include viral protease and viral RNA-dependent RNA polymerase. The virus replicates in the cytoplasm like other positive-sense RNA viruses by using its viral RNA polymerase for transcription and replication, and virus assembly in the cytoplasm and release upon cell lysis. At present, two genera of caliciviruses that cause diarrhea are noroviruses (the family prototype) and sapoviruses. *Norovirus* particles are round, whereas other calicivirus particles are star-shaped. The viruses appear to be extremely hardy; their infectivity persists after exposure to acid, ether, and heat (60°C for 30 minutes). After 48 years of the identification of norovirus as a causative agent of diarrhea, it can now be grown in intestinal epithelial cells in the laboratory.

Five different *Norovirus* serotypes or genotypes (GI-GV) have been identified, with three genotypes (GI, GII, and GIV) infecting humans, as demonstrated by immunoelectron microscopy with convalescent sera from affected patients and genetic analysis. Knowledge of the antigenic characteristics and biology of these viruses was hampered by the inability to grow them in the laboratory. However, development of the new tissue culture system to grown norovirus in the laboratory may enhance the knowledge about the genetics and pathogenesis of noroviruses.

Small, round, naked, icosahedral capsid RNA viruses are hardy

Two genera: *Norovirus* and *Sapovirus* cause diarrhea in humans

✳ Several serotypes/genotypes can be grown in the laboratory

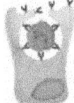 ## CALICIVIRUS INFECTIONS

EPIDEMIOLOGY

Calicivirus (norovirus) infection occurs worldwide with an estimated 685 million cases, including 200 million in children below age 5 years and 50,000 child deaths every year mainly in developing countries. In the United States, between 19 and 21 million cases of noroviruses are reported annually, including 2.3 million outpatient visits, 46,5000 emergency room visits, 56,000 to 109,000 hospitalizations, and 900 deaths mostly among adults aged 65 years and older. Generally, they are the most common cause of nonbacterial gastroenteritis in adults. However, with the implementation of the rotavirus vaccine in the United States, norovirus has become the leading cause of viral gastroenteritis in children below 5 years of age. They can infect any time of the year but are most common during the winter months. Sharp family and community outbreaks are common and can occur in any season. The noroviruses have been particularly a major issue in closed settings, such as cruise ships, hospitals, nursing homes, and schools. Moreover, norovirus is responsible for causing more

Transmission is by fecal–oral route

685 million cases, 50,000 deaths in developing countries

20 million infections, 900 deaths in the United States

✽ Norovirus common in older adults spreads in community centers, hospitals, nursing homes, cruise ships

✽ Now leading cause of viral gastroenteritis in infants children in the United States

than 90% of the diarrhea outbreaks on the cruise ships. The major sources of transmission include contaminated food, person to person, water, and unknown source. Caliciviruses are much more common causes of gastrointestinal illness in older children and adults. This difference in age-specific predilection is perhaps reflected in serosurveys, which have shown that the prevalence of antibodies rises slowly, reaching approximately 50% by the fifth decade of life, a striking contrast to the frequent acquisition of antibodies to rotaviruses early in life. Because rotavirus infection has significantly reduced due to vaccination, norovirus has now become a leading cause of viral diarrhea in infants and children in the United States. Transmission is primarily by fecal–oral route; outbreaks have also been associated with consumption of contaminated water, uncooked shellfish, and other foods. Sharp outbreaks include older children and adults.

PATHOGENESIS

Enterotoxic features are not present

Both the pathogenesis and the pathology are similar to those described for rotaviruses, except that no enterotoxic features have yet been described for caliciviruses. Biopsy of the intestinal tissue shows that the intestinal mucosa is intact but there are histological changes such as broadening and blunting of the villi, shortening of the microvilli, enlarged and pale mitochondria, increased cytoplasmic vacuolization, and intercellular edema. These mucosal changes usually revert to normal within 2 weeks of onset of illness. Virus shedding in the feces generally lasts no more than 3 to 4 days.

IMMUNITY

Reinfection can occur with same serotypes

Patients and experimentally infected volunteers respond to infection with the production of humoral antibodies, which persist for a long time; their role in protection from reinfection, however, appears minimal. Reinfection and illness with the same serotype occur, and the role of local (mucosal) antibody (IgA) has not been well defined. It is possible that nonimmune or genetic factors are essential for protection.

 CLINICAL ASPECTS

Clinical picture and diagnostic tests similar to those for Rotavirus

No treatment or vaccine exists

The incubation period is 12 to 48 hours (0.5-2 days), followed by abrupt onset of vomiting and diarrhea, a syndrome clinically indistinguishable from that caused by rotaviruses. Patients infected with noroviruses experience more vomiting than sapoviruses. The most common complication is dehydration. Respiratory symptoms rarely coexist, and the duration of illness is relatively brief (usually 1-2 days). These viruses can be detected by electron microscopy or immunoelectron microscopy in stools during the acute phase of illness. In addition, EIA and PCR methods have been developed. As with rotavirus infection, there is no specific treatment other than fluid and electrolyte replacement. Prevention requires good hygienic measures such as washing hands with soap and water, especially before eating or handling food, using toilet or changing diapers, etc. Currently, there is no vaccine available.

 While norovirus causes gastroenteritis in adults, why it has now become a leading cause of diarrheal disease in infants and children?

● ASTROVIRUSES

Star-shaped virus

Illness is often, but not always mild

Astroviruses belong to the family Astroviridae. Astroviruses have a shape that resembles a five- or six-pointed star (Figure 15–1C). These have been known since 1975. In recent years, astroviruses have been acknowledged as causes of often-mild gastroenteritis outbreaks, primarily among toddlers, school children, and elderly nursing home residents. Eight human serotypes, 1 to 8, of astroviruses have been identified.

 Think ▸▸ Apply 15-3: Because rotavirus, which used to cause diarrhea in infants/children, is now prevented by vaccination, therefore, norovirus has also become a leading cause of diarrhea in infants and children.

Astroviruses are star-shaped, 28 to 38 nm, naked capsid, icosahedral, positive-sense RNA viruses. The virions are spherical, and the shape and genome resemble that of some calicivirus members. The genome of 6.8 to 7.9 nucleotides encodes a full length and a subgenomic RNA. Subgenomic RNA encodes structural proteins, whereas full-length RNA encodes RNA-dependent RNA polymerase. Astroviruses are acid stable, heat resistant for a short period of time, and resistant to a range of detergents and lipid solvents. The replication cycle of the astroviruses is not fully characterized because of the lack of a reliable cell culture system. However, astroviruses have been propagated in primary human embryonic kidney cells with fecal extracts containing astroviruses. The virus most likely replicates similar to other positive-sense RNA viruses in the cytoplasm by first translating the RNA genome into a polyprotein followed by proteolytic cleavage into individual proteins, including RNA-dependent RNA polymerase, which then transcribes mRNA and genomic RNA. Virus assembly takes place in the cytoplasm and release upon cell lysis.

Small, naked capsid, icosahedral, positive-sense RNA viruses

Similar to other viruses of diarrhea, astroviruses are also transmitted via fecal–oral route through contaminated food, water, or fomites and are spread worldwide. The incubation period is 1 to 2 days and the virus is shed in feces. Symptoms include copious, watery diarrhea, nausea, vomiting, fever, malaise, anorexia, and abdominal pain for up to 2 to 3 days, especially in toddlers, children, and elderly. Adults generally do not get sick until they are infected with a very high dose of the virus. The virus was identified in intestinal epithelial cells, suggesting that the virus probably replicates in these cells. Viral pathogenesis data from humans are limited. The virus is shed for a long time in immunocompromised individuals. Viral RNA can be detected by RT-PCR and antibodies by EIA. There is no specific treatment or vaccine. Similar measures such as those taken for other diarrheal viruses are required.

Fecal–oral transmission

Virus shed in feces

Identified in intestinal epithelial cells

● ADENOVIRUSES AND "CANDIDATE" VIRUSES

Some enteric adenoviruses serotypes (double-stranded DNA, naked capsid virus), most of which were exceedingly difficult to cultivate *in vitro* (in contrast to those associated with respiratory diseases and discussed in Chapter 9), but now have been cultured in some cell lines, are recognized as significant intestinal pathogens. These adenovirus serotypes may account for an estimated 5% to 15% of all viral gastroenteritis in young children. These include serotypes 40, 41, and perhaps 3, 2, 1, 5, and 57. These adenoviruses mainly infect infants aged around less than 2 years. They are transmitted by fecal–oral route and the incubation period is 8 to 10 days and the symptoms of gastroenteritis last for 5 to 12 days. The diagnosis can be done by antigen detection, PCR, virus isolation, and serology. Treatment and prevention strategies are similar to those of other diarrheal viruses.

Serotypes 40 and 41 associated with viral gastroenteritis

Infects infants less than 2 years old

Incubation 8 to 10 days, symptoms 5 to 12

Other agents that have been associated with gastrointestinal diseases include coronavirus-like agents, toroviruses (coronavirus), and some group A coxsackieviruses (the latter primarily cause gastrointestinal symptoms in severely immunocompromised patients). This list may grow in the future; however, until more is learned about their biology, epidemiologic behavior, and impact on human health, they remain "candidate" viruses for now.

Some coronavirus-like agents, toroviruses may cause diarrhea

Group A coxsackieviruses cause gastroenteritis in immunocompromised

KEY CONCLUSIONS

- Worldwide, rotavirus diarrheal disease deaths in 2016 dropped to 128,500 in children below 5 years of age, whereas rotavirus-related deaths are rare in the United States due to rotavirus vaccination.

- Rotavirus has a naked capsid, icosahedral, wheel-shaped, 11 segments double-stranded RNA genome that replicates in the cytoplasm by using viral RNA-dependent RNA polymerase.

- Following fecal–oral transmission and incubation of 1 to 3 days, rotavirus causes vomiting and watery diarrhea that can lead to dehydration, including death, particularly in malnourished infants below 5 years of age with severity in 3 to 35 months of age during winter months.

- Rotavirus can be prevented by two live, attenuated oral vaccines given in two or three doses before 8 months of age, which has significantly reduced the number of infections and hospitalizations, and death a rarity in the United States.

- Norovirus, a member of calicivirus (a naked capsid, positive-sense RNA virus), causes diarrheal disease generally in adults in institutionalized settings and cruise ships; however, in the post-rotavirus vaccine era, norovirus has become a leading cause of viral diarrhea in children below 5 years of age.

- Worldwide 685 million Norovirus cases and 50,000 deaths in developing countries, whereas 20 million infections and 900 deaths in the United States.

- Other diarrhea-causing viruses include astroviruses (naked capsid, positive-sense RNA virus), adenoviruses serotypes (naked capsid, double-stranded DNA virus), and some candidate viruses.

CASE STUDY

An Unscheduled Tour Stop

A 20-year-old man was on a 3-week tour of Italy with 14 other college students. On the way to Florence, he abruptly became ill with nausea and vomiting, followed by abdominal cramps and watery diarrhea 5 hours later. No fever was noted.

QUESTIONS

1. Which of these viruses is the most likely cause of the patient's illness?
   A. Calicivirus
   B. Rotavirus
   C. Parvovirus
   D. Adenovirus
   E. Astrovirus

2. His illness might have been prevented by any of the following, *except*:
   A. Avoidance of raw fruits
   B. Live, reassortant vaccine
   C. Careful handwashing
   D. Avoidance of local drinking water
   E. Avoidance of raw oysters

3. Infection by which of the following is localized to the duodenum and upper jejunum?
   A. Rotavirus
   B. Norovirus
   C. Sapovirus
   D. Astrovirus
   E. Adenovirus

ANSWERS

1. (A)

2. (B)

3. (A)

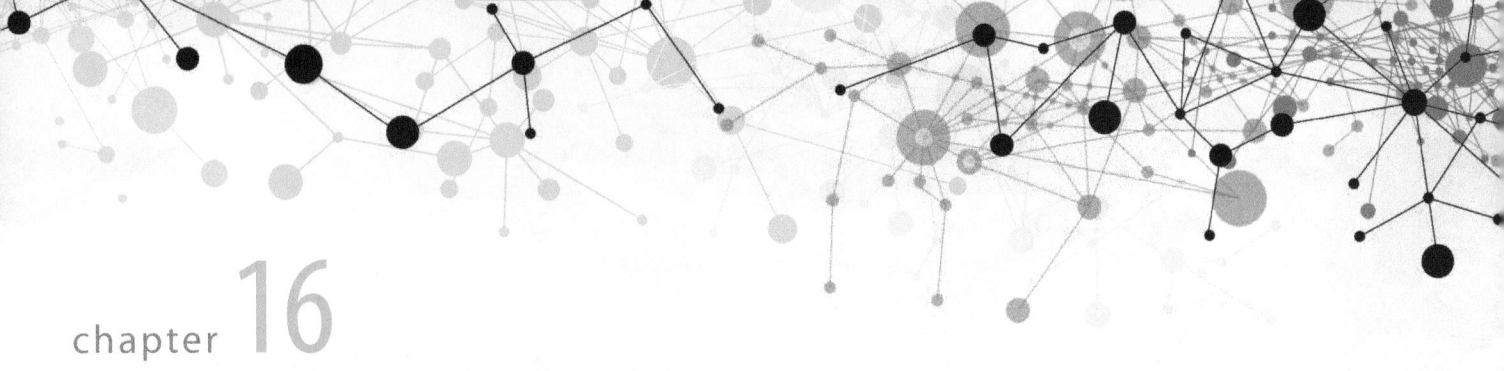

chapter 16

Arthropod-Borne and Other Zoonotic Viruses

Togavirus · Flavivirus · Reovirus · Western Equine Encephalitis · Eastern Equine Encephalitis · St. Louis Encephalitis ·

California (La Crosse) Virus · Japanese B Encephalitis · West Nile Virus · Yellow Fever Virus · Dengue Virus · Zika Virus ·

Chikungunya Virus · Colorado Tick Fever Virus · Hantavirus · Arenavirus · Ebola Virus

The zoonotic viruses comprise of more than 400 viral agents, one or more of which occur in most parts of the world. Members of the group have their ultimate reservoirs in insects or lower vertebrates. They are from diverse families of RNA viruses that primarily include the togaviruses, flaviviruses, bunyaviruses, reoviruses, arenaviruses, and filoviruses. The zoonotic viruses discussed here are divided into two groups: Arthropod-borne (arboviruses) and nonarthropod-borne zoonotic viruses. The arthropod-borne or arboviruses are transmitted to humans by infected blood-sucking insects, such as mosquitoes, ticks, and *Phlebotomus* flies (sandflies). The other zoonotic RNA viruses are generally believed to be transmitted by inhalation of infected animal excretions, by the conjunctival route, or occasionally by direct contact with infected animals (nonarthropod zoonotic viruses). Rabies virus, which is commonly transmitted by animal bites, is discussed separately in Chapter 17. Certain DNA viruses (poxviruses) are also transmissible from animals to humans, which are described in Chapter 11.

Arthropod-borne zoonotic virus transmitted by insects

Nonarthropod zoonotic viruses transmitted by inhalation of animal's excreta or contact

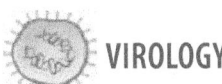 VIROLOGY

In most cases, the zoonotic viruses were first named after the place or region of initial isolation or reported infection (eg, St. Louis encephalitis virus, West Nile virus [WNV], Zika virus) or after the disease produced (eg, yellow fever). More recent studies have assigned the majority to families and genera on the basis of properties including morphologic and genetic features, geographic distribution, and disease spectrum summarized in **Table 16–1**. The major characteristics of these arboviral families, including togaviruses, flaviviruses, bunyaviruses, and reoviruses are summarized in the following discussion.

Often named after place of initial isolation

ARTHROPOD-BORNE ZOONOTIC ARBOVIRUSES

Overview

Arboviruses are transmitted to humans through insects (arthropods) bite tropic to central nervous system (CNS), liver or small blood vessels and cause encephalitis, meningitis, hemorrhage, or febrile illness. These RNA viruses come from viral families such as togaviruses, flaviviruses, bunyaviruses, and reoviruses. In case of CNS infection, there is a severe inflammation of the brain (encephalitis) with damage or destruction of neural cells that may be fatal or lead to permanent neurologic damage in survivors. These viruses include WNV, St. Louis encephalitis virus, California virus, and Japanese B encephalitis virus. One of these viruses, WNV, has a wide disease spectrum, including no symptoms, flu-like symptoms, gastrointestinal symptoms to CNS infection such as meningitis, meningoencephalitis, and poliomyelitis. Some viruses such as dengue viruses can produce illnesses that range from mild flu-like symptoms to overwhelming shock with widespread hemorrhage into tissues, whereas others such as yellow fever virus primarily attack liver cells leading to extensive destruction and sometimes fatal liver failure. Immunity is serotype specific. Diagnosis is done by RT-PCR or enzyme immunoassay (EIA). There is no specific treatment or vaccine for most of these viral infections. However, vaccines for yellow fever virus, Japanese encephalitis virus, and western and eastern equine encephalitis viruses are available in the United States but not routinely used.

TABLE 16-1	Arboviruses of Major Importance to Humans		
GENUS AND MEMBER	**MAJOR GEOGRAPHIC DISTRIBUTION**	**PRIMARY ARTHROPOD VECTOR**	**USUAL DISEASE EXPRESSION**
TOGAVIRUSES			
Alphavirus			
Western equine encephalitis virus	North America	Mosquito	Encephalitis
Eastern equine encephalitis virus	North America	Mosquito	Encephalitis
Venezuelan equine encephalitis virus	Central and South America	Mosquito	Encephalitis
Chikungunya virus	Africa and Asia	Mosquito	Febrile illness
Ross River virus	Australia	Mosquito	Febrile illness
FLAVIVIRUSES			
Flavivirus			
St. Louis encephalitis virus	North America	Mosquito	Encephalitis
Japanese B encephalitis virus	Asia and Western Pacific	Mosquito	Encephalitis
Dengue virus	All tropical zones	Mosquito	Febrile illness or hemorrhagic fever
Yellow fever virus	Africa, South America, and the Caribbean	Mosquito	Hepatic necrosis, hemorrhage
West Nile virus	Africa, Eastern Europe, Middle East, Asia, North America	Mosquito	Febrile illness or encephalitis
Zika virus	Americas, Southeast Asia, the Caribbean, Pacific Islands, Africa	Mosquito	Febrile illness, birth defects
Murray Valley encephalitis virus	Australia	Mosquito	Encephalitis
Powassan virus	North America, Russia	Tick	Encephalitis
Tick-borne encephalitis viruses (TBEVs): Far Eastern, European/ Western, and Siberian	Eastern Former Soviet Union and Central Europe	Tick	Encephalitis

(Continued)

TABLE 16–1	Arboviruses of Major Importance to Humans (Continued)		
GENUS AND MEMBER	MAJOR GEOGRAPHIC DISTRIBUTION	PRIMARY ARTHROPOD VECTOR	USUAL DISEASE EXPRESSION
BUNYAVIRUSES			
Bunyavirus			
California (La Crosse) virus	North America	Mosquito	Encephalitis
Bunyamwera virus	Africa	Mosquito	Febrile illness
Phlebovirus			
Rift Valley fever virus	Africa	Mosquito	Febrile illness
Sandfly fever virus	Mediterranean	*Phlebotomus*	Febrile illness
Heartland virus	North America	Tick	Febrile illness
Nairovirus			
Crimean-Congo hemorrhagic fever virus	Asia, Africa, Europe	Tick	Febrile illness
REOVIRUSES			
Coltivirus			
Colorado tick fever virus	North America	Tick	Febrile illness

TOGAVIRUSES

Togaviruses are from Togaviridae family and *Alphavirus* genus includes arboviruses within this family that infect humans. The other genus, *Rubivirus* that includes rubella virus is discussed in Chapter 10. Alphaviruses have enveloped virions that measure 70 mm in external diameter and contain a positive-sense single-stranded, linear RNA genome. The RNA genome is encapsidated in an icosahedral capsid that measures approximately 40 nm. The lipid bilayer envelope contains viral-encoded glycoproteins (GPs), E1 and E2. Alphaviruses have the ability to hemagglutinate via fusion of E1 glycoprotein to lipids in erythrocyte membrane and E2 also participates in this process. The structure of an alphavirus virion is shown in **Figure 16–1.** Replication occurs in the cytoplasm of the cells of infected arthropods and in vertebrate hosts. Virus enters via receptor-mediated endocytosis by interacting with a variety of cellular receptors, depending on the host and the cell type. The positive-sense genomic RNA serves as the mRNA for the translation of nonstructural proteins, including viral RNA-dependent RNA polymerase. The RNA-dependent RNA polymerase synthesizes negative-sense RNA intermediates, which is used for the synthesis

Alphavirus genus Togaviruses includes most arboviruses

✴ Positive-sense RNA, icosahedral, enveloped viruses

Envelope GPs; hemagglutinin, lipoproteins

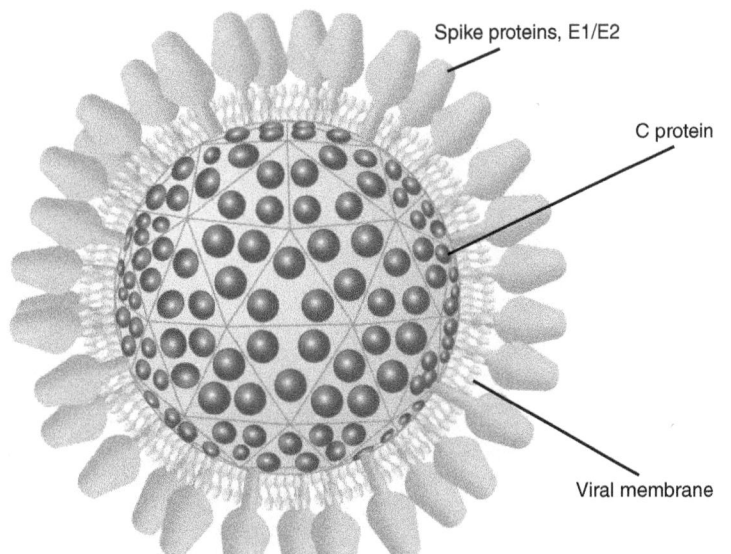

Spike proteins, E1/E2

C protein

Viral membrane

FIGURE 16–1. **Virion structure of alphavirus.** The single-stranded, positive-sense RNA genome is encapsidated into an icosahedral capsid (C protein) wrapped by a lipid bilayer envelope (viral membrane) containing viral-encoded glyco-proteins (spikes), E1 and E2 with an external diameter of 70 nm. E1 has the ability to hemagglutinate via fusion to lipids on erythrocyte membrane and E2 also participates in this process.

Full-length RNA and subgenomic RNA encodes nonstructural, structural proteins

✳ Persistent infection in arthropods, acute infection in humans

Flavivirus **genus comprises arboviruses**

✳ Enveloped, positive-sense RNA, icosahedral capsid viruses

Replicates in cytoplasm

Genomic RNA translated into polyprotein, cleaved into individual proteins

✳ Lytic in humans, sustained viremia in lower vertebrates, persistent in invertebrates

of both subgenomic RNA (mRNA for synthesis of structural proteins) and new positive-sense, full-length genomic RNA. Virus assembly takes place in the cytoplasm. Virions mature by budding from cellular membranes. The effect of viral replication on invertebrate and vertebrate hosts is variable, with usually a persistent infection in invertebrate (arthropod) hosts. Viruses within the *Alphavirus* genus are frequently serologically related to one another but not to others. Representatives are listed in Table 16–1.

FLAVIVIRUSES

Flaviviruses come from Flaviviridae family and *Flavivirus* genus includes arboviruses transmitted through mosquitoes to humans. The other genus of Flaviviridae is *Hepacivirus* (hepatitis C virus) that is a blood-borne virus and causes hepatitis C (discussed in Chapter 13). Flaviviruses are similar to togaviruses in several respects such that they are positive-sense, single-stranded RNA, icosahedral capsid, enveloped viruses. However, the virions of flaviviruses are smaller than those of togaviruses, ranging from 40 to 50 nm in diameter. The RNA genome is surrounded by multiple copies of small basic proteins; the capsid (C) protein that covers the core and makes it icosahedral. The lipid bilayer envelope membrane contains the membrane (M) protein and envelope (E) protein, which is glycosylated in many flaviviruses. An example of a flavivirus virion is shown in **Figure 16–2**. *Flavivirus* members are serologically related, and there is cross-reactivity among members. Virus replication starts with virus entering the target cells via receptor-mediated endocytosis; flaviviruses can also bind to Fc receptors on macrophages, monocytes, and other cells coated with antibody. The enhancing antibody enhances viral adsorption and infectivity. The virus replicates like positive-sense RNA viruses in the cytoplasm, and the full-length positive-sense RNA genome is translated into a polyprotein (like picornaviruses), which is cleaved into individual mature proteins, including a protease, an RNA-dependent RNA polymerase, a capsid, and envelope proteins. Virus assembly takes place in the cytoplasm and the envelope is acquired by budding into intracellular vesicles and released upon cell lysis. Like alphaviruses, flaviviruses also cause a lytic response in vertebrate hosts and a persistent infection in invertebrate hosts. However, the virus uses lower vertebrates as host reservoir with sustained viremia in some on the flaviviruses.

FIGURE 16–2. Virion structure of flavivirus. Two types of virions, intracellular and extracellular virions, are shown. The positive-sense, single-stranded RNA genome is packaged into an icosahedral capsid wrapped into a lipid bilayer envelope containing membrane (M) protein and spike glycoprotein (E). The prM is the precursor to M protein. The size of flavivirus virion ranges from 40 to 50 nm in diameter. There are two major differences between intracellular and extracellular virions; intracellular virions have only prM and E as monomer, whereas extracellular virions have prM and M and E as dimer.

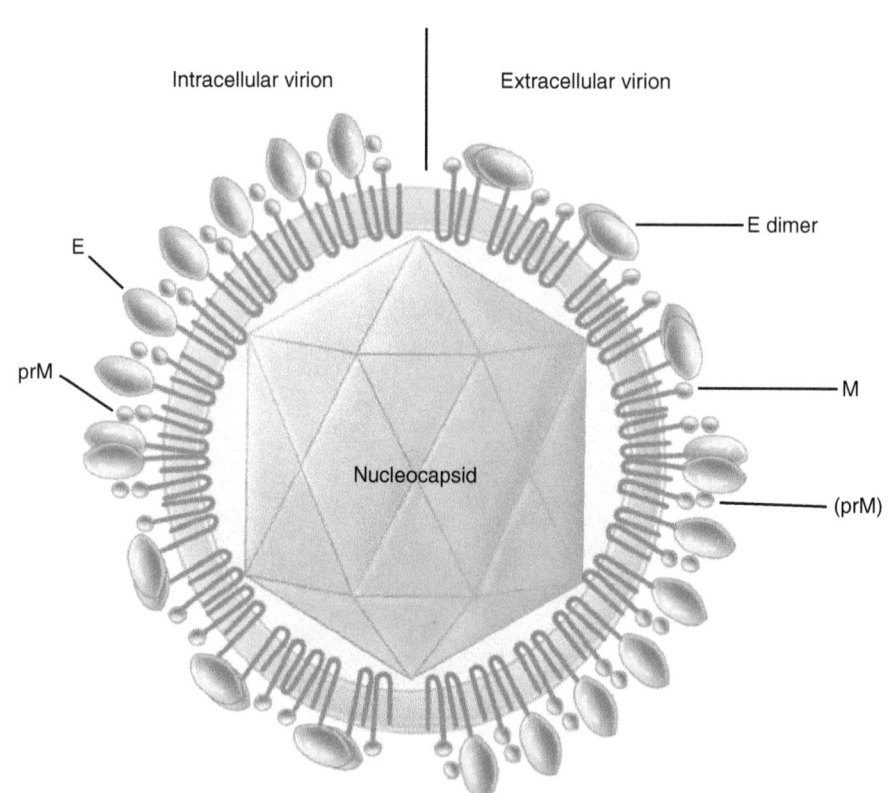

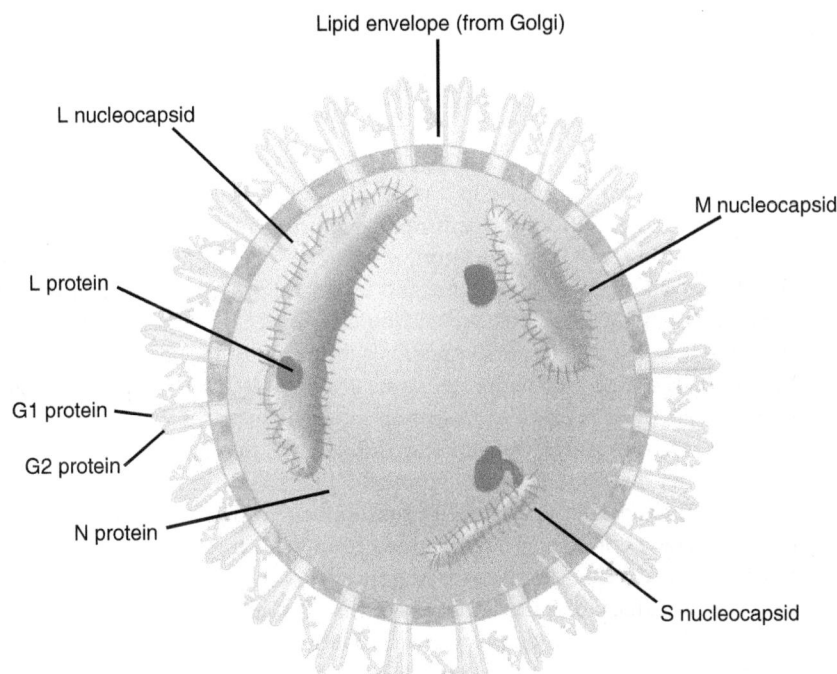

Lipid envelope (from Golgi)

L nucleocapsid

L protein

G1 protein

G2 protein

N protein

M nucleocapsid

S nucleocapsid

FIGURE 16–3. **Bunyavirus virion structure.** The virions of bunyaviruses contain single-stranded, negative-sense RNA viruses that are spherical and enveloped with an external diameter of 90 to 100 nm. The envelope contains two glycoproteins, G1 and G2, and encloses three helical nucleocapsids containing RNA, namely, large (L), medium (M), and small (S), associated with an RNA-dependent RNA polymerase (L) and nonstructural proteins (N).

BUNYAVIRUSES

There are four genera of Bunyaviridae family: *Bunyavirus* (–) RNA, *Phlebovirus* (–) RNA, *Nairovirus* (+/–) ambisense RNA, and *Hantavirus* (–) RNA. All bunyaviruses are arboviruses, except *Hantavirus*, which is a nonarthropod zoonotic virus and discussed in the next section. Bunyaviruses are morphologically spherical, enveloped virions of 90 to 100 nm in external diameter containing two envelope GPs, G1 and G2. Inside the virion, the single-stranded, negative-sense, or ambisense RNA genome forms three helical nucleocapsids containing RNA, namely, large (L), medium (M), and small (S), associated with an RNA-dependent RNA polymerase (L) and nonstructural proteins (N) (**Figure 16–3**). Unlike enveloped RNA viruses, bunyaviruses are devoid of a matrix protein. The viral attachment protein (G1) interacts with cellular receptors, and the virus enters the cell via receptor-mediated endocytosis. After lysis of endosomal vesicles and release of the nucleocapsids in the cytoplasm, the negative RNA strands (L, M, S) transcribe to synthesize mRNA using virion-associated RNA-dependent RNA polymerase. The M strand encodes G1 and G2 envelope, a nonstructural protein; L strand encodes the L protein (RNA-dependent RNA polymerase); and the S strand encodes the nucleocapsid protein (NP) and a nonstructural protein. They mature by budding into smooth-surfaced vesicles in or near the Golgi region of the infected cell. The major disease-causing bunyaviruses in North America are California virus La Crosse virus subtype and others (arbovirus) and Hantavirus (nonarthropod zoonotic virus).

Four genera, three arboviruses, and one nonarthropod zoonotic virus

Enveloped, single-stranded, negative-sense, or ambisense RNA viruses

✳ Ambisense (+/-) RNA uses negative-sense RNA strategies for replication in cytoplasm

Helical nucleocapsids RNA: large, medium, small

REOVIRUSES

Reoviruses are spherical, naked capsid icosahedral, double-stranded segmented RNA viruses that measure about 80 nm in diameter. The details about virus structure and replication of another member of the Reoviridae family, *Rotavirus*, are described in Chapter 15. The double-stranded segmented RNA genome of reoviruses replicates in the cytoplasm by utilizing the negative-stranded RNA of the double strand for transcription and replication using their virion-associated RNA-dependent RNA polymerase. However, the reoviruses described here are arboviruses that are transmitted through insect (tick) bites. The most important North American arbovirus of this family, which is a member of the genus *Coltivirus*, causes Colorado tick fever (CTF) in humans. The other arboviruses from the Reoviridae family are *Orbivirus* which includes African horse sickness and bluetongue viruses, mainly causing disease in animals.

✳ Colorado tick fever transmitted by ticks to humans, prominent in North America

Naked capsid, double-stranded RNA viruses replicate in the cytoplasm

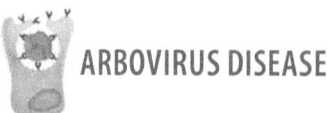

ARBOVIRUS DISEASE

EPIDEMIOLOGY

Arboviruses of major importance in human disease are listed in Table 16–1 with summaries of their geographic distribution, the arthropod vectors that transmit them, and the usual disease syndromes that can result from infection.

With the exception of urban dengue and urban yellow fever, in which the virus may simply be transmitted between humans and mosquitoes, other arboviral diseases involve nonhuman vertebrates. These are usually small mammals, birds, or, in the case of jungle yellow fever, monkeys. Infection is transmitted within the host species by arthropods (eg, mosquitoes or ticks) that become infected. In some cases, the infection can be maintained from generation to generation in the arthropod by transovarial transmission. Infection in the arthropod usually does not appear to harm the insect; however, a period of virus multiplication (termed **extrinsic incubation period**) is required to enhance the capacity to transmit infection to vertebrates by bite.

The consequences of infection transmitted from the arthropod to susceptible vertebrate hosts are variable; some develop illness of varying severity with viremia, whereas others have long-term viremia without clinical disease. Vertebrate hosts are then a source of further spread of the virus by amplification, in which noninfected arthropods feeding on viremic hosts acquire the virus, thereby increasing the risk of transmission. The general features of this overall transmission cycle are illustrated in the following discussion.

Transient viremia is a feature of many of these infections in hosts other than their reservoir; those affected, including humans and higher vertebrates (eg, horses and cattle), are often referred to as blind-end hosts. In contrast, if viremia is sustained for longer periods (eg, weeks to months in a variety of togavirus, flavivirus, and bunyavirus infections of lower vertebrates), the vertebrate host becomes highly important as a reservoir for continuing transmission. Viremia may last a week or more in human dengue and yellow fever infections, and humans may then serve as a reservoir in urban disease.

Sometimes maintained by vertical transmission in vector

Multiplication in vector required before transmission

Sustained viremia required in vertebrate host for reservoir and transmission

Season-to-season survival has multiple mechanisms

✳ Basic specific cycles of arbovirus transmission include urban, sylvatic, arthropod sustained

 Why are arboviruses not pathogenic in insects or some lower vertebrate reservoirs but pathogenic in humans?

Obviously, the typical arthropod vectors are rarely present during all seasons. The question then arises as to how the arboviruses survive between the time the vector disappears and the time it reappears in subsequent years. Several mechanisms can operate to sustain the virus between transmission periods (often referred to as **overwintering**): (1) sustained viremia in lower vertebrates such as small mammals, birds, and snakes, from which newly mature arthropods can be infected when taking a blood meal; (2) hibernation of infected adult arthropods that survive from one season to the next; and (3) transovarial transmission, whereby the infected female arthropod can transmit virus to its progeny.

■ Urban

As the term suggests, the urban cycle is favored by the presence of relatively large numbers of humans living in close proximity to arthropod (usually mosquito) species capable of virus transmission. The cycle is:

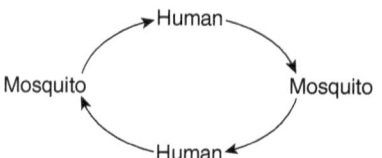

 Think ▸▸ Apply 16-1: **Arboviruses are less pathogenic in insects and some lower vertebrates than humans because of low level of viral replication and less cytopathic effects in these reservoirs probably due to differences in host factors.**

Examples of the urban cycle include urban dengue, urban yellow fever, and occasional urban outbreaks of St. Louis encephalitis.

Urban cycle exists with dengue and yellow fever

■ Sylvatic

In the sylvatic cycle, a single nonhuman vertebrate reservoir may be involved.

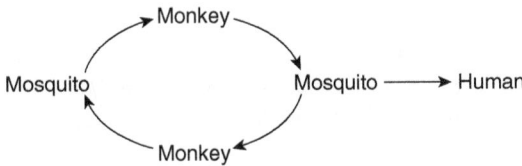

In this situation, the human, who becomes a tangential host through accidental intrusion into a zoonotic transmission cycle, is not important in maintaining the infection cycle. An example of this cycle is jungle yellow fever.

In other sylvatic cycles, multiple vertebrate reservoirs may be involved:

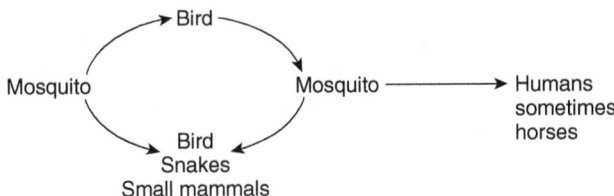

Examples include western equine encephalitis, eastern equine encephalitis, and California viruses. In some situations, such as St. Louis encephalitis and yellow fever, the urban and sylvatic cycles may operate concurrently. WNV uses lower vertebrates such as birds as a principal host and reservoir.

Sylvatic cycle occurs with many viruses

Humans are incidental or dead-end hosts

■ Arthropod Sustained

Arthropods, especially ticks, may sustain the reservoir by transovarial (via ovaries) transmission of virus to their progeny, with amplification of the cycle by spread to and from small mammals:

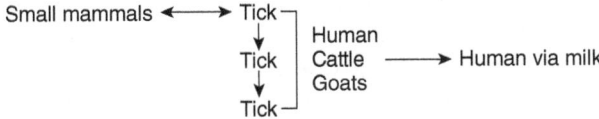

Tick-borne encephalitis in Russia is transmitted by the arthropod-sustained cycle. In temperate climates such as the United States, arboviruses are major causes of disease during the summer and early fall months, the seasons of greatest activity of arthropod vectors (usually mosquitoes or ticks). When climatic conditions and ecologic circumstances (eg, swamps and ponds) are optimal for arthropod breeding and egg hatching, arbovirus amplification may begin.

An example of amplification is provided by western equine encephalitis. When the mosquito vectors become abundant, the level of transmission among the basic reservoir hosts (birds and small mammals) increases, and the mosquitoes also turn to other susceptible species such as the domestic fowl. These hosts experience a rapidly developing asymptomatic viremia, which permits still more arthropods to become infected on biting. At this point, spread to blind-end hosts such as humans or horses and the development of clinical disease become likely. This occurrence depends on the accessibility of the host to the infected mosquito and on mosquito feeding preferences which, for unknown reasons, vary from one season to another.

Arthropod sustained by tick transovarial transmission

✳ Weather, swamps, and ponds alter conditions

Mosquito population increase creates risk for blind-end human infection

PATHOGENESIS

There are three major manifestations of arbovirus diseases in humans associated with different tropisms of various viruses for human organs, although overlap can occur. In some, the CNS is primarily affected, leading to aseptic meningitis or meningoencephalitis. A second syndrome involves many major organ systems, with damage to the liver, as in yellow fever. The third syndrome is manifested by hemorrhagic fever, in which damage is particularly severe to the small blood vessels, with skin petechiae and intestinal and other hemorrhages.

✳ CNS, visceral, and hemorrhagic fever are major syndromes

Infection of the human by a biting of an infected arthropod is initiated by viral replication at the site of bite probably in Langerhans cells of the skin and mononuclear cells followed by viremia, which is apparently amplified by extensive virus replication in the reticuloendothelial system and vascular endothelium. After replication, the virus becomes localized in various target organs, depending on its tropism, and illness results. The viruses produce cell necrosis with resultant inflammation, which leads to fever in nearly all infections. If the major viral tropism is for the CNS, then the virus reaching this site by crossing the blood–brain barrier or along neural pathways can cause meningeal inflammation (aseptic meningitis) or neuronal dysfunction (encephalitis). The CNS pathology consists of meningeal and perivascular mononuclear cell infiltrates, degeneration of neurons with neuronophagia, and occasionally destruction of the supporting structure of neurons.

> **How do arboviruses cause viremia in humans after a mosquito bite?**

In some infections, especially yellow fever, the liver is the primary target organ. Pathologic findings include hyaline necrosis of hepatocytes, which produces cytoplasmic eosinophilic masses called **Councilman bodies.** Degenerative changes in the renal tubules and myocardium may also be seen, as may microscopic hemorrhages throughout the brain. Hemorrhage is a major feature of yellow fever, largely because of the lack of liver-produced clotting factors because of liver necrosis.

Hemorrhagic fevers other than those related to primary hepatic destruction have a somewhat different pathogenesis, which has been studied most extensively in dengue infections. In uncomplicated dengue fever, which is associated with a rash and influenza-like symptoms, there are changes in the small dermal blood vessels. These alterations include endothelial cell swelling and perivascular edema with mononuclear cell infiltration. More severe infection, as in dengue hemorrhagic fever, often complicated by shock, is characterized by perivascular edema and widespread effusions into serous cavities such as the pleura and by hemorrhages. The spleen and lymph nodes show hyperplasia of lymphoid and plasma cell elements, and there is focal necrosis in the liver. The pathophysiology seems related to increased vascular permeability and disseminated intravascular coagulation, which is further complicated by liver and bone marrow dysfunction (eg, decreased platelet production and decreased production of liver-dependent clotting factors). The major vascular abnormalities may be provoked by circulating virus–antibody complexes (immune complexes), which mediate activation of complement and subsequent release of vasoactive amines. The precise reason for this phenomenon is not clear; it may be related to intrinsic virulence of the virus strains involved and to host susceptibility factors.

Two hypotheses are based on the existence of four distinct but antigenically related serotypes of dengue virus, DEN1, DEN2, DEN3, and DEN4, any of which can generate group-specific cross-reacting antibodies that are not necessarily protective against other serotypes. One possibility is that preexisting group-specific antibody at a critical concentration serves as "enhancing" rather than neutralizing antibody. In the presence of enhancing antibody, virus–antibody complexes are more efficiently adsorbed to and engulfed by monocytes and macrophages. Subsequent replication leads to extensive spread throughout the host. Alternatively, or in concert with this, activation of previously sensitized T cells by viral antigen present on the surfaces of macrophages may result in the release of cytokines, which mediate the development of shock and hemorrhage.

IMMUNITY

The usual humoral responses (hemagglutination inhibition, IgM, neutralization) in relation to onset of illness are illustrated in **Figure 16–4.** The rise in antibody titer generally correlates with recovery from infection. Neutralizing antibodies, which are the most serotype-specific, generally

Sidebar notes

After bite and initial viral replication, viremia and viral tissue tropism define disease

✳ In CNS, aseptic meningitis and encephalitis follow cell injury

Liver often the target, with necrosis of hepatocytes

✳ Dengue hemorrhagic fevers involve perivascular and endothelial injury, may progress to shock

Lymphoid hyperplasia seen

Virus–antibody complexes trigger complement activation

✳ Antigenically related cross-reacting antibodies not protective against other serotypes but may enhance infection and disease severity

✳ Serotype specific neutralizing antibodies protective, last years

---

 Think ▸▸ Apply 16-2: Arbovirus is transmitted through mosquito bite and replicates at the site of bite in the skin Langerhans cells to amplify its inoculum followed by replication in mononuclear cells and viremia.

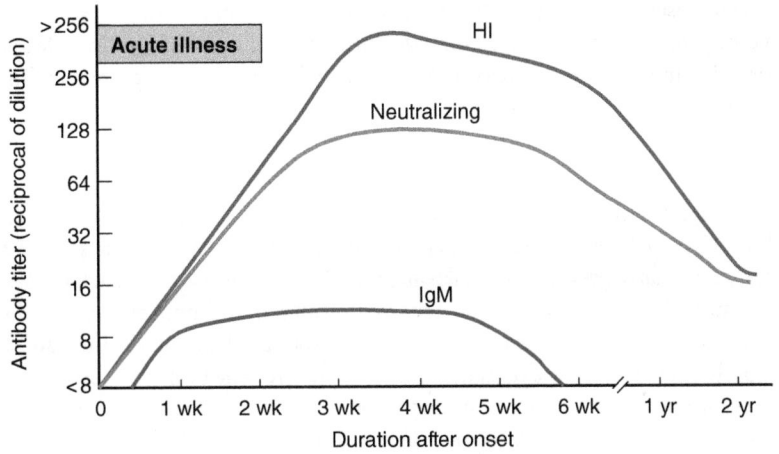

FIGURE 16–4. Typical patterns of antibody response after arbovirus infection. These patterns begin to appear about 3 days after onset and decline after about 6 weeks. HI, hemagglutination inhibition antibodies; IgM, immunoglobulin M antibodies.

persist many years after infection. The presence of IgM-specific antibodies indicates that primary infection likely occurred within the previous 2 months. In cell-mediated immunity, the CD8 T cells control viral replication by eliminating infected cells. Neutralizing antibodies prevent further infection of uninfected cells. Cellular immunity and humoral immunity to reinfection are serotype specific and appear to be permanent.

Cell-mediated immunity contains viral infection

SPECIFIC ARBOVIRUS DISEASES

■ Western Equine Encephalitis

Western equine encephalitis virus (*Alphavirus*/Togavirus) causes western equine encephalitis that is prevalent in the central valley of California, eastern Washington (Yakima Valley), Colorado, and Texas. It has also been responsible for outbreaks in Midwestern states (Minnesota, Wisconsin, Illinois, Missouri, and Kansas) and as far east as New Jersey. The virus is transmitted through mosquito (*Culex tarsalis*) bites. Horses and humans represent blind-end hosts; both are susceptible to infection and illness, commonly manifested as encephalitis. Although human infection in endemic areas is commonplace, overall only 1 of 1000 infections causes clinical symptoms. However, in young infants, 1 of every 25 infections may produce severe illness. The attack rates are therefore far higher in young infants than in other groups. The disease spectrum may range from mild, nonspecific febrile illness to aseptic meningitis or severe, overwhelming encephalitis. Mortality rate is estimated at 5% for cases of encephalitis. It is a very serious disease in infants less than 1 year of age; as many as 60% of survivors have permanent neurologic impairment.

Human and equine illness

Prevalent in the Western United States, outbreaks in the Midwestern United States

✳ Encephalitis more likely in young infants

■ Eastern Equine Encephalitis

The eastern equine encephalitis virus (*Alphavirus*/Togavirus) is largely confined to the Atlantic Seaboard states from New England down the coasts of Central America and South America. The mosquito vector (principally *Culiseta melanura*) generally restricts its feeding to horses and birds, although occasional outbreaks among humans have occurred. Increasing numbers of human infections have been observed from 2010 to 2019, which is a cause of concern and most of the cases were reported from Massachusetts, Michigan, Florida, Georgia, New York, and North Carolina. The virus can cause severe encephalitis in horses and also in wild birds. The mortality rate for eastern equine encephalitis among humans is estimated at 33% for individuals of all ages, especially below 15 years and above 50 years and the incidence of severe sequelae among survivors is high. In the United States, an average of 11 cases are reported annually.

New England to South America

Mosquito vector feeds on horses and birds

Outbreaks with encephalitis in all ages

■ St. Louis Encephalitis

The St. Louis encephalitis virus (*Flavivirus*) is a major cause of arbovirus encephalitis in the United States. Its major mosquito vector is *C tarsalis* similar to those of western equine encephalitis, but St. Louis encephalitis has been much more prevalent in eastern and central states and in Texas, Mississippi, and Florida. The incubation period is from 5 to 15 days. Most people infected with the virus have no symptoms and less than 1% develop clinical symptoms. Symptoms include fever, headache, dizziness, nausea, and malaise. However, some infected people develop CNS symptoms such as stiff neck, confusion, disorientation, dizziness, and tremors, including coma in

✳ Major cause of encephalitis in the United States, highest attack rates above age 40

severe cases. The highest attack rates are among adults more than 40 years of age. Infants and young children are relatively spared. About 40% of infected children develop fever and headache or mild meningitis, whereas 90% of infected elderly develop encephalitis. Overall mortality is between 5% and 15%.

Prevalent in eastern, central, and southern United States

California Virus or La Crosse Virus Encephalitis

＊ La Crosse distributed in Midwestern United States

Virus and vector in suburban, rural areas

Mosquito vector and chipmunk reservoir host

＊ Highest attack rate at 5 to 18 years

＊ Abrupt onset of encephalitis, frequent seizures

Although California virus (*bunyavirus*) was first isolated in the State of California, its major distribution in the United States has been in the Midwest; outbreaks due to the **La Crosse virus** subtype are particularly prevalent in Wisconsin, Ohio, Minnesota, Indiana, and West Virginia. In Wisconsin and Minnesota, California virus is considered an important cause of encephalitis. However, studies elsewhere in North America and throughout the world indicate that California virus or closely related agents are present nearly everywhere. The primary mosquito vector (*Aedes triseriatus*) is commonly encountered in suburban or rural environments. The reservoir host is the chipmunk; transovarial transmission by mosquitoes to their larvae also serves to sustain the virus in nature. Unlike western equine, eastern equine, and St. Louis encephalitis viruses, the highest attack rates of California virus are seen in children below age 16 years. The incubation period is 5 to 15 days followed by symptoms such as fever (2-3 days duration), headache, nausea, vomiting, tiredness, and lethargy. Severe neuroinvasive diseases are often characterized by abrupt onset of encephalitis and may include seizures, coma, and paralysis. Survivors have neurologic sequalae.

Japanese B Encephalitis

Transmission by mosquito bites similar to St. Louis and western equine encephalitis

Less than 1% of infected develop disease

Japanese B encephalitis virus (*Flavivirus*) causes Japanese B encephalitis that is prevalent on the eastern coast of Asia, on its offshore islands (Japan, Taiwan, and Indonesia), and in India. Its transmission cycle resembles that of the St. Louis encephalitis and western equine encephalitis viruses in the sense that the mosquito vector is from the genus *Culex* but more specifically, *Culex tritaeniorhynchus*. The virus uses pigs and birds as vertebrate hosts. A high proportion of human infections are subclinical, especially in children; less than 1% of the infected people develop clinical disease and when encephalitis does develop, it is severe and often fatal. After infection, the virus generally multiplies for 5 to 15 days (incubation period) followed by initial symptoms such as fever, headache, and vomiting. In the next few days, other symptoms develop that include mental status changes, neurologic issues, weakness, movement disorders, and seizures (common in children). Twenty to thirty percent fatality among patients who develop encephalitis and 30% to 50% survivors have neurologic sequalae.

There is no specific treatment. However, avoiding mosquito bites may reduce the risk of transmission. Inactivated Japanese encephalitis virus vaccine is licensed and available for use in the United States for people above 2 months of age. The vaccine is given in two doses, 28 days apart, and may need a booster after 1 year for those above 17 years of age. This vaccine is recommended for travelers in endemic area.

West Nile Virus (Febrile Illness or Encephalitis)

First appeared in the United States in 1999

Most important arbovirus in North America

Distributed in many parts of the world

WNV, a member of flaviviruses, was first detected in 1937 in Uganda, Africa. During the summer of 1999 in the Northeastern United States, human WNV infections appeared for the first time in the Western Hemisphere. A subsequent outbreak occurred again in 2000. Together, these outbreaks resulted in 78 hospitalized patients and 9 deaths, mostly among the elderly. More widespread activity was observed in 2001 (66 human cases); then in 2002 (4156 cases) and 2003 (9862 cases) saw a dramatic increase in virus spread across the United States (in 46 states) and 4 Canadian provinces. WNV has now been detected in all states in the continental United States, except Alaska. In the last 10 years, between 2000 and 3000 cases of WNV are reported every year in the United States, of which more than 50% are neuroinvasive diseases. Before 1999, outbreaks of human WNV infections were primarily confined to eastern Africa, the Middle East, eastern Europe, west Asia, and Australia. Now it is distributed throughout Africa, the Middle East, parts of Europe, the former USSR, North America, South America, Asia, India, and Indonesia. Since 2010, WNV infections have also been emerged in Australia.

Transmission vector: mosquito; principal vertebrate host: Bird

＊ Transmitted from mosquitoes to humans, other animals

WNV is antigenically related to St. Louis encephalitis and Japanese encephalitis. The vector for transmission is mosquito and the principal vertebrate host is bird. Crows are particularly affected; virus has been detected in dead crows found as far south as Florida, and more recently in the Midwestern United States. Transmission is from infected mosquitoes that feed on infected birds and then transmit the virus to humans and other animals. WNV can also be spread through transfusion, transplants, breastfeeding, and from mother to child. After mosquito bite, the virus multiplies in Langerhans cells of skin with an incubation period of 2 to 14 days (average 2-6 days) followed by viremia and spread of the virus to the peripheral organs and in some cases the CNS.

Three outcomes of the infection have been observed: asymptomatic, West Nile fever, or severe West Nile disease. **(1) Asymptomatic:** Approximately 80% of WNV-infected people do not get any symptoms. **(2) West Nile fever:** 20% of the infected people develop WNV fever. The typical case is mild, characterized by fever, headache, backache, muscle pain, joint pain, generalized myalgia, and chills. Rash appears in half of the cases, involving the chest, back, and upper extremities. Generalized lymphadenopathy is a common finding. Pharyngitis and gastrointestinal symptoms (nausea, vomiting, abdominal pain, diarrhea) may occur. The disease runs its course from 3 to 6 days, followed by recovery. Children generally experience milder illness than adults. **(3) Severe West Nile Disease:** About 1 in 150 people infected with WNV develop severe West Nile disease. The virus, in this case, evades the nervous system causing aseptic meningitis, meningoencephalitis, encephalitis, or West Nile poliomyelitis, especially in the elderly, and in some cases may result in death. Symptoms of severe disease include headache, high fever, stiff neck, disorientation, coma, tremors, convulsions, muscle weakness, and paralysis. Severe disease may last for weeks and cause permanent injury or, in some cases, death. The symptoms may last for several weeks; neurologic effects may be permanent and may also result in death. The fatality rate is 10% in people with severe disease affecting the CNS. Serious illness can occur in people over the age of 50 years and the immunocompromised. In addition, people with other medical conditions such as cancer, diabetes, hypertension, kidney disease, and organ transplant recipients have also risk of serious disease. Chemokine receptor, CCR5 that acts as a coreceptor to HIV, provides resistance to WNV infection, whereas Δ32CCR5 homozygosity that provides resistance to HIV is significantly associated with severe West Nile disease.

 How does West Nile virus damage the CNS?

Clinical laboratory findings include leukopenia and, in cases with CNS signs, cerebrospinal fluid (CSF) pleocytosis, and elevated protein. Diagnosis: serology (antibody to WNV) or reverse transcriptase-polymerase chain reaction (RT-PCR) to detect viral RNA in serum or CSF. The treatment is supportive and several vaccine candidates are under development.

■ Yellow Fever

Geographically, yellow fever virus (*Flavivirus*) is distributed throughout the Caribbean and Central America, the Amazon valley in South America, and a broad central zone in Africa from the Atlantic Coast to the Sudan and Ethiopia. Thirty-four countries in Africa and 13 countries in Central and South America have endemic areas. In 2013, 84,000 to 170,000 severe cases and 29,000 to 60,000 deaths were estimated in an African modeling study. In November 2016, an outbreak of yellow fever started in Brazil that continued toward Brazil's Atlantic coast in early 2017. It continues to be a potential threat to the Southeastern United States because of an urban vector (*Aedes aegypti*) in that area. The incubation period is 3 to 6 days, and majority of infected people are either asymptomatic or have mild symptoms. The clinical disease is characterized by abrupt onset of fever, chills, headache, back pain, body ache, nausea, vomiting, fatigue, and weakness. After a short remission of hours to a day, 15% of cases develop serious diseases such as high fever, jaundice, bradycardia, hemorrhage, bleeding, shock, and failure of multiple organs. Severe vomiting sometimes causes gastric hemorrhage. If the patient recovers from the acute episode, there are no long-term sequelae. However, the fatality of the severe disease is 30% to 60%. Diagnosis can be done by detecting IgM antibody in serum or sometimes viral RNA can be detected in blood if samples are taken early in infection. Treatment is supportive and medications such as aspirin and nonsteroidal anti-inflammatory drugs (NSAID) should be avoided because these drugs may

Dead crows herald spread of virus

❋ Incubation period: 2 to 14 days

❋ WNV infection asymptomatic (80%), West Nile fever (20%), or severe West Nile disease (~ 1%)

❋ Rash in half of the cases of West Nile fever, disease runs its course (3-6 days)

❋ Severe West Nile includes aseptic meningitis, meningoencephalitis, encephalitis, West Nile poliomyelitis

❋ Serious illness above age of 50 years and immunocompromised

Δ32CCR5 homozygosity associated with severe West Nile

Widespread in tropical areas

Vector persists in the United States

❋ Sudden fever, chills, headache, hemorrhage

❋ May progress to vomiting, bradycardia, jaundice, shock

 Think ▶▶ Apply 16-3: The CNS inflammation due to West Nile virus may be due to viral-induced cytopathic effects and cytokines-mediated damage.

increase the risk of bleeding. A live, attenuated vaccine (17-D) is available and recommended for travelers to endemic areas.

■ Dengue

Distributed worldwide

400 million infected annually

Mosquito vector (*A aegypti*) same as yellow fever

✳ High fever, rash, severe pain in back, head, eye, muscles, joints

Dengue virus (*Flavivirus*) has four related serotypes (DEN 1-4), any of which may exist concurrently in a given endemic area. There are more than 100 countries where dengue has become endemic. These viral agents are widespread throughout the world, particularly in Africa, the Americas, the Eastern Mediterranean, South Asia and the Indian subcontinent, South-east Asia and the Western Pacific, the Middle East, Africa, the Far East, and the Caribbean Islands. Globally, 400 million people are infected with dengue, 100 million people become sick, and 22,000 die with severe dengue disease every year. They have invaded the United States in the past with an outbreak in south Texas in 2005. All dengue cases in the continental United States are imported, but it is common is the U.S. territories of Puerto Rico, the U.S. Virgin Island, and American Samoa. People above 60 years of age also have severe dengue disease and deaths. The mosquito vector (*A aegypti*) is the same as the domestic vector of yellow fever. The known transmission cycle is human–mosquito–human, although a sylvatic cycle involving monkeys may also exist. The incubation period is 4 to 7 days.

Severe form: shock, pleural effusion, abdominal pain, hemorrhage

✳ Lifelong immunity serotype specific

Cross-immunity to other serotypes short-term and incomplete

✳ Subsequent infections with other serotypes increase severity

The symptoms last for 3 to 10 days. The characteristic clinical illness usually results in high fever, an erythematous rash, and severe pain in the back, head, eyes (retro-orbital—behind eyes), muscles, bone, and joints. There is also sometimes mild bleeding such as nose or gum bleed, petechiae, or bruising. Especially in the Far East (Philippines, Thailand, and India), dengue has periodically assumed a severe form characterized by shock, pleural effusion, severe abdominal pain and vomiting, and hemorrhage often followed by death.

Severity of the dengue disease is seen more in children but also in elderly people. The treatment is supportive and there is no vaccine available for protection. Avoiding mosquito bites is the best preventive measure. Protection after recovery is serotype specific. People who recover from infection of a serotype are protected for life against the same serotype. There is some cross-reactive immunity to other serotypes, which is only temporary and partial. More importantly, subsequent infections with other serotypes increase the risk of developing severe dengue disease, most likely by antibody-dependent enhancement (enhancing antibodies) that do not neutralize the virus rather enhance viral entry into the host cells.

 How does reinfection with a different serotype cause severe disease and not cross protection?

■ Zika Virus

Zika virus identified in a monkey in 1947 and in humans in 1952

Zika is distributed in Central and South America, the Caribbean, the Pacific Islands, Puerto Rico, and the United States

Transmitted through mosquito bite

Zika virus, a *Flavivirus*, was discovered in 1947 in a monkey in the Zika forest, Uganda and in 1952 in humans. Before 2015, Zika virus outbreaks occurred in Africa, Southeast Asia, and the Pacific Islands. In 2015, Zika virus cases were reported in Brazil, and since then Zika is now distributed in Central and South America, the Caribbean, Cape Verde (Africa), Singapore and Vietnam (Southeast Asia), the Pacific Island, Puerto Rico, and all states of the United States. In the United States, 5109 Zika cases were reported between January 2015 and March 2016, whereas 38,099 cases were reported in the U.S. territories (American Samoa, Puerto Rico, U.S. Virgin Islands). Since 2017, Zika cases (travelers) started declining and in 2020, three Zika cases were reported in the United States and 57 cases in U.S. territories.

Zika virus is transmitted to humans through mosquito (*Aedes agypti*) bite, mother-to-child (during pregnancy), sexual, and blood transfusion. The incubation period is 2 to 14 days. Many

 Think ►► Apply 16-4: **While there is cross reactivity among four dengue serotypes, the enhancing antibodies made during the first infection cause antibody-dependent enhancement of viral entry into the host cells rather neutralize the virus.**

people infected with Zika virus do not develop any symptoms. However, the most common symptoms include fever, rash, joint pain, muscle pain, headache, conjunctivitis. Symptoms last for several days to a week (2-7 days). The severity in Zika virus infection during pregnancy can cause brain defects such as microcephaly and other fetal brain defects and defects of the eye, hearing deficits, and impaired growth. Infants born with microcephaly has been linked with several problems such as seizures, developmental delay, intellectual disability, problems with movement and balance, feeding problems, hearing loss, visual problems. In adults, Zika infection may also cause Guillain-Barré syndrome (GBS).

The pathogenesis of Zika infection is not understood but believed to involve an interaction with the immune cells. After the mosquito bite, the virus probably replicates in the skin cells such as Langerhans cells, dendritic cells, and other cells. The virus interacts with innate immune cells molecules (TLR-3, RIG-1) causing stimulation of IFN-α/β and IFN-γ and several other proinflammatory cytokines. The mechanism of Zika's association with microcephaly is not known but the possibility could be the cytotoxic effects of viral replication in neural progenitor cells.

The diagnosis of Zika virus infection is done by detecting viral RNA by RT-PCR (blood and other bodily secretions) and/or IgM antibody. Supportive treatment is indicated. Aspirin and NSADs are contraindicated unless dengue is ruled out, to reduce the risk of bleeding. There is no vaccine, but development is underway.

■ Chikungunya Fever

Chikungunya (a native term for "that which bends up") is an *Alphavirus* (Togaviruses) transmitted by mosquitoes (*A aegypti* and some other species), particularly in urban areas of Asia, Africa, Europe, and the Indian and Pacific Oceans. In 2013, chikungunya virus was found in the Americas, the Caribbean islands. The virus may be maintained in a sylvatic subhuman primate reservoir. The incubation period is between 2 and 12 (average 3-7) days and a majority of infected people develop some symptoms. Illness is characterized by an abrupt onset of fever, accompanied by excruciating myalgia and polyarthritis. Infected people may experience additional symptoms such as headache, myalgia, arthritis, joint swelling, conjunctivitis, nausea, vomiting, or maculopapular rash. Symptoms usually last 1 week, but the musculoskeletal complaints can sometimes persist for weeks to months. Higher risk groups for severe disease include newborns, older adults more than 65 years, and people with comorbidities such as hypertension, diabetes, or heart disease. The disease is usually not fatal. Imported cases have been diagnosed in the United States and the number has been increasing every year, but there is no evidence that the virus has established itself in North America. Diagnosis is done by detecting IgM or RNA by RT-PCR. There is no specific treatment or vaccine.

■ Powassan Virus

Powassan virus is the only known tick-borne *Flavivirus* species of North America. First isolated in the town of Powassan, Ontario from a fatal human case of encephalitis, it has been found in infected ticks in Ontario, British Columbia, and Colorado. Powassan virus infection in humans has been found in the United States, Canada, and Russia. In the United States, Powassan virus cases have been reported from the states in the northeastern and the Great Lakes regions mainly from the late spring to early summer because of the activity of ticks. Although, Powassan virus cases are rare, the numbers have been on rise in recent years with such 33 cases in 2017, 21 in 2018, and 39 in 2019. Most infected people are asymptomatic; however, symptomatic people may have fever, headache, vomiting, and weakness 1 week to 1 month after the tick bite. Severe disease includes encephalitis or meningitis and 1 in 10 people with severe disease may die. Diagnosis can be done by detecting IgM antibody and/or viral RNA by RT-PCR in blood or CSF. No treatment or vaccine is available.

■ Colorado Tick Fever

CTF virus is transmitted by infected Rocky Mountain wood ticks, which belong to *Coltivirus* genus of Reoviridae family that causes CTF and has been found throughout the western United States and western Canada. In the United States, 59 cases were reported between 2009 and 2019 in the western United States. It is frequently found in *Dermacentor andersoni,* which are also vectors for *Rickettsia rickettsii.* The typical illness, which occurs 3 to 6 days average (range 1 to 14 days) after the tick bite, is characterized by a sudden onset with headache, muscle pains, fever, and some patients may have sore throat, vomiting, abdominal pain or rash, and occasionally encephalitis or meningitis. Leukopenia is a consistent feature of infection.

Many asymptomatic

✳ Symptoms include fever, rash, joint pain, muscle pain, headache, conjunctivitis

✳ Vertically infected infants may have birth defects such as microcephaly

✳ Risk of GBS in infected adults

✳ Pathogenesis involves interaction with immune cells

✳ Diagnosis by RT-PCR (viral RNA) and/or IgM (serology)

Major problem in Asia and Africa

Risk to tourists traveling in endemic areas

✳ Fever, accompanied by excruciating myalgia and polyarthritis

Tick borne, rare, cases on rise in the northeastern United States

Asymptomatic, severe disease may be encephalitis or meningitis

Tick borne, throughout western United States

Most infections asymptomatic

It is estimated that no more than one clinical illness occurs for every 100 infections with this agent. Diagnosis is done by IgM antibody or viral RNA by RT-PCR. No treatment or vaccine is available.

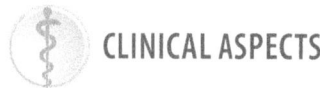 ## CLINICAL ASPECTS

DIAGNOSIS

Blood best source but must be early in disease

Diagnosis by IgM followed by IgG in acute and convalescent serum

Viral RNA by RT-PCR is detected for diagnosis and/or confirmation

Arboviral infection diagnosis is mainly done by detecting IgM antibody by enzyme-linked immunosorbent assay (ELISA) or EIA within 1 to 2 weeks and IgG after 2 to 4 weeks of infection in serum or CSF of symptomatic people, which will differentiate between acute versus convalescent serum. Because of cross reactivity among arboviruses, antibody tests require confirmation. Therefore, RT-PCR is utilized to detect viral RNA in serum or CSF depending on the type of specific arbovirus being sought. The viruses may be found in the blood (viremia) from a few days before the onset of symptoms through the initial 1 to 2 days of illness. The arboviruses may be isolated in various culture systems. Attempts at isolation from the blood are generally useful only when viremia is prolonged, as in dengue, CTF, and some of the hemorrhagic fevers. Virus is not present in the stool and is rarely found in the throat; viral recovery from CSF is also difficult, although virus can be detected in CSF or affected tissue by RT-PCR, and sometimes by culture during the acute phase of illness.

TREATMENT AND PREVENTION

Treatment supportive only

Protection from bites, vector control primary prevention

There is generally no specific treatment for arboviral infections other than supportive care; ribavirin has been used on occasion, but controlled studies have not been reported to support or refute its effectiveness. Prevention is primarily avoidance of contact with potentially infected arthropods, a task that can be extremely difficult even with the use of adequate screening and insect repellents. In some settings, vector control can be accomplished by elimination of arthropod-breeding sites (stagnant pools and the like) and sometimes by attempts to eradicate the arthropods with careful use of insecticides. Such measures have been highly effective in the control of urban yellow fever, in which elimination of urban breeding sites and other measures to eradicate the principal mosquito vector species (*A aegypti*) have been used. Viruses maintained in complex sylvatic cycles are infinitely more difficult to control without risking major environmental disruption and inestimable expense.

Yellow fever, TBEV, and Japanese B encephalitis vaccines are available

Vaccines are available for immunization of horses against western, eastern, and Venezuelan equine encephalitis virus infections, and the latter has also been used for some laboratory personnel who work with the virus. Another arbovirus vaccine in general use for humans is a live attenuated yellow fever virus vaccine (17-D strain), which is used to protect rural populations exposed to the sylvatic cycle and international travelers to endemic areas. In fact, many countries in tropical Africa, Asia, and South America require proof of yellow fever vaccination before allowing travelers to enter. There is also a vaccine for human tick-borne encephalitis virus (TBEV), which is endemic in areas of Western Europe; inactivated Japanese B encephalitis vaccines are widely used in endemic areas of eastern Asia and adjacent southern Pacific countries and are also licensed in the United States.

KEY CONCLUSIONS

- Arboviruses, transmitted through insect (mosquitoes, ticks) bites, cause encephalitis, hemorrhage, hepatitis, or febrile illness. These viruses are distributed in different parts of the world, including the United States.
- Encephalitis-causing arboviruses in the United States include togaviruses (Western and Eastern and equine encephalitis viruses), flaviviruses (St. Louis encephalitis viruses, WNV), and bunyavirus (California/La Crosse virus).
- Some arboviruses such as yellow fever cause hepatitis, hemorrhage, others such as dengue causes a wide range of spectrum from febrile illness to hemorrhage to shock. Reinfection with different but closely dengue serotype does not provide protection but enhances the infection.

- Several arboviruses such as chikungunya, dengue, West Nile, Zika virus have symptoms of polyarthritis and joint pain.
- WNV that is distributed in the United States causes West Nile fever in 20% of the infected people and CNS-associated diseases such as meningitis, encephalitis, meningoencephalitis, and poliomyelitis in less than 1% of the infected people. Older people above age 50 years of age and those with weakened immune system have severe disease.
- Zika virus, which emerged in 2015 in South America, was also reported in the United States from 2016 to 2017. Infection is asymptomatic or mild in most people, whereas some people have febrile illness. Infection during pregnancy is associated with birth defects, especially microcephaly.

NONARTHROPOD-BORNE VIRUSES OF ZOONOTIC ORIGIN

Overview

The nonarthropod-borne zoonotic viruses are those that are not transmitted through arthropod vectors but transmitted through small mammals and rodents. These viruses include Hantaviruses (bunyavirus), arenaviruses, and filoviruses, and their characteristics are summarized in **Table 16–2.** Hantavirus is the only nonarthropod zoonotically transmitted bunyavirus whose some species cause Hantavirus pulmonary syndrome (HPS) in the United States, whereas other species cause hemorrhagic fever and renal syndrome (HFRS) in Asia and Europe. Arenaviruses that are associated with hemorrhagic fevers include South American hemorrhagic fever (Junín virus, Machupo virus, Sabia virus) and West African Lasa fever (Lassa virus). In addition, another arenavirus of animals, lymphocytic choriomeningitis virus (LCMV) may cause infection in humans associated with CNS disease. Two members of Filovirus, *Marburgvirus* and *Ebolavirus*, are known to cause Marburg and Ebola fevers, the highly fatal hemorrhagic fevers. Both innate and adaptive immunity is suppressed in Ebola virus infection most likely due to infection of monocytes/macrophages. The fatality rate is very high in Ebola virus infection. There is neither any specific treatment nor vaccine available for these infectious agents. These viral diseases will be discussed in this section. Rabies virus is transmitted to humans through animal bites such as dogs and wild animals and is described in Chapter 17. Some other viruses that are occasionally transmitted by animals including orthomyxoviruses (birds, pigs), henipaviruses (horses, pigs, dogs), and vesicular stomatitis virus (VSV) (cattle, pigs, horses) are briefly mentioned here.

HANTAVIRUSES

Hantavirus, a negative-sense RNA, helical, enveloped virus (virion structure shown in Figure 16–3), is the only Bunyavirus that is a nonarthropod-transmitted zoonotic virus. Other bunyaviruses are arboviruses that are discussed in the previous section. Hantaviruses have several species that cause different diseases based on geographic distribution, including the **old world Hantavirus** such as Hantaan and others causing the HFRS found across the world (Asia, parts of Europe) and the **new world Hantavirus** species such as Sin Nombre virus causing HPS found in the United States.

■ Old World Hantavirus Species: HFRS

The Hantavirus causing HFRS includes diseases such as Korean hemorrhagic fever (KHF), epidemic hemorrhagic fever, and nephropathia epidemica. These Hantavirus species are Hantaan, Dobrava, Saaremaa, Seoul, and Puumala. These viruses are distributed or are endemic in various countries, including Asia, Western and Central Europe, Scanvandia, and the Balkins (Table 16-2). Hantaan virus is distributed in eastern Asia, mainly China, Russia, and Korea. Seoul virus is found worldwide carried and spread by brown or Norway rats. In 2017, there was an outbreak of Seoul virus that infected 17 people and found in 31 ratteries in 11 states of the United States. It is an important cause of hemorrhagic fever, often complicated by varying degrees of acute renal failure. In the 1950s, thousands of military personnel developed the disease during the Korean War and given the name KHF. The first reported isolation of KHF was in 1978, when the antigen was detected in the lung tissues of wild rodents (*Apodemus* species) by indirect immunofluorescence

Causes of hemorrhagic fever during the Korean War

Other viruses similar to KHF throughout northern Eurasia

TABLE 16–2   Selected Nonarthropod Zoonotic Viruses of Major Importance to Humans

GENUS AND MEMBER	MAJOR GEOGRAPHIC DISTRIBUTION	PRIMARY VECTOR	USUAL DISEASE EXPRESSION
BUNYAVIRUSES			
Hantavirus			
Hantavirus (Sin Nombre virus)	United States (Southwest)	Deer mouse (*Peromyscus maniculatus*)	Hantavirus pulmonary syndrome (HPS)
Hantavirus virus (Andes virus)	South America	Rodents (various species)	HPS
Hantaan virus	Eastern Asia, China, Russia, Korea	*Apodemus species* (rodent)	Hemorrhagic fever with renal syndrome (HFRS)
Puumala virus	Scandinavia, western Europe, western Russia	*Clethrionomys* (bank vole)	HFRS
Dobrava virus	Balkans	*Apodemus species*	HFRS
Seoul virus	Worldwide	*Rattus* (brown rat)	HFRS
Saaremaa virus	Central Europe, Scandinavia	*Apodemus species*	HFRS
ARENAVIRUSES			
Junin virus	Argentina	Drylands Vesper Mouse (*Calomys musculinus*)	Argentinean hemorrhagic fever
Lassa virus	West Africa	Natal Multimammate Mouse (*Mastomys natalensis*)	Lassa fever
Machupo virus	Bolivia	Larger vasper mouse (*Calomys callosus*)	Bolivian hemorrhagic fever
Whitewater Arroyo virus	United States (Southwest)	Woodrat (*Neotoma*)	Hemorrhagic fever
Chapare virus	Bolivia	Rodent	Hemorrhagic fever
Lugo virus	South Africa	Rodent	Hemorrhagic fever
Lymphocytic choriomeningitis virus (LCMV)	Worldwide	House mouse, hamsters	CNS infections
FILOVIRUSES			
Marburg virus	Africa	African monkeys	Hemorrhagic fever
Ebola virus (Zaire, Sudan, Tai-Forest)	Africa	Fruit bats, apes, monkeys, duikers	Hemorrhagic fever

using convalescent sera from affected patients. No illness was apparent in the rodents, suggesting a reservoir mechanism and mode of transmission like those described for the arenaviruses.

The virus is transmitted through inhalation of excreta of the rodents by the conjunctival route or by direct contact with skin breaks. People may also be infected with aerosolized urine, droppings, or saliva of infected rodents or after exposure to dust from their nests. Rodents' bite has also been reported to transmit the virus. The incubation period is 1 to 2 weeks (in rare cases up to 8 weeks), and initial symptoms are headaches, back and abdominal pain, fever, chills, nausea, flushing of the face, redness of the eyes, and blurred vision. Patients later develop low blood pressure, acute shock, vascular leakage, and acute renal failure. The severity of the disease also depends on the species, with Hantaan and Dobrava causing severe disease, whereas Seoul, Saaremaa, and Puumala cause moderate disease. Recovery takes weeks or months. The fatality rate for Hantaan is 5% to 15% and for other species is less than 1%.

Diagnosis is performed through serology (IgM), viral antigen, or viral RNA (RT-PCR). Treatment is supportive with fluid and electrolyte balance and management of other underlying conditions. Dialysis maybe required to correct fluid overload. Intravenous ribavirin has shown some benefits, if used early in infection. There is no vaccine. Contact with rodents should be avoided to prevent infection.

■ **New World Hantavirus Species: HPS**

It was known for some time that rodents in the United States are infected with a *Hantavirus*, but no associated human disease was recognized. In early 1993, an outbreak of fulminant respiratory disease

Margin notes

Detected in lungs of wild rodents

✳ Transmission through inhalation of rodent excreta or direct skin contact

✳ Severe disease; hypotension, acute shock, vascular leakage, acute renal failure

✳ Diagnosis by serology (IgM) or RT-PCR (viral RNA)

Supportive treatment, no vaccine

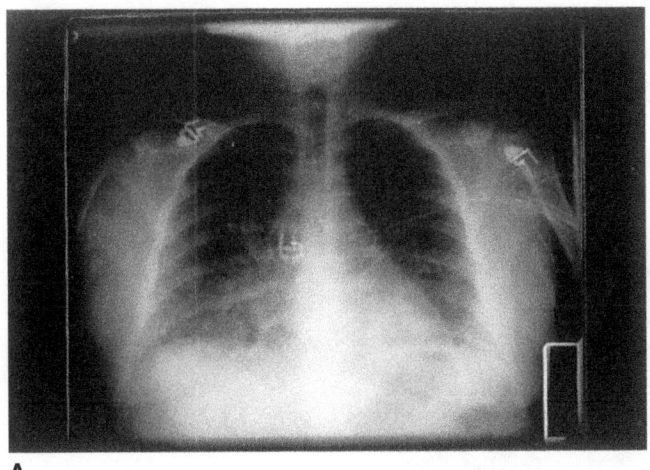
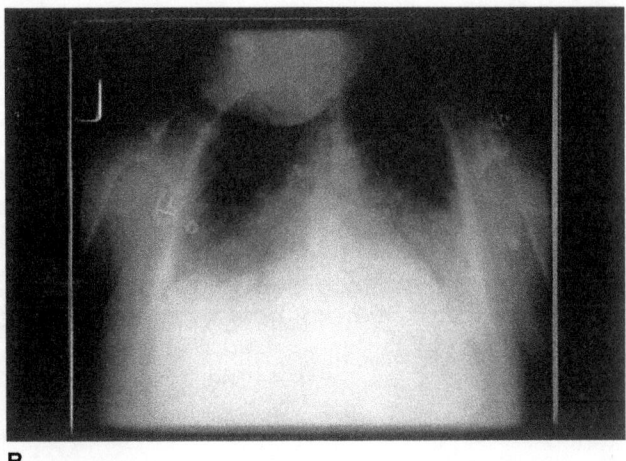

A

B

FIGURE 16–5. **A and B.** Serial radiographs obtained over 48 hours in a patient with Hantavirus pulmonary syndrome (HPS). (Reproduced with permission from Connor DH, Chandler FW, Schwartz DQ, et al: *Pathology of Infectious Diseases.* Stamford CT: Appleton & Lange; 1997.)

with high mortality (around 56%) occurred in the Southwestern United States at the Four Corners shared by Arizona, Colorado, New Mexico, and Utah. This syndrome (HPS) has been related to at least three Hantaviruses, of which Sin Nombre virus is the most common. The host of the Sin Nombre virus is the deer mouse (*Peromyscus maniculatus*) found in the western and central United States and Canada. Several other species of Hantaviruses can cause HPS in the United States, including the New York Hantavirus (host: white-footed mouse) in the Northeastern United States, Black Creek Hantavirus (host: cotton rat) in the Southeastern United States, and Bayou Hantavirus (host: rice rat). There is another species of hantavirus, Andes virus, that causes HPS in South America. Infections are associated with an increased population of infected mice in and around human habitations.

From 1993 to 2018, active surveillance in the United States has documented over 751 cases that have occurred in residents of 34 states, with most having been acquired in the Southwest region. Overall, the average mortality rate is around 38%. Hantaviruses causing HPS has been reported in Canada and South America, including Argentina, Bolivia, Brazil, Chile, Panama, Paraguay, and Uruguay.

The virus is believed to be transmitted to humans most often by inhalation of infectious rodent excreta, by the conjunctival route, or by direct contact with skin breaks. Human-to-human spread has not been encountered in the United States. However, rare cases of person-to-person transmission have occurred in people with close contacts with Andes hantavirus, in Chile and Argentina. The incubation period may be between 1 and 5 weeks followed by early symptoms, including fever, fatigue, chills, headaches, aches in large muscle group (thighs, hips, back, shoulder), abdominal problems (vomiting, diarrhea). The second phase of the HPS starts 4 to 10 days after early symptoms that include coughing, shortness of breath, and heaviness around the chest as lungs fill with fluid (**Figure 16–5**). The diagnosis is done on clinical grounds based on a history of potential rural rodent exposure, severe pulmonary syndrome, and lung imaging. There is no specific treatment or vaccine for HPS. Treatment has involved aggressive respiratory support in intensive care unit. Public health measures to inform inhabitants of routes of spread and to reduce the rodent population appear to have controlled the outbreak. Intravenous ribavirin has shown some benefit in HFRS (KHF), but no evidence of efficacy in U.S. strains causing HPS. As noted, the mortality rate is high, around 38%.

Hantavirus among rodents in the United States

Southwestern U.S. outbreak related to deer mice

✳ Humans infected by inhalation of rodent excreta or direct contact with skin breaks

No human-to-human transmission in the United States

✳ Hantavirus pulmonary syndrome in the United States

● ARENAVIRUSES

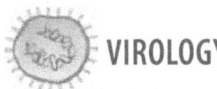 ## VIROLOGY

The arenaviruses of the family Arenaviridae are enveloped, bisegmented, containing a large (L), single-stranded, negative-sense (–) and a small (S) ambisense (–/+) RNA genome with pleomorphic morphology ranging in size from 50 to 300 (mean 110-130) nm in diameter (**Figure 16–6**). There are two separate helical nucleocapsids, L and S, encapsidating L and S RNA segments,

FIGURE 16-6. **Virion structure of arenavirus.** Arenaviruses are enveloped containing two surface glycoproteins, G1 and G2, and the RNA genome comprises large (L) single-stranded, negative-sense (–) and a small (S) ambisense (–/+) RNA that form L and S nucleocapsids. The size of virions ranges from 50 to 300 nm in diameter. The virion contains host cell ribosomes inside the virus particle. These ribosomes confer a granular or sandy appearance to the virions; hence their name (from the Latin *arenosus* for "sandy").

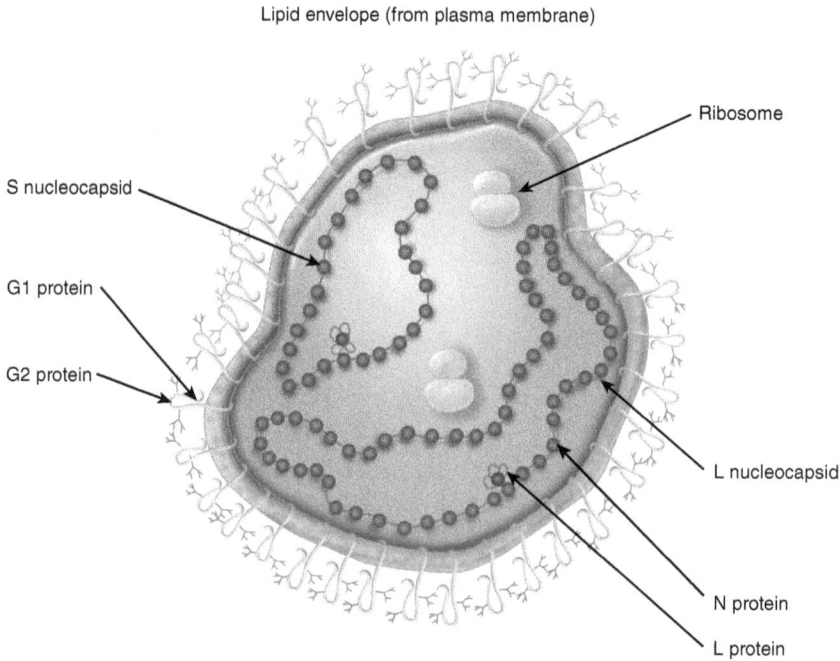

Lipid envelope (from plasma membrane)

Ribosome

S nucleocapsid

G1 protein

G2 protein

L nucleocapsid

N protein

L protein

✳ Pleomorphic, enveloped viruses with two RNA-helical nucleocapsids and host ribosomes

Two RNA segments, L (negative sense) and S (ambisense)

Replicate in the cytoplasm of infected cells

respectively. The envelope contains two viral surface GPs, G1 and G2. The virion contains host cell ribosomes in its interior. These ribosomes confer a granular appearance to the viruses; hence their name (from the Latin *arenosus* for "sandy"). The most significant arenavirus infections in humans are the hemorrhagic fevers caused by Lassa virus in West Africa. In addition, the South American hemorrhagic fevers are caused by arenaviruses, including Junín virus, Machupo virus, Guanarito virus, and Sabia virus. Another arenavirus, Lujo virus was identified in South Africa. In the United States, Whitewater Arroyo arenavirus (WAV) recovered from white-throated woodrat from New Mexico in 1990s), caused infection in humans in 2000. LCMV is occasionally transmitted to humans from infected mice and other rodents, and associated with CNS infection that may persist for several months.

Arenaviruses replicate in the cytoplasm of the infected host cell using the strategy of negative-sense RNA genomes. Viral attachment protein G1 interacts with a cell surface receptor (αDG), and the virions are internalized in vesicles. Viral fusion protein G2 mediates fusion, resulting in the release of nucleocapsids. Virion-associated RNA-dependent RNA polymerase (L protein, Figure 16–5) mediates transcription, and the L RNA segment encodes the polymerase (L) protein and a Z protein, which may help the virus in assembly and release. The S RNA segment, which has ambisense (–/+) polarity, encodes NP and envelope GPs G1 and G2, using a negative-sense RNA strategy for transcription. The ambisense RNA strategy allows arenaviruses to regulate their gene expression, first encoding the N and later the G proteins. Like bunyaviruses, arenaviruses also lack a matrix protein, a characteristic of enveloped viruses. They mature by budding from the host cell plasma membrane. Arenaviruses cause persistent infection in rodents and are also transmitted to humans from the excreta of infected rodents.

EPIDEMIOLOGY

A common feature of the arenaviruses is their zoonotic reservoir, particularly small rodents, in which they may be sustained for long periods. Primary infection (horizontal transmission) in mature rodents often results in disease and death, whereas intrauterine or perinatal infection (vertical transmission) usually leads to chronic lifelong viremia with persistent shedding of virus into the feces, urine, and respiratory secretions. Although chronically infected rodents are somewhat tolerant to the virus (ie, infection is persistent without causing illness), they produce antibodies, and evidence of deleterious effects can be found in older hosts, usually in the form of immune complex glomerulonephritis. The viruses are perpetuated by vertical transmission from infected mothers to their offspring. When environmental contact becomes close, spread from the rodent reservoir to humans (and, in some instances, subhuman primates) can occur via aerosols; through exposure to infective urine, feces, or tissues; or directly by rodent bites. This contrasts with the arthropod spread of arboviruses.

Sustained in small rodent reservoirs

Vertical transmission in rodents

✳ Spread to humans by aerosols and close contact

CLINICAL DISEASE

■ Arenaviruses Associated with Hemorrhagic Fevers

The agents of arenavirus hemorrhagic fevers are transmitted from infected rodents to humans in the manner described earlier, although person-to-person spread by contact with secretions and body fluids also occurs readily. The viruses in this group include the South American hemorrhagic fever agents (the Junín virus, the cause of Argentinean hemorrhagic fever, and the Machupo virus, the cause of Bolivian hemorrhagic fever), Sabia virus (Brazilian hemorrhagic fever), Lassa virus, the cause of **Lassa fever** in West Africa, Chapare virus, the cause of Chapare (Bolivia) hemorrhagic fever and Lugo virus, the cause of Lujo (South Africa) hemorrhagic fever.

Arenaviruses have pathogenic and pathologic features similar to those described for the arboviruses that cause hemorrhagic fevers; however, the mechanism involved in the coagulation abnormalities is not understood. All are characterized by fever, usually accompanied by hemorrhagic manifestations, shock, neurologic disturbances, and bradycardia. Lassa fever also frequently causes hepatitis, myocarditis, exudative pharyngitis, and acute deafness. The last deficit may persist after recovery. Mortality rate is estimated to be 10% to 50% for Lassa fever and 5% to 30% for the other viruses. All are considered highly dangerous in terms of infectivity. Importation of cases to nonendemic areas has occurred, with significant risk of spread to medical and laboratory personnel.

The diagnosis of an arenavirus infection is suggested primarily by the recent travel history of the patient and the clinical syndrome. Although viral antibodies (IgM, IgG) and viral antigens (in some cases) by ELISA, viral RNA by RT-PCR, and virus isolation diagnosis may be performed, these procedures should not be attempted in a hospital diagnostic laboratory but in a containment laboratory facility. Any patient suspected of having such an infection should be immediately isolated and public health authorities should be notified. Because of the high risk of spread of infection from body fluids and excreta, even routine laboratory studies are best deferred until the diagnosis and proper disposition of specimens can be resolved. Viremia can persist 1 month, and virus shedding in the urine may continue more than 2 months after the onset of illness. Treatment is primarily supportive; however, intravenous ribavirin, if begun within 6 days of illness onset, has been shown to be helpful in Lassa fever.

■ Arenaviruses Associated with CNS Infections—LCMV

Infection with LCMV is particularly common in hamsters and mice. In the United States, most human illnesses have been traced to contact with rodent breeding colonies in research or pet supply centers and to pet hamsters in the home. The illness usually consists of fever, headache, and myalgia, although meningitis or meningoencephalitis also occurs occasionally. Such CNS infections may persist as long as 3 months. There is also evidence that transplacental infection can occur in humans, resulting in fetal death, hydrocephalus, or chorioretinitis. No person-to-person transmission of infection has been documented.

The diagnosis of lymphocytic choriomeningitis is suggested by a history of rodent contact. The virus may be isolated in the early stages of disease by cell culture or intracerebral inoculation of blood or CSF into weanling mice or young guinea pigs. Serologic testing of acute and convalescent sera is usually performed by indirect immunofluorescence. RT-PCR to detect viral RNA is also available.

● FILOVIRUSES

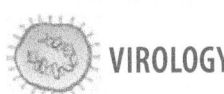 **VIROLOGY**

Filoviruses come from the virus family Filoviridae that have two genera, *Marburgvirus* and *Ebolavirus* that cause Marburg and Ebola fevers, the two known highly fatal hemorrhagic fevers. Although no subtypes or species of Marburg virus has been found, Ebola virus exits as six subtypes (species), including Zaire, Sudan, Tai Forest (formerly known as Ivory Coast), Bundibugyo, Bombali (identified in bats, no known disease in humans), and Reston (no known disease in humans). Filoviruses are enveloped, helical, single-stranded, negative-sense RNA viruses with filamentous and highly pleomorphic virions, averaging 80 nm in diameter and 300 to 14,000 nm

---

Side notes:

❋ Person-to-person spread occurs by contact with body fluids

❋ Arenaviruses cause fever, shock, and hemorrhage

Hepatitis, myocarditis with Lassa fever

High mortality, risk of further transmission

Suggested by clinical findings, travel history

Diagnosis by antibody, antigen, viral RNA (RT-PCR) done in containment labs

Viremia may be prolonged

Transplacental infection in humans

Mice and hamsters in pet stores

❋ Meningitis may persist for months

Two filoviruses: Marburg and Ebola cause hemorrhagic fevers

Single subtype for Marburg, six subtypes for Ebola

Enveloped, filamentous, helical negative-sense RNA viruses

FIGURE 16–7. **Morphology of filovirus virion.** Filoviruses are enveloped, single-stranded, negative-sense RNA viruses with filamentous and highly pleomorphic virions, averaging 80 nm in diameter and 300 to 14,000 nm in length. The nucleocapsid protein (NP) has a helical symmetry and the envelope is derived from plasma membrane containing 10 nm peplomers or spikes, the (GP) glycoprotein, which mediate virus entry into susceptible cells.

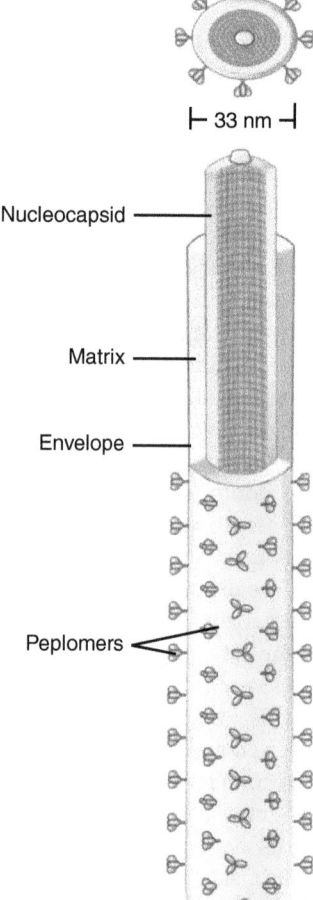

Replicate in the cytoplasm

in length (**Figure 16–7**). There are seven viral genes that are sequentially arranged on a 19 kb RNA genome. The NP has a helical symmetry, and the envelope is derived from the plasma membrane as a result of budding. The envelope contains 10 nm peplomers or spikes, and the GP, which mediates virus entry into susceptible cells.

Viral GP surface protein mediates virus entry into target cells. RNA-dependent RNA polymerase directs the synthesis of mRNA from a linear negative-sense RNA genome, like other negative-sense RNA viruses (rhabdoviruses, paramyxoviruses). Seven monocistronic mRNAs are generated followed by translation of viral proteins. Translation of NP triggers the switch from transcription to genome replication. The NP binds to the RNA genome to form the nucleocapsid, which is enclosed in a matrix protein and buds from plasma membrane containing viral GPs.

EPIDEMIOLOGY AND CLINICAL DISEASE: MARBURG AND EBOLA VIRUSES

Initial cases transmitted from monkeys

The association of the Marburg virus with serious disease did not become apparent until 1967, when 31 cases of hemorrhagic fever and 7 deaths occurred among persons in Germany and former Yugoslavia who were handling a group of African monkeys imported from central Uganda. The agent was later identified as Marburg virus (named after Marburg, Germany) and was apparently transmitted by the infected monkeys. In 1975, the virus was associated with a similar disease in three travelers in South Africa, and in 1980 in Kenya.

In 1976, severe outbreaks of hemorrhagic fever occurred in northern Zaire (now the Democratic Republic of Congo) and southern Sudan, with case fatality rates of 90% and 50%, respectively. The illnesses were similar to those described for Marburg virus, but were later shown to be caused by an antigenically different agent known as Ebola virus, named after a river in Zaire. In 1990, another filovirus (Reston) serologically related to Ebola virus was isolated from monkeys during an epizootic of simian hemorrhagic fever at a U.S. quarantine facility with no human infection. The reservoir was determined to be monkeys imported from the Philippines. However, in 1990 and 2008, few human asymptomatic cases with evidence of antibodies against the virus were reported. Reston-Ebola does not cause any disease in humans but could be the cause of disease in monkeys. In 1994, a scientist was infected with a new strain of Ebola virus, Ebola-Ivory Coast (Cote d'Ivoire), in Tai Forest (Cote d'Ivoire) from a chimpanzee's autopsy and was successfully treated and survived. The latest and the largest outbreak in history started in West Africa in March 2014 that severely affected countries such as Guinea, Liberia, and Sierra Leone. It also affected several other countries with few cases through travelers such as Nigeria, Senegal, Spain, United States, Mali, United Kingdom, and Italy. In this long outbreak or epidemic that lasted almost 2 years reported 28,652 estimated and confirmed cases, 15,261 laboratory-confirmed cases, and 11,325 deaths. In March 31, 2016, WHO terminated the public health emergency concern for the Ebola outbreak in West Africa. The average fatality rate is around 50% but has varied from 25% to 90% in previous outbreaks. Since then, cases of Ebola virus have been reported in Democratic Republic of Congo with eight cases and four deaths (61%) in 2017, 3470 cases and 2287 deaths (66%) in 2018, and 138 cases and 55 deaths (42.3%) in 2020.

Ebola subtypes (species) differ antigenically

Ebola subtype specificity associated with fatality

While filoviruses are zoonotic, it is not known how these viruses are primarily transmitted from infected animals (fruit bats or primates like apes or monkeys or duikers) to humans. The reservoir, though uncertain, is thought to be in bats. After the virus is transmitted from animals to humans, person-to-person transmission is probably the way by which further infections occur (secondary transmission), most likely through direct contacts such as broken skin or mucous membranes in eyes, nose, or mouth to blood or body fluids (urine, saliva, sweat, feces, vomit, breast milk, semen, and others) of infected, sick, or deceased persons. Sexual transmission (oral, vaginal, or anal) and contaminated objects like needles and syringes have been shown. The incubation period is between 2 and 21 days (average 4-10 days) followed by flu-like illness characterized by fever, headache, joint and muscle pain, sore throat, diarrhea, vomiting, and stomach pain. In some patients, a purplish-red, maculopapular rash, hiccups, and internal and external bleeding are seen. Patients who develop severe disease have hemorrhages of the gastrointestinal tract and other sites, including shock and multiorgan failure. Numerous patients who die do not have a significant immune response at the time of death. However, some people recover from Ebola infection and mechanisms of recovery are not known; recovery is most likely related to patient's immune response. Survivors had Ebola antibody response for up to 10 years with some protective immunity. Some survivors have long-term complications like joint and eye problems. Ebola virus persists in semen for 3 to 9 months in some men and also in eye, amniotic fluid, placenta, breast milk, and CNS.

✳ Reservoir may be bats

✳ Primary transmission from animals to humans

✳ Secondary and further infections through direct contacts to blood and bodily fluids

✳ Symptoms start with flu-like illness leading to hemorrhage, bleeding, shock, multiorgans failure

✳ Mortality high in symptomatic infection

How does Ebola virus cause hemorrhage?

The reasons why these viruses can cause such fulminant, lethal hemorrhagic disease with shock in humans are not entirely clear. There is evidence that Marburg virus replicates in vascular endothelial cells, with subsequent necrosis. Ebola virus replicates at a remarkably high rate shutting off the host cell synthesis and immune responses. Both innate and adaptive immunity is suppressed most likely due to infection of monocytes/macrophages and dendritic cells. Some studies have shown that Ebola virus may exert its effects via its GP, synthesized in either a secreted or transmembrane form. The secreted GP interacts with neutrophils to inhibit early activation of the inflammatory response and alter the innate immune response. The GP allows the virus to infect monocytes/macrophages and dendritic cells causing cell damage and cytokine release associated with inflammation and fever. Viral entry into reticuloendothelial cells causes damages to vascular integrity, including cytokines release, which contributes to exaggerated inflammatory responses that are not protective. There is damage to the liver, combined with massive viremia, leading to disseminated intravascular coagulopathy. The virus eventually infects microvascular endothelial cells and compromises vascular integrity. This contributes to the hemorrhagic fever because the

✳ Fulminant and lethal effects in Ebola due to lytic infection of monocytes, macrophages, dendritic cells, and reticuloendothelial cells

✳ Cytokines released cause inflammation and damage

 Think ▸▸ Apply 16-4: Ebola virus infection and cytokine damage the endothelial cells leading to loss of vascular integrity, bleeding, and hemorrhage.

✳ Damage to vascular integrity caused by viral cytopathic effects, cytokines leading to hemorrhage, shock

✳ Humoral immunity detected in Ebola

Diagnosis by IgM or RT-PCR of viral RNA, precautions similar to arenavirus hemorrhagic fevers

Monoclonal antibodies against surface GP approved for treatment

Single-dose Ebola virus vaccine (rVSV-ZEBOV) approved

Henipaviruses spread by aerosols from bats

virus targets the reticuloendothelial network and the lining of blood vessels. The terminal stages of Ebola virus infection usually include diffuse bleeding, and hypotensive shock accounts for many fatalities. Antibody titers against Ebola virus GPs are readily detectable in patients who recover from Ebola virus infection. Serosurveys of humans residing in the areas where outbreaks have occurred suggest that human infections may be relatively common; as much as 7% of the survey group had antibodies, indicating past infection. In symptomatic infections, the mortality rate for both Marburg and Ebola viruses is extremely high but higher for Zaire-Ebola virus (50-90%) than other species of Ebola viruses or Marburg viruses.

The diagnosis of infection by these agents is suggested by symptoms and recent travel history. Person-to-person transmission occurs in Ebola virus infections and may be possible with Marburg virus. Diagnosis can be confirmed in a reference center by isolation of virus, antigen capture by ELISA, IgM antibody detection by ELISA, and genome amplification by RT-PCR. The virus can be identified in specimens from deceased patients by immunofluorescence or RT-PCR. However, as with the arenavirus-associated hemorrhagic fevers, utmost care in isolation precautions and prompt notification of public health authorities are mandatory for suspected cases before any diagnostic attempts are made. Supportive care is recommended. However, U.S. Food and Drug Administration (FDA) approved two treatments in 2020 for Zaire Ebola infection in adults and children: (1) Inmazeb (a combination of 3 monoclonal antibodies against Ebola surface GP) and (2) Ebanga (a single monoclonal antibody against GP). These treatments are combined with supportive care.

Prevention can be done by avoiding contacts with infected person's bodily fluids and objects and animals and bushmeat of animals in the endemic area. In December 2019, U.S. FDA approved a single dose protective and safe Ebola virus vaccine called Ervebo, which is a VSV (a rhabdovirus) vector expressing Ebola virus surface GP, recombinant vesicular stomatitis-Zaire Ebola virus vaccine (rVSV-ZEBOV).

ORTHOMYXOVIRUSES

Avian and animal (pigs and horses) influenza viruses may infect humans. In the past 10 years, avian influenza viruses (bird flu), including H5N1, H7N2, H7N3, H7N7, H7N9, H9N2, and H9N7, and pig reassortant influenza virus (H1N1 in 2009) have been documented to cause infections in humans. See Chapter 9 for avian influenza virus pathogenesis.

HENIPAVIRUSES

Two zoonotic paramyxoviruses involving humans and animals appeared in Australia and Southeast Asia during the late 1990s. These are Hendra and Nipah viruses, now classified in the *Henipavirus* genus of the Paramyxoviridae family.

Hendra virus has been detected in Australia in two small outbreaks involving horses that also affected humans. The human cases were characterized by pneumonia and encephalitis. However, large Nipah virus outbreaks have occurred in India, Bangladesh, Malaysia, and Singapore, affecting pigs, dogs, and humans. The human illnesses were similar to Hendra virus, as were outcomes (more than 50% fatality rate for both). The reservoir of henipaviruses is the *Pteropus* species of fruit bats ("flying foxes") and spread to humans and animals occurs via aerosols.

VESICULAR STOMATITIS VIRUS

A rhabdovirus, VSV causes outbreaks of disease in cattle, pigs, and horses that can be transmitted between animals by arthropods. Human infection is acquired by contact with infected animals but is unusual; it consists of a self-limited febrile illness and occasional herpes-like eruptions over the lips and oral mucosa. VSV vector has been used to make Ebola virus vaccine approved in 2019.

KEY CONCLUSIONS

- Hantavirus, a negative-sense RNA, helical, enveloped bunyavirus, is transmitted through inhalation of rodents' excreta and causing HPS in the United States (Sin Nombre virus), and HFRS in Asia and some parts of Europe (Hantaan virus).
- Arenaviruses are enveloped, bisegmented, ambisense RNA viruses that replicate in the cytoplasm using viral RNA-dependent RNA polymerase.
- Arenaviruses are transmitted via aerosols; through exposure to infective urine, feces, or tissues; or directly by rodent bites.

- Arenaviruses cause hemorrhagic fevers with manifestations such as shock, neurologic disturbances, and bradycardia. In addition, Lassa fever frequently causes hepatitis, myocarditis, exudative pharyngitis, and acute deafness. Another arenavirus, LCMV causes CNS infection that may persist for months.

- Ebola virus has six subtypes but only four subtypes cause infection in humans: Zaire, Sudan, Tai-Forest, and Bundibugyo. Zaire Ebola virus is the major virus in Ebola epidemics with a very high fatality rate (50-95%).

- Ebola virus is enveloped, filamentous, helical nucleocapsid, and a negative-sense RNA virus, which replicates in the cytoplasm by using viral RNA-dependent RNA polymerase.

- Ebola virus is primarily transmitted to humans by infected animals and then person to person by direct contact with blood or body fluids of infected, sick, or deceased persons.

- Ebola virus disease includes initially flu-like illness after 2 to 21 days of exposure to the virus further leading to hemorrhage, bleeding, shock, and multiorgan failure.

- Ebola virus pathogenesis includes infection and lysis of monocytes/macrophages, dendritic cells, reticuloendothelial cells, and release of inflammatory cytokines causing damage to vascular integrity leading to hemorrhage and shock.

- Two monoclonal antibodies against Ebola surface GP for treatment and an Ebola virus vaccine (rVSV-ZEBOV) for prevention/protection were approved by the U.S. FDA.

CASE STUDY

An Acute Case of Confusion

This 70-year-old woman, who lives in a rural area in the Midwestern United States, developed an illness in August that progressed over 3 days to include a moderate fever, headache, lower extremity weakness, and lethargy progressing to severe confusion.

On examination, she is unresponsive to verbal stimuli, and both pupils respond sluggishly to light. No other neurologic abnormalities are apparent. She lives with her husband on an old farm, and rodents and mosquitoes have been frequently seen around the house and barn.

QUESTIONS

1. Which one of the following would be the most probable viral cause?
   A. Western equine encephalitis
   B. California (La Crosse strain) encephalitis virus
   C. Colorado tick fever virus
   D. West Nile virus
   E. Lymphocytic choriomeningitis virus

2. Which one of the following viruses is primarily transmitted by mosquitoes?
   A. Ebola virus
   B. *Hantavirus*
   C. Yellow fever virus
   D. *Orbivirus*
   E. *Henipavirus*

3. Which one of the following features is the best predictor of suggesting the possible cause of a severe arboviral illness?
   A. Cerebrospinal fluid pleocytosis
   B. Patient age
   C. Season of occurrence
   D. Knowledge of environmental reservoirs
   E. Travel history

ANSWERS

1. (D)

2. (C)

3. (B)

chapter 17

Rabies

Rabies virus

The dog was certainly rabid. Joseph Meister had been pulled out from under him covered with foam and blood.

—Louis Pasteur, describing the 9-year-old boy he successfully immunized against rabies in July 1885

OVERVIEW

Rabies is an acute fatal viral illness of the central nervous system (CNS) commonly resulting in encephalitis. Rabies virus is a bullet-shaped, enveloped, helical nucleocapsid containing a negative-sense RNA genome of the Rhabdoviridae family. The word rabies is derived from the Latin verb "to rage," which suggests the appearance of the rabid patient. It can affect all mammals and is transmitted between them by infected secretions, most often by bite. It was first recognized more than 3000 years ago and has been the most feared of infectious diseases. It is said that Aristotle recognized that rabies could be spread by a rabid dog. Rabies involves the development of severe neurologic symptoms and signs in a patient who was previously bitten by an animal (a rabid dog or wild animals). The incubation period is 10 days to 1 year. The virus replicates at the site of bite followed by entry into the peripheral nervous system at the neuromuscular junctions and spreads to the CNS, where it replicates exclusively within the gray matter and then spreads centrifugally to the autonomic nervous system. The neurologic manifestations are very characteristic, with a relentlessly progressive excess of motor activity, agitation, hallucinations, and salivation. The patient appears to be foaming at the mouth and has severe throat contractions if swallowing is attempted. Involvement of the respiratory center produces respiratory paralysis, the major cause of death. Recovery is rare. The postexposure prophylaxis and treatment include cleansing the wound with soap and water, instilling hyperimmune globulin in and around the wound and administering IM to neutralize the virus, and vaccinating with inactivated rabies vaccine at days 0, 3, 7, and 14. The hyperimmune globulin and the vaccine should be given at two different sites.

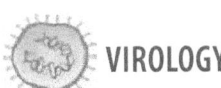 VIROLOGY

The rabies virus is a rhabdovirus, which is a bullet-shaped, enveloped, helical, RNA virus, 70 nm in diameter × 180 nm in length, of the *Lyssavirus* genus and Rhabdoviridae family (**Figure 17–1**). The helical nucleocapsid (N) is composed of a single-stranded, negative-sense RNA genome and an RNA-dependent RNA polymerase enclosed in a matrix (M) protein covered by a lipid bilayer envelope containing knob-like glycoprotein (G). The knob-like glycoprotein excrescences, which elicit neutralizing and hemagglutination-inhibiting antibodies, cover the surface of the virion. In the past, a single antigenically homogeneous virus was believed to be responsible for all rabies; however, differences in cell culture growth characteristics of isolates from different animal sources (bats, cats, dogs, foxes, and skunks), some differences in virulence for experimental animals, and antigenic differences in surface glycoproteins have indicated strain heterogeneity among rabies virus isolates. These studies may help to explain some of the biologic differences as well as the occasional case of "vaccine failure." Other pathogens in the rhabdovirus group include vesicular stomatitis virus (VSV), which is an animal virus but may also occasionally infect humans (see Chapter 16).

✳ Bullet-shaped, enveloped, helical nucleocapsid, and a negative-sense RNA virus

Knob-like envelope glycoproteins elicit neutralizing and hemagglutination antibodies

Strains from different animals antigenically heterogeneous

FIGURE 17–1. **Electron micrograph of the rabies virus (yellow) (×36 700).** Note the bullet shape. The external surface of the virus contains spike-like glycoprotein projections that bind specifically to cellular receptors. (Reproduced with permission from Willey JM: *Prescott, Harley, & Klein's Microbiology*, 7th ed. New York, NY: McGraw Hill; 2008.)

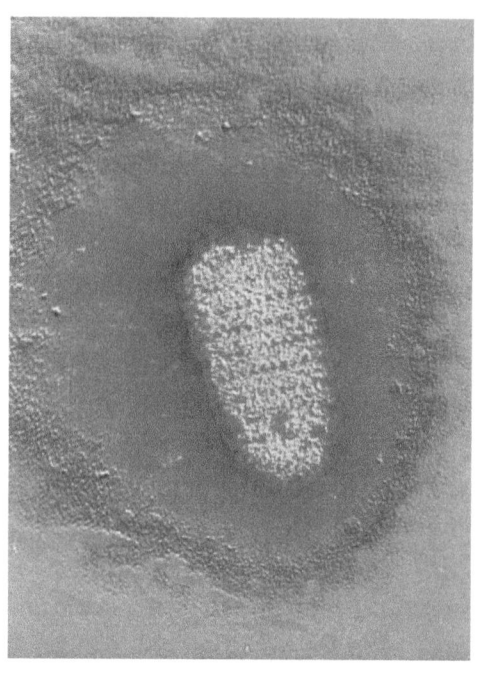

Rabies virus is transmitted from the bite of an animal (usually a rabid dog or wild animal) and multiplies initially at the site of entry in muscle cells, and then the virus travels to the CNS to replicate in the brain cells. Rabies virus G protein binds to the acetylcholine or neural cell adhesion molecule (NCAM) receptor present on the cell surface. The virus is internalized followed by fusion of the viral envelope with the endosomal membrane and uncoating and release of the nucleocapsid in the cytoplasm. Because rabies virus is a negative-sense RNA virus, virion-associated RNA-dependent RNA polymerase transcribes the genome to make several mRNAs in the cytoplasm. These mRNAs are translated into various proteins, including nucleocapsid, matrix, RNA polymerase, and G glycoproteins. The G glycoproteins are expressed on the infected cell surface membranes. After replication of viral RNA genomes directed by the viral RNA-dependent RNA polymerase, the progeny virions are assembled in the cytoplasm. The nucleocapsid protein binds the RNA genome and packages the viral RNA-dependent RNA polymerase. This nucleocapsid complex associates with the matrix protein, and the lipid bilayer envelope containing G protein is acquired as the progeny virions bud through the plasma membrane.

G protein binds to acetylcholine or NCAM receptor on target cells

✳ (-) RNA genome replicates in the cytoplasm using viral RNA polymerase

G protein-containing lipoprotein envelope acquired from plasma membrane

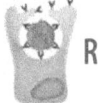 RABIES

EPIDEMIOLOGY

Rabies exists in two epizootic forms, urban and sylvatic. The urban form is associated with unimmunized dogs or cats, and the sylvatic form occurs in wild skunks, foxes, wolves, raccoons, and bats, but not rodents or rabbits. While these wild animals associated with rabies are distributed in distinct geographic regions of the United States, bats are distributed throughout the country. Introduction of an infected animal into a different geographic area can lead to infection of many new members of that species (**Figure 17–2**). For example, due to raccoon hunting, there was a sudden appearance of raccoon rabies in West Virginia and Virginia in 1977. Before that time, the nearest cases of raccoon rabies were found several hundred miles away in South Carolina. The hunters are believed to have imported infected raccoons from another state. Since 1977, raccoon rabies has spread from West Virginia and Virginia to 12 northeastern states. In the United States, raccoon rabies is found in the northeast and southeast, skunk rabies in Midwest, fox rabies in southwest, and skunk in California area. Rabies virus exists in several variants. There are five distinct antigenic rabies virus variants associated with eight terrestrial reservoir species and more than 13 rabies virus variants associated with bats.

Human infection, or the much more common infection of cattle, is incidental, is blind ended, and does not contribute to maintenance or transmission of the disease. In the United States, an

Two epizootic forms: urban (dogs and cats) and sylvatic (wild animals)

Several rabies virus variants associated with wild animals

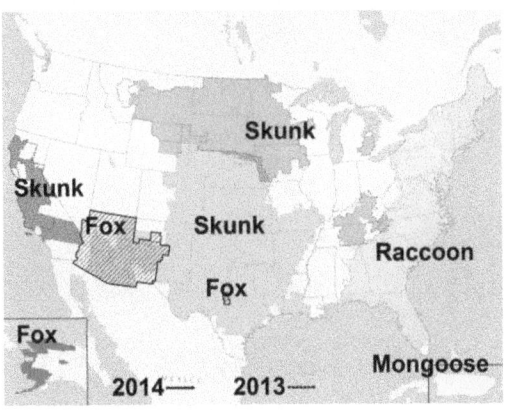

FIGURE 17–2. In the United States, rabies is found in terrestrial animals in 10 distinct geographic areas. In each area, a particular species is the reservoir, and one of five antigenic variants of the virus predominates as illustrated by the five different colors.

estimated 92.6% of reported cases of rabies in animals occur among wildlife, with raccoons accounting for 30.2%, bats 29.1%, skunks 26.3%, foxes 5.15%, cats 5.51%, cattle 1.29%, and dogs 0.98% cases in 2014. Human exposures may be from wild animals or from unimmunized dogs or cats. In the United States, 127 cases of rabies were reported between 1960 and 2018, 70% from bat exposure and about 25% from dog bites during international travel. In recent years, there has been a decrease in the US cases, one to three cases per year but 55,000 people getting postexposure prophylaxis for suspected infection, and bat exposure has been the source in almost all cases despite a resurgence of rabies in skunks and raccoons. An occasional case has resulted from aerosol exposure (eg, bat caves and no bite). Domestic animal bites are very important sources of rabies in developing countries because of lack of enforcement of animal immunization. Infection in domestic animals usually represents a spillover from infection in wildlife reservoirs. Human infection tends to occur where animal rabies is common and where there is a large population of unimmunized domestic animals. Worldwide, the occurrence of human rabies is estimated to be more than 59,000 fatal cases per year mostly in Asia and Africa, with the highest attack rates in Southeast Asia, the Philippines, and the Indian subcontinent. Almost all of these cases result from dog bites. Human-to-human transmission of rabies has been documented via transplanted corneas and solid-organ transplantation. In theory, infected humans could potentially transmit rabies to uninfected humans via bite or nonbite, but such cases have not been reported.

* Risks to humans in the United States from wild animal bites (bats, coyotes, foxes, raccoons, skunks, wolves)

More than 59,000 deaths mostly in Asia and Africa

Highest attack rates in Southeast Asia and Indian subcontinent, mostly from dog bites

PATHOGENESIS

The sequence of events of the pathogenesis of rabies virus infection is depicted in **Figure 17–3**. The essential first event in human or animal rabies infection is the inoculation of virus through the epidermis, usually as a result of an animal bite. Inhalation of heavily contaminated material, such as bat droppings, can also cause infection. The incubation period is between 10 days and 1 year (average 20-90 days). Rabies virus first replicates in striated muscle tissue at the site of inoculation. Immunization at this time is presumed to prevent migration of the virus into neural tissues. In the absence of immunity, the virus then enters the peripheral nervous system at the neuromuscular junctions and spreads to the CNS, where it replicates exclusively within the gray matter. It then passes centrifugally along autonomic nerves to reach other tissues, including the salivary glands, adrenal medulla, kidneys, and lungs. Passage into the salivary glands in animals facilitates further transmission of the disease by infected saliva. The neuropathology of rabies resembles that of other viral diseases of the CNS, with infiltration of lymphocytes and plasma cells into CNS tissue and nerve cell destruction. The pathognomonic lesion is the Negri body (**Figure 17–4**), an eosinophilic cytoplasmic inclusion distributed throughout the brain, particularly in the hippocampus, cerebral cortex, cerebellum, and dorsal spinal ganglia.

Replicates at site of entry, enters peripheral nervous system

* Spreads to CNS, replicates in gray matter

* Passes centrifugally along autonomic nerves reaching salivary glands, adrenal medulla, kidneys, lungs

Virus in salivary glands of animals facilitates transmission

 How does rabies reach from the animal bite site in the muscles to the brain and why does it replicate in the brain?

 Think ▶▶ Apply 17-1: **Rabies virus initially replicates in the muscles and enters the peripheral nervous system at the neuromuscular junctions and spreads to the CNS. Rabies is tropic to the brain because of the presence of its receptors.**

FIGURE 17-3. Sequential steps (1-8) in the pathogenesis of rabies virus infection are shown in the diagram.

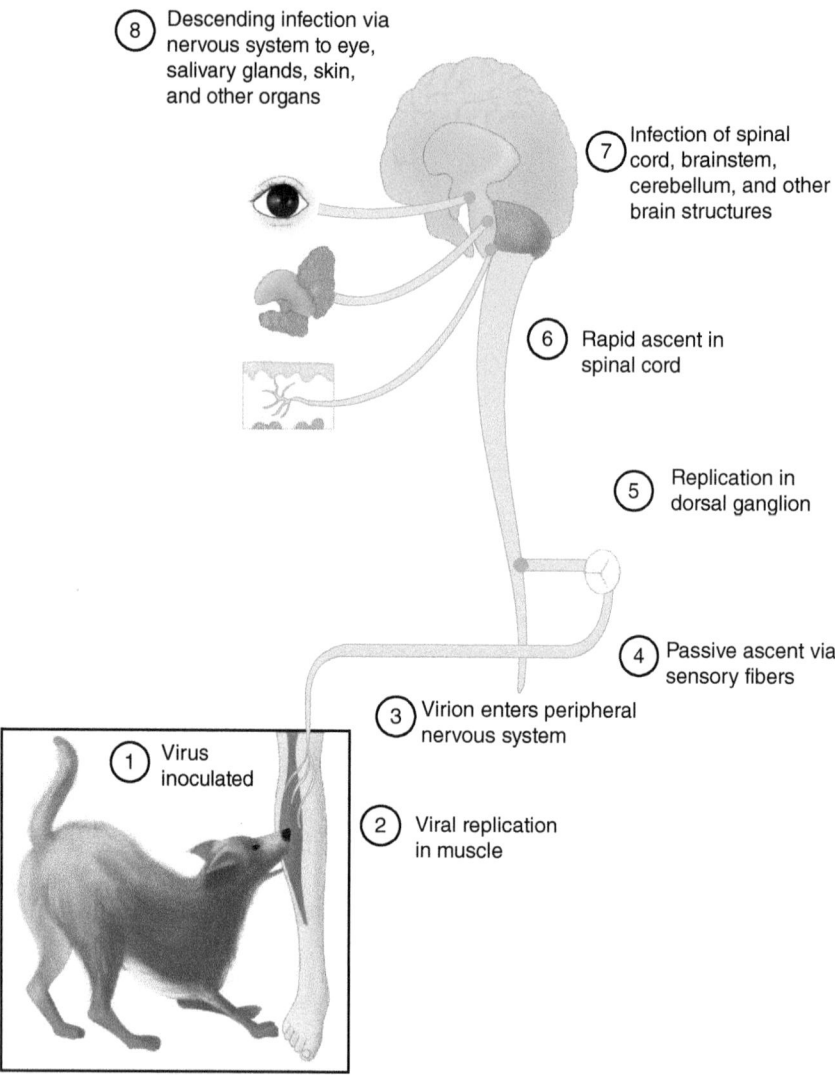

⑧ Descending infection via nervous system to eye, salivary glands, skin, and other organs

⑦ Infection of spinal cord, brainstem, cerebellum, and other brain structures

⑥ Rapid ascent in spinal cord

⑤ Replication in dorsal ganglion

④ Passive ascent via sensory fibers

③ Virion enters peripheral nervous system

① Virus inoculated

② Viral replication in muscle

Incubation period can be prolonged for months

✳ Immunization early in incubation period aborts infection

The incubation period for rabies ranges from 10 days to 1 year, depending on the amount of virus introduced, the amount of tissue involved, the host immune mechanisms, the innervation of the site, and the distance that the virus must travel from the site of inoculation to the CNS. Thus, the incubation period is generally shorter with face wounds than with leg wounds. Immunization early in the incubation period frequently aborts the infection.

FIGURE 17-4. The Negri body in cytoplasm of neuron. (Used with permission from Dr. Daniel P. Perl.)

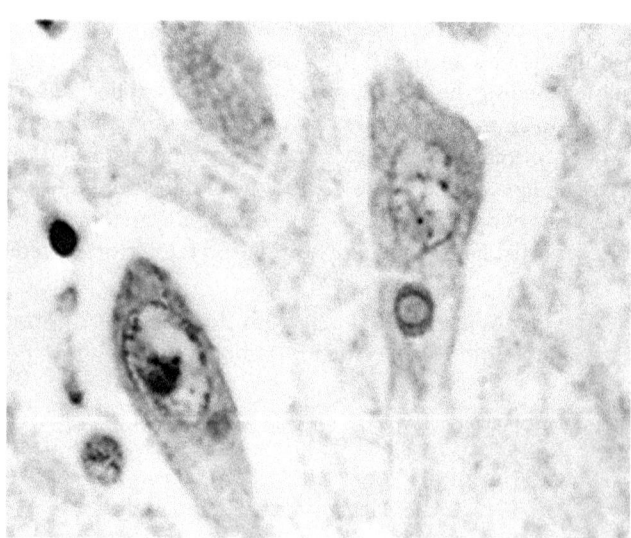

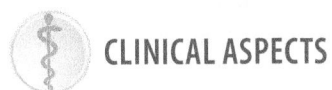 **CLINICAL ASPECTS**

MANIFESTATIONS

Rabies in humans usually results from a bite by a rabid animal or contamination of a wound by its saliva. It presents as an acute, fulminant, fatal encephalitis; human survivors have been reported only occasionally. The clinical stages of rabies infection are summarized in **Table 17–1.** After an average incubation period of 20 to 90 days (range 10 days to 1 year), the disease begins as a non-specific flu-like illness marked by fever, headache, malaise, nausea, and vomiting known as pro-drome stage. Abnormal sensations at or around the site of viral inoculation occur frequently and probably reflect local nerve involvement. In the acute neurologic stage, the onset of encephalitis is marked by periods of excess motor activity and agitation. Hallucinations, combativeness, mus-cle spasms, signs of meningeal irritation, seizures, and focal paralysis occur. Periods of mental dysfunction are interspersed with completely lucid periods; however, as the disease progresses, the patient lapses into coma. Autonomic nervous system involvement often results in increased salivation. Brainstem and cranial nerve dysfunction is characteristic, with double vision, facial palsies, and difficulty in swallowing. The combination of excess salivation and difficulty in swal-lowing produces the fearful picture of "foaming at the mouth." Hydrophobia, the painful, violent involuntary contractions of the diaphragm and accessory respiratory, pharyngeal, and laryngeal muscles, initiated by swallowing liquids including water, is seen in about 50% of the cases. Involve-ment of the respiratory center produces respiratory paralysis, the major cause of death. Occasion-ally, rabies may appear as an ascending paralysis resembling Guillain-Barré syndrome. Once symptoms have developed, no drug or vaccine administration can improve survival. The median survival after onset of symptoms is 4 days, with a maximum of 20 days unless artificial supportive measures are instituted. Recovery is exceedingly rare.

✻ Four phases; Incubation period, prodrome stage, acute neurologic stage, and coma

✻ Encephalitis common, sometimes with ascending paralysis

Almost uniformly fatal

DIAGNOSIS

There are several tests that are performed from different sources, including saliva, neck biopsy, serum, and CSF in human ante mortem to rule out rabies. Viral RNA can be detected by RT-PCR in saliva, neck biopsy, and brain biopsy (if taken for other tests). Viral antigen can be detected by immunofluorescent staining in neck biopsy. Rabies antibody can be detected by immuno-fluorescence test in serum and CSF. Rabies antibody in the CSF regardless of immunization his-tory suggests a rabies virus infection. Virus culture can also be performed from a saliva sample. The CSF of a rabies patient shows minimal reaction with some patients exhibiting a lymphocytic pleocytosis (5-30 cells/mm^3), mainly monocytosis with normal glucose and protein. Laboratory diagnosis of rabies in animals or deceased patients is accomplished by demonstration of virus

Viral RNA, antigen and antibody detected ante mortem in saliva, neck biopsy, serum, CSF, and brain biopsy

Viral antigen detected postmortem in brain tissue of humans or animals

TABLE 17–1	Clinical Stages of Rabies Virus Infection		
STAGES OF INFECTION	**TIME FRAME**	**SYMPTOMS**	**SITE OF VIRUS REPLICATION**
Incubation period	10-365 days Average: 20-90 days	No symptoms	Site of bite, muscle cells
Prodrome stage	2-10 days	Nonspecific symptoms, malaise, headache, fever, nausea, vomiting, upper respiratory distress, subtle mental changes (insomnia), pain, itching, tingling at the site of bite	Virus replication in the CNS
Acute neurologic stage	2-7 days	Furious or dumb presentation *Furious:* Hyperactivity, excitement, disorienta-tion, hallucination, bizarre behavior, hydropho-bia, convulsions, aggressive *Dumb (paralytic phase):* Lethargy, paralysis, (respiratory)	Virus replication in brain and transported to other sites (salivary glands and other organs)
Coma	0-14 days	Patient in coma; respiratory paralysis, cardiac arrest, drop in blood pressure, secondary infections	Virus replication in brain and transported to other organs
Death		Extremely rare survival	

Negri bodies in histologic examinations

in brain tissue. Viral antigen can be demonstrated rapidly by immunofluorescence procedures. Intracerebral inoculation of infected brain tissue or secretions into suckling mice results in death in 3 to 10 days. Histologic examination of their brain tissue shows the Negri bodies in 80% of the cases; electron microscopy may demonstrate both the Negri bodies and rhabdovirus particles. Specific antibodies to rabies virus can be detected in serum, but generally only late in the disease.

TREATMENT

No specific treatment is available

✱ **Vaccination immediately after animal bites prevents rabies disease**

Prevention is the mainstay of controlling rabies in humans immediately after exposure by starting the rabies vaccination process. With symptomatic rabies, intensive supportive care has resulted in four or five long-term survivals; despite the best modern medical care, however, the mortality rate still exceeds 90%. In addition, because of the infrequency of the disease, many patients die without definitive diagnosis. Human hyperimmune antirabies globulin, interferon, and vaccine do not alter the disease once the symptoms have developed. Postexposure prophylaxis is considered as a treatment for rabies exposure to humans after bites from rabid or wild animals.

 How is rabies vaccine successful in treating and/or preventing rabies if given soon after exposure?

In a controversial experimental treatment strategy in 2004, known as the Wisconsin or Milwaukee protocol, a 15-year-old patient with rabies symptoms was placed in a chemically induced coma to protect her brain from rabies virus and treated with antivirals (ribavirin and amantadine). The coma was reversed in the patient after 6 days when her immune system started making rabies antibodies. The patient became free of rabies virus and survived.

PREVENTION

In the late 1800s, Pasteur, noting the long incubation period of rabies, suggested that a vaccine to induce an immune response before the development of disease might be useful in prevention. He apparently successfully vaccinated Joseph Meister, a boy severely bitten and exposed to rabies, with multiple injections of a crude vaccine made from dried spinal cord of rabies-infected rabbits. This treatment emerged as one of the best-known and most noteworthy accomplishments in the annals of medicine. It is now believed that vaccination induces antibody that is either neutralizing or inhibits cell-to-cell spread of virus. Natural infection does not lead to an early immune response and limitation of viral migration because the virus is replicating in muscle or neural tissue and lymphocytes do not access these sites.

Vaccine-induced antibody inhibits viral spread

Currently, the prevention of rabies is divided into **preexposure prophylaxis (PreEP)** and **postexposure prophylaxis (PEP).** There are currently two inactivated (killed) vaccines licensed in the United States: human diploid cell vaccine (an attenuated strain of rabies virus grown in human diploid cell culture and inactivated by β-propiolactone) and purified chick embryo cell vaccine (fixed rabies virus strain grown in primary cultures of chicken fibroblasts and inactivated by β-propiolactone). Rabies vaccine made by Novartis is called "RabAvert" and by Sanofi Pasteur "IMOVAX" used for PreEP and PEP.

High-risk individuals include veterinarians, spelunkers, laboratory workers, animal handlers

Preexposure prophylaxis is recommended for individuals with high risk of contact with rabies viruses, such as veterinarians, spelunkers, laboratory workers, and animal handlers. Preexposure prophylaxis consists of three doses of intramuscular injections (deltoid area) of vaccine on days 0, 3, and 21 or 28. A booster dose is needed to maintain a neutralizing antibody titer of 1:5 in high-risk people (researchers working with rabies vaccine, veterinarians) after testing 6 months later.

Postexposure prophylaxis requires careful evaluation and judgment. Every year, more than 1 million people are bitten by animals in the United States, and approximately 55,000 receive

 Think ▸▸ Apply 17-2: Postexposure prophylaxis through rabies vaccine is both treatment and prevention if given soon after infections, including on days 0, 3, 14, and 28. Because the incubation period of rabies is from 10 days to 1 year (average 20-90 days), it is sufficient to elicit neutralizing antibodies to prevent travel of the virus to the CNS.

postexposure rabies prophylaxis. Worldwide, more than 29 million people receive rabies vaccine after rabid animal bites (postexposure) that prevents thousands of deaths annually worldwide. The physician must consider (1) whether the individual came into physical contact with saliva or another substance likely to contain rabies virus; (2) whether there was significant wound or abrasion; (3) whether rabies is known or suspected in the animal species and area associated with the exposure; (4) whether the bite was provoked or unprovoked (ie, the circumstances surrounding the exposure); and (5) whether the animal is available for laboratory examination.

Any wild animal or ill, unvaccinated, or stray domestic animal involved in a possible rabies exposure, such as an unprovoked bite, should be captured and removed from the community through the assistance of veterinary services and either quarantined for observation (for healthy dogs or cats) or examined by an appropriate laboratory (dead or euthanized animals with signs of rabies), usually at the state health department, to search for rabies antigen by immunofluorescence. If examination of the brain by this technique is negative for rabies virus, it can be assumed that the saliva contains no virus and that the exposed person may discontinue postexposure prophylaxis treatment. If the test is positive, the patient should continue postexposure prophylaxis. It should be noted that rodents and rabbits are not important vectors of rabies virus. There have been no rabies deaths in the United States when postexposure prophylaxis was given promptly after exposure.

Careful history and studies of biting animal are important in decision making

Postexposure prophylaxis is based on immediate, thorough washing of the wound with soap and water (to kill the virus around the wound); passive immunization with antirabies hyperimmune globulin (RIG) by intramuscular injection, including a portion instilled around the wound site (to neutralize the virus); and active immunization with killed/inactivated rabies vaccine on days 0, 3, 7, and 14. The RIG and the vaccine should be administered at two different sites. For individuals who were previously immunized, the postexposure prophylaxis includes wound cleansing with soap and water and rabies vaccination on days 0 and 3 (hyperimmune globulin should not be given). Physicians should always seek the advice of the local health department when the question of rabies prophylaxis arises.

✳ Rabies immune globulin plus vaccine necessary in postexposure management

KEY CONCLUSIONS

- Rabies virus is a bullet-shaped rhabdovirus, which is a negative-sense RNA, helical nucleocapsid, enveloped with knob-like glycoproteins and replicates in the cytoplasm by using viral RNA-dependent RNA polymerase.
- Rabies virus is transmitted to humans through animal bites from dogs, cats, wild animals, and bats generally in the United States, and rabid dogs in developing countries.
- Four phases of rabies infection; incubation period (10 days-1 year, average 20-90 days), prodrome phase (2-10 days) with nonspecific flu-like illness, acute neurological phase (2-7 days) with furious (hyperactivity, excitement, disorientation, hallucination, bizarre behavior, hydrophobia, convulsions, aggressive) or dumb (lethargy and respiratory paralysis) presentations, and coma phase (0-14 days) with respiratory paralysis, hypotension, and cardiac arrest. This acute encephalitis results in death with rare survival.
- The most important conclusion is that rabies is a highly preventable disease. Postexposure prophylaxis is part of the treatment plan, where rabies vaccination (killed or inactivated vaccine) is started immediately after exposure with intramuscular shots given on days 0, 3, 7, and 14. In addition, the wound must be cleaned with soap and water and hyperimmune antirabies immunoglobulin is instilled at the wound site and given intramuscularly at a different site than the vaccine shot.

CASE STUDY

The Friendly Boy and the Unfriendly Dog

A 15-year-old boy in San Francisco reaches into a car to pet another family's dog and is bitten on the finger.

QUESTIONS

1. What is the next course of action?
   A. Obtain documentation of the dog's immunization status
   B. Give rabies immune globulin
   C. Give rabies immune globulin plus rabies vaccine
   D. Give interferon-γ
   E. Examine the dog's brain for rabies antigen

2. Six weeks after the bite, the child develops fever, headache, and a seizure. He becomes combative and hallucinates. The best diagnostic test to perform on the patient to rule in rabies as a cause of his 3-day illness is:
   A. Detection of serum antirabies antibody
   B. Culture of CSF for virus
   C. Immunofluorescence of a biopsy from the nape of the neck
   D. Brain biopsy
   E. CSF antirabies antibody

3. Which type of rabies vaccine is used for postexposure prophylaxis in the United States?
   A. Rabies virus glycoprotein vaccine
   B. Live attenuated rabies vaccine
   C. Inactivated rabies vaccine
   D. Conjugated rabies vaccine
   E. DNA vaccine

ANSWERS

1. **(A)**

2. **(C)**

3. **(C)**

chapter 18

Human Retroviruses: HTLV, HIV, and AIDS

Human Immunodeficiency Virus type 1 (HIV-1) · Human Immunodeficiency Virus type 2 (HIV-2) ·

Human T-Lymphotropic Virus type I (HTLV-I) · Human T-Lymphotropic Virus type II (HTLV-II)

Retroviruses are enveloped, icosahedral, single-stranded, positive-sense RNA viruses. These viruses are known as retroviruses because they encode an enzyme called **reverse transcriptase** (RT), which converts the RNA genome into a double-stranded DNA copy that subsequently becomes integrated into the host chromosome. The discovery of RT in 1970 by two American virologists, David Baltimore and Howard Temin, earned them a Nobel Prize in Medicine. There are two major groups of retroviruses that infect humans: the **oncoretroviruses** (*onco-*, "related to a tumor") and the **lentiviruses** (*lenti-*, "slow"). There are several other groups of retroviruses that infect animals. Endogenous retrovirus sequences are found throughout the human genome. Like most enveloped viruses, all retroviruses are highly susceptible to factors that affect surface tension and are thus not transmissible through air, dust, or fomites under normal conditions, but instead require intimate contact with the infecting sources, such as bodily fluids, blood, and blood-derived products.

※ Enveloped (+) RNA viruses, RT enzyme converts RNA genome to DNA

Members of the oncoretrovirus, a subgroup of retroviruses, have long been associated with a variety of cancers in animals, including leukemias, lymphomas, and sarcomas. However, an oncoretrovirus was discovered in the late 1970s that infects humans known as human T-cell lymphotropic virus type I (HTLV-I). It causes adult T-cell leukemia and lymphoma (ATLL), a rare malignancy found only in Japan, Africa, and the Caribbean, although serologic evidence shows that it also occurs in the United States and has raised the possibility of an association with some chronic neurologic conditions. A relative of HTLV-I, HTLV-II has been associated with a few rare cases of T-cell malignancies, including hairy cell leukemia, but its precise role in these diseases remains unclear.

Oncoretroviruses cause tumors in animals

※ HTLV-I and HTLV-II associated with human leukemias/lymphomas

The most important disease resulting from a human retrovirus infection is called **acquired immunodeficiency syndrome (AIDS),** which is caused by a lentivirus known as **human immunodeficiency virus (HIV).** There are two types: HIV-1 and HIV-2, and HIV-1 is the major cause of AIDS. A devastating disease worldwide, for which there is no permanent cure or preventive vaccine for protection, AIDS has spurred unprecedented research efforts to determine the nature and immunopathogenic mechanisms of the virus in the hope of finding more and new effective drugs and a preventive AIDS vaccine. Most of our present knowledge of HIV is derived from studies on HIV-1, which is the major cause of AIDS worldwide. In 2008, two French virologists, Françoise Barré-Sinoussi and Luc Montagnier, shared the Nobel Prize in Medicine for their work on the discovery of HIV-1, the virus that causes AIDS.

HIV-1 and HIV-2 are lentiviruses; HIV-1 is the major cause of AIDS worldwide

Oncoretroviruses are not cytolytic in the sense that they do not kill the cells that they infect, but rather they transform the cells by different mechanisms (see Chapter 7 and HTLV section of this chapter) and continue to produce low levels of new virus indefinitely. With lentivirus infections,

Usually not cytolytic; transform cells

Lentiviruses cause a long latency with viremia before disease

the host cell–virus relationship is different. Lentiviruses can apparently persist in infected hosts for long periods of time in a clinically latent state. Over time, the virus becomes highly cytopathic and kills CD4+ T-cells (lymphocytes), causing impairment of the host immune defenses followed by development of opportunistic infections and AIDS. The prototype of this type of lentivirus is HIV-1. The second type of HIV, HIV-2, also causes immunodeficiency in humans that develops slowly and tends to be milder and mainly found in West Africa. HIV-1 is the causative agent of AIDS and found in most of the HIV-infected people worldwide.

RETROVIRUSES

Overview

Retroviruses such as HIV-1 have two copies of positive-sense RNA genome (diploid) complexed with nucleocapsid (NC) protein and packaged in an icosahedral capsid protein (CA, p24), matrix (MA) protein, and lipid bilayer envelope containing two surface glycoproteins, gp120 and gp41. The virus particles also carry three viral enzymes protease (PR), RT, and integrase (IN). HIV-1 mainly infects CD4+ T-lymphocytes but also other cell types with a lower efficiency, including monocytes/macrophages, Langerhans cells, dendritic cells, and some brain cells. HIV-1 enters target cells by binding to CD4 receptor and CCR5 or CXCR4 coreceptor and gp41 helps the viral envelope to fuse with plasma membrane of host cell. After partial uncoating in the cytoplasm, the RT (viral RNA-dependent DNA polymerase) enzyme converts the viral RNA into complementary DNA (cDNA) and double-stranded DNA as well as degrades the viral RNA. The double-stranded viral DNA with the help of viral IN enzyme moves into the nucleus and integrates in the host chromosome at random sites, making the host cell permanently infected with HIV-1. With the help of host RNA polymerase, viral mRNAs and genomic RNA are made followed by protein synthesis, first of regulatory proteins such as Tat, Rev. Tat increases viral transcription, whereas Rev exports mRNA/RNA for structural proteins. Once all the viral proteins are made, NC binds to viral genomic RNA for packaging in CA and MA protein helps to bring the complex near the plasma membrane and buds out acquiring plasma membrane expressing gp120 and g41. The maturation of HIV-1 takes place in the virions when viral PR cleaves Gag and Pol into several mature proteins to make the infectious virus particles. Several antiretroviral therapy (ART) agents have been developed against specific steps of HIV-1 life cycle such as entry (CCR5 and gp41 inhibitors) and viral enzymes (RT, IN, and protease inhibitors [PIs]), which are being successfully used to treat HIV-infected patients.

⁎ HIV-1 attacks and destroys CD4+ T-lymphocytes

⁎ Infects monocytes/ macrophages, dendritic cells, Langerhans cells, CNS cells

HIV-1 can remain clinically latent in most infected patients without causing viral latency in untreated patients, which means that virus is produced at low levels without serious disease, but when allowed to replicate in the absence of effective immune response and other factors, high levels of virus are produced causing CD4+ T-lymphocyte cell death and AIDS. Although HIV-1 can infect a variety of human cell types, such as T-lymphocytes, monocytes/macrophages, dendritic cells, Langerhans cells, and microglia/glial cells, its most drastic effects appear to result from destruction of the CD4+ T-lymphocytes, which play a central role in the capacity of the host to mount effective and protective immunologic responses, cell-mediated and humoral, to a wide range of infections.

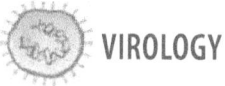 VIROLOGY

STRUCTURE

Virion contains two (+) RNA genome, icosahedral capsid and lipid bilayer envelope with surface glycoproteins

All retroviruses are remarkably similar in their basic virion composition and structure. The virion structure of HIV-1 is depicted in **Figure 18–1.** The virion size is about 100 nm in diameter, and because it contains two copies of the RNA genome, it is diploid. The RNA genome is coated with the NC protein, and the RNA–protein complexes are enclosed in a capsid (CA, also called p24) composed of multiple subunits in an icosahedral symmetry, which is covered by a membrane-associated matrix (MA, also called p17) protein. Like most enveloped viruses, the lipid

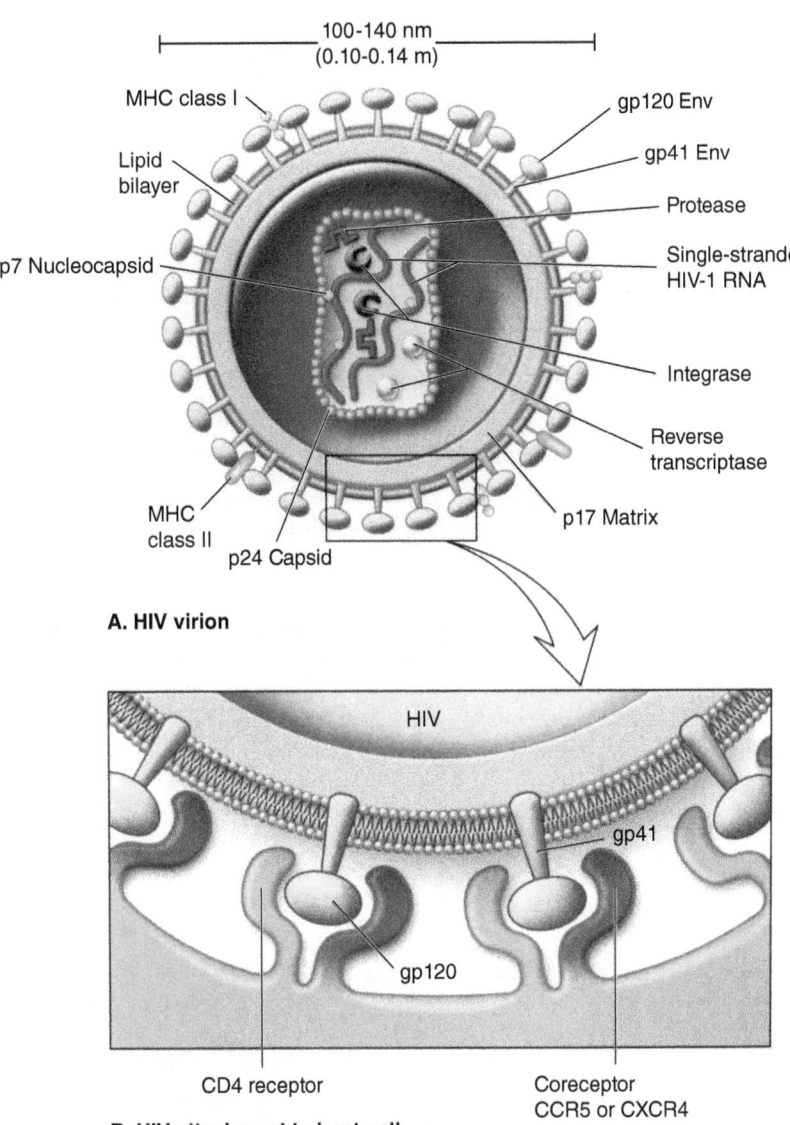

100-140 nm
(0.10-0.14 m)

MHC class I
Lipid bilayer
p7 Nucleocapsid
MHC class II
p24 Capsid

gp120 Env
gp41 Env
Protease
Single-stranded HIV-1 RNA
Integrase
Reverse transcriptase
p17 Matrix

A. HIV virion

HIV

gp41

gp120

CD4 receptor

Coreceptor CCR5 or CXCR4

B. HIV attachment to host cell

FIGURE 18–1.
particle. A. T
cules enclosed
coated with the
tein. The matrix pr
the membrane ....pe. **B.** The
envelope contains two membrane
glycoproteins, gp41 and gp120, also
called transmembrane protein and
surface protein, respectively. CCR5;
CXCR4, chemokine receptors, acting
as coreceptors.

320

bilayer membrane is acquired during budding from the host cell plasma membrane, but the surface (SU, also called gp120) and transmembrane (TM, also called gp41) glycoproteins found in the envelope are virally encoded. Gp120 binds to CD4 receptor and coreceptor CCR5 or CXCR4 (chemokine receptor) binds on CD4+ T-cells and other cells. In addition to the structural proteins shown in Figure 18–1, the virion core contains three virus-specific proteins (enzymes) that are essential for viral replication: RT, PR, and IN. The relation between the viral genes found in all retroviruses (*gag*, *pol*, and *env*) and the proteins they encode are presented in **Table 18–1.** Some retroviruses, including HTLV and HIV-1, encode additional regulatory and accessory proteins. Based on SU gp120 variable region/loop 3 (V3 loop) sequence, HIV-1 that binds to CD4 and CXCR4 is called X4 (T-lymphotropic) HIV-1, whereas HIV-1 that binds to CD4 and CCR5 is called R5 (Macrophage tropic) HIV-1. Some HIV-1 isolates are also X4/R5 HIV-1 (dual tropic).

＊Three critical viral enzymes RT, PR, IN

RETROVIRAL REPLICATION CYCLE

Figure 18–2 depicts the life cycle of a typical retrovirus (eg, HIV-1) and serves to illustrate the many unique aspects of retroviral replication that are targets for current antiviral agents and could be potential targets of new and effective therapeutic interventions.

Viral Entry

Retroviral virions are adsorbed to cellular membrane receptors through an interaction of viral surface protein and cellular receptors and enter the cell by direct fusion of the viral envelope with

TABLE 18–1	Major Retroviral Genes and Proteins	
GENE[a]	PROTEIN PRODUCTS	FUNCTION
gag	Matrix (MA)	Structural, matrix protein of the virion
	Capsid (CA)	Structural, capsid protein of the virion
	Nucleocapsid (NC)	Structural, forms complex with viral RNA
	Protease[b] (PR)	Gag-Pol protein processing
pol	Protease[b] (PR)	Gag-Pol protein processing
	Reverse transcriptase (RT)	Viral DNA synthesis
	Integrase (IN)	Integration of viral DNA in host chromosome
env	Surface glycoprotein (SU)	Adsorption, binding to the receptor
	Transmembrane protein (TM)	Fusion of envelope with plasma membrane

[a]Each gene encodes a polyprotein that is subsequently processed by proteolysis to yield the individual proteins.
[b]The protease is encoded in either the gag gene or the pol gene, depending on the virus.

✳ HIV-1 gp120 attaches to CD4 receptor and CCR5 or CXCR4 coreceptor

the plasma membrane of the host cell. For HIV-1, the virion attachment protein is the SU glycoprotein, gp120, and the cellular receptor is the CD4 molecule with one of the chemokine receptors, CXCR4 or CCR5, acting as a coreceptor. These receptors and coreceptors are expressed primarily on the plasma membrane of CD4+ T-lymphocytes, but also on cells of the monocyte–macrophage lineage, and some other target cells, such as Langerhans cells, dendritic cells, and

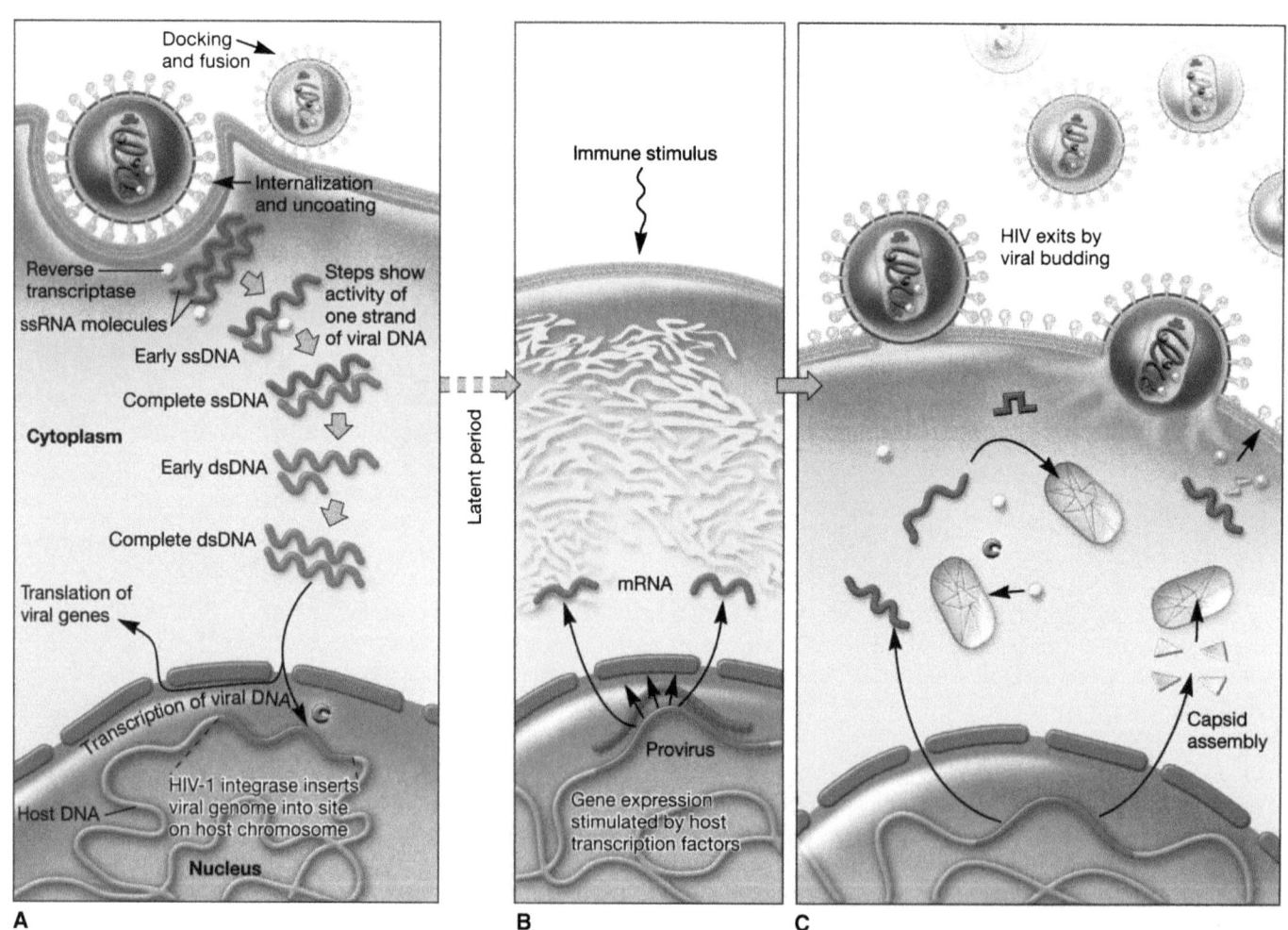

FIGURE 18–2. **Retroviral (HIV-1) life cycle. A.** Viral entry and postentry (reverse transcription, DNA synthesis, and integration) events; **B.** Viral gene expression (transcription and protein synthesis); **C.** Virus assembly and release.

certain brain cells. The naïve CD4+ T-lymphocytes express higher levels CXCR4 and somewhat lower levels of CCR5. However, the mucosal memory CD4+ T-lymphocytes, monocytes/macrophages, Langerhans cells and others express higher levels of CCR5 but lower levels of CXC4. Inhibitors of CCR5 coreceptor are available to be used in combination HIV-1 therapy. Early in infection, the HIV-1 isolates in infected patients are R5 because R5 viruses that use CCR5 coreceptor are predominantly transmitted to recipients. The emergence of syncytia-forming HIV-1 variants that use the CXCR4 coreceptor are X4 viruses that appear to correlate with rapid advancement to AIDS. The HIV-1 transmembrane TM protein gp41 is responsible for the fusion of the viral and cell membranes, leading to entry of the virion core complex into the cytoplasm of the cell. Fusion inhibitor to gp41 function is a peptide-based antiviral agent approved as a part of combination therapy when other first-line drugs have failed.

* R5 HIV-1 binds to CD4, CCR5, X4 HIV-1 interacts with CD4, CXCR4

Gp41 protein mediates fusion of viral and cellular membranes

Inhibitors to CCR5 and gp41 approved for ART

 How can the same region (V3 loop) of Env gp120 bind to both CCR5 and CXCR4?

HIV-1 can also infect cells that lack the CD4 surface molecule such as certain brain cells and other cells types with a low efficiency, apparently because the chemokine receptors in combination with the fusion-inducing activity of the TM protein is sufficient in these cases to promote entry. Fusion activity may also play an important role in amplification of the effects of the virus infection, particularly during the later stages of the infection, because infected cells expressing viral glycoproteins in their membranes readily fuse with uninfected CD4+ T-lymphocytes to form large syncytia. This process appears to provide a means for cell-to-cell transmission of the virus that bypasses the usual extracellular phase and may contribute to the overall depletion of CD4+ T-lymphocytes in an infected person.

HIV-1 infects CCR5 or CXCR4 positive cells without CD4 with low efficiency

Fusion provides cell-to-cell transmission

■ Viral Postentry Events

Among the RNA viruses, retroviral replication is unique because it involves reverse transcription. Soon after the entry of the viral core into the cytoplasm of the infected cell, there is partial uncoating and the viral RNA is reverse transcribed (converted) into a cDNA by the action of RT enzyme, the virion-associated RNA-dependent DNA polymerase. The cDNA is then converted into double-stranded DNA by the action of the DNA-dependent DNA polymerase activity of the same RT enzyme. The viral RNA template is removed from the RNA–DNA hybrid by RNAase H activity of the same RT enzyme. The overall process is referred to as **reverse transcription.** Currently, there are several antiviral agents that are inhibitors of RT enzyme (nucleoside [NRTIs] and nonnucleoside reverse transcriptase inhibitors [NNRTIs]) used in combination therapy (as the first line of drugs) to treat HIV-1 infection. Following RT, the resultant linear DNA molecule circularizes and makes a preintegration complex with the help of viral and host factors, including viral IN enzyme and Vpr protein. The preintegration complex enters the nucleus and integrates more or less at random sites into the host cell chromosome catalyzed by viral IN enzyme. The integration process is highly specific with respect to the viral DNA, and two base pairs are generally lost from each end of the viral DNA LTR (long terminal repeat). The choice of a target site for integration into the cellular DNA appears, however, to be nearly random but preferably in actively transcribed host genes. Once the viral genetic information has been converted to DNA and integrated, it essentially becomes part of the cellular genome, and the cell is permanently infected. The viral DNA genome, called the **provirus,** is therefore replicated and faithfully inherited as long as the infected cell continues to divide. IN inhibitors have been developed and approved as a part of combination HIV-1 therapy currently used as the first line of therapy.

RT enzyme copies RNA to double-stranded DNA

RNase H activity degrades original RNA genome

DNA integrates into the host chromosome, replicates as a provirus

* IN -catalyzed integration random in host DNA

* RT and IN inhibitors used in combination ART

Special sequences contained within the RNA are duplicated during the reverse transcription process so that the integrated provirus contains identical LTRs at its ends (**Figure 18–3**). The LTR sequences contain the appropriate promoter, enhancer, and other signals required for transcription of the viral genes by the host RNA polymerase II. Transcription produces a full-length RNA

LTR promoter and enhancer signals required for transcription and regulation

 Think ►► Apply 18-1: The V3 loop gp120 is a hypervariable region that changes more rapidly due to error-prone reverse transcriptase and immune pressure generating two different variants of V3 loop, one binding to CCR5 and the other to CXCR4.

FIGURE 18–3. **Retroviral RNA replication.** LTR, long terminal repeat.

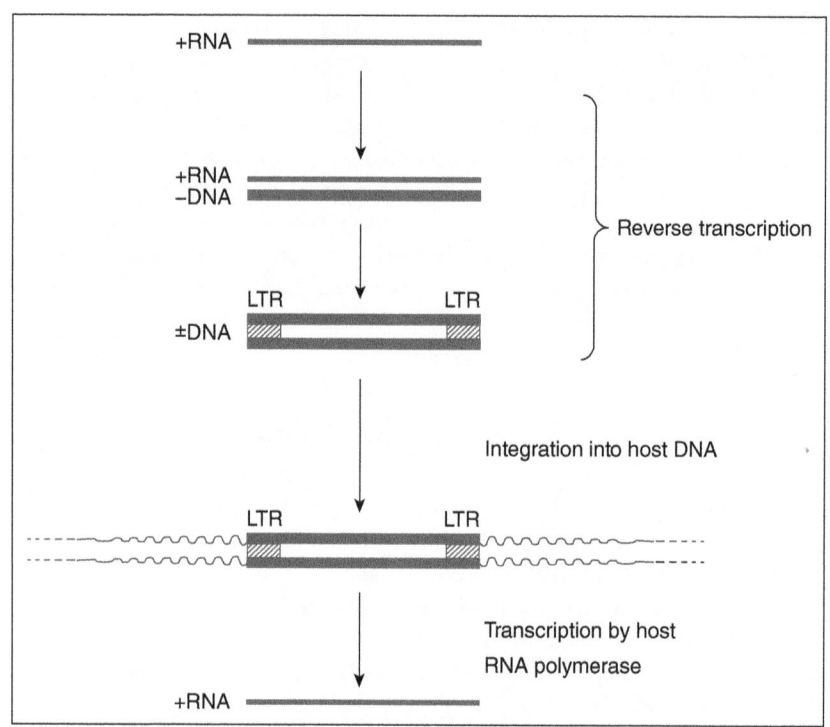

* Integrated HIV-1 DNA is transcribed by host RNA polymerase

Genomic RNA and spliced mRNAs encode structural and regulatory proteins

HIV-1 controls genomic or spliced mRNA production

genome and one or more spliced mRNAs. For HIV-1, a series of spliced mRNAs are produced that encode envelope proteins and a series of viral regulatory and accessory proteins. Gag and Gag-Pol precursors are encoded by full-length RNA. Unlike most retroviruses, HIV-1 and the other lentiviruses apparently exert considerable control over whether the primary transcripts are allocated to full-length RNA or are spliced to produce mRNAs (see text that follows). With the exception of these regulatory and accessory proteins, all retroviral proteins are initially translated as polyproteins that are subsequently processed by proteolysis into the individual protein molecules. Although the HIV-1 envelope precursor proteins (gp160) are cleaved into gp120 and gp41 by host cell PR, the enzyme responsible for cleavages of Gag and Gag-Pol precursors into capsid proteins and enzymes, respectively, is the virus-specific PR that is encoded by the *pol* gene of HIV-1. HIV-1 PIs are approved for use as part of combination HIV-1 therapy.

 While reverse transcriptase converts HIV RNA to a cDNA, how does it become double-stranded DNA in the cytoplasm?

* Error-prone RT generates viral quasispecies or variants

Isolates from the same patient differ in genotypic, phenotypic properties

Of all the known retroviruses, HIV-1 possesses the most error-prone RT. The consequence of this high error rate is that each time the viral RNA is reverse transcribed, three to four new mutations are introduced into the resulting DNA. In addition, the process of transcription of the integrated proviral DNA to produce new viral genomes may also make errors, mutant genomes accumulate rapidly over the course of an infection. The end result is a quasispecies that accounts for the many nucleotide differences observed between different isolates (even from the same infected individual) and for the variability of the SU envelope protein gp120. It may explain, in part, the failure of the immune system to control the infection, the increases in viral virulence that appear to occur during the course of the infection, and the difficulty of developing an effective vaccine.

RETROVIRAL GENES

The genome organization of different types of retroviruses is shown in **Figure 18–4** (see also Table 18–1). All retroviruses contain the same structural genes in the order of *gag–pol–env* genes. The *gag* (group-specific antigen) gene encodes the structural proteins (matrix-MA, capsid-CA,

 Think ▸▸ Apply 18-2: **The DNA-dependent DNA polymerase activity of reverse transcriptase enzyme converts cDNA to dsDNA.**

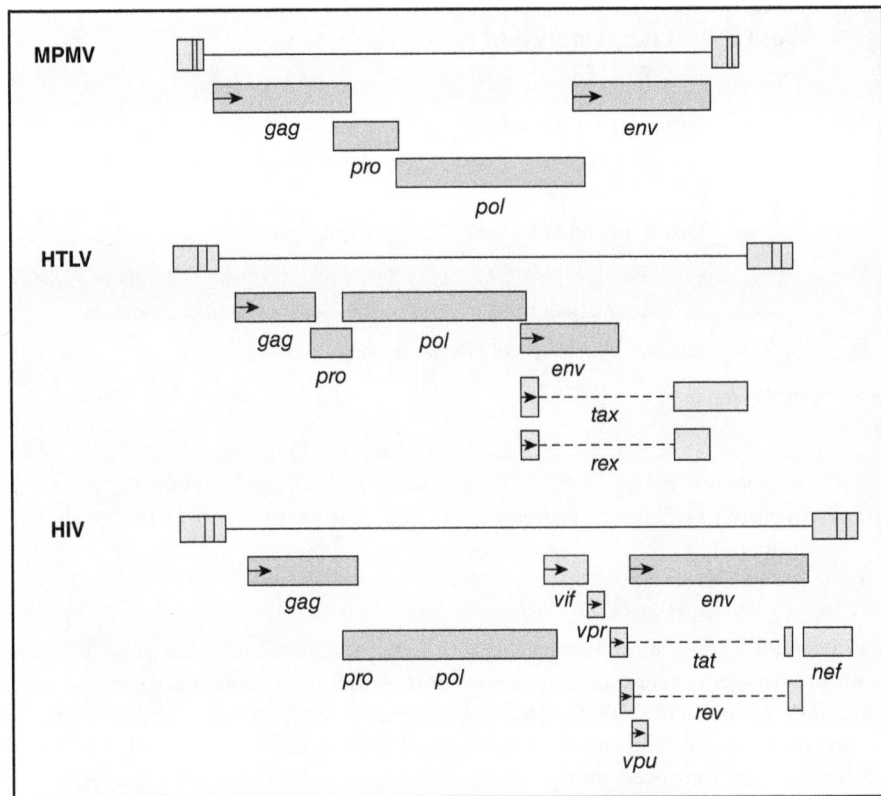

FIGURE 18–4. **Structure of retroviral genes of a mouse retrovirus (MPMV), HTLV, and HIV-1.**

nucleocapsid-NC) of the virus and, in some animal retroviruses, the PR. The *pol* (polymerase) gene in human retroviruses and HIV-1 encodes the PR, RT, and the IN. The *env* (envelope) gene encodes the two membrane glycoproteins found in the viral envelope, SU gp120 and TM gp41. HIV-1 gp120 has five variable regions (V1-V5) and several constant regions (C1-C5). The CD4-binding domains on gp120 are localized in the constant regions, whereas the coreceptor (CXCR4/CCR5) binding regions on gp120 are confined in the variable region 3 (V3 loop). The V3 region is also the principal neutralizing domain of the virus, and therefore contributes to antigenic variation and varying degrees of neutralization. However, gp41 is embedded in the envelope and mediates fusion of the viral envelope with the plasma membrane at the time of viral infection and less variable than gp120.

Genome is organized into *gag*, *pol*, and *env* genes

A comparison of the genetic makeup of HIV-1 with that of a typical retrovirus (Figure 18–4) reveals a larger number of genes and a much more complex organization. HIV-1 contains, in addition to the *gag*, *pol*, and *env* genes, an array of other genes (*tat*, *rev*, *nef*, *vif*, *vpr*, and *vpu*). Expression of these genes requires mRNA splicing, and all apparently encode proteins that serve regulatory or accessory roles during the infection (see text that follows). HTLV-I encodes the regulatory proteins, Tax and Rex, which are analogous to the HIV-1 Tat and Rev proteins. The names of the genes that have been best characterized and the proteins and functions they determine are listed in **Table 18–2.**

HIV-1 has multiple regulatory and accessory genes; *tat*, *rev*, *nef*, *vif*, *vpu*, and *vpr*

VIRUS ASSEMBLY AND RELEASE

Once all the viral proteins are made, the process of virus assembly proceeds. The Env gp120 and gp41 are expressed on cell surface. The nucleoprotein complexes of the Gag and Gag-Pol polyproteins with viral genomic RNA are created, where NC protein of Gag polyprotein binds to packaging site on the 5′ end of viral RNA. The MA protein of Gag polyprotein interacts with its C terminus to the NC-RNA-Gag-Gag-Pol complex and on the N terminus to the C terminus of gp41 that is expressed in conjunction gp120 onto plasma membrane. This NC-RNA-Gag-Gag-Pol complex buds out of the plasma membrane with gp120 and gp41 on cell surface. The next step includes the morphogenesis involving proteolytic processing of Gag and Gag-Pol polyproteins by HIV-1 PR enzyme into various Gag proteins (MA, CA, NC) and Pol enzymes (PR, RT, IN),

Assembly by formation of NC-RNA complex with Gag, Gag-Pol polyproteins

Release by budding from plasma membrane

TABLE 18–2		Roles of HIV-1 Regulatory and Accessory Proteins
GENE	PROTEIN	FUNCTION
tat	Tat	Transcriptional activator
rev	Rev	Promotes transport of unspliced and singly spliced mRNAs from nucleus to cytoplasm
nef	Nef	Downregulation of cellular CD4 and MHC I proteins
vpu	Vpu	Facilitates virus assembly and release. HIV-2 encodes Vpx instead of Vpu
vpr	Vpr	Facilitates nuclear entry in nondividing cells, arrests dividing cells
vif	Vif	Increases viral infectivity in certain cell types

MHC, major histocompatibility complex.

Gag-Pol proteins make infectious particles, can be inhibited by PIs in ART

making it a complete infectious virus particle. If PIs are used as part of combination therapy, then Gag and Gag-Pol polyproteins will not be processed, and mature infectious virus particles will not be made.

ROLES OF HIV-1 REGULATORY AND ACCESSORY PROTEINS

HIV-1 encodes a complex array of regulatory and accessory proteins that appear to be involved in viral replication, pathogenesis, and disease progression. Antivirals against these proteins may aid in improving HIV-1 treatment. These proteins also appear to interact with cellular factors to modulate the infection differently in different host cells. The roles of the two HIV-1 regulatory genes, *tat* and *rev*, and the four accessory genes, *nef*, *vpu*, *vpr*, and *vif*, are discussed later and summarized in Table 18–2.

✳ Tat promotes synthesis of viral full-length and spliced RNAs

Tat and Rev proteins are essential for viral replication by playing a positive role in promoting viral gene expression. Tat is a transcriptional activator that acts at a sequence near the beginning of the viral mRNA in the LTR, called Tat-acting responsive (TAR) element, to recruit cellular proteins to help the host RNA polymerase to complete efficient transcription and make HIV-1 RNA of the HIV-1 proviral genome. In the absence of Tat, the host RNA polymerase initiates the transcription at the LTR promoter, but transcription is prematurely terminated leading to the production of a short, dead-end RNA.

✳ Rev promotes export of unspliced and singly spliced RNAs to cytoplasm

The Rev protein is posttranscriptional transactivator that acts at the level of mRNA splicing and transport. Normally, unspliced and singly spliced RNAs are retained in the nucleus, and only multiply spliced mRNAs that encode Tat, Rev, and Nef are transported to the cytoplasm for translation. For the synthesis of proteins such as Env, Vif, Vpr, and Vpu that are made from singly spliced mRNAs, and the Gag and Pol polyproteins from the unspliced genomic RNA, it is necessary to transport these proteins mRNAs to the cytoplasm. Transport of these singly spliced mRNAs or unspliced RNAs is accomplished by Rev binding to an RNA sequence within the *env* gene called the Rev-responsive element (RRE). The Rev-RRE interaction exports the singly spliced mRNAs or unspliced RNAs from the nucleus to cytoplasm for translation. By promoting translation of the virion structural proteins and some of the accessory proteins, Rev turns up late gene expression that leads directly to a high rate of virus production.

✳ Nef downregulates CD4 and MHC I to interfere with immune recognition

The Nef accessory protein interferes with immune recognition of infected cells. Nef causes the internalization and degradation of the CD4 protein, which likely prevents superinfection and the formation of complexes between the cellular receptor and newly synthesized virions. Nef also downregulates the cell surface major histocompatibility complex (MHC) I molecules, which may prevent killing of infected cells by cytotoxic T-lymphocytes (CTLs). In addition, virions produced in the absence of the Nef protein are at least partially blocked at some step before integration. The combination of these and perhaps other effects allows the Nef protein to play an essential pathogenic role in an infected individual.

Vpu targets CD4 destruction and virion release

✳ BST-2 antiviral activity neutralized by Vpu to facilitate virus release

The Vpu protein of HIV-1 appears to play two separate roles during the late stages of infection. In the absence of Vpu, the Env protein forms complexes with CD4 in the endoplasmic reticulum and fails to reach the plasma membrane of the cell. One of the roles of Vpu is to target the destruction of CD4 in the endoplasmic reticulum to allow for incorporation of Env into newly synthesized virions. The second role of Vpu is to promote the release of virions from the infected cell. The most likely mechanism is that Vpu counteracts the function of a host factor, BST-2 (bone marrow stromal antigen 2, CD137, or tetherin). BST-2 tethers HIV-1 to the cell and prevents virus release, and thus has antiviral activity.

The Vpr protein is required for efficient viral replication in resting T-cells and monocytes/macrophages. Several possible roles for Vpr in HIV-1 replication have been suggested, including modest transactivation of HIV-1 LTR, enhancement of the nuclear migration of the preintegration complex in the newly infected nondividing cells, inhibition of establishment of chronic infection, arrest of cells in the G2/M phase of the cell cycle, and inducing latent cells into a high level of virus production. Furthermore, successful infection of nondividing cells such as macrophages and resting T-lymphocytes requires Vpr to allow the newly synthesized viral DNA to reach the nucleus and be integrated into the cellular DNA.

✽ Vpr promotes preintegration complex into nucleus

✽ Vpr arrests cells in G2/M cell cycle

HIV-2 encodes Vpx instead of Vpu. Vpx has homology to Vpr and shares the functions of Vpr. The functions of Vpr and Vpx have been segregated, including Vpr maintaining the ability to induce G2 arrest, whereas Vpx retains the ability to enhance infection of nondividing cells such as macrophages.

HIV-2 encode Vpx instead of Vpu

Vif (virion infectivity factor) increases the infectivity of HIV-1 in primary T-cells and monocytes/macrophages in culture. In the absence of Vif, the virus fails to complete reverse transcription in these cell types. Vif also inhibits an RNA editing enzyme, APOBEC3G (apolipoprotein B, a member of innate immune system), which causes hypermutation in HIV-1 DNA after reverse transcription and inhibiting viral replication.

Vif increases efficiency and yield

APOBEC3G disrupted by Vif

Superimposed on this complex regulatory network is the fact that the viral promoter contains elements that are sensitive to specific cellular transcription factors. This observation may help explain why virus production in CD4+ T-lymphocytes is greatly increased when the cells are activated. Clearly, the outcome of an HIV-1 infection is determined by a complex interplay among very large number of different factors.

Activation of CD4+ T-lymphocytes increases virus production

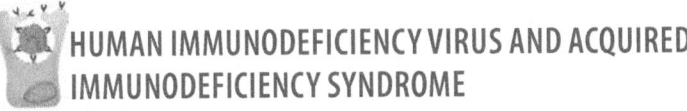

HUMAN IMMUNODEFICIENCY VIRUS AND ACQUIRED IMMUNODEFICIENCY SYNDROME

OVERVIEW

HIV is a pandemic infection affecting more than 38 million people worldwide, with 67% of the infected people living in Sub-Saharan Africa. In the United States, there are 1.2 million people living with HIV. New rates of infection and death have declined. HIV infection is transmitted through anal or vaginal sex, mother-to-child, and by exposure to contaminated bodily fluids, blood or blood-products. The acute phase of the infection, 2 to 4 weeks after infection, involves intense viral replication causing a high viremia (within 7-28 days) and dissemination to lymphoid tissues followed by flu- or mononucleosis-like symptoms such as fever, chills, night sweats, sore throat, lymphadenopathy, arthralgias, fatigue, hepatosplenomegaly, and rash, the acute retroviral syndrome. Upon activation of innate and adaptive immune response, the viral replication is brought to a set-point by the immune response but never eliminated. HIV-1 antibodies appear in 3 to 12 weeks after infection. The virus then enters in a chronic or clinical latency phase (asymptomatic phase) that lasts in a majority of the patients for 8 to 10 years. HIV-1 also establishes reservoirs in GALT and lymph nodes and resting T-cells and monocytes/macrophages. There is continued viral replication, declining CD4 T-cell counts and immune activation followed by an advanced phase of marked depletion of CD4 T cells leading to immune deficiency and development of AIDS with opportunistic infections in untreated patients. Patients with AIDS may experience many symptoms such as recurring fever, night sweats, rapid weight loss, diarrhea, sores in mouth or genitals, thrush, pneumonia, and some neurological disorders. This AIDS phase also causes an extensive array of viral, bacterial, fungal, and parasitic opportunistic infections and malignancies that may result in death, if untreated. HIV-1 diagnosis is done by a fourth-generation HIV-1 test that detects both HIV-1 antigen and antibodies, which may be confirmed by HIV-1 RNA (PCR). Current HIV-1 ART regimens include two NNRTIs plus one INSTI and other combinations, which reduce viral load to undetectable levels, improve the CD4 T-cells count, prevent AIDS and opportunistic infections and improve longevity and quality of patients' lives. There is no cure or vaccine available at this time.

EPIDEMIOLOGY

AIDS was first recognized in the United States in 1981, when it became apparent that an unusual number of rare skin cancers (Kaposi sarcoma) and opportunistic infections were occurring among men who have sex with men (MSM). These patients were found to have a marked

t recognized in MSM,
hemophiliacs, and drug
abusers

HIV-1 major cause of AIDS
worldwide

HIV-2 endemic in West Africa

✳ Transmission through anal
and vaginal sex, intravenous
drug use, body fluids

✳ Highest risk in receptive anal
sex, MSM

Mother-to-child transmission
reduced by ART during
pregnancy

✳ Condom usage, circumcision,
ART reduce risk

Risk increases due to disruption
of mucosal integrity in
traumatic sex

HIV recognizes Langerhans
cells dendrites, transferred to
submucosal macrophages,
dendritic cells, CD4 T-cells

reduction in CD4+ T-lymphocytes and were subject to a wide range of opportunistic infections normally controlled by an intact immune system. The disease was found to progress relentlessly to a fatal outcome and was first identified in MSM, hemophiliacs, who were receiving blood-derived coagulation factors, and injection drug users.

Retrospective serologic studies with specimens saved from patients in various studies indicate that HIV-1 infection was already occurring in Africa in the 1950s and in the United States in the 1970s. In 1985, HIV-2 was found to be endemic in parts of West Africa and to cause a milder immunodeficiency at a slower pace. To date, this virus has been relatively restricted geographically, although HIV-2 infections have occurred in the Western Hemisphere. Therefore, HIV-1 will be referred as HIV in this section, as it is the major cause of AIDS worldwide.

■ Transmission

HIV is transmitted between humans in several ways: sexually, parenterally, vertically, and by exposure to contaminated bodily fluids, blood or blood-derived products. The virus has been demonstrated in bodily fluids particularly in high titers in semen, vaginal and cervical secretions, rectal fluids, and breast milk. HIV is mainly transmitted in the United States through anal or vaginal sex, the highest risk is through receptive anal sex (risk 1.38%), although insertive anal sex (risk 0.11%) also spread the virus. In vaginal sex, both partners have risk of transmission, but the receptive partner (female) has a higher risk (0.08%) than insertive partner male (risk 0.04%), although the risk is lower than receptive anal sex. Worldwide, penile-vaginal sex is the major route of transmission. People sharing needles or syringes for intravenous drug use can spread the virus at a higher risk of 0.63%, whereas percutaneous needle-stick risk is 0.23% and exposure of HIV-infected blood and fluids to mouth, eye, nose, or nonintact skin risk is 0.1%. The risk of HIV transmission through contaminated blood transfusion is extremely high (risk 92.5%), but the blood supply in the United States and other developed countries is rigorously tested. HIV is less commonly transmitted through needle stick or sharp objects for health-care workers. In extremely rare cases, HIV has been shown to be transmitted by oral sex, receiving blood and blood products (prescreened for HIV) or organs, contact with broken skin, biting, deep mouth kissing with sores. HIV transmission can be reduced by condom usage, circumcision, and ART in infected people. Mother-to-child transmission can occur prepartum (via transplacental route), intrapartum (through birth canal), and postpartum (through breast milk). It is important to note that ART during pregnancy has significantly reduced the risk of mother-to-child transmission of HIV by less than 1%.

Infection is facilitated by breaks in epithelial surfaces, which provide direct access to the underlying tissues or bloodstream. The relative fragility of the rectal mucosa and the large numbers of sexual contacts are probable contributing factors to the predominance of the disease among promiscuous MSM. HIV is transmitted in penile to vaginal sex to females by vaginal or cervical routes, despite natural barriers, such as multicellular layers of squamous epithelial cells of vaginal mucosa and antimicrobial activity of cervicovaginal secretions. The risk of transmission further increases with the disruption of integrity of the vaginal or rectal mucosa because of dry or traumatic sex and other infectious and inflammatory diseases. Once the virus is deposited in the vaginal or rectal mucosa, the virus can also traverse the mucous layer and probably reach the dendritic projections of Langerhans cells followed by infection of submucosal cells such as macrophages, T-lymphocytes, and dendritic cells.

 How does HIV establish infection in vaginal or rectal mucosa which is devoid of CD4+ cells?

Transmission due to blood or blood-products transfusion and organ transplantation has been significantly reduced in the United States and other developed countries due to rigorous HIV testing and screening for infectious agents. However, transmission by blood is now largely

 Think ►► Apply 18-3: **The submucosal layer has cells such as Langerhans cells (CD4+/CCR5+) whose dendrites are recognized by HIV or submucosal CD4 cells contact HIV due to disruption of mucosal integrity in traumatic sex.**

associated with sharing of needles and syringes by injecting drug users, and this has been an increasing source of the disease. In some areas of the world, the seroprevalence of HIV positivity among injecting drug users has been as high as 70%. Transmission of infection to healthcare workers through accidental needle-sticks that are potentially contaminated is very low (~ 0.23%). Nevertheless, transmission has occurred from both clinical and laboratory exposure, and extreme care in handling needles, sharps, and so on, is necessary. Transmission does not occur through day-to-day nonsexual contact with infected individuals or through insect vectors because of the fragility of the virus and the need for direct mucosal or blood contact. As described earlier, HIV can be found in most bodily fluids. While HIV is found in saliva, transmission has not been documented, whereas HIV found in breast milk is readily transmitted to infants in the absence of ART.

Testing blood supply reduces risk

Intravenous drug abusers at high risk

Needlesticks mandate extreme care

Shed in breast milk may infect breastfeeding infants

Occurrence

Globally by the end of 2019, 38 million (31.6-44.5 million) people, including 20.1 million women and 1.8 million children, were living with HIV, 1.7 million people (150,000 children, 52% lower than 2010) were newly infected with HIV in 2019 (23% decline since 2010), and 690,000 people died of AIDS in 2019 (39% decline since 2010 and 60% since the peak in 2004). Since the start of the epidemic until the end of 2019, 76 million people have been infected and 33 million people have died. More importantly, 26 million people with HIV (68%) globally have access to ART by June 2020. In 2019, 85% of pregnant women with HIV had access to antiretroviral treatment to prevent transmission to their child. Although sub-Saharan Africa has 25.6 million or 67% of all HIV-infected people in the world, about 5.8 million or 15% people are living with HIV in South, Southeast, and East Asia, 2.2 million or 6% in Western and Central Europe and North America and 2.1 million or 6% in Latin America at the end of 2019. After sub-Saharan Africa and Asia and Pacific, the most heavily affected area regions where 1% of the people are living with HIV in 2019 are the Caribbean, Eastern Europe, and Central Asia. By the end of 2019, 240,000 people were living with HIV in the Middle East and North Africa. One of the striking trends of the HIV epidemic is that 45% of infected people are between the ages of 15 and 24 years. Due to the COVID-19 pandemic, HIV-related services such as testing and ART were disrupted that may increase AIDS-related deaths and new infections.

Thirty-eight million with HIV worldwide

Infection in children declined 52%, adult 23%

Deaths decreased 39% since 2010, 60% since 2004

Sixty-eight percent of infected have access to ART

In the United States, approximately 1.2 million people are living with HIV in 2018, including 41% blacks/African American, 29% whites, 23% Hispanics, 1.5% Asians, 0.3% American Indians/Alaska Native, and 0.09% Native Hawaiians and Other Pacific Islanders. Males accounted for 76.4% of the HIV-infected population, and 0.7 million people have died with HIV/AIDS. New HIV infections were 37,968 in 2018 in the United States, which is a 7% decline between 2014 and 2018. The highest prevalence rates (66%) have been in MSM followed by high-risk heterosexual contact (23.8%), intravenous drug users (6.6%), and those infected with both male-to-male and injection drug use (3.6%). The overall rate of HIV perinatal (mother-to-child) transmission with ART in the United States has been less than 1%. In 2018, 15,500 people with HIV died (HIV-related and unrelated causes) in the United States, a 37% decrease between 2010 and 2018, and this decline is attributed to the success of ART.

United States has 1.2 million with HIV

41% black/African American

Males 76% of all HIV

Highest rates in MSM

New infections declined by 7%, deaths 37%

Drop in mother-to-child transmission

In contrast to the situation in the United States and Western Europe, heterosexual transmission is the primary route of transmission in Africa and Asia, where there is an approximately equal distribution of infection and disease between the sexes. This may be due to a high incidence in these areas of ulcerative genital lesions caused by other sexually transmitted diseases. These lesions facilitate passage of virus into the tissues of others during intercourse. In central and eastern Europe, where there is an emerging epidemic, the most common risk factor is intravenous drug use.

AIDS has been reported in more than 186 countries. The rate of new infection has dropped by 23% in 2019 compared with 2010 and HIV-related deaths by 39% and 60% in 2019 compared with 2010, and the peak in 2004, respectively. The sharpest decline in new infection by 38% was observed in the Eastern and Southern African and 25% in Western and Central African countries. However, the epidemics in Americas have declined modestly. In Eastern Europe and Central Asia, the number of newly HIV-infected people has increased by 72% between 2010 and 2019. The number of people living with HIV in Russia is estimated to be 1 to 1.5 million, about 1% of its population. In the Middle East and North Africa, the number of newly HIV-1 infected people has increased by 25% between 2010 and 2019. In Asia and the Pacific region, where HIV infection was exploding until 2009, the number of new HIV-1 infection has decreased by 12% since 2010. In China, there are 1.5 million people living with HIV in 2018 and new 400 people were diagnosed per day in 2018. In India, 2.1 million people living with HIV in 2017, and new infections

Men and women equally infected in Africa and Asia

Infection declined in Africa, Asia, Pacific

Increased in Eastern Europe, Central Asia, Middle East, North Africa

declined by 27% between 2010 and 2017. The declining or stabilizing infections in various regions of the world are attributed to access to ART.

■ HIV-1 Clades or Subtypes and Geographic Distribution

Based on genetic variation, four classes of HIV-1 have developed worldwide, including M (major), O (outlying), N (new), and P (pending identification). However, class M accounts for more than 90% of all HIV-1 cases globally and is further classified into nine **subtypes** or **clades,** including A to K and their circulating recombinants form such as clades and recombinants (CRF). In addition, the demographic distribution of individuals infected with particular clades is becoming heterogeneous with the progressing pandemic. Among all subtypes circulating worldwide, subtype C is found in more than 47%, subtype B 12%, subtype A 10%, CRF02_AG 8%, and CRFG01_AE 5% of HIV-1–infected people. However, several subtypes predominate in a given region of the world, including clade B (Americas, Europe, and Australia), clade C (India and South Africa), clade E (Southeast Asia), most major CRFs (Africa), and subtypes B, A, and CRF (Eastern Europe and Central Asia). In addition, several CRFs are also found in various countries and regions. The interclade variation in the envelope gene is in the range of 20% to 30%, whereas intraclade variation is 10% to 15%. There is also some argument that certain clades may have an increased risk of transmission and progress to AIDS more rapidly than others. Understanding the immunopathogenesis of the emerging HIV-1 clades is key to vaccine development.

PATHOGENESIS

HIV infection is typically characterized by: (1) an inefficient transmission of HIV (common route: anal or vaginal sex); (2) an acute phase of intense viral replication and dissemination to lymphoid tissues (acute retroviral syndrome; flu- or mononucleosis-like illness in infected individuals); (3) activation of innate and adaptive immune response but unable to contain the highly replicating and mutating virus; (4) a chronic (persistent) asymptomatic phase (clinical latency) of continued viral replication and immune activation; and (5) an advanced phase of marked depletion of CD4 T-lymphocytes (immune deficiency) leading to development of AIDS (opportunistic infections). **Figure 18–5** summarizes the immunopathogenic events of HIV infection. Although the pathogenesis of HIV infection is very complex, the following factors are likely to be important in the disease-causing process.

■ Infection

Sexual transmission of HIV following exposure to infectious virus in semen or mucosal surfaces represents the common route of HIV transmission worldwide (other routes of HIV transmission are discussed earlier). The initial target of HIV is the CD4 molecule and a chemokine receptor

Class M most common

Clade or subtype B found in the United States

Several CRFs in Africa, Asia

Clade C in half of infected

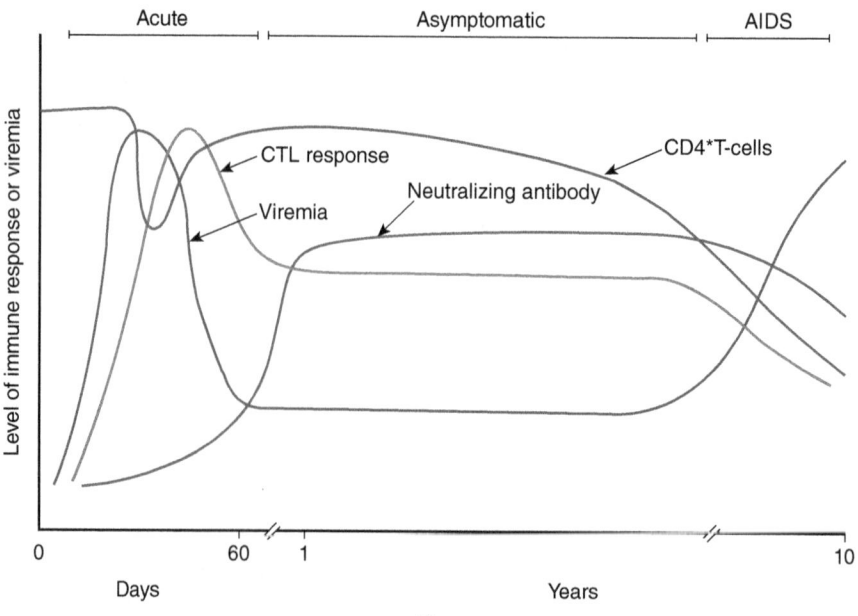

FIGURE 18–5. Temporal changes in viral load, anti-HIV-1 immune responses, and total CD4 T-cell counts during various stages of HIV-1 infection.

(CCR5), particularly on the surface of monocytes/macrophages, Langerhans cells, and mucosal CD4+ helper T-lymphocytes, as a minor genotype of HIV (single founder virus) with R5 phenotype is predominantly transmitted from person to person. The first cell type to be infected is most likely the Langerhans cell or macrophages via CD4 and CCR5. The virus replicates in these cells, which could also serve as a reservoir for continued expansion of the infection to other cell types, especially CD4 T-lymphocytes (the major target cells) by cell-to-cell fusion. In addition, dendritic cells (DC-SIGN) also play an important role in transferring HIV to CD4 T-lymphocytes. HIV productively replicates in the genital mucosal CD4 T-lymphocytes (CD4+/CCR5+) and migrates via draining lymph nodes to gut-associated lymphoid tissue (GALT) and replicates and depletes memory CD4+ T-lymphocytes (CD4+/CCR5+) in intestinal lamina propria. HIV then disseminates to other secondary lymphoid tissue to establish stable viral reservoirs. At this time (2-4 weeks after transmission), a majority of patients experience flu- or mononucleosis-like illness (acute retroviral syndrome). During the early phase of infection, aggressive viral replication occurs in the absence of immune response and the concentration of HIV reaches 10 million copies per milliliter, which can be detected in blood as early as 7 to 28 days after transmission. There is a depletion of CD4+ T-lymphocytes in the peripheral blood and a massive depletion of CD4+ T-lymphocytes in the GALT, which results in damage of gut immunity, loss of gut barrier integrity and permeability of microbial products (such as lipopolysaccharide or LPS and others) and dysbiosis. The immune system mounts a response that lags behind the high viral load and is unable to completely control viral replication. However, the viral load decreases by the action of CD8 cytotoxic T lymphocytes (CTL) activity and later neutralizing antibodies, and the virus establishes a set point in infected patients, which means the virus continues to replicate and mutate while avoiding the immune response. There is also a rebound of CD+ T-lymphocytes in the peripheral blood. This asymptomatic phase is also referred to as clinical latency.

The virus can also more efficiently infect T-lymphocytes, cells that express CD4 and CXCR4, which is seen in late stages of HIV disease. HIV can infect a wide range of CD4+ cells, including renal and gastrointestinal epithelium and brain astrocytes. The mechanism for infection of non–CD4-bearing cells is not clearly understood but may involve coreceptors such as CCR5 or CXCR4.

Infected monocytes may participate in the breakdown of the blood–brain barrier, allowing monocytes to infiltrate the central nervous system (CNS). These infected monocytes differentiate into perivascular macrophages and become the resident cells harboring HIV in the CNS. Although CNS disturbance is a part of fully developed AIDS, it is not clear whether they are a direct result of infection of these cells or mediated by cytokines from infected macrophages and T-lymphocytes.

Following transmission, HIV replicates in CD4+/CCR5 cells and the predominant phenotype of HIV is R5 in infected people initially, whereas the highly replicating and mutating virus late in infection becomes X4, which replicates more efficiently in CD4 T-lymphocytes, causing cytopathic effects.

Kinetic studies of changes in viral load with antiviral therapy demonstrated that the half-life of HIV in plasma is 5 to 6 hours and an estimated 10 billion HIV particles are produced every day in an infected individual. In other words, more than 50% of the viral load measured on any given day has been produced in the last 24 hours. Because 99% of the viral load is produced by cells that were infected within the last 48 to 72 hours, cell turnover must be equally rapid. Indeed, when similar kinetic studies are performed on changes in CD4 cell counts, it is estimated that up to 1 billion CD4+ cells are produced per day in response to the infection and that the half-life of these cells is only 1.6 days.

■ Clinical Latency or Chronic Phase

Following infection and establishment of a viral set point, the long asymptomatic period (clinical latency or chronic phase) occurs despite active virus replication in the host. Several factors can terminate the long clinical latency period of HIV. Mutations occur during viral replication, which appear to enhance induction of virulent forms of the virus (conversion of R5 to X4), with increased cytopathic capacity and altered cell tropisms. Thus, the mutated forms of HIV isolated from later stages of disease (X4 HIV-1) infect a broader range of cell types and grow more rapidly than those isolated in the asymptomatic period (R5). Initially, it was believed that little or no viral replication occurred during this clinically latent period, but studies of lymph nodes of individuals with early asymptomatic disease have shown a significantly higher level of virus and intense immunologic

Margin notes:
* Target cells CD4+/CCR5, most Langerhans or macrophages

Cell-to-cell fusion transfers HIV to CD4+/CCR5 mucosal CD4 T-lymphocytes

Dendritic cells participate in transfer to CD4 T-lymphocytes

* Massive depletion of mucosal CD4+ T-lymphocytes in GALT

* Partial control by immune response

T-lymphocytes expressing CD4+/CXCR4 infected

Non-CD4+ infected through CCR5 or CXCR4

Infected monocytes infiltrate CNS, differentiate into perivascular macrophages that harbor HIV

* R5-HIV in early infection, X4-HIV emerges late

X4-HIV replicates and depletes T-lymphocytes

Ten billion HIV particles produced every day

Rapid turnover of CD4+ cells

Mutation results in altered phenotype and tropisms

Immune control of virus is seen during clinical latency, later lost

reactions within the lymphoid tissue at early stages of disease. This implies that the immune system is capable of controlling the virus to some degree early in the course of disease, an ability that is later lost as the disease progresses over time. Figure 18–5 shows the temporal changes in viral load, anti-HIV immune responses, and total CD4+ T-cell counts during various stages of HIV infection.

* Viremia correlates with progression

* Higher the viral load, faster the progression

Following clinical latency, various studies have shown that the level of free HIV in the plasma increases in direct relation to the stage of disease. Individuals with early-stage disease have less than 10 infectious virions per milliliter of plasma, whereas those in late-stage disease have between 100 and 1000/mL. These studies imply that either viral replication was increasing during later stages of disease as a result of more virulent mutations and/or the immune system had lost its ability to clear free virus as the disease progresses. However, current HIV treatment has changed these scenarios.

■ Immune Activation

Immune activation result of proinflammatory cytokines and chemokines

HIV infection causes a generalized immune activation, including production of proinflammatory cytokines (TNF-α, interleukin-1 [IL-1], IL-6, IL-12) and chemokines, INF-α and lipopolysaccharides (LPS). One of these factors, LPS, is a potent activator of macrophages and dendritic cells to release proinflammatory cytokines during acute infection, most likely by translocation of microbial product (LPS) by disruption of intestinal barrier of GALT infection by HIV-1. The role of INF-α and TNF-α is described later.

■ Immune Response and Its Failure to Eliminate HIV

Early control of infection by innate immunity through TLR and induction of INF-α

HIV interferes with the components of innate immunity

Early control of HIV infection is achieved by innate immunity. Soon after infection, dendritic cells respond through recognition of viral products (viral RNA) by pattern recognition receptors (toll-like receptors and/or RIG-1-like receptors) and releasing antiviral cytokines, INF-α and TNF-α, which inhibit viral replication and promote activation of immune response. Recent studies suggest that dendritic cells from females produce a higher level of INF-α than males probably resulting in a lower viral load set point in females compared with males. HIV Env gp120 binds to TLR9 causing activation of INF-α/β and NK cells that also provide early control of infection. Several other innate immune cells respond to HIV infection by releasing antiviral cytokines or factors through their distinct set of innate immune receptors. These cells include phagocytes (monocytes, macrophages, and dendritic cells that clear antigens), cytolytic cells (NK cells and neutrophils that destroy the pathogen or pathogen-infected cells), and professional antigen-presenting cells (APCs; dendritic cells that present antigens to adaptive immunity). Moreover, NK cells are activated by INF-α and IL-15 made by dendritic cells and kill HIV-infected cells to control early infection. However, HIV has found ways to interfere with the components of innate immunity and the infection proceeds.

* HIV specific CTLs control viremia by killing infected cells

INF-γ and β-chemokines reduce viral spread

* Neutralizing antibodies also control viremia

* CTL and neutralizing antibody escape variants emerge due to mutation that allows continued viral replication

The professional APCs, dendritic cells, make the transition from innate to adaptive immunity by presenting antigens to T-lymphocytes. HIV-specific CD8+ CTLs are generated that control plasma viremia by killing HIV-infected cells. The function of CTL is mediated by perforin that makes holes in the target cell through which granzyme can enter and destroy the infected cells. In addition, CD8+ T-lymphocytes express Fas ligand that can bind to Fas (CD95) on infected cells resulting in apoptosis-induced cell death. CD8+ T-lymphocytes produce INF-γ that creates an antiviral state and β-chemokines (MIP 1-α, MIP 1-β, and RANTES) that bind to CCR5 and reduce the ability of HIV to infect other uninfected cells. However, the emergence of CTL escape mutants, because of mutations generated due to continued viral replication, are unable to sustain suppression of viral replication. The B lymphocytes respond to HIV antigens by making neutralizing antibodies after the decline in the level of viremia. The B lymphocytes see antigens in the native form initially and make IgM and later interact with HIV-specific CD4+ T-lymphocytes to class switch to IgG generating neutralizing antibodies. These neutralizing antibodies neutralize cell-free virions. However, viral variants emerge that escape neutralization from antibody response allowing continued viral replication. HIV antibodies can be detected between 3 and 12 weeks after infection.

Lack of help to B- and T-lymphocytes due to CD4 T-lymphocytes killing

The CD4+ T-lymphocytes that make cytokines (especially IL-2) to help B lymphocytes and both CD4+ and CD8+ T-lymphocytes are impaired because CD4+ T-lymphocytes are infected and killed by HIV. In early infection, memory CD4+ T-lymphocytes are depleted; however, both memory and naïve CD4+ T-lymphocytes are depleted as the infection progresses.

Despite a robust immune response, the immune system fails to eliminate HIV from infected individuals. Several reasons could be attributed, including cell-to-cell spread of the virus that avoids recognition by the neutralizing antibodies; high mutation rates resulting in antigenic variation causing CTL and antibody escape variants; interference with cytokine production; suppression of MHC I and II; integration of proviral DNA into the host chromosome; establishment of persistent infection; and diminished ability of T-lymphocyte precursor to generate mature CD4+ and CD8+ T-lymphocytes. The immune system is unable to keep up with the pace of mutating virus, resulting in impaired T- and B-lymphocyte functions and immune deficiency.

Immune system fails to eliminate HIV from infected hosts

 Why does the viral load in HIV-infected individuals only drop to a set point, never eliminated, and become a lifelong infection, despite a robust CTL and antibody response?

■ Immune Deficiency

The primary immune deficiency in AIDS results from the reduction in the numbers and effectiveness of CD4+ helper T-lymphocytes, both in absolute numbers and relative to CD8+ T-lymphocytes. This is due to direct killing of CD4+ T-lymphocytes by the virus, but also involve other mechanisms. These include secondary killing of uninfected (bystander) cells during cell fusion and syncytia formation, apoptosis, interference with T-cell maturation, autoimmune processes that lead to the elimination of CD4+ T-lymphocytes by opsonophagocytosis, and antibody-dependent cell-mediated cytotoxicity (ADCC) directed at gp120 expressed on the CD4+ cell surface. There are also functional defects in CD4+ T-lymphocytes affecting cytokine production and leading to inhibition of some macrophage functions.

Immune deficiency related to reduction in numbers and normal functions of CD4+ T-lymphocytes

Effects on CD4+ T-lymphocytes thus lead to a generalized failure of cell-mediated immune responses, but there is also an effect on antibody production, including lack of class switching in response to antigens of newly generated variants as well as due to polyclonal activation of B cells, possibly associated with other viral infections of these cells. This overwhelms the capacity of infected individuals to respond to specific antigens. The end result of these processes is a disturbance of immune balance that can give rise to malignancies as well as the susceptibility of AIDS patients to a range of opportunistic viral, fungal, and bacterial infections.

✳ *Infected individuals are susceptible to other infections and malignancies due to immune suppression*

■ HIV Reservoirs

Following infection, HIV establishes persistent infection even in the presence of a competent immune system. Whereas in the absence of ART (described later), infected individuals develop immune deficiency (described earlier) and opportunistic infections (described later), HIV persists in reservoirs (cells or tissues that harbor HIV) in the presence of effective ART. HIV reservoirs are the biggest hurdle in eradicating HIV from infected individuals by effective ART. There are two types of HIV reservoirs: lymphoid tissues (GALT and lymph nodes: many target cells for HIV and low penetration of ART) and cellular reservoirs (resting T-lymphocytes and monocytes/macrophages). In HIV-infected individuals undergoing successful viral suppression with ART, a small pool of resting CD4+ T-lymphocytes remain silently infected with HIV provirus that also provides a long-lived source of rebound viremia. The phenotype of these CD4+ T-lymphocytes includes central memory CD4+ T-lymphocytes (T_{CM}), transitional memory CD4+ T-lymphocytes (T_{TM}), and effector memory CD4+ T-lymphocytes (T_{EM}). Whereas T_{CM} that are long-lived quiescent T-lymphocytes present in lymph nodes might represent a latent reservoir for HIV-1, T_{EM} that are present in a high frequency in GALT may provide residual viral replication. Recent studies suggest that HIV can persist latently in CD34 stem cells in bone marrow, especially in those patients who do not start ART early following infection. Research continues to find ways to destroy HIV from these reservoirs.

HIV persists in reservoirs during treatment

Lymphoid tissues and cellular reservoirs (resting T-lymphocytes, monocytes/macrophages)

HIV persists in CD4 central, transitional, effector memory T-lymphocytes

HIV DNA found in bone marrow, CD34 stem cells

 Think ▸▸ Apply 18-4: HIV is never eliminated from infected people because HIV mutates more rapidly and escapes immune response, suppresses immune system, integrates in the DNA of host cells, and establishes reservoirs without being recognized.

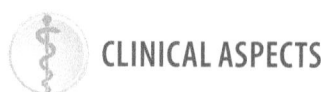 CLINICAL ASPECTS

MANIFESTATIONS

In 1993, the CDC definition of AIDS stated that all patients who are HIV antibody positive (currently HIV test includes HIV-antigen/antibody or HIV-RNA) and have CD4+ T-lymphocyte counts lower than 200/mm³ or less than 14% of total T-lymphocytes have the disease. HIV-1 infection is characterized as a three-stage process: (1) acute phase (flu- or mononucleosis-like illness, also known as acute retroviral syndrome), (2) clinical latency or chronic phase (asymptomatic with low level of HIV production), and (3) AIDS phase (immune deficiency, opportunistic infections). However, use of ART in infected people will slow down disease progression and stage 3 may not usually be seen.

Stage 1: Acute Phase. After 2 to 4 weeks of infection, some infected individuals are asymptomatic, while other infected individuals develop a flu- or mononucleosis-like illness with many symptoms such as fever, chills, night sweats, sore throat, lymphadenopathy, arthralgias, fatigue, hepatosplenomegaly, and rash that lasts about 2 to 6 weeks. Sometimes a mild aseptic meningitis is also present. During this time, HIV RNA and antigen can be detected. Whether these early manifestations of infection occur or do not occur, the virus rapidly invades, persists, and integrates into the genome of some host cells, and the individual is thus infected for life.

Stage 2: Clinical Latency or Chronic Phase. The initial infection is followed by an asymptomatic period (clinical latency, during which a low level of virus is produced) that, in most cases, continues for years before the disease becomes clinically apparent. During this time, the virus can be isolated from blood, semen, and other bodily fluids and tissues. More than 60% of infected individuals remain in clinical latency for about 8 to 10 years after infection before they develop significant disease, and the number continues to increase thereafter if untreated. It is expected that nearly all HIV-infected persons eventually develop some clinical aspects of this infection if left untreated, although long-term (>10 years) nonprogressors are well documented. Some infected individuals (5-10%) develop significant clinical diseases within few years after infection, if untreated, are referred as rapid progressors. Approximately 5% of infected, untreated patients show no decrease in CD4 counts over a period of more than 10 years, but ultimately many of these individuals begin to progress. Based on the availability of more specific and sensitive tests, HIV can be detected early in infection and potent ART can be initiated to suppress viral load, improve CD4 T-cell counts, and prevent infected patients developing clinical HIV disease, symptomatic AIDS.

Stage 3: AIDS. As the disease progresses in untreated patients, the number of CD4+ T-lymphocytes declines. An increasing immunodeficiency, and opportunistic infections becoming more frequent, severe, and difficult to treat is considered AIDS. One of the best markers of the severity of AIDS is the absolute number of CD4+ T-lymphocytes. Those individuals with overt AIDS almost always have fewer than 200 CD4+ T-lymphocytes/mm³ of blood (normal = 500-1600/mm³), although opportunistic infections may occur with CD4+ T-cells greater than 200/mm³. Patients with AIDS at the late stage of HIV infection may experience many symptoms such as recurring fever, night sweats, rapid weight loss, diarrhea (for more than a week), sores in mouth or genitals, white patches on the tongue or oral mucous membranes (thrush), pneumonia, and some neurological disorders. Many infected people are tested for HIV-1 after experiencing these symptoms. If they are tested positive, viral load and CD4 T-cell counts, in addition to other blood work, are ordered, and treatment is initiated. Viral load and CD4 T-cells count are monitored to assess the progress of the treatment.

✴ Early symptoms may include flu or mononucleosis-like illness

✴ HIV infection is lifelong

✴ Progression to AIDS is highly variable among individuals

HIV treatment prevents progression to AIDS

Individuals with overt AIDS usually have fewer than 200 CD4+ lymphocytes/mm³

 Why do symptomatic AIDS patients develop other viral, bacterial, and fungal infections more frequently than asymptomatic patients?

 Think ▸▸ Apply 18-5: Because the CD4 T-cell count falls below 200 in symptomatic AIDS patients resulting in depressed cell-mediated immunity allowing many pathogens infect these patients easily because of impaired immunity.

Patients with full-blown AIDS, who were untreated (no ART), experience a wide spectrum of infections depending on the severity of their immune deficiency and on the opportunistic organisms in their normal flora or those with which they come in contact (**Table 18–3**). Some clinical manifestations of AIDS may thus vary by locale. For example, disseminated histoplasmosis was a common complication in the Midwestern United States and disseminated coccidioidomycosis in the Southwestern United States, as was disseminated toxoplasmosis in France. These infections are uncommon in areas where the diseases are not endemic. The diversity and anatomic sites of infection vary among patients, and any one patient may have several infections. The most common infection is pneumocystosis, and approximately 50% of the AIDS patients who do not receive ART or prophylaxis for pneumocystosis develop *Pneumocystis jirovecii* pneumonia. In the past, about 25% of all patients with AIDS developed Kaposi sarcoma, but the number of cases has been falling in the United States. The apparent explanation is that Kaposi sarcoma is due to a transmitted agent different from HIV, the Kaposi sarcoma herpesvirus (KSHV) or HHV-8.

Pneumocystosis, candidiasis, mycobacteriosis, and CMV are common

TABLE 18–3	Common Opportunistic Infections and Malignancies in Patients with Untreated AIDS (Without Antiretroviral Therapy). The CD4 T cell counts are a general but not an absolute indicator of appearance of opportunistic infections because several of these infections can be seen at any CD4 T cell count.
INFECTION/DISEASE	**PATHOGEN/CONDITION**
CD4 T cell counts <500/mL	
Candidiasis (Thrush)	*Candida albicans*—**Fungal**
Coccidioidomycosis (disseminated).	*Coccidioides immitis*—**Fungal**
Herpes zoster (shingles)	Varicella-zoster virus (reactivation)—**Viral**
Histoplasmosis (disseminated).	Histoplasma capsulatum—**Fungal**
Kaposi sarcoma	HHV-8—**Viral**
Lymphoma (Hodgkin and Non-Hodgkin)	Due to Immune suppression, EBV?
Opportunistic malignancies.	Due to immune suppression
Oral hairy leukoplakia.	EBV—**Viral**
Persistent mucocutaneous herpes simplex.	Herpes simplex virus—**Viral**
Pneumonia, recurrent	*Streptococcus pneumoniae*—**Bacterial**
Tuberculosis (reactivation)	*Mycobacterium tuberculosis* -**Bacterial**
CD4 T cell counts <200/mL	
Invasive cervical cancer	HPV—**Viral**
HIV-related encephalopathy.	HIV—**Viral**
HIV-related Wasting syndrome.	HIV—**Viral**
Pneumocystis pneumonia.	*Pneumocystis jirovecii*—**Fungal**
Progressive multifocal leukoencephalopathy	JC virus (Polyomavirus)—**Viral**
Salmonella septicemia, recurrent.	Salmonella—**Bacterial**
Tuberculosis (primary)	*Mycobacterium tuberculosis*—**Bacterial**
CD4 T cell counts <100/mL and <50/mL	
Bacillary angiomatosis.	*Bartonella henselae/quintana* -**Bacterial**
CMV retinitis, gastrointestinal, or disseminated infection.	CMV—**Viral**
Cryptococcosis	*Cryptococcus neoformans*—**Fungal**
Cryptosporidiosis (diarrhea)	*Cryptosporidium* spp—**Protozoa/Parasitic**
Esophageal candidiasis.	*Candida albicans*—**Fungal**
Isospora belli (diarrhea)	*Cystisospora belli*—**Protozoa/ Parasitic**
Mycobacterium avium–intracellulare complex (MAC)	*Mycobacterium avium*—**Bacterial**
Toxoplasmosis (CNS)	*Toxoplasma gondii*—**Protozoa/ Parasitic**
Pulmonary aspergillosis.	Aspergillus fumigatus—**Fungal**

❊ Most common opportunistic
infection is *P jirovecii*
pneumonia

Disease due to mycobacteria of the *Mycobacterium avium–intracellulare* complex is common, and patients with AIDS are also highly susceptible to *Mycobacterium tuberculosis* infection. Oral thrush and esophagitis due to *Candida albicans* and meningitis due to *Cryptococcus* are commonly encountered fungal infections. Persistent progressive mucocutaneous herpes simplex and herpes zoster infections are common. Cytomegalovirus (CMV) chorioretinitis is one of the most common opportunistic infections seen at very low CD4 T-cells count (~50) and may result in unilateral or bilateral blindness. Disseminated CMV infection is also seen, and patients present with fever and visceral (eg, gastrointestinal) organ involvement.

Specific opportunistic infections are associated with differing levels of CD4+ T-lymphocyte counts. For example, fungal and tuberculous pneumonia may occur with CD4+ T-lymphocyte counts of 200 to 500 cells/mm³, whereas CMV and *M avium–intracellulare* disease are seen almost exclusively in those whose counts are lower than 50 to 100 cells/mm³. Patients with opportunistic infections are treated for specific infections or conditions. However, with current ART regimens and patient management, the number of opportunistic infections has significantly reduced in the United States and other developed countries.

CMV retinitis, mycobacterial
dissemination with extremely
low CD4+ counts

HIV treatment prevents
development of opportunistic
infections

The CDC Classification of Clinical Categories of HIV-1 Disease was revised in 2014 that could be used to clinically categorize a confirmed case of HIV-1 based on the positivity of HIV-1 antigen/antibody or HIV RNA in one of five stages of HIV-1 infection, including 0, 1, 2, 3, or unknown. If an individual was tested negative for HIV within 6 months of the first HIV infection diagnosis, the stage is 0 and remains 0 until 6 months after diagnosis. If an individual is diagnosed with stage 3 defining opportunistic illness, the stage is 3. Otherwise, the stage of infection is determined based on CD4 T cell counts for different age groups.

Stage 0: HIV test negative for the first time within 6 months, remains stage 0 until 6 months.

Stage 1: ≥1500 CD4 counts (age <1 year), ≥1000 (age 1-5 years), ≥500 (age 6 years-adult).

Stage 2: 750-1499 CD4 counts (age <1 year), 500-999 (age 1-5 years), 200-499 (age 6 years-adult).

Stage 3: <750 CD4 counts (age <1 year), <500 (age 1-5 years), <200 (age 6 years-adult).

Unknown: If none of the stages apply because of missing information on CD4 results.

CDC clinical classification of
HIV disease used in clinical
evaluation of patients

These stages of HIV infection can be found on www.cdc.gov/hiv.

As the duration of survival of patients with HIV became longer as a result of ART with the earliest drugs, an increased number of patients developed neurologic manifestations of the disease and lymphoid neoplasms, especially non-Hodgkin lymphomas. HIV is a neurotropic virus and can be isolated from the cerebrospinal fluid (CSF) of 50% to 70% of patients. CNS involvement may be asymptomatic, but many patients develop a subacute neurologic illness that produced clinical symptoms varying from mild cognitive dysfunction to severe dementia. Loss of complex cognitive function is usually the first sign of illness. Progression to severe memory loss, depression, seizures, and coma may ensue. Cerebral atrophy involving primarily cortical white matter can be demonstrated by computed tomography or magnetic resonance imaging. Histologically, focal vacuolation of the affected brain tissue with perivascular infiltration of macrophages is noted. Multinucleated giant cells with syncytium formation surround the perivascular infiltrates. Neurologic symptoms do not usually occur until CD4+ T-lymphocyte counts are lower than 200 cells/mm³.

HIV is also neurotropic and can
lead to dementia

The disease spectrum in Africa is similar in many respects to that in the Western world, but many more patients present with severe intractable wasting (involuntary loss of more than 10% of body weight), diarrhea, and weakness, known as **wasting syndrome** or **slim disease.** Tuberculosis is also more commonly encountered in AIDS patients in Africa, reflecting the higher incidence of the disease in the population in general. The 2-year mortality rate of persons with AIDS, once the disease has been fully established, was initially 75%, with nearly all persons eventually dying of opportunistic infections or neoplasms. However, with the accessibility of ART and other preventive measures, HIV-related deaths and new infections have declined in these countries.

DIAGNOSIS

The diagnosis of HIV infection can be done by three major types of available tests, including (1) HIV antigen/antibody combination test (4th-generation HIV test), (2) nucleic acid amplification tests based on PCR, and (3) antibody tests. Some of these tests differentiate between HIV-1 and HIV-2:

1. **HIV Antigen/Antibody Combination Test (4th-Generation HIV Test):** This test detects HIV-1 antigens and HIV-1 and HIV-2 antibodies in blood within 2 to 6 weeks after infection. HIV virions appear in 1 to 4 weeks after infections, which means HIV antigens such as p24 (capsid protein) can be detected early in infection before the development of antibodies. Antibodies will be produced within a week after the appearance of antigens. This sensitive and specific test can detect both HIV antigen and antibody in 2 to 6 weeks after infection. Antigen and antibody detection in this combination utilizes ELISA-based technology. There are three steps involved in this test. If a patient tests positive in Step 1 it means HIV-1 p24 antigen is present, Step 2 differentiates between HIV-1 and HIV-2 antibodies, and if positive for either antibodies, confirms HIV-1 infection. However, if Step 2 is negative or indeterminate, Step 3, the nucleic acid test by PCR to detect HIV-1 RNA is performed, and if positive, confirms HIV-1 infection. If Step 3 is negative, then Step 1 was a false positive and result is HIV negative. The fourth-generation test is now widely used in the United States and many countries. There is a rapid version available that uses blood or saliva samples.

2. **Nucleic Acid Test (NAT):** More practical approaches include nucleic acid-based assays such as the polymerase chain reaction (PCR) for plasma HIV-1 RNA (RT-PCR) or HIV-1 DNA (in peripheral blood mononuclear cells) and the branched-chain DNA (bDNA) assay. HIV-1 RNA in the plasma of infected individuals can be detected 7 to 28 days after infection. These nucleic acid detection methods are also useful in assessing the benefits of antiviral therapy, as well as in determining whether infants born to seropositive mothers are infected or simply demonstrating passively transmitted transplacental antibody.

    Quantitation of plasma HIV RNA plays an especially important part in management. For example, if a patient's HIV RNA copy number rises during therapy, or fails to fall to low levels (eg, lower than 50 copies/mL), this signals that the antiviral efficacy of the drug regimen is inadequate. The most likely explanation is mutational resistance that either preexisted or developed during treatment. Other explanations to be considered include patient noncompliance and inadequate dosing.

3. **Antibody Test:** The HIV antibody test is done to demonstrate antibody to HIV antigens. Initial screening tests are performed using whole viral lysates as the target antigens in enzyme-linked immunosorbent assay (ELISA) test. This test has a high level of sensitivity, but because false-positive results occur, all positive ELISA antibody tests must be confirmed. The confirmatory test used to be a western blot analysis that detects antibodies to specific HIV-1 proteins but is no longer used or recommended. The ELISA antibody-positive results are confirmed by the nucleic acid test or PCR of HIV genome. The ELISA tests give a high degree of specificity to test results, but antibody is detectable by these procedures in the first 3 to 12 weeks after infection. This is called window period and 97% of infected people are likely to develop antibody during this period. If a suspected individual test is negative during window period, the test should be repeated 3 months after exposure. During this window period, the individual can still transmit the infection to others by sexual contact or blood donation. Therefore, the nucleic acid test is performed for blood transfusion.

    The FDA has also approved several rapid HIV antibody tests that can be performed in 30 minutes and used in both clinical and nonclinical settings, including home and can help to overcome some of the barriers to early diagnosis. These screening tests use oral swabs (saliva) or blood and are interpreted visually and require no instrumentation. Like the ELISA test, all require confirmation if reactive. In these rapid tests, HIV antigens are affixed to the test membrane and if HIV antibodies are present in the specimen being tested, they bind to the affixed antigen. The colorimetric reagent provided in the kit binds to these immunoglobulins and is visually detected.

4. **HIV diagnosis in infants born to infected mothers:** Since maternal IgG is transferred to the fetus, antibody tests will not diagnose HIV infection in infants. Therefore, HIV diagnosis in infants is confirmed by HIV-1 culture or HIV DNA/RNA PCR and positive results are confirmed repeating the test. HIV DNA PCR positivity is 38% for 48 hours of life, 93% for 14 days, and 98% for 4 weeks.

※ Fourth-generation HIV test detects both HIV antigen and HIV antibody 2 to 6 weeks after infection

※ Nucleic acid test detects HIV RNA by PCR in 7 to 28 days after infection

※ HIV RNA levels important to assess ART efficacy

Antibodies detected 3 to 12 weeks after infection

HIV rapid tests screen for HIV antibodies but require confirmation

Risk of transmission during window period

※ HIV DNA/RNA PCR used to diagnose HIV infection in infants

SCREENING

The CDC and US Preventive Task Force (USPTF) recommend that clinicians screen all adolescents and adults aged 13 to 64 years for HIV infection at least once as part of routine annual. The screening should be repeated annually for those who are at increased risk of HIV infection. In addition, MSM and bisexual men and those who inject drugs could benefit for more frequent testing like every 3 to 6 months. HIV screening should also be included in the routine panel of prenatal screening for all pregnant women. This recommendation is in line with the CDC guidelines of 2006 that HIV testing should be a part of routine healthcare for all adolescents and adults. While 1.2 million people are infected with HIV, 1 in 7 or 15% are unaware of their HIV status. More than 40% of HIV infections are transmitted by those who are unaware of their HIV status. Screening and diagnosing people early would allow starting treatment and further reducing HIV transmission and new cases in the United States.

TREATMENT

Currently, there are six classes of antiretroviral agents, including NRTIs, NNRTIs, PIs, integrase strand transfer inhibitors (INSTIs), the CCR5 antagonist, and the gp41 fusion inhibitor. These anti-HIV-1 agents are listed in **Table 18–4.** These inhibitors are used in a combination therapy (at least three separate inhibitors from two different classes) known as ART. In addition, in some combinations, a pharmacokinetic enhancer is added to increase its effectiveness of HIV-1 regimen. Several of these combinations are available is a single pill. Data to use two drugs combination is also supported for initial treatment under certain conditions.

The Department of Health and Human Services (HHS) has a working group (panel) for developing guidelines for antivirals use in adults and adolescents in the office of AIDS Research Advisory Council (OARAC). The current guidelines were updated on December 18, 2019 and are updated periodically (www.clinicalinfo.hiv.gov). The recommendation is to use ART for all HIV-infected individuals regardless of CD4 T-cell count to reduce morbidity and mortality associated with HIV infection. For treatment of naïve patients, ART generally consists of two NRTIs and a third antiviral that could be either an INSTI, an NNRTI, or a PI with a pharmacokinetic (PK) enhancer (booster) such as cobicistat or ritonavir.

The panel recommended the following HIV regimens (recommended regimen) for ART in adults and adolescents for most patients with HIV in no order of preference. **For INSTI-based regimens:** (1) Biktarvy–a single pill combination containing one INSTI (Bictegravir) and two NRTIs (Tenofovir TAF and Emtricitabine), (2) one INSTI (Dolutegravir) plus two NRTIs (Tenofovir TAF or Tenofovir TDF) or (Emtricitabine or Lamivudine), (3) one INSTI (Dolutegravir) plus two NRTIs (Abacavir and Lamivudine)—for HLA-B*5701-negative patients and without chronic hepatitis B infection, and (4) one INSTI (Raltegravir) plus two NRTIs (Emtricitabine or Lamivudine) plus (Tenofovir TAF or Tenofovir TDF). A two-drug regimen can also be used for initial treatment with one INSTI (Dolutegravir) plus one NRTI (Lamivudine)—except for patients with HIV RNA >500,000 copies/mL, HBV coinfection or ART needs to be started before genotypic testing or HBV testing are available. Also, two NRTIs (Tenofovir TAF and Emtricitabine) plus an INSTI (Elvitegravir) with a PK enhancer (Cobicistat); or two NRTIs (Tenofovir TDF and Emtricitabine) plus an INSTI (Raltegravir). **For PI-based regimens:** two NRTIs (Tenofovir TDF and Emtricitabine) plus a PI (Darunavir) with a PK enhancer (Ritonavir). The alternative regimens are two NRTIs (in similar combinations listed earlier) plus one NNRTI (Efavirenz or Rilpivirine). The alternate regimens are effective but have limitations for certain patient population. Several other combinations, alternative regimen options and other regimen options for clinical conditions are available on www.clinicalinfo.hiv.gov. Several of these combinations are available in a single pill listed in Table 18–4. Tenofovir TAF has fewer bone and kidney toxicities than TDF, while TDF is associated with lower lipid levels. Within 6 weeks of ART, many patients see plasma HIV RNA reduction by more than 1 log, and by 6 months of treatment, HIV RNA should be almost undetectable (less than 50 copies of HIV-1 RNA/mL). With the suppression of HIV load, patients should see their CD4 T-cells count increasing. ART must be continued indefinitely to keep the viral load suppressed. On January 21, 2021, U.S. FDA approved monthly injectable nanoformulations of an HIV regimen Cabenuva, a combination of two drugs, one INSTI inhibitor (Cabotegravir) and one NNRTI inhibitor (Rilpivirine), for HIV treatment in virally suppressed patients. Before starting injectable Cabenuva, the patient should orally take Cabotegravir and Rilpivirine for a month to ensure that these medications are well tolerated. This monthly treatment would be most useful for those patients who have difficulty with adherence.

TABLE 18-4 Currently FDA-approved and DHHS-recommended Antiretroviral Agents Belonging to Six Different Classes of Antiretroviral Drugs

NUCLEOSIDE REVERSE TRANSCRIPTASE INHIBITORS (NRTIs)	NONNUCLEOSIDE REVERSE TRANSCRIPTASE INHIBITORS (NNRTIs)	PROTEASE INHIBITORS (PIs)	INTEGRASE INHIBITORS	CCR5 ANTAGONISTS	GP41 FUSION INHIBITOR	FIXED COMBINATIONS
Abacavir (ABC)	Delavirdine (DLV)	Atazanavir (ATV)	Bictegravir (BIC)	Maraviroc (MVC)	Enfuvirtide (T-20)	Abacavir, lamivudine (Epzicom)
Didasosine (ddI)	Efavirenz (EFV)	Darunavir (DRV)	Cabotegravir (CAB)			Abacavir, dolutegravir, lamivudine (Triumeq)
Emtricitabine (FTC)	Etravirine (ETR)	Fosamprenavir (FPV)	Dolutegravir (DTG)			Abacavir, lamivudine, zidovudine (Trizivir)
Lamivudine (3TC)	Nevirapine (NVP)	Indinavir (IDV)	Elvitegravir (EVG)			Bictegravir/tenofovir TAF/emtricitabine (Biktarvy)
Stavudine (D4T)	Rilpivirine (RPV)	Nelfinavir (NFV)	Raltegravir (RAL)			Darunavir, cobicistat[a] (Prezcobix)
Tenofovir DF (TDF, TAF)		Ritonavir (RTV)[a]				Efavirenz, emtricitabine, tenofovir DF (Atripla)
Zidovudine (ZDV, AZT)		Saquinavir (SQV)				Elvitegravir, cobicistat, emtricitabine, tenofovir AF (Genoya)
		Tipranavir (TPV)				Emtricitabine, rilpivirine, tenofovir DF (Complera)
						Emtricitabine, tenofovir (Descovy)
						Emtricitabine, tenofovir DF (Truvada)
						Lamivudine, zidovudine (Combivir)
						Lopinavir, ritonavir (Kaletra)

[a]Cobicistat, Ritonavir: Pharmacokinetic (PK) enhancer which may be used in ART to increase its effectiveness.

Monthly ART regimen approved for virally suppressed patients

HIV regimens recommended for PEP and PrEP in high-risk individuals

ART during pregnancy reduces mother-to-child transmission by less than 1%

ART reduced risk of opportunistic infections

Reconstitution of immune system due to ART causes IRIS

Complications include body fat accumulation, dyslipidemia, abnormal glucose metabolism, cardiovascular disease, bone disorders

❋ Antiretroviral treatment is recommended for HIV infected regardless of CD4 T-cell count

❋ Viral load and CD4 T-cell count monitored to determine ART efficacy, immune deficiency

HIV genotyping to determine ART resistance done before therapy

 How does ART suppress viral load to undetectable or very low levels and reduce the risk of resistance in many patients and prevent opportunistic infections?

HIV regimen is also recommended for HIV-suspected occupational and nonoccupational postexposure prophylaxis (PEP). For **PEP**, INSTI-based regimen should be started as soon as possible but before 72 hours postexposure, and should be given for 28 days followed by regular testing for HIV by a fourth-generation HIV test. ART has also shown to prevent HIV transmission and can be used as preexposure prophylaxis (PrEP) by HIV-negative partners of HIV-positive partners. For **PrEP**, the FDA-approved daily dose of two NRTIs, Tenofovir and Emtricitabine (Truvada), in combination with safer sex practices, can reduce the risk of HIV-1 transmission by 90% from sex and 70% from injection drug use. For prevention of **mother-to-child transmission** during pregnancy, the preferred regimens in treatment-naïve pregnant women are: two NRTIs (Abacavir and Lamivudine or Emtricitabine and Tenofovir or Tenofovir and Lamivudine) plus one PI (Atazanavir or Darunavir) or one INSTI (Raltegravir or Dolutegravir). The use of ART during pregnancy has reduced the mother-to-child transmission rates by less than 1% in the United States.

Recent advances in HIV therapy have slowed the progression of the HIV disease and appear to be responsible for dramatic improvement in many patients' lives, but toxicity or the development of resistance remains the concern. However, successful suppression of HIV by ART can reconstitute CD4 T-lymphocyte numbers that cause an inflammatory response known as immune reconstitution inflammatory syndrome (IRIS). Some of the common coinfections that may be exacerbated by IRIS are tuberculous and nontuberculous mycobacteria, CMV retinitis, cryptococcal meningitis, hepatitis B, and hepatitis C. In addition to side effects of antiretrovirals, several complications of ART include lipoatrophy (visceral fat accumulation), hypercholesterolemia, low HDL, hypertriglyceridemia, insulin resistance, impaired glucose tolerance, cardiovascular disease, lactic acidosis, osteopenia, osteoporosis, osteonecrosis, and others.

■ Initiation of Treatment

Because HIV replication proceeds at such a phenomenal rate, it seems most rational to begin treatment as soon as HIV infection is detected. Therefore, ART is recommended by HHS panel for all HIV-infected individuals regardless of CD4 T-cell count to reduce the morbidity and mortality related to HIV infection. ART is also recommended to prevent adult HIV transmission and mother-to-child transmission. In some instances, ART may be deferred because of clinical and/or psychological factors but should be started as soon as possible. In addition, several conditions increase the urgency to start ART, including pregnancy of HIV-infected women, AIDS-defining illness, acute opportunistic infections and malignancies, CD4 T-cell counts of lower than 200 cells/mm³, HIV-associated nephropathy, acute HIV infections (acute retroviral syndrome), coinfection with HBV or HCV. However, considerations of toxicity, resistance development, quality of life, cost, and patient wishes are extremely important additional determinants. Before the initiation of ART, plasma HIV RNA (viral load), CD4 T-cell count, HIV genotyping (to determine ART resistant mutants), and other laboratory parameters should be performed. The efficacy of ART should be followed by performing viral load and CD4 T-cell count and the adverse effects of the ART should also be evaluated. Because current therapy is unlikely to eradicate HIV infection, most patients are likely to stay on therapy for life.

■ Resistance

HIV error-prone reverse transcriptase enzyme and high rates of viral replication contribute to frequent mutations. As a result, resistance to an antiviral is a regular and often rapid development. Use of antiviral therapies that maximally suppress HIV viral load appears to diminish the appearance of resistant virus, especially combination therapy. The emergence of resistance occurs at a

 Think ▸▸ Apply 18-6: **ART includes three drugs from two different classes, which suppress viral replication at multiple steps and becomes undetectable. The risk of resistance is reduced due to lack of viral replication and mutation. The rise in CD4 T-cell count prevents opportunistic infections.**

rate proportional to the frequency of preexisting variants and their relative growth benefit in the presence of antiviral. Antiviral resistance is determined before the start of therapy and during the therapy if viral suppression is not achieved. In addition to the primary antiviral treatment of HIV, patients with CD4+ counts of less than 200/mm³ should begin prophylactic regimens to prevent *P jirovecii* pneumonia. When CD4+ counts are less than 75 to 100/mm³, they should receive prophylaxis for mycobacterial and fungal infection.

Drug resistance is expected

Prophylaxis of opportunistic infections important

PREVENTION

There are many tools available to prevent HIV transmission starting from education about the means of transmission and strategies such as abstinence (not having sex), using condoms in a proper way during every sex, never sharing needles, and using safe and clean needles for every injection. Latex condoms, properly used, do prevent HIV transmission bidirectionally, and with efficacy rates up to 98% to 99%. Circumcision of males decreases the risk of acquisition of HIV by 60% in men, but has not been clearly shown to reduce transmission to women. There are several communities that have syringe service programs (SSPs) that provide new needles and syringes and dispose the used ones. Screening and testing are another important part of HIV preventive strategies. CDC recommends that adolescents and adults between the ages of 13 and 64 should be tested for HIV infection at least once as part of routine annual and high-risk people should be tested frequently to know their HIV status, and if positive, can be started on ART. HIV-infected individuals who have undetectable or suppressed viral load (<200 HIV RNA copies/mL) because of ART can live longer and have a significantly reduced risk of transmitting to other individuals, including HIV-negative partners through sex, sharing needles and syringes, and from mother to child through vertical transmission. ART is recommended to prevent HIV transmission in high-risk groups known as PrEP. PrEP includes two combinations of HIV regimens, Truvada and Descovy (described above), that reduce the risk of getting HIV through sex by 99%, although its effectiveness for people who inject drugs is not well known but reduces the risk at least by 74%. Truvada ART using combinations of agents should be given as part of PEP to prevent infection of accidentally exposed individuals (eg, healthcare workers) or nonoccupational exposure within 72 hours of an exposure. Detection and treatment of HIV-infected pregnant women are very effective in reducing perinatal infection. Cesarean section delivery, particularly that which is elective rather than emergent, is also preventive, as is the avoidance of breastfeeding by HIV-positive mothers. Screening of blood supplies for HIV by nucleic acid testing by PCR is very effective.

Education cornerstone of prevention

✱ Condoms, properly used, can prevent transmission

Male circumcision decreases HIV transmission in men

Screening for infection in pregnancy aids effective prophylaxis

PeEP and PEP reduce risk of transmission

 What are the hurdles for HIV vaccine development?

Several other preventive measures are under development and in clinical trials such as microbicides to be used as vaginal or rectal microbicides for HIV prevention. Four long-acting HIV preventive strategies are under trial, including an intravaginal ring that would be inserted in the vagina and release antiretroviral drug over time, implant (a device implanted that would release antiretroviral drugs over time, a long-acting drug injected into the body and broadly neutralizing antibodies (bNAbs) infused or injected in the body. For treatment, a monthly infectable combination of antiretroviral regimens (Cabenuva) and a monoclonal antibody (ibalizumab directed against membrane-bound CD4) were recently approved.

Currently, there is no vaccine approved for HIV. One of the hurdles to develop HIV vaccines has been the marked mutability of HIV and generation of several subtypes/CRFs. However, several candidates are under development and in clinical trials, including two multinational HIV vaccine clinical trials; Imbokodo (in sub-Saharan African countries) in men and women and Mosaico (in North and South America and Europe) in MSM and transgender people. These vaccines are adenovirus vector–based HIV antigens. There are several other candidates that are under development.

Currently no HIV vaccines approved

Vaccine candidates in clinical trial

 Think ▸▸ Apply 18-7: The major hurdle is extensive genetic variation in HIV that is caused by a highly replicating and rapidly mutating virus.

HUMAN T-LYMPHOTROPIC OR T-CELL LEUKEMIA VIRUS

Human T-lymphotropic virus or human T-cell leukemia virus (HTLV) has two members, HTLV-I and HTLV-II, which cause disease in humans. HTLV-I causes two distinct diseases: ATLL (adult T cell leukemia and lymphoma) and HTLV-associated myelopathy (HAM, a neurologic disease). HTLV-II may also cause these diseases but has been primarily linked to variant hairy cell leukemia.

HTLV-I causes ATLL, myelopathy; HTLV-II causes variant hairy cell leukemia

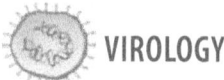 **VIROLOGY**

Similar to other retroviruses, HTLV has the usual retroviral *gag*, *pol*, and *env* genes but also encode two regulatory proteins: Tax and Rex. Tax is a transcriptional activator of HTLV LTR and is also required for transformation. However, Rex, similar to HIV-1 Rev, is a posttranscriptional activator that increases transport of structural protein mRNAs from nucleus to cytoplasm. In addition, other HTLV proteins are similar to HIV-1 proteins but differ in sequence and antigenicity. The HTLV envelope glycoproteins are gp46 and gp21, whereas the capsid protein is p24. Several cellular factors interact with HTLV LTR and activate transcription. Unlike HIV-1, the receptors for HTLV-I and HTLV-II have not been fully biochemically identified. However, the receptors are found in a wide variety of human and animal cells. In recent years, some receptors have been suggested, including glucose transporter (GLUT1), neuropilin (NRP-1), and heparin sulfate proteoglycans (HSPGs). HTLV-I and HTLV-II probably use the same receptor. HTLV is able to penetrate and infect a number of cell types; however, productive infection is observed in only a few cell types such as CD4 T-lymphocytes. The replication cycle of HTLV is very similar to that of HIV-1. Syncytia formation has been demonstrated in T-lymphocytes.

Similar retroviral genes with Tax and Rex proteins

HTLV-I and HTLV-II use the same receptor

Preferentially infects CD4 T-lymphocytes

TRANSMISSION

Transmission of HTLV occurs via blood to blood, including anal and vaginal sex and intravenous drug use. Mother-to-child transmission of HTLV has also been documented. Unlike HIV-1, HTLV is not transmitted through cell-free fluids but through cell-associated fluids.

✳ **Transmission via cell-associated fluids**

EPIDEMIOLOGY

HTLV is more prevalent in the Caribbean, Japan, and Hawaii, sub-Saharan Africa, and South America. In addition, the incidence of HTLV is increasing in Western Europe and the United States among intravenous drug users. In some of these endemic areas, the rate of HTLV infection is more than 20%. It is estimated that 5 to 10 million people are infected with HTLV worldwide.

PATHOGENESIS

ATLL is caused by HTLV-I infection of CD4 T-lymphocytes leading to malignant transformation. HTLV-encoded Tax protein that binds to HTLV LTR and increases transcription of HTLV genes is also responsible for enhancing the transcription of protooncogenes resulting in transformation (see later under "Transformation by animal and human oncoretroviruses" section). In addition, Tax increases the production of IL-2 (T-cell growth factor) and IL-2 receptor that cause uncontrolled growth of T cells resulting in transformation. The transformed cells typically do not produce HTLV progeny viruses. The other disease caused by HTLV is called HAM, or tropical spastic paraparesis (TSP), which is a demyelinating disease of the brain and spinal cord, especially the motor neurons. It is believed that the mechanisms of HAM/TSP are immune-mediated, including an autoimmune reaction-induced damage of the neurons as well as cytotoxic T-cell–induced killing of neurons. The virus becomes latent for a long period of time (approximately 20-30 years) or slowly replicates to transform cells without causing cytopathic effects. In terms of immunity, antibodies are elicited against gp46 and other HTLV proteins that neutralize the slowly replicating virus and prevent cell-mediated killing of HTLV-infected cells.

✳ **HTLV Tax increases the transcription of protooncogenes resulting in oncogenesis**

HLLV-associated HAM/TSP is immune-mediated

MANIFESTATIONS

HTLV-I causes ATLL, which is a highly malignant disease. There is a long period of latency (about 20-30 years) before the onset of ATLL. Only 1% to 2.5% of infected people progress to ATLL disease, and their survival is often in months. ATLL patients present with lymphadenopathy, hepatosplenomegaly, and skin and bone lesions. The malignant T cells have a flower-shaped nucleus and are

Long latency period of 20 to 30 years

pleomorphic. Fungal and viral opportunistic infections are commonly seen in ATLL patients, especially those treated with aggressive chemotherapy. In HAM/TSP patients, gait stiffness/spasticity, lower limb weakness, and low back pain are generally seen. The flower-shaped T cells can be found in the CSF. The CSF shows lymphocytic pleocytosis, and the protein level is elevated. In addition, hematologic malignancies, B-cell chronic lymphocytic leukemia, and immunosuppression are found in patients infected with HTLV-I. HTLV-II causes a T-cell variant hairy cell leukemia, which resembles hairy cell leukemia of B-cell origin.

1% to 2.5% of HTLV-infected patients progress to ATLL

CSF finding abnormal in HAM/TSP

DIAGNOSIS

HTLV infection is diagnosed by detection of antibodies against HTLV by ELISA; however, there is cross-reactivity with HTLV-I and HTLV-II antigens. PCR can specifically differentiate between HTLV-I and HTLV-II. ATLL is diagnosed by the presence of malignant T cells in the lesions. HAM/TSP is diagnosed by the presence of HTLV antibody in the CSF or HTLV nucleic acid in the CSF.

Diagnosis by EIA or PCR

TREATMENT

In some patients with HAM/TSP, a combination of antiretrovirals and interferon has shown benefit, and corticosteroids may relieve symptoms. ATLL is generally treated by anticancer chemotherapy.

PREVENTION

Screening for HTLV antibodies, using condoms, and not breastfeeding babies by HTLV-infected mothers can reduce the risk of HTLV transmission. Currently, there is no vaccine to prevent HTLV infection.

TRANSFORMATION BY ANIMAL AND HUMAN ONCORETROVIRUSES

Oncoretroviruses cause a variety of cancers in animals and humans, including leukemia, lymphoma, and sarcoma. Oncogenic retroviruses appear to transform cells to an oncogenic state by three distinct mechanisms: by acquiring a cellular oncogene (acute transforming animal retroviruses), by insertional mutagenesis (animal retrovirus), and by transforming cells by continual expression of viral regulatory Tax protein for human retrovirus, HTLV (see Chapter 7). The genomes of acute transforming oncoviruses have one feature common to nearly all of them: Some viral genes are replaced by host genes derived from their hosts that render them oncogenic (see later in the text). In every case, the signals required for reverse transcription and for transcription of the provirus, which are located near the ends of the RNA, are retained in the infecting virus. In the example shown in **Figure 18–6**, the *pol* gene and parts of both the viral *gag* and *env* genes are deleted, but other configurations are possible. Such oncoviruses are defective and replicate only in the presence of a helper virus that can supply the missing functions.

Defective transforming oncogenic animal viruses require helper virus

Some animal retroviruses carry host genes rendering them oncogenic

First, the defective acute transforming viruses (Figure 18–6) have acquired a cellular gene (thereafter called an **oncogene**), which, when expressed in the infected cell, results in loss of normal growth control. On infection, the transduced oncogene is expressed from the viral LTR promoter, resulting in a rapid and acute onset of malignant disease. Persistent transformation by oncogene transduction is possible only for retroviruses that are not cytocidal. More than 30 oncogenes have been identified in a variety of animal retroviruses, but no human retroviruses are known that transform by this mechanism.

Noncytocidal animal viruses carrying cellular oncogenes can produce persistent transformation

The second mechanism is called **insertional mutagenesis.** Integration of an animal retrovirus in the vicinity of particular cellular genes can cause inappropriate expression of the gene, resulting

Typical retrovirus

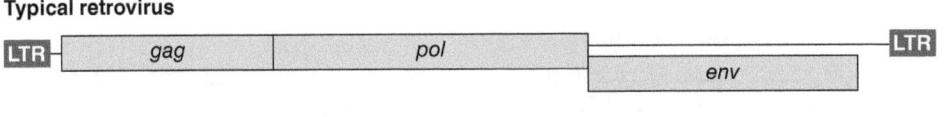

Defective acute transforming retrovirus

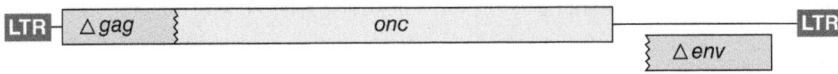

FIGURE 18–6. Comparison of a typical retrovirus with a defective acute transforming retrovirus. Onc, cellular oncogene.

Integration adjacent to cellular protooncogenes can activate them in animal retroviruses

in uncontrolled cell growth. These cellular genes are called **protooncogenes,** and insertional activation by the virus is apparently due to the close proximity of the integrated viral promoter or enhancer to the gene. Cancers that are caused by this mechanism have very long latent periods, because integration is random and only rarely occurs near a cellular protooncogene in case of animal retrovirus infection.

The causative agent of ATLL, HTLV-I, exemplifies the third mechanism. In this case, the integrated provirus in the leukemic cells from any one patient is found at a unique location on a particular chromosome. Thus, the tumors are probably monoclonal. The cancer is not the result of insertional activation, however, because the chromosomal location of the provirus is never the same in any two patients. Instead, transformation results from the continual expression of the viral *tax* gene (the HTLV-I homolog of the HIV *tat* gene; Table 18–2). Apparently, the Tax protein not only can transactivate viral transcription in the same manner as HIV Tat, but Tax can also **transactivate** the expression of one or more cellular genes (possibly protooncogenes), resulting in malignant transformation.

✳ HTLV-1 transforms by production of Tax, which activates cellular transforming genes

KEY CONCLUSIONS

- Two types of human retroviruses, oncoretroviruses (HTLV) that do not kill but transform cells and can cause cancer, whereas lentiviruses (HIV) that infect, persist, and kill CD4 T-cells and cause immune deficiency.

- Retrovirus such as HIV has two copies of positive-sense RNA genome bound to nucleocapsid protein and packaged in an icosahedral capsid (p24) and a matrix protein surrounded by lipid bilayer membrane containing gp120 and gp41. Three enzymes are also packaged in the virus particles, protease, reverse transcriptase, and integrase.

- All retroviruses have *gag* (matrix, capsid, nucleocapsid), *pol* (protease, reverse transcriptase, integrase), and *env* (SU, TM) genes; however, HTLV has two additional regulatory genes, *tax* and *rex*, and HIV has two regulatory, *tat* and *rev*, and four accessory genes, *vif, vpr, vpu,* and *nef*.

- HIV enters host cells through gp120 binding to CD4 receptor and CXCR4 or CCR5 coreceptor and gp41 facilitating the fusion of viral envelope to host cell membrane. Based on HIV gp120 (V3 loop) specificity with CCR5 or CXCR4, HIV can be either R5 when it binds to CCR5 (expressed mainly on monocytes/macrophages, dendritic cells, and mucosal CD4 T-cells) or X4 when it binds to CXCR4 (expressed mainly on T cells).

- After uncoating in the cytoplasm, RT converts RNA into ds DNA which then moves in the nucleus and integrates into the host chromosome by IN enzyme. Host RNA polymerase transcribes viral DNA into mRNAs that are translated into various viral proteins. Virus assembles in the cytoplasm and buds out of plasma membranes containing gp120 and gp41. PR matures the virions by processing Gag and Pol polyproteins.

- Tat increases HIV transcription, Rev exports structural proteins mRNAs from nucleus to cytoplasm, Vif increases virus infectivity, Vpr arrests cell cycle and promotes viral replication in resting cells, Vpu helps in virus release, and Nef downregulates CD4 and MHC 1. HIV-2 encodes Vpx instead of Vpu.

- HIV can be transmitted mainly through anal or vaginal sex, mother-to-child, and intravenous drug use but also through percutaneous needle-stick and exposure of infected bodily fluids and blood to eyes, nose, mouth, broken skin, or other mucous areas.

- More than 38 million people are living with HIV infection worldwide, 67% in sub-Saharan Africa. New infections and HIV-related deaths have decreased due to accessibility of ART to more than 68% of the infected people worldwide.

- In the United States, 1.2 million people are living with HIV (66% MSM), new infections have slightly declined, and death rates have significantly declined due to ART.

- While HIV can be transmitted from mother to child at a rate of 30%, use of ART during pregnancy has reduced the rate to less than 1%.

- HIV infection can be characterized into three stages—acute phase, clinical latency or chronic phase, and AIDS phase with opportunistic infections.

- During the first 2 to 4 weeks of infection, there is extensive HIV replication in genital mucosal Langerhans cells, macrophages, and CD4 T-cells and the virus migrates to GALT and replicates and depletes mucosal memory CD4 T-cells. It disseminates to other lymphoid tissues, establishes reservoirs, and causes a high viremia that could be detected in blood in 1 to 4 weeks. Many infected patients experience flu or mononucleosis-like illness, also referred as acute retroviral syndrome.

- The innate and adaptive immunity control HIV replication. DCs make cytokines such as IL-12. CD8 T-cells kill HIV-infected cells. CD4 T-cells make cytokines such as IFN-γ and TNF-α. B cells secrete antibodies. The concerted effort of the immune system brings the viremia to a set point. HIV then enters in clinical latency or chronic phase, which is asymptomatic for 8 to 10 years in a majority of patients with a low level of HIV production.

- Due to a constant fight between the rapidly mutating HIV and the deteriorating immune system damaged by HIV proteins, the impaired immune system is unable to keep up with the changing pace of the virus, resulting in unrestricted viral replication, depletion of CD4 T-cells and causing immune deficiency, AIDS, and opportunistic infections, if untreated.

- During the AIDS phase, patients experience symptoms such as recurring fever, night sweats, rapid weight loss, diarrhea, sores in mouth or genitals, thrush, pneumonia, and some neurological disorders. There is an extensive array of viral, bacterial, fungal, and parasitic opportunistic infections and malignancies that may result in death, if untreated.

- HIV diagnosis is done by a fourth-generation test that detects both HIV antigen and antibody in 2 to 6 weeks after infection. PCR-based nucleic acid test can detect HIV RNA in 1 to 4 weeks after infection.

- Six classes of ART agents have been developed targeting reverse transcriptase (NRTI and NNRTI agents), IN, PR, CCR5, and gp41.

- Current HHS recommendation for HIV treatment, ART, is to include three drugs from two different classes: two NRTIs plus one INSTI or one NNRTI or one PI with a PK enhancer. The goal of ART is to bring viral load down to undetectable levels in less than 6 months, including elevation of CD4 T-cell counts and prevention of AIDS and opportunistic infections. ART is recommended for all HIV-infected individuals regardless of CD4 T cell counts and should be taken indefinitely.

- Long-term use of ART causes IRIS and other complications such as lipid deposition, insulin resistance, cardiovascular problems, and bone disorders.

- HTLV-1 transforms cells by its Tax regulatory protein, which increases the transcription of protooncogenes. HLTV-1 causes ATLL in 20 to 30 years in 1% to 2.5% of infected people. It is seen in intravenous drug users, mainly in the Caribbean and Japan, but cases are increasing in America and Europe.

CASE STUDY
A Month-Long Multisystem Illness

A 25-year-old man comes to a clinic accompanied by his girlfriend, complaining of increased dyspnea, fevers, and chills. He also complains of having watery diarrhea and has lost weight over the last month. His chest X-radiograph reveals a bilateral reticular infiltrate. Further laboratory testing reveals that he is positive for HIV-1 antigen/antibody; his CD4 count is 200/mm³ and viral load is more than 200,000 copies/mL. He was born in the United States and lives in Ohio. He was placed on ART. His viral load and CD4 counts will be followed every 3 to 6 months.

QUESTIONS

1. Which of the following is true of HIV-1 viral load/CD4 lymphocyte count?
   A. HIV-1 viral load is the better indicator of the risk of opportunistic infections.
   B. The CD4 count assesses lymphocyte quantitation and functions.
   C. Recovery of the CD4 count in response to ART is a better indicator of clinical outcome than viral load results.
   D. Decrease in viral load in response to antiviral therapy is generally not associated with increase in CD4 lymphocyte counts in most patients.

2. What is the most likely cause of pulmonary infection in this patient?
   A. Cytomegalovirus
   B. Coccidioidomycosis
   C. Herpes simplex
   D. *Mycobacterium tuberculosis*
   E. *Pneumocystis jirovecii*

3. Which one of the following statements about HIV-1/AIDS is true?
   A. Presence of HIV-1 antibodies in this patient indicates that the infection will be cleared.
   B. Antibodies to HIV-1 generated in infected patients are unable to eliminate the infection.
   C. HIV-1 arose as an endogenous virus because HIV-1 DNA is found in normal cells.
   D. If treatment reduces the plasma viral load to undetectable, the patient is cured.

4. Since the patient's girlfriend is tested for HIV infection, which of the following is true in her case?
   A. If she is negative for HIV-1 antibody, there is no need to test her again.
   B. The risk of HIV-1 transmission from male to female is remote, and she should not be concerned.
   C. If she is negative now, she should be tested for HIV-1 antigen/antibody in 3 months and if negative, then she is not infected.
   D. Circumcision of her male partner would reduce her risk of HIV-1 transmission by 50-fold.

ANSWERS

1. (C)
2. (E)
3. (B)
4. (C)

chapter 19

Papilloma and Polyoma Viruses

Human Papilloma Viruses (HPV) • Human Polyomaviruses (JC Virus and BK Virus)

Historically, the papillomaviruses and polyomaviruses have been discussed together in microbiology textbooks, lumped under the category of papovaviruses. Papovaviruses are now split into two separate families: Papillomaviridae and Polyomaviridae. The unique characteristics that distinguish them from each other are shown in **Table 19–1.**

● PAPILLOMAVIRUSES

OVERVIEW

Human papillomaviruses (HPVs) are the most common sexually transmitted infections in the United States. HPVs are naked capsid, icosahedral, double-stranded circular DNA viruses that replicate in the nucleus of the infected cell by using host RNA polymerase for transcription and host DNA polymerase for genome replication. More than 100 genotypes of HPVs have been identified in human specimens. The genotypes are antigenically different, and groups of genotypes are associated with specific lesions, and low-risk or high-risk genotypes for cancers. HPVs are transmitted through skin-to-skin contact and through vaginal, anal, or oral sex. HPVs have been identified in common hand warts, plantar warts, flat cutaneous warts of other skin areas (HPV 1-4, 7, 10); in juvenile laryngeal papillomas (HPV 6, 11); and in a variety of genital hyperplastic epithelial lesions, including cervical, vulvar, and penile warts and papillomas (HPV 6, 11, 16, 18). In addition, they are associated with premalignant cervical intraepithelial neoplasia (CIN) and malignant disease, cervical cancer (HPV 16, 18). Lesions comparable to those occurring in the cervix are now recognized in the anus, especially among men who have sex with men (MSM) and those who are infected by HIV. HPV 6 and 11 (low risk) are the most common genotypes associated with genital infections and cause benign condylomas, condylomata acuminata, HPV 16 and 18 are considered the high-risk genotypes because of their potential to cause malignant cancers such as cervical cancer in women and oropharyngeal cancer mainly in men. While a majority of HPV-associated infections are benign and cleared by the immune system over time, some progress to malignancies. HPV can be detected on regular pap smear test, which is a screening test for cervical cancer recommended in vaccinated and unvaccinated women. A safe and effective recombinant protein vaccine, Gardasil-9 (HPV types 6, 11, 16, 18, 31, 33, 45, 52, and 58) is used in the United States recommended for routine immunization in ages 11 to 12 years for girls and boys, but can be given until age 26 years and in some high-risk people up to age 45 years. Since the introduction of the HPV vaccine, HPV-associated cancers have dropped in the United States.

TABLE 19–1	Characteristics of Papilloma and Polyoma Viruses				
VIRUS SIZE	**HUMAN SUBTYPES**	**TRANSMISSION**	**DISEASE**	**TREATMENT**	**PREVENTION**
Papillomavirus 55 nm	HPV-1-4, 7, 10	Close skin-to-skin contact, occupational exposure, public shower/ swimming pool	Skin warts Common warts Plantar warts Flat cutaneous warts Meat/fish handler warts	Topical cytotoxins or surgical removal	
Papillomavirus 55 nm	HPV-6, 11	Close contact, sexual contact	Oral, laryngeal papillomatosis Genital warts (condylomata accuminata)	Treatment of laryngeal lesions is complex, varied	HPV vaccine
Papillomavirus 55 nm	HPV-16, 18 31, 33, 45, 52, and 58	Sexual (anal, vaginal, oral)	Cervical, oropharyngeal, other neoplasias	May be removed by electrocautery	HPV vaccine
Polyomavirus 45 nm	BKV	Respiratory, oral, contaminated food or water (?)	Hemorrhagic cystitis in transplant recipients; postrenal transplantation nephropathy	Cidofovir maybe used, but is not proven	
Polyomavirus 45 nm	JCV	Respiratory/oral contaminated food or water (?)	Progressive multifocal leukoencephalopathy (PML)	Reduce immune suppression	

BKV, BK virus; HPV, human papillomavirus; JCV, JC virus.

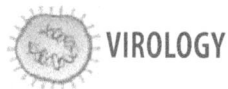 VIROLOGY

Papillomaviruses are small, naked capsid, icosahedral, double-stranded, circular DNA viruses of 55 nm in diameter (**Figure 19–1**). The icosahedral capsid comprises of two capsid (structural) proteins, L1 (major capsid protein) and L2 (minor capsid protein). The 8 kb, circular, double-stranded DNA genome of human papillomavirus (HPV) encodes seven or eight early genes (E1-E8) and two late structural capsid genes (L1 and L2). The early genes are required for regulation of viral replication and transformation. Two of the early genes such as E1 is involved in viral DNA replication and E2 in the regulation of viral transcription and DNA replication. The other two early genes, including E6 and E7 play important roles in transformation and oncogenesis by interacting with tumor suppressor genes. The virus does not encode any RNA or DNA polymerases and, therefore, is dependent on host cell transcription (host RNA polymerase) and replication machinery (host DNA polymerase). L1, the major capsid protein, is involved in binding to the

✳ Naked capsid, icosahedral, double-stranded, circular DNA viruses

L1 major capsid protein interacts with receptor on host cells

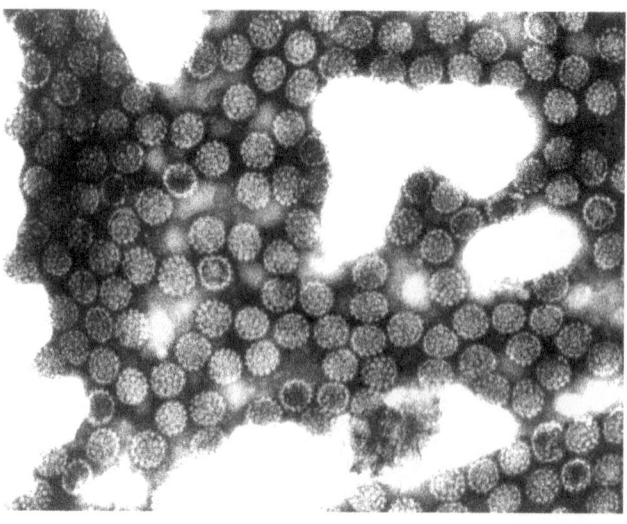

FIGURE 19–1. Electron micrograph of human papillomavirus (HPV) particles isolated from a plantar wart (×300,000). (Reproduced with permission from Connor DH, Chandler FW, Schwartz DQ, et al: *Pathology of Infectious Diseases*. Stamford CT: Appleton & Lange; 1997.)

receptor on host cells. L1 is also a highly immunogenic protein and contains epitopes that induce neutralizing antibodies, and assembles into virus-like particles (VLPs) and is, therefore, the antigen for HPV vaccine. L2, the minor capsid, may transport viral DNA to nucleus. Based on DNA homology, there are over 100 genotypes of HPVs. Papillomaviruses cause epidermal papillomas and warts in a wide range of higher vertebrates. Different members of the group are generally species specific. For example, bovine papillomaviruses and HPVs infect only the hosts reflected in their names. In some cases, lesions caused by these agents can become malignant, and the role of these agents as causes of certain human cancers is increasingly recognized. While papillomaviruses were difficult to grow in tissue culture and many virologic information were derived from molecular and gene expression studies, several cell lines–based cultures, including keratinocyte cell line and new differentiating skin system, have been developed that are being used to study the biology of HPV.

The genomes of many of the papillomaviruses have now been cloned and compared by restriction endonuclease and DNA homology procedures. These studies have shown a wide genomic diversity among papillomaviruses that infect different species and also among those that infect humans. This has led to the allocation of numbers for the different genotypes important in human diseases.

HPV targets stratified squamous epithelium through the damaged area of the epithelium and infects the basal cells. The replication cycle of HPV was reproduced in cultured cells by using a raft culture system made up of stratified squamous epithelial cells. Moreover, in infected human tissue, infectious particles are found. HPV infects the basal layer of squamous epithelium by the initial interaction of L1 major capsid protein probably to heparin sulfate proteoglycan, α-6 β-4 integrin, or other receptors on the basal membrane and then transfer to the receptor expressed on keratinocytes moving on the basal membrane in wound healing process of the damaged epithelium. After the virus is internalized by viropexis and uncoated, the viral DNA is transported to the nucleus probably aided by L2 minor capsid protein. Host RNA polymerase transcribes early (E) genes followed by early protein synthesis. Some of the early genes, E1 and E2, are synthesized that regulate viral transcription and initial replication. Transcription factor, E2, regulates the expression of E6 and E7 that are involved in the transformation that causes an increase in cell division. E6 binds to p53 (tumor suppressor) and E7 p105RB (retinoblastoma) proteins and abrogate cell cycle regulation. The dividing cells carry viral genome as extrachromosomal DNA (episomal DNA) allowing HPV genome to persist in these cells. As the infected cells differentiate to early terminal stages, other viral early genes, in addition to E1 and E2, are expressed which further regulate viral transcription and replication. Viral DNA synthesis occurs at two levels directed by host cell DNA polymerase: (1) in the lower portion of the epidermis to maintain a stable multicopy viral DNA for latent infection, and (2) in the more differentiated epithelial cells to synthesize genomic DNA (known as vegetative DNA replication) to be packaged in daughter virions. In some cases, papillomavirus DNA can integrate into the host chromosomes. The infected cells further differentiate to a terminal stage (keratinocytes), wherein late gene expression synthesis of late (L) capsid structural proteins and vegetative DNA synthesis take place. At this stage, there is a burst of viral DNA synthesis followed by virus assembly in the nucleus and virus release by cell lysis.

* L1 elicits neutralizing antibodies and is the antigen for HPV vaccine

Devoid of viral RNA or DNA polymerase uses host RNA and DNA polymerase

Genomic diversity important in humans

* High-risk HPV-associated cancers with HPV genotypes

HPV infects and initially replicates in basal epidermis

* E6 and E7 early proteins transform cells by abrogating cell cycle control

* Transcription by host RNA polymerase, genome replication by DNA polymerase

Viral DNA replication, assembly in keratinocytes

Latent viral DNA maintained in basal layer of epithelium

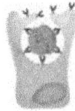 **How does HPV infect basal squamous epithelium when it transmitted through skin-to-skin contact?**

 PAPILLOMAVIRUS DISEASE

EPIDEMIOLOGY

Nearly 80 million Americans are infected with some type of HPV, including common and genital warts, and more than 80% of the people will have HPV at some point in their lives. HPV is the most common sexually transmitted infection in the United States. In 2018, there were 43 million people with genital HPV infections and 13 million new infections occurred in the United States mostly among people in late teens and early 20s. About 340,000 to 360,000 genital warts in women and men were reported every year in the United States. In addition,

* Most common sexually transmitted infection in the United States

Think ►► **Apply 19-1:** After skin-to-skin contact, HPV may reach the basal squamous epithelium probably through some damage or abrasions.

80 million have HPV, 43 million genital HPV, 14 million annual infections

✳ Major cause of cervical cancers

✳ About 12,000 cases, 4000 deaths every year

✳ Globally 570,000 cases and 311,000 deaths

✳ About 16,200 cases in men, 3500 in women of HPV-associated oropharyngeal cancer in the United States

more than 31,000 women and men are diagnosed with cancer caused by HPV, including 12,000 cases and 4000 deaths due to cervical cancer in women. Furthermore, 16,200 new HPV-associated oropharyngeal cancer cases in men and 3500 in women are diagnosed every year in the United States. The rates of cervical cancers are higher in black women than white woman as well as in Hispanics than non-Hispanics. On the contrary, the rates of oropharyngeal cancer are higher in whites than blacks and in non-Hispanics than Hispanics. Many types of cancers are caused by HPV including 70% of vulvar and vaginal cancer, 60% of penile cancer, 90% of anal and cervical cancers, and 70% of oropharyngeal cancer. It is believed that tobacco and alcohol also play a role in oropharyngeal cancers. Globally, an estimated 570,000 new cases and 311,000 deaths due to cervical cancer occurred in 2018, and nearly 90% of these cases/deaths are in developing countries, which account for 7.5% of all female cancer deaths.

HPV GENOTYPES, RISK FACTORS, AND DISEASES

HPV genotypes are important in disease spectrum and severity. The genotypes causing genital lesions are different from those causing cutaneous, nongenital warts. Cutaneous, nongenital warts usually occur in children and young adults; presumably, immunity to the HPV genotypes causing these lesions develops and provides subsequent protection. Common warts that grow generally on hands are caused by HPV types 1 and 2; plantar warts that grow on soles of feet are caused by types 1, 2, and 4; flat cutaneous warts by types 3 and 10; meat and fish handlers are prone to HPV type 7. Over 40 HPV genotypes have been identified in genital lesions of humans, and there are many apparently silent infections with these viruses. Cross-immunity does not occur, and sequential infection with multiple genotypes does take place. A single sexual exposure to an infected person may transmit the infection 60% of the time; usually the infected person is asymptomatic. Having multiple sex partners is the major risk factor for acquiring HPV infection. From 20% to 60% of adult women in the United States are infected with one or another of the genotypes. In addition, more than 50% of sexually active people become infected with HPV at least once in their lifetime. HPV types 6 and 11 are most commonly transmitted HPV genital infection mainly associated (about 90%) with benign genital warts (condylomata acuminata) in males and females and with some cellular dysplasias of the cervical epithelium, but these lesions rarely become malignant. These genotypes are considered **low-risk**. HPV types 6 and 11 have been associated with nasal, oral, conjunctival, and laryngeal warts. They can be perinatally transmitted from mother to child and cause infantile laryngeal papillomas. HPV types 16, 18, 31, 33, 45, 52, and 58 may cause lesions of the vulva, cervix, and penis and may become malignant. These genotypes are considered **high risks**. HPV types 16 and 18 are also associated with oropharyngeal cancer. Several other types have also been implicated such as 35, 39, 56, 59, 66, and 68 in dysplasia and carcinoma. Clinically, these HPV genotypes are considered high risk for the development of cervical cancer and its precursor lesion, cervical intraepithelial neoplasia (CIN). Infections with these viral types, especially types 16 and 18, may progress to malignancy. In addition, HPV-16 is probably the most carcinogenic genotype because of its association with 60% of cervical cancers, whereas HPV-18 association is about 10% to 15%. Furthermore, 80% of the HPV-associated cancers are caused by HPV-16 and 18 and 12% by HPV-31, 33, 45, 52, and 58, and these genotypes are part of Gardasil 9-valent vaccine. Viral genomes of at least one of these genotypes are found in the majority—but not all—of markedly dysplastic uterine cervical cells, in carcinoma *in situ*, and in cells of frankly malignant lesions.

✳ HPV types 6 and 11 common; mainly benign, rarely lead to malignancy

✳ Types 16, 18, 31, 33, 45, 52, and 58 are associated with dysplasia and malignancy

HPV-associated oropharyngeal cancer is on the rise, especially in men. While 7% of people have oral HPV, only 1% have HPV-16 associated with oropharyngeal cancer in the United States. The high risk (HPV-16) is associated with cancers of head and neck and low risk (HPV 6, 11) with mouth or oral warts.

Type 16 60% and type 18 10% to 15% cervical cancers and CIN

Type 16 associated with head and neck (oropharyngeal) carcinoma

 Why are HPV 16 and 18 more oncogenic than HPV 6 and 11?

HPV infection is now considered to be a contributory cause of most carcinomas of the cervix. HPV infection of the anus is a clinical problem in men having sex with men (MSM), especially those with human immunodeficiency virus (HIV), and it is related to the subsequent development of anal neoplasia in these individuals.

TRANSMISSION

HPV causing common warts are transmitted through skin-to-skin contact and spreads through damaged, broken skin, fingernail biting, etc. People can spread the virus to other parts of their body. The virus can also be transmitted by touching anything that was touched by a person with wart, including public showers, swimming pools, occupational tools, recreational and sports tools. In addition, meat and fish handlers are prone to hand warts. HPV is transmitted sexually during intimate sexual contact through vaginal and/or anal sex. It can also be transmitted through oral sex or other sex play. HPV is the most common sexually transmitted infection in the United States. HPV can be transmitted perinatally from mother to child causing recurrent respiratory papillomatosis (RRP) in the baby.

Common hard warts transmitted through skin-to-skin contact, public showers, swimming pools, occupational tools

Sexual transmission through anal and/or vaginal sex; oral sex also transmits HPV

PATHOGENESIS

Papillomaviruses have a predilection for infection at the junction of squamous and columnar epithelium (eg, in the cervix and anus). Papillomaviruses were the first DNA viruses linked to malignant changes. In the mid-1930s, Shope demonstrated that benign rabbit papillomas were due to filterable agents (older terminology for viruses) and could advance to become malignant squamous cell carcinomas. External cofactors, such as coal tar, could hasten this process. However, work on the biology and mechanism by which these agents foster malignant transformation has been impeded by the inability to cultivate papillomaviruses *in vitro*. Molecular probes to detect viral products *in vivo* indicate that replication and assembly of these viruses take place only in the differentiating layers of squamous epithelia, a situation that has not been reproduced *in vitro*.

Replication in squamous epithelium

The first evidence that HPVs could be associated with human malignant disease came from observations on epidermodysplasia verruciformis. This disease has a genetic basis that results in unusual susceptibility to HPV types 5 and 8, which produce multiple flat warts. About one-third of affected patients develop squamous cell carcinoma from these lesions.

HPV 16 and 18 are associated with most of the cervical cancers in women. However, the mechanism of oncogenicity of HPV is less clear. Cells infected with genomes of several papillomaviruses can transform cells and produce tumors when injected into nude (T lymphocyte–deficient) mice. The viral genome exists as multiple copies of a circular episome within the nucleus of transformed cells but is not integrated into the cellular genome. This also appears to be the case with benign human lesions. In malignant tumors, part of the viral genome may be integrated into the cellular genome, but integration is not site-specific. Both the integrated viral genome and the extrachromosomal form carry their own transforming genes. Host cells normally produce a protein that inhibits expression of papillomavirus transforming genes, but this can be inactivated by products of the virus and possibly by other infecting viruses, thus allowing malignant transformation to occur. HPV early gene products, E6 and E7, have been implicated in oncogenicity. E6 accelerates the degradation of p53, a tumor suppressor protein, and reduces its stability. E7 interacts with pRB, retinoblastoma protein, to abrogate cell cycle regulation. The inhibition of p53 and pRB functions results in cell transformation by E6 and E7, causing tumors. Another HPV gene product, E5, has been found to function in benign papillomas. HPV DNA is found in more than 95% of cervical carcinoma specimens when tested by polymerase chain reaction (PCR). The discovery that HPV causes most cervical cancers earned the 2008 Nobel Prize in Medicine for the German researcher, Harald zur Hausen.

✳ Viral genomes carry their own transforming genes, E6 and E7

✳ E6 degrades p53 and E7 interacts with pRB to abrogate cell cycle causing transformation

✳ HPV is the major cause of cervical cancer

IMMUNITY

Immunity is generally limited due to localized infection in basal epithelial cells that are probably shielded by circulating immune cells and the nonlytic nature of virus replication. Innate immunity controls infection to some extent but down regulated by early protein of HPV. In the later stages of infection, immune cells can detect viral proteins when the virus replication moves to suprabasal keratinocytes, leading to a strong localized cell-mediated immunity and, in most cases, clearance of viral infection. Antibody response against L1 major capsid protein is

Effective localized cell-mediated immunity eliminates infection, depressed immunity allows persistence

 Think ►► Apply 19-2: **E6 and E7 are the major oncogenic proteins of HPV. The probability could be that E6 and E7 of high risk (HPV 16 and 18) have a higher affinity for pRb and p53 leading to abrogation of cell cycle than E6 and E7 of low risk (HPV 6 and 11).**

Antibody response generated during infection

detected in infection. In regressing warts, infiltrating T lymphocytes and macrophages are seen. However, in some people, the virus is not cleared and persists, which increases the risk of cancer.

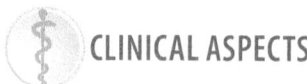

CLINICAL ASPECTS

MANIFESTATIONS

Oral or laryngeal papillomatosis in infants infected during delivery

Cutaneous warts develop at the site of inoculation within 1 to 3 months and can vary from flat to deep plantar growths (**Figure 19–2**A-C). Common warts are caused by HPV-1, 2; plantar warts on soles of feet are caused by types 1, 2, and 4; flat cutaneous warts by types 3 and 10; and meat and fish handlers are infected with HPV type 7. Although they can persist for years, they ultimately spontaneously regress. Respiratory papillomatosis due most often to types 6 and 11 occurs as intraoral or laryngeal lesions. These tend to occur in infants as a result of natal exposure or in adults. Treatment is varied and complex.

Anal carcinoma due to HPV is on rise

Oropharyngeal cancer four times common in men than women

External genital HPV infection occurs as exophytic genital warts (condylomata acuminata) caused most often by types 6 or 11 HPV (**Figures 19–2D** and **19–3**). They are often found on the head or shaft of the penis, at the vaginal opening, or perianal 4 to 6 weeks after exposure. Lesions may increase in size to cauliflower-like appearance during pregnancy or immunosuppression. Genital HPV infection is most often benign, and many lesions reverse spontaneously. However, they may become dysplastic and proceed through a continuum of CIN, CIN 1 (mild dysplasia), CIN 2 (moderate dysplasia) to CIN 3 (severe dysplasia), and/or carcinoma (**Figure 19–4**). Type 16, 18, and other higher genotypes are associated with genital infections and the most common HPV in the malignant lesions is type 16, although this genotype, as well as the others, is most pertinent to cause lesions that regress spontaneously. Higher-grade malignancy is most pertinent to occur in the cervix, but the rate of anal carcinoma related to HPV appears to be increasing, especially in AIDS patients. In oral HPV that is mainly HPV 6 and 11, the oropharyngeal cancer of head and neck (in the back of the throat and base of tongue and tonsils) is caused by HPV 16, which is four times more common in men than women, and the initial symptoms in some people may include persistent sore throat, ear pain, hoarseness, enlarged lymph nodes, pain when swallowing, and unexplained weight loss. In most instances these symptoms may go, whereas in some cases it may lead to malignancy. Several factors such as tobacco chewing, smoking, and alcohol may increase the risk of HPV-associated oropharyngeal cancer.

FIGURE 19–2. **Warts. A.** Common warts on fingers. **B.** Flat warts on the face. **C.** Plantar warts on the feet. **D.** Perianal condylomata acuminata. (Reproduced with permission from Willey JM: *Prescott, Harley, & Klein's Microbiology*, 7th ed. New York, NY: McGraw Hill; 2008.)

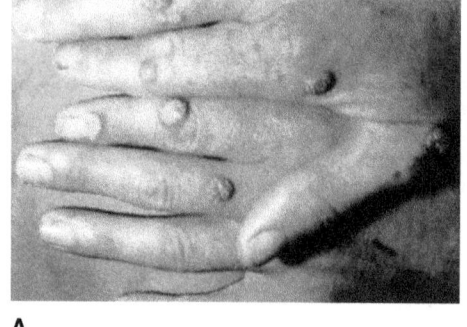

A

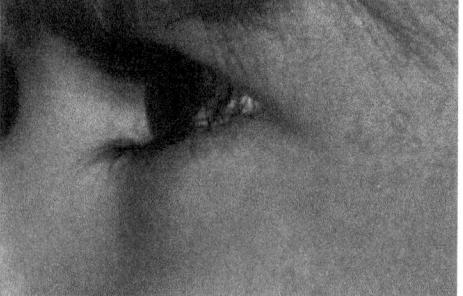

B

C

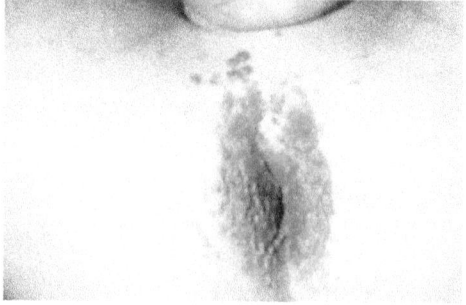

D

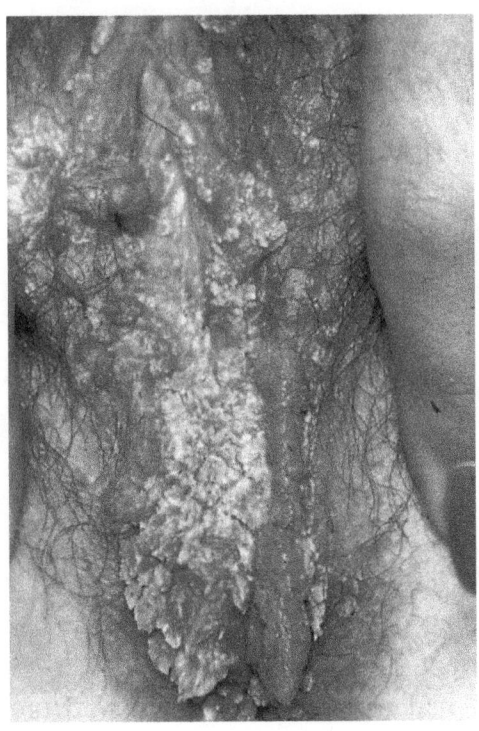

FIGURE 19-3. Extensive condylomata of vulva caused by HPV-6. (Reproduced with permission from Connor DH, Chandler FW, Schwartz DQ, et al: *Pathology of Infectious Diseases.* Stamford CT: Appleton & Lange; 1997.)

DIAGNOSIS

HPV is not routinely propagated in tissue culture, and antibody tests are rarely used, since results remain positive after the first HPV genotype infection. Papillomavirus infection leads to perinuclear cytoplasmic vacuolization and nuclear enlargement, referred to as "koilocytosis," in epithelial cells of the cervix or vagina. These changes can be seen in a routine Papanicolaou (Pap) smear (**Figure 19-5**). The use of immunoassays to detect viral antigen and *in situ* nucleic acid hybridization or PCR to detect specific viral DNA in cervical swabs or tissue is more sensitive (**Figure 19-6**) than Pap smear. Four diagnostic tests have been approved by the FDA in the United States, including HC II High-Risk test (Qiagen), HC II Low-Risk HPV test (Qiagen), Cervista HPV 16/18 test, and Cervista HPV High-Risk test (Hologics). Detection of an abnormal cytology due to HPV should prompt colposcopy to assist in following up or treating patients with abnormal lesions.

❋ Koilocytosis can be seen in cytologic specimens

Molecular methods to detect specific genotypes in biopsies of cervical swabs are available

TREATMENT

Currently, there is no antiviral against HPV; however, HPV-caused warts or growth is usually treated either by cytotoxic or surgical means. Among the topical cytotoxins are podophyllin, podophyllotoxin, 5-fluorouracil, and trichloroacetic acid. Systemic and local interferon-alpha; may provide some benefit. Warts can also be removed by laser or freezing with liquid nitrogen. Loop electrosurgical excision procedure (LEEP) can be used to remove abnormal cells with an

Recurrences are common after topical treatment

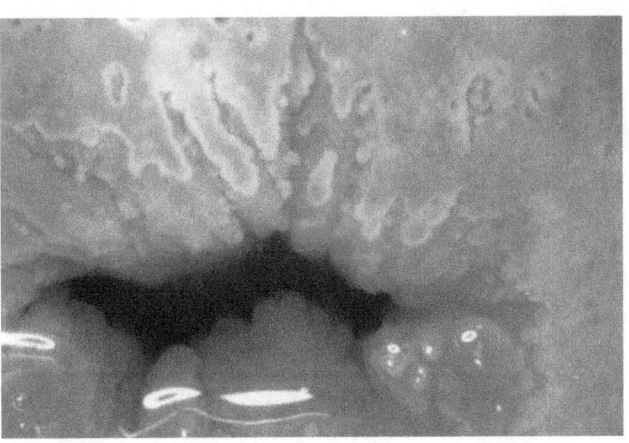

FIGURE 19-4. Colposcopic photograph of cervical transformation zone with diffusely scattered acetowhite staining, characteristic of HPV infection. (Reproduced with permission from Connor DH, Chandler FW, Schwartz DQ, et al: *Pathology of Infectious Diseases.* Stamford CT: Appleton & Lange; 1997.)

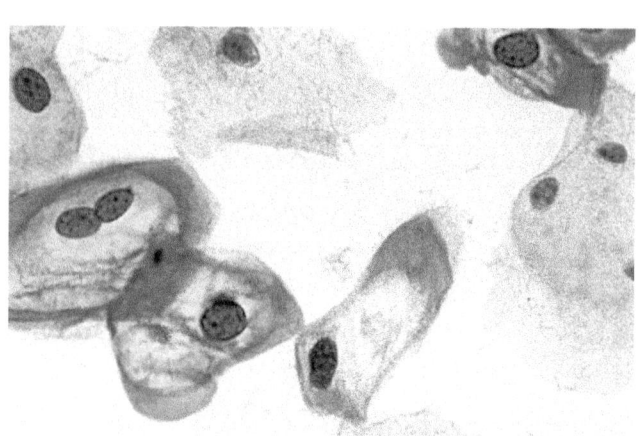

FIGURE 19–5. **Abnormal Pap smear.** The pink and blue objects are squamous epithelial cells; abnormalities include the doubling of the nuclei and a clear area around them. Most abnormal smears in young women are due to human papillomavirus (HPV) infection; when persistent, it is considered an important factor in the development of cancer of the cervix.

Removal of warts by cryosurgery or other methods

electric current. Another procedure called conization, also known as cone biopsy, removes abnormal cells. Recurrences are common after cessation of treatment because of the survival of virus or viral DNA in the basal layers of the epithelium. Cervical and anal lesions may be treated with electrocautery, but carcinoma may require chemotherapy, radiation therapy, or radical surgery.

 Why have HPV vaccines have added more HPV genotypes over time?

PREVENTION

Condom usage encouraged to prevent transmission

Three recombinant VLP vaccines comprising HPV viral major capsid L1 protein including, Cervarix bivalent (HPV types 16 and 18), Gardasil quadrivalent vaccine (HPV types 6, 11, 16, and 18), and Gardasil 9-valent vaccine (HPV types 6, 11, 16, 18, 31, 33, 45, 52, and 58) are licensed in the United States. These vaccines are subunit recombinant protein vaccines that are noninfectious and elicit neutralizing antibodies that provide protection against commonly prevalent HPV that cause cervical, anal, genital, and oropharyngeal cancers. However, Gardasil quadrivalent vaccine was discontinued in 2017 in the United States. Since late 2016, Gardasil 9-valent is the only vaccine used in the United States. HPV vaccine is recommended for routine vaccination at ages 11 to

FIGURE 19–6. Human papillomavirus (HPV) type 16 DNA demonstrated in a cervical smear by *in situ* hybridization. The dark dots represent detection of HPV DNA sequences by the DNA probe.

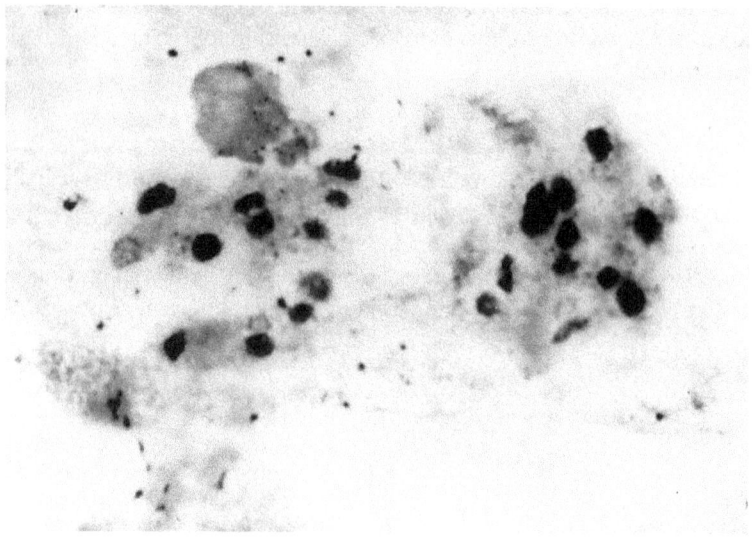

 Think ►► Apply 19-3: **Different HPV genotypes are associated with different lesions and cancers. The vaccine started with the high-risk genotypes for cancer (types 16 and 18) and then additional genotypes were based on epidemiological evidence of their prevalence with HPV-associated diseases. The current vaccine Gardasil-9 has types 6, 11, 16, 18, 31, 33, 45, 52, and 58.**

12 for both girls and boys (can be started at age 9 years), given in two doses (IM injection) 6 to 12 months apart. For children 15 years of age or above, three doses over a 6-month period should be given. HPV vaccine is also recommended for everyone through 26 years, if not fully vaccinated previously. Vaccination is not recommended for everyone above 26 years; however, high-risk adults for HPV infection between ages 27 and 45 years may take the vaccine in consultation with their healthcare provider. HPV vaccine is not recommended during pregnancy. HPV vaccines are safe, effective, and provide long-term protection against cancer-causing HPVs. Vaccinated females should continue Pap smear and HPV screening, because other HPV genotypes than those included in the vaccine can cause cervical cancer. Pap smear test for cervical cancer screening is recommended in women aged 21 to 65 years in the United States. People with a history of abnormal Pap or HPV infection should receive the Gardasil-9 vaccine because it will protect them and their partners with several other types of HPV included in the vaccine. Condom usage is encouraged to prevent sexual transmission of HPV, including vaginal, anal, and oral sex. The National Health and Nutrition Examination Survey data on the impact of HPV vaccines demonstrate reductions of the prevalence of HPV types 6, 11, 16, and 18 and the prevalence of anogenital warts. HPV-associated cancers and genital warts have dropped by 86% in teens and 71% in young adult women and cervical precancers by 40% among vaccinated women.

✳ Cervical Pap smears done regularly to detect early HPV lesions

Gardasil-9 includes 9 HPV types used in the United States

Vaccine recommended at 11 to 12 years

KEY CONCLUSIONS

- HPV is the most common sexually transmitted infection in the United States. It is the major cause of cervical cancer in women worldwide as well as anal and genital cancers in men. It also causes oropharyngeal cancer in men four times higher than women in the United States.

- HPV is a naked capsid, icosahedral, double-stranded circular DNA virus that replicates in the nucleus by using host RNA and DNA polymerases.

- HPV enters through direct skin-to-skin contact and through vaginal, anal, and oral sex.

- HPV targets stratified squamous epithelium through the damaged area of the epithelium and infects the basal cells, and then gets transferred to a receptor expressed on keratinocytes moving on the basal membrane in wound healing process of the damaged epithelium.

- HPV genotypes are clinically relevant because of their association with different types and location of lesions and with low-risk and high-risk probability with cancer.

- While the HPV types 6 and 11 are most common genital infections (low risk) and cause benign genital warts (condylomata acuminata), types 16, 18, and higher genotypes are considered high-risk types in causing cervical, anal, and oropharyngeal cancers. Type 16 is the most malignant type because of its association to 60% of cervical cancers, whereas HPV 18 association is about 10% to 15%.

- More than 80% of the HPV-associated cancers are caused by HPV 16 and 18, whereas 12% by HPV 31, 33, 45, 52, and 58, and these genotypes are part of Gardasil 9-valent vaccine.

- HPV early proteins E6 and E7 are involved in transformation and oncogenesis, including E6 degradation of p53 and E7 binding with pRB to abrogate cell cycle.

- HPV Gardasil-9 vaccine is recommended for routine immunization between 11- and 12-year-old girls and boys but can be given until age 26 years and in some cases up to 45 years. The vaccines have shown reduction in HPV-associated cancers.

POLYOMAVIRUSES

Overview

Human polyomaviruses, closely related to HPVs structurally, are also naked capsid, icosahedral, circular double-stranded DNA viruses that replicate in the nucleus of infected cells by using host RNA and DNA polymerases. They have cellular transforming ability *in vitro* but do not cause cancer in humans. Two members, JC virus (JCV) and BK virus (BKV), infect a large population but only cause clinical disease in immunocompromised patients. JCV can cause a rare, slow, progressive multifocal leukoencephalopathy (PML), whereas BKV can cause hemorrhagic cystitis/nephropathy in immunocompromised patients and those receiving immunosuppressive drugs.

FIGURE 19–7. JC virus (arrow) among debris of cells from a brain biopsy of a case of progressive multifocal leukoencephalopathy (PML). (Reproduced with permission from Palmer E, Martin ML. *An Atlas of Mammalian Viruses.* Boca Raton, FL: CRC Press; 1982.)

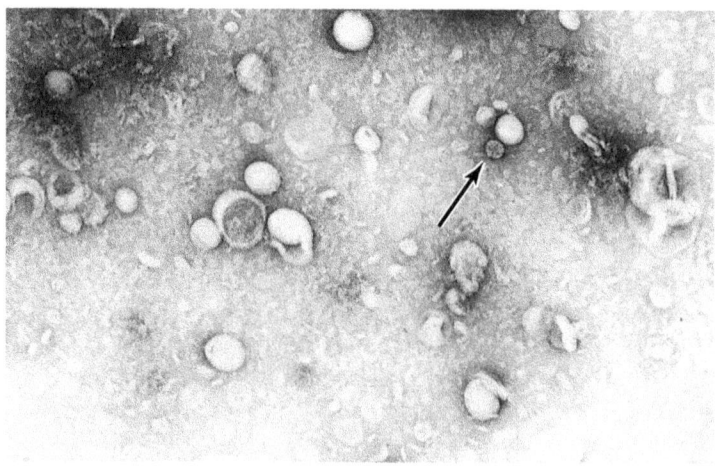

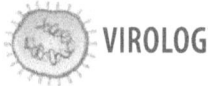 ## VIROLOGY

* Naked capsid, icosahedral, double-stranded, circular DNA virus

Early proteins and late capsid proteins (VP1-VP3)

Can transform cells *in vitro* but do not cause cancer in humans

Polyomaviruses are classified in a new family known as Polyomaviridae, which are widely distributed in humans and among various animal species, usually without causing apparent disease. However, these viruses are able to transform cells of a variety of heterologous cell lines in culture. Polyomaviruses are naked capsid, icosahedral, double-stranded circular DNA genome of 5 kb and virion size of 45 nm in diameter. Like papillomaviruses, polyomaviruses also encode early and late genes. Early genes encode the large, middle, and small T antigens that are involved in mRNA transcription, DNA replication, cell growth, and transformation. Late proteins are structural capsid proteins, namely VP1, VP2, and VP3. The virus does not encode or carry RNA or DNA polymerase. An electron micrograph of a human polyomavirus, JCV is shown in **Figure 19–7.**

Thirteen human polyomaviruses have been identified to date. In 1971, JCV and BKV were identified (named after patients' initials) and were linked with progressive PML and hemorrhagic cystitis, respectively. In 2007, two additional human polyomaviruses were isolated from pediatric respiratory samples, namely, Karolinska Institute virus (KIV) and Washington University virus (WUV). Another human polyomavirus was identified in 2008 in the form of viral transcripts from a patient with an uncommon but aggressive form of Merkel cell carcinoma (MCC) skin cancer, and therefore, named as Merkel cell polyomavirus (MCV). In 2010, three new human polyomaviruses, including human polyomaviruses 6 and 7 and trichodysplasia spinulosa-associated polyomavirus (TSPyV) from the skin samples were identified. In 2010, human polyomavirus 9 (HPyV9) was identified in human blood and skin samples. Four more polyomaviruses have been identified in humans, including MWPyV in the stool (2012), STLPyV in the stool (2013), HPy12 in gastrointestinal tract (2013), NJPyV in muscle biopsy (2014).

Thirteen human polyomaviruses have been identified

* JCV and BKV more studied and associated with human disease

Viral assembly and release from the nuclei of infected cells

* Host cell RNA and DNA polymerase direct virus RNA and DNA synthesis

Viral replication in nucleus

The polyomaviruses including the JCV and BKV of humans that are known to cause diseases and the simian virus 40 (SV40) of monkeys have been studied in detail and are described in this section.

Viral VP1 protein binds to host cell receptors containing sialic acid and enters the cell through receptor-mediated endocytosis (viropexis) and transported to the nucleus. Viral replication takes place in the nucleus of the infected cells. Transcription of early genes is performed by host RNA polymerase, which leads to synthesis of early proteins, including large, middle, and small T antigens. The early proteins regulate viral transcription, DNA replication, cell division, and transformation. Viral DNA genomes for progeny viruses are synthesized by host cell DNA polymerase. Late mRNAs are translated into capsid proteins (VP1, VP2, VP3) that are translocated in the nucleus, where assembly of progeny viruses takes place. These progeny viruses are released upon cell death or lysis.

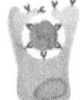 ## POLYOMAVIRUS DISEASE

EPIDEMIOLOGY

Routes of transmission unclear

Respiratory, oral transmission suspected

The exact routes of polyomavirus transmission in humans are not known. However, respiratory or oral transmission (due to contaminated food or water) is suspected. Viruses are excreted in the urine. Approximately 80% of adults show serologic evidence of JCV and BKV infections, all of which are usually asymptomatic. However, the viruses remain latent and may reactivate and cause disease in immunocompromised patients. BKV is estimated to cause renal disease, including graft failure in 2% to 5% of renal transplant recipients, and JCV is the cause of an uncommon neurologic disorder, PML.

PATHOGENESIS

Polyomaviruses can produce malignant tumors in certain experimental animals but not in their natural hosts (human). For example, SV40 can produce lymphocytic leukemia and a variety of reticuloendothelial cell sarcomas in baby hamsters but is not oncogenic in its natural monkey host. Fortunately, even though it can transform some human cells *in vitro*, SV40 fails to produce disease in humans, a fact that became apparent on follow-up of recipients of early batches of poliomyelitis vaccine produced in monkey kidney cell cultures that were contaminated with live SV40.

Do not cause malignancies in their natural hosts

 Why do human polyomaviruses not cause cancer in humans but transform cells *in vitro*?

The reason polyomaviruses fail to produce tumors in their natural hosts is uncertain, but it may be because these viruses are usually cytocidal under these conditions. From a biologic point of view, the polyomaviruses are particularly useful models of oncogenicity because they can be readily studied *in vitro* and interact with cells in different ways. In some, they produce lytic infections and cell death with the production of complete virions. In others, they integrate randomly into the cell genome and cause transformation by the expression of one or more of the viral genes. No human tumor has been shown to be associated with polyomaviruses, such as JCV or BKV. However, recent identification of MCV from patients with MCC raises an interesting question of the association of a human polyomavirus with cancer, although this information needs more scientific evaluation and confirmation because MCV DNA is also found in non-MCC (lower DNA numbers in non-MCC than MCC).

Interact with cells in a variety of ways

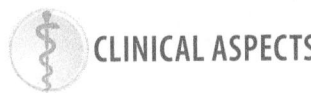

CLINICAL ASPECTS

MANIFESTATIONS

■ Progressive Multifocal Leukoencephalopathy

PML is a rare, subacute, degenerative disease of the brain found primarily in adults with immunosuppressive diseases, especially HIV/AIDS and hematologic malignancies, or those receiving immunosuppressive agents such as autoimmune disease and transplant patients. PML is one of the AIDS-defining illnesses or opportunistic infection as a result of CD4 T-cell depletion in untreated patients. However, HIV patients receiving ART treatment with successful viral suppression and improvement in CD4 T cell counts do not experience JCV reactivation. PML disease is characterized by the development of impaired memory, confusion, and disorientation, followed by a multiplicity of neurologic symptoms and signs that include hemiparesis, visual disturbances, incoordination, seizures, and visual abnormalities. PML is progressive, with death usually occurring 3 to 6 months after the onset of symptoms.

In PML, CT scan or MRI shows single or multiple confluent lesions without mass effects, most frequently in the parieto-occipital white matter. The cerebrospinal fluid (CSF) findings are often normal, although some patients show a slight increase in lymphocytes, and protein levels may be elevated. Pathologically, foci of demyelination are found, surrounded by giant, bizarre astrocytes containing intranuclear inclusions. The demyelination is due to viral damage to oligodendroglial cells, which synthesize and maintain myelin. Abundant JCV particles can be seen in the brain by electron microscopy (Figure 19–7) and maybe concentrated within the nuclei of

JCV in cell nuclei, with demyelination

 Think ▸▸ Apply 19-4: Probably due to their cytocidal effects on cells and weak interaction of human polyomavirus T antigens with cellular proteins and/or tumor suppressors in abrogating cell cycle.

No specific treatment, reducing immune suppression have clinical benefits

oligodendrocytes. JCV DNA sequences have been demonstrated by PCR in the brain of patients without PML or demyelinating lesions, suggesting that the virus may be latent in the brain before immunosuppression. There is no specific treatment for PML, although reducing the immunosuppression, if possible, may have some clinical benefit.

 Why does JCV cause PML in older people or immunocompromised patients?

■ Urinary Tract Infection

✳ **BKV causes hemorrhagic cystitis and nephritis**

Infection of the urinary tract with JCV and BKV can be demonstrated frequently in immunocompromised patients, but usually without symptoms or evidence of renal injury. BKV is associated with a hemorrhagic cystitis, particularly in bone marrow and renal transplant recipients. In addition, BKV is also the cause of a severe nephropathy and vasculopathy, which may lead to kidney loss in renal transplant recipients. The disease develops months after renal transplantation. Treatment consists of reducing immunosuppression, but up to 50% of the patients with this syndrome may require nephrectomy. Cidofovir (a nucleotide analog) is a possible antiviral treatment for BKV disease.

DIAGNOSIS

BKV can be isolated in cell culture

JCV and BKV can be detected by PCR

Urine from patients excreting these polyomaviruses may contain "decoy" cells similar to those from patients excreting cytomegalovirus, but they can be distinguished cytologically. BKV can be isolated by routine culture in diploid fibroblast or Vero monkey kidney cells, but nephropathy is usually preceded by plasma PCR positivity, which can be monitored. At present, a kidney biopsy is required for a definitive diagnosis. Viral antigens can be demonstrated in tissue by a variety of immunoassays. JCV DNA has been demonstrated in the brains of PML patients by PCR, and PCR of CSF is a diagnostic test for PML.

KEY CONCLUSIONS

- Two members of human polyomaviruses, JCV and BKV, cause disease in humans under immune suppressive conditions.
- JCV and BKV are naked capsid, icosahedral, double-stranded circular DNA viruses that replicate in the nucleus of the infected cell by employing host RNA and DNA polymerases.
- About 80% of the population is seropositive for JCV and BKV. JCV persists in the CNS and JCV and BKV in the kidneys or urinary tract. Reactivation occurs under immune suppression or other infections like HIV resulting in JC-mediated PML and BK-induced hemorrhagic cystitis, nephropathy, and vasculopathy.
- PML is a subacute, degenerative disease of the brain found primarily in adults with immunosuppressive diseases, especially HIV patients with low CD4 counts and hematologic malignancies, or those receiving immunosuppressive agents. In brain biopsy, icosahedral JCV is seen.

CASE STUDY

Postcoital Concerns

A 19-year-old woman had her first and only intercourse 6 months ago and is concerned whether she has genital HPV infection. Pelvic examination reveals normal genitalia.

 Think ►► Apply 19-5: JCV persists in the CNS in a huge population. Immune system probably controls this persistent infection. Once there is immune suppression due to aging, diseases, or drugs, JCV is reactivated and may cause disease. Same concept is true for BKV.

QUESTIONS

1. What would be the best test for this purpose?
   A. Serology for HPV IgG antibody
   B. Serology for HPV IgM antibody
   C. Cervical "Pap" smears
   D. *In situ* hybridization or PCR of HPV DNA in cervical sample

2. Her test for HPV infection is positive. Which of the following is most appropriate?
   A. Cervical "Pap" smears every other year
   B. Gardasil 9-valent HPV vaccine
   C. Topical trichloroacetic acid treatment of the cervix
   D. Determination whether her HPV infection is oncogenic genotype
   E. Prophylactic radiation treatment of cervix

3. Her sex partner should:
   A. Be counseled to practice "safe sex" and receive Gardasil-9.
   B. Have HPV *in situ* hybridization assay on urethral swab.
   C. Have HPV *in situ* hybridization assay on anal swab.
   D. Receive quadrivalent HPV vaccine.

ANSWERS

1. (D)
2. (B)
3. (A)

chapter 20

Persistent Viral Infections of the Central Nervous System

Measles Virus · Rubella Virus · JC Virus · HIV · Enterovirus · Herpes Simplex Virus Types 1 and 2

Varicella-Zoster Virus · Prions

OVERVIEW

Persistent viral infections are those in which termination of early symptoms and disease is not accompanied by elimination of the virus from the host but by the persistence of viral genome in the host. Persistent viral infections could be latent infection, in which viral genome is maintained without making any infectious virus particles or chronic infection, where a low level of virus is made without causing any or little damage to the target tissue. Three main conditions must be fulfilled for a virus to cause persistent infection, including little to no cytopathic effect of the virus to the host cells, maintenance of viral genome in the host cell, and avoid elimination by the immune system. Several viruses have utilized these strategies to persist in an immune-privileged site, the central nervous system (CNS), and over time after reactivation cause rare disease in the CNS or distant sites. These viruses include measles, rubella, enterovirus, HIV, JCV, HSV 1, 2, and VZV. In addition, nonconventional agents such as prions (infectious prion proteins, PrPsc) cause slow degenerative diseases of the CNS such as Creutzfeldt-Jakob disease (CJD) and others. These persistent viral agents and prions and the diseases they cause will be discussed in this chapter.

The molecular mechanisms of persistent viral infections are not clearly understood, but three broad conditions must be satisfied for a virus to establish a persistent infection in a host:

1. Virus must be able to infect host cells without being cytolytic or cytopathic. Viruses have found various cell types such as nonpermissive cells in a host to infect and remain less cytopathic or noncytolytic to maintain persistence. For example, herpes simplex virus (HSV) remains latent in sensory neurons; HIV is less cytopathic to resting T cells or monocytes/macrophages.

2. Viral genome must be maintained by various mechanisms. Viral genomes can be maintained in several ways, including integration of retroviral DNA (HIV) and extrachromosomal episomes for DNA viruses (HSV). However, the mechanisms of viral RNA genome maintenance are not known.

3. Virus must avoid detection and elimination by the host's immune system. Viruses have evolved several evasion strategies such as infection of immunologically privileged sites that are not easily accessible to the immune system such as the central nervous system (CNS) and

∗ Viruses must be less cytolytic to cells in which they persist

∗ DNA genomes either integrate or persist as episomes

Persistence of RNA genomes not understood

TABLE 20–1	Conventional Viruses Causing Persistent CNS Infections
DISEASE/INFECTION	**AGENT**
Subacute sclerosing panencephalitis (SSPE)	Measles virus
Progressive panencephalitis following congenital rubella	Rubella virus
Progressive multifocal encephalopathy	Polyoma virus (JC virus)
AIDS dementia complex (ADC)	Human immunodeficiency virus (HIV)
Persistent enterovirus infection of the immunodeficient	Enteroviruses
Latent/persistent herpes simplex virus infection	Herpes simplex virus types 1 and 2
Latent/persistent varicella-zoster virus infection	Varicella-Zoster virus

＊ Antigenic variation, immune components downregulation, infection of immune-privileged sites such as CNS allow viral persistence

other sites, antigenic variation, downregulation of immune components, and others. Several viruses cause persistent infection of the CNS because they are not easily detected and eliminated by the host immune response. Many of the persistent viruses employ some or all strategies to avoid elimination by the immune system.

 How does antigenic variation allow the virus to escape elimination?

Evidence has accumulated that a variety of progressive neurologic diseases in both humans and animals are caused by viral or other filterable agents that share some of the properties of viruses (**Tables 20–1, 20–2,** and **20–3**). These illnesses have been termed "slow viral diseases" because of the protracted period between infection and the onset of disease as well as the prolonged course of the illness, but a better term is "persistent viral infection."

Progressive neurologic diseases in humans and animals

Most persistent viral infections involve well-differentiated cells, such as lymphocytes and neuronal cells. They can be classified as (1) diseases associated with "conventional" viral agents that possess nucleic acid genomes and protein capsids and/or envelopes induce immune responses and can be grown in cell culture systems; and (2) diseases associated with "unconventional" agents that are small, filterable infectious agents, known as "prions," which are transmissible to certain experimental animals, but do not contain nucleic acids, do not appear to be associated with immune or inflammatory responses by the host, and have not been cultivated in cell culture.

Include conventional viruses, unconventional agents, prions

＊ "Prions" do not produce immune or inflammatory responses

Persistence due to a variety of mechanisms

Persistence of conventional viruses can result from infection of a nonpermissive cell in the host with restrictive cytolytic effects, preservation of viral nucleic acid in infected host's cells, and mutations that interfere with or severely limit viral replication or antigenicity.

DISEASES ASSOCIATED WITH CONVENTIONAL AGENTS

The following conditions are the major persistent infections caused by conventional viral agents. They are summarized in Table 20–1.

TABLE 20–2	Unconventional Virus (Prion) Diseases[a]
HUMANS	**ANIMALS (PRIMARY HOSTS)**
Creutzfeldt-Jakob disease[b]	Scrapie (sheep)
Variant Creutzfeldt-Jakob disease	Transmissible mink encephalopathy (mink)
Gerstmann-Sträussler-Scheinker syndrome	Chronic wasting disease (mule deer, elk)
Kuru	Bovine spongiform encephalopathy (BSE; cows)[b]
Fatal familial insomnia	Inherited, no animal host

[a]Subacute spongiform encephalopathies.
[b]Prion agents of variant Creutzfeldt-Jakob disease and bovine spongiform encephalopathy (BSE) are identical.

 Think ▸▸ Apply 20-1: **Antigenic variation occurs due to random mutations; however, due to immune pressure, mutations occur in immunogenic epitopes resulting in immune escape.**

TABLE 20–3	Biological and Physical Properties of Prions

- Chronic progressive pathology without remission or recovery
- No inflammatory response
- No alteration in pathogenesis by immunosuppression or immunopotentiation
- Estimated diameter of 5 to 100 nm
- No virion-like structures visible by electron microscopy
- Transmissible to experimental animals
- No interferon production or interference by conventional viruses
- Unusual resistance to ultraviolet irradiation, alcohol, formalin, boiling, proteases, and nucleases
- Can be inactivated by prolonged exposure to steam autoclaving or 1N or 2N NaOH

■ Subacute Sclerosing Panencephalitis

Subacute sclerosing panencephalitis (SSPE) is discussed in Chapter 10. It is a rare chronic measles virus infection of children that usually appears 2 to 10 years after measles virus infection and produces progressive neurologic disease characterized by an insidious onset of personality change, progressive intellectual deterioration, and both motor and autonomic nervous system dysfunctions.

✳ Persistence of measles virus after childhood infection, causing SSPE after many years

 How does measles or rubella virus (RNA virus) persist in the brain for many years before causing SSPE?

■ Progressive Postrubella Panencephalitis

Even more rarely, a degenerative neurologic disorder similar to SSPE is associated with persistent rubella virus infection of the CNS. This condition is seen most often in adolescents who have had the congenital rubella syndrome. Rubella virus has been isolated from brain tissue in these patients using cocultivation techniques.

Can be a late sequela of congenital rubella infection

■ Progressive Multifocal Leukoencephalopathy

Progressive multifocal leukoencephalopathy (PML) is a subacute, degenerative disease of the brain found primarily in adults with (1) immunosuppressive diseases, especially HIV infection with low CD4 counts and hematologic malignancies; or (2) diseases requiring therapy with immunosuppressive agents such as transplant and autoimmune disease patients. PML is due to a polyomavirus (JC virus) and is described in Chapter 19.

✳ Progressive neurologic disease of immunocompromised

■ Persistent Enterovirus Infection

Persons with congenital or severe acquired immunodeficiency, especially those with agamma-globulinemia, may develop a chronic CNS infection due to an echovirus or other enterovirus. Headache, confusion, lethargy, seizures, and cerebrospinal fluid (CSF) pleocytosis are common manifestations. The virus can be isolated from the CSF. Clinical improvement may be achieved by the administration of human hyperimmune globulin to the infecting virus type. Relapse, however, occurs when therapy is discontinued, indicating persistence of virus despite the therapy.

Associated with humoral immunodeficiencies

Temporary improvement with virus type-specific hyperimmune globulin

■ AIDS Dementia Complex or HIV-Associated Dementia

Human immunodeficiency virus (HIV) causes a persistent infection of the CNS in many patients with symptomatic AIDS known as AIDS dementia complex (ADC) or HIV-associated dementia (HAD). The virus does not directly infect the nerve cells, but the virus produced by perivascular macrophages and/or microglia may produce a bystander effect causing inflammation that may

 Think ▸▸ Apply 20-2: Measles or Rubella virus most likely persists in the CNS (neuron and glial cells) as nucleocapsids (viral RNA complexed with protein) inside the cells with little to no virus replication, and over a long time in rare cases continue causing chronic damage resulting in SSPE.

ADC or HAD seen in patients with symptomatic AIDS

damage brain and spinal cord. The clinical course may vary from a mild subacute illness (early stage of HIV infection) to severe progressive dementia (symptomatic AIDS, HIV infection with low CD4 counts). HAD primarily occurs with more advanced HIV infection and symptoms include encephalitis, behavioral changes, and a gradual decline in cognitive function. HAD is more common in HIV-infected infants than infected adults. For more on HIV/AIDS, see Chapter 18.

■ Latent Herpes Simplex Virus Infection

HSV persists in ganglia

Reactivation by sunlight, stress, trauma, immune suppression

Herpes simplex viruses, HSV-1 and HSV-2, following primary infection ascend in the trigeminal and sacral root ganglia, respectively, and establish persistent/latent infection. HSV DNA persists in the ganglia but then it becomes latent without making infectious viruses. Reactivation of HSV due to sunlight, stress, immune suppression, trauma, etc. passes viral genome anterograde in axons to the epithelium to cause replication and disease (see Chapter 14 for details).

■ Latent Varicella-Zoster Virus Infection

VZV persists in dorsal root ganglia

Reactivation occurrence increases with age

Varicella-Zoster virus (VZV) causes primary chickenpox and after recovery from acute infection, the virus establishes latency in dorsal root ganglia. After some time, several years or in many instances above age 50, the virus is reactivated and the skin lesions are seen in the same area of the dermatome. Clinically, this disease is called shingles and it is usually unilateral. In immunocompromised patients, the reactivated form could disseminate and cause serious diseases. Details are described in Chapter 14.

HUMAN DISEASES CAUSED BY UNCONVENTIONAL AGENTS: SUBACUTE SPONGIFORM ENCEPHALOPATHIES

Prions affect animals and humans

✳ **Cause neuronal loss and spongiform changes in brain**

A group of progressive degenerative diseases of the CNS has been shown to be caused by **prions** that are proteinaceous infectious agents without any genome or nucleic acid and have unusual physical and chemical properties. Since the prions lack genome or nucleic, they cannot multiply or grow in culture. The Nobel Prize in Medicine for 1997 was awarded to Stanley Prisoner for his work in identifying the role of prions in disease. Prions cause five CNS diseases in animals such as bovine spongiform encephalopathy (BSE) in cattle, scrapie in sheep, and others, and five fatal CNS diseases in humans, such as Creutzfeldt-Jakob disease (CJD), variant CJD (vCJD), and others listed in **Table 20–2**. Prions can be the etiologic agents of inherited, communicable, or sporadic diseases. The pathogenesis of these illnesses is not well understood, but the pathologic and clinical features are similar. Varying degrees of neuronal loss and astrocyte proliferation occur. The diseases are known as "spongiform" encephalopathies or transmissible spongiform encephalopathies (TSE) because of the vacuolar changes in the cortex and cerebellum (**Figures 20–1** and **20–2**). The incubation periods for these diseases are months to years, and their courses are protracted and inevitably fatal.

A prion is a "small proteinaceous infectious particle" that is not inactivated by procedures that destroy nucleic acids (Table 20–3). They have diameters of 5 to 100 nm or less and can remain viable even in formalinized brain tissue for many years. They are resistant to ionizing radiation,

FIGURE 20–1. Appearance of brain with spongiform encephalopathy. (*Left*) Normal brain. (*Right*) Brain infected with a prion. Note the sponge-like appearance. (Reproduced with permission from Nester EW, Anderson DG, Roberts CE Jr, et al: *Microbiology: A Human Perspective*, 6th ed. New York, NY: McGraw Hill; 2008.)

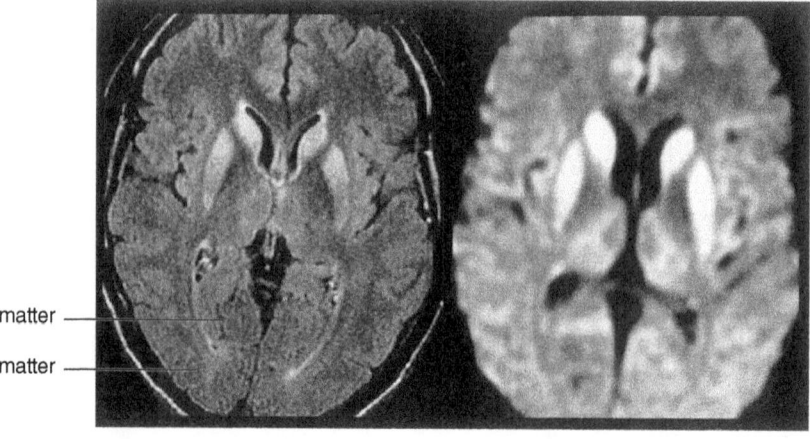

White matter ——

Gray matter ——

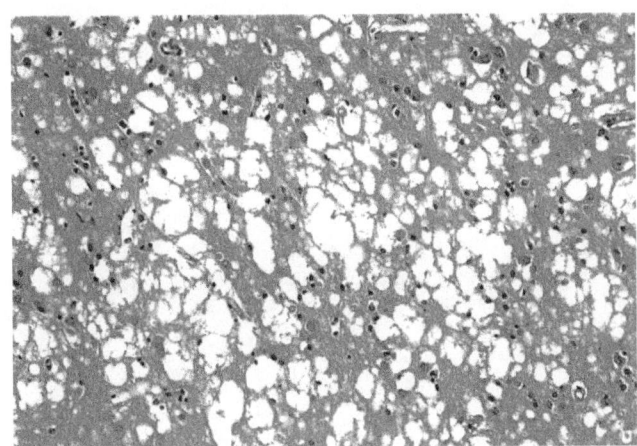

FIGURE 20–2. Spongiform changes. (Reproduced with permission from Connor DH, Chandler FW, Schwartz DQ, et al: *Pathology of Infectious Diseases.* Stamford CT: Appleton & Lange; 1997.)

boiling, and many common disinfectants. Recognizable virions have not been found in tissues by electron microscopy, and the agents have not been grown in cell culture.

A prion is composed of a protein encoded by a normal cellular gene, *PrP*, in the brain which is located on chromosome 20. The normal prion protein designated as prion protein cellular (PrPc) or normal prion (NP) in **Figure 20–3** is converted into a disease-causing form by a change in posttranslational conformational process probably by misfolding to an abnormal infectious protein designated as prion protein scrapie (PrPsc) or abnormal infectious prion protein (PP) (Figure 20–3). Brain extracts from scrapie-infected animals contain PrPsc, which is not found in the brains of normal animals, and it is the PrPsc which is the infectious prion that is responsible for transmission and infection and causing diseases of the CNS. Furthermore, the conformational change is also the way in which infectious prions PrPsc or PP increase their numbers by interacting with normal prions, PrPc or NP and conformational changing the normal prion host cell protein, PrPc or NP into additional abnormal or infectious prion protein, PrPsc or PP (Figure 20–3). Production of infectious PrPsc prions or PP and the consequent pathology result from this process. During PrPsc infection, PP may aggregate into amyloid-like birefringent rods and filamentous structures termed scrapie-associated fibrils (**Figure 20–4**), which are found in membranes of scrapie-infected brain tissues. The amino acid sequence of different PPs in different animal species differ from one another and transmission across species usually does not occur. Specifically, ingestion of tissue from sheep or elk infected with abnormal prions has not been documented to lead to human disease. Tissue from infected cows did, however, transmit variant CJD (see the following text).

* Prion is an infectious agent comprised of protein without any nucleic acids

Infectious agents resist inactivation

Prion, PrPc, encoded by a normal cellular gene

* Conformational changes convert normal prion proteins to infectious prion proteins

How does few infectious prion become many infectious prions and cause CJD without any replication?

Kuru

Kuru was a subacute, progressive neurologic disease of the Fore people of the Eastern Highlands of New Guinea. The disease was brought to the attention of the Western world by Gadjusek and Zigas in 1957. Although the illness was localized and decreasing in incidence, its study has thrown light on the transmissibility and infectious nature of similar encephalopathies. Epidemiologic studies indicated that kuru usually afflicted adult women or children of either sex. The disease was rarely observed outside the Fore region, and outsiders in the region did not contract the disease. The symptoms and signs were ataxia, hyperreflexia, and spasticity, which led to

Women and children of the Fore people of New Guinea

Transmissible to primates

Think ▶▶ Apply 20-3: **Infectious prions interact with normal prions to change their conformation and make them infectious prions in a long duration and causing varying degrees of neuronal loss and astrocyte proliferation occurs resulting in spongiform encephalopathies.**

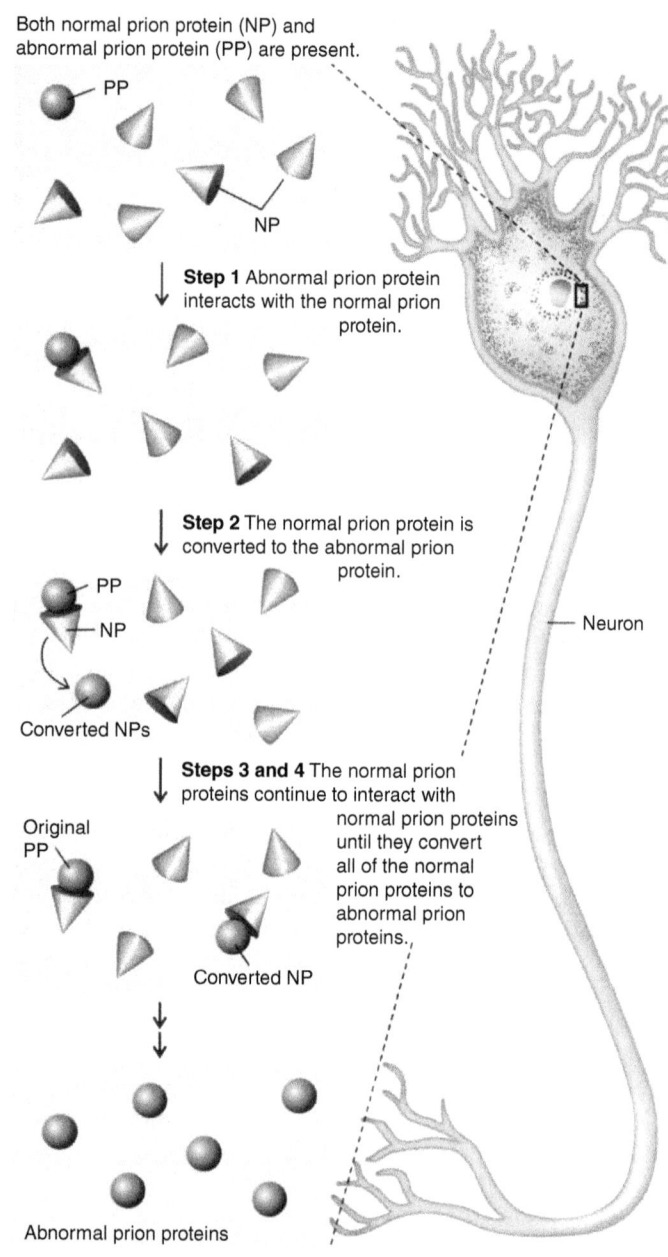

FIGURE 20-3. **Proposed mechanism of how prions are converted to abnormal proteins.** The normal and abnormal prion proteins differ in their tertiary structures. (Reproduced with permission from Nester EW, Anderson DG, Roberts CE Jr, et al: *Microbiology: A Human Perspective*, 6th ed. New York, NY: McGraw Hill; 2008.)

Both normal prion protein (NP) and abnormal prion protein (PP) are present.

PP

NP

Step 1 Abnormal prion protein interacts with the normal prion protein.

Step 2 The normal prion protein is converted to the abnormal prion protein.

PP

NP

Converted NPs

Steps 3 and 4 The normal prion proteins continue to interact with normal prion proteins until they convert all of the normal prion proteins to abnormal prion proteins.

Original PP

Converted NP

Abnormal prion proteins

Neuron

Associated with cannibalism

progressive dementia, starvation, and death. Pathologic examination revealed changes only in the CNS, with diffuse neuronal degeneration and spongiform changes of the cerebral cortex and basal ganglia. No inflammatory response was apparent. Inoculation of infectious brain tissue into primates produced a disease that caused similar neurologic symptoms and pathologic

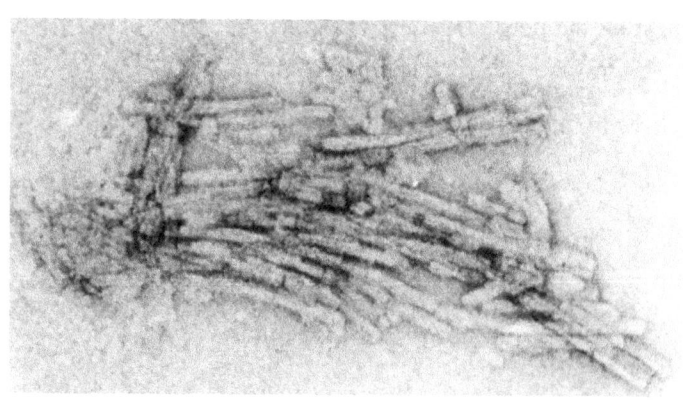

FIGURE 20-4. Amyloid-like fibrils (scrapie-associated fibrils) observed in brain extract of a patient with Creutzfeldt-Jakob disease. (Reproduced with permission from Bockman JM, Kingsbury DT, McKinley MP, et al. Creutzfeldt-Jakob disease prion proteins in human brains. *N Engl J Med* 1985; Jan 10;312(2):73–82.)

manifestations after an incubation period of approximately 40 months. Epidemiologic studies indicated that transmission of the disease in humans was associated with ingestion of a soup made from the brains of dead relatives and eaten in honor of the deceased. Clinical disease developed 4 to 20 years after exposure. Since the elimination of cannibalism from the Fore culture, kuru has disappeared.

Creutzfeldt-Jakob Disease

CJD is a progressive, fatal illness of the CNS that is seen most frequently in the sixth and seventh decades of life. The initial clinical manifestations are a change in cerebral function, usually diagnosed initially as a psychiatric disorder. Forgetfulness and disorientation progress to overt dementia and the development of changes in gait, increased tone in the limbs, involuntary movement, and seizures. These manifestations resemble those of kuru. The disorder usually runs a course of 4 to 7 months, eventually leading to paralysis, wasting, pneumonia, and death.

CJD is found worldwide, including the United States, with an incidence of disease of one to two case(s) per million per year. The risk of CJD increases with age (median age 68 years). Between 1979 and 2018, an annual average rate of 3.6 cases per million people above age 50 years has been reported in the United States. The mode of acquisition is unknown, but it occurs both **sporadically** (85%) with no recognizable pattern of transmission and in a **familial pattern** (15%) such as Gerstmann-Straüssler-Scheinker and fatal familial insomnia probably due to mutations in normal prion PP. Infection has also been transmitted by dura mater grafts and corneal transplants, by contact with contaminated electrodes or instruments used in neurosurgical procedures, and by pituitary-derived human growth hormone. The latter was responsible for more than 100 cases. The incubation period of the disease is approximately 3 years to more than 20 years. The agent of CJD has not been transmitted to animals by inoculation of body secretions, and no increased risk of disease has been noted in family members or medical personnel caring for patients.

It has been transmitted to chimpanzees, mice, and guinea pigs by inoculation of infected brain tissue, leukocytes, and certain organs. High levels of infectious agents have been found, especially in the brain, where they may reach 107 infectious doses per gram of brain tissue. Nonpercutaneous transmission of CJD has not been observed, and there is no evidence of transmission by direct contact or airborne spread.

Brains from patients with CJD have the birefringent rods and fibrillar structures noted in kuru and scrapie (Figure 20–4). Identification of PrPsc and antibodies directed against it may become a useful diagnostic adjunct to neuropathologic examination of brain tissue. Pathologic examination of brain tissue is the only definitive diagnostic test. Additional studies can be done such as presence of 14-3-3 protein (expressed at higher levels in the brain in several neurological orders) and/or finding a typical electroencephalogram (EEG) pattern.

Therapy

There is no effective therapy for CJD, and all cases have been fatal.

Prevention

The small risk of nosocomial infection is related only to direct contact with infected tissue. Stereotactic neurosurgical equipment, especially which was used in patients with undiagnosed dementia, should not be reused. In addition, organs from patients with undiagnosed neurologic disease should not be used for transplants. Growth hormone from human tissue has now been replaced by a recombinant genetically engineered product. Recommendations for disinfection of potentially infectious material include treatment for 1 hour with 2N NaOH or by autoclaving at 132°C for 60 to 90 minutes. Others recommend even more extensive treatment such as combining these two procedures to ensure inactivation.

Bovine Spongiform Encephalopathy "Mad Cow Disease") and "Variant vCJD"

BSE was identified in 1986 in cows in the United Kingdom, causing them to become uncoordinated and unusually apprehensive. The source of the emerging epidemic was soon traced to a food supplement that included meat and bone meal from dead sheep. Between 1986 and 2004, 180,000 cases of BSE in cattle were confirmed in the United Kingdom. To combat BSE, the British government banned the use of animal-derived feed supplements in 1988, and the epidemic among cattle, which peaked at nearly 40,000 cases in 1992, decreased to less than 4000 new cases in 1997.

Marginal notes:

* Progressive disease among elderly

* Altered cerebral functions; changes in gait, increased tone in limbs, involuntary movement, seizures

* Course 4 to 7 months leading to paralysis, wasting, pneumonia, death

* One to two case(s) of CJD per million people annually in the United States

* Mode of acquisition of CJD; sporadic: 85%; familial: 15%

Pathology identical to kuru

Scrapie-like structures seen in brain

Nosocomial infections preventable by avoidance of potentially infectious materials, careful sterilization

Source was meat and bone meal from sheep in cattle feed

By February 2002, most European countries had reported cases of BSE, but new infections have ceased as a result of imposing tight controls on cattle feed. The United States had been spared, as measured by over 19,000 cattle brain examinations. From 1993 to 2018, 26 cases of BSE were reported in North America, including six in the United States and 20 in Canada. The incubation period in cattle was determined to be 2 to 8 years. In addition to the incoordination and apprehension, the cows exhibited hyperesthesia, hyperreflexia, muscle fasciculations, tremors, and weight loss. Autonomic dysfunction was frequently manifested as reduced rumination, bradycardia, and other cardiac arrhythmias. Unfortunately, the prion that causes BSE survived the heat of cooking and was transmitted to humans who inadvertently consumed infected bovine neural tissue or bone marrow (both are sometimes found in processed meats, depending on the rendering procedures used). There is strong evidence that infectious prions transmitted from cattle with BSE to humans caused vCJD.

Globally, over 229 humans with "variant CJD" have been reported, with a majority of them, 177 cases, in the United Kingdom, 27 cases in France, and four cases in the United States. In all the four cases reported in the United States, infection most likely occurred outside the United States, including United Kingdom (two cases), Saudi Arabia (one case), and Europe and/or the Middle East (one case). The cases frequently present in young adults (median age 28 years) as psychiatric problems progressing to neurologic changes and dementia, with death in an average of 13-14 months. It appears that destruction of diseased cattle and the changes in livestock feeds have prevented further cases.

■ Gerstmann-Straüssler-Scheinker Disease

Gerstmann-Straüssler-Scheinker (GSS) disease is similar to CJD but occurs at a younger age (fourth to fifth decade). Cerebellar ataxia and paralysis are common, but dementia is less often seen. The disease evolves over an average of 5 years. It was originally thought to be familial, but it also occurs sporadically, very rarely. GSS has been transmitted to experimental animals. The familial nature of this disease raises the question of vertical transmission versus inherited susceptibility.

■ Fatal Familial Insomnia

This is a recently recognized familial (inherited) prion disease in which a syndrome of sleeping difficulty is followed by progressive dementia. It occurs in patients aged 35 to 61 years, culminating in death within 13 to 25 months. In almost all cases, this disease is caused by a specific mutation in the PP. The infectious agent has been transmitted to experimental animal models.

Margin notes:

❊ BSE prion survived heat during cooking

Transmitted to humans by consuming prion contaminated bovine neural tissue, bone marrow, meat, processed meat

❊ vCJD apparently transmitted by infected bovine tissues to humans

❊ Clinical manifestations, outcome similar to CJD

GSS disease similar to CJD but evolves more slowly

Sleeping difficulties progressing to dementia

KEY CONCLUSIONS

- Persistent viral infections of the CNS include some rare infections such as measles (causing SSPE) and rubella (progressive postrubella panencephalitis).
- Some other persistent CNS infections such as enterovirus (due to congenital or acquired immunodeficiency), HIV-associated dementia (HIV/AIDS), JC virus (PML, HIV/AIDS, immune suppression).
- Some viruses persist their genomes in the CNS, such as herpes simplex virus, VZV, JC virus.
- Infectious prions (PrPsc) are protein molecules that are made due to conformational changes (misfolding) of a normal prion protein (PrPc). Mode of acquisition is sporadic (85%), including ingesting infectious prion-contaminated meats and familial (15%).
- Infectious prion causes altered cerebral functions with progressive neurologic diseases such as CJD, vCJD, and other familial disorders.
- CJD is characterized by changes in gait, increased tone in the limbs, involuntary movement, and seizures and runs its course in 4 to 7 months leading to paralysis, wasting, pneumonia, and death.
- CJD occurs in older people (median age 68 years) with shorter duration of illness (4-7 months) and vCJD is seen in younger people (median age 28 years) with 13 to 14 months of duration of illness.

Progressive Forgetfulness

During the last 3 months, a previously healthy 50-year-old man has become increasingly forgetful. Last week he was unable to find his home when returning from a walk. His walking has become unsteady, and yesterday he had a first grand mal seizure. He has not traveled outside the United States and takes no medications. Neurologic examination reveals cerebellar ataxia and spastic reflexes in his lower extremities.

QUESTIONS

1. This man's most likely diagnosis is:
   A. Alzheimer disease
   B. Progressive multifocal leukoencephalopathy
   C. Creutzfeldt-Jakob disease
   D. Mad cow disease
   E. AIDS dementia

2. The most useful diagnostic test would be:
   A. PCR of CSF
   B. PCR of plasma
   C. Brain biopsy
   D. X-ray of brain

3. Which of the following is true regarding therapy of this disease?
   A. There is no therapy proven to be effective.
   B. Immunosuppressive therapy would be effective.
   C. Cidofovir is effective.
   D. Antiretroviral therapy (ART) is effective.

ANSWERS

1. (C)

2. (C)

3. (A)

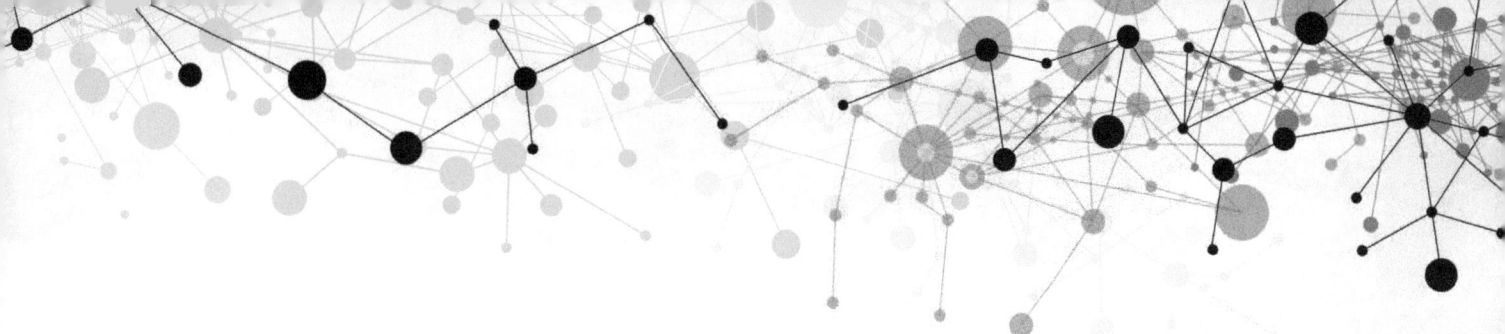

PART III
Pathogenic Bacteria

Paul Pottinger · L. Barth Reller · Kenneth J. Ryan · Gayatri Vedantam · Scott Weissman

chapter 21

Bacteria—Basic Concepts

OVERVIEW

Bacteria are the smallest and most versatile independently living cells. This chapter examines the structural, metabolic, and genetic features that contribute to the ubiquity and diversity of this large group of microorganisms. The discussion which follows focuses on the characteristics of the tiny sliver of the bacterial world which causes disease in humans. The goal is to provide the background and vocabulary fundamental to understanding how bacterial pathogens deploy their structural and metabolic products to confound the immune system and produce injury to the human hosts they invade. These mechanisms will then be explained in the 20 chapters that follow.

● BACTERIAL STRUCTURE

As discussed in Chapter 1, in the hierarchy of infectious agents, bacteria are the smallest organisms capable of independent existence. In the wider microbial world, their prokaryotic cell plan is still considered to provide the minimum possible size for an independently reproducing organism. Individuals of different bacterial species that colonize or infect humans range from 0.1 to 10 μm in their largest dimension (however, the largest bacteria described can reach 300 μm). As shown in Figure 1–2, bacteria overlap in at least one dimension with large viruses and some eukaryotic cells, but they are the sole possessors of the 1 μm size.

Bacteria are in the range of 1 to 10 μm

The small size and nearly colorless nature of bacteria require the use of stains for visualization with a light microscope or the use of electron microscopy. The major morphologic forms are spheres, rods, bent or curved rods, and spirals (**Figure 21–1A-E**). Spherical or oval bacteria are called **cocci** (singular: coccus) and are typically arranged in clusters or chains. Rods are called **bacilli** (singular: bacillus) and may be straight or curved. Bacilli that are small and pleomorphic to the point of resembling cocci are often called coccobacilli. Spiral-shaped bacteria may be rigid or flexible and undulating.

Bacteria exhibit sphere, rod, and spiral shapes

Whatever the overall shape of the cell, a 1 μm size cannot accommodate eukaryotic mitochondria, nucleus, Golgi apparatus, lysosomes, and endoplasmic reticulum in a cell that is itself only as large as an average mitochondrion. The solution is in the unique **prokaryotic** design of the bacterial cell. A generalized bacterial cell is shown in **Figure 21–2.** The major structures of the cell belong either to the multilayered **envelope** and its **appendages** or to the interior core consisting of the **nucleoid** (or nuclear body) and the **cytoplasm.** The cytoplasm is analogous to that of eukaryotic cells, but because there is no nucleus it is not clearly separated from the genetic material. The general chemical nature of the bacterial design includes the familiar macromolecules of life (DNA, RNA, protein, carbohydrate, and phospholipids) in addition to some macromolecules unique to bacteria such as the peptidoglycan, lipopolysaccharide (LPS), and lipoteichoic acid found in bacterial cell walls. The smallness and simplicity of the bacterial design contribute to the ability of metabolic activities in the cytosol to allow growth much faster than eukaryotic cells, a significant feature in producing disease.

✳ **Prokaryotic design includes envelope, appendages, cytosol, nucleoid**

Chemically similar to eukaryotic cells plus unique components

Design facilitates rapid growth

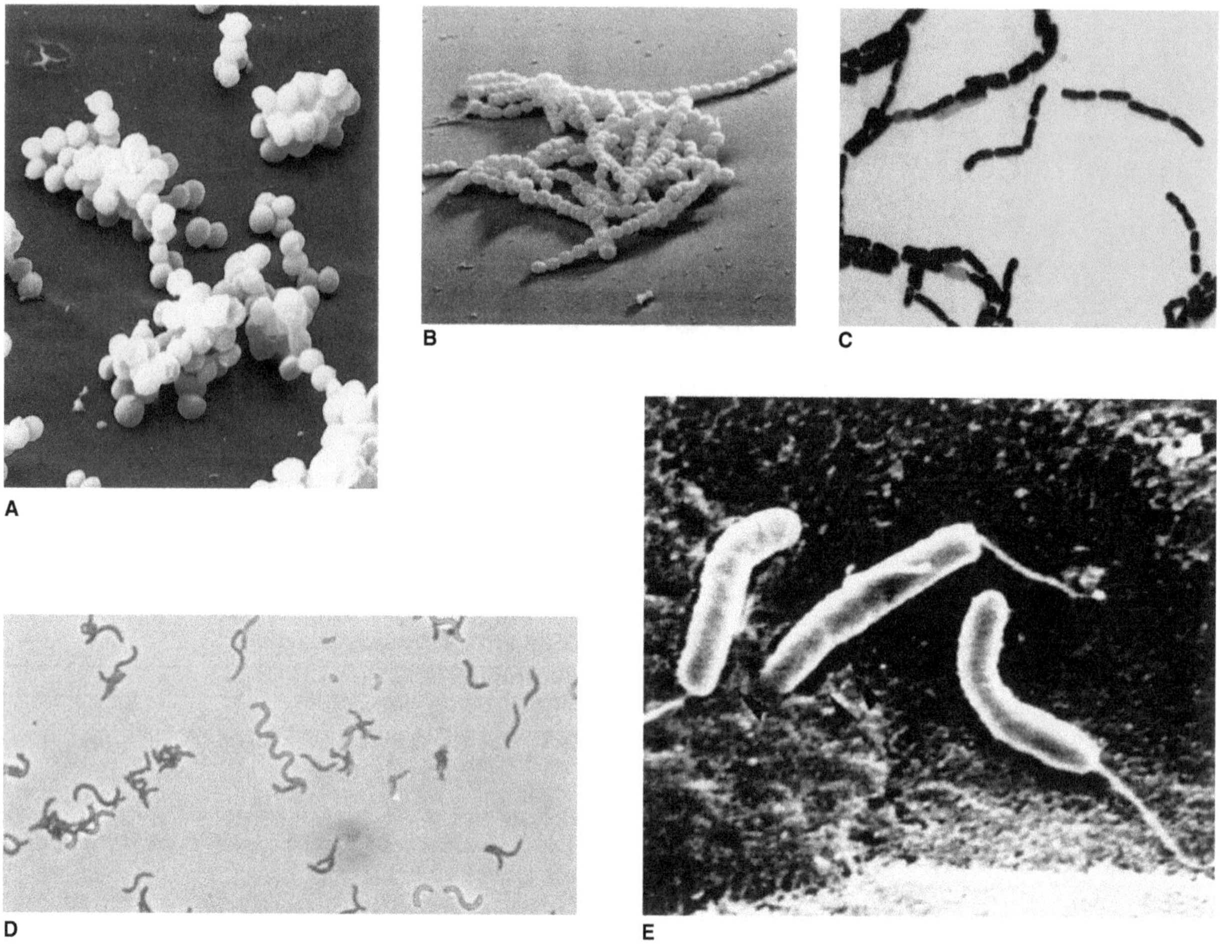

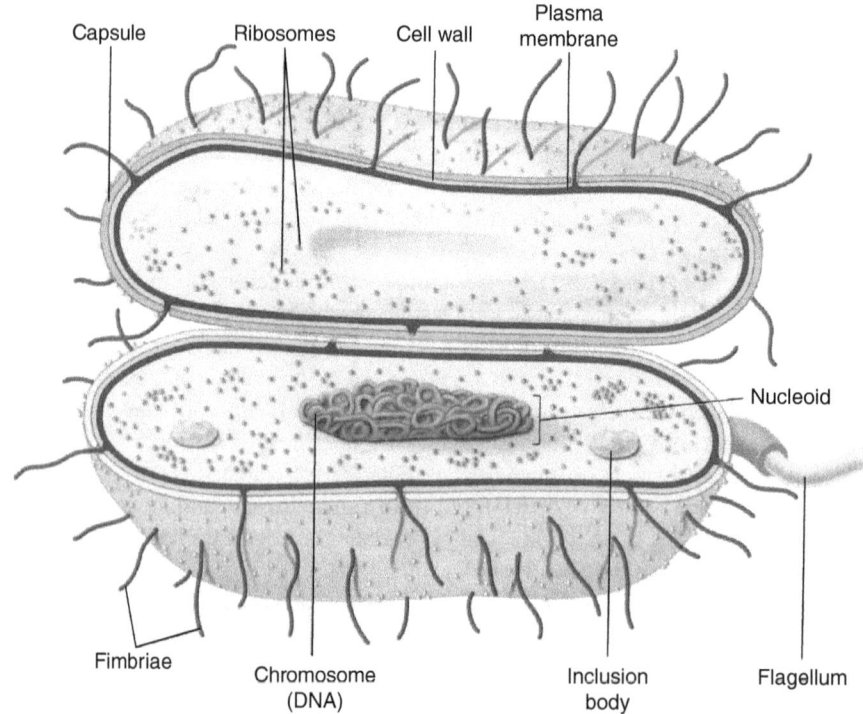

FIGURE 21-1. Shapes of bacteria. A. *Staphylococcus aureus,* cocci arranged in clusters; scanning electron micrograph (SEM). **B.** Group B streptococci, cocci arranged in chains; SEM. **C.** *Bacillus* species, straight rods; Gram stain. **D.** Spirochete, phase contrast, SEM. **E.** Vibrio, curved rods, SEM. (Reproduced with permission from Willey JM: *Prescott, Harley, & Klein's Microbiology,* 7th ed. New York, NY: McGraw Hill; 2008.)

FIGURE 21-2. The prokaryotic bacterial cell. (Reproduced with permission from Willey JM: *Prescott, Harley, & Klein's Microbiology,* 7th ed. New York, NY: McGraw Hill; 2008.)

Capsule   Ribosomes   Cell wall   Plasma membrane

Nucleoid

Fimbriae   Chromosome (DNA)   Inclusion body   Flagellum

ENVELOPE AND APPENDAGES

Bacteria have a very plain interior but a complex, even baroque, exterior. This can be readily understood by appreciating that the envelope not only protects the cell against chemical and biologic threats in its environment but is also the location for many metabolic processes that are the province of the internal organelles of eukaryotic cells. Structures in the envelope and certain appendages also mediate attachment to human cell surfaces, the first step in disease. Some of these features are presented in **Table 21–1** in relation to the major bacterial cell wall types.

Envelope and appendages carry out multiple functions

■ Capsule

Many bacterial cells surround themselves with some kind of hydrophilic gel. This layer is often thick; commonly it is thicker than the diameter of the cell. Because it is transparent and not readily stained, this layer is usually not appreciated unless made visible by its ability to exclude particulate material, such as India ink or Ruthenium Red, or by special capsular stains (**Figure 21–3**). If the material forms a reasonably discrete layer, it is called a **capsule;** if it is amorphous, it is referred to as a **slime layer.** Most capsules are **polysaccharide-rich,** consisting of single or multiple types of sugar residues; a few are simple polypeptides. Capsules provide some general protection for bacteria, but their major function in pathogenic bacteria is protection from the immune system attack.

✳ Hydrophilic capsules usually polysaccharides

✳ Protect from immune system

■ Cell Wall

Internal to the capsule (if one exists) but still outside the cell proper, a rigid **cell wall** surrounds all bacterial cells except wall-less bacteria such as the mycoplasmas and *Chlamydia* sp. The structure and function of the bacterial wall is a hallmark of the prokaryotes; nothing like it is found elsewhere. This wall protects the cell from mechanical disruption and from lysis caused by the turgor

TABLE 21–1	Components of Bacterial Cells			
		CELL WALL TYPE[a]		
STRUCTURE	**COMPOSITION**	**GRAM NEGATIVE**	**GRAM POSITIVE**	**NONE[b]**
Envelope				
Capsule (slime layer)	Polysaccharide or polypeptide	+ or −	+ or −	−
Wall		+	+	−
Outer membrane	Proteins, phospholipids, and lipopolysaccharide	+	−	−
Peptidoglycan layer	Peptidoglycan (+ teichoic acid in gram positive)	+	+[c]	−
Periplasm	Proteins and oligosaccharides in solution	+	−	−
Cell membrane	Proteins, phospholipids	+	+	+
Appendages				
Pili (fimbriae)	Protein (pilin)	+ or −	+ or −	−
Flagella	Proteins (flagellin plus others)	+ or −	+ or −	−
Core				
Cytosol	Polyribosomes, proteins, carbohydrates (glycogen)	+	+	+
Nucleoid	DNA with associated RNA and proteins	+	+	+
Plasmids	DNA	+ or −	+ or −	+ or −
Endospore				
	All cell components plus dipicolinate and special envelope components	−	+ or −	−

[a]"+" indicates that the structure is invariably present, "−" indicates it is invariably absent, and "+ or −" indicates that the structure is present in some species or strains and absent in others.
[b]Mycoplasma and *Ureaplasma*.
[c]In *Mycobacterium* complexed with mycolic acids and other lipids.

FIGURE 21-3. **Bacterial capsule.** This capsule surrounding the cells of *Klebsiella pneumoniae* has been stained red. (Reproduced with permission from Willey JM: *Prescott, Harley, & Klein's Microbiology*, 7th ed. New York, NY: McGraw Hill; 2008.)

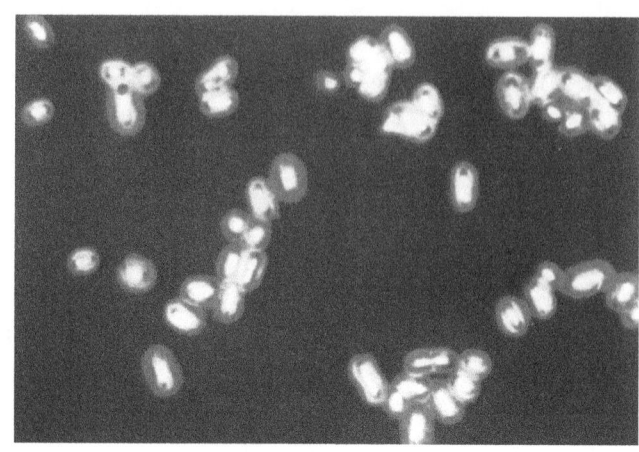

✳ Cell wall structure prevents osmotic lysis, determines the shape

pressure resulting from the hypertonicity of the cell interior relative to the environment. It also provides a barrier against certain toxic chemical and biologic agents. Its form is responsible for the shape of the cell. Overall, a well-constructed wall protects these minute, fragile cells from chemical and physical assault, while still permitting the rapid exchange of nutrients and metabolic byproducts required for rapid growth.

Bacterial evolution has led to two major solutions to cell wall structure. Although the detailed structural basis of the two is now well known, the separation derives from their reaction to the Gram stain (see Chapter 4). Virtually all bacteria with walls can now be assigned a Gram category even if they cannot be visualized with the stain itself for technical reasons. Examples include the causative agents of tuberculosis and syphilis. *Mycobacterium tuberculosis* (Gram positive) has lipids in its cell wall that resist the uptake of most stains. *Treponema pallidum* (Gram negative) stains poorly and is also too thin to be resolved in the light microscope without special illumination. In these cases, the Gram categorization is based on electron microscopy (**Figure 21-4**) and chemical analysis of the cell wall.

Poorly staining bacteria still have a Gram category

Gram-positive Cell Wall

The gram-positive cell wall contains two major components, peptidoglycan and teichoic acids, plus additional carbohydrates and proteins, depending on the species. A generalized scheme illustrating the arrangement of these components is shown in **Figure 21-5.** The chief component is

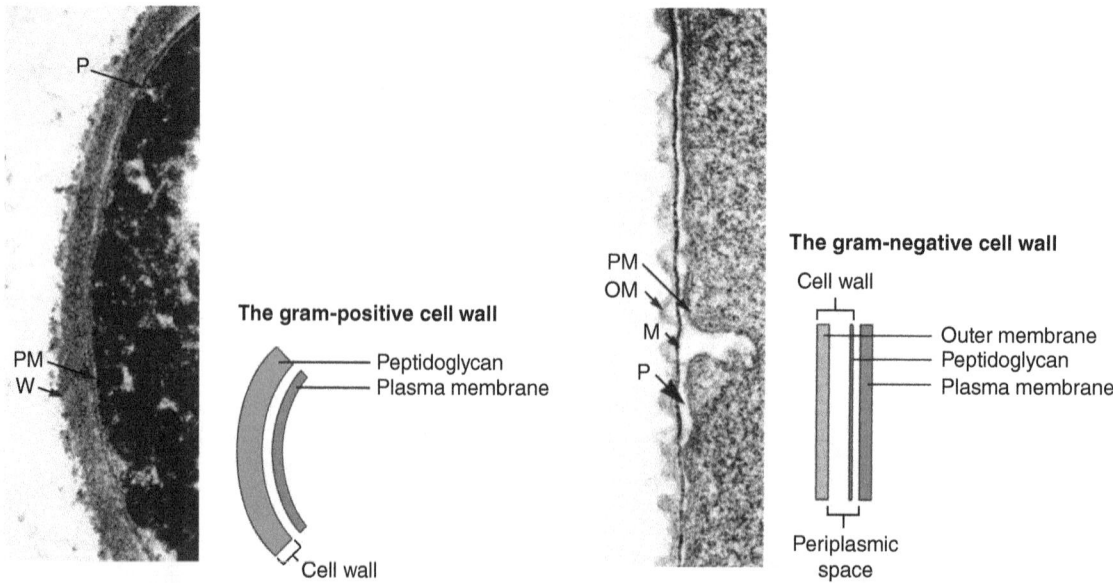

FIGURE 21-4. **Gram-positive and Gram-negative cell walls.** M, peptidoglycan or murein layer; OM, outer membrane; P, periplasmic space; PM, plasma membrane; W, Gram-positive peptidoglycan wall. (Reproduced with permission from Willey JM: *Prescott, Harley, & Klein's Microbiology*, 7th ed. New York, NY: McGraw Hill; 2008.)

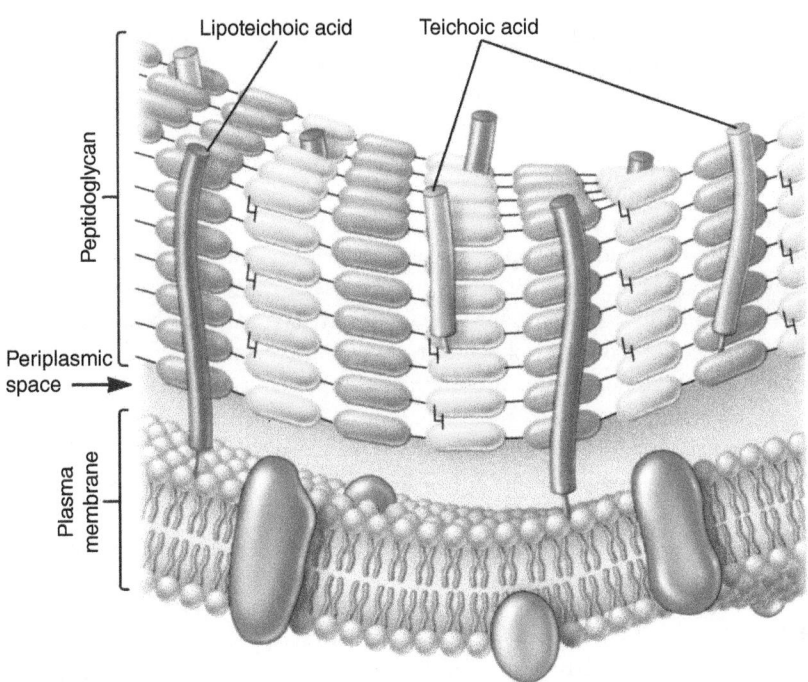

FIGURE 21-5. Gram-positive envelope. (Reproduced with permission from Willey JM: *Prescott, Harley, & Klein's Microbiology*, 7th ed. New York, NY: McGraw Hill; 2008.)

peptidoglycan, which is found only in prokaryotes. Peptidoglycan consists of a linear glycan chain of two alternating sugars, *N*-acetylglucosamine (NAG) and *N*-acetylmuramic acid (NAM) (**Figure 21–6**). Adjacent glycan chains are cross-linked into sheets by peptide bonds between peptide amino acid side chains. The same cross-links between other peptides connect the sheets to form a three-dimensional, rigid matrix. The cross-linking extends around the cell, producing a scaffold-like giant molecule. Peptidoglycan is much the same in all bacteria, except that there is diversity in the nature and frequency of the cross-linking bridge and in the nature of the amino acids at certain positions of the peptide.

The peptidoglycan sac derives its great mechanical strength from the fact that it is a single, covalently bonded structure. Most enzymes found in mammalian hosts and other biologic systems do not degrade peptidoglycan; one important exception is **lysozyme,** the hydrolase in tears and other secretions, which cleaves the bonds between muramic acid and glucosamine residues. The role of the peptidoglycan component of the cell wall in conferring osmotic resistance and shape on the cell is easily demonstrated by removing or destroying it. Treatment of a Gram-positive cell with penicillin (which blocks formation of the peptide cross-links) destroys the

Gram-positive walls have peptidoglycan, teichoic acid

✳ Peptidoglycan glycan chains cross-linked by peptide chains

Scaffold-like sac surrounds cell

Peptidoglycan components provide resistance to mammalian enzymes

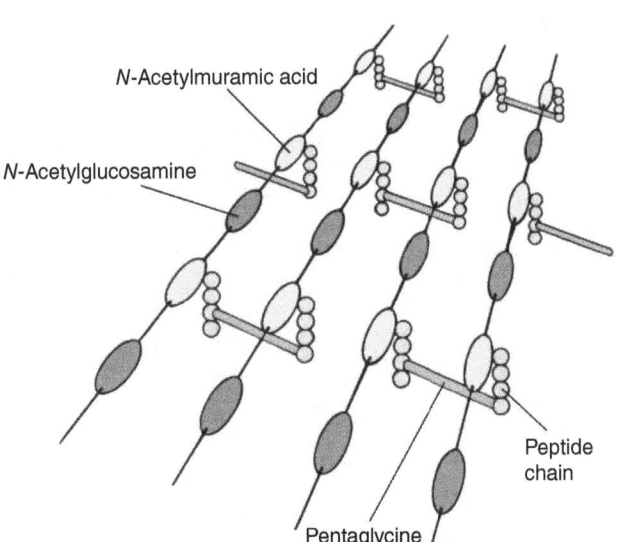

FIGURE 21–6. **Peptidoglycan structure.** A schematic diagram of one model of peptidoglycan. Shown are the polysaccharide chains, tetrapeptide side chains, and peptide bridges. (Reproduced with permission from Willey JM: *Prescott, Harley, & Klein's Microbiology*, 7th ed. New York, NY: McGraw Hill; 2008.)

* Loss of cell wall leads to lysis or protoplasts

peptidoglycan sac, and the wall is lost. Prompt lysis of the cell ensues. If the cell is protected from lysis by suspension in a medium approximately isotonic with the cell interior, the cell becomes round and forms a sphere called a **protoplast.**

A second component of the Gram-positive cell wall is **teichoic acid.** These compounds are polymers of either glycerol phosphate or ribitol phosphate, with various sugars, amino sugars, and amino acids as substituents. The lengths of the chain and the nature and location of the substituents vary from species to species and sometimes among strains within a species. A type of teichoic acid called **lipoteichoic acid** appears to play a role in anchoring the wall to the cell membrane and as an epithelial cell adhesin. Besides the major wall components—peptidoglycan and teichoic acids—Gram-positive walls usually contain diminished amounts of other molecules characteristic of their species. Some are polysaccharides, such as the group-specific antigens of streptococci; others are proteins, such as the M protein of group A streptococci.

* Teichoic and lipoteichoic acids promote adhesion and anchor wall to membrane

Other cell wall components related to species

Gram-negative Cell Wall

The second kind of cell wall found in bacteria, the Gram-negative cell wall, is depicted in **Figure 21–7.** Except for the presence of peptidoglycan, there is little chemical resemblance to cell walls of Gram-positive bacteria, and the architecture is fundamentally different. In Gram-negative cells, the amount of peptidoglycan has been greatly reduced, with some of it forming a single-layered sheet around the cell and the rest in a gel-like substance, the periplasm, with little cross-linking. External to this **periplasm** is an elaborate outer membrane. The proteins in solution in the periplasm consist of enzymes with hydrolytic functions, sometimes antibiotic-inactivating enzymes, and various proteins with roles in chemotaxis, transport, secretion, and surface-molecule anchoring.

* Thin peptidoglycan sac is imbedded in periplasmic gel

Periplasmic proteins have transport, chemotactic, hydrolytic roles

The periplasm is an intermembrane structure, lying between the cell membrane and a special membrane unique to Gram-negative cells, the **outer membrane.** This has an overall structure similar to most biologic membranes with two opposing phospholipid–protein leaflets. However, in terms of its chemical composition, the outer membrane is unique. Its inner leaflet consists of ordinary phospholipids, but these are replaced in the outer leaflet by a special molecule called **lipopolysaccharide,** which is extremely toxic to humans and other animals, and thus commonly

Gram-negative outer membrane is phospholipid-protein bilayer

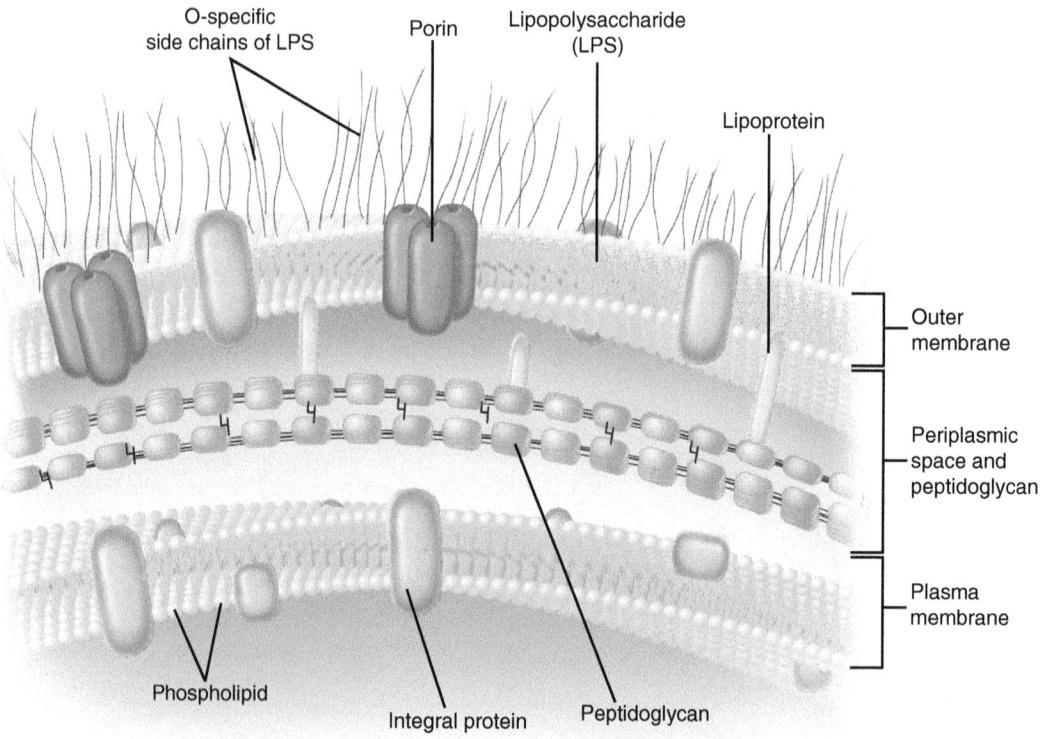

FIGURE 21–7. Gram-negative envelope. (Reproduced with permission from Willey JM: *Prescott, Harley, & Klein's Microbiology,* 7th ed. New York, NY: McGraw Hill; 2008.)

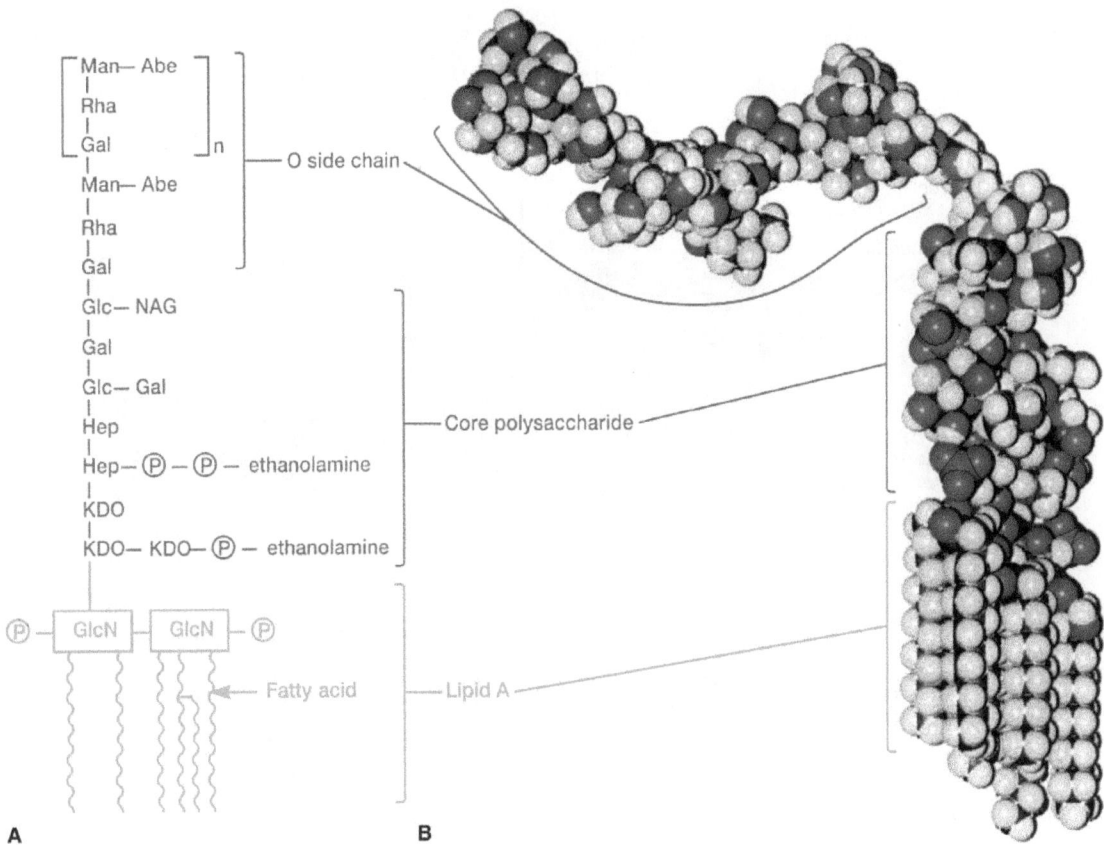

A

B

FIGURE 21–8. **Lipopolysaccharide structure. A.** O side chain—formed by linked sugars. Core polysaccharide—sugars linked to *N*-acetylglucosamine (NAG) and keto-deoxycholate (KDO). Lipid A—buried in the outer membrane. **B.** Molecular model. (Reproduced with permission from Willey JM: *Prescott, Harley, & Klein's Microbiology*, 7th ed. New York, NY: McGraw Hill; 2008.)

called **endotoxin.** Even in minute amounts, such as the amounts released to circulation during the course of a Gram-negative infection, this substance can produce a fever and shock syndrome called Gram-negative or **endotoxic shock.**

LPS consists of a toxic **lipid A** (a phospholipid-containing glucosamine rather than glycerol), a **core polysaccharide** (containing some unusual carbohydrate residues and fairly constant in structure among related species of bacteria), and **O antigen polysaccharide side chains** (**Figure 21-8A** and **B**). The last component constitutes the major surface antigen of Gram-negative cells.

The presence of the outer membrane results in the covering of Gram-negative cells that create a formidable permeability barrier. For whatever benefit is afforded by possessing a wall with an outer membrane, Gram-negative bacteria must make provision for the entry of nutrients. Special structural proteins, called **porins,** form pores through the outer membrane that makes it possible for hydrophilic solute molecules to diffuse through it and into the periplasm.

* Outer membrane leaflet contains LPS endotoxin

* Lipid A is the toxic moiety of LPS

* Impermeability of outer membrane overcome by porins

■ Cell Membrane

Generally, the cell (plasma) membrane of bacteria (**Figure 21-9**) is similar to the familiar bi-leaflet membrane of most cells, containing phospholipids and proteins, and which is found throughout the living world. However, there are important differences. The bacterial cell membrane is exceptionally rich in proteins and does not contain sterols (except mycoplasmas). The bacterial chromosome is attached to the cell membrane, which plays a role in the segregation of daughter chromosomes at cell division, analogous to the role of the mitotic apparatus of eukaryotes. The membrane is the site of synthesis of DNA, cell wall polymers, and membrane lipids. It contains the entire electron transport system of the cell (and, hence, is functionally analogous to the mitochondria of eukaryotes). It contains receptor proteins that function in chemotaxis. Similar to the cell membranes of eukaryotes, it is a permeability barrier and contains proteins involved in the selective and active transport of solutes. It is also involved in secretion to the exterior of proteins

Phospholipid–protein bilayer lacking sterols

* Roles in synthetic, homeostatic, secretory, and electron transport processes

FIGURE 21–9. Bacterial cell membrane. (Reproduced with permission from Willey JM: *Prescott, Harley, & Klein's Microbiology*, 7th ed. New York, NY: McGraw Hill; 2008.)

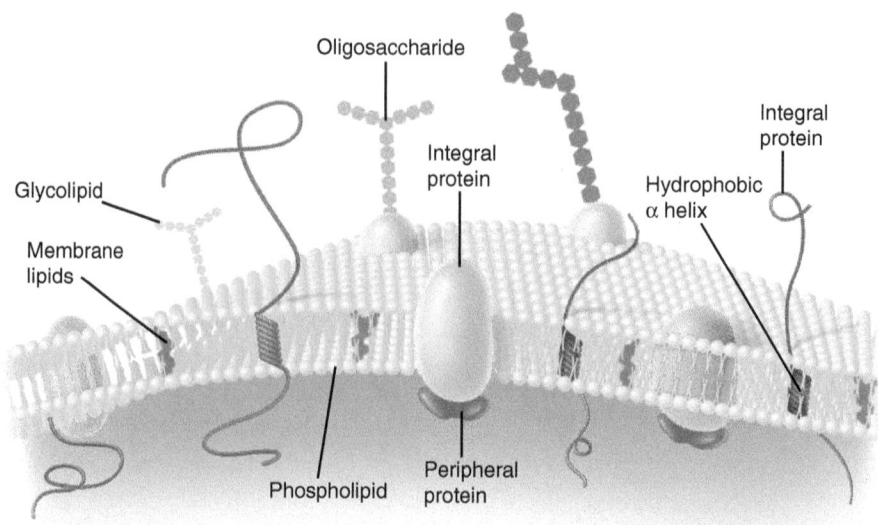

FIGURE 21–9. Bacterial cell membrane. (Reproduced with permission from Willey JM: *Prescott, Harley, & Klein's Microbiology*, 7th ed. New York, NY: McGraw Hill; 2008.)

including exotoxins and hydrolytic enzymes involved in the pathogenesis of disease. The bacterial cell membrane is therefore the functional equivalent of most of the organelles of the eukaryotic cell and is vital to the growth and maintenance of the cell.

Functional equivalent of eukaryotic organelles

■ Flagella

Flagella are molecular organelles of motility found in many species of bacteria, both Gram-positive and Gram-negative. These filamentous organelles may be distributed around the cell, at one pole or at both ends of the cell. Flagella propel the cell by rotating at the point of insertion in the cell envelope. Directionality is achieved via clockwise or counterclockwise rotation ("swimming" and "tumbling"), an energy-consuming process. The presence or absence of flagella and their cellular position (peritrichous, polar, bundled) are important taxonomic characteristics. The flagellar apparatus is complex but consists entirely of proteins attached to the cell by a basal body consisting of several proteins organized as rings on a central rod. Other structures include a hook that acts as a universal joint and ring-like bushings. Many flagella are "capped" by a unique protein that protects the organelle tip and controls filament length.

✳ **Flagella are rotating helical protein structures responsible for locomotion**

Have bushing rings in cell envelope

■ Pili

Pili (also called fimbriae) are hair-like projections found on the surface of cells of many Gram-positive and Gram-negative species. They are composed of molecules of a protein called **pilin** arranged to form a tube with a minute, hollow core. There are two general classes, common pili and sex pili (see Figure 21–33). Up to a thousand **common pili** cover the surface of the cell (**Figure 21–10**). They are, in many cases, adhesins, which are responsible for the ability of bacteria to colonize surfaces and cells. These processes are not always passive, since some pili can retract mediating movement across cell surfaces. Some pili are specialized for adherence to certain cell types such as enterocytes or uroepithelial cells. The same cell may have common and specialized pili. The **sex pilus** contributes to Gram-negative bacterial conjugation (exchange of genetic material) by potentiating cell-cell juxtaposition and DNA transfer.

Pili are tubular hair-like projections

Pili have adherence roles and can retract

✳ **Specialized pili mediate selective attachment or genetic transfer**

CORE

In contrast to the structural richness of the layers and appendages of the cell envelope, the interior appears relatively simple in transmission electron micrographs of thin sections of bacteria. There are two clearly visible regions, one granular (the cytoplasm) and one fibrous (the nucleoid).

■ Cytoplasm

The dense cytoplasm (cytosol) is bounded by the cell membrane. It appears granular because it is densely packed with ribosomes, which are much more abundant than in the cytoplasm

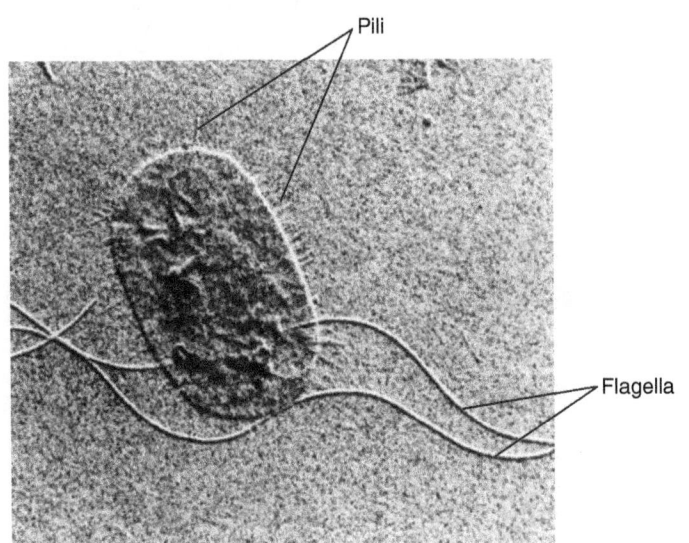

Pili

Flagella

FIGURE 21–10. Flagella and pili. The long flagella and numerous shorter pili are evident in this electron micrograph of *Proteus mirabilis.* (Reproduced with permission from Willey JM: *Prescott, Harley, & Klein's Microbiology,* 7th ed. New York, NY: McGraw Hill; 2008.)

of eukaryotic cells. This is a reflection of the higher growth rate of bacteria. Each ribosome is a ribonucleoprotein particle consisting of three species of rRNA and over 50 proteins. The overall subunit structure of the 70S bacterial ribosome resembles that of eukaryotic ribosomes, but is smaller and differs sufficiently in function that a very large number of antimicrobial agents have the prokaryotic ribosome as their target.

> ✳ Cytoplasm is packed with ribosomes

The bacterial cytoplasm has a **cytoskeleton** which localizes proteins, participates in cell division, and along with the cell wall peptidoglycan, gives shape to the cell. The bacterial cytoskeleton elements are chemical and structural homologs of the microfilaments, microtubules, and intermediate filaments of eukaryotic cells. In the bacterial cell, the microfilaments are made from **actin** and the microtubules from **tubulin.** Multiple counterparts of intermediate filaments are formed from a mixture of proteins, some of which are unique to bacteria. Modification of the cytoskeleton is a major mechanism of bacterial virulence.

> ✳ Actin, tubulin, intermediate filaments form cytoskeleton

Nucleoid

The nucleoid is a region of the cytoplasm which contains the genome and a collection of related proteins. The bacterial genome resides on a single chromosome and bacterial pathogens contain between 600 and 6000 genes encoded in one large, circular molecule of double-stranded DNA. This molecule is more than 1 mm long exceeding the length of the cell by about 1000 times. Tight packing displaces ribosomes and other cytosol components, creating regions that contain a chromosome, coated usually by polyamines and some specialized DNA-binding proteins. The double-helical DNA chain is twisted into supercoils and attached to the cell membrane and/or some central structure at a large number of points. The absence of a nuclear membrane confers on the prokaryotic cell a great advantage for rapid growth in changing environments. Ribosomes can be translating mRNA molecules even as the latter are being made; this is called "coupled transcription-translation" and is unique to bacteria. Importantly, this implies that no transport of the mRNA is required from sites of synthesis to those of function.

> ✳ Circular chromosome of supercoiled double-stranded DNA
>
> **No mRNA transport required**

Plasmids

Many bacteria contain small, usually circular, covalently closed, double-stranded DNA molecules, invariably separate from the chromosome ("extra-chromosomal"). Individual species have regulatory systems controlling plasmids, and more than one type or multiple copies (more than 100) of a single plasmid may be present in the same cell. Plasmids typically contain up to 30 genes and replicate independent of the chromosome. They are unlikely to contain genes essential for survival of the cell but may have specialized genes such as those mediating virulence or resistance to antimicrobial agents. In fact, many attributes of virulence, including production of pili and exotoxins, and the complex apparatus for the myriad secretion systems elaborated by bacteria, may be plasmid-encoded.

> ✳ Plasmids are small, circular, double-stranded DNA molecules
>
> **Virulence and resistance genes are present**

SPORES

Endospores, commonly called **spores,** are small, dehydrated, metabolically quiescent morphotypes that are produced by some bacteria in response to nutrient limitation or a related signal that tough times are coming. Very few species produce spores but they are invariably Gram-positive, and prevalent in the environment. Some spore-forming bacteria are of great importance in medicine, causing such diseases as anthrax, gas gangrene, tetanus, and botulism. All medically important spore-formers are Gram-positive rods. The bacterial endospore is not a reproductive structure. One cell forms one spore under adverse conditions in a process called **sporulation.** The spore may persist for a long time (centuries) and then, on appropriate stimulation, germinates into a single vegetative bacterial cell. Spores, therefore, are survival rather than reproductive forms.

Spores of some species can withstand extremes of pH and temperature, including boiling water and disinfectants, for surprising periods of time. The thermal resistance is brought about by the low water content and the presence of a large amount of a substance found only in spores, **calcium dipicolinate.** Resistance to chemicals and, to some extent, radiation, is aided by extremely tough, special coats (cortex) surrounding the spore.

The molecular process by which a cell produces a highly differentiated product that is incapable of immediate growth but is able to sustain growth after prolonged periods of nongrowth under extreme conditions of heat, desiccation, and starvation is of great interest. In general, the process involves the initial walling-off of a nucleoid and its surrounding cytosol by invagination of the cell membrane, with later additions of special spore layers (**Figure 21–11**). Thus, the spore develops inside the "mother cell." This entire cell fate decision is made at the end of the bacterial rapid growth phase (logarithmic growth) and is exquisitely controlled by multiple, hierarchical molecular signals and signaling proteins.

Germination begins with activation by heat, acid, reducing conditions, or small molecules. Following a massive influx of water into the spore, the interior is hydrated, and prepackaged proteins are able to recommence function. Completion of germination eventually leads to the outgrowth of a new vegetative cell of the same genotype as the cell that produced the spore.

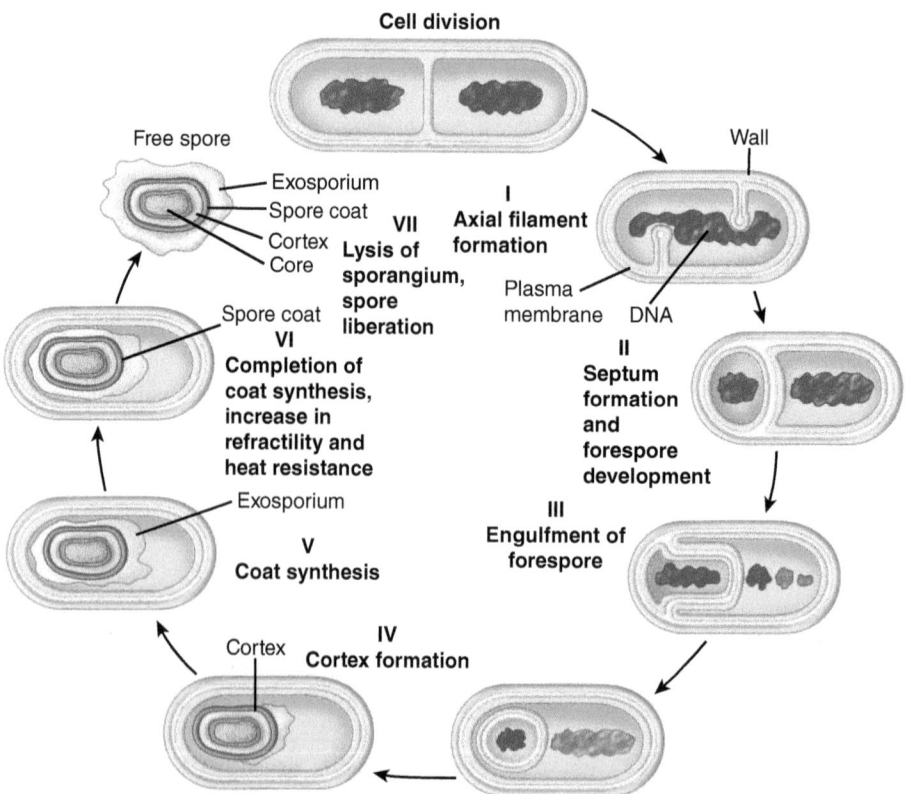

FIGURE 21–11. Stages of bacterial spore formation. (Reproduced with permission from Willey JM: *Prescott, Harley, & Klein's Microbiology*, 7th ed. New York, NY: McGraw Hill; 2008.)

KEY CONCLUSIONS

KEY CONCLUSIONS

- The prokaryotic bacterial cell plan is simple, unique, and facilitates very rapid growth.
- Cell wall rigidity is provided by peptidoglycan, a polymer of sugars molecules and peptides cross-linked by transpeptidases.
- In addition to peptidoglycan, Gram-negative bacteria have an outer membrane containing proteins, porins, and LPS endotoxin.
- Polysaccharide capsules provide protection from immune responses.
- Filamentous flagella are organelles of locomotion.
- Hair-like pili mediate attachment to human cells.
- The cell membrane is a site for metabolic activity like the eukaryotic cell mitochondria.
- The cytoplasm is packed with ribosomes and contains a single double-stranded DNA chromosome.
- Plasmids are small DNA units replicating independent of the chromosome.
- Spores are dehydrated survival forms which may germinate to metabolically active vegetative cells.

● BACTERIAL GROWTH AND METABOLISM

Growth of bacteria is accomplished by an orderly progress of metabolic processes followed by cell division by binary fission. This requires metabolism, which produces cell material from the nutrient substances in the environment; regulation, which coordinates the progress of the hundreds of independent biochemical processes in an orderly way; and, finally, cell division, which produces two independent living units from one.

Growth requires metabolism, regulation, and division by binary fission

BACTERIAL METABOLISM

Many of the principles of metabolism are universal. This section focuses on the unique aspects of bacterial metabolism that are important in medicine. The need to compare bacterial and mammalian pathways is muted by the fact that much of what we understand about human metabolism is derived from work with *Escherichia coli*. The broad differences between bacteria and human eukaryotic cells can be summarized as follows:

Speed. Bacteria metabolize at a rate 10 to 100 times faster.

Versatility. Bacteria use more varied compounds as energy sources and are much more diverse in their nutritional requirements.

Simplicity. The prokaryotic body plan makes it possible for bacteria to synthesize macromolecules in a streamlined way.

Uniqueness. Some biosynthetic processes, such as those producing peptidoglycan, LPS, and toxins, are unique to bacteria.

Bacterial metabolism is highly complex. The bacterial cell synthesizes itself and generates energy by as many as 2000 chemical reactions. These reactions can be classified according to their function in the metabolic processes of fueling, biosynthesis, polymerization, and assembly.

■ Fueling Reactions

Fueling reactions provide the cell with energy and with precursor metabolites used in biosynthetic reactions (**Figure 21–12**). The first step is the capture of nutrients from the environment. Other than water, oxygen, and carbon dioxide, almost no important nutrients enter the cell by **simple diffusion** because the cell membrane is too effective a barrier. Some transport occurs by **facilitated diffusion** in which a protein carrier in the cell membrane, specific for a given compound, participates in the shuttling of molecules of that substance from one side of the membrane to the other (**Figure 21–13A and B**). Because no energy is involved, this process can work only with, never against, a concentration gradient of the given solute.

Active transport mechanisms involve specific protein molecules as carriers of particular solutes, but the process is energy linked and can therefore establish a concentration gradient. That is, active transport can pump "uphill." Bacteria have multiple systems of active transport, some of

Substrates enter despite permeability barriers

✳ Facilitated diffusion involves shuttling by carrier protein

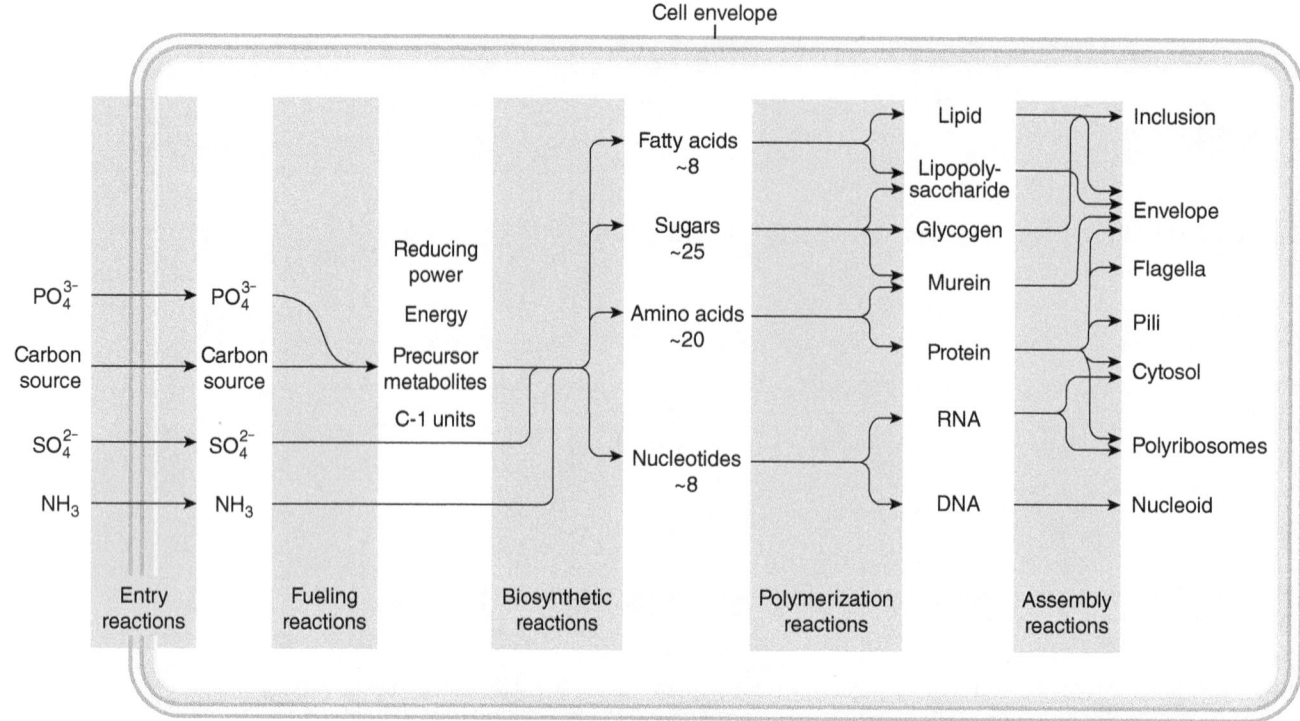

FIGURE 21–12. Bacterial metabolism. General pattern of metabolism leading to the synthesis of a bacterial cell from glucose.

※ Active transport involves binding proteins and ATP

Bacterial siderophores chelate iron and are actively transported into cell

Central fueling pathways produce biosynthetic precursors

※ Fermentation and respiration pathways each regenerate ATP and NAD⁺

which involve ATP-dependent binding proteins (**Figure 21–14**) and others that require proton pumps driven by electron transport within the energized cell membrane.

The transport of iron is of particular importance in virulence. There is little free Fe^{3+} in human blood or other body fluids, because it is sequestered by iron-binding proteins (eg, **transferrin** in blood and **lactoferrin** in secretions). Bacteria must have iron to grow, and their colonization of the human host requires capture of iron. Bacteria secrete **siderophores** (iron-specific chelators) to trap Fe^{3+}; the iron-containing chelator is then transported into the bacterium by specific active transport.

Once inside the cell, sugar molecules or other sources of carbon and energy are metabolized by the Embden–Meyerhof glycolytic pathway, the pentose phosphate pathway, and the Krebs cycle to yield the carbon compounds needed for biosynthesis.

Working in concert, the central fueling pathways produce the precursor metabolites. Connections to **fermentation** and **respiration** pathways allow the reoxidation of reduced coenzyme nicotinamide adenine dinucleotide (NAD) to NAD⁺ and the generation of ATP. Bacteria make ATP

FIGURE 21–13. **Facilitated diffusion. A.** The membrane carrier can change conformation after binding an external molecule and subsequently releasing the molecule to the cell interior. **B.** It then returns to the outward oriented position and is ready to bind another solute molecule. Because there is no energy input, molecules continue to enter only as long as their concentration is greater on the outside. (Reproduced with permission from Willey JM: *Prescott, Harley, & Klein's Microbiology,* 7th ed. New York, NY: McGraw Hill; 2008.)

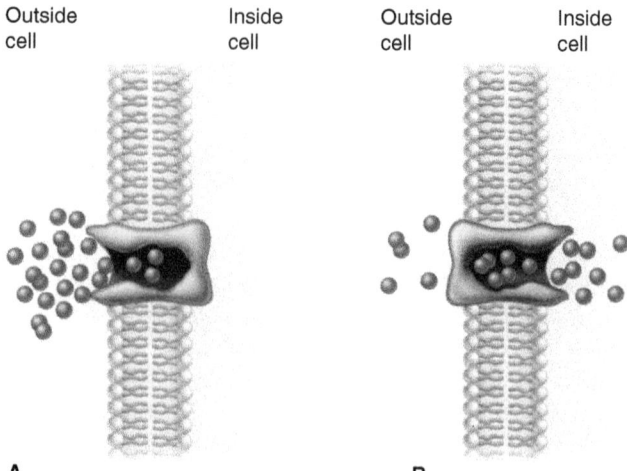

A   B

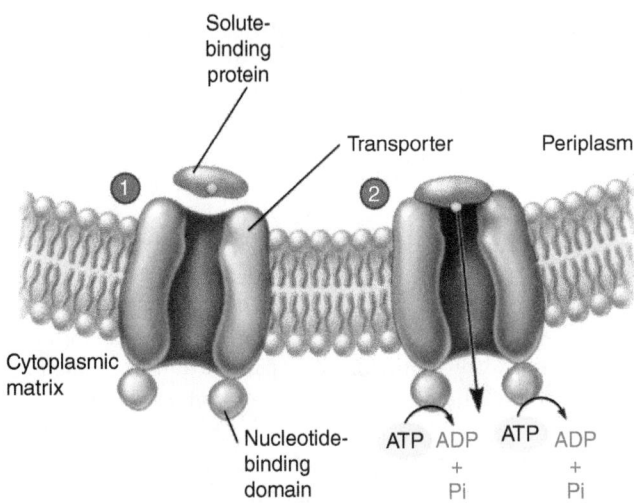

Solute-binding protein

Transporter

Periplasm

Cytoplasmic matrix

Nucleotide-binding domain

ATP   ADP + Pi   ATP   ADP + Pi

FIGURE 21–14. Active transport. 1. The solute-binding protein binds the substrate to be transported and approaches the transporter complex. **2.** The solute binding which is moved across the membrane with the aid of ATP hydrolysis. (Reproduced with permission from Willey JM: *Prescott, Harley, & Klein's Microbiology*, 7th ed. New York, NY: McGraw Hill; 2008.)

by substrate phosphorylation in fermentation or by a combination of substrate phosphorylation and oxidative phosphorylation in respiration.

Fermentation is the transfer of electrons and protons via NAD$^+$ directly to an organic acceptor. Pyruvate occupies a pivotal role in fermentation (**Figure 21–15**). Fermentation is an inefficient way to generate ATP, and consequently huge amounts of sugar must be fermented to satisfy the growth requirements of bacteria anaerobically. Large amounts of organic acids and alcohols are produced in fermentation. Which compounds are produced depends on the particular pathway of fermentation used by a given species, and therefore the profile of fermentation products is a diagnostic aid in the clinical laboratory.

Respiration involves fueling pathways in which substrate oxidation is coupled to the transport of electrons through a chain of carriers to some ultimate acceptor, which is frequently, but not

Fermentation involves direct transfer of proton and electron to organic acceptor

ATP-generating efficiency is low

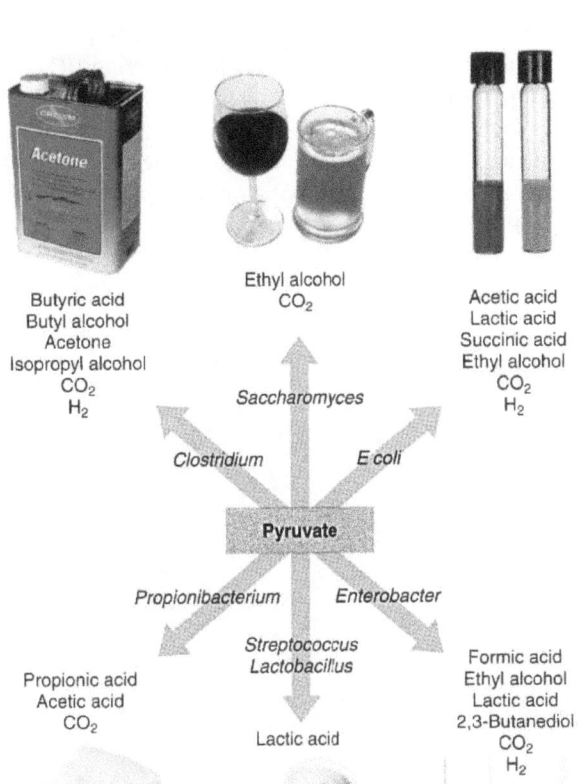

Butyric acid
Butyl alcohol
Acetone
Isopropyl alcohol
CO_2
H_2

Ethyl alcohol
CO_2

Acetic acid
Lactic acid
Succinic acid
Ethyl alcohol
CO_2
H_2

Saccharomyces

Clostridium   *E coli*

Pyruvate

Propionibacterium   *Enterobacter*

Streptococcus
Lactobacillus

Propionic acid
Acetic acid
CO_2

Lactic acid

Formic acid
Ethyl alcohol
Lactic acid
2,3-Butanediol
CO_2
H_2

FIGURE 21–15. End products of fermentation pathways. Because a given type of organism uses a characteristic fermentation pathway, the end products can also be used as an identifying marker. (Reproduced with permission from Nester EW, Anderson DG, Roberts CE Jr, et al: *Microbiology: A Human Perspective*, 6th ed. New York, NY: McGraw Hill; 2008.)

always, molecular oxygen. Other inorganic (eg, nitrate) as well as organic compounds (eg, succinate) can serve as the final electron acceptor, and therefore many organisms that cannot ferment can live in the absence of oxygen. Respiration is an efficient generator of ATP. Respiration in prokaryotes as in eukaryotes occurs by membrane-bound enzymes, but in prokaryotes the cell membrane rather than mitochondrial membranes provide the physical site.

■ Aerobes and Anaerobes

In evolving to colonize every conceivable nook and cranny on this planet, bacteria have developed distinctive responses to oxygen. Bacteria are conveniently classified according to their fermentative and respiratory activities but much more generally by their overall response to the presence of oxygen. The response depends not only on their genetic ability to ferment or respire but also on their ability to protect themselves from the deleterious effects of oxygen.

Oxygen, though itself only mildly toxic, gives rise to at least two extremely reactive and toxic substances, **hydrogen peroxide** (H_2O_2) and the **superoxide anion** (O^{2-}). Peroxide is produced by reactions in which electrons and protons are transferred to O_2 as the final acceptor. The superoxide radical is produced as an intermediate in most reactions that reduce molecular O_2. Superoxide is partially detoxified by an enzyme, **superoxide dismutase,** found in all organisms (prokaryotes and eukaryotes) that survive the presence of oxygen. Bacteria that lack the ability to make superoxide dismutase and catalase are exquisitely sensitive to the presence of molecular oxygen and, in general, must grow anaerobically using fermentation. Bacteria that possess these protective enzymes can grow in the presence of oxygen, but whether they use oxygen in metabolism or not depends on their ability to respire. Whether these oxygen-resistant bacteria can grow anaerobically depends on their ability to ferment.

Various combinations of these two characteristics (oxygen resistance and the ability to use molecular oxygen as a final acceptor) are represented in different species of bacteria, resulting in the four general classes shown in **Table 21–2. Aerobes** require oxygen and metabolize by respiration. **Anaerobes** are inhibited or killed by oxygen and utilize fermentation exclusively. **Facultative** bacteria (the majority of pathogens) grow well under aerobic or anaerobic conditions. If oxygen is available they respire, if not they use fermentation. Some facultative bacteria ferment even if oxygen is available. **Microaerophilic** bacteria sit in the middle requiring 5% to 10% oxygen for optimal growth. There are important pathogens within each class. Although most anaerobes in the microbial world strictly follow the criteria in Table 21–2, many of the pathogenic anaerobes are in fact moderately aerotolerant and possess low levels of superoxide dismutase and peroxidases. Although they prefer anaerobic growth conditions, this allows them to survive the brief exposure to oxygen that is inherent to initiating disease.

TABLE 21–2	Classification of Bacteria by Response to Oxygen				
	GROWTH RESPONSE				
TYPE OF BACTERIA	**AEROBIC**	**ANAEROBIC**	**POSSESSION OF CATALASE AND SUPEROXIDE DISMUTASE**	**COMMENT**	**EXAMPLE**
Aerobe	+	−	+	Requires O_2; cannot ferment	*Mycobacterium tuberculosis, Pseudomonas aeruginosa, Bacillus anthracis*
Anaerobe	−	+	−[a]	Killed by O_2; ferments in absence of O_2	*Clostridium botulinum, Bacteroides melaninogenicus*
Facultative	+	+	+	Respires with O_2; ferments in absence of O_2[c]	*Escherichia coli, Shigella dysenteriae, Staphylococcus aureus*
Microaerophilic	+[b]	+[b]	+	Grows best at low O_2 concentration; can grow without O_2	*Campylobacter jejuni*

[a]Many pathogenic anaerobes produce catalase and/or superoxide dismutase.
[b]Optimal growth at 5% to 10% O_2.
[c]Some ferment in the presence or absence of O_2.

■ Biosynthesis

Biosynthetic reactions form a network of pathways that lead from precursor metabolites (provided by the fueling reactions) to the many amino acids, nucleotides, sugars, amino sugars, fatty acids, and other building blocks needed for macromolecules (Figure 21–12). In addition to the carbon precursors, large quantities of reduced nicotinamide adenine dinucleotide phosphate (NADPH), ATP, amino nitrogen, and some source of sulfur are needed for biosynthesis of these building blocks. These pathways are similar in all species of living things, but bacterial species differ greatly as to which pathways they possess. Because all cells require the same building blocks, those that cannot be produced by a given cell must be obtained preformed from the environment.

There are relatively few biosynthetic pathways that are unique to bacteria, but some form a basis for bacterial vulnerability or bacterial pathogenicity. Because bacteria must synthesize folic acid rather than use it preformed from their environment, inhibition of those pathways is the basis of the antibacterial action of sulfonamides and trimethoprim. Catalyzing ADP-ribosylation (**Figure 21–16**), a unique enzymatic reaction, is the mechanism of action of multiple bacterial toxins including diphtheria toxin (DT) and cholera toxin (CT). To accomplish this, the active unit of the toxin binds both NAD from body fluids and its target protein. This catalyzes the transfer of an ADP-ribose group to the protein rendering it inactive. The biologic outcome of this inactivation depends on the function of the target protein. If it is crucial for a process like protein synthesis the result is cell death. If it is a regulatory protein, the process it controls may be up- or downregulated.

■ Polymerization Reactions

Polymerization of DNA is called **replication.** Replication always begins at special sites on the chromosome and then precedes bidirectionally around the circular chromosome (**Figure 21–17**). Some chemotherapeutic agents derive their selective toxicity for bacteria from the unique features of prokaryotic DNA replication. The synthetic quinolone compounds inhibit DNA gyrase, one of the many enzymes participating in DNA replication.

Transcription is the synthesis of RNA. Transcription in bacteria differs from that in eukaryotic cells in several ways. One difference is that all forms of bacterial RNA (mRNA, tRNA, and rRNA) are synthesized by the same enzyme, **RNA polymerase.** RNA polymerase is a large, complicated molecule that locates specific DNA sequences, called promoters, which precede all transcriptional units. Remarkably, bacterial mRNA is synthesized, used, and degraded, all in a matter of a few minutes. Bacterial RNA polymerase is the target of the antimicrobial **rifampin,** which blocks the initiation of transcription.

Translation is the name given to protein synthesis. Bacteria activate the 20 amino acid building blocks of protein in the course of attaching them to specific transfer RNA molecules.

Biosynthesis requires precursor metabolites, energy, amino nitrogen, sulfur, and reducing power

Nutritional requirements differ depending on synthetic ability

Few pathways are unique to bacteria

✳ ADP-ribosylation is the action of multiple toxins

Bidirectional, semiconservative replication occurs at replication forks

Bidirectional, replication occurs at replication forks

DNA gyrase inhibitors selectively toxic for bacteria

✳ Single RNA polymerase makes all forms of bacterial RNA

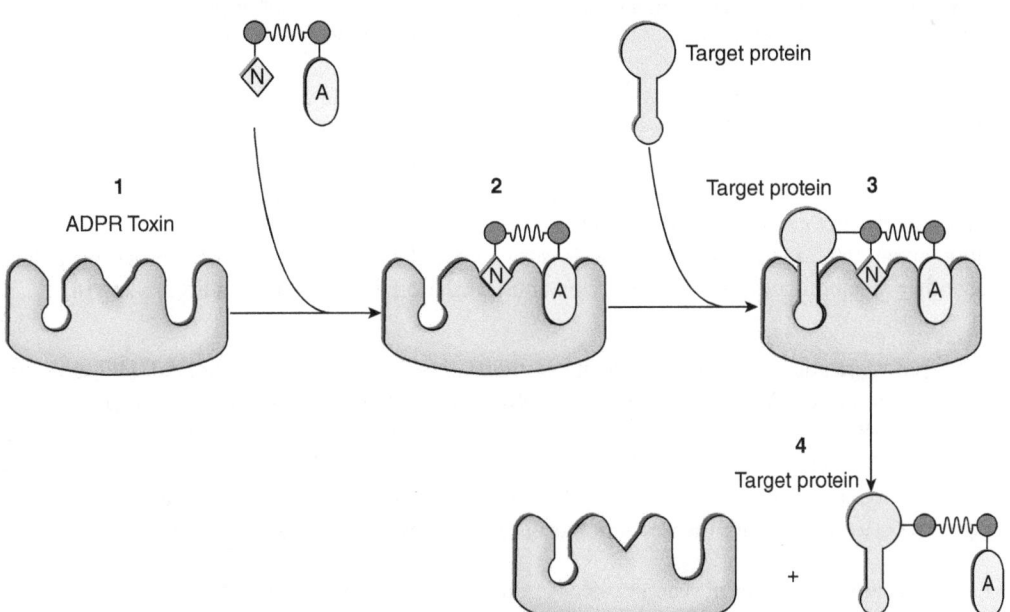

FIGURE 21–16. ADP-ribosylation (ADPR). 1. The active toxin unit binds NAD that is present in fluids. **2.** The toxin also binds a cell protein, its target protein. **3.** An ADP-ribose group is transferred to the protein rendering it inactive. **4.** The toxin is released free to repeat the process.

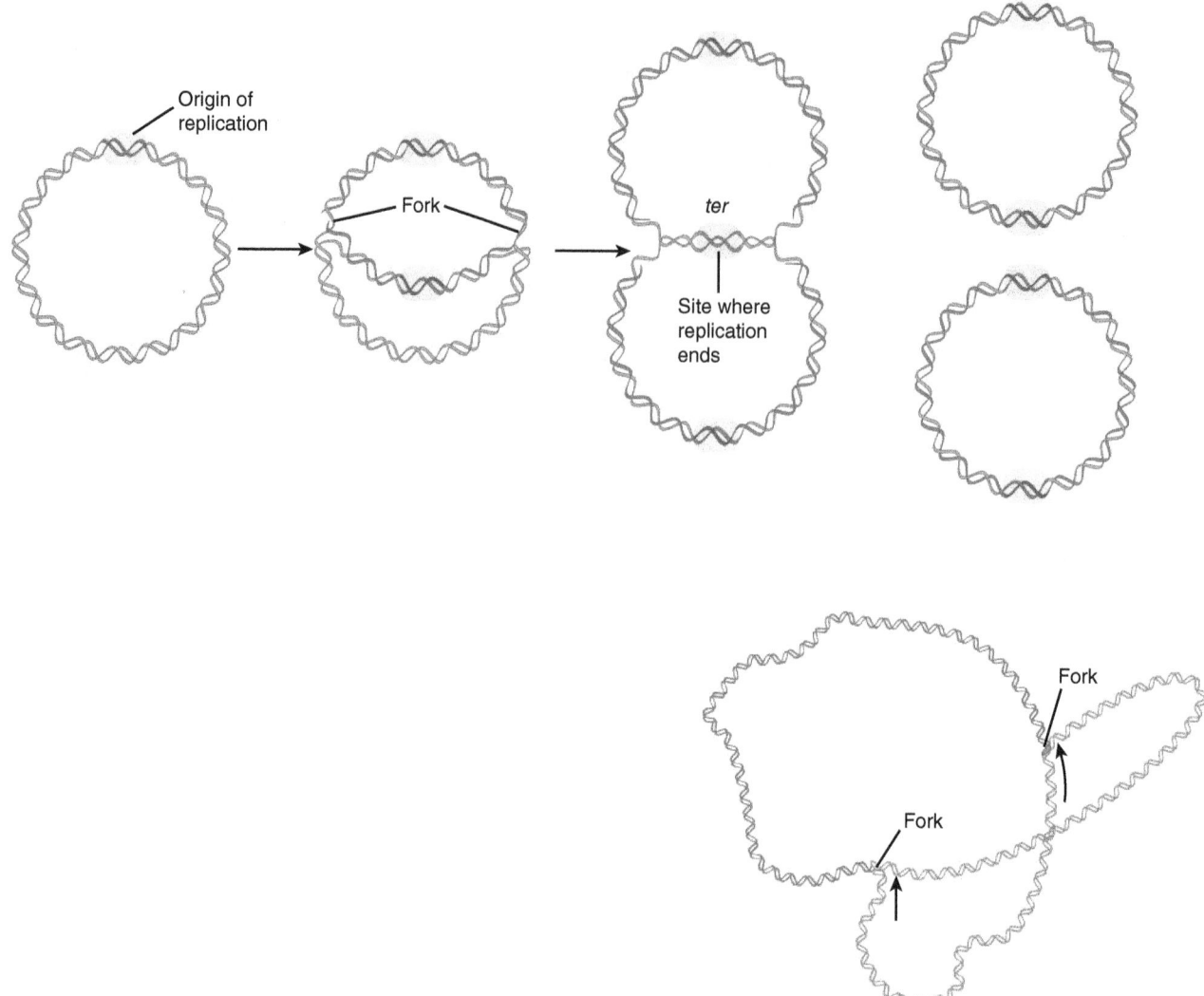

FIGURE 21–17. DNA replication in bacteria. Replication begins at the origin of replication. Two replication forks proceed in opposite directions until they meet at the replication termination site (*ter*). (Reproduced with permission from Willey JM: *Prescott, Harley, & Klein's Microbiology*, 7th ed. New York, NY: McGraw Hill; 2008.)

Amino acid residues polymerized from specific tRNAs

Antimicrobials act on translation machinery

mRNA translation simultaneous with transcription

The aminoacyl-tRNAs are brought to the ribosomes by soluble protein factors, and there the amino acids are polymerized into polypeptide chains according to the sequence of codons in the particular mRNA that is being translated. Having donated its amino acid, the tRNA is released from the ribosome to return for another aminoacylation cycle. Many antimicrobial agents derive their selective toxicity for bacteria from the unique features and proteins of the prokaryotic translation apparatus. In fact, protein synthesis is the target of a greater variety of antimicrobials than any other metabolic process. Transcription and translation are illustrated in **Figure 21–18.**

Peptidoglycan Synthesis

Other polymerization reactions involve the synthesis of peptidoglycan, phospholipid, LPS, and capsular polysaccharide. All of these reactions involve activated building blocks that are polymerized or assembled within or on the exterior surface of the cytoplasmic membrane. The most unique of these is the **peptidoglycan,** which is completely absent from eukaryotic cells. Peptidoglycan synthesis takes place in three compartments of the cell. The steps involved are summarized below and illustrated in **Figure 21–19** together with the attack points of some antimicrobials that block steps in the process.

1. **In the cytosol,** a series of reactions leads to the synthesis, on a nucleotide carrier (UDP), of an *N*-acetylmuramic acid (NAM) residue bearing a pentapeptide.

2. This precursor is then attached, with the release of UMP, to a special lipid-like carrier in the cell membrane called **bactoprenol.** Within the cell membrane, *N*-acetylglucosamine (NAG)

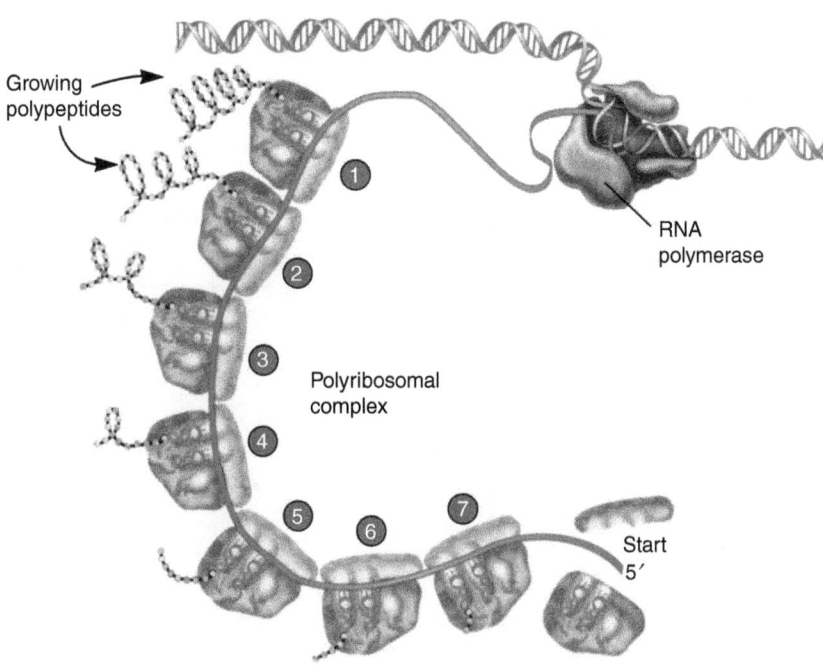

Growing
polypeptides

RNA
polymerase

①

②

③

Polyribosomal
complex

④

⑤ ⑥ ⑦

Start
5′

FIGURE 21–18. **Coupling of transcription and translation in bacteria.** As the DNA is transcribed, ribosomes bind the free 5′ end of the mRNA. Thus, translation is started before transcription is completed. Note multiple ribosomes are bound to the mRNA, forming a polyribosome. (Reproduced with permission from Willey JM: *Prescott, Harley, & Klein's Microbiology*, 7th ed. New York, NY: McGraw Hill; 2008.)

① UDP derivatives of NAM and NAG are synthesized (not shown).

② Sequential addition of amino acids to UDP-NAM to form the NAM-pentapeptide. ATP is used to fuel this, but tRNA and ribosomes are not involved in forming the peptide bonds that link the amino acids together.

③ NAM-pentapeptide is transferred to bactoprenol phosphate. They are joined by a pyrophosphate bond.

④ UDP transfers NAG to the bactoprenol-NAM-pentapeptide. If a pentaglycine interbridge is required, it is created using special glycyl-tRNA molecules, but not ribosomes. Interbridge formation occurs in the membrane.

⑤ The bactoprenol carrier transports the completed NAG-NAM-pentapeptide repeat unit across the membrane.

UDP — NAM
│
L-Ala
↓
D-Glu
↓
② L-Lys (DAP)
↓
D-Ala — D-Ala

L-Ala
⊖
↓
D-Ala
⊖   Cycloserine

Lipid I   UDP — NAG   **Lipid II**

Pentapeptide   Pentapeptide

Ⓟ Ⓟ — NAM   Ⓟ Ⓟ — NAM — NAG

Cytoplasm

UDP — NAM — pentapeptide
Ⓟ
│   UMP
③

Bactoprenol   →   Bactoprenol   →   Bactoprenol

Pᵢ

④   UDP

Membrane

Bacitracin

⑦   ⑤

Bactoprenol   Bactoprenol

Periplasm

Ⓟ Ⓟ   Ⓟ Ⓟ — NAM — NAG

Peptidoglycan — NAM — NAG   Peptidoglycan   Pentapeptide

Pentapeptide   ⊖   Vancomycin
⑥

⑧ Peptide cross-links between peptidoglycan chains are formed by transpeptidation (not shown).

⑦ The bactoprenol carrier moves back across the membrane. As it does, it loses one phosphate, becoming bactoprenol phosphate. It is now ready to begin a new cycle.

⑥ The NAG-NAM-pentapeptide is attached to the growing end of a peptidoglycan chain, increasing the chain's length by one repeat unit.

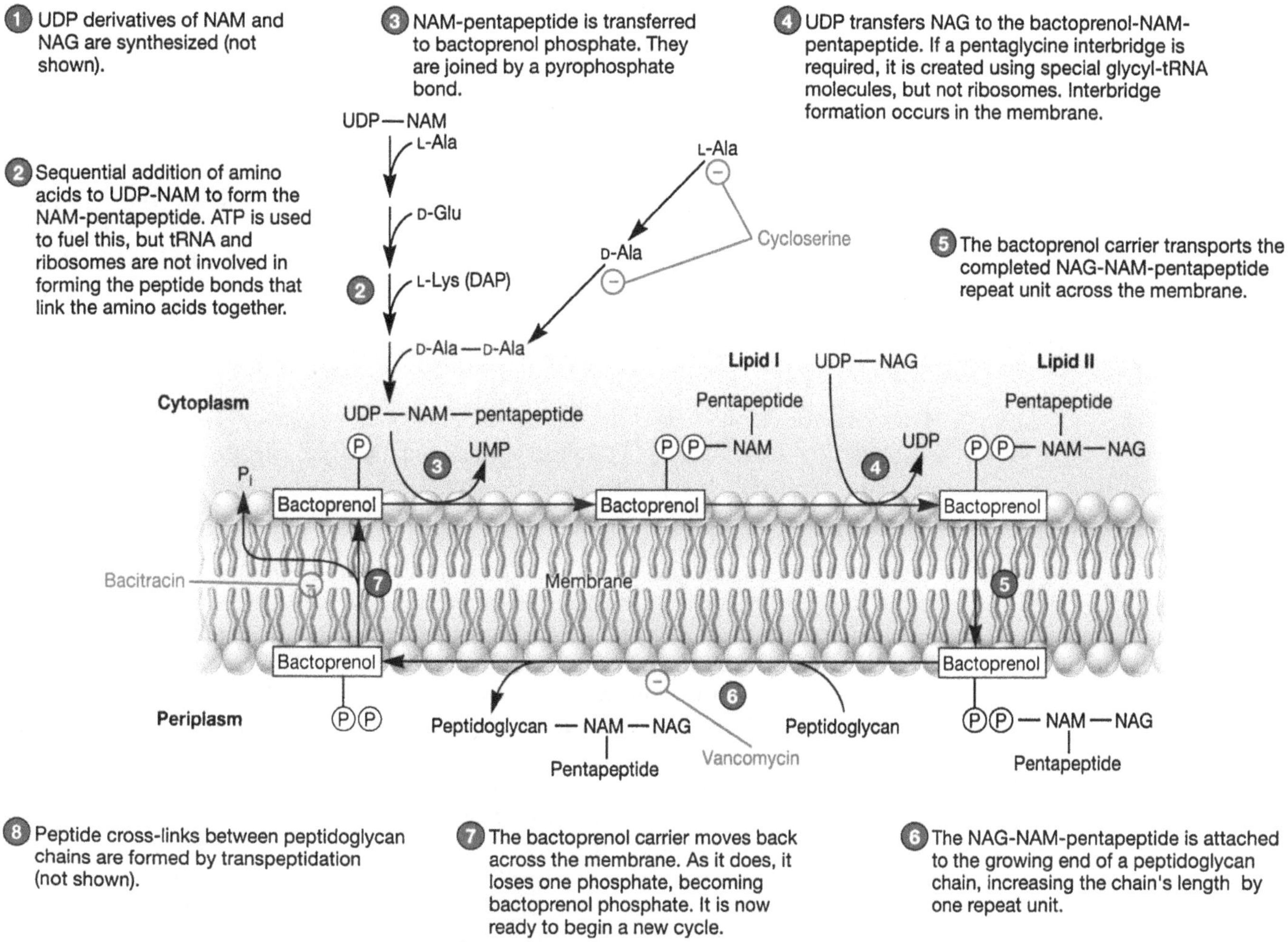

FIGURE 21–19. **Peptidoglycan synthesis.** NAM is *N*-acetylmuramic acid and NAG is *N*-acetylglucosamine. The pentapeptide contains L-lysine in *Staphylococcus aureus* and diaminopimelic acid in *Escherichia coli*. Inhibition by bacitracin, cycloserine, and vancomycin are shown. Transpeptidation and the action of penicillins are shown in **Figure 21–20**. (Reproduced with permission from Willey JM: *Prescott, Harley, & Klein's Microbiology*, 7th ed. New York, NY: McGraw Hill; 2008.)

FIGURE 21–20. **Transpeptidation.** The transpeptidation reactions in the formation of the peptidoglycan of *Escherichia coli* and *Staphylococcus aureus* are shown. β-Lactam antibiotics bind the transpeptidases and block cross-linking of the peptidoglycan backbone molecules. (Reproduced with permission from Willey JM: *Prescott, Harley, & Klein's Microbiology,* 7th ed. New York, NY: McGraw Hill; 2008.)

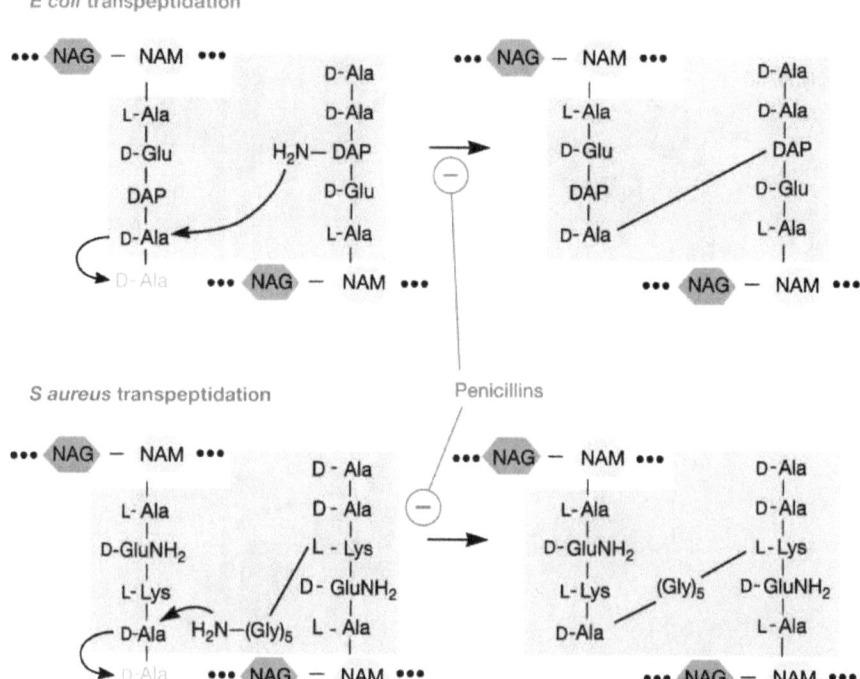

is added to the precursor, along with any amino acids that in this particular species will form the bridge between adjacent tetrapeptides.

3. **Outside the cell membrane,** this disaccharide subunit is attached to the end of a growing glycan chain, and then the cross-links between chains that give the macromolecule its strength are formed by **transpeptidases (Figure 21–20).** These enzymes are also called **penicillin-binding proteins (PBPs)** for their property of binding to this antibiotic. These transpeptidases are involved in forging, breaking, and reforging the peptide cross-links between glycan chains necessary to permit expansion of the peptidoglycan sac during cellular growth. Details of the cross-linking process vary among bacterial species.

■ Protein Secretion

Proteins transported to locations in the cell structure or exterior

In Gram negatives, the periplasm and outer membrane are additional barriers

GSP uses signal peptide and chaperone proteins

Six systems transport across the outer membrane

Moving macromolecules out of the cell interior and into their proper place in the wall, outer membrane, and capsule is a complex process. Moreover, many proteins are translocated through all layers of the cell envelope to the exterior environment. The latter instance is of particular medical interest when the protein is an exotoxin or other protein involved in virulence. Protein secretion has become the general term to designate all these instances of translocation of proteins out of the cytosol (ie, whether the protein is to leave the cell or become part of the envelope). The process is relatively simple in Gram-positive bacteria in which proteins, after export across the cytoplasmic membrane, have only to move through the relatively porous peptidoglycan layer. In Gram-negative bacteria, the periplasmic space and the outer membrane must also be traversed.

The simplest and most common mechanism for protein secretion called the **general secretory pathway (GSP)** is used by both Gram-positive and Gram-negative bacteria. Proteins secreted by the GSP are called preproteins because they have a signal peptide at their leading end that allows them to be guided by cytosolic chaperone proteins through the transport machinery **(Figure 21–21).** Once through the GSP, the signal peptide is removed and the mature protein folds into its final shape.

In Gram-negative species, additional pathways have been discovered that accomplish the export of proteins across the outer membrane into the environment **(Figure 21–22).** Currently, at least eight different bacterial secretion systems are known. Two of these (types II and V) provide a second step for proteins that have already been secreted by the GSP. The others extend across both membranes, and two of these (types III and IV) have an elaborate syringe-like apparatus, which literally injects the proteins across yet a third membrane—that of a host cell.

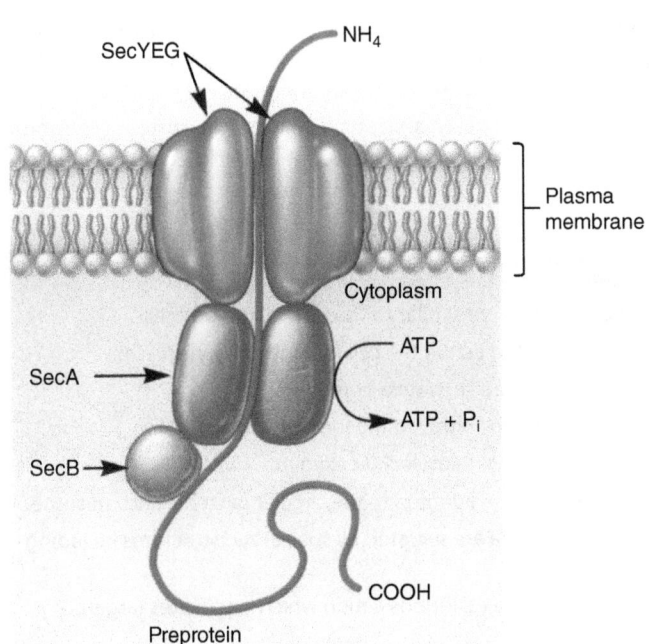

SecYEG

NH₄

Plasma membrane

Cytoplasm

ATP

SecA

ATP + P$_i$

SecB

COOH

Preprotein

FIGURE 21–21. General secretion pathway. The amino-terminal end of the preprotein has a signal peptide that facilitates transport through the apparatus by chaperone (SecB) and proteins that form channels (SecY, SecE, SecG) or have propelling functions (SecA). The signal peptide is removed on the outside. Energy is required in the form of ATP (adenosine triphosphate) hydrolysis. (Reproduced with permission from Willey JM: *Prescott, Harley, & Klein's Microbiology*, 7th ed. New York, NY: McGraw Hill; 2008.)

Type I   Type III   Type II   Type V   Type IV

Cell exterior

TolC

Yop

Outer membrane

YscJ

Periplasmic space

PulS

Tat

SecD EFGY

Sec

ADP + P$_i$

ATP

Plasma membrane

ATP   ADP + P$_i$ ATP   ADP + P$_i$ ATP   ADP + P$_i$ ATP   ADP + P$_i$

Chaperone

Cytoplasm

Chaperone

Protein

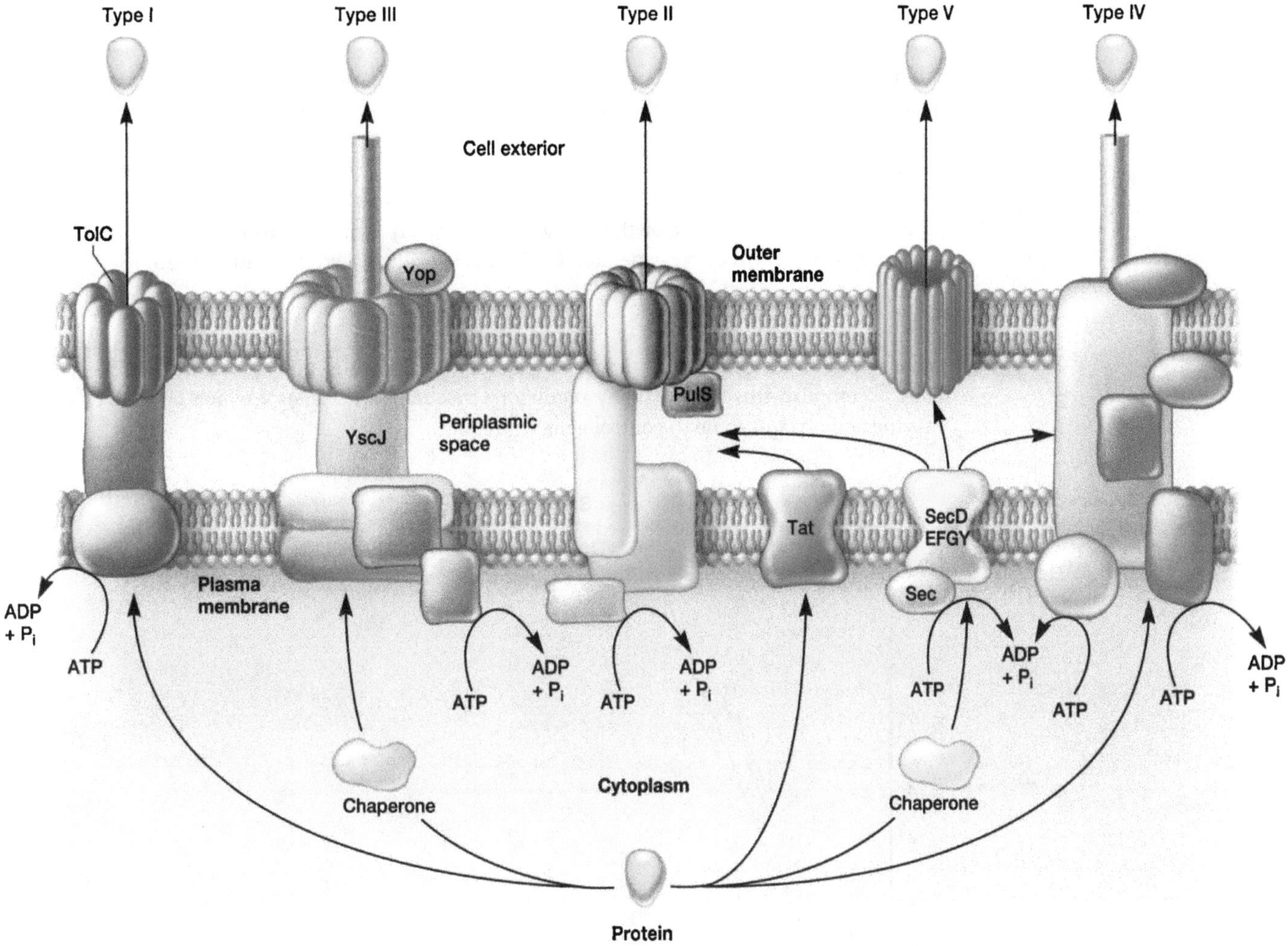

FIGURE 21–22. Gram-negative secretion systems. Type I. Proteins are exported directly across the cytoplasmic and outer membranes (OM) without use of the GSP. **Type II.** GSP or another system called Tat secrete into the periplasmic space and proteins are then transported across the OM. **Type III.** Proteins are transported across both membranes and then injected by a syringe apparatus. **Type IV.** Similar to type III but also injects DNA. **Type V.** Similar to type II except the protein is auto-transported across the OM. (Reproduced with permission from Willey JM: *Prescott, Harley, & Klein's Microbiology*, 7th ed. New York, NY: McGraw Hill; 2008.)

These nanosyringe injection systems are a major mechanism for the delivery of exotoxins and other proteins important in the pathogenesis of human infections. Type IV systems have the additional property of being able to inject DNA as well as proteins and are important in gene transfer as discussed in the following text. A recently discovered sixth type of secretion system resembles the cell-puncturing devices of bacteriophages and thus can inject into bacteria as well as eukaryotic cells. Functionally, it appears similar to the type III and IV injection secretion systems.

KEY CONCLUSIONS

- Except for speed, bacterial metabolic processes are similar to those of eukaryotic cells.
- Nutrients must diffuse or be actively transported across the cell wall into the cytoplasm.
- Porin channels facilitate transport across the Gram-negative outer membrane.
- Fermentation and oxidative respiration generate energy in the form of ATP.
- Anaerobic bacteria only ferment and are sensitive to molecular oxygen.
- DNA replication, transcription, and translation are adapted to the circular bacterial chromosome.
- Proteins including toxins synthesized by bacteria are secreted by specialized structures including syringe-like injectors.
- Toxins stimulate unique enzymatic reactions like ADP-ribosylation which inactivates targeted proteins.

CELL GROWTH AND REGULATION

After lag period, cultures exhibit exponential growth

Nutrient depletion, waste accumulation terminate growth

Bacteria multiply by binary fission. The time needed for a bacterial culture to double its mass or cell number is in the range of 30 to 60 minutes for most pathogenic bacteria in nutrient-replete media. Some species can double in 20 minutes (*E coli* and related organisms), and some (eg, some mycobacteria) take almost as long as mammalian cells—20 hours. When first inoculated, liquid cultures of bacteria characteristically exhibit a **lag period** followed by a phase of constant, maximal cell doubling, called **exponential** or **logarithmic growth.** As nutrients are depleted and waste products are accumulated, growth becomes progressively limited (**stationary** phase) and eventually stops. The growth curve generated by this cycle is illustrated in **Figure 21–23.**

REGULATION AND ADAPTATION

Bacteria can do little to control their environment, so they must adjust to it in a flexible manner. They accomplish this feat by many regulatory mechanisms, some of which operate to control enzyme activity and some to control gene expression.

FIGURE 21–23. Growth curve. The phases of bacterial growth in liquid medium.

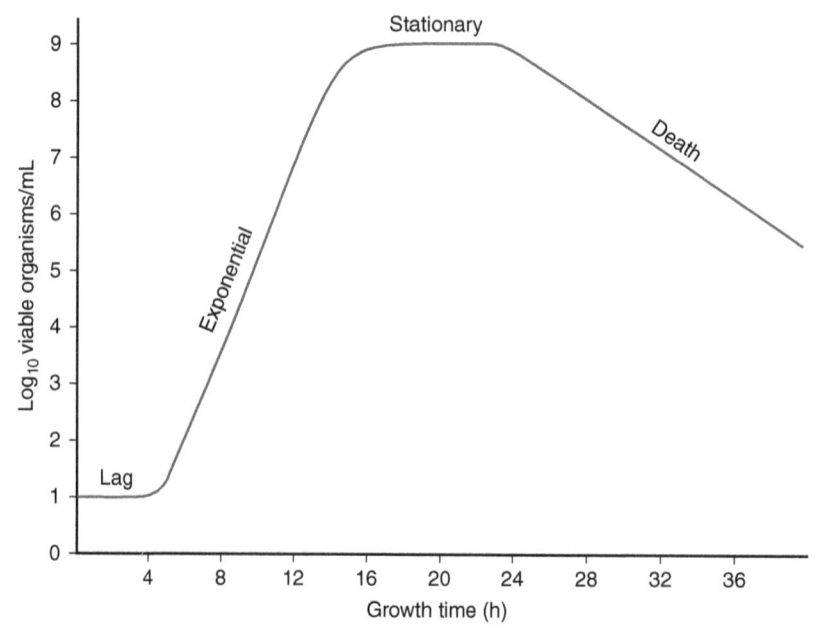

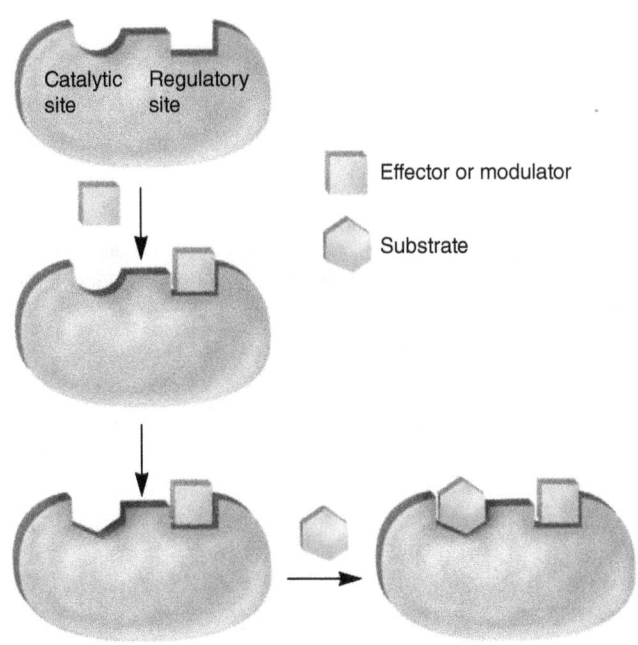

FIGURE 21-24. **Allosteric regulation.** In this example of the structure and function of an allosteric enzyme, the effector or modulator first binds to a separate regulatory site and causes a change in enzyme conformation that results in an alteration in the shape of the active site. The active site can now more effectively bind the substrate. This effector is a positive effector because it stimulates substrate binding and catalytic activity. (Reproduced with permission from Willey JM: *Prescott, Harley, & Klein's Microbiology*, 7th ed. New York, NY: McGraw Hill; 2008.)

Control of Enzyme Activity

By far the most prevalent means by which bacterial cells modulate the flow of material through fueling and biosynthetic pathways is by changing the activity of allosteric enzymes through the reversible binding of low molecular weight ligands (**Figure 21-24**). In fueling pathways, it is common for AMP, ADP, and ATP to control the activity of enzymes by causing conformational changes of **allosteric enzymes,** usually located at critical branch points where pathways intersect. By this means, the flow of carbon from the major substrates through the various pathways is adjusted to be appropriate to the demands of biosynthesis. In biosynthetic pathways, it is common for the end product of the pathway to control the activity of the first enzyme in the pathway. This pattern, called **feedback inhibition** or end-product inhibition, ensures that each building block is made at exactly the rate it is being used for polymerization (**Figure 21-25**). It also ensures that building blocks supplied in the medium are not wastefully duplicated by synthesis.

Metabolic pathways controlled by allosteric enzymes

Feedback inhibition provides economy and efficiency

Control of Gene Expression

To a far greater extent than eukaryotic cells, bacteria regulate their metabolism by changing the amounts of different enzymes. This is accomplished chiefly by governing their rates of synthesis,

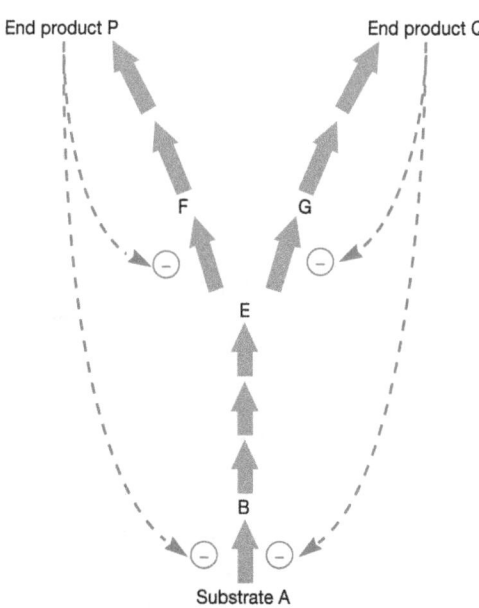

FIGURE 21-25. **Feedback inhibition.** Feedback inhibition in a branching pathway with two end products. The branch-point enzymes, those catalyzing the conversion of intermediate E to F and G, are regulated by feedback inhibition. Products P and Q also inhibit the initial reaction in the pathway. A colored line with a minus sign at one end indicates that an end product, P or Q is inhibiting the enzyme catalyzing the step next to the minus. (Reproduced with permission from Willey JM: *Prescott, Harley, & Klein's Microbiology*, 7th ed. New York, NY: McGraw Hill; 2008.)

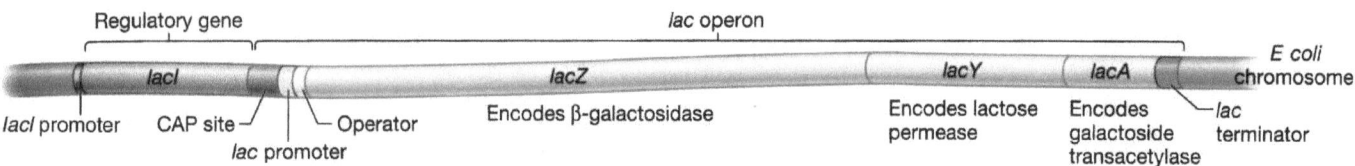

FIGURE 21–26. The *lac* operon. The *lac* operon consists of three genes: *lacZ*, *lacY*, and *lacA*, which are transcribed as a single unit from the *lac* promoter. The operon is regulated both negatively and positively. Negative control is brought about by the *lac* repressor, which is the product of the *lacI* gene. The operator is the site of *lac* repressor binding. Positive control results from the action of CAP. CAP binds the CAP site located just upstream from the *lac* promoter. CAP is, in part, responsible for a phenomenon called catabolite repression, an example of a global control network, in which numerous operons are controlled by a single protein. (Reproduced with permission from Willey JM: *Prescott, Harley, & Klein's Microbiology*, 7th ed. New York, NY: McGraw Hill; 2008.)

Changes in gene expression change enzyme synthesis

Genes organized as transcriptional units called operons

RNA polymerase binds to promoter

Activator and repressor proteins regulate transcription by binding to the operator region of operons

Two-component systems link environmental sensing with regulation

Formation of a stationary phase cell produces latency

that is, by controlling gene expression. This works rapidly for bacteria because of their speed of growth; shutting off the synthesis of a particular enzyme results in short order in the reduction of its cellular level owing to dilution by the growth of the cell.

Most of the genes we know about in bacteria are organized as **multicistronic operons**. A **cistron** is a segment of DNA encoding a polypeptide. An **operon** is the unit of transcription; the cistrons that it comprises are co-transcribed as a single mRNA. The structure of a typical operon (**Figure 21–26**) consists of a **promoter** region, an **operator** region, component cistrons, and a **terminator(s)**. RNA polymerase recognizes the promoter region and binds to the DNA.

Near the promoter in many operons is an operator to which a specific **regulator protein** or **transcription factor** can bind. In some cases the binding of this regulator blocks initiation; in such a case of negative control, the regulator is invariably called a **repressor**. The functioning of both positive and negative types of regulation on transcription initiation is illustrated in **Figure 21–27**. Some regulatory systems are able to act in multiple stages. The two-component system illustrated in **Figure 21–28** shows an environmental signal sensed in the cytoplasmic membrane leading to the activation of a separate regulon. This linking of environmental sensing with regulation is taken to another level with two-component systems used by pathogens for the deployment of virulence factors. *Bordetella pertussis* uses such a system to produce attachment proteins and toxins at just the right time during the production of whooping cough.

■ Stationary Phase Cells

For some bacteria, adaptation to a nongrowing state involves formation of a differentiated cell called the stationary phase cell. Its envelope is made tougher by many modifications of its structure, its chromosome is aggregated, and its metabolism is adjusted to a maintenance mode. Such states may be important in diseases such as tuberculosis, which have long latent periods after primary infection, or in cholera in which cells persist in a dormant state in the environment between epidemics.

KEY CONCLUSIONS

- Bacterial growth is related to nutrients and controlled activation and repression of gene operons.
- Two-component regulatory systems respond to environmental signals.
- A stationary phase may lead to prolonged latency in humans or the environment.

● BACTERIAL GENETICS

No feature is more central to bacterial diversity and power to produce disease than their genetic mechanisms. The news media now deliver a constant stream of reports of new antibiotic resistance and emerging pathogens. Bacteria treated successfully with an antimicrobial for decades suddenly develop resistance; diseases seemingly under control reappear; new diseases (at least new to us) emerge and spread. When traced to their origin most of these involve the speed and breadth of bacterial genetic mechanisms. Bacteria use mutation and recombination for genomic change, as do eukaryotic cells. In addition, they have powerful mechanisms for exchange of genes between cells that do not even have to be closely related. Combined with the so-called "jumping genes" (transposons [Tn]), which seem to be able to go anywhere, bacteria present an astonishing array of genetic tools. The mechanisms of mutation, recombination, transformation, transduction, conjugation, and transposition form the basis of this genetic power and are discussed in the text that follows.

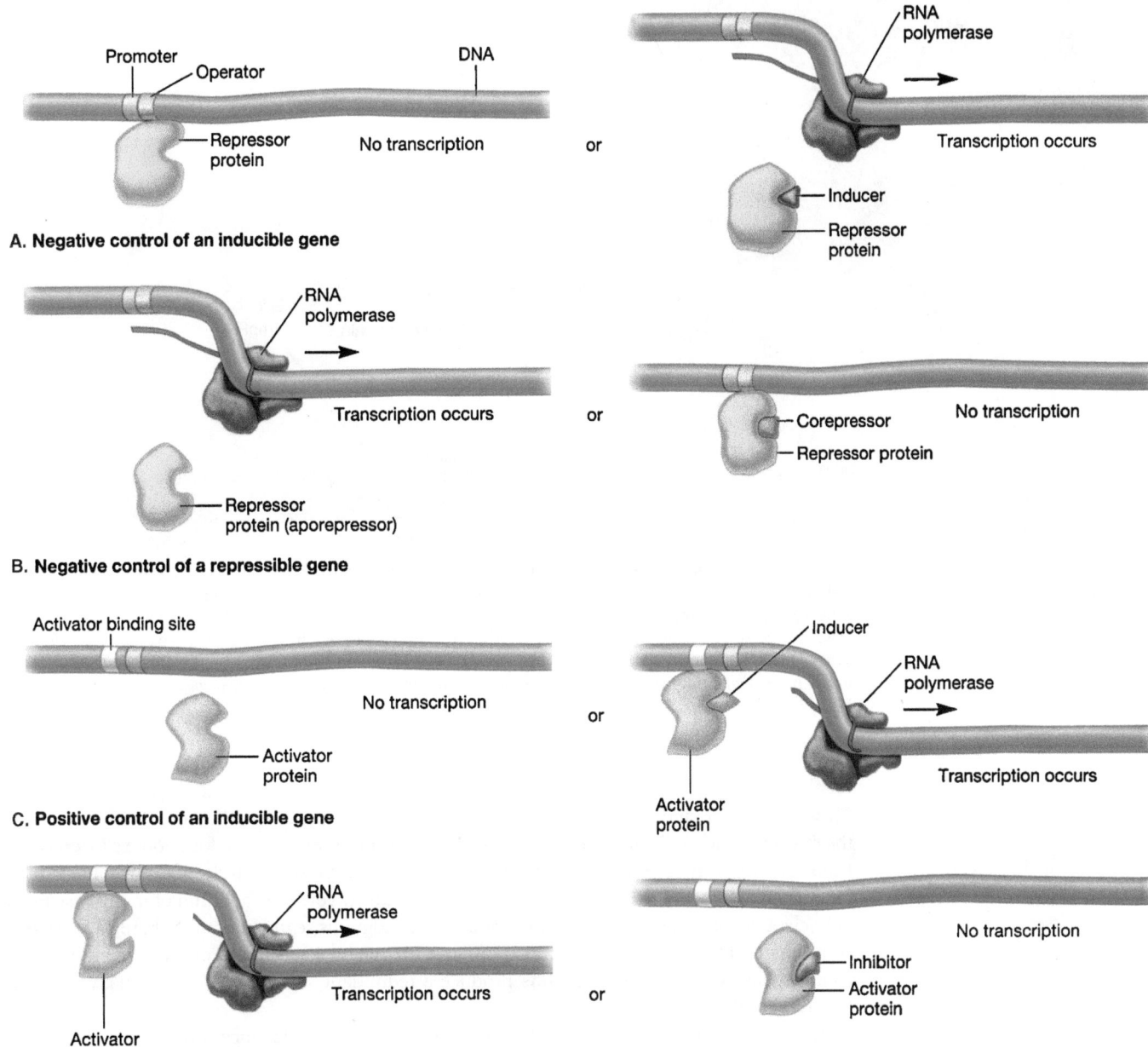

A. **Negative control of an inducible gene**

B. **Negative control of a repressible gene**

C. **Positive control of an inducible gene**

D. **Positive control of a repressible gene**

FIGURE 21–27. **Bacterial regulatory proteins.** Bacterial regulatory proteins have two binding sites—one for a small effector molecule and one for DNA. The binding of the effector molecule changes the regulatory protein's ability to bind DNA. **A.** In the absence of inducer, the repressor protein blocks transcription. The presence of inducer prevents the repressor from binding DNA, and transcription occurs. **B.** Without a corepressor, the repressor is unable to bind DNA, and transcription occurs. When the corepressor is bound to the repressor, the repressor is able to bind DNA and transcription is blocked. **C.** The activator protein is able to bind DNA and activate transcription only when it is bound to the inducer. **D.** The activator binds DNA and promotes transcription unless the inhibitor is present. When inhibitor is present, the activator undergoes a conformational change that prevents it from binding DNA; this inhibits transcription. (Reproduced with permission from Willey JM: *Prescott, Harley, & Klein's Microbiology*, 7th ed. New York, NY: McGraw Hill; 2008.)

MUTATION

The spontaneous development of mutations is a major factor in the evolution of bacteria. Mutations occur in nature at a low frequency, on the order of one mutation in every million cells for any one gene, but the large size of microbial populations ensures the presence of many mutants. Because bacteria are haploid, the consequences of a mutation, even a recessive one, are immediately evident in the mutant cell. Because the generation time of bacteria is short, it does not take many hours for a mutant cell that has arisen by chance to grow to the dominant cell type if the mutation gives it a survival advantage.

✳ Mutations rapidly expressed and predominate under selective conditions

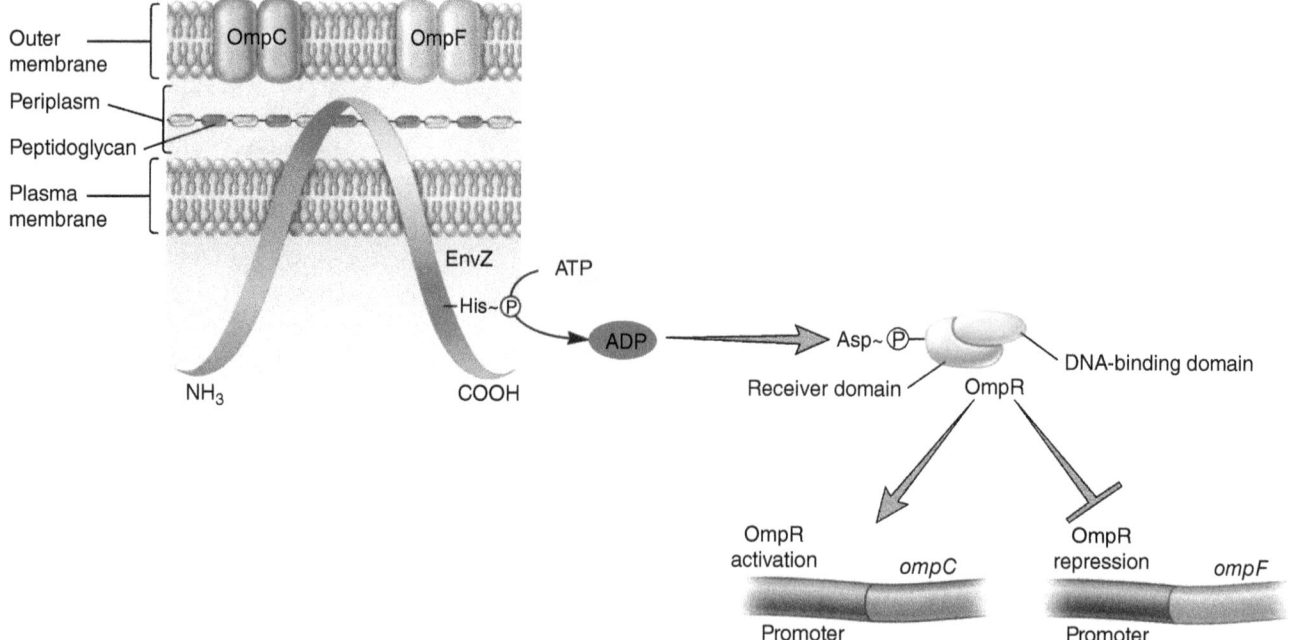

FIGURE 21-28. Two-component signal transduction system and the regulation of porin proteins. In this system, the sensor kinase protein EnvZ loops through the cytoplasmic membrane so that both its C- and N-termini are in the cytosol. When EnvZ senses an increase in osmolarity, it autophosphorylates a histidine residue at its C-terminus. EnvZ then passes the phosphoryl group to the response regulator OmpR, which accepts it on an aspartic acid residue located in its N-terminus. This activates OmpR so that it is able to bind DNA, repress *ompF* expression, and enhance that of *ompC*. (Reproduced with permission from Willey JM: *Prescott, Harley, & Klein's Microbiology*, 7th ed. New York, NY: McGraw Hill; 2008.)

■ Kinds of Mutations

There are several kinds of mutations, based on the nature of the change in nucleotide sequence of the affected gene(s). **Replacements** involve the substitution of one base for another. **Microdeletions** and **microinsertions** involve the removal and addition, respectively, of a single nucleotide (and its complement in the opposite strand). **Insertions** involve the addition of many base pairs of nucleotides at a single site. **Deletions** remove a contiguous segment of many base pairs. **Inversions** change the direction of a segment of DNA by splicing each strand of the segment into the complementary strand. **Duplications** produce a redundant segment of DNA, usually adjacent (tandem) to the original segment.

By recalling the nature of genes and how their nucleotide sequence directs the synthesis of proteins, one can understand the immediate consequence of each of these biochemical changes. If a replacement mutation in a codon changes the mRNA transcript to a different amino acid, it is called a **missense mutation** (eg, an AAG [lysine] to a GAG [glutamate]). The resulting protein may be enzymatically inactive or very sensitive to environmental conditions, such as temperature. If the replacement changes a codon specifying an amino acid to one specifying none, it is called a **nonsense mutation** (eg, a UAC [tyrosine] to UAA [STOP]). Microdeletions and microinsertions cause **frameshift mutations,** changes in the reading frame by which the ribosomes translate the mRNA from the mutated gene (**Figure 21-29**). Frameshifts usually result in polymerization of a stretch of incorrect amino acids until a nonsense codon is encountered, so the product is usually a truncated polypeptide fragment with an incorrect amino acid sequence at its N-terminus. Deletion or insertion of a segment of base pairs from a gene shortens or lengthens the protein product if the number of base pairs deleted or inserted is divisible evenly by three; otherwise, it also brings about the consequence of a frameshift. Mutations are summarized in **Table 21-3.**

RECOMBINATION

Recombination is the process in which nucleic acid molecules from different sources are combined or rearranged to produce a new nucleotide sequence. In eukaryotes, this occurs by crossing over during meiosis. Since bacteria do not reproduce sexually or undergo meiosis, it might seem that this mechanism would be limited. In fact, it can occur any time there is a source of

---

Margin notes:

✳ Mutations involve changes in nucleotide sequence

Changes in nucleotide sequence affect the synthesis of the protein products

Frameshift mutations affect mRNA translation

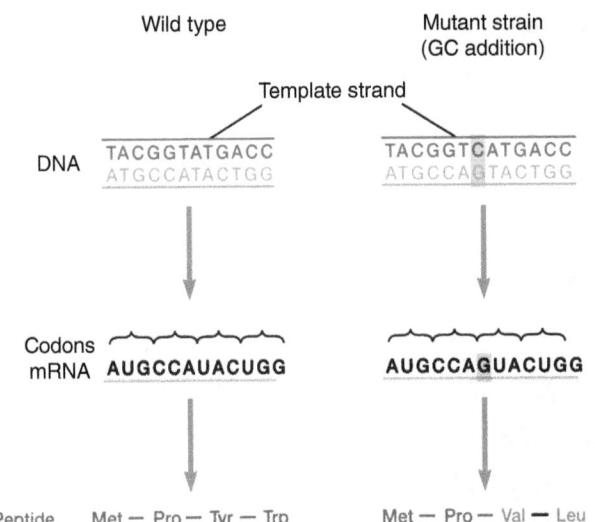

Wild type

Mutant strain
(GC addition)

Template strand

DNA

`TACGGTATGACC`
`ATGCCATACTGG`

`TACGGTCATGACC`
`ATGCCAGTACTGG`

Codons
mRNA

AUGCCAUACUGG

AUGCCAGUACUGG

Peptide   Met — Pro — Tyr — Trp   Met — Pro — Val — Leu

FIGURE 21–29. Frameshift mutation. A frameshift mutation resulting from the insertion of a GC base pair. The reading frameshift translates to different amino acids after the frameshift producing a different peptide. (Reproduced with permission from Willey JM: *Prescott, Harley, & Klein's Microbiology*, 7th ed. New York, NY: McGraw Hill; 2008.)

recombinant DNA and strand breaks in the bacterial chromosome. This creates stretches of single-stranded DNA with nucleotides exposed for potential pairing. The source of recombinant DNA may be another part of the same chromosome or from outside the cell from one of the genetic transfer mechanisms described later. If successful, a new hybrid chromosome is formed. In bacteria, there are two major molecular mechanisms of recombination, homologous recombination (**Figure 21–30**) and site-specific recombination.

■ Homologous Recombination

This term homologous recombination reflects one of the two requirements for this process: (1) the donor DNA must possess reasonably large regions of nucleotide sequence identity or similarity to segments of the host chromosome because extensive base-pairing must occur between strands of the two recombining molecules; and (2) the recipient cell must possess the genetic ability to make a set of enzymes that can bring about the covalent substitution of a segment of the donor DNA for the homologous region of the host. A protein known as RecA (recombination)

＊ Homologous recombination involves nucleotide similarity

TABLE 21–3	Mutations	
TYPE	**CAUSATIVE AGENT**	**CONSEQUENCES**
Replacement		
Transition: pyrimidine replaced by a pyrimidine or a purine by a purine	Base analogs, ultraviolet radiation, deaminating and alkylating agents, spontaneous	Transitions and transversions: if nonsense codon formed, truncated peptide; if missense codon formed, altered protein
Transversion: purine replaced by a pyrimidine or vice versa	Spontaneous	
Deletion		
Macrodeletion: large nucleotide segment deleted	HNO_2, radiation, bifunctional alkylating agents	Truncated peptide; other products possible, such as fusion peptides
Microdeletion: one or two nucleotides deleted	Same as macrodeletions	Frameshift, usually resulting in nonsense codon and truncated peptide
Insertion		
Macroinsertion: large nucleotide segment inserted	Transposons or insertion sequence (IS) elements	Interrupted gene yielding truncated product
Microinsertion: one or two nucleotides inserted	Acridine	Frameshift, usually resulting in nonsense codon yielding a truncated product
Inversion	IS or IS-like elements	Many possible effects

FIGURE 21–30. **The double-stranded break model of homologous recombination.** (Reproduced with permission from Willey JM: *Prescott, Harley, & Klein's Microbiology*, 7th ed. New York, NY: McGraw Hill; 2008.)

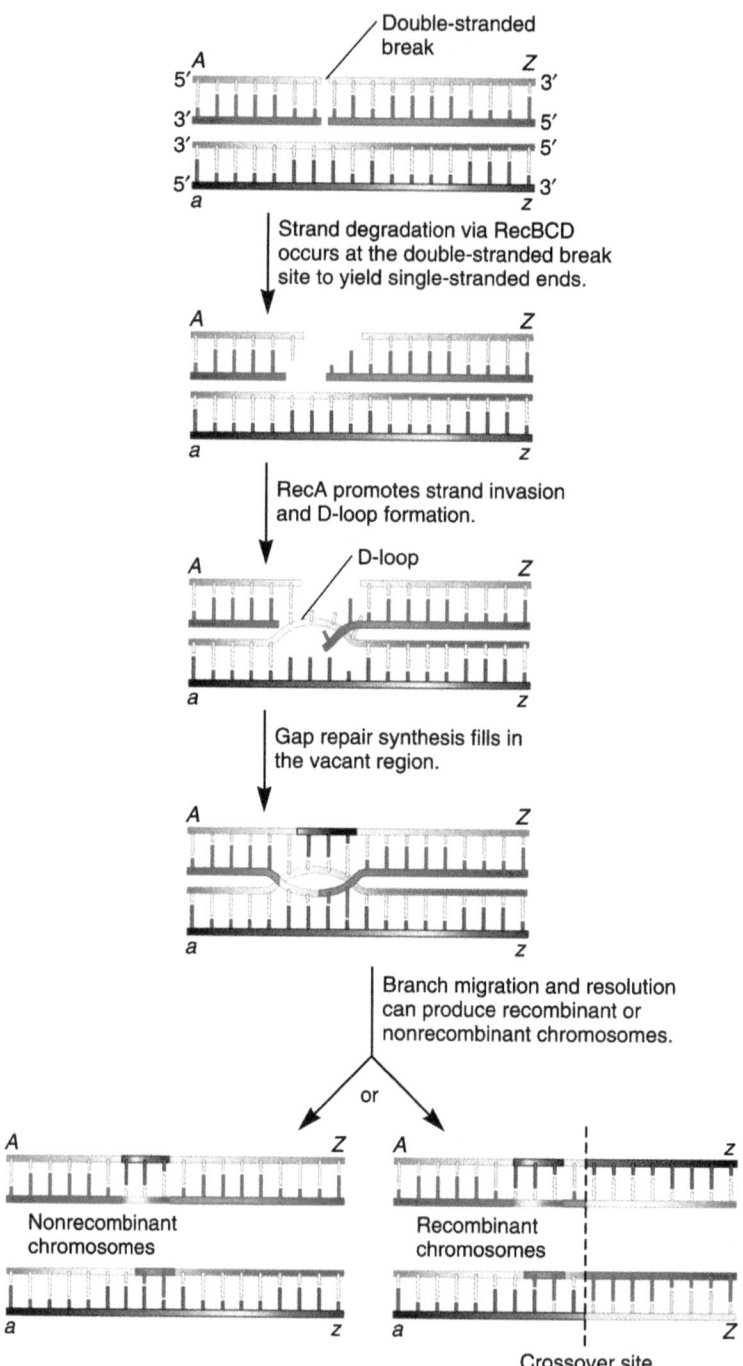

controls the entire process. The same breakage and reunion process then links the second strand of each recombining DNA molecule. This crossover event repeated farther down the chromosome results in the substitution of the donor segment between the two crossovers for the homologous segment of the host.

■ Site-Specific Recombination

The second major type of recombination is site-specific recombination, which is particularly important in the integration of virus genomes into host chromosomes. Site-specific recombination relies on only limited DNA sequence similarity at the sites of crossover mediated by different sets of specialized enzymes designed to catalyze recombination of only certain DNA molecules. These recombinational events are restricted to specific sites on one or both of the recombining DNA molecules. The enzymes that bring about site-specific recombination operate not on the basis of DNA homology, but on recognition of unique DNA sequences that form the borders of the specific sites.

✳ Site-specific recombination operates only on unique sequences

■ Recombination and Antigenic Variation

A fascinating aspect of DNA rearrangements brought about by genetic recombination is that the expression of some chromosomal genes important in virulence can be controlled by recombinational events. In *Salmonella* species an **invertible element** lying between the two flagellin genes can switch between them. In one orientation, the promoter initiates transcription of one flagellar type; in the other orientation, transcription proceeds in the opposite direction to transcribe the other. These kinds of antigenic variations provide a selective advantage to the bacteria by allowing invading populations to include individuals that can escape the developing immune response of the host and thus continue the infectious process.

Antigenic variation brought about by recombinational event

Invertible elements act as a genetic switch

TRANSPOSITION

Transposition involves transposable elements that are genetic units capable of mediating their own transfer from one chromosome to another, from one location to another on the same chromosome, or between chromosome and plasmid. This transposition relies on their ability to synthesize their own site-specific recombination enzymes, called **transposases.** The major kinds of transposable elements are **insertion sequence** (IS) elements and **transposons** (**Figure 21–31**).

Genetic units move within and between chromosomes and plasmids

■ Insertion Sequences

IS elements are segments of DNA that encode enzymes for site-specific recombination and have distinctive nucleotide sequences at their termini. Different IS elements have different termini, but as illustrated, a given IS element has the same sequence of nucleotides at each end but in an inverted order. Only genes involved in transposition (eg, one encoding a transposase) and in the regulation of its frequency are included in IS elements, and they are, therefore, the simplest transposable elements. Because IS elements contain only genes for transposition, their presence in a chromosome is not easy to detect unless they insert within a gene. Such an insertion is actually a mutation that alters or destroys the activity of the gene.

IS elements encode only proteins for their own transposition

Insertion of IS elements into a gene causes mutation

■ Transposons

IS elements are components of **transposons** that are transposable segments of DNA-containing genes beyond those needed for transposition. The general structure of these composite Tn consist of a central area of genes bordered by IS elements. The genes may code for such properties as antimicrobial resistance, substrate metabolism, or other functions. Composite Tn translocate by what is called simple or **direct transposition,** in which the Tn is excised from its original location and inserted in a simple cut-and-paste manner into its new site without replication (**Figure 21–32**). Another mechanism called **replicative transposition** leaves a copy of the replicative Tn at its original site.

Transposons encode functions beyond those needed for transposition

✻ Direct transposition moves the transposon to a new site

✻ Replicative transposition leaves a copy behind

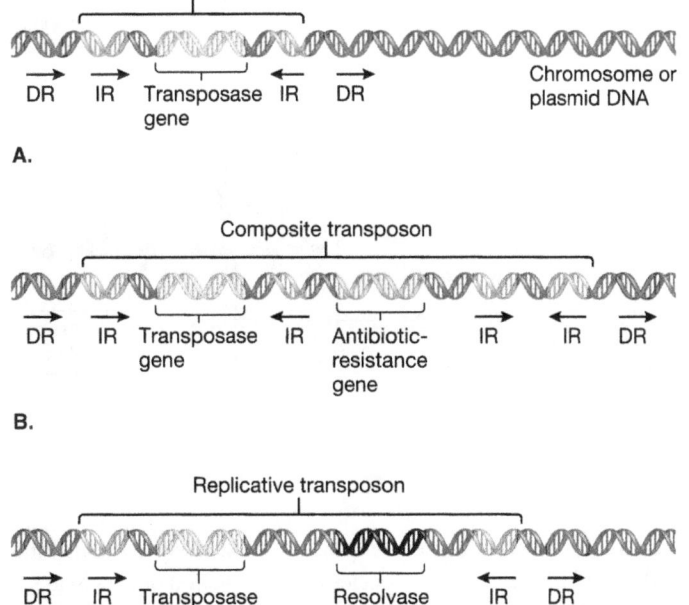

Insertion sequence

DR   IR   Transposase gene   IR   DR   Chromosome or plasmid DNA

A.

Composite transposon

DR   IR   Transposase gene   IR   Antibiotic-resistance gene   IR   IR   DR

B.

Replicative transposon

DR   IR   Transposase gene   Resolvase gene   IR   DR

C.

FIGURE 21–31. Transposable elements. All transposable elements contain common elements. These include repeating sequences, usually inverted repeats (IRs), at the ends of the elements and a transposases gene. **A.** Insertion sequences consist only of the IRs on either side of the transposases gene. **B.** Composite transposons and **C.** genes. Insertion sequences and composite transposons move by simple cut-and-paste transposition. Replicative transposons move by replicative transposition. Direct repeats (DRs) in host DNA flank a transposable element. (Reproduced with permission from Willey JM: *Prescott, Harley, & Klein's Microbiology,* 7th ed. New York, NY: McGraw Hill; 2008.)

FIGURE 21–32. **Simple transposition.** IR, inverted repeat; TE, transposable element. (Reproduced with permission from Willey JM: *Prescott, Harley, & Klein's Microbiology*, 7th ed. New York, NY: McGraw Hill; 2008.)

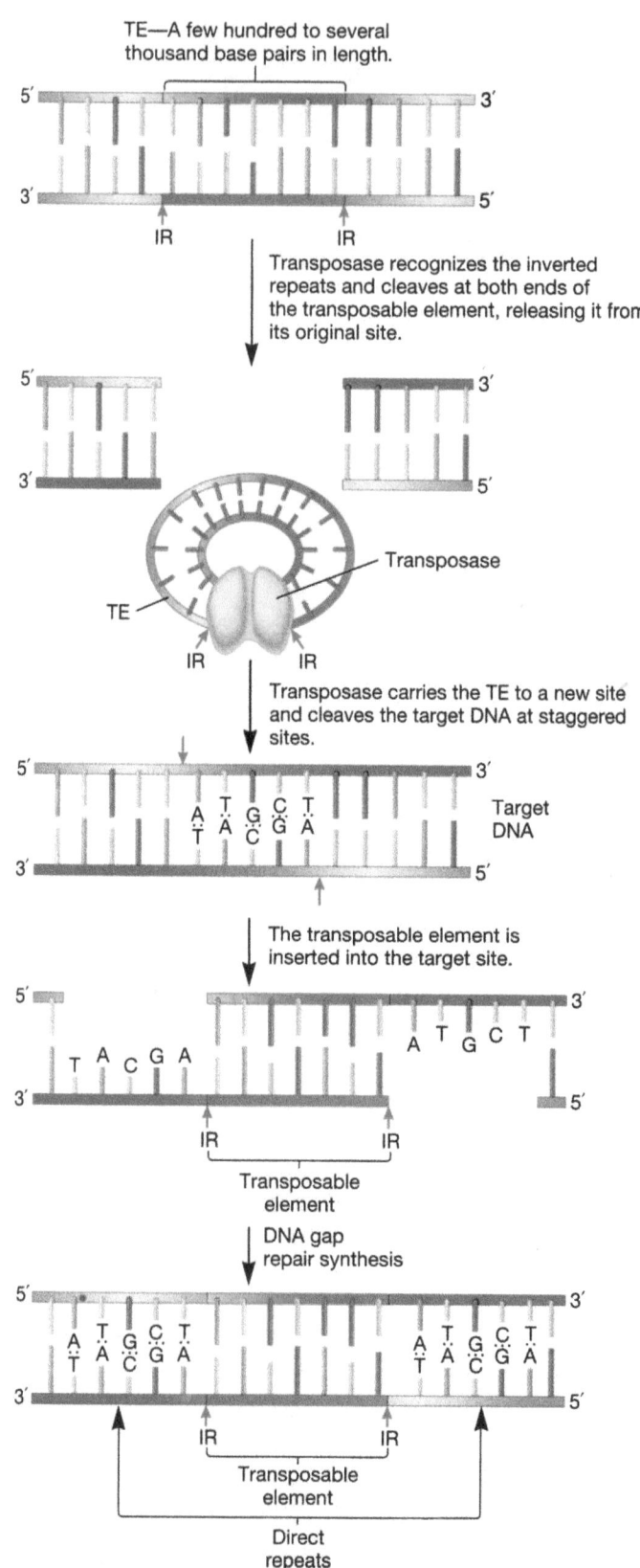

GENETIC EXCHANGE

✳ One-way passage of DNA from a donor to a recipient adds an exogenote to the recipient endogenote

Despite the fact that bacteria reproduce exclusively asexually, the sharing of genetic information within and between related species is common and occurs in at least three fundamentally different ways. All three processes involve a one-way transfer of DNA from a donor cell to a recipient cell.

One process of DNA transfer, called **transformation,** involves the release of DNA into the environment by the lysis of some cells, followed by the direct uptake of that DNA by the recipient cells. In **transduction,** the DNA is introduced into the recipient cell by a bacteriophage that has infected the bacterial cell. The third process, called **conjugation,** involves an actual contact between a donor and recipient cell during which the autonomously replicating, extrachromosomal DNA of a plasmid is transferred.

> Transformation, transduction, and conjugation are the major processes of DNA transfer

■ Transformation

The ability to take up DNA from the environment is called **competence,** and in many species of bacteria, it is encoded by chromosomal genes that become active under certain environmental conditions. Any DNA present in the medium is bound indiscriminately. The fate of the internalized DNA fragment then depends on whether it shares homology (the same or similar base sequences) with a portion of the recipient cell's DNA. If so, recombination can occur, but heterologous DNA is degraded and causes no heritable change in the recipient (**Figure 21–33**). Other species do not naturally enter the competent state but can be made permeable to DNA by treatment with agents that damage the cell envelope, making an **artificial transformation** possible.

> Competence is the ability to take in DNA from the environment
>
> ✳ Internalized DNA either recombines or is degraded

■ Transduction

Transduction is the transfer of genetic information from donor to recipient cell by viruses of bacteria called **bacteriophages** or simply phages. The phages infect sensitive cells by adsorbing to specific receptors on the cell surface and then injecting their DNA or RNA. Phages come in two functional varieties according to what happens after injection of the viral nucleic acid. **Virulent (lytic) phages** cause lysis of the host bacterium as a culmination of the synthesis of many new virions within the infected cell. **Temperate phages** may initiate a lytic growth process of this sort or can enter a quiescent form (called a **prophage**), in which the phage DNA integrates into the bacterial chromosome. The infected host cell is permitted to proceed about its business of growth and division, but passes on to its descendants a prophage genome capable of being **induced** to produce phage in a process nearly identical to the growth of lytic phages. The bacterial cell that

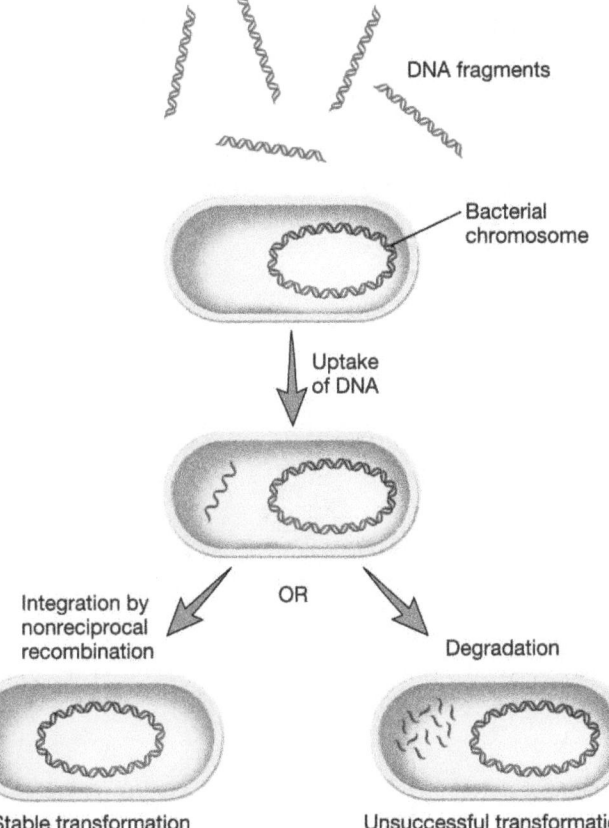

FIGURE 21–33. Bacterial transformation. The bacterial cell is transformed with DNA fragments (*purple*), which are either integrated into the chromosome (*blue*) by recombination or degraded by nucleases in the cytosol. (Reproduced with permission from Willey JM: *Prescott, Harley, & Klein's Microbiology*, 7th ed. New York, NY: McGraw Hill; 2008.)

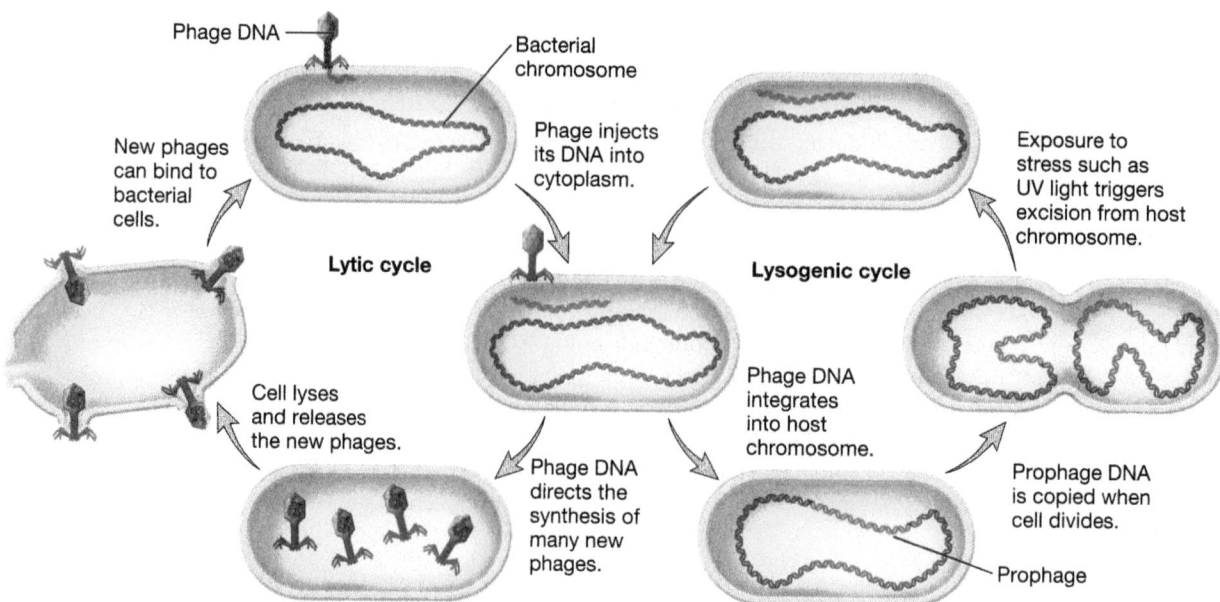

Phage DNA

Bacterial chromosome

Phage injects its DNA into cytoplasm.

New phages can bind to bacterial cells.

Lytic cycle

Lysogenic cycle

Exposure to stress such as UV light triggers excision from host chromosome.

Cell lyses and releases the new phages.

Phage DNA integrates into host chromosome.

Phage DNA directs the synthesis of many new phages.

Prophage DNA is copied when cell divides.

Prophage

FIGURE 21–34. Transduction: lytic and lysogenic cycles of temperate phages. Temperate phages have two phases to their life cycles. The lysogenic cycle allows the genome of the virus to be replicated passively as the host cell's genome is replicated. Certain environmental factors such as UV light can cause a switch from the lysogenic cycle to the lytic cycle. In the lytic cycle, new virus particles are made and released when the host cell lyses. Virulent phages are limited to just the lytic cycle. (Reproduced with permission from Willey JM: *Prescott, Harley, & Klein's Microbiology*, 7th ed. New York, NY: McGraw Hill; 2008.)

Temperate phages either lyse the bacterial host cell or lysogenize it

harbors a latent prophage is said to be a lysogen (capable of producing lytic phages), and its condition is referred to as **lysogeny.** Steps in this process are illustrated in **Figure 21–34.**

■ Conjugation

One need only look at **Figure 21–35** and add the title "Sexuality in Bacteria" (as has often been done) to grasp the idea that bacteria have something special going for them in the way of gene exchange. This process called conjugation is the transfer of genetic information from the donor to a recipient bacterial cell in a process that requires intimate cell contact. By themselves, bacteria cannot conjugate. Only when a bacterial cell contains a self-transmissible **plasmid** (see later for definition) or a **conjugative transposon** does DNA transfer occur. In most cases, conjugation involves transfer only of plasmid DNA; transfer of chromosomal DNA is a rarer event and is mediated by specialized elements including plasmids. Plasmids are of enormous importance in medical microbiology. They are discussed in detail later in this chapter, but to understand conjugation, we should first introduce some of their features.

✳ Conjugation is plasmid-encoded and requires cell contact

FIGURE 21–35. **Bacterial conjugation with sex pilus.** On the left-hand side is a "donor" *Escherichia coli* cell exhibiting many common (somatic) pili and a sex pilus by which it has attached itself to a "recipient" cell, which lacks the plasmid encoding the sex pilus. The sex pilus facilitates exchange of genetic material between the male and female *E coli*. In this micrograph preparation, the sex pilus has been labeled with a bacterial virus that attaches to it specifically. (Used with permission from Charles C. Brinton and Judith Carnahan.)

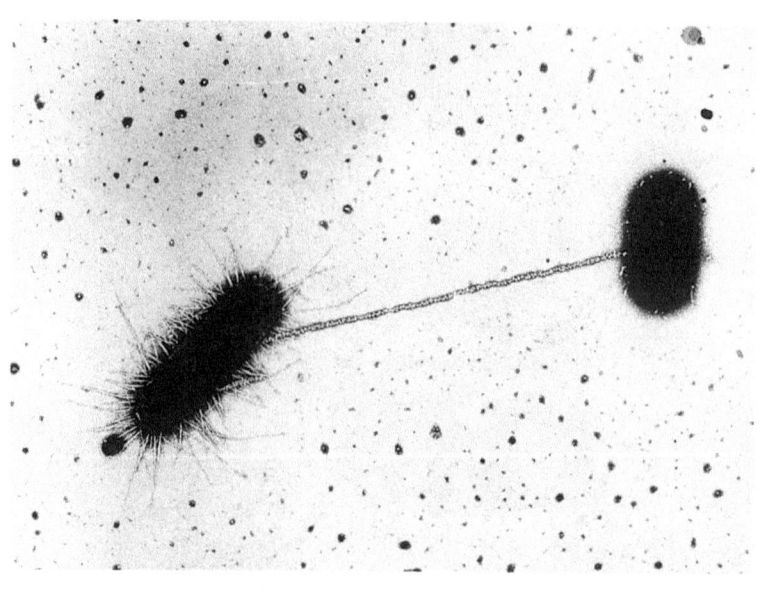

Plasmids are autonomous extrachromosomal elements composed of circular double-stranded DNA; a few rare linear examples have also been found. A single organism can harbor several distinct plasmids and single or multiple copies of each. Plasmids are found in most species of Gram-positive and Gram-negative bacteria in most environments. They replicate within the host cell (and only within the host cell) and are partitioned between daughter cells at the time of cell division. In addition, many plasmids facilitate their own transfer from one bacterial cell to another by encoding proteins that permit passage of their, and nonrelated, DNA from donor to recipient. Such plasmids are **conjugative plasmids** and those that lack the full compendium of transfer proteins are either **mobilizable** (depend on a conjugative plasmid for cell-cell passage) or **nontransferable.**

Conjugation is a highly evolved and efficient process. Suitable mixtures of donor and recipient bacteria can lead to near-complete conversion of all the recipients into donor, plasmid-containing cells. Furthermore, although some conjugative plasmids can transfer themselves only between cells of the same or closely related species, others are promiscuous, promoting conjugation across a wide variety of (usually Gram-negative) species. Conjugation is time-sensitive, and exquisitely controlled process, normally kept in check by the production of multiple positive and negative regulators. Some conjugative elements, especially those harbored by the Bacteroidetes, also respond to subinhibitory concentrations of antibiotics (especially the tetracycline family) by enhancing DNA transfer frequency.

Plasmids usually include a number of genes in addition to those required for their replication and transfer to other cells. The variety of cellular properties associated with plasmids is very great and includes production of toxins, pili and other adhesins, and resistance to antimicrobials. However, plasmids can add a small metabolic burden to the cell, and in many cases, a slightly reduced growth rate results. Unless this excess genetic content provides the cell with some advantage, plasmids tend to be lost during prolonged growth. Conversely, when the property conferred by the plasmid is advantageous (eg, in the presence of the antimicrobial to which the plasmid determines resistance), selective pressure favors the plasmid-carrying strain.

Conjugation in Gram-negative Species

Conjugative plasmids in Gram-negative bacteria contain a set of genes which encode the structures and enzymes required to potentiate DNA transfer between cells. These include bridging structures such as a type IV secretion system (Figure 21–22) or in *E coli* the **sex pilus,** shown in Figure 21–35. The sex pilus has the ability to draw the donor and recipient cell into an intimate contact needed to form a conjugal bridge and support assembly of a distinct portal through which DNA can pass. The plasmid DNA is enzymatically cleaved, and one strand is guided through the conjugation structure into the recipient cell by the action of various proteins (**Figure 21–36**). Both the introduced strand and the strand remaining behind in the donor cell direct the synthesis of their complementary strands, resulting in complete copies in both donor and recipient cells. Finally, circularization of the double-stranded molecules occurs, the conjugation bridge is broken, and both cells can now function as donor cells. An alternative outcome is the recombination of fragments of the transferred plasmid with the chromosome.

Conjugation in Gram-positive Species

Plasmids carrying genes encoding antimicrobial resistance, common pili and other adhesins, and some exotoxins are readily transferred by conjugation among Gram-positive bacteria. However, Gram-positive species may involve chromosomal genes in the process. In *Enterococcus faecalis*, one of the most resistant Gram-positive species, donor and recipient cells do not couple by means of a secretion system or sex pilus but rather by the clumping of cells that contain a plasmid with those that do not. This clumping is the result of interaction between a proteinaceous adhesin or "aggregation substance" on the surface of the donor (plasmid-containing) cell and a receptor on the surface of the recipient (plasmid-lacking) cell. Both types of cells make the receptor, but only the plasmid-containing cell can make the adhesin, presumably because it is encoded by a plasmid gene.

R Plasmids

Plasmids that include genes conferring resistance to antimicrobial agents or virulence factors such as toxins are of great significance in medicine. One class of antibiotic resistance-encoding plasmids are the **R plasmids** or **R factors** (**resistance factors**). The genes responsible for resistance usually code for enzymes that mediate many of the resistance mechanisms discussed in Chapter 23. R plasmids of Gram-negative bacteria can be transmitted across species boundaries

---

Plasmids are small, circular DNA molecules

* Conjugative plasmids contain the genes for transfer

Conjugation may cross species lines

Many plasmid genes promote survival and pathogenesis

Without selection pressure, plasmids may be lost

Secretion systems or sex pili form bridges between cells

Replication or recombination follows transfer

Coupling results from adhesin–receptor interaction

FIGURE 21-36. **Conjugation.** A conjugative plasmid in **A** is donating a strand of its DNA to cell **B.** The transferred DNA either synthesizes a complementary strand and re-circularizes as in **C** and **D** or remains in fragments as in **E.** The fragments either recombine with the recipient cell chromosome as in **F** or are digested by nucleases in the cytosol.

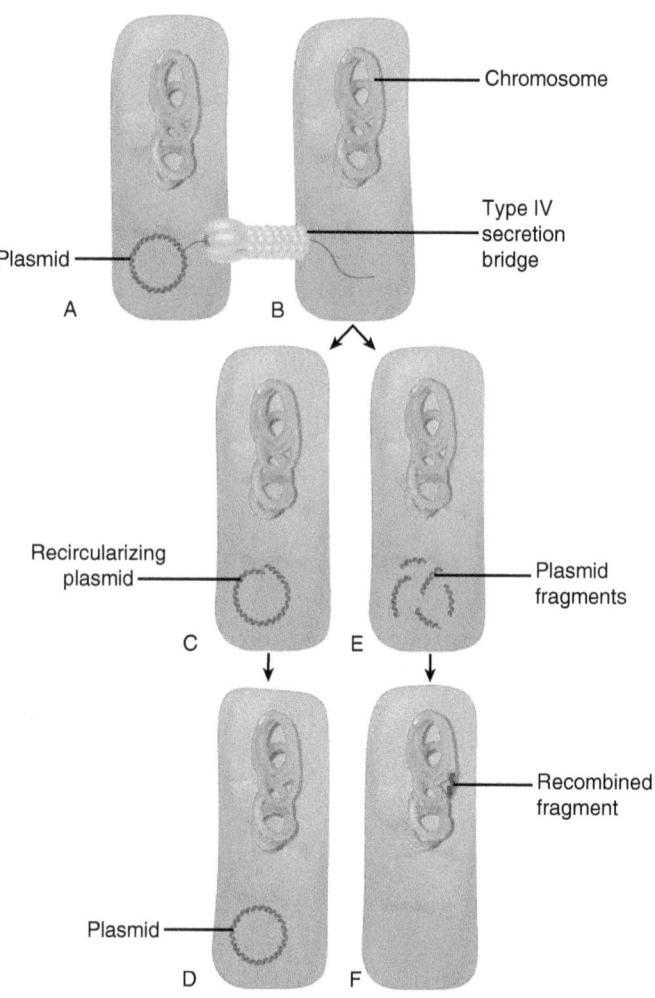

and, at lower frequency, even between genera. Many encode resistance to several antimicrobial agents and can thus spread multiple resistance through a diverse microbial population under selective pressure of only one of those agents to which they confer resistance. Nonpathogenic bacteria can serve as a natural reservoir of resistance determinants on plasmids that are available for spread to pathogens. It is increasingly becoming appreciated that the Bacteroidetes which are predominant human gut commensals, are a gastrointestinal tract reservoir for antibiotic resistance genes.

R plasmids can encode and transfer multiresistance

Resistance genes are acquired by plasmids from Tn

Spread is facilitated by plasmid–chromosome Tn hopping

Widespread antimicrobial use selects R plasmids

R plasmids evolve rapidly and can easily acquire additional resistance-determining genes from fusion with other plasmids or acquisition of mobile genetic elements such as Tn. Most plasmids, and all R factors, contain many IS elements and Tn. In fact, almost all the resistance-determining genes on plasmids are harbored as Tn. As a result, these genes can be amplified by tandem duplications on the plasmid and can insert into coresident plasmids (or to the bacterial chromosome) in the same cell. Combined with the natural properties of many plasmids to transfer themselves by conjugation (even between dissimilar bacterial species), the rapid evolutionary development of multiple drug resistance plasmids and their spread through populations of pathogenic bacteria is a predictable result of the widespread use of antimicrobials in our society.

KEY CONCLUSIONS

- Mutations are caused by replacements, insertions, deletions, and other rearrangements of the nucleotides in genes. They most often inactivate the gene but may change its product.
- Recombination occurs when homologous pairing takes place between DNA strands changing sections of the gene sequence.
- Transposition involves insertion of genes into plasmids and chromosomes in the same cell by recognition of nucleotide sequences.

- Genetic exchange takes place when DNA from one bacterial cell is transferred from a donor to a recipient cell by transformation, transduction, or conjugation. These one-way exchanges may include virulence or antimicrobial resistance genes.

- In transformation, naked DNA is passed across the donor and recipient's cell wall.

- In transduction a bacteriophage injects its DNA which may contain virulence genes into the recipient cell.

- In conjugation plasmid DNA is transferred through a bridge by direct contact between donor and recipient cells.

● BACTERIAL CLASSIFICATION

Bacteria are classified into genera and species according to a binomial scheme similar to that used for higher organisms. For example, in the case of *Staphylococcus aureus*, *Staphylococcus* is the **genus** and *aureus* is the **species** designation. Some genera with common characteristics are further grouped into **families.** However, morphologic descriptors are not as abundant as in higher plants and animals, there is little readily interpreted fossil record to help establish phylogeny, and there is no elaborate developmental process to recapitulate the evolutionary path from ancestral forms. These problems are minor compared with others: bacteria mutate and evolve rapidly, they reproduce asexually, and they exchange genetic material over wide boundaries. The single most important test of species—the ability of individuals within a species to reproduce sexually by mating and exchanging genetic material—cannot be applied to bacteria. As a result, bacterial taxonomy developed pragmatically by determining multiple characteristics and weighting them according to which seemed most fundamental; for example, shape, spore formation, Gram's reaction, aerobic or anaerobic growth, and temperature for growth were given special weighting in defining genera. Additionally, properties as ability to ferment particular carbohydrates, production of specific enzymes and toxins, and antigenic composition of cell surface components were often used in defining species. As presented in Chapter 4, such properties and their weighting continue to be of importance in the identification of unknown isolates in the clinical laboratory, but these approaches are much less sound in establishing taxonomic relationships based on phylogenetic principles.

Weighted classification schemes are more valuable for identification than for taxonomy

NEW TAXONOMIC METHODS

The recognition that sound taxonomy ought to be based on the genetic similarity of organisms and to reflect their phylogenetic **relatedness** has led in recent years to the use of new methods and new principles in taxonomy. The most direct approach available in recent years involves analysis of chromosomal DNA. Analysis can be somewhat crude, such as the overall ratio of A–T to G–C base pairs; differences of greater than 10% in G–C content are taken to indicate unrelatedness, but closely similar content does not imply relatedness. Closer relationships can be assessed by determining base sequence similarity, as by DNA–DNA hybridization (see Chapter 4). However, overwhelmingly, the molecular genetic technique that is introducing the greatest insights into infectious disease is the comparison of nucleotide sequences of genes highly conserved in evolution, such as 16 S ribosomal DNA genes. With the widespread availability of the entire genome sequence for most human pathogens, relatedness can be accessed in silico methods alone. So can the presence of virulence genes in the absence of their products, even for bacteria never isolated in culture.

Phylogenetic relationships are assuming greater significance as the result of DNA sequence analysis

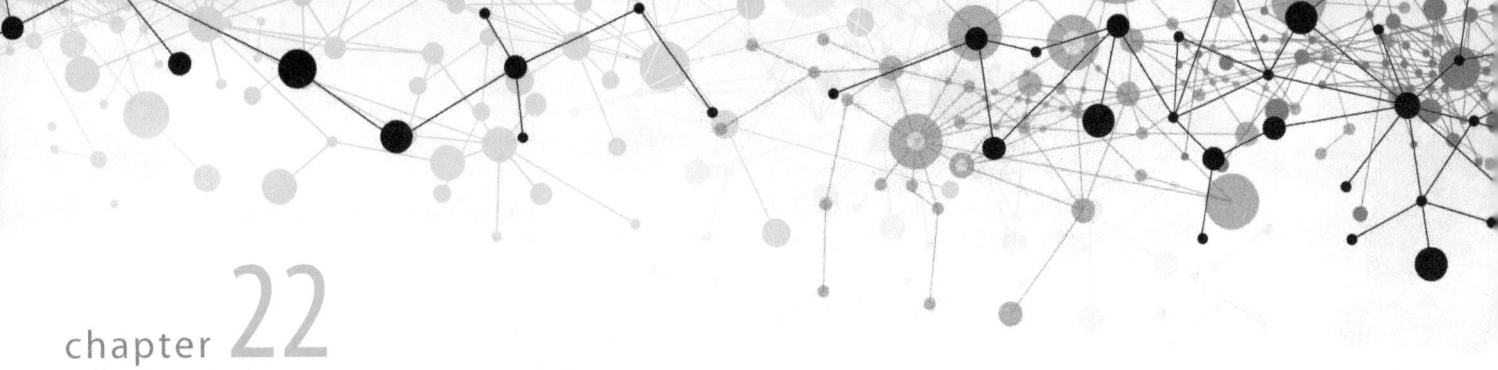

chapter 22

Pathogenesis of Bacterial Infections

Pathogenicity is, in a sense, a highly skilled trade, and only a tiny minority of all the numberless tons of microbes on the earth has ever involved itself in it; most bacteria are busy with their own business, browsing and recycling the rest of life. Indeed, pathogenicity often seems to me a sort of biological accident in which signals are misdirected by the microbe or misinterpreted by the host.

—Lewis Thomas, *The Medusa and the Snail*

OVERVIEW

Chapter 21 describes the astounding diversity and adaptability of bacteria made possible by simplicity, speed, and robust genetic exchange mechanisms. When antibiotics came into use in the middle of the last century, it was supposed to be the end for the bacteria. How wrong we were! Except for those prevented by immunization, bacterial pathogens occupy as prominent a position as at any time since the widespread implementation of public health measures a century ago. The emergence of new pathogens and the resistance of familiar ones to the antimicrobial agents developed in the "arms race" against them are primarily responsible. This chapter lays out the basic mechanisms that bacteria use to produce disease and the genetic mechanisms involved in their deployment. The purpose is to provide a foundation for explaining how these mechanisms are used by specific bacterial pathogens described in Chapters 24 to 41.

DEFINITIONS

Pathogenicity—The ability of any bacterial species to cause disease in a susceptible human host.

Pathogen—A bacterial species able to cause such disease when presented with favorable circumstances (for the organism).

Virulence—A term which presumes pathogenicity, but allows expression of degrees from low to extremely high, for example:

- **Low virulence**—*Streptococcus salivarius* is universally present in the oropharyngeal flora of humans. On its own, it seems incapable of disease production, but if during a transient bacteremia it lands on a damaged heart valve, it can stick and cause slow but steady destruction.

- **Moderate virulence**—*Escherichia coli* is universally found in the colon, but if displacement to other sites such as adjacent tissues or the urinary bladder regularly causes acute infection.

- **High virulence**—*Bordetella pertussis*, the cause of whooping cough, is not found in the resident flora, but if encountered it is highly infectious and causes disease in almost every nonimmune person it contacts.

- **Extremely high virulence**—*Yersinia pestis*, the cause of plague, is also highly infectious, but in addition leads to death in a few days in over 70% of cases.

HUMANS AND BACTERIA

As discussed in Chapter 1, humans have a rich microbiota, and the composition of that flora is mostly bacterial. Long-term survival for a primary pathogen is absolutely dependent on its ability to replicate, survive, and be transmitted to another host. To accomplish this, primary pathogens have evolved the ability to breach human cellular and anatomic barriers that ordinarily restrict or destroy commensal and transient microorganisms. Thus, pathogens can inherently cause damage to cells to gain access by force to a new unique niche that provides them with less competition from other microorganisms, as well as a ready new source of nutrients. Thus, pathogens have not only acquired the capacity to breach cellular barriers, but they also have, by necessity, learned to circumvent, exploit, subvert, and even manipulate our normal cellular mechanisms for their own selfish need to multiply at our expense.

For pathogens not adapted to humans, other animals, or insects, survival in the environment is a requirement for continued disease production. As the most adaptable living forms on the planet, it is not surprising that pathogens are part of the free-living forms common among bacteria. Extended survival is often enhanced by the formation of biofilms in which an extracellular polysaccharide-rich matrix binds an entire bacterial community to an environmental site, for example, water pipes, or a prosthesis. Endospores provide the most extended survival form for Gram-positive bacteria.

The emergence of many seemingly new bacterial diseases has as much to do with human behavior as bacterial adaptability. The Legionnaires disease outbreak of 1976 was eventually traced to *Legionella pneumophila*, which is widely found in aquatic environments as an infectious agent of amoebae. However, without the aerosolization created by modern systems (cooling towers) designed to humidify large buildings, transmission to humans would not have occurred. The development of super-absorbent tampons had the unintended consequence of providing conditions favorable for the production of a toxin by some strains of *S aureus*. The result was a national outbreak of toxic shock syndrome. Food poisoning by *E coli* O157:H7, *Campylobacter*, and *Salmonella* arise as much from food technology and modern food distribution networks as from any fundamental change in the virulence properties of the bacteria in question. No part of our planet is more than 3 days away by air travel, a fact known and feared by all public health officials.

Pathogens must move on to another host

Survival enhanced by biofilms, endospores

Aerosols spread *Legionella*

Tampons enhance toxin production

***E coli* O157:H7 is spread by food processing**

● ATTRIBUTES OF BACTERIAL PATHOGENICITY

Whether a microbe is a primary or opportunistic pathogen, it must be able to enter a host; find a unique niche; avoid, circumvent, or subvert normal host defenses; multiply; and injure the host. For long-term success as a pathogen, it must also establish itself in the host or somewhere else long enough to eventually be transmitted to a new susceptible host. This competition between the pathogen and the host can be viewed as similar to the more familiar military or athletic struggles—that is, the offense against the defense. The more we learn about bacterial pathogens, the more it seems that the most successful ones not only have an excellent offense; they are also particularly able to confound the host defense.

✳ Pathogens must establish a niche and persist

Success involves offense and confounding host defenses

ENTRY: BEATING INNATE HOST DEFENSES

Each of the portals in the body that communicates with the outside world becomes a potential site of microbial entry. Human and other animal hosts have various protective mechanisms to prevent microbial entry (**Table 22–1**). A simple, though relatively efficient, mechanical barrier to microbial invasion is provided by the epithelial borders of the internal and external body surfaces. Of these, the skin is the most formidable with its tough keratinized superficial layer. Organisms can gain access to the underlying tissues only by breaks or by way of hair follicles, sebaceous glands, and sweat glands that traverse the stratified layers. The surface of the skin continuously desquamates and thus tends to shed contaminating organisms. The skin also inhibits the growth of most extraneous microorganisms because of low moisture, low pH, and the presence of substances with antibacterial activity. Bacteria have no known mechanism for passing the unbroken skin.

For the internal surfaces viscous layers of thin and thick **mucin** secreted by goblet cells protect the epithelium lining of the respiratory tract, the gastrointestinal tract, and the urogenital system. Microorganisms become trapped in this thick network of protein and polysaccharide and may be swept away before they reach the epithelial cell surface. Secretory IgA (sIgA) secreted into the mucus and other secreted antimicrobials such as lysozyme and lactoferrin aid this cleansing process. Some bacteria excrete an enzyme **sIgA protease,** which cleaves human sIgA1 in the hinge

Microbes gain access from the environment

✳ Skin is a major protective barrier

TABLE 22-1   Innate Defenses Against Colonization with Pathogens

SITE	MECHANICAL BARRIER	CILIATED EPITHELIUM	COMPETITION BY NORMAL FLORA	MUCUS	SigA	LYMPHOID FOLLICLES	LOW PH	FLUSHING EFFECTS OF CONTENTS	PERISTALSIS	SPECIAL FACTORS
Skin	+++	-	+	-	-	-	++	-	-	Fatty acids from action of normal flora on sebum
Conjunctiva	++	-	-	-	+	-	-	+++	-	Lysozyme
Oropharynx	+++	-	+++	-	+	Yes	-	++	-	
Upper respiratory tract	++	+	+++	++	++	Yes	-	++	-	Turbinate baffles
Middle ear and paranasal sinuses[a]	++	+++	-	++	?	-	-	+	-	
Lower respiratory tract[a]	++	+++	-	++	++	Yes	-	-	-	Mucociliary escalator, alveolar macrophages; cough reflex
Stomach	++	-	-	++	-	-	+++	+	+	Production of hydrochloric acid
Intestinal tract	++	-	+++	+++	+++	Yes	-	+	+++	Bile; digestive enzymes
Vagina	+++	-	+++	+	+	-	+++	-	-	Lactobacillary flora ferments
Urinary tract[a]	++	-	-	-	+	-	+	+++	-	

[a]Sterile in health.

+, ++, +++, relative importance in defense at each site; -, unimportant.

TABLE 22–2	Dose of Microorganisms Required to Produce Infection in Human Volunteers		
MICROBE		**ROUTE**	**DISEASE-PRODUCING DOSE**
Salmonella serotype Typhi		Oral	10^5
Shigella spp.		Oral	10-1000
Vibrio cholerae		Oral	10^8
V cholerae		Oral + HCO_3^-	10^{4a}
Mycobacterium tuberculosis		Inhalation	1-10

[a]Lower dose reflects bicarbonate neutralizing the acid barrier of the stomach.

Mucin coats mucosal epithelium

✳ sIgA protease aids survival

Acids and enzymes aid in cleansing

✳ Infection may be dose related

region to release the Fc portion from the Fab fragment. This enzyme may play an important role in establishing microbial species at the mucosal surface. Ciliated epithelial cells constantly move the mucin away from the lower respiratory tract. In the respiratory tract, particles larger than 5 μm are trapped in this fashion. The epithelium of the intestinal tract below the esophagus is a less efficient mechanical barrier than the skin, but there are other effective defense mechanisms. The high level of hydrochloric acid and gastric enzymes in the normal stomach kill many ingested bacteria. Other bacteria are susceptible to pancreatic digestive enzymes or to the detergent effect of bile salts.

How efficiently bacterial pathogens navigate all these barriers before their initial encounter with their target cell type is, in many cases, determined by their infecting dose. How many organisms must be given to a host to ensure infection in some proportion of the individuals? Estimates of the infectious doses for several pathogens are shown in **Table 22–2.** In general, pathogens that have environmental or animal reservoirs can overwhelm innate defenses with large numbers. Those that are amplified by growth in food may also deliver high numbers with or without a reservoir. Pathogens with no reservoir or amplification mechanism must be transmitted human to human and thus require the lowest infecting doses. Without this advantage, these pathogens would eventually die out in the population.

ADHERENCE: THE SEARCH FOR A UNIQUE NICHE

The first major interaction between a pathogenic microorganism or its virulence factor(s) and its host entails contact with a eukaryotic cell surface. When the offending organism itself engages with the host cell, the process is called "adherence" and it requires the participation of two sets of factors: **adhesins** on the invading microbe and **receptors** on the host cell (**Figure 22–1**).

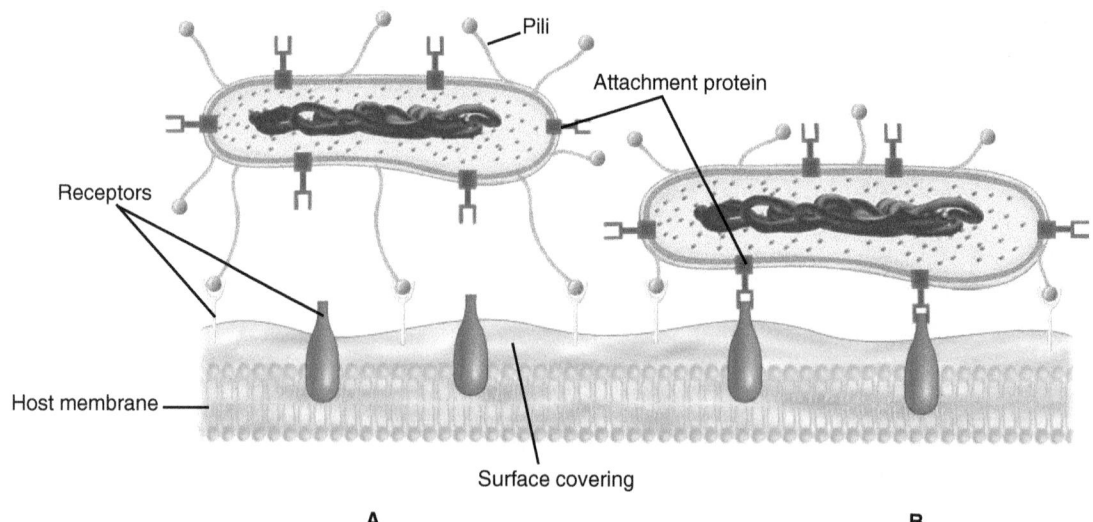

FIGURE 22–1. Bacterial attachment. A. The bacterial cell has both adhesive pili and another protein adhesin protruding from its surface. The pili are binding to a receptor present in material covering the cytoplasmic membrane. **B.** The pili have pulled the organism into closer contact allowing the second adhesin to bind its receptor, which extends from the cytoplasmic membrane through the surface coating.

Pili

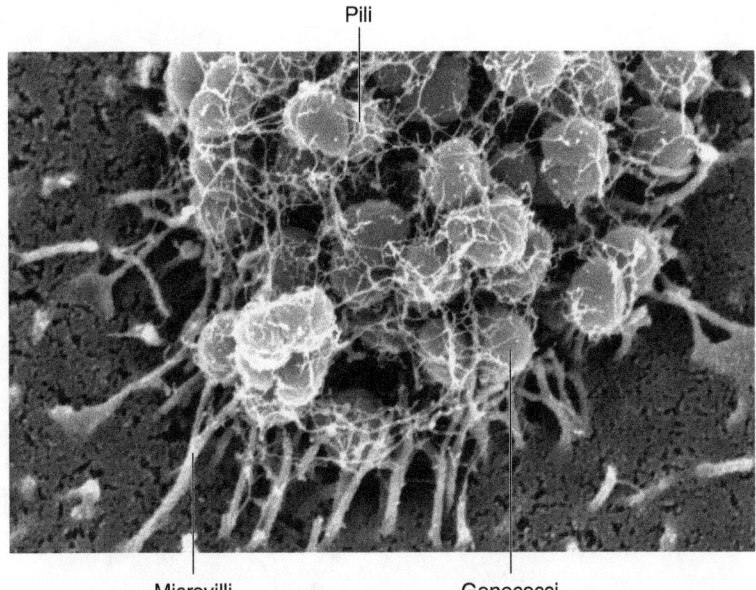

Microvilli   Gonococci

FIGURE 22–2. **Pili.** Pili extending from a microcolony of *Neisseria gonorrhoeae* (gonococci) are shown attaching the microvilli of an epithelial cell. The pili actively retract and mediate a movement of the colony across the cell surface called twitching motility. (Used with permission from Dustin L. Higashi and Magdalene So.)

The adhesin must be exposed on the bacterial surface either alone or in association with appendages like pili. Pili seem to be "sticky" by themselves which may be enhanced by specific adhesin/receptor molecular relationships mediated by molecules at their tips. In Gram-negative bacteria, the outer membrane is a major site for adhesins. Most adhesins are proteins, but carbohydrates and teichoic acids may also be involved. The chemical nature of host receptors is less well known because of the greater difficulty in their isolation (bacteria can be grown by the gallon), but they may be thought of as general or specific. For example, two of the most common receptors, mannose and fibronectin, are widely present on human epithelial cell surfaces. Pili that bind to them can mediate attachment at many sites. Specific receptors are those unique to a particular cell type such as human enterocytes or uroepithelial cells. Where known, these receptors are usually sugar residues that are part of glycolipids or glycoproteins on the host cell surface.

> **Adhesin and receptor are required**
>
> ✳ Pili often bind mannose, fibronectin
>
> **Receptors may be specific to host cell type**

Many bacteria have more than one mechanism of host cell attachment. In some instances, pili mediate initial attachment, which is followed by a stronger, more specific binding mediated by another protein. This may allow implementation of a second function such as cytoskeleton rearrangement or invasion. Multiple adhesins may also allow bacteria to use one set at the epithelial surface but a different set when encountering other cell types or the immune system. The role of pili may be more than a simple adhesive one. The pili of *Neisseria gonorrhoeae*, the etiologic agent of gonorrhea, mediate an active twitching motility on the cell surface with the formation of mobile microcolonies (**Figure 22–2**). Biofilms may also act as an adherence mechanism by binding to catheters, prosthetic devices, or mucosal surfaces.

> **Many have multiple attachment mechanisms**
>
> ✳ Biofilms can mediate adherence

■ **Strategies for Survival**

Once the bacterial pathogen attaches, it must persist if it is to produce disease. Survival is less complicated if the organism can produce injury without being displaced from its initial niche. This is the case with some exotoxin-mediated bacterial diseases (diphtheria, whooping cough), but most pathogens must either enter into the cell or traverse beyond it. To do so requires a new set of survival strategies which include either multiplying in the intracellular milieu or avoiding the attack of complement and phagocytes in the submucosa.

INVASION: GETTING INTO CELLS

A few bacteria, like viruses, are obligate intracellular pathogens. Other bacteria are facultative intracellular pathogens and can grow as free-living cells in the environment as well as within host cells. Generally, invasive organisms adhere to host cells by one or more adhesins but use a class of molecules, called **invasins,** which interact with integrins or other families of cell adhesion molecules. The integrins in turn interact with elements of the cell cytoskeleton stimulating modifications which end in uptake of the bacterial cell. Invasive bacteria seem to be exploiting cell uptake mechanisms that are there for other purposes such as nutrition.

> ✳ Invasins interact with cytoskeleton

FIGURE 22–3. **Bacterial invasion. A.** The bacterial cell has an injection secretion system that is injecting multiple proteins into the host cell. Some of these cause cytoskeletal reorganization, which engulfs the bacteria. In the cytosol, the bacteria lyse the vacuolar membrane, escape, and move about. **B.** A bacterial surface protein binds to the cell surface and induces its own endocytosis. In the cell, some escape (as in A), and others multiply in the phagosome. Another bacterium is seen invading between cells A and B by disrupting intercellular attachment molecules.

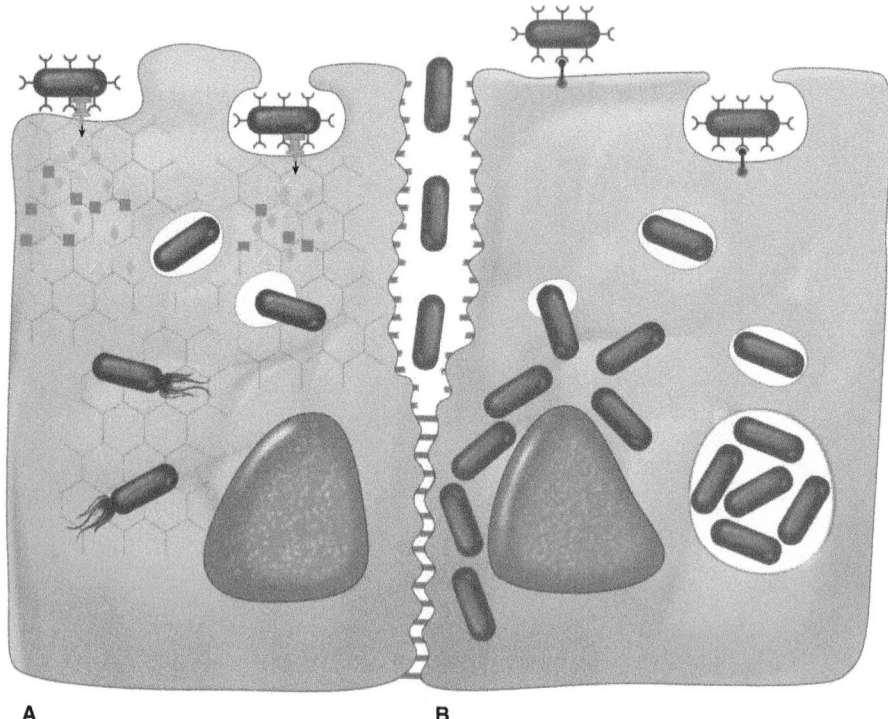

A   B

Enter phagosome or cytoplasm

✱ Pathogens can block phagosome killing

✱ Injection secretion systems trigger invasion or tight binding

Subepithelial environment is different

✱ Siderophores compete for iron sources

Bacteria enter cells initially within a membrane-bound, host-vesicular structure but then follow one of two pathways (**Figure 22–3**). Some bacteria (*Listeria, Shigella*) enzymatically lyse the phagosome membrane and escape to the nutrient-rich safe haven of the host cell cytoplasm. These bacteria may continue to multiply there, infect adjacent cells, or move through the cell to the submucosa. Other invasive pathogenic species (*Salmonella* serotype Typhi, *Mycobacterium tuberculosis*) remain in the phagosome and replicate even in professional phagocytes. Their survival in this usually perilous location is due to thwarting of normal host cell trafficking patterns and avoidance of the killing action of the phagolysosome. There are multiple known mechanisms for this including preventing phagosome–lysosome fusion or, if fused, blocking acidification to the optimum pH for digestive enzyme activity. Some bacteria are able to neutralize the phagocytes' oxidative burst by the production of neutralizing enzymes (catalase, superoxide dismutase).

In Gram-negative bacteria with injection secretion systems (types III, IV, VI), a variation on the above scenarios is possible. The secretion systems inject many proteins, some of which disrupt cellular signaling and the cell's cytoskeleton. The cytoskeleton rearrangements may leave the bacteria tightly bound to an altered surface or trigger invasion. Enteropathogenic *E coli* even injects its own receptor, which is processed to the outer membrane where it mediates tight binding of its parent bacterial strain.

PERSISTING IN A NEW ENVIRONMENT

Bacteria that reach the subepithelial tissues are immediately exposed to the extracellular tissue fluids, which have defined properties that inhibit multiplication of many bacteria. For example, most tissues contain lysozyme in sufficient concentrations to disrupt the cell wall of Gram-positive bacteria. Tissue fluid itself is a suboptimal growth medium for most bacteria and is deficient in free iron. In humans, the iron not found in hemoglobin is chelated to a series of iron-binding proteins (lactoferrin, transferrin). Because virtually all pathogenic bacteria require iron, they have evolved their own set of iron-binding proteins called **siderophores** which effectively compete with the human proteins for available iron.

CONFOUNDING THE IMMUNE SYSTEM

The host immune system evolved in large part because of the selective pressure of microbial attack. To be successful, microbial pathogens must escape this system at least long enough to be transmitted to a new susceptible host or to take up residence within the host in a way that is compatible with mutual coexistence.

INNATE IMMUNITY

Manipulating PAMPs and AMPs

The early warning and response system in which pathogen-associated molecular patterns (PAMPs) are recognized by Toll-like receptors (TLRs) (see Chapter 2) is subject to evasion by successful pathogens. This has been studied in regard to Gram-negative bacterial lipopolysaccharide (LPS) whose pattern is typically detected by TLR-4. In some pathogens (*Helicobacter, Legionella, Yersinia*), the lipid A (toxic) component of LPS is simply a variant poorly recognized by TLR-4; other pathogens (*Salmonella, Pseudomonas*) are able to modulate their lipid A pattern. The result of both is a head start by evading a major innate immune mechanism. Modification of lipid A in a way that modifies their surface charge is also a mechanism by which Gram-negative bacteria escape the action of antimicrobial peptides (AMPs) which attack bacterial membranes by electrostatic force. Gram-positive bacteria may similarly accomplish this by altering their cell wall teichoic acids.

✴ LPS modifications disrupt PAMPs and AMPs

Disrupting Complement

A fundamental requirement for many pathogenic bacteria is escape from phagocytosis by macrophages and polymorphonuclear leukocytes. The most common bacterial means of avoiding phagocytosis is an antiphagocytic capsule, which is possessed by almost all principal pathogens that cause pneumonia and meningitis. These polysaccharide capsules of pathogens interfere with effective complement deposition on the bacterial cell surface by binding regulators of C3b that are present in serum. When one of these, serum factor H, is concentrated on the capsular surface, it accelerates the degradation of C3b deposited from the host's serum. This negates both direct complement injury and makes the receptors recognized by phagocytes unavailable (**Figure 22–4**). This mechanism is not restricted to polysaccharide capsules. Surface proteins able to bind factor H have the same biologic effect. Antibody directed against the capsular antigen reverses this effect because C3b can then bind in association with IgG. Another mechanism for complement disruption is through surface acquisition of sialic acid, a common component of capsular polysaccharides. Some bacteria are able to incorporate sialic acid from the host on their surfaces with an effect similar to capsules.

Polysaccharide capsules and surface proteins may be antiphagocytic

✴ Binding serum factor H to the surface interferes with C3b deposition

■ Adaptive Immunity

Antigenic Variation

Another method by which microorganisms avoid host immune responses is by varying surface antigens. Gonorrhea is a disease in which there appears to be no natural immunity and

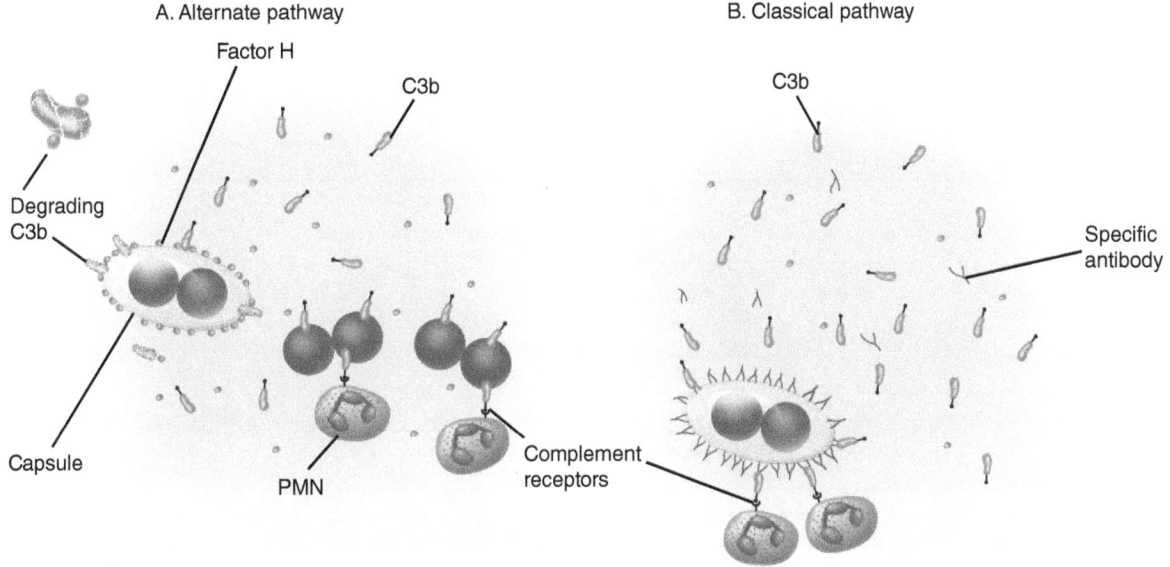

FIGURE 22–4. Bacterial resistance to opsonophagocytosis. A. Alternate pathway. In the alternate complement pathway, C3b binds to the surface of bacteria, providing a recognition site for professional phagocytes and sometimes causing direct injury. Bacteria with special surface structures such as capsules or protein are able to bind serum factor H to their surface. This interferes with complement deposition by accelerating the breakdown of C3b. **B.** Classical pathway. Specific antibody binding to an antigen on the surface provides another binding site for C3b. Phagocyte recognition may occur even if factor H is present.

reinfections are common. In fact, an immune response can be mounted to the pathogenically significant surface pili and outer membrane proteins (OMPs) of *N gonorrhoeae*, but the organism is continuously varying them. This can happen even in the course of a single acute infection. The genetic mechanism for antigenic variation of pili involves recombination between multiple silent and expressing genes in the gonococcal chromosome. For OMPs multiple genes are turned on and off by the status of a frame-shift mutation. These mechanisms are illustrated in **Figure 22–5** and discussed further in Chapter 30. The effect is that when the immune system delivers specific IgG to the site of infection, it will bind its homologous antigen, but a subpopulation with an antigenically different surface can multiply and continue the infection. Therefore, the pathogen escapes immune surveillance. A number of other bacteria and parasites also undergo antigenic variation.

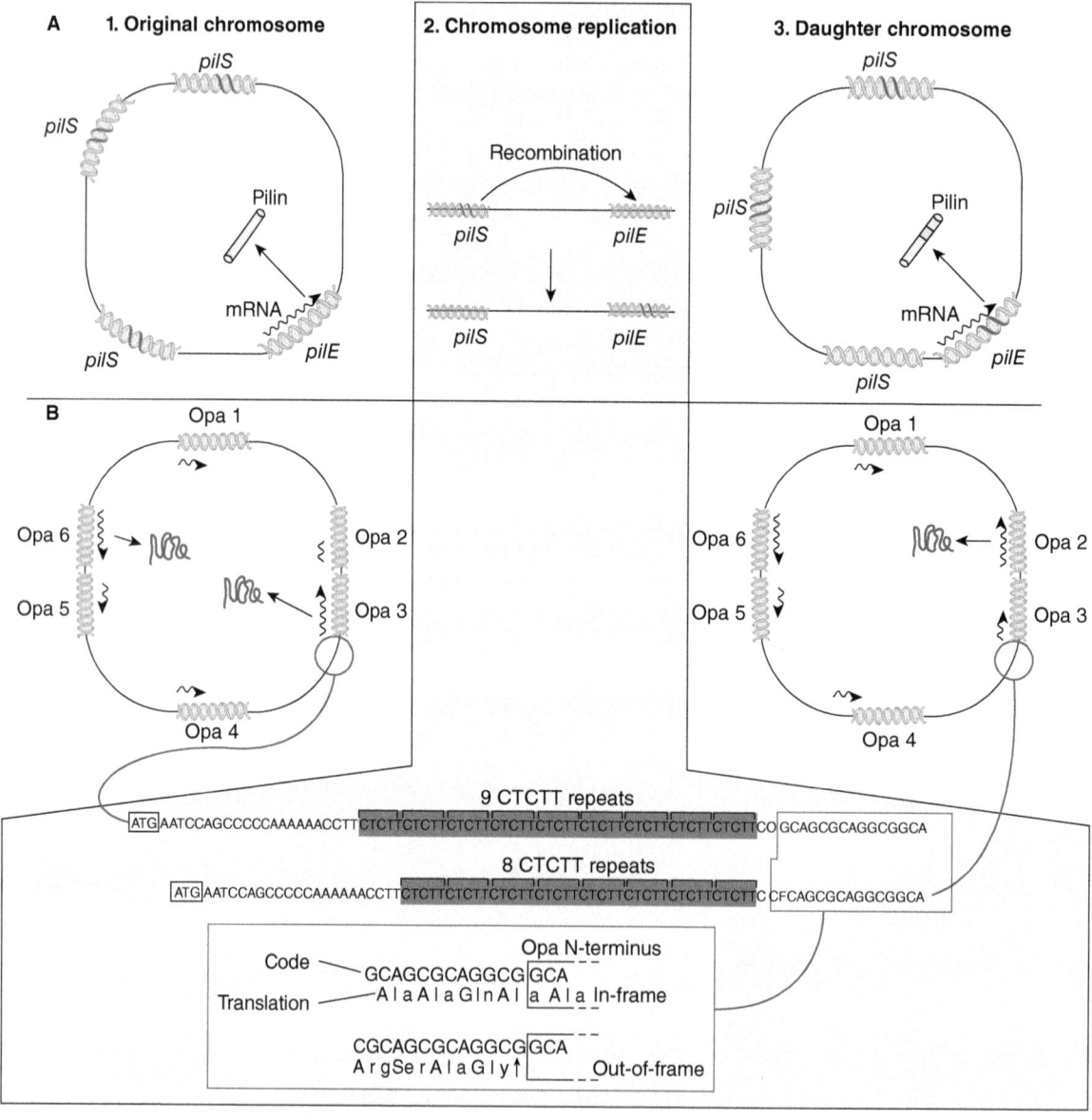

FIGURE 22–5. Antigenic variation. Mechanisms for change in the antigenic makeup of both pili and outer membrane Opa proteins of *Neisseria gonorrhoeae* are shown. **A.** The chromosome contains multiple unlinked pilin genes, which are either expressing (*pilE*) or silent (*pilS*). The expressing gene is transcribing a mature pilin protein subunit. During chromosome replication, one of the *pilS* genes recombines with one of the *pilE* genes, donating some of its DNA (red). The new daughter chromosome now produces an antigenically different pilin based on transcription of the donated (red) sequences into protein. **B.** The chromosome contains multiple Opa genes. Opa 3 and Opa 6 are "on" (producing protein), and the others are "off." During chromosome replication, replicative slippage in the leader peptide causes a five-base sequence (CTCTT) to be repeated variable numbers of times. Translation of the Opa will remain in-frame only if the number of added CTCTT nucleotides is evenly divisible by 3. For the Opa gene in **B1**, the triplet code for alanine (GCA) is in-frame (9 × 5 = 45. 45 ÷ 3 = 15) but in **B3** it is out-of-frame.

INJURY

The successful pathogen must survive and multiply in the face of multiple host defenses. Although this is a formidable achievement, by itself it is not enough to cause disease. Disease requires some disruption of host function by the bacteria. Bacterial toxins are the most obvious mechanism of injury and are exported by the secretion systems described in Chapter 21 often along with multiple other virulence factors. In some diseases the only injury appears to be due to the inflammatory response to the invader.

Disease requires injury to the host

■ Exotoxins

The longest known and best-studied virulence factors are bacterial exotoxins. They are proteins toxic to the human host which are secreted by the bacteria into the surrounding body fluids. Their action may be local or systemic if absorbed into the bloodstream. These exotoxins usually possess some degree of host cell specificity, which is dictated by the nature of the binding of one or more toxin components to a specific host cell receptor. The distribution of host cell receptors often dictates the degree and nature of the toxicity.

A–B Exotoxins

The best-known pathogenic exotoxin theme is represented by the A–B exotoxins. These toxins are divided into two general domains. The B subunit(s) contains the binding specificity of the holotoxin to the host cell. In general, the B region binds to a specific host cell surface glycoprotein or glycolipid. The specificity of this binding determines the host cell specificity of the toxin. The A (active) subunit catalyzes an enzymatic reaction specific to the toxin. After attachment of the B domain to the host cell surface, the A domain is transported by direct fusion or by endocytosis into the host cell. In the cell, the A unit carries out the enzymatic modification of a protein called its **target protein.** The most common enzymatic reaction is **ADP-ribosylation,** which attaches the ADP-ribose moiety from nicotinamide adenine dinucleotide (NAD) to the target protein. The ADP-ribosylated host protein is then unable to carry out its function or behaves abnormally. There are multiple other enzymatic reactions carried out by A–B exotoxins.

✳ B unit binds to cell receptor

✳ A unit acts on target protein

The net effect of the toxin depends on the intracellular function of the target protein and the biologic function of the cell in humans. If it is crucial for the protein-synthesizing apparatus of the cell (diphtheria toxin), protein synthesis ceases and the cell dies (see Figure 1–7). However, cell death is not the inevitable outcome of toxin action. One of the major targets of the ADP-ribosylating A–B toxins are guanine nucleotide-binding proteins (G proteins), which are involved in signal transduction in eukaryotic cells. In this case, the inactivation of the regulatory G protein can inhibit or stimulate some activity of the cell. Cholera toxin inactivates a G protein that downregulates a secretory pathway. If the cell is an intestinal enterocyte, the end result is hypersecretion of electrolytes and diarrhea. Cholera toxin applied to cells from the adrenal gland stimulates steroid production.

Biologic effect depends on function of target protein

Toxin effect may be inhibitory, stimulatory, or fatal

Membrane-Active Exotoxins

Some exotoxins act directly on the surface of host cells to lyse or to kill them. Many were first observed in the laboratory by their ability to cause hemolysis of erythrocytes. The most common action is to create pores by direct insertion into eukaryotic membranes of a wide range of cells including phagocytes (**Figure 22-6**). These **pore-forming toxins** are produced by some of the

✳ Insertion in cytoplasmic membrane creates a leaking pore

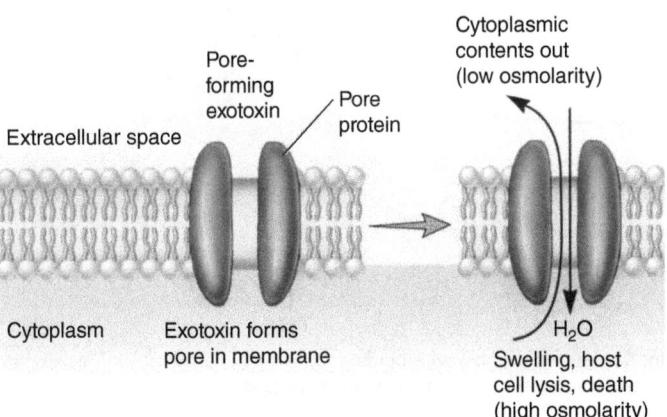

FIGURE 22–6. **Pore-forming exotoxin.** The pore protein has inserted itself into the host cell membrane making an open channel. Formation of multiple such pores causes cytoplasmic contents to leave the cell and water to move in. This ultimately leads to cell lysis and death. (Reproduced with permission from Willey JM: *Prescott, Harley, & Klein's Microbiology*, 7th ed. New York, NY: McGraw Hill; 2008.)

most aggressive pathogens (*S aureus*, group A streptococcus, *E coli*) and cause cellular death by loss of cellular integrity and leakage through the pore. The α-toxin of *Clostridium perfringens* is a lecithinase causing hemolysis of RBCs.

Superantigen Exotoxins

Some microbial exotoxins have a direct effect on cells of the immune system, and this interaction leads to disease. The most dramatic of these are the toxins causing the toxic shock syndromes of *S aureus* and group A streptococci. These syndromes are evoked when toxin is produced at an infected site and absorbed into the circulation. These toxins are able to bind directly to class II major histocompatibility complex (MHC) molecules on antigen-presenting cells (without processing) and directly stimulate production of cytokines such as interleukin 1 (IL-1) and tumor necrosis factor (TNF) (**Figure 22–7**). These molecules are called superantigens because they act as polyclonal stimulators of T cells. This means a significant proportion of all T cells respond by dividing and releasing cytokines, which makes the cytokine release massive enough to cause systemic effects such as shock. When ingested preformed in food, some of these toxins cause diarrhea and vomiting.

■ Endotoxin

In many infections caused by Gram-negative bacteria, the LPS endotoxin of the outer membrane is a significant component of the disease process. LPS can cause local injury, but the major effects are manifested when Gram-negative bacteria enter the bloodstream and circulate. The lipid A portion causes fever through the release of IL-1 and TNF from macrophages and dramatic physiologic effects associated with inflammation. These include hypotension, lowered

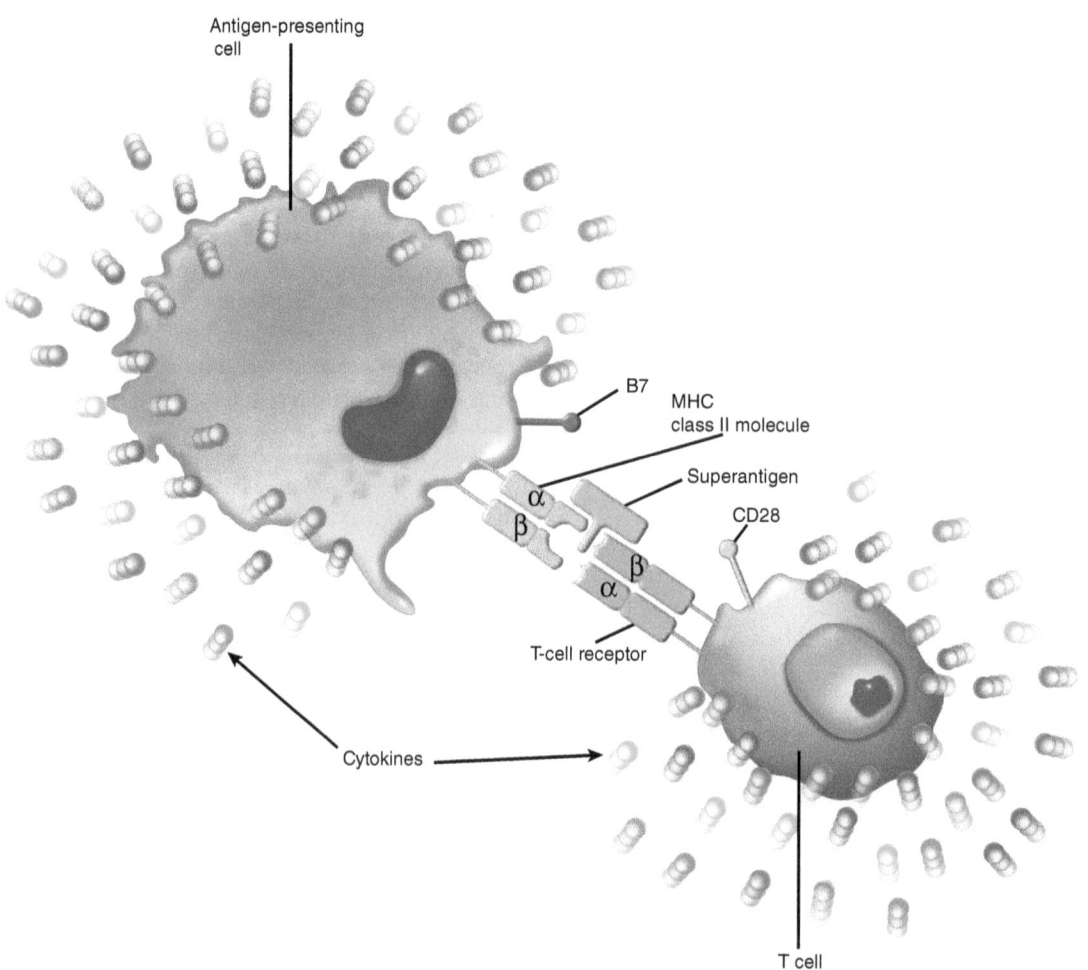

FIGURE 22–7. Superantigen exotoxin. A superantigen (*yellow*) is binding to the MHC class II molecular complex outside the groove for antigen presentation. This causes a massive secretion of cytokines.

polymorphonuclear leukocyte and platelet counts from increased margination of these cells to the walls of the small vessels, hemorrhage, and sometimes disseminated intravascular coagulation (DIC) from the activation of clotting factors. Rapid and irreversible shock may follow passage of endotoxin into the bloodstream.

The term "endotoxin" comes from the fact that LPS is an inherent structural component of the Gram-negative cell wall, not a secreted product of the bacteria. A comparable event with Gram-positive and Gram-negative bacteria can occur with the release and circulation of peptidoglycan cell wall fragments. This also leads to cytokine release and systemic manifestations. Although the biology is similar, the terms "endotoxin" or "endotoxemia" are not used because they have long been reserved for the LPS endotoxin of Gram-negative bacteria.

Lipid A is toxic portion

Peptidoglycan fragments are not called endotoxin

■ Damage Caused by Inflammation and Immune Responses

Many successful pathogens produce disease without using any of the known virulence factors just described. In these instances, injury can still be produced by acute or chronic inflammation or a misdirected immune response triggered by antigenic components of the pathogen.

Persistent Inflammation

The normal inflammatory response is a two-edged sword in both acute and chronic infections. Although the enzymes of PMNs are killing the invader, they still cause some damage to host tissues or compromise organ function. Pulmonary alveoli filled with PMNs and macrophages are not effective in the absorption of oxygen. In the closed space of the central nervous system, the swelling caused by inflammation may directly lead to brain injury. In some chronic infections, the pathologic and clinical features are due largely to delayed-type hypersensitivity (DTH) reactions to the organism or its products. In tuberculosis, if the host is unable to halt the growth of *M tuberculosis* by activation of cell-mediated immunity, persistent growth of the pathogen will continue to stimulate DTH-mediated injury.

✱ PMNs cause swelling, occupy space

✱ Prolonged DTH is destructive

Misdirected Immune Responses

Reactions between high concentrations of antibody, soluble microbial antigens, and complement can deposit immune complexes in tissues and cause acute inflammatory reactions and immune complex disease. In poststreptococcal acute glomerulonephritis, for example, the complexes are sequestered in the glomeruli of the kidney, with serious interference of renal function from the resulting complement deposition and tissue reaction. Antibodies produced against bacterial antigens can cross-react with certain host tissues and initiate an autoimmune process. This molecular mimicry is felt to be the explanation for poststreptococcal rheumatic fever.

Bacterial antigens trigger autoimmune cross-reactions

KEY CONCLUSIONS

- Bacteria use pili and surface proteins to adhere to mannose, fibronectin, and other receptors on the surface of epithelial cells.
- Cell invasion and cytoskeleton modification are triggered by surface "invasins." This allows residence in the cytoplasm, progress to adjacent cells, or exit to the submucosa.
- Survival in professional phagocytes is achieved by multiple mechanisms which defeat steps in their bacterial killing processes.
- Survival in the submucosa and beyond requires nutrient scavenging and defense against the innate and adaptive immune systems.
- Capsules and surface proteins interfere with complement C3b deposition by binding serum factor H.
- Specific humoral immunity is confounded by antigenic variation of surface virulence factors.
- Superantigens cause massive cytokine release.
- Pore-forming toxins punch holes in cells.
- Protein exotoxins catalyze enzymatic reactions which inactivate or disrupt key metabolic processes of the cell. LPS endotoxin causes shock.
- Acute and chronic inflammation compromise organ function. Prolonged DTH is destructive.

● GENETICS OF BACTERIAL PATHOGENICITY

PLASMIDS

Many of the essential determinants of pathogenicity are actually replicated as part of the bacterial chromosome, but a surprising number are carried in plasmids. This often includes multiple virulence factors in the same plasmid. For example, one type of diarrhea-causing *E coli* carries the genes for pili mediating adherence to enterocytes, and for the enterotoxin, it delivers to those enterocytes on the same plasmid. The term **virulence plasmid** has been used for plasmids whose loss or modification causes loss of pathogenicity for the host strain. Since plasmids are inherently a less secure home for genes than the chromosome, this location must provide some efficiency for the pathogen. Perhaps the excess baggage of the plasmid is a trade-off for avoiding disruption of the organization of the bacterial chromosome.

REGULATION OF VIRULENCE GENES

In addition to the multiple steps of pathogenesis, some pathogens lurk in locations like seawater (cholera) or fleas (plague) until their opportunity to cause human disease presents itself. As it is not economical to produce virulence factors when they are not needed, it is not surprising that bacteria have evolved mechanisms for their timely deployment. The control involves regulatory genes and their products activating genes, operons, regulons (see Chapter 21), and more complex systems. One of the longest known of these are the "on" and "off" states of flagellar genes explaining their phase variation. It turns out that the motility mediated by these flagella is a virulence factor in *E coli* urinary tract infections. Many pathogens have evolved regulatory systems, which link sensing of environmental cues (temperature, osmolarity, iron concentration) to activation of their virulence apparatus. These signals can "tell" the pathogen whether it is in a benign environment, inside an insect vector, in body fluids, or even inside a phagocyte. The virulence factor deployment then proceeds often in a multistep manner, synthesizing the adhesin or toxin just at the time it is needed. An example of this is shown in **Figure 22–8,** which illustrates the two-component regulatory system used by *B pertussis* in whooping cough. In the resting state *B pertussis* produces no virulence factors. Sensing a physiologic temperature, it starts to produce its multiple virulence factors in two stages. The first is the factors needed in the early stages of infection such as the adherence protein Fha. After a delay the toxins which mediate the disease itself (pertussis toxin, adenylate cyclase) are produced. This just-in-time production is energy-efficient and effective in producing disease.

QUORUM SENSING

The quantitative aspects of pathogenicity suggest there could be value in timing the deployment of virulence factors in relation to the size of the population ready to attack. Success may depend on a cell population large enough to produce disease before the host mounts an effective defense. For bacteria this would require the cell to be able to sense the local presence of other members of the same species and respond accordingly. Such cell-to-cell communication systems have been described. This communication is called **quorum sensing.** It has been shown to regulate the expression of adherence factors, toxin production, secretion systems, and biofilm formation. In the species studied, the communication is by secretion of small **autoinducer** molecules which can readily diffuse and cross cell membranes much like hormones in higher organisms. In Gram-negative bacteria acylated homoserine lactones and ketones (α-hydroxyketone) have been shown to carry out these functions. In Gram-positive bacteria small peptides are more common. The sending and receiving cells have transcription regulators, which modulate the product of the target gene. Each cell in the population has a synthesis/receptor pair that generates and responds to the autoinducer molecule. The end result is transcription of the relevant virulence factor proteins by the entire bacterial population in unison.

PATHOGENICITY ISLANDS

In recent years, large blocks of genes found on the bacterial chromosome have been given the name pathogenicity island (PAI) to describe unique regions exclusively associated with virulence (**Figure 22–9**). The "island" component of the name comes from the fact that the PAI regions themselves usually have fundamental characteristics such as guanine + cytosine content, codon

Margin notes

*Genes on plasmids are multiple and related

Loss of virulence plasmids negates pathogenicity

Pathogens can sense their environment

*Virulence factors are produced "just in time"

Auto inducers are like hormones

Transcription regulators modulate virulence factors

*Toxins, biofilms, secretion systems activated in unison

Large genomic segments transferred from an unrelated species

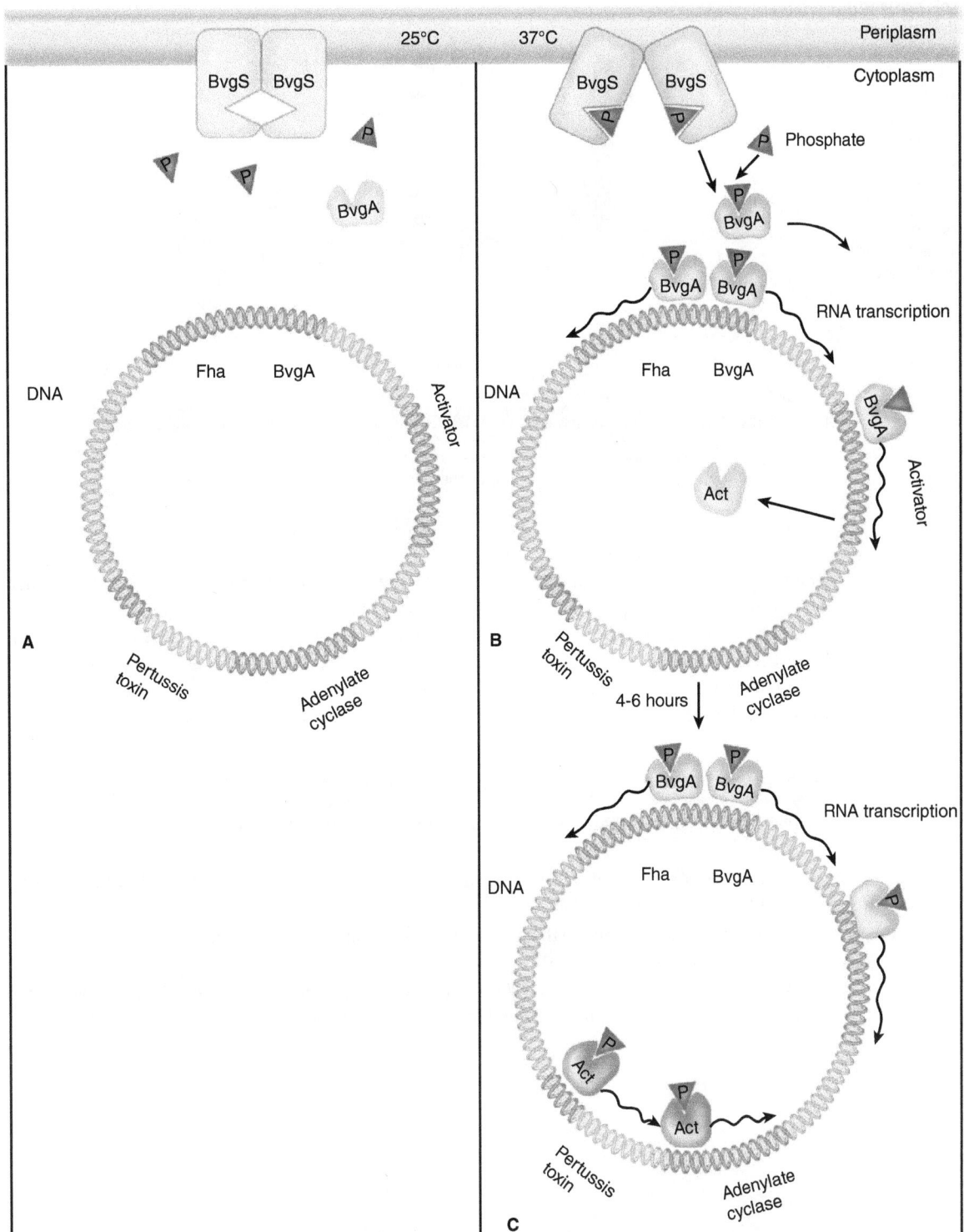

FIGURE 22–8. **Regulation of virulence factors. A.** At 25°C, the membrane-associated regulatory protein BvgS is inactive as are the genes for virulence factors filamentous hemagglutinin (Fha), pertussis toxin, and adenylate cyclase. **B.** At 37°C, BvgS autophosphorylates and activates a cytoplasmic regulatory protein, BvgA, by phosphorylation. BvgA activates transcription of genes for production of BvgS, BvgA, Fha, and a postulated second regulator, Act. **C.** Hours later, transcription of the pertussis toxin and adenylate cyclase is activated by Act. (Adapted with permission from Melton, AR, Weiss AA.)

usage, and tRNA genes that are different from the rest of the genome of the current host organism. This suggests that gene transfer from a foreign species sometime in the distant past is the likely origin. Many PAIs have strikingly similar homologs in bacteria that are pathogenic for plants and animals. The PAIs typically contain the complete package required for delivery of the pathogenic trait, even those that are the most complex involving 20 to 30 genes. In organisms that

✴ Genes for all components of virulence are included

FIGURE 22–9. **Pathogenicity island (PAI). A.** Two bacterial strains are engaged in genetic exchange by one of the mechanisms described in Chapter 21. The recipient (right) has incorporated a large segment of the donor DNA into its chromosome. **B.** The chemical makeup of the donated segment is different from that of the host chromosome. This PAI contains genes for adhesins, toxins, and a secretion system all for the production of the same disease.

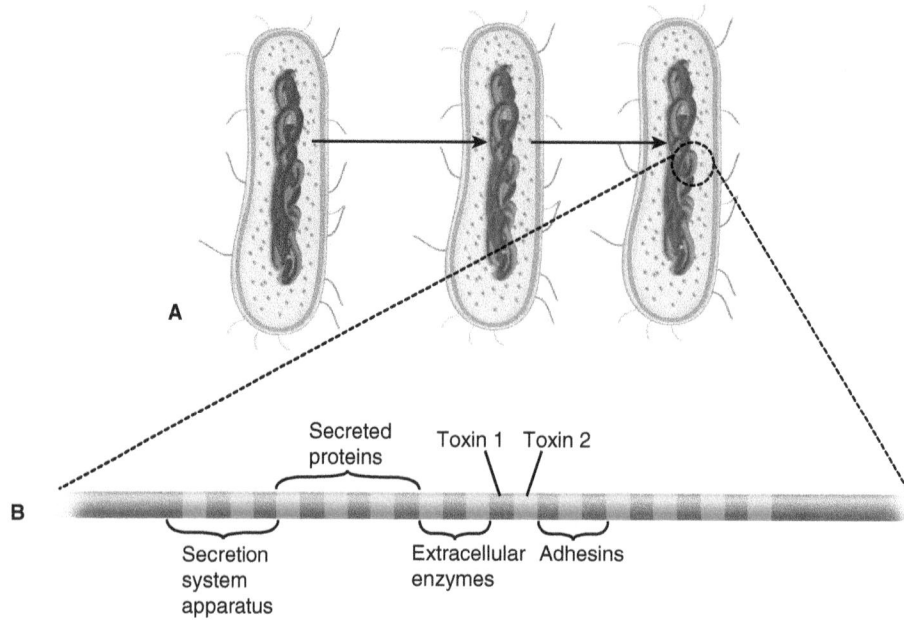

deploy injection secretion systems, the genes for the injection apparatus, the secreted proteins, and regulatory elements are all included in the PAI.

Although human bacterial pathogens represent only a tiny percentage of the microbial world, they are among the most ingenious in the ways they produce disease. The independence and power of the bacterial cell are translated into some of the most feared of all diseases. The bacteriology, disease mechanisms, and clinical aspects of these diseases are explored in the following chapters.

KEY CONCLUSIONS

- Plasmids are common carriers of single or multiple virulence and/or antimicrobial resistance genes.
- Environmental sensors allow complex regulation of multiple virulence factors orchestrating their production only when needed.
- Pathogenicity islands contain the genes for multiple components needed for execution of virulence factors for one disease.
- Quorum sensing involves cell-to-cell communication in a growing bacterial population allowing production of virulence produce when reaching a threshold (the quorum).

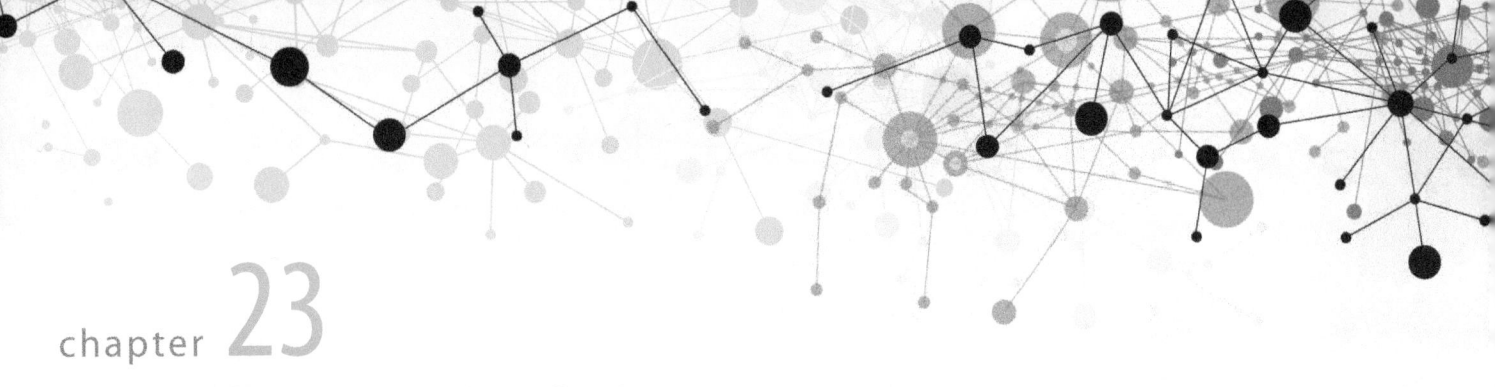

chapter 23

Antibacterial Agents and Resistance

This chapter explains how antibacterials work, the ways in which bacteria become resistant, and strategies we can take to minimize that resistance. Specific information about pathogenic bacteria can be found in Chapters 24 to 41; a complete guide to the treatment of infectious diseases is beyond the scope of this book.

Natural materials with some activity against microbes were used in folk medicine in earlier times. Rational approaches to chemotherapy began with Ehrlich's development of arsenical compounds for the treatment of syphilis early in the 20th century. Years elapsed before the next major development, which was the discovery of the therapeutic effectiveness of a sulfonamide (prontosil rubrum) by Domagk in 1935. Penicillin had been discovered in 1929 by Fleming but could not be adequately purified at that time; this was accomplished later, and penicillin was produced in sufficient quantities so that Florey and colleagues could demonstrate its clinical effectiveness in the early 1940s.

Sulfonamides, penicillin first effective antibacterial agents

Since that time, numerous new antimicrobial agents have been discovered or developed, and many have found their way into clinical practice. Thanks to these medicines, the human experience in industrialized nations is dramatically different today than it was in the pre-antibiotic era. However, this success has come at the cost of rising antimicrobial resistance. In order to be good antimicrobial stewards, all clinicians must understand the ways in which these drugs work, the ways in which bacteria evolve in response to antibiotics, and strategies for their judicious use.

Antimicrobial resistance a critical challenge for modern medicine

ANTIBACTERIAL AGENTS AND THERAPY

Overview

Antibacterial medications attack a variety of bacterial targets. In this chapter, we will classify these drugs by their mechanisms of action. In clinical practice, antibacterials may also be grouped by their spectrum of activity, tissue penetration, route of administration, process of metabolism and elimination, toxicity, drug interactions, and cost.

GENERAL CONSIDERATIONS

Clinically effective antimicrobial agents exhibit selective toxicity toward the microbe rather than the host, a characteristic that differentiates them from the disinfectants (see Chapter 3). In most cases, selectivity is explained by action on microbial processes or structures that differ from those of mammalian cells. For example, some agents inhibit the synthesis of the bacterial cell wall (an organelle not present in eukaryotes), and others act on the 70S bacterial ribosome (but not the 80S eukaryotic ribosome). Some antimicrobials, such as penicillin, are usually nontoxic to the host, unless hypersensitivity develops. For others, such as the aminoglycosides, the effective therapeutic dose is relatively close to the toxic dose; as a result, control of dosage and blood levels must be much more precise.

Selective toxicity based on ability to attack a target present in bacteria not humans

■ Definitions

- **Antibiotics**—antimicrobials of microbial origin, many of which are produced by fungi or by bacteria of the genus *Streptomyces*.
- **Antimicrobials**—substances used in the treatment of infectious diseases, including antibiotics and other antibacterials, antifungals, antiparasitics, and antivirals.
- **Bactericidal**—potent antimicrobial activity that is highly lethal to bacterial growth.
- **Bacteriostatic**—weaker antimicrobial activity than bactericidal agents. Ultimately, host defense mechanisms are responsible for eradication of infection whether bactericidal or bacteriostatic drugs are used.
- **Minimal inhibitory concentration (MIC)**—a laboratory term that defines the lowest concentration (µg/mL) able to inhibit growth of the microorganism *in vitro*.
- **Resistant, nonsusceptible**—microorganisms are not inhibited by clinically achievable concentrations of an antimicrobial agent.
- **Sensitive, susceptible**—microorganisms will be inhibited by concentrations of the antimicrobial that can be achieved clinically.
- **Spectrum**—an expression of the categories of microorganisms against which an antimicrobial is typically active. A narrow-spectrum agent has activity against only a few organisms. A broad-spectrum agent has activity against diverse types of organisms (eg, both Gram-positive and Gram-negative bacteria).

■ Sources of Antimicrobial Agents

There are three main sources of antimicrobial agents.

First are antibiotics, which are molecules of biological origin. They probably play an important part in microbial ecology in the natural environment. Penicillin, for example, is produced by several molds of the genus *Penicillium*, and the first cephalosporin antibiotics were derived from other molds. These substances provide fungi with a selective advantage by protecting them from environmental bacteria, and we can harvest these molecules for clinical use. Another source of naturally occurring antibiotics is the genus *Streptomyces*, which are Gram-positive, branching bacteria found in soil and freshwater sediments. Streptomycin, the tetracyclines, chloramphenicol, erythromycin, and many other antibiotics were discovered by screening large numbers of *Streptomyces* isolates from different parts of the world. Antibiotics are mass-produced by techniques derived from the procedures of the fermentation industry.

Second are the chemically synthesized antimicrobial agents. These were initially discovered among compounds synthesized for other purposes and tested for their therapeutic effectiveness in animals. The sulfonamides, for example, were discovered as a result of routine screening of aniline dyes. More recently, active compounds have been synthesized with structures tailored to be effective inhibitors or competitors of known metabolic pathways. Trimethoprim, which inhibits dihydrofolate reductase, is an excellent example. "Structure-based drug design" involves the use of X-ray crystallography and *in silico* simulations to understand the three-dimensional molecular conformation of potential drug targets, then synthesizing small molecules to bind those targets. This technique holds great promise, although relatively few antimicrobials have yet been developed in this manner.

A third source of antimicrobials arises from the molecular manipulation of previously discovered antibiotics to broaden their range and degree of activity against microorganisms or to improve their pharmacologic characteristics. Examples include the development of penicillinase-resistant and broad-spectrum penicillins, as well as a large range of aminoglycosides and cephalosporins of increasing activity, spectrum, and resistance to inactivating enzymes.

■ Spectrum of Action

The **spectrum** of activity of each antimicrobial agent describes the genera and species against which it is typically active. See **Table 23–1** for the most common antimicrobial agents and bacteria. Spectra overlap but are usually characteristic for each broad class of antimicrobial. Some antibacterial antimicrobials are known as **narrow-spectrum agents;** for example, benzyl penicillin is highly active against many streptococci but has little activity against enteric Gram-negative

---

* Antibiotics synthesized by molds or bacteria

Produced in quantity by industrial fermentation

Chemicals discovered by screening programs or via molecular drug design

Antibiotics can be chemically modified

* Spectrum = range against which agent is typically active

TABLE 23–1	Characteristics of Antibacterial Drugs
TARGET/REPRESENTATIVE DRUGS	**CHARACTERISTICS**
Cell Wall Synthesis	
β-Lactams	Bactericidal against a variety of bacteria; inhibit penicillin-binding proteins
Penicillins	
Natural penicillins: penicillin G, penicillin V	Active against Gram-positive bacteria and some Gram-negative cocci
Penicillinase-resistant: methicillin, dicloxacillin	Similar to the natural penicillins, but resistant to inactivation by the penicillinase of staphylococci
Broad-spectrum: ampicillin, amoxicillin	Similar to the natural penicillins, but more active against Gram-negative organisms
Extended-spectrum: ticarcillin, piperacillin	Increased activity against Gram-negative rods, including *Pseudomonas* species, and anaerobes including *Bacteroides fragilis*. Usually combined with β-lactamase inhibitors
Cephalosporins	Some are more effective against Gram-negative bacteria and less susceptible to destruction by β-lactamases. Generally, newer generations have enhanced Gram-negative coverage, often at expense of Gram-positive coverage.
Cephalexin, cefoxitin, ceftriaxone, cefepime, ceftaroline, ceftolozane, cefiderocol	
Carbapenems	Resistant to inactivation by β-lactamases. Many Gram-positive and Gram-negative bacteria including anaerobes are susceptible
Imipenem, meropenem, doripenem, ertapenem	
Monobactams	Resistant to β-lactamases. Purely Gram-negative coverage, primarily active against members of the family Enterobacteriaceae
Aztreonam	
Non–β-Lactams	
Vancomycin, teicoplanin, telavancin, dalba-vancin, oritavancin	Bactericidal against most staphylococci, but less so than β-lactams; bacteriostatic against most enterococci
Bacitracin	Bactericidal against Gram-positive bacteria
Protein Synthesis	
Aminoglycosides	Bactericidal against Gram-negative aerobic and facultative bacteria
Gentamicin, tobramycin	
Tetracyclines	Bacteriostatic against some Gram-positive and Gram-negative bacteria
Tetracycline, doxycycline, minocycline, tigecycline, omadacycline, eravacycline	
Chloramphenicol	Bacteriostatic and broad spectrum
Pleuromutilins	Bacteriostatic against many Gram-positive and some Gram-negative bacteria
Retapamulin, lefamulin	
Macrolides	Bacteriostatic against many Gram-positive bacteria as well as some mycobacteria
Erythromycin, clarithromycin, azithromycin	
Lincosamides	Bacteriostatic against a variety of Gram-positive and Gram-negative bacteria, including anaerobes
Clindamycin	
Oxazolidinones	Bacteriostatic against a variety of Gram-positive bacteria and mycobacteria
Linezolid	
Nitrofurans	Bacteriocidal in the urinary bladder; concentrations elsewhere too low
Nitrofurantoin	
Streptogramins	A synergistic combination of two drugs that bind to two different ribosomal sites. Individually each drug is bacteriostatic, but together they are bactericidal. Effective against a variety of Gram-positive bacteria, including *Enterococcus faecium*
Quinupristin, dalfopristin	

(Continued)

TABLE 23–1	Characteristics of Antibacterial Drugs (*Continued*)
TARGET/REPRESENTATIVE DRUGS	**CHARACTERISTICS**
Nucleic Acid Synthesis	
Fluoroquinolones	Bactericidal against a wide variety of Gram-positive and Gram-negative bacteria
Ciprofloxacin, levofloxacin, moxifloxacin, delafloxacin	
Rifamycins	Bactericidal against Gram-positive and some Gram-negative bacteria. Often used to treat infections caused by *Mycobacterium tuberculosis* and as prophylaxis for close exposure to *Neisseria meningitidis*
Rifampin, rifaximin, rifapentine	
Folate Biosynthesis	
Sulfonamides	Bacteriostatic against a variety of Gram-positive and Gram-negative bacteria
Trimethoprim	Often used in combination with a sulfa drug for a synergistic effect
Cell Membrane Integrity	
Polymyxin B colistin	Bactericidal against Gram-negative cells by damaging cell membranes
Daptomycin	Bactericidal against Gram-positive bacteria

✳ Broad-spectrum inhibit Gram positive and Gram negative

bacilli. The tetracyclines, the cephalosporins, and the carbapenems, on the other hand, are **broad-spectrum agents** that inhibit a wide range of Gram-positive and Gram-negative bacteria.

SELECTED ANTIBACTERIAL AGENTS

The major antimicrobials are now considered in more detail, with emphasis on their modes of action and spectrum. Details on specific antimicrobial agent use, dosage, and toxicity should be sought in a specialized text or handbook written for that purpose.

■ Antimicrobials That Act on Cell Wall Synthesis

Cross-linking of peptidoglycan target of β-lactams and glycopeptides

Without an intact wall, bacteria become fragile, subject to osmotic stress, and are more easily eliminated by the immune system. The peptidoglycan component of the bacterial cell wall provides its shape and rigidity. This giant molecule is formed by weaving the linear glycans *N*-acetylglucosamine and *N*-acetylmuramic acid into a basket-like structure. Mature peptidoglycan is held together by cross-linked short peptide side chains hanging off the long glycan molecules. This cross-linking process is the target of two of the most important groups of antimicrobials, the β-lactams and the glycopeptides (including vancomycin) (**Figure 23–1**). Peptidoglycan is unique to bacteria and its synthesis is described in more detail in Chapter 21.

FIGURE 23–1. **Action of antimicrobials on peptidoglycan synthesis.** The glycan backbone and the amino acid side chains of peptidoglycan are shown. The transpeptidase enzyme catalyzes the cross-linking of the amino acid side chains. Penicillin and other β-lactams bind to the transpeptidase, preventing it from carrying out its function. Vancomycin binds directly to the amino acids, preventing the binding of transpeptidase.

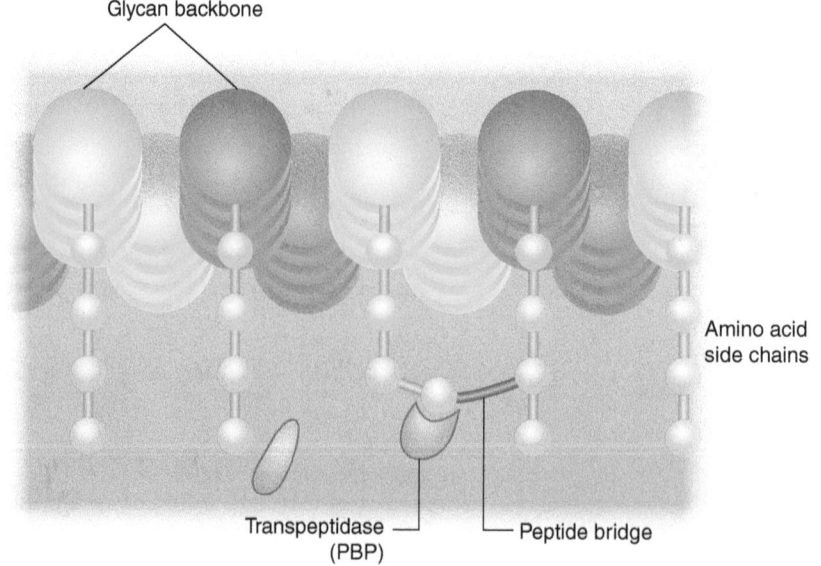

Glycan backbone

Amino acid side chains

Transpeptidase (PBP)

Peptide bridge

β-Lactam Antimicrobials

The β-lactam antimicrobial agents comprise the penicillins, cephalosporins, carbapenems, and monobactams. They are named after the β-lactam ring in their structure; this ring is essential for their antibacterial activity. Penicillin, the first member of this class, was derived from molds of the genus *Penicillium*. Later, β-lactams were derived from both *Cephalosporium* molds (now called *Acremonium*) and bacteria of the genus *Streptomyces*. Today it is possible to synthesize β-lactams, but most are derived from semisynthetic processes involving chemical modification of the products of fermentation.

The β-lactam antibacterial agents interfere with the transpeptidation enzymes that seal peptide crosslinks between glycan chains. These targets of all the β-lactams are commonly called penicillin-binding proteins (PBPs). Several distinct PBPs occur in any one strain and vary in their avidity of binding to different β-lactam drugs.

The β-lactams are classified by chemical structure (**Figure 23–2**). They may have one β-lactam ring (monobactams), or a β-lactam ring fused to a five-member thiazolidine penem ring (penicillins, carbapenems) or a six-member dihydrothiazine cephem ring (cephalosporins). Within these major groups, differences in the side chain(s) attached to the single or double ring can have a significant effect on the drug's pharmacologic properties and spectrum. These properties include resistance to gastric acid, which allows oral administration and their pattern of distribution into body compartments (eg, blood, cerebrospinal fluid, joints). The features that alter their spectrum include permeability into the bacterial cell, affinity for PBPs, and vulnerability to the various bacterial mechanisms of resistance.

β-Lactam antimicrobials are usually highly bactericidal, but only to growing bacteria synthesizing new cell walls. Killing involves attenuation and disruption of the developing peptidoglycan "basket," liberation or activation of autolytic enzymes that further disrupt weakened areas of the wall, and finally osmotic lysis due to passage of water through the cytoplasmic membrane to the hypertonic interior of the cell. Cell wall–deficient organisms, such as *Mycoplasma*, are not susceptible to β-lactam antimicrobials.

Penicillins. Penicillin G is the oldest penicillin. It remains active primarily against certain Gram-positive organisms, many Gram-negative cocci, and some spirochetes, including *Treponema pallidum*, the cause of syphilis. It has little action against most Gram-negative bacilli, because their outer membrane prevents passage of these antibiotics to their sites of action on cell wall synthesis. Penicillin G is the least toxic of the penicillins. Its modification as penicillin V confers acid stability, so it can be given orally.

Three major strategies in drug development have allowed penicillins to remain an important antibiotic class. First, semisynthetic penicillins were developed to cope with staphylococcal penicillinase. This penicillinase is one of a family of bacterial enzymes called β-lactamases that inactivate β-lactam antimicrobials. The penicillinase-resistant penicillins (**methicillin, nafcillin, oxacillin, dicloxacillin**) have narrow spectra but are active against penicillinase-producing *Staphylococcus aureus* (although methicillin is no longer in use, these bacteria are still commonly referred to as "methicillin-susceptible *S aureus*," or "MSSA").

Second, a group of broader spectrum penicillins was created, which owe their expanded activity to their ability to traverse the outer membrane of some Gram-negative bacteria, and in some cases to their resistance to hydrolysis by Gram-negative β-lactamases. Some, such as the

β-lactam ring structure in all β-lactams

✳ **Interfere with PBPs**

Differ in structures fused to the β-lactam ring

β-Lactams kill by lysing weakened cell walls

✳ **Penetration of outer membrane limited**

✳ **Resistance to β-lactamases determines spectrum**

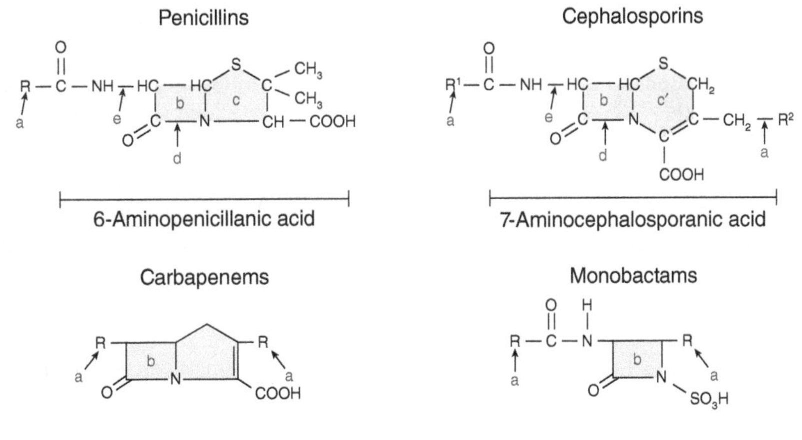

Penicillins

6-Aminopenicillanic acid

Cephalosporins

7-Aminocephalosporanic acid

Carbapenems

Monobactams

FIGURE 23–2. **Structure of β-lactam antibiotics. A.** Different side chains determine degree of activity, spectrum, pharmacologic properties, resistance to β-lactamases. **B.** β-Lactam ring. **C.** Thiazolidine ring; c′ dihydrothiazine ring. **D.** Site of action of β-lactamases. **E.** Site of action of amidase.

aminopenicillins **ampicillin** and **amoxicillin,** have excellent activity against a range of Gram-negative pathogens but not against *Pseudomonas aeruginosa*, an important opportunistic pathogen. Others, such as the ureidopenicillin **piperacillin,** are active against *Pseudomonas* when given in high dosage. These penicillins with enhanced Gram-negative spectrum are slightly less active than penicillin G against Gram-positive organisms. Finally, in order to combat bacterial β-lactamases, penicillins are sometimes dosed with β-lactamase inhibitors (see later).

Cephalosporins.   The structure of the cephalosporins confers resistance to hydrolysis by staphylococcal penicillinase and to varying degrees the β-lactamases of groups of Gram-negative bacilli. The cephalosporins are classified by generation—first, second, third, fourth, fifth, or "unclassified." The "generation" term relates to historical breakthroughs in expanding their spectrum through modification of the side chains. In general, a cephalosporin of a higher generation has a wider spectrum, and in some instances, more quantitative activity (have a lower MIC) against Gram-negative bacteria. As the Gram-negative spectrum increases, these agents typically lose some of their potency (have a higher MIC) against Gram-positive bacteria.

The first-generation cephalosporins **cefazolin** and **cephalexin** have a spectrum of activity against Gram-positive organisms that resembles that of the penicillinase-resistant penicillins. In addition, they are active against some of the Enterobacteriaceae (see Table 23–1). These agents continue to have therapeutic value because of their high activity against Gram-positive organisms, because they are well tolerated, and because a broader spectrum is unnecessary in many infections due to methicillin-susceptible staphylococci and streptococci.

Second-generation cephalosporins such as **cefoxitin** and **cefaclor** are resistant to β-lactamases of some Gram-negative organisms that inactivate first-generation compounds. Of particular importance is their expanded activity against Enterobacteriaceae species, although in theory this comes at the cost of reduced effectiveness against certain Gram positives.

Third-generation cephalosporins, such as **ceftriaxone, cefotaxime,** and **ceftazidime,** have an even wider spectrum; they are active against Gram-negative organisms, often at MICs that are 10- to 100-fold lower than first-generation compounds. Of these three agents, only ceftazidime is active against *P aeruginosa*. The potency, broad spectrum, and low toxicity of the third-generation cephalosporins have made them preferred agents in life-threatening infections in which the causative organism has not yet been isolated. Selection depends on the clinical circumstances. For example, ceftriaxone or cefotaxime are preferred for bacterial meningitis because they have the highest activity against the three major causes, *Neisseria meningitidis*, *Streptococcus pneumoniae*, and *Haemophilus influenzae*. For a febrile stem cell transplant patient, ceftazidime might be chosen because of the higher likelihood of *P aeruginosa* involvement in these very immunosuppressed and healthcare exposed patients.

Fourth-generation cephalosporins retain much of the Gram-positive coverage of ceftriaxone, and have enhanced ability to cross the outer membrane of Gram-negative bacteria. Compounds such as **cefepime** have activity against a wider spectrum of Enterobacteriaceae as well as *P aeruginosa*. These cephalosporins retain the high affinity of third-generation drugs and activity against *Neisseria* and *H influenzae*. In effect, these drugs can be conceptualized as having the activity of ceftriaxone plus ceftazidime. They are also relatively unaffected by the production of bacterial ampC β-lactamases by certain Gram-negative bacteria (see later). The antibiotic **cefiderocol** share structural similarities with cefepime and ceftazidime, but is designed to take advantage of bacteria's hunger for iron by binding to iron ions, in effect tricking the germ into importing the antibiotic (see Figure 23–8D). This makes cefiderocol an important option for treating Gram-negatives resistant to most other agents (see later).

Ceftaroline has the unique ability to bind avidly to PBP-2A, the altered PBP that confers resistance to other β-lactam antibiotics in methicillin-resistant *S aureus* (MRSA). See Chapter 24 for information on MRSA. Ceftaroline retains some activity against Enterobacteriaceae, although it should be thought of primarily as an anti–Gram-positive agent. For this reason, some prefer to categorize ceftaroline as "unclassified" rather than as "fifth generation," because it bucks the trend of adding Gram-negative coverage as is seen when comparing fourth-generation cephalosporins to first generation ones. In effect, think of ceftaroline as having a similar spectrum of activity as ceftriaxone *plus* coverage of MRSA.

Fifth-generation cephalosporins such as **ceftolozane** are built to kill highly drug-resistant Gram-negative bacteria, including *P aeruginosa*. Ceftolozane is dosed in combination with the β-lactamase inhibitor **tazobactam** to partially protect it from the activity of these hydrolytic enzymes (see section on β-lactamase inhibitors). Ceftolozane has less activity against Gram-positive bacteria than earlier generation cephalosporins.

Carbapenems. The carbapenems **imipenem, meropenem,** and **doripenem** have the broadest spectrum of all β-lactam antibiotics. This is due to their combination of easy penetration of Gram-negative and Gram-positive bacterial cells and high level of resistance to β-lactamases. All three agents are active against streptococci, retain some antistaphylococcal activity, and are highly active against both β-lactamase-positive and negative strains of *N gonorrhoeae* and *H influenzae*. In addition, they are as or more active than third-generation cephalosporins against Gram-negative rods. They are highly effective against obligate anaerobes such as *Bacteroides fragilis*. A closely related drug, **ertapenem,** is ineffective against *Pseudomonas*, and less reliable against EBSL-producing Enterobacteriaceae (see later), but is otherwise similar. Imipenem is the carbapenem of choice against Gram-positive pathogens, but it is rapidly hydrolyzed by renal tubular dehydro-peptidase-1; therefore, it is administered together with an inhibitor of this enzyme (cilastatin), which greatly improves its urine levels and other pharmacokinetic characteristics. Meropenem, doripenem, and ertapenem are not significantly degraded by dehydropeptidase-1 and do not require coadministration of cilastatin. None of the carbapenems available in the United States today are administered orally.

> Carbapenems have very broad spectra

Monobactams. **Aztreonam,** the first monobactam licensed in the United States, has a spectrum limited to aerobic and facultatively anaerobic Gram-negative bacteria, including Enterobacteriaceae, *P aeruginosa*, *Haemophilus*, and *Neisseria*. Monobactams have poor affinity for the PBPs of Gram-positive organisms and strict anaerobes and thus demonstrate little activity against them. However, they are highly resistant to hydrolysis by β-lactamases of Gram-negative bacilli.

> ✳ Active exclusively against Gram negatives

β-Lactamase Inhibitors. A number of β-lactams with little or no antimicrobial activity are capable of binding irreversibly to β-lactamase enzymes and, in the process, rendering them inactive. Three such compounds, **clavulanic acid, sulbactam,** and **tazobactam,** are referred to as suicide inhibitors, because they must first be hydrolyzed by a β-lactamase before becoming effective inactivators of the enzyme. They are highly effective against staphylococcal penicillinases and broad-spectrum β-lactamases; however, their ability to inhibit cephalosporinases is significantly less. Combinations of one of these inhibitors with an appropriate β-lactam antimicrobial agent protect the therapeutic agent from destruction by many β-lactamases and significantly enhances its spectrum. Four such combinations are now available in the United States: amoxicillin/clavulanate, ampicillin/sulbactam, ceftolozane/tazobactam, and piperacillin/tazobactam. Bacteria that produce certain chromosomally encoded inducible β-lactamases are not susceptible to these combinations. To address the limitations of β-lactamase inhibitors, a new class has been developed: Non–β-lactam β-lactamase inhibitors. **Avibactam, vaborbactam,** and **relebactam** are now available in combination with various β-lactam antibiotics. They are not β-lactam molecules, and thus do not require bacteria to hydrolyze them. Rather, they are ready to inhibit broad-spectrum β-lactamases as soon as they are infused, via a reversible rather than via suicide process. They provide superior blockade of certain β-lactamases found in difficult-to-treat Gram-negative infections, such as those caused by KPC and ampC producers. See the following section on enzymatic inactivation as a resistance mechanism for more information on β-lactam resistance.

> ✳ Activity enhanced in presence of β-lactamase inhibitors
>
> ✳ Clavulanate, sulbactam, tazobactam inhibit via irreversible binding
>
> Avibactam, vaborbactam, relebactam inhibit a wider range of β-lactamases

Clinical Use. The β-lactam antibiotics are usually the drugs of choice for infections caused by susceptible organisms because of their bactericidal action and low toxicity. They also have great value in the prevention of many infections, such as surgical site infections. Most are excreted by the kidney and achieve high urinary levels. Penicillins reach the cerebrospinal fluid when the meninges are inflamed and are effective in the treatment of meningitis, whereas first- and second-generation cephalosporins are not. In contrast, the third-generation cephalosporins penetrate the blood–brain barrier well and have become the agents of choice in the treatment of most causes of bacterial meningitis.

> Low toxicity favors use of β-lactams

Glycopeptide Antimicrobials

Vancomycin and **teicoplanin** belong to this group. Each of these antimicrobials inhibits assembly of the linear peptidoglycan molecule by binding directly to the terminal amino acids of the peptide side chains. The effect is the same as with β-lactams: interruption of peptidoglycan cross-linking. Both agents are bactericidal but are primarily active only against Gram-positive bacteria. Their main use has been against multidrug-resistant Gram-positive infections including those caused

Glycopeptide antimicrobics bind directly to amino acid side chains

by strains of staphylococci that are resistant to the penicillinase-resistant penicillins and most cephalosporins, especially MRSA. Neither agent is absorbed by mouth; this feature allows these medications to be given orally to treat *Clostridioides difficile* infections of the bowel (see Chapter 29). A related drug, **telavancin,** was created by adding a lipid tail onto a glycopeptide backbone, thus giving it the theoretical advantage of cell membrane activity and cell wall activity, although its clinical usefulness remains to be firmly established. Semi-synthetic lipoglycopeptides **dalbavancin** and **oritavancin** are structurally similar to vancomycin but have been modified to greatly increase their half-lives, such that they may be dosed once per *week* for certain Gram-positive infections, which provides certain clinical benefits.

KEY CONCLUSIONS

- Cell walls provide bacteria with essential structural stability.
- Cell walls are comprised of glycan molecules with amino acid side chains, which are cross-linked by peptide bridges.
- The transpeptidase molecules that form these cross-links are the target of β-lactam antibiotics, thus we call them "penicillin-binding proteins (PBPs)."
- Glycopeptides treat only Gram-positive bacteria. They interfere with cell wall integrity by attaching directly to the amino acid side chains. They tend to be less bactericidal than β-lactam antibiotics.
- Organisms without a cell wall, such as *Mycoplasma*, will not be affected by these drugs.
- Bacteria may resist the activity of β-lactam antibiotics by producing altered target sites (eg, PBP-2A in MRSA) or by producing hydrolytic enzymes called β-lactamases (eg, ampC).
- We, in turn, combat this resistance by either modifying the β-lactam antibiotic to attack the altered target (eg, ceftaroline) or add a β-lactamase inhibitor to block the hydrolytic enzyme (eg, adding clavulanate to amoxicillin).

■ Inhibitors of Protein Synthesis (Figure 23–3)

Aminoglycosides

✳ Must be transported into cell by oxidative metabolism

All members of the aminoglycoside group of antibacterial agents have a six-member aminocyclitol ring with attached amino sugars. The individual agents differ in terms of the exact ring structure and the number and nature of the amino sugar residues. Aminoglycosides are active against a wide range of bacteria, but only those organisms that are able to transport them into the cell by a mechanism that involves oxidative phosphorylation. Thus, they have little or no activity against

FIGURE 23–3. **Action of antimicrobials on protein synthesis.** Aminoglycosides (A) bind to multiple sites on both the 30S and 50S ribosomes in a manner that prevents tRNA from forming initiation complexes. Tetracyclines (T) act in a similar manner, binding only to the 30S ribosomes. Chloramphenicol (C) blocks formation of the peptide bond between the amino acids. Macrolides (M), lincosamides (L), Oxazolidinones (O), and pleuromutilins (P) block the translocation of tRNA from the acceptor to the donor side on the ribosome.

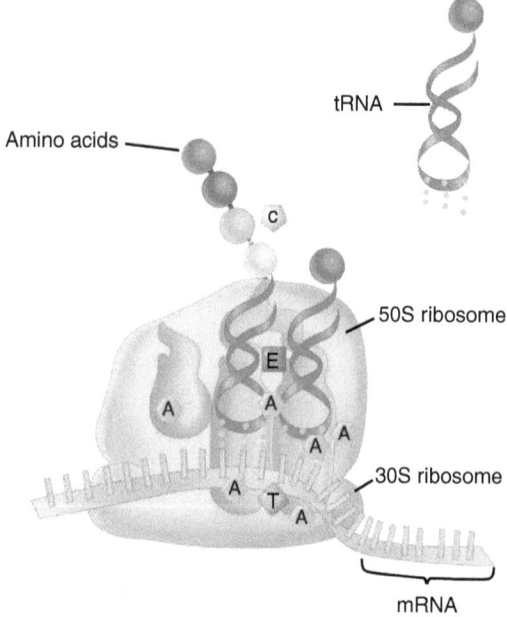

strict anaerobes or facultative organisms that metabolize only fermentatively (eg, streptococci). It appears highly probable that aminoglycoside activity against facultative organisms is similarly reduced *in vivo* when the oxidation–reduction potential is low, as in abscesses.

* Not active against anaerobes

Once inside bacterial cells, aminoglycosides inhibit protein synthesis by binding to the bacterial ribosomes either directly or by involving other proteins. This binding destabilizes the ribosomes and blocks initiation complexes, thus preventing the elongation of polypeptide chains. The agents may also cause distortion of the site of attachment of mRNA, mistranslation of codons, and failure to produce the correct amino acid sequence in proteins. The first aminoglycoside, streptomycin, binds to the 30S ribosomal subunit, but the newer and more active aminoglycosides bind to multiple sites on both 30S and 50S subunits. This gives the newer agents broader spectra and less susceptibility to resistance caused by binding site mutation.

* Ribosome-binding disrupts initiation complexes

* Newer agents bind to multiple ribosome sites

Eukaryotic ribosomes are resistant to aminoglycosides, and the antimicrobials are not actively transported into eukaryotic cells. These properties account for their selective toxicity and also explain their ineffectiveness against intracellular bacteria such as *Rickettsia* and *Chlamydia*.

No entry into human cells

Gentamicin and **tobramycin** are the major aminoglycosides; they have an extended spectrum, which includes Enterobacteriaceae, and of particular importance, *P aeruginosa*. They are sometimes beneficial in treating serious infections caused by Gram-positive pathogens such as *S aureus* and enterococci, but only when combined with other drugs. **Streptomycin** and **amikacin** are now primarily used in combination with other antimicrobial agents in the therapy of tuberculosis and other mycobacterial diseases. **Neomycin,** the most toxic aminoglycoside, is used in topical preparations and as an oral preparation before certain types of intestinal surgery, because it is poorly absorbed.

* Gentamicin and tobramycin spectrum includes *P aeruginosa*

All of the aminoglycosides are toxic to the vestibular and auditory branches of the eighth cranial nerve to varying degrees; this damage can lead to complete and irreversible loss of hearing and balance. These agents may also be toxic to the kidneys. The difference between a drug's effective concentration and its toxic concentration is called its "therapeutic index," and aminoglycosides have a narrower therapeutic index than most other antibiotics. It is essential to monitor blood levels during therapy to ensure adequate yet nontoxic doses, especially when renal impairment diminishes excretion of the drug. Patients with cystic fibrosis may benefit from inhaled tobramycin when treating *P aeruginosa* lung infections because high concentrations are achieved and there is little if any absorption into the bloodstream in these patients, thus reducing toxicity risk.

Renal and vestibular toxicity must be monitored

The clinical value of the aminoglycosides is a consequence of their rapid bactericidal effect, their broad spectrum, and the slow development of bacterial resistance, including retained action against *Pseudomonas* strains that resist many other drugs. They cause fewer disturbances of the resident microbiota than most other broad-spectrum antimicrobials, probably because of their lack of activity against the predominantly anaerobic flora of the bowel, and because they are only used parenterally for systemic infections. The β-lactam antibiotics may act synergistically with the aminoglycosides, most likely because their action on the cell wall facilitates aminoglycoside penetration into the bacterial cell. This effect is most pronounced with organisms such as streptococci and enterococci, which lack the metabolic pathways required to transport aminoglycosides to their interior. However, because of the risk of toxicity even at smaller synergistic doses, even this use is restricted to the most serious cases, such as prosthetic heart valve infections due to certain difficult-to-treat bacteria.

Broad spectrum and slow development of resistance

Cautiously combined with β-lactams

Tetracyclines

Tetracyclines are composed of four fused benzene rings. Substitutions on these rings provide differences in pharmacologic features of the major members of the group, **doxycycline** and **minocycline.** The tetracyclines inhibit protein synthesis by binding to the 30S ribosomal subunit at a point that blocks attachment of aminoacyl-tRNA to the acceptor site on the mRNA ribosome complex. Unlike the aminoglycosides, their effect is reversible. They are bacteriostatic rather than bactericidal. **Tigecycline** belongs to a related class, the glycylcyclines. It covers anaerobes aggressively and thus may be used for treating polymicrobial intraabdominal infections and other complicated deep-tissue infections. Because it is poorly tolerated from a gastrointestinal standpoint, and because of concerns for clinical failure when used for bloodstream infections, this drug's most useful role may be in the treatment of nontuberculous mycobacterial infections. The most recent members of this larger family are the semisynthetic **omadacycline** and fully synthetic **eravacycline**. Although their spectrum is similar to that of tigecycline, some patients tolerate them better from a gastrointestinal perspective.

* Block tRNA attachment

* Activity is bacteriostatic

The tetracyclines are broad-spectrum agents with a range of activity that encompass most common pathogenic species, including Gram-positive and Gram-negative rods and cocci and both aerobes and certain anaerobes. They are also active against cell wall-deficient organisms, such as *Mycoplasma*, and against some obligate intracellular bacteria, including members of the genera *Rickettsia* and *Chlamydia*. Acquired resistance to one may confer resistance to others; however, tigecycline, eravacycline, and omadacycline appear to overcome the major resistance mechanisms to other tetracyclines, and thus may be useful alternatives in select cases.

The tetracyclines and omadacycline are absorbed orally, whereas tigecycline and eravacycline are not. Tetracyclines are chelated by divalent cations, which may reduce their absorption and activity. Thus, they should not be taken with dairy products or many antacid preparations. Tetracyclines are excreted in the bile and urine in active form.

The original tetracycline drug had a strong affinity for developing bone and teeth, to which it gave a yellowish color and enamel damage, and thus it was avoided in children up to 8 years of age. But, this is less of a problem with doxycycline. For life-threatening infections such as Rocky Mountain spotted fever (RMSF), patients should be treated with doxycycline regardless of their age. Common complications of tetracycline therapy include photosensitivity, nausea, and esophagitis.

Chloramphenicol

Chloramphenicol has a simple nitrobenzene ring structure that can be mass produced by chemical synthesis. It influences protein synthesis by binding to the 50S ribosomal subunit and blocking the action of peptidyl transferase, which prevents formation of the peptide bond essential for extension of the peptide chain. Its action is reversible in most susceptible species; thus, it is bacteriostatic. It has little effect on eukaryotic ribosomes, which explains its selective toxicity.

Like tetracycline, chloramphenicol is a broad-spectrum antibiotic with a wide range of activity against both aerobic and anaerobic species (see Table 23–1). Chloramphenicol is readily absorbed from the upper gastrointestinal tract and diffuses readily into most body compartments, including the cerebrospinal fluid. It also permeates readily into mammalian cells and is active against obligate intracellular pathogens such as *Rickettsia* and *Chlamydia*. It is poorly concentrated in urine.

The major drawback to this inexpensive, broad-spectrum antimicrobial with almost ideal pharmacologic features is a rare but serious toxicity. Between 1 in 100,000 and 1 in 1,000,000 patients treated with even low doses of chloramphenicol have an idiosyncratic reaction that results in aplastic anemia. The condition is irreversible and, before the advent of stem cell transplantation, was universally fatal. In high doses, chloramphenicol also causes a reversible depression of the bone marrow and, in neonates may cause abdominal, circulatory, and respiratory dysfunction. The inability of the immature infant liver to conjugate and excrete chloramphenicol aggravates this latter condition.

In the United States, chloramphenicol use is now restricted to the treatment of rickettsial or ehrlichial infections in which tetracyclines are relatively contraindicated because of hypersensitivity or pregnancy. In some developing countries, chloramphenicol is used more extensively because of its low cost and proven efficacy in diseases such as typhoid fever and bacterial meningitis.

A related class of drugs, the pleuromutilins, also blocks peptidyl transferase at the 50S ribosomal subunit. **Retapamulin** is used topically for relatively superficial streptococcal and staphylococcal skin infections. **Lefamulin** is the first orally absorbed pleuromutilin, making it an attractive option for certain multidrug-resistant Gram-positive infections.

Macrolides

The macrolides **erythromycin, azithromycin,** and **clarithromycin** differ in their composition of a large 14- or 15-member ring structure. They impair protein synthesis at the ribosomal level by binding to the 50S subunit and blocking the translocation reaction. Their effect is primarily bacteriostatic. Macrolides, which are concentrated in phagocytes and other cells, are effective against some intracellular pathogens.

Erythromycin, the first macrolide, has a spectrum of activity that includes many pathogenic Gram-positive bacteria and some Gram-negative organisms. Its Gram-negative spectrum includes *Neisseria*, *Bordetella*, *Campylobacter*, and *Legionella*, but not the Enterobacteriaceae. Erythromycin and related drugs are also effective against *Chlamydia* and *Mycoplasma*.

Bacteria that have developed resistance to erythromycin are usually resistant to the newer macrolides azithromycin and clarithromycin as well. These newer agents have the same spectrum as erythromycin, with some significant additions. Azithromycin has quantitatively greater activity

---

Spectrum includes some intracellular bacteria

Chelated by some calcium-rich foods

Dental staining, enamel damage limit use in children

✳ Blocks peptidyl transferase

Readily diffuses into body compartments

✳ Marrow suppression, aplastic anemia serious toxicities

Use sharply restricted

Lefamulin, retapamulin block ribosomal translocation

✳ Erythromycin active against Gram positives and *Legionella*

(lower MICs) against most of the same Gram-negative bacteria. Clarithromycin is the most active of the three against both Gram-positive and Gram-negative pathogens, and it is also active against mycobacteria, but drug–drug interactions limit its usefulness. Both azithromycin and clarithromycin may have undesirable side effects, including GI upset and cardiac arrhythmias. Erythromycin is sometimes used not as antibiotic but to stimulate stomach contractions in patients with diabetic gastroparesis. Azithromycin may benefit patients with cavitary lung disease due in part to its anti-inflammatory effects. A related drug, **telithromycin,** belongs to the ketolide class; it is less susceptible to bacterial resistance mechanisms but has been associated with liver toxicity and is thus rarely used.

✳ Azithromycin and clarithromycin have enhanced Gram-negative spectrum

Clindamycin

Clindamycin is a lincosamide, chemically unrelated to the macrolides but with a similar mode of action and spectrum. It has greater activity than the macrolides against Gram-negative anaerobes, including the important *B fragilis* group. Although clindamycin is a perfectly adequate substitute for a macrolide in many situations, its primary use is in instances where anaerobes are or may be involved. In addition, there is experimental evidence that clindamycin may mitigate toxin production by highly virulent *S aureus* and *Streptococcus pyogenes* strains. For this reason, many clinicians add it to a bactericidal agent such as nafcillin or vancomycin for treatment of serious deep-tissue infections caused by these organisms. Unfortunately, clindamycin tends to cause more diarrhea than many other antibiotics, presumably because of its collateral damage to healthy colonic microbiota.

✳ Spectrum similar to macrolides plus anaerobes

May mitigate toxin production

Oxazolidinones

Linezolid is the most widely used of a class of antibiotics that act by binding to the bacterial 50S ribosome of Gram-positive organisms and many mycobacteria and anaerobes. It does not cover aerobic Gram negatives. Oxazolidinones are clinically useful in pneumonia and soft tissue infections, particularly those caused by resistant strains of staphylococci and enterococci. Risk of bone marrow suppression is notorious for linezolid, especially when dosed for more than 2 weeks. Optic and peripheral neuropathy have been reported. It is also a monoamine oxidase inhibitor, and thus may precipitate a systemic reaction called the serotonin syndrome when given to patients simultaneously taking certain antidepressants. **Tedizolid,** a related drug, may have a lower risk of this complication.

Active against Gram-positive bacteria resistant to other agents

Nitrofurans

Nitrofurantoin is a unique antibiotic which interrupts bacterial ribosomal function in a variety of ways. It is well absorbed when taken by mouth, concentrates heavily in the urinary stream, and is effective at killing most uropathogenic *E coli*, which makes it ideally suited to treat urinary tract infections; its use in other syndromes is limited.

Streptogramins

Quinupristin and **dalfopristin** are used in a synergistic combination known as synercid. They inhibit protein synthesis by binding to different sites on the 50S bacterial ribosome of certain Gram positives, including MRSA and vancomycin-resistant enterococci (VRE); quinupristin inhibits peptide chain elongation, and dalfopristin interferes with peptidyl transferase. Muscle pain is a common and often-limiting side effect. Their clinical use thus far has been limited generally to the treatment of VRE.

Useful against vancomycin-resistant enterococci

KEY CONCLUSIONS

- Protein synthesis blockers are a diverse group of medications.
- They may be active against a wide array of bacteria, including intracellular organisms and those lacking a cell wall.
- Toxicity potential ranges from negligible to severe.

■ Inhibitors of Nucleic Acid Synthesis (Figure 23–4)

Quinolones

The quinolones have a nucleus of two fused six-member rings that when substituted with fluorine become fluoroquinolones, which are now the dominant quinolones for the treatment of bacterial infections. The fluoroquinolones now in use are **ciprofloxacin, levofloxacin, gemifloxacin, moxifloxacin,** and **delafloxacin.** The addition of a piperazine ring and its methylation alter the activity and pharmacologic properties of each individual compound. The target of the quinolones

✳ Fluorinated quinolone derivatives now dominant

FIGURE 23-4. **Antimicrobials acting on nucleic acids.** Sulfonamides block the folate precursors of DNA synthesis, metronidazole inflicts breaks in the DNA itself, rifampin inhibits the synthesis of RNA from DNA by inhibiting RNA polymerase, and quinolones inhibit DNA topoisomerase and thus prevent the supercoiling required for the DNA to "fit" inside the bacterial cell.

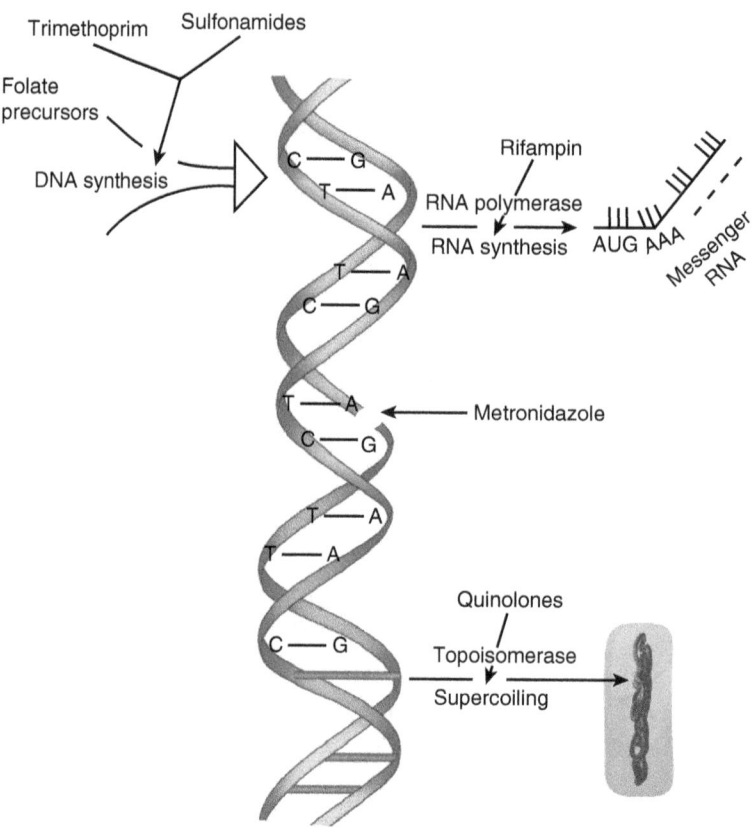

* Inhibition of gyrase and topoisomerase blocks supercoiling

* Fluoroquinolones broad spectrum, including *Pseudomonas*

Well distributed after oral administration

* Bacteria must synthesize folate that humans acquire in their diet

are DNA gyrase and topoisomerase IV, the enzymes responsible for nicking, supercoiling, and sealing bacterial DNA during replication. Binding to two enzymes reduces the chance a single mutation can lead to resistance, which was a problem with the first quinolone, nalidixic acid, a single binding-site agent.

The fluoroquinolones are highly active and bactericidal against a wide range of aerobes and facultative anaerobes. However, strict anaerobes are generally resistant. Levofloxacin and moxifloxacin have significant activity against *S pneumoniae* and *Chlamydia*, whereas ciprofloxacin is more useful against *P aeruginosa*. Fluoroquinolones have several favorable pharmacologic properties in addition to their broad spectrum. These include oral administration, low protein binding, good distribution to all body compartments, penetration of phagocytes, and a prolonged serum half-life that allows once- or twice-a-day dosing. Levofloxacin and ciprofloxacin are excreted primarily by the kidney, resulting in high drug concentrations in the urine, making them suitable for the treatment of many urinary tract infections. Moxifloxacin is secreted to a smaller degree into the urine.

Because of their broad spectrum and oral administration, fluoroquinolones have been prescribed heavily for many years. This has both increased bacterial resistance and unmasked concerning potential side effects, including tendon injury, diarrhea, cardiac arrhythmias, aortic injury, and peripheral and central neuropathy. For these reasons, fluoroquinolones are no longer first-line treatment for common problems such as urinary tract infections or bacterial sinusitis.

Folate Inhibitors

Agents that interfere with the synthesis of folic acid by bacteria have selective toxicity because mammalian cells acquire preformed folate from dietary sources. Folic acid is derived from *para*-aminobenzoic acid (PABA), glutamate, and a pteridine unit. In its reduced form, it is an essential coenzyme for the transport of one-carbon compounds in the synthesis of purines, thymidine, and some amino acids; thus, folic acid is indirectly essential for the synthesis of nucleic acids and proteins. The major inhibitors of the folate pathway are the sulfonamides, trimethoprim, *para*-aminosalicylic acid, and the sulfones.

Sulfonamides. Sulfonamides are structural analogs of PABA and compete with it for the enzyme (dihydropteroate synthetase) that combines PABA and pteridine in the initial stage of folate synthesis. This blockage has multiple effects on the bacterial cells; the most important of these is disruption of nucleic acid synthesis. The effect is bacteriostatic, and the addition of PABA to a medium that contains sulfonamide neutralizes the inhibitory effect and allows growth to resume.

When introduced in the 1940s, sulfonamides had a very broad spectrum, but resistance developed quickly. Now their primary use is for uncomplicated urinary tract infections caused by members of the Enterobacteriaceae, particularly *Escherichia coli*. Sulfonamides are convenient for this purpose because they are inexpensive, well absorbed by the oral route, and excreted in high levels in the urine. They also have a role in some skin infections due to MRSA.

Trimethoprim-Sulfamethoxazole. Trimethoprim acts on the folate synthesis pathway but at a point after sulfonamides. It competitively inhibits the activity of bacterial dihydrofolate reductase, which catalyzes the conversion of folate to its reduced active coenzyme form. When combined with sulfamethoxazole, a sulfonamide, trimethoprim leads to a two-stage blockade of the folate pathway, which often results in synergistic bacteriostatic or bactericidal effects. This quality is exploited in therapeutic preparations that combine both agents in a fixed proportion designed to yield optimum synergy.

Trimethoprim-sulfamethoxazole (TMP-SMX) has a spectrum that is much broader and more stable than either of its components alone; this includes most of the common pathogens, whether they are Gram-positive or Gram-negative, cocci or bacilli. Anaerobes and *P aeruginosa*, however, are not covered. It is also active against some uncommon agents such as *Nocardia*. TMP-SMX is widely and effectively used in the treatment of urinary tract infections, otitis media, sinusitis, prostatitis, and MRSA skin infections. Interestingly, its spectrum expends beyond bacteria. It is useful for the treatment of certain protozoan causes of diarrhea and is the agent of choice for pneumonia caused by *Pneumocystis jirovecii*, a fungus.

Metronidazole

Metronidazole is a nitroimidazole, a family of compounds with activity against bacteria, fungi, and parasites. The antibacterial action requires reduction of the nitro group under anaerobic conditions, which explains the limitation of its activity to bacteria that prefer anaerobic or at least microaerophilic growth conditions. The reduction products act on the cell at multiple points; the most lethal of these effects is induction of breaks in DNA strands.

Metronidazole is active against a wide range of anaerobes, including *B fragilis*. Clinically, it is useful for any infection in which anaerobes may be involved, especially those in the gastrointestinal tract. Because these infections are typically polymicrobial, a second antimicrobial (eg, β-lactam) is usually added to cover aerobic and facultative bacteria. Toxicity includes nausea, a metallic taste perversion, and—less commonly—peripheral neuropathy. Alcohol consumption may trigger an unpleasant disulfiram-like reaction for the patient.

Rifamycins

Rifampin binds to the β-subunit of DNA-dependent RNA polymerase, which prevents the initiation of RNA synthesis. This agent is active against most Gram-positive bacteria and selected Gram-negative organisms, including *Neisseria* and *Haemophilus*. The most clinically useful property of rifampin is its antimycobacterial activity, which includes *Mycobacterium tuberculosis* and the other species that infect humans. Because resistance by mutation of the polymerase readily occurs, rifampin is combined with other agents in the treatment of active infections. It is only used alone for chemoprophylaxis of *N meningitidis* and *H influenzae* in close contacts of infected patients, and in the treatment of latent tuberculosis infection. When given for prolonged courses, rifampin may radically alter the metabolism of other medications via induction of hepatic cytochrome enzyme expression. A related drug, **rifaximin,** is not absorbed when taken by mouth and has reasonable *E coli* coverage, making it ideal for the treatment and prevention of certain causes of bacterial diarrhea.

* Competition with PABA disrupts nucleic acids

Major use is urinary tract infections

* Dihydrofolate reductase inhibition is synergistic with sulfonamides

Activity against common bacteria plus some protozoa and fungi

* Action requires anaerobic conditions

Blocking of RNA synthesis occurs by binding to polymerase

KEY CONCLUSIONS

- Nucleic acid synthesis blockers are a diverse group of medications with a variety of spectra.
- Differences between microbial and human synthesis apparatuses allow for an acceptable toxicity profile; nevertheless, side effects may happen with any of these medications, and they should be used judiciously.

■ Antimicrobials Acting on the Outer and Cytoplasmic Membranes

Broad Gram-positive spectrum

Reduced efficacy in lungs

Daptomycin is a lipopeptide antimicrobial. This drug's molecular structure mimics that of the bacterial cell membrane phospholipid bilayer; it inserts itself into this membrane and forms pores that allow efflux of ions, thus killing the cell. Its spectrum is limited to Gram-positive organisms, including multidrug-resistant strains of *Enterococcus* and *S aureus*. Surfactant molecules in the lung bind to this molecule, rendering it unreliable for the treatment of pneumonia.

❋ **Bind to cytoplasmic membrane**

Toxic when administered systemically

The polypeptide antimicrobial agents **polymyxin B** and **colistin** have a cationic detergent-like effect. They bind to the cell membranes of susceptible Gram-negative bacteria and alter their permeability, resulting in the loss of essential cytoplasmic components and bacterial death. These agents react to a lesser extent with cell membranes of the host, resulting in nephrotoxicity and neurotoxicity. Their spectrum is essentially Gram-negative; they act against *P aeruginosa* and other Gram-negative rods. Although these antimicrobials were used for systemic treatment in the past, their use was subsequently limited to topical applications because of their toxicity; with the rise in Gram-negative resistance to first-line drugs, these medications are once again being used more by the intravenous route. They have an advantage: resistance to them rarely develops.

■ Other Agents

Several other effective antimicrobials are in use almost exclusively for a single infectious agent or types of infections such as tuberculosis, urinary tract infections, and anaerobic infections. Where appropriate, these agents will be discussed in the relevant chapter. It is beyond the scope and intent of this book to provide comprehensive coverage of all available agents.

ANTIMICROBIAL RESISTANCE

Overview

The continuing success of antimicrobial therapy depends on keeping ahead of the ability of the microorganisms to develop resistance to antimicrobial agents. New antimicrobials are key to this effort, although at times, resistance seems to occur at a rate equal to that of the development of new drugs. Judicious use of these precious resources should benefit the individual patient and also reduce the pace of resistance generally. This section covers common mechanisms of resistance and the ways in which laboratory tests are used to guide clinicians through the uncertainties of modern treatment.

SUSCEPTIBILITY AND RESISTANCE

❋ **MICs must be below achievable blood, tissue, or body fluid levels**

Clinical experience must validate *in vitro* data

Deciding whether any bacterium should be considered susceptible or resistant to an antimicrobial involves an integrated assessment of *in vitro* activity, pharmacologic characteristics, and clinical factors. Any agent approved for clinical use has demonstrated *in vitro* its potential to inhibit the growth of some target group of bacteria at concentrations that can be achieved with acceptable risks of toxicity. That is, the **minimum inhibitory concentration (MIC)** can be comfortably exceeded by doses tolerated by the patient. Use of the antimicrobial in animal models and then human infections must also have demonstrated a therapeutic response. Because the influence of antimicrobials on the natural history of different infections (eg, pneumonia, meningitis, diarrhea) varies, clinical trials may include both a range of bacterial species and different infected sites (eg, lung, bone, CSF). These clinical studies are important to determine whether what *should* work actually *does* work and, if so, to define the parameters of success and failure. Physicians must decide whether the evidence used to earn FDA approval for a new antimicrobial applies to the particular circumstances of the case before them.

❋ **Susceptible bacteria inhibited at achievable nontoxic levels, resistant strains are not**

Once these factors are established, the routine selection of therapy can be based on known or expected characteristics of organisms and pharmacologic features of antimicrobial agents. With regard to organisms, use of the term **susceptible** (sensitive) implies that their MIC is at a concentration attainable in the blood or other appropriate body fluid (eg, urine) using recommended doses. **Resistant,** the converse of susceptible, implies that the MIC is not exceeded by normally attainable levels. As in all biological systems, the MIC of some organisms lies in between the susceptible and resistant levels. Borderline strains are called **intermediately sensitive.** The antimicrobial in question may still be used to treat these organisms but at increased doses. For example, less toxic antibiotics such as the penicillins and cephalosporins can be administered in massive amounts and may thereby inhibit some pathogens that would normally be considered resistant *in vitro*. Furthermore, in urinary infections, urine levels of some antimicrobial agents may be very high (eg, fluoroquinolones), and organisms that are resistant *in vitro* may be eliminated in the patient.

Important pharmacologic characteristics of antimicrobial agents include dosage as well as the routes and frequency of administration. Other characteristics include whether the agents are absorbed from the upper gastrointestinal tract, whether they are excreted and concentrated in active form in the urine, whether they can pass into cells, whether and how rapidly they are metabolized, and the duration of effective antimicrobial levels in blood and tissues. Most agents are bound to some extent to serum albumin, and the protein-bound form is usually unavailable for antimicrobial action. The amount of free to bound antibiotic can be expressed as an equilibrium constant, which varies for different antibiotics. In general, high degrees of binding lead to more prolonged but lower serum levels of an active antimicrobial after a single dose.

LABORATORY TESTING OF ANTIMICROBIAL SUSCEPTIBILITY

A unique feature of laboratory testing in bacteriology is that the individual patient's isolate is routinely tested against a battery of antimicrobial agents. These tests are built around the common theme of placing the organism in the presence of varying concentrations of the antimicrobial in order to determine the MIC. The methods used are standardized, including a measured inoculum of the bacteria and controlled growth conditions (eg, medium, temperature, atmosphere, and time).

In selecting therapy, clinicians must consider more than the results of laboratory tests. The clinical pharmacology of the drug, the cause of the disease, the site of infection, the immune function of the patient, and the pathology of the lesion must be taken into account as well. For example, the antimicrobial must reach the subarachnoid space and cerebrospinal fluid in meningitis. Similarly, treatment may be ineffective for an infection that has resulted in abscess formation unless the abscess is surgically drained. Previous clinical experience is also critical. In typhoid fever, for instance, azithromycin may be effective while aminoglycosides are not, even though the typhoid bacillus may be equally susceptible to both *in vitro*. This is due to the aminoglycosides' failure to achieve adequate concentrations inside the macrophages where *Salmonella enterica* serovar Typhi multiplies.

■ Dilution Tests

Dilution tests determine the MIC directly by using serial dilutions of the antimicrobial agent in broth that span a clinically significant range of concentrations. The dilutions are prepared in tubes or microdilution wells, and by convention, their concentrations are doubled using a base of 1 μg/mL (0.25, 0.5, 1, 2, 4, 8, and so on). The bacterial inoculum of the patient's isolate is adjusted to a standard density (10^5 to 10^6 bacteria/mL) and added to the broth. After incubation overnight (or other defined time), the tubes are examined for turbidity produced by bacterial growth. The first tube in which visible growth is absent (clear) is the MIC for that organism (**Figure 23-5**).

Margin notes

* Borderline isolates called intermediate

Pharmacologic properties (absorption, distribution, metabolism, elimination) affect usefulness

Bacteria tested against antimicrobials over a range of concentrations

* Drug selection should include susceptibility, pharmacology, and clinical experience

Penetration inside cells may be important

* MIC endpoint is the lowest concentration that inhibits growth

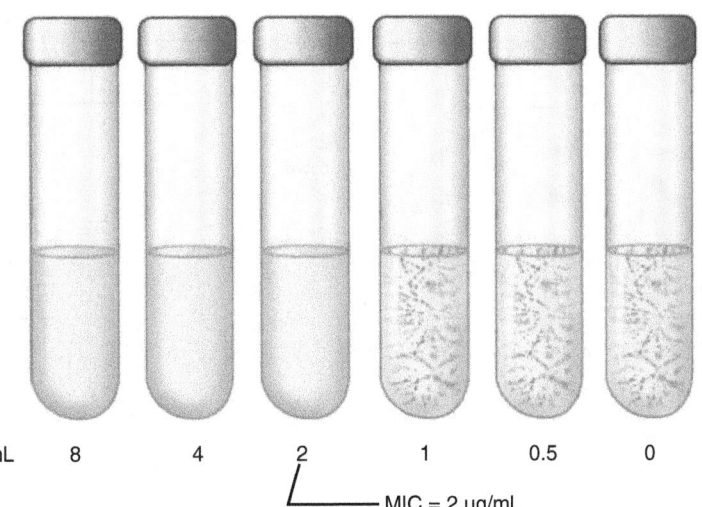

FIGURE 23-5. **Broth dilution susceptibility test.** The stippled tubes represent turbidity produced by bacterial growth. The MIC is 2 μg/mL.

μg/mL   8   4   2   1   0.5   0

MIC = 2 μg/mL

Automated Tests

Instruments are now available that carry out rapid, automated variants of the broth dilution test. In these systems, the bacteria are incubated with the antimicrobial in specialized modules that are read automatically on a frequent basis. The multiple readings and the increased sensitivity of determining endpoints by turbidimetric or fluorometric analysis make it possible to generate MICs in as little as 4 hours. In laboratories with sufficient volume, these methods are no more expensive than manual methods, and the rapid results have enhanced potential to influence clinical outcome, particularly when interfaced with computerized hospital information systems.

Automated methods read dilution tests in a few hours

Diffusion Tests

In diffusion testing (often called the Kirby-Bauer technique), the inoculum is seeded onto the surface of an agar plate, and filter paper disks containing defined amounts of antimicrobials are applied. While the plates are incubating, the antimicrobial diffuses from the paper into the medium to produce a circular gradient around the disk. After incubation overnight, the size of the zone of growth inhibition around the disk (**Figure 23–6A**) can be used as an indirect measure of the MIC of the organism. Zone size is also influenced by the growth rate of the organism, the diffusibility of the drug, and other technical factors. The diameters of the zones of inhibition obtained with the various antibiotics are interpreted as "susceptible," "intermediate," or "resistant" by referring to an interpretive table. This method is convenient and flexible for rapidly growing aerobic and facultative bacteria such as the Enterobacteriaceae, *Pseudomonas*, and staphylococci. Another diffusion procedure uses gradient strips to produce elliptical zones that can be directly correlated with the MIC. This method, the epsilometer or "E-test" (**Figure 23–6B**), can also be applied to slow-growing, fastidious, and anaerobic bacteria. This approach is slower and more laborious than automated broth systems, but it has the advantage of revealing the presence of multiple colony morphologies, mixed infections, or resistant subpopulations that appear as "inner colonies" within an otherwise clear zone of inhibition.

✳ **Antimicrobial in disks produces a circular concentration gradient, or in strips an elliptical gradient**

Inhibition zone is a measure of the drug's effect

Molecular Testing

The molecular techniques of nucleic acid hybridization, sequencing, and amplification (see Chapter 4) have been applied to the detection and study of resistance. The strategy is to detect the resistance gene rather than to measure the phenotypic expression of that gene's product. These methods offer the prospect of automation and rapid results, but they can only detect genes already known to science, although some forms of resistance do not yet have well-defined genetic causes. Phenotypic gene expression remains the "bottom line" that guides most resistance testing today.

Molecular methods detect known resistance genes

Bactericidal Testing

The above methods do not distinguish between inhibitory and bactericidal activity. Doing so requires quantitative subculture of the clear tubes in the broth dilution test and comparison of the number of viable bacteria at the beginning and end of the test. The least amount required to kill a predetermined portion of the inoculum (usually 99.9%) is called the **minimal bactericidal concentration (MBC)**. Direct bactericidal testing is important in the initial characterization and

Quantitation of the bactericidal effect determines the MBC

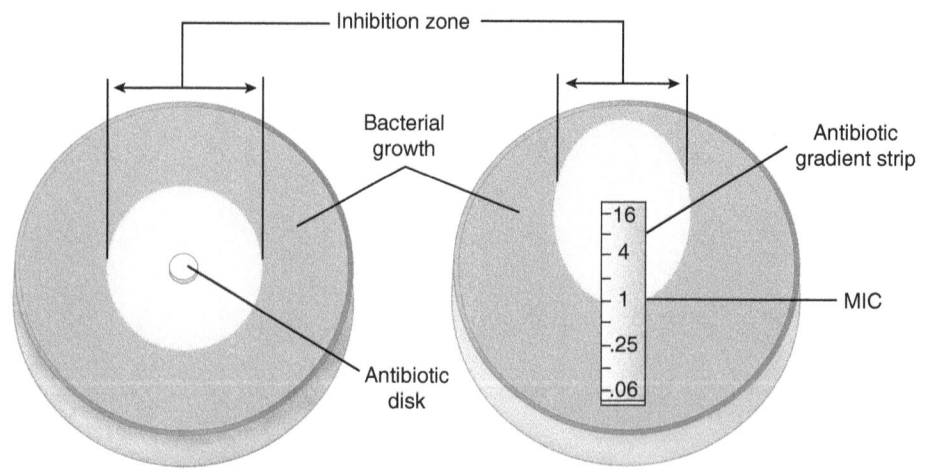

FIGURE 23–6. **Diffusion tests. A.** Disk diffusion. The diameter of the zone of growth inhibition around a disk of fixed antimicrobial content is inversely proportional to the minimum inhibitory concentration (MIC) for that antimicrobial, that is, the larger the zone, the lower the MIC. **B.** The E test. A strip containing a gradient of antimicrobial content creates an elliptical zone of inhibition. The conditions are empirically adjusted so that the MIC endpoint is where the growth intersects the strip.

clinical evaluation of antimicrobial agents but is rarely used clinically. Most of the antimicrobials used for acute and life-threatening infections (eg, β-lactams, aminoglycosides) act by bactericidal mechanisms.

■ Antimicrobial Assays

For antimicrobials with a narrow therapeutic index, meaning toxicity is near the therapeutic range, monitoring the concentration in the serum or other body fluid is sometimes necessary. Therapeutic monitoring may also be required when the patient's pharmacologic handling of the agent is unpredictable, as in renal failure. A variety of biologic, immunoassay, and chemical procedures have been developed for this purpose. The drugs most commonly measured are vancomycin and the aminoglycosides.

Pharmacologic monitoring necessary in some situations

BACTERIAL RESISTANCE TO ANTIMICROBIALS

Antimicrobial agents were originally hailed as "wonder drugs." Unfortunately, their effectiveness has been steadily eroded by the appearance of resistant bacterial strains. This resistance may be inherent to the organism or appear in a previously susceptible species by mutation or the acquisition of new genes. Keeping ahead of the microbes requires that we understand the mechanisms by which bacteria develop resistance and the ways this resistance spreads. The following sections discuss the biochemical mechanisms of resistance, how resistance is genetically controlled, and how resistant strains survive and spread in our society. How these features relate to the antimicrobial groups is summarized in **Table 23–2** and further discussed in the chapters on specific bacteria (see Chapters 24-41).

Resistance has eroded the effectiveness of many agents

Antimicrobial resistance has survival value for the organism, and its expression in the medical setting requires that virulence be retained despite the change that mediates resistance. There are no direct connections between resistance and virulence: some highly drug-resistant bacteria may cause relatively indolent infections, whereas exquisitely susceptible organisms may cause severe infections. Resistant bacteria have increased opportunities to produce disease, but the disease itself is the same as that produced by the bacterium's susceptible counterpart. Although uncommon, it is possible for enhanced virulence traits to be added to resistant strains by linkage with virulence genes on plasmids or other genetic elements. This appears to have occurred with the emergence of MRSA clones with enhanced potential to infect skin and soft tissues (see Chapter 24). The term "superbug," increasingly used to describe multiresistant bacteria, implies this linkage is more common than it actually is.

Resistance and virulence are separate properties but may be linked

■ Mechanisms of Resistance

The major mechanisms of bacterial resistance (**Figure 23–7**) are (1) Exclusion of the antimicrobial from the bacterial cell due to impermeability or active efflux; (2) alterations of an antimicrobial target, which render it insusceptible; and (3) inactivation of the antimicrobial agent by an enzyme produced by the microorganism.

Exclusion (Figure 23–8)

An effective antimicrobial must enter the bacterial cell and achieve concentrations sufficient to act on its target. The cell wall, particularly the outer membrane of Gram-negative bacteria presents a formidable barrier for access to the interior of the cell (see Figure 21–4). Inability to traverse the outer membrane is the primary reason most β-lactams are less active against Gram-negative than Gram-positive bacteria. Outer membrane protein porin channels may allow drug penetration depending on their size, charge, degree of hydrophobicity, or general molecular configuration. This is a major reason for inherent resistance to antimicrobial agents, but these transport characteristics may change even in typically susceptible species due to mutations in the porin proteins. For example, strains of *P aeruginosa* may develop resistance to carbapenems due to loss of the outer membrane protein most important for their penetration.

Cell wall and outer membrane barriers to antimicrobials

✳ Outer membrane protein porins restrict access to interior

Some antimicrobials must be actively transported into the cell. For example, bacteria lacking the metabolic pathways required to transport aminoglycosides across the cytoplasmic membrane (streptococci, enterococci, anaerobes) are intrinsically resistant. Conversely, other antimicrobials are actively transported *out* of the cell. A number of bacterial species have energy-dependent efflux mechanisms that literally pump antimicrobial agents which have entered the cell back out. The membrane transporter systems that drive these efflux pumps often affect antimicrobials of several classes.

✳ Active transport required for some drugs to enter cell

✳ Efflux pumps push antimicrobials back out

TABLE 23–2	Features of Bacterial Resistance to Antimicrobial Agents			
	MECHANISM[a]			
ANTIMICROBIAL	ENTRY BARRIER (EB)	ALTERED TARGET (AT)	ENZYMATIC INACTIVATION (EI)	EMERGING RESISTANCE[b] (ORGANISM/ ANTIMICROBIC/MECHANISM)
β-Lactams	Variable outer membrane[c] penetration	Mutant and new PBPs	β-lactamases	*Staphylococcus aureus*/penicillin/EI *S aureus*/methicillin/AT *Streptococcus pneumoniae*/penicillin/AT *Haemophilus influenzae*/ampicillin/AT, EI *Neisseria gonorrhoeae*/penicillin/AT, EI *Pseudomonas aeruginosa*/ceftazidime/EB *Klebsiella, Enterobacter*/third-generation cephalosporins/EI
Glycopeptides	Thickened cell wall	Amino acid substitution	–	*Enterococcus* (VRE)/*S aureus* (VRSA)/ vancomycin/AT *S aureus* (VISA)/vancomycin/EB
Aminoglycosides	Oxidative transport required	Ribosomal binding site mutations	Adenylases, acetylases, phosphorylases	*Klebsiella, Enterobacter*/gentamicin/EI *P aeruginosa*/gentamicin/EB
Macrolides, clindamycin	Minimal outer membrane[c] pene- tration, efflux pump	Methylation of rRNA	Phosphotransferase, esterase	*Bacteroides fragilis*/clindamycin/AT *S aureus*/ erythromycin/AT
Chloramphenicol	–	–	Acetyltransferase	*Salmonella*/chloramphenicol/EI
Tetracycline	Efflux pump	New protein protects ribosome site	–	
Fluoroquinolones	Efflux pump, per- meability mutation	Mutant topoisomerase	–	*Escherichia coli*/ciprofloxacin/AT *P aeruginosa*/ ciprofloxacin/AT *N gonorrhoeae*/EB/AT
Rifampin	–	Mutant RNA polymerase	–	*Mycobacterium tuberculosis*[d]/rifampin/AT *Neisseria meningitidis*/rifampin/AT
Daptomycin	Membrane charge alteration	–		*S aureus*/EB *Enterococcus*/EB
Folate inhibitors	–	New dihydropteroate synthetase, altered dihydrofolate reductase	–	Enterobacteriaceae/sulfonamides/AT

[a]Only primary mechanisms of resistance are listed.
[b]A highly selective list of resistance emergence that has altered or threatens a major clinical use of the agent.
[c]Outer membrane of Gram-negative bacteria.
[d]See Chapter 27.
Abbreviations: PBP, penicillin-binding protein; VRE, vancomycin-resistant enterococci; VISA, vancomycin intermediate *Staphylococcus aureus*; VRSA, vancomycin-resistant *S aureus*.

Altered Target (Figure 23–9)

Once in the cell, antimicrobials act by binding and inactivating their target, which is typically a crucial enzyme or ribosomal site. If the target is altered in a way that decreases its affinity for the antimicrobial, the inhibitory effect will be proportionately decreased. Substitution of a single amino acid at a certain location in a protein may alter its binding to the antimicrobial without affecting its function in the bacterial cell.

✳ Binding affinity for enzymes and ribosomes can change

If an alteration at a single site on the target renders it nonsusceptible, mutation to resistance can occur in a single step, even during therapy. This occurred with the early aminoglycosides (strep-tomycin), which bound to a single ribosomal site, and the first quinolone (nalidixic acid), which attached to only one of four possible topoisomerase subunits. Newer agents in each class bind at multiple sites on their target, making mutation to resistance less probable.

Multiple binding sites reduce chances for resistance

One of the most important examples of altered target involves the β-lactam family and the peptidoglycan transpeptidase PBPs on which they act. In Gram-positive and Gram-negative spe-cies, changes in one or more of these proteins correlate with decreased susceptibility to multiple β-lactams. These alterations were initially detected as changes in electrophoretic migration of one or more PBPs using radiolabeled penicillin (hence the origin of the term PBP). These changes have now been traced to point mutations and substitutions of amino acid sequences.

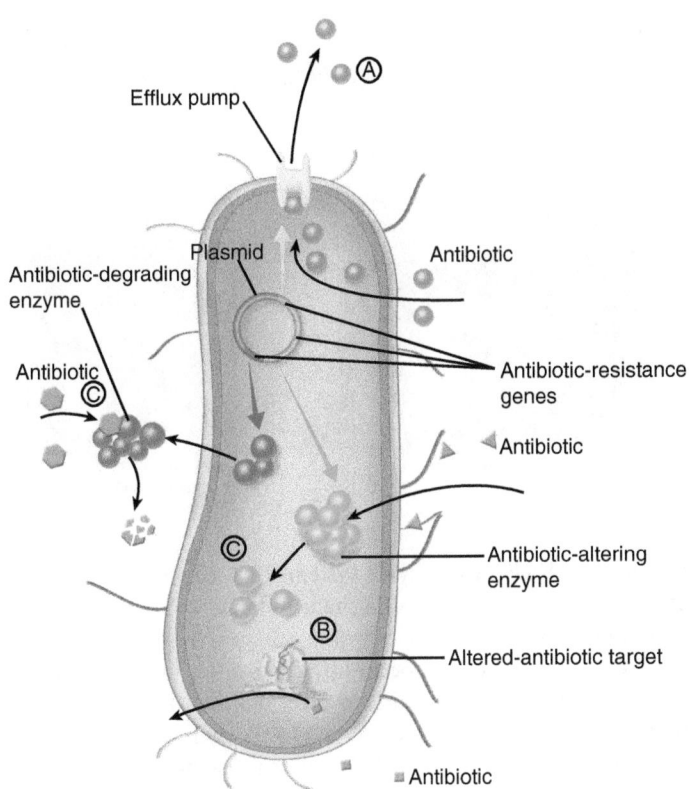

FIGURE 23-7. **Antimicrobial resistance mechanisms. A.** Exclusion barrier. **B.** Altered target. **C.** Enzymatic inactivation. (Reproduced with permission from Willey JM: *Prescott, Harley, & Klein's Microbiology*, 7th ed. New York, NY: McGraw Hill; 2008.)

Because the altered binding may not be absolute, decreases in susceptibility may be incremental. Wild-type pneumococci and gonococci are inhibited by 0.06 μg/mL of penicillin, while those with altered PBPs have MICs of 0.1 to 8.0 μg/mL. At the lower end, these MICs still appear to be within therapeutic range but are associated with treatment failures, even when dosage is increased. Altered PBPs may affect some or all β-lactams. Although the exact MICs vary, a strain with a 10-fold decrease in susceptibility to penicillin has decreased susceptibility to cephalosporins similarly. In some cases, the alteration is significant enough to render an entire class useless against the bacteria, such as the production by *S aureus* of PBP-2A, which renders it resistant to all β-lactams (except ceftaroline). PBP alterations are one of multiple mechanisms of resistance in a variety of other bacteria including enterococci, gonococci, *H influenzae*, and many other Gram-positive and Gram-negative species.

✳ Altered PBPs have reduced affinity for β-lactams

✳ Pneumococci and MRSA have altered PBPs

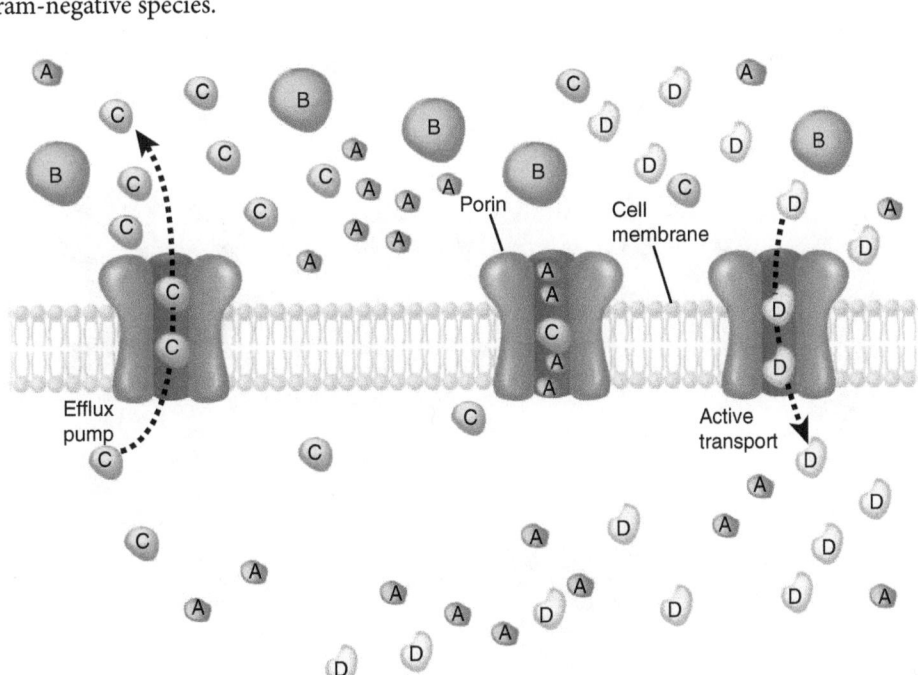

FIGURE 23-8. **Exclusion barrier resistance.** A, B, C, and D molecules are external to the cell wall here shown as what could be either the outer membrane (Gram negatives) or the cytoplasmic membrane. **A molecules** pass through and remain inside the cell, **B molecules** are unable to pass due to their size, **C molecules** pass through but are transported back out by an efflux pump, and **D molecules** must be pulled through by an active process.

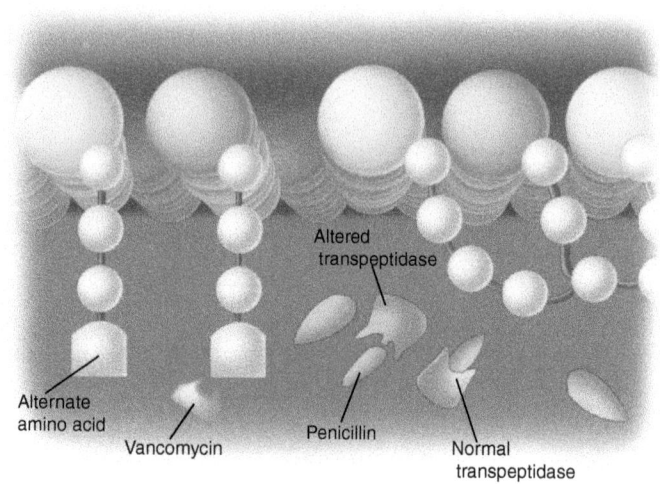

FIGURE 23-9. **Altered target resistance.** (Compare with Figure 23–1A, B.) A normal transpeptidase or penicillin-binding protein (PBP) is inactivated by penicillin, but penicillin no longer binds to the PBP with altered binding sites. This PBP is still able to carry out its cross-linking function so the β-lactam is no longer effective. Also shown is a terminal amino acid substitution which will no longer bind vancomycin (see Figure 23–1C).

✳ Mutation or acquisition of a new enzyme occurs

Alteration of other targets happens, too. VRE have enzyme systems that substitute a different amino acid in the terminal position of the peptidoglycan side chain (often alanyl lactate instead of alanyl alanine). Vancomycin does not bind to the alternate amino acid, rendering these strains resistant. Resistance to sulfonamides and trimethoprim occurs by acquisition of new enzymes with low affinity for these agents but still allows bacterial cells to carry out their respective functions in the folate synthesis pathway. Clindamycin resistance involves an enzyme that methylates ribosomal RNA, preventing attachment. This modification also confers resistance to erythromycin and other macrolides, because they share binding sites. Interestingly, induction with erythromycin leads to clindamycin resistance, although the reverse is unusual.

Enzymatic Inactivation (Figure 23–10)

✳ Enzymes disrupt or chemically modify antimicrobials

Enzymatic inactivation of antimicrobial agents is the most powerful and robust resistance mechanism. Literally hundreds of distinct enzymes produced by resistant bacteria may inactivate antimicrobials in the cell, in the periplasmic space, or outside the cell. They may act on the antimicrobial molecule by disrupting its structure or by catalyzing a reaction that chemically modifies it.

β-Lactamases. β-Lactamase is a general term referring to any one of many bacterial enzymes able to break open the β-lactam ring and inactivate various members of the β-lactam group. The

FIGURE 23-10. **Enzymatic inactivation resistance.** (See Figure 23–1.) The bacterium is producing a β-lactamase enzyme, which destroys penicillin by breaking open the β-lactam ring. If intact penicillin reaches a PBP, it can still bind and inactivate it; the more β-lactamase produced, the higher the level of resistance.

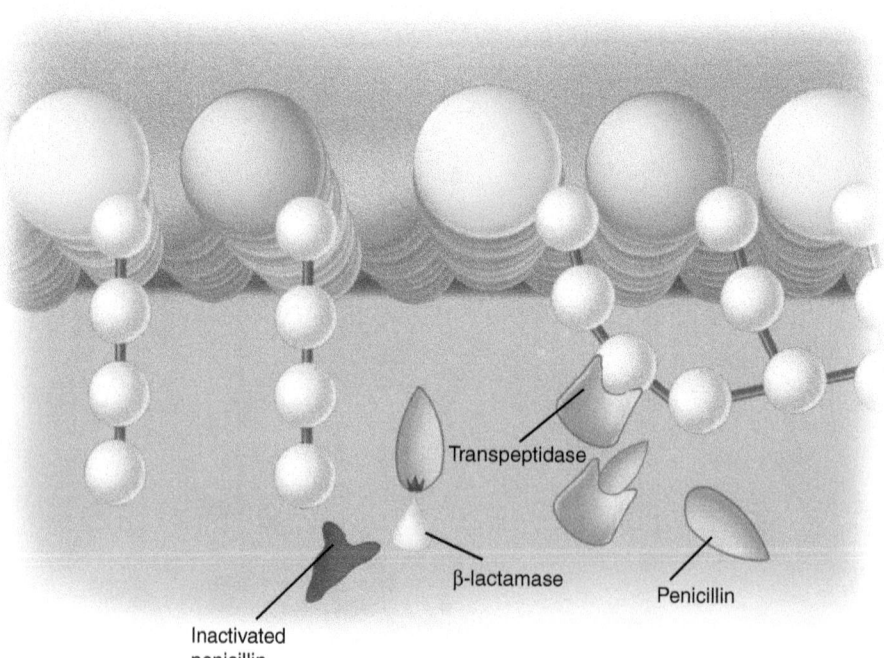

first was discovered when penicillin-resistant strains of *S aureus* emerged and were found to inactivate penicillin *in vitro*. The enzyme was called penicillinase, but with expansion of the β-lactam family and concomitant resistance, it has become clear that the situation is quite complex. Each β-lactamase is a distinct enzyme with its own physical characteristics and substrate profile. For example, the original staphylococcal penicillinase is also active against ampicillin but not against methicillin or any cephalosporin. β-Lactamases produced by *E coli* may have some cephalosporinase activity but vary in their potency against individual first-, second-, third-, and fourth-generation cephalosporins. Some β-lactamases are bound by the β-lactamase inhibitor clavulanic acid, while others are not.

٭ Enzymes break open the β-lactam ring

Activity variable against β-lactam substrates

Bacteria that produce β-lactamases typically demonstrate high-level resistance with MICs far outside the therapeutic range. But even weak β-lactamase producers are considered resistant because the outcome of susceptibility tests (and presumably infected sites) is strongly influenced by the number of bacteria present. Large bacterial populations may secrete enough β-lactamase to inactivate the antimicrobial before it even reaches the organisms.

Weak β-lactamase producers still considered resistant

A full discussion of β-lactamase classification is beyond the scope of this book, but some understanding of the major types is useful.

- Most Gram-positive β-lactamases are exoenzymes with little activity against cephalosporins or the antistaphylococcal penicillins (methicillin, oxacillin). They are bound by β-lactamase inhibitors such as clavulanic acid.

- Some Gram-positive β-lactamases, such as Type A β-lactamase, selectively hydrolyze cefazolin and cephalexin, while remaining ineffective against the antistaphylococcal penicillins.

- Most Gram-negative β-lactamase enzymes concentrate in the periplasmic space (Figure 21–4) and may have penicillinase and/or cephalosporinase activity. They may or may not be inhibited by clavulanic acid. Many of the Gram-negative β-lactamases are constitutively produced at low levels but can be induced to high-level expression by exposure to a β-lactam agent. The resistance gene *ampC* is a notorious member of this group. *AmpC* is concerning because its expression may not be induced during routine laboratory testing, but may subsequently be induced *in vivo*, leading to clinical failure during treatment with penicillins or first- and third-generation cephalosporins.

- Even more worrisome is another class of Gram-negative resistance genes, called extended-spectrum β-lactamases (ESBLs) because their substrates include multiple cephalosporins. The laboratory detection of ESBLs is complex, as is their naming scheme (CTX-M, TEM, OXA, SHV, etc). From a clinical perspective, they are significant because treatment with any generation of cephalosporin may lead to clinical failure. Carbapenems are an excellent drug class for treating infections caused by ESBL-producing organisms.

٭ ESBLs have broad activity against cephalosporins

- Most concerning of all among the Gram-negative resistance genes are the carbapenemases. Although carbapenems still provide reliable coverage of Enterobacteriaceae in most circumstances, enzymes which specialize in hydrolyzing these drugs—and usually penicillins and cephalosporins at the same time—are on the rise. New Delhi metallo-beta lactamase (NDM-1) and *Klebsiella pneumoniae* carbapenemase (KPC) are but two troubling members of a larger family of such genes. These genes have made carbapenem-resistant Enterobacteriaceae (CRE) one of the most important challenges facing infectious diseases medicine today. The newer non–β-lactam β-lactamase inhibitors were designed with these enzymes in mind (see above).

Carbapenemases may lyse all known β-lactams

Modifying Enzymes. The most common cause of acquired bacterial resistance to aminoglycosides is through the production of one or more of over 50 enzymes that acetylate, adenylate, or phosphorylate hydroxyl or amino groups on the aminoglycoside molecule. The modifications take place in the cytosol or in close association with the cytoplasmic membrane. The resistance conveyed by these actions is usually high level; the chemically modified aminoglycoside no longer binds to the ribosome. As with the β-lactamases, the aminoglycoside-modifying enzymes represent a large and diverse group of bacterial proteins, each with its characteristic properties and substrate profile. Inactivating enzymes have been described for a number of other antimicrobials. Most act by chemically modifying the antimicrobial molecule in a manner similar to the aminoglycoside-modifying enzymes. The most clinically significant enzymes convey resistance to erythromycin (esterase, phosphotransferase) and chloramphenicol (acetyltransferase).

٭ Chemically modified aminoglycosides do not bind to ribosomes

■ Genetics of Resistance

Intrinsic Resistance

For any antimicrobial, there are bacterial species that are typically within its spectrum and those which are not (see **Appendix 23–1**). The resistance of the latter group is referred to as **intrinsic** or **chromosomal** to reflect its inherent nature. The resistant species have features such as permeability barriers, a lack of susceptibility of the cell wall, or ribosomal targets that make them inherently insusceptible. Some species constitutively produce low levels of inactivating enzymes, particularly the β-lactamases of Gram-negative bacteria. The chromosomal genes encoding these β-lactamases may be under repressor control and subject to induction by certain β-lactam antimicrobials. This leads to increased production of β-lactamase, which usually results in resistance not only to the inducer but other β-lactams to which the organism would otherwise be susceptible. AmpC β-lactamases operate in this manner.

Permeability barriers, enzyme production

Inducible enzymes

Acquired Resistance

A species may initially be susceptible to an antibiotic but subsequently develop resistance. Such acquired resistance may be due to a genetic mutation within that organism or may be derived from another organism by the acquisition of new genes.

Mutational Resistance

Acquired resistance may occur when there is a crucial mutation in the target of the antimicrobial or in proteins related to access to the target (ie, reduced permeability). Mutations in regulatory proteins can also lead to resistance. Mutations take place at a regular but low frequency and are expressed only if they are not associated with other effects that are disadvantageous to the bacterial cell. Mutational resistance can emerge in a single step or evolve slowly, requiring multiple mutations before clinically significant resistance is achieved. Single-step mutational resistance is most likely when the antimicrobial agent binds to a single site on its target. Resistance can also emerge rapidly when it is related to gene regulation, such as mutational derepression of a chromosomally encoded cephalosporinase. A slow, progressive resistance evolving over the years, even decades, is typical for β-lactam resistance related to altered PBPs.

Mutations in structural or regulatory genes

Mutations low frequency

Genetic Exchange

Of the four major mechanisms of genetic exchange among bacteria described in Chapter 21 and illustrated in **Figure 23–11** (transformation, transduction, conjugation, transposition), conjugation and transposition are the most important clinically and often work in tandem.

Conjugation and transposition most important

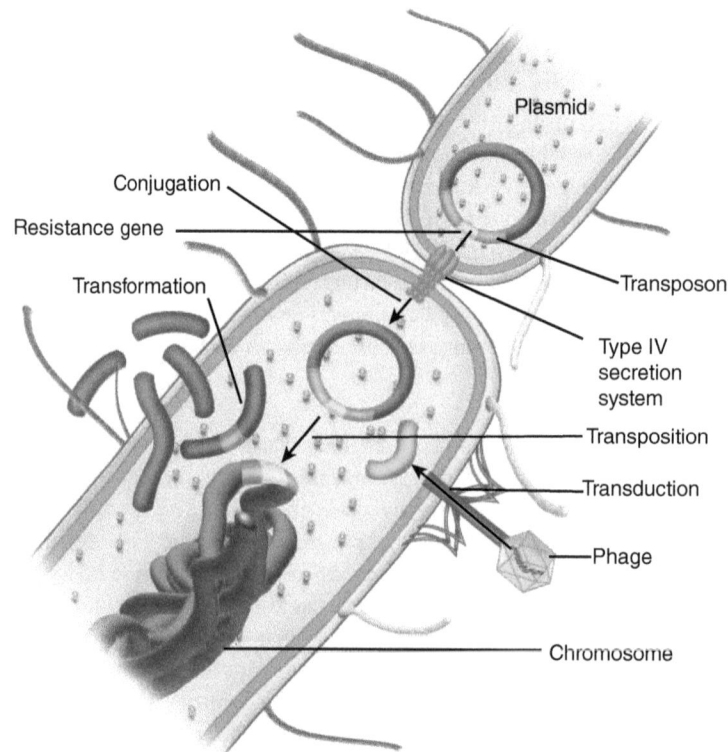

FIGURE 23–11. **Genetic mechanisms of acquired resistance.** Bacteria are shown exchanging genetic information by transformation, transduction, conjugation, and transposition. Conjugation and transposition are the most common in human infections and are often combined. (Reproduced with permission from Willey JM: *Prescott, Harley, & Klein's Microbiology*, 7th ed. New York, NY: McGraw Hill; 2008.)

Plasmids and Conjugation

The transfer of plasmids by conjugation was the first discovered mechanism for the acquisition of new resistance genes, and it continues to be the most important. Resistance genes on plasmids (R plasmids) can determine resistance to one or more antimicrobials, even ones that act by different mechanisms. After conjugation, the resistance genes may remain on a recircularized plasmid or, less often, become integrated into the chromosome by recombination. A single cell may contain more than one distinct plasmid and/or multiple copies of the same plasmid. Although most resistance mechanisms have been linked to plasmids in one species or another, plasmid distribution among the bacterial pathogens is by no means uniform. The compatibility systems that maintain plasmids from one bacterial cell generation to the next are complex. Some species of bacteria are more likely than others to contain plasmids. For example, *Neisseria gonorrhoeae* typically has multiple plasmids, whereas closely related *N meningitidis* rarely has any.

* Plasmid conjugation allows multidrug resistance

Species carry multiple or no plasmids

Plasmids are most likely to be transferred to another strain if they are conjugative, that is, if the resistance plasmid also contains the genes mediating conjugation. Another factor in the spread of plasmids is their host range. Some plasmids can be transferred only to closely related strains; others can be transferred to a broad range of species within and beyond their own genus. A conjugative plasmid with a broad host range has great potential to spread any resistance genes it carries.

* Conjugation genes, host range enhance spread

Transposons and Transposition

Transposons containing resistance genes can move from plasmid to plasmid or between plasmid and chromosome. Most of the resistance genes carried on plasmids are transposon insertions that can be carried along with the rest of the plasmid genome to another strain by conjugation. Once there, the transposon is free to remain in the original plasmid, insert into a new plasmid, insert into the chromosome, or any combination of these (Figure 23–11). Theoretically, plasmids can accomplish the same events by recombination, but the nature of the transposition process is such that it is much more likely to result in the transfer of an intact gene. Transposons also have a variable host range which in general is even broader than plasmids. Together, conjugation and transposition provide extremely efficient means for spreading resistance genes.

* Transposon genes move between chromosomes and plasmids

Transposition and conjugation combine

Other Genetic Mechanisms

Transduction is the process in which viral bacteriophages inject genetic material into bacteria. Although the transfer of resistance genes by transduction has been demonstrated in the laboratory, its association with clinically significant resistance has been uncommon. Transduction of imipenem resistance by wild-type bacteriophages carried by *P aeruginosa* to other strains of the same bacteria is one such example. Because of the high specificity of bacteriophages, transduction is typically limited to bacteria of the same species. Transformation is the insertion of DNA directly across the cell membrane. This is the most common way genes are manipulated in the laboratory, but detecting its occurrence in the environment or human hosts is particularly difficult, because naked DNA lacks the signatures that flag the presence of plasmids and transposons. Molecular epidemiologic studies suggest that the spread of PBP mutations in *S pneumoniae* is due to transformation, and there may be more examples awaiting discovery.

* Transduction limited by bacteriophage specificity

Transformation may be underappreciated

■ Epidemiology of Resistance

It seems that sooner or later, microorganisms will develop resistance to any antimicrobial agent to which they are exposed. Since the start of the antibiotic era, each new antimicrobial has tended to go through a remarkably similar sequence. When an agent is first introduced, its spectrum of activity is highly predictable; some species are naturally resistant, and others are susceptible, with few exceptions. With clinical use, resistant strains of previously susceptible species begin to appear and become increasingly common.

Clinical use followed by resistance

In some situations, resistance develops rapidly; in other cases it takes years, or even decades. For example, when penicillin was first introduced in 1944, all strains of *S aureus* appeared to be fully susceptible, but by 1950, less than one-third of isolates remained susceptible. We now know that strains containing the penicillinase plasmid existed long before and were selected when penicillin use became widespread. These plasmids likely conferred a survival benefit to strains of *S aureus* in the environment, where they live in competition with *Penicillium* and other molds. However, the discovery of *H influenzae* (meningitis) and *N gonorrhoeae* (gonorrhea) strains resistant to ampicillin and penicillin did not occur until those antibiotics had been used heavily for a decade or more. In these instances, resistance genes apparently not present in the species initially

* Preexisting resistance selected by antimicrobial use

Resistance rapid or acquired after long delays

were acquired from other bacterial species, either directly or through recombination of plasmids. There are small enclaves of bacteria that have not developed resistance. After almost a century, the causes of syphilis (*Treponema pallidum*) and strep throat (group A streptococcus) have thus far retained their susceptibility to penicillin.

Whatever the genetic mechanism, the persistence and spread of resistance requires an environment in which the resistant strain pays little or no price in terms of fitness, or has a selective advantage. The primary human factors that favor this selection are the overuse of antimicrobial agents in medicine and the inclusion of antimicrobials in livestock feed. Any use of antimicrobial agents by physicians—whether appropriate or not—has the potential for the unintended consequence of selecting for resistance. This includes prescribing antibacterial agents for viral infections or using a broad-spectrum agent when a narrower drug would work just as well—if not better. Exceeding guidelines for prophylactic use of antimicrobials (see later) also contributes. In many nations, physician prescriptions are not required for the use of antibiotics, and self-prescription of antibiotics is common, which may accelerate resistance. Microorganisms do not respect geopolitical boundaries, and the effect of antibiotic misuse in one region can have profound impacts thousands of miles away. As with any intervention in medicine, the use of antimicrobial agents carries benefits and risks for the patient. The difference with antimicrobials is that the risk of resistance is for the population at large, not just the individual patient.

Antimicrobial use creates selection for resistance

✳ Overuse increases risk for patients and population at large

The addition of antimicrobials to animal feeds for their prophylactic or growth-promoting effects is a concerning source of resistant strains of bacteria. Cattle or poultry that consume feed supplemented with antimicrobials develop resistant enteric flora that spreads throughout the herd. Resistant strains can then appear in the microbiota of humans living in proximity or handling animal products, including consumers at home. Links from farm to human disease have been established in multiple outbreaks. As a consequence, some countries tightly regulate the use of antimicrobial agents which are used in humans unless necessary for the treatment or prevention of livestock infections. Because microbes may carry resistance genes from person to person, to and from animals, and into the environment, physicians and scientists must rise to the challenge by collaborating cooperating with each other. Doctors, veterinarians, dentists, microbiologists, pharmacists, nurses, epidemiologists, ecologists, ranchers, farmers, civil engineers, public health officers, policy makers, and members of the general public are all key stakeholders in the antimicrobial resistance crisis. Recognition of this fundamental truth has led to an exciting field called One Health, which acknowledges our interconnectedness—as professionals and as dwellers in a fragile, threatened environment.

✳ Antimicrobials in animal feeds increase resistant population

Outbreaks traced from patients back to farms

KEY CONCLUSIONS

- Antimicrobial resistance genes may be present in bacteria and unmasked under selective pressure induced by medications.
- Resistance may also evolve from mutations within a bacterial population.
- Some resistance genes may be shared between bacteria, even between different species.

ANTIMICROBIAL STEWARDSHIP

Ultimately, bacteria will always evolve in response to selective pressure. Because this has the potential to happen much more rapidly than we can develop new antibiotics, we must defend the current armamentarium. Just as we must protect our natural environment, so too must we protect this precious resource of antimicrobials by using them wisely.

A coordinated, sustained effort will be required to minimize the spread of antimicrobial resistance. Everyone shares responsibility for the current crisis of resistance—the veterinarians who use it in farm animals, the politicians who regulate and set priorities in healthcare, the insurance companies that dictate access to certain medications for reasons of cost, the drug manufacturers who choose which drugs to focus on, the patients who ask for antibiotics even when they are not necessary, and of course the providers who prescribe these vital medications. A coordinated response to antibiotic resistance is called "antimicrobial stewardship." Many hospitals now have formal stewardship programs, closely integrated with infection prevention teams. Most antibiotics are prescribed in the outpatient setting where there is a pressing need for better stewardship. As a future prescriber, you bear a professional responsibility to become an antimicrobial steward for the benefit of the individual patient, and for the benefit of society. The mantra is "Together, we can reduce antimicrobial resistance."

✳ Antimicrobial stewardship is the rational, optimal use of antimicrobials

Medical providers should behave as stewards

Learning to prescribe antibiotics effectively and safely takes practice. Some fundamental principles are included in the following discussion, and in **Appendix 23-2.**

■ Empiric Therapy

Unfortunately, definitive microbiological data are rarely available when patients first present with an infection. Because time is usually of the essence, providers must make their best guess and start with "empiric therapy." These first decisions are based on the physician's assessment of the probable microbial etiology of the patient's infection. Variables involved in choosing the best empiric drug include the site of infection (eg, throat, lung, urine, bone) and epidemiologic factors such as season, geography, patient age, pregnancy status, drug allergies, prior antibiotic exposure, other medications being taken, and predisposing conditions. This list of individual factors must then be matched with their probable microbiology and antimicrobial susceptibilities as shown in Table 23-1 and **Appendix 23-1.** Local antibiograms provide "batting averages" for each antimicrobial against common bacterial pathogens. These are available from hospital laboratories and infection control committees; note that, depending on the technique used to create the antibiogram, these resources may be more suitable for inpatients than outpatients, because resistance to broad-spectrum agents may be less rampant in the community than in the hospital.

✳ Probable etiology and susceptibility statistics guide initial selection

This process may be as simple as selecting penicillin to treat an ambulatory patient with suspected group A streptococcal pharyngitis, or as complex as resorting to a combination of broad-spectrum antibacterial, antifungal, and antiviral agents to treat a critically ill inpatient who has undergone stem cell transplantation. In general, the risks of broad-spectrum treatment (eg drug toxicity and selection of resistant microbiota) become more acceptable as the severity of the infection increases. When the risk of not "covering" an improbable pathogen is death, as may be the case in critically ill or immunosuppressed patients, it is more difficult to prescribe narrow coverage initially. But, empiric therapy should be converted to specific therapy within a few days, once microbiology data are available, although in some instances this is not possible. For example, in otitis media, there is no easy way to culture the middle ear, so empiric therapy must be continued for a defined duration, and the outcome evaluated on clinical grounds.

✳ Narrow versus broad empiric spectrum influenced by likelihood of resistance, severity of illness

SPECIFIC THERAPY

Specific therapy is that directed only at the known pathogen, based on isolation and susceptibility testing of the patient's organism in the laboratory. This is possible for most bacterial infections—if microbiological testing is performed. As the results of Gram stains, cultures, and susceptibility tests are reported, unnecessary antimicrobials must be discontinued and the spectrum of therapy narrowed. For example, a patient with suspected staphylococcal or streptococcal infection might be empirically started on vancomycin, which covers both possibilities. Once MRSA has been excluded, a more specific β-lactam is substituted for the broader spectrum treatment. Usually this is a single best agent, but sometimes combinations of antimicrobials that have different modes of action are used for enhanced effect. The major indications for combinations are to reduce the probability of emergence of resistance (which is important in chronic infections like tuberculosis and lung infections in cystic fibrosis), and taking advantage of known synergy between two antimicrobials. Synergy happens when the activity of a drug combination is far greater than would be expected from the individual MICs of the two antimicrobials.

✳ Isolation of the causative agent allows deescalation to specific coverage

✳ Susceptibility tests provide final guidance

Combinations may be synergistic

■ Prophylaxis

The use of antimicrobials to prevent infection is a tempting but potentially hazardous endeavor. The risk for the individual patient: toxicity, side effects, reduced healthy gastrointestinal microbiota, and subsequent infection with a different, more resistant organism. The risk for the whole population: increased risk for the spread of resistance. After many years of experience, the indications for antimicrobial prophylaxis have been narrowed to a small number of situations in which antimicrobials have been shown to decrease infection during a period of high risk. For example, persons known to have been exposed to highly infectious and virulent pathogens like *N meningitidis* (meningitis), *Bacillus anthracis* (anthrax), or *Yersinia pestis* (plague) can abort an infection during the incubation period by the administration of ciprofloxacin. Prophylaxis can also reduce the risk in certain patients of endogenous infection associated with certain surgical and dental procedures if given during the procedure. The practice of administering prophylactic penicillin during labor to mothers with demonstrated vaginal group B streptococcal (GBS) colonization dramatically decreases the leading cause of sepsis and meningitis in neonates.

✳ High-risk exposures, some surgical procedures merit prophylaxis

GBS reduced in neonates

APPENDIX 23–1 Usual Susceptibility Patterns of Common Bacteria to Some Commonly Used Bacteriostatic and Bactericidal Antimicrobial Agents

Antimicrobial	Bactericidal	Bacteriostatic	Staphylococcus aureus	Enterococci	Other Streptococci	Neisseria	Haemophilus	Legionella	Mycoplasma	Escherichia coli	Proteus mirabilis	Other Proteus spp	Klebsiella	Enterobacter	Serratia	Pseudomonas aeruginosa	Bacteroides fragilis	Other gram-negative anaerobes	Clostridium	Rickettsia	Chlamydia	
Benzyl penicillin	+		1 ◔	C ⊙	1 ◔	1 ◔	⊙	●	●	⊙	●	●	●	●	●	●	1 ◔	○	1 ○	●	●	Narrow-spectrum agents
Penicillinase-resistant penicillins	+		1 ◔	●	2 ◔	●	●	●	●	●	●	●	●	●	●	●	●	●	●	●	●	
Erythromycin	±	+	2 ◑	2 ◑	2 ◑	◔	1 ○	1 ○	○	●	●	●	●	●	●	–	–	–	–	●	2 ○	
Clindamycin	±	+	2 ◔	–	◔	●	●	–	–	●	●	●	●	●	●	●	◔	◑	◔	–	–	
Daptomycin	+		○	○	○	●	●	●	●	●	●	●	●	●	●	●	●	●	●	●	●	
Linezolid		+	○	○	○	●	●	●	●	●	●	●	●	●	●	●	◑	◑	◔	●	●	
Vancomycin	+		2 ○	1 ◔	2 ○	●	●	●	●	●	●	●	●	●	●	●	–	–	1 ○	–	–	
Ampicillin	+		2 ●	1 ◔	2 ◔	1 ◔	◔	●	●	1 ◑	1 ◔	●	●	●	●	●	1 ◕	–	○	●	●	
Piperacillin	+		–	○	○	–	◔	●	●	1 ◔	1 ◔	1 ◔	1 ◔	1 ◔	1 ◔	2 ◔	1 ○	–	●	●	●	Broad-spectrum agents
Cefazolin	+		◑	●	◔	●	●	●	●	◔	◔	◑	◔	●	●	●	●	●	●	●	●	
Ceftriaxone	+		C ◑	●	◔	○	○	●	●	○	○	○	○	◔	◔	●	●	●	●	●	●	
Cefepime	+		◑	–	◔	◔	○	●	●	○	○	○	○	○	○	◔	●	●	●	●	●	
Ceftaroline	+		C ○	◔	◔	–	○	●	●	–	–	–	–	–	–	●	●	–	●	●	●	
Cefotetan	+		–	●	1 ○	1 ◔	–	●	●	1 ○	1 ○	1 ○	1 ○	●	◔	●	2 ◔	○	–	●	●	
Ceftazidime	+		–	–	–	–	○	●	●	1 ◔	1 ◔	1 ◔	1 ◔	2 ◔	2 ◔	◔	●	–	●	●	●	
Imipenem	+		2 ○	2 ○	2 ○	1 ○	1 ○		●	1 ○	1 ○	1 ○	1 ○	1 ○	1 ○	1 ◔	1 ○	○	1 ○	–	–	
Aztreonam	+		●	●	●	1 ◔	1 ◔	●		1 ○	1 ○	1 ○	1 ○	1 ◔	1 ◔	●	●	●	●	–	–	
Gentamicin	+		C ◔	●	●	–	–	●	–	1 ◔	1 ◔	1 ◔	1 ◔	1 ◔	1 ◔	●	●	●	●	–	–	
Tetracycline		+	◔	●	◑	◔	2 ○	1 ○	◔	●	◔	◑	●	●	●	◑	◑	●	1 ○	1 ○	
Ciprofloxacin	+		◑	◑	⊙	2 ○	–	–	●	1 ◔	1 ◔	1 ◔	1 ◔	1 ◔	1 ◔	2 ◔	●	●	–	–	⊙	
Moxifloxacin	+		◔	◑	◔	◑	○	○	○	◔	○	○	◑	◔	◔	●	●	◑	●	–	○	
Sulfamethoxazole + trimethoprim	±	+	◔	–	–	–	1 ◔	–	–	1 ○	◔	◔	◔	◔	◔	●	◔	–	–	–	3 –	

Proportions of susceptible and resistant strains: ○, 100% susceptible   ◔, 25% resistant   ●, 100% resistant   ⊙, intermediate susceptibility.

Abbreviations: – = no present indication for therapy or insufficient data   1 = antimicrobic of choice for susceptible strains   2 = second-line agent
3 = c trachomatis-sensitive, c psittaci-resistant   C = Useful in combinations with other antibiotics such as β-lactams + aminoglycosides or other β-lactams

APPENDIX 23–2 Principles of Effective Antimicrobial Stewardship

- **Maintain Meticulous Infection Control.** Minimize the risk of passing resistance genes to bystander bacteria by keeping drug-resistant pathogens away from other patients—and yourself. Clean hands before and after every encounter, obey other special precaution protocols, and maintain a clean examination area or hospital room. (See Chapter 3.)

- **Say NO to Antibiotics for Viral Rhinosinusitis.** The common cold is due to viral infection approximately 95% of the time. Encourage patients to "get smart" about antibiotics, treat their symptoms, and emphasize the importance of maintaining the effectiveness of antimicrobials if they should eventually require them.

- **Establish a Firm Diagnosis.** Is the patient truly infected with a bacterial pathogen? Some diseases mimic infection but do not respond to antibiotics. If a serious bacterial infection is present, culture data are extraordinarily helpful, because they will reveal not only the pathogen but also its susceptibility profile. Ideally, cultures should be obtained before antimicrobials are started. But, for patients who have a severe infection such as sepsis or meningitis, delays in starting treatment may have grave consequences; start antibiotics immediately and send specimens for culture as soon as possible.

- **De-escalate When Possible.** If broad-spectrum empiric treatment was initiated for severe infection, be willing to trust the results of positive cultures and focus treatment. More expensive, newer drugs may not be superior to tried and true therapies. In fact, narrower spectrum agents are often more bactericidal—and cause less collateral damage to helpful commensal microbiota—than broad-spectrum drugs.

- **Shorter May Be Better.** Using the briefest duration of therapy possible may reduce selective pressure on bystander, normal microbes. Subtherapeutic doses or intermittent, haphazard administration are bad practice, but treating at a full dose for a short period may have benefits for resistance—so long as the underlying infection has been adequately treated.

- **Collaborate with Experts.** Specialists in the field of infectious diseases (ID) are always eager to work with other physicians, both to generate protocols and to care for specific patients. Consult ID specialists when patients are severely ill, when they fail to improve as expected, when the resistance profile is unexpectedly challenging, or when treatment involves multiple or toxic drugs.

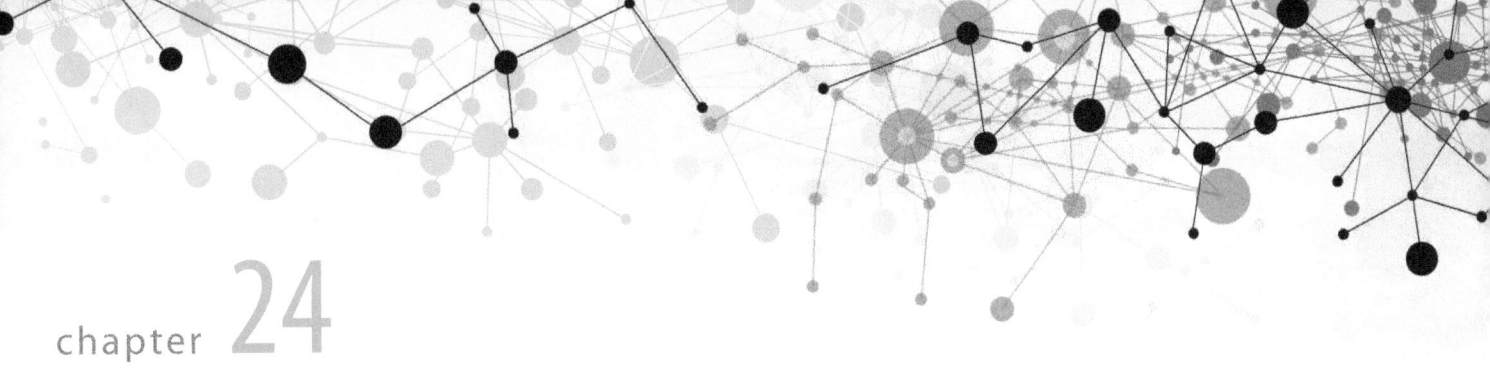

chapter 24

Staphylococci

Staphylococcus aureus • Staphylococcus epidermidis • Staphylococcus saprophyticus

Thou art a boil,

A plague sore, an embossed carbuncle

In my corrupted blood.

—Shakespeare: *King Lear*

OVERVIEW

Members of the genus *Staphylococcus* (staphylococci) are Gram-positive cocci that tend to be arranged in grape-like clusters (**Figure 24–1**). Infections produced by *Staphyloccocus aureus* are typified by acute, aggressive, locally destructive purulent lesions. The most familiar of these is the common boil, a painful lump in the skin that has a necrotic center and fibrous reactive shell. Infections in organs other than the skin such as the lung, kidney, or bone are also focal and destructive, but have greater potential for extension within the organ and beyond to the blood and other organs. Such infections typically produce high fever and systemic toxicity and may be fatal in only a few days. The major virulence factors for these effects are surface attachment proteins, fibrinogen-binding proteins, and a pore-forming exotoxin. A subgroup (less than 10%) of *S aureus* infections has manifestations produced by secreted toxins in addition to those associated with the primary infection. Symptoms include diarrhea, rash, skin desquamation, and multiorgan effects as in staphylococcal toxic shock syndrome (TSS). Superantigen toxins are involved in these diseases. Ingestion of preformed staphylococcal enterotoxin causes a form of food poisoning in which vomiting begins in only a few hours. *Staphylococcus epidermidis* and other non-*aureus* species produce less aggressive disease typically associated with biofilm-mediated attachment to medical devices such as indwelling catheters and biomedical implants like heart valves and artificial joints.

● STAPHYLOCOCCI: GROUP CHARACTERISTICS

Although staphylococci have a marked tendency to form clusters, some single cells, pairs, and short chains are also seen. Staphylococci have a typical Gram-positive cell wall structure. In contrast to streptococci, staphylococci produce catalase. Of the 40+ known species of staphylococci, more than a dozen are known to colonize humans; of these, *S aureus* is by far the most virulent. In the clinical laboratory the ability of *S aureus* to form coagulase separates it from other, less virulent species (**Table 24–1**). It is common to lump the other species together as coagulase-negative staphylococci (CoNS).

※ Form clusters and catalase-positive

※ Coagulase distinguishes *S aureus*

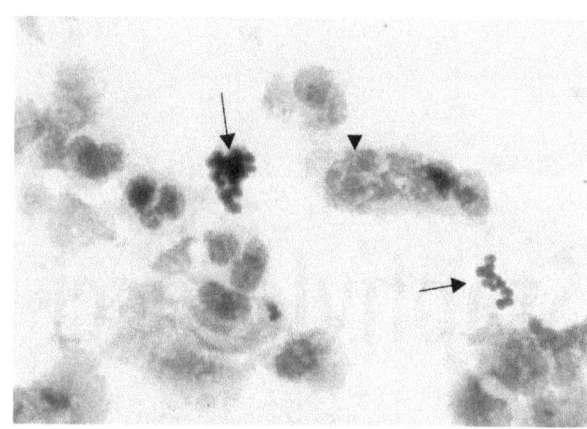

FIGURE 24–1. *Staphylococcus aureus.* Gram stain showing the Gram-positive cocci in clusters resembling bunches of grapes (arrows) and neutrophils (arrowhead). (Used with permission from Professor Shirley Lowe, University of California, San Francisco School of Medicine.)

● *STAPHYLOCOCCUS AUREUS*

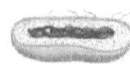 **BACTERIOLOGY**

STRUCTURE

The cell wall of *S aureus* consists of a typical Gram-positive peptidoglycan interspersed with considerable amounts of teichoic acid. The peptidoglycan of the cell wall is commonly overlaid with polysaccharide and surface proteins. Polysaccharide capsules are present in many strains, but their significance in human infections is unknown. Surface proteins such as clumping factors (ClfA, ClfB), which bind to fibrinogen, and fibronectin-binding proteins (FnBPA, FnBPB) likely play a role in the early stages of infection. Another protein, surface Protein A, is unique in that it binds the Fc portion of IgG molecules, leaving the antigen-reacting Fab portion directed externally (turned around). It is present in most clinical isolates of *S aureus*.

✳ Clumping factor binds fibrinogen, FnBP fibronectin

✳ Protein A binds Fab portion of IgG

■ Metabolism

After overnight incubation on blood agar, *S aureus* produces white colonies that tend to turn a buff-golden color with time. The most important laboratory test used to distinguish *S aureus* from other staphylococci is the production of **coagulase,** an enzyme which binds prothrombin in a manner that provides for the cleavage of fibrinogen to fibrin. It is demonstrated by incubating staphylococci in plasma where its growth produces a fibrin clot in a few hours.

✳ Coagulase converts fibrinogen to fibrin

TABLE 24–1	Features of Human Staphylococci							
SPECIES	COAGULASE	α-TOXIN	SAgs	HABITAT	BIOFILM	BOILS	UTI[a]	DEEP INFECTIONS
Staphylococcus aureus	+	+	+	Anterior nares, perineum	+	+	–	Pneumonia, osteomyelitis, abscesses, TSS
S epidermidis	–	–	–	Anterior nares, skin	+	–	–	Device colonization
S saprophyticus	–	–	–	Gastrointestinal tract	–	–	+	None
S lugdunensis	–[b]	–	–	Skin, mucous membranes	Variable	+/–	–	Endocarditis, osteomyelitis, abscesses
S haemolyticus	–	–	–	Anterior nares, skin	Variable	–	–	Device colonization, sepsis, meningitis, endocarditis

SAgs, superantigens; TSS, toxic shock syndrome; UTI, urinary tract infection.
[a]Significant cause of urinary tract infection (UTI).
[b]May test positive depending on laboratory method.

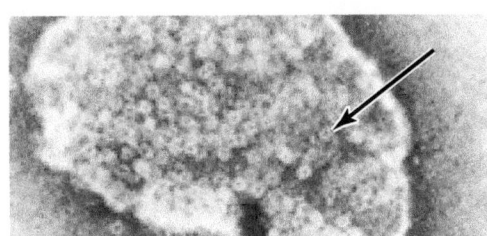

FIGURE 24–2. *Staphylococcus aureus* α-toxin. A fragment of a rabbit erythrocyte lysed with α-toxin is shown. Note the ring-shaped pores in the membrane created by insertion of the toxin. (Reproduced with permission from Bhakdi S, Tranum-Jensen J: Mechanism of complement cytolysis and the concept of channel-forming proteins, *Philos Trans R Soc Lond B Biol Sci* 1984 Sep 6;306(1129):311–324.)

TOXINS AND BIOLOGICALLY ACTIVE EXTRACELLULAR ENZYMES

■ Toxins

← break red blood cells (A)

S aureus produces a number of named cytolytic hemolysins (toxins) (α, β, δ, γ), of which α-Hemolysin is the most important. α-Hemolysin, is a protein secreted by almost all strains of *S aureus*, but not by CoNS. It is a pore-forming cytotoxin (see Figure 22-6) that lyses the cytoplasmic membranes by direct insertion into the lipid bilayer to form transmembrane pores (**Figure 24-2**). The resultant egress of vital molecules leads to cell death. This action is similar to complement, streptolysin O, and the effector proteins of cytotoxic T-lymphocytes. α-Hemolysin is not active against neutrophils but does lyse a wide variety of other cells including keratinocytes. Another pore-forming toxin is active against neutrophils and thus long ago named Panton-Valentine leukocidin (PVL). PVL is also active against platelets. It causes tissue necrosis but until recently was found in only a small portion of clinical isolates (less than 10%).

✱ α-Toxin inserts in lipid bilayer forming transmembrane pores

PVL attacks neutrophils, platelets

← feast on contents of red blood cells

■ Exfoliatin

Exfoliatin is produced by a small proportion of *S aureus* strains. It binds to a specific cell membrane ganglioside found only in the stratum granulosum of the keratinized epidermis of the skin. There it causes intercellular splitting of the epidermis between the stratum spinosum and stratum granulosum, presumably by disruption of intercellular junctions. The toxin itself is a protease which acts on desmosomes important to adhesion between keratinocytes.

✱ Splits intraepidermal junctions

■ Staphylococcal Superantigen Toxins

The superantigens (SAgs) are a family of secreted proteins that are able to stimulate systemic effects as a result of absorption from the gastrointestinal tract after ingestion or at a site where they are produced *in vivo* by multiplying bacteria. Details of the SAg mechanism are described in Chapter 22. Although first described in the 1920s, interest in SAgs erupted during a large outbreak of what we now call staphylococcal toxic shock syndrome (TSS) in the 1980s. In the end, we not only discovered a new SAg, but that SAgs are important in staphylococcal and group A streptococcal diseases we already knew but did not completely understand. There are now more than 15 described SAgs the most important of which are the causes of staphylococcal TSS (TSST-1), staphylococcal enterotoxin diarrhea, and streptococcal TSS. An individual strain may produce one or more toxins, but less than 20% of *S aureus* strains produce any SAg. As SAgs they are strongly mitogenic for T cells and do not require proteolytic processing before binding with class II major histocompatibility complex (MHC) molecules on antigen-presenting cells. This process not only bypasses the specificity of antigen processing but results in massive cytokine release due to the ability of these SAgs to activate up to 20% of the total T-cell pool. The staphylococcal and streptococcal SAg toxins share physiochemical and biologic activity similarities with each other.

✱ Staphylococcal SAgs bind MHC II without processing

✱ SAgs cause massive cytokine release

Staphylococcal Enterotoxins

The ability of *S aureus* enterotoxins to stimulate gastrointestinal symptoms (primarily vomiting) in humans and animals has long been known. Once formed, these toxins are quite stable, retaining activity even after boiling or exposure to gastric and jejunal enzymes. In addition to their superantigen actions, they appear to act by stimulating reflexes in the abdominal viscera, which are transmitted to medullary emetic centers in the brain stem via the vagus nerve. The mechanism of the SAg action on the intestinal mucosa is unknown.

✱ Enterotoxins stable to boiling, digestive enzymes

Vomiting stimulated in brain stem

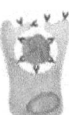

STAPHYLOCOCCAL DISEASE

In many ways, *S aureus* is the "all-time champion" of microbial pathogens. Although tuberculosis and malaria have greater global prevalence and the spread of AIDS and COVID-19 are more ominous, the ferocity of staphylococcal infections has remained constant for as long as we can tell. In Shakespeare's King Lear (1606), quoted above, Lear is not himself infected. He has just chosen two prototype staphylococcal lesions (boil, carbuncle) as the vilest of symbols to characterize his ungrateful daughters and his treatment at their hands. Today, in virtually any hospital in the world *S aureus* heads the list of pathogens isolated from the bloodstream of seriously ill patients.

EPIDEMIOLOGY

The basic human habitat of *S aureus* is the anterior nares. Ten to thirty percent of the population carry the organism at this site at any given time, and rates among hospital personnel and patients may be much higher. From the nasal site, the bacteria are shed to the exposed skin and clothing of the carrier and others with whom they are in direct contact. Spread is augmented by touching the face and, of course, nose picking. It is blocked by handwashing. Once present on the skin, even transiently, *S aureus* can gain deeper access either through skin appendages or trauma (**Figure 24–3**).

Most *S aureus* infections acquired in the community are autoinfections with strains that the subject has been carrying in the anterior nares, on the skin, or both.

> Does a physician colonized with *S aureus* need to suspend practice and/or be treated?

Community outbreaks are usually associated with poor hygiene and fomite transmission from individual to individual. Unlike many pathogenic bacteria, *S aureus* can survive periods of drying;

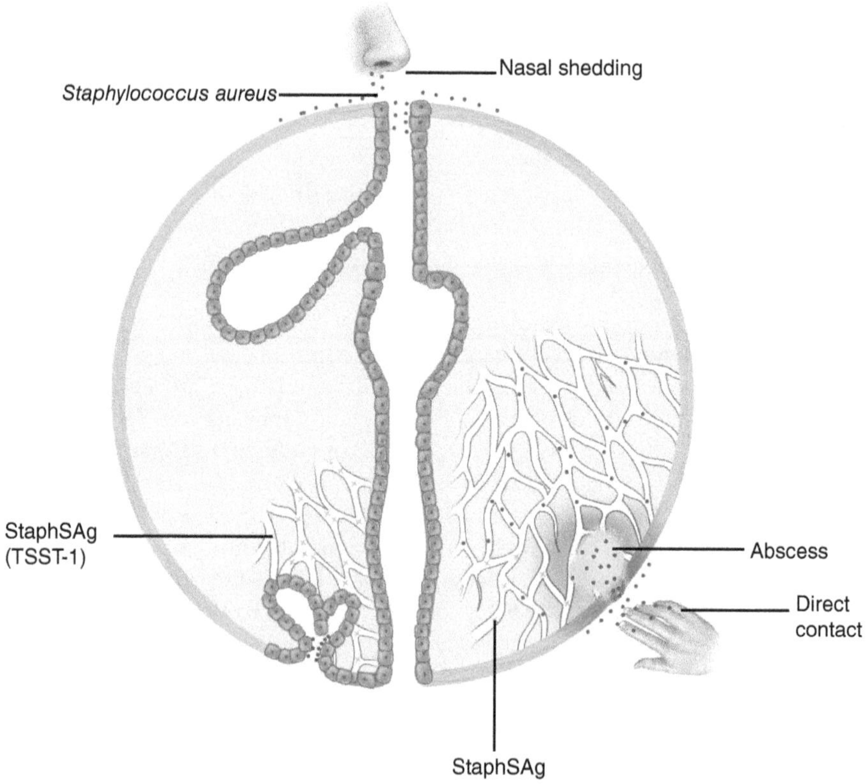

* Anterior nares colonization

* Handwashing blocks transmission

Community infections endogenous

FIGURE 24–3. **Staphylococcal disease.** The source of infection is most commonly endogenous from colonized anterior nares or by direct contact with someone carrying *Staphylococcus aureus*. An abscess (boil) is the typical lesion. In a small proportion of cases, the strain may produce a circulating exotoxin similar to the staphylococcal superantigens, which can produce toxic shock syndrome (TSS) in association with a local infection (*lower right*) or with menses (*lower left*). For details of menstrual-associated TSS, see Figure 24–8.

Think ▸▸ Apply 24-1: **No. Colonization is too common for this to be practical or an accurate measure of risk unless there is laboratory evidence fingerprinting the physician's isolate as the one causing the outbreak. This evidence could be bacteriophage typing, molecular testing, or a distinctive antimicrobial resistance profile.**

for example, recurrent skin infections can result from the use of clothing contaminated with pus from a previous infection.

Hospital outbreaks caused by a single strain of *S aureus* most commonly involve patients who have undergone surgical or other invasive procedures. The source of the outbreak may be a patient with an overt or unapparent staphylococcal infection (eg, decubitus ulcer), which is then spread directly to other patients on the hands of hospital personnel. A nasal or perineal carrier among medical, nursing, or other hospital personnel may also be the source of an outbreak, especially when carriage is heavy and numerous organisms are disseminated. The most hazardous source is a medical attendant who works despite having a staphylococcal lesion such as a boil.

Staphylococcal food poisoning is one of the most common foodborne illnesses in the world. It has been an unhappy and embarrassing sequel to innumerable group picnics and wedding receptions in which gastronomic delicacies have been exposed to temperatures that allow bacterial multiplication. Characteristically, the food is moist and rich (eg, red meat, poultry, creamy dishes). The food becomes contaminated by a preparer who is a nasal carrier or has a staphylococcal lesion. If the food is left unrefrigerated for hours between preparation and serving, the staphylococci are able to multiply and produce enterotoxin in the food. Because of the heat resistance of the toxin, toxicity persists even if the food is subsequently cooked before eating.

S aureus survives drying

Spread on hands of medical personnel

＊ Outbreaks involve nasal carrier or worker with lesion

＊ Enterotoxin produced in rich foods before ingestion

PATHOGENESIS

◾ Primary Infection

A boil (furuncle) is an abscess and a prototype for the purulent lesions produced by many other bacteria. The initial stages of attachment by *S aureus* are mediated by a number of surface proteins, which bind to elements on the host cell to their surface. Proteins that bind to the glycoprotein fibronectin that is ubiquitous on mucosal surfaces are of particular importance in the early stages of infection. The staphylococcal fibronectin-binding proteins (FnBPs) mediate adhesion to and perhaps invasion of mammalian cells. This allows *S aureus* to persist and to produce α-Hemolysin and other cytolysins, which injure the cell (**Figure 24–4**). As the lesions become

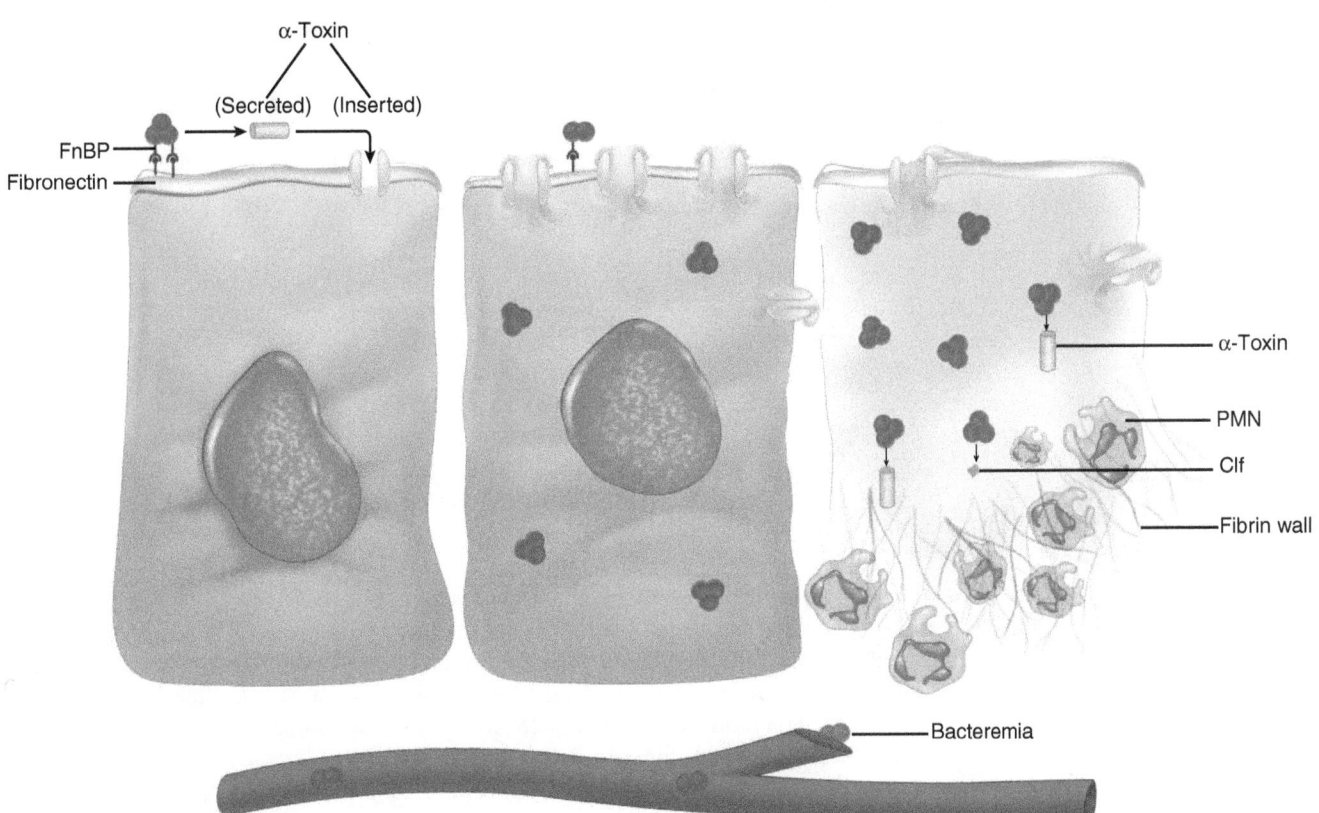

FIGURE 24–4. Staphylococcal disease cellular view. Initial attachment to fibronectin is mediated by fibronectin-binding proteins, and the major injury is caused by the pore-forming α-toxin. Cells are destroyed by leaking their cytosol. The α-toxin also inserts into the polymorphonuclear neutrophils. Resistance to phagocytosis and the formation of a wall are aided by fibrinogen-binding Clf.

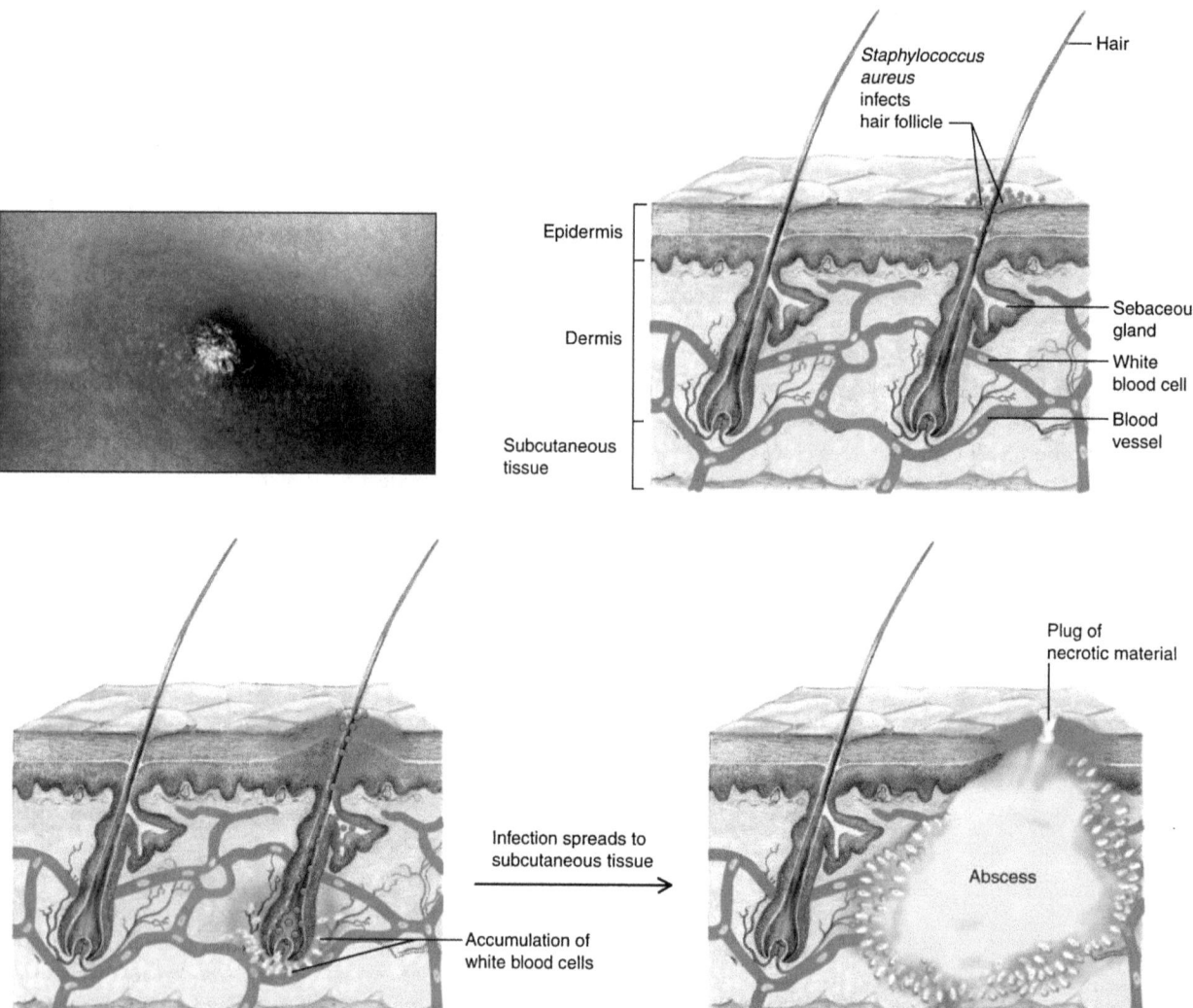

FIGURE 24–5. **Furuncle (boil).** Note the focal nature of the lesion. This one appears about to "point" and drain its walled-off pus externally. (Reproduced with permission from Nester EW, Anderson DG, Roberts CE Jr, et al: *Microbiology: A Human Perspective*, 6th ed. New York, NY: McGraw Hill; 2008.)

✳ FnBPs bind cell surface fibronectin

✳ Coagulase, Clf, protein A, compromise defenses

✳ α-Hemolysin destroys cells, platelets

destructive and spread below the surface, other proteins that bind to collagen and other elements of the extracellular matrix may play a role. At this stage, actions of coagulase and Clfs on fibrinogen-binding, and the antiphagocytic effect of protein A binding to IgG, all combine to limit the effectiveness of host phagocytes. The continued production of α-Hemolysin destroys keratinocytes, other cells, and platelets thus compromising repair and allowing the lesion to expand. The inflammatory cells, fibrin, and other tissue components form a wall, which becomes the painfully familiar boil (**Figure 24–5**). A carbuncle (**Figure 24–6**) is an extension of this process in which, rather than discharging at the surface, the process forms multiple compartments.

Exotoxins add to primary disease

■ Toxin-mediated Disease

If the strain of *S aureus* causing any of the effects described above also produces one or more of the exotoxins, those actions are added to those of the primary infection. The primary infection serves as a site for absorption of the toxin and need not be extensive or even clinically apparent for the toxic action to occur. In staphylococcal food poisoning, there is no infection at all. The contaminating bacteria produce SAg toxin in the food, which can initiate its enterotoxic action on the intestine within hours of its ingestion.

✳ Exfoliative toxin causes blisters or scalded skin syndrome

The *in vivo* production of exfoliative toxin takes at least a few days and may exert its effect locally or systemically. Toxin absorbed at the infection site reaches its infant stratum granulosum binding site through the circulation causing widespread desquamation by its action on the stratum granulosum of the epidermis as in the staphylococcal scalded skin syndrome (**Figure 24–7A** and **B**). The molecular target of the toxin is a transmembrane desmosomal glycoprotein which

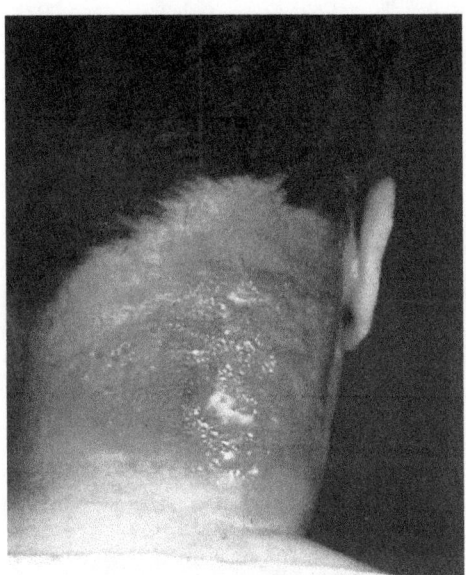

FIGURE 24-6. **Staphylococcal carbuncle.** Multiple abscesses have coalesced to form this angry cellulitis with draining sinuses. (Reproduced with permission from Connor DH, Chandler FW, Schwartz DQ, et al: *Pathology of Infectious Diseases.* Stamford CT: Appleton & Lange; 1997.)

Boils back of neck/back shaving and waxing can carry staph inwards. Capsule inside must get peeled out.

mediates interkeratinocyte adhesion. In older children, exfoliative toxin-producing strains may also directly cause a localized blister-like lesion called **bullous impetigo** at the site of infection.

In staphylococcal TSS, TSST-1 is produced during the course of a staphylococcal infection with systemic disease as a result of absorption of toxin from the local site. In comparison with other SAgs, TSST-1 is more readily adsorbed across mucosal membranes. Menstruation-associated TSS requires a combination of improbable events. At any one time, less than 15% of women carry *S aureus* in their vaginal flora, and less than 20% of these have the potential to produce TSST-1. During menstruation, the relatively high protein level and pH in the vagina favor accelerated growth of these staphylococci. In the presence of such a strain, the combination of menstruation and the composition of high-absorbency tampons provide the relatively neutral pH (6.5-8) and ionic conditions (elevated pCO_2 and pO_2) that enhance both the growth of the staphylococci and the production of TSST-1. Toxin absorbed from the vagina can then circulate to produce the multiple effects of massive superantigen-mediated cytokine release (**Figure 24–8**).

＊ TSST-1-producing strain colonizes vagina

＊ Menstruation, tampons enhance local toxin production

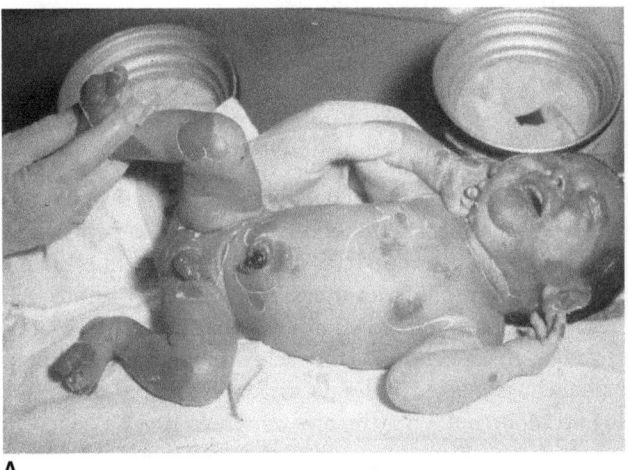

A

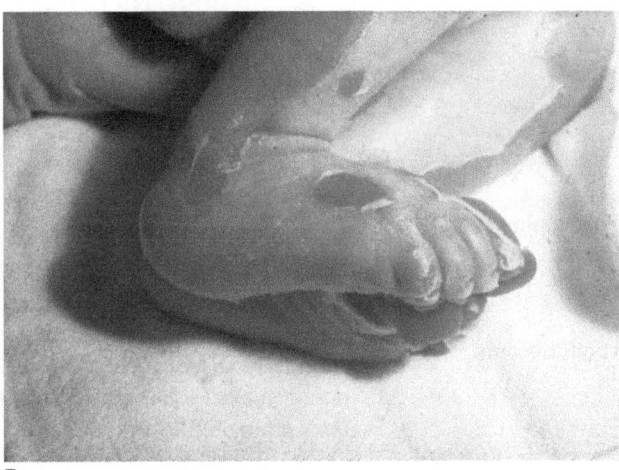

B

FIGURE 24-7. **Staphylococcal scalded skin syndrome in a neonate. A.** This infant has a small focal staphylococcal breast abscess and looks as if he has been sunburned or dipped in boiling water. **B.** Note the peeling of the superficial layers of the skin as a result of the action of circulating exfoliatin.

FIGURE 24–8. **Pathogenesis of staphylococcal toxic shock syndrome. A.** The vagina is colonized with normal flora and a strain of *Staphylococcus aureus* containing the staphylococcal superantigen toxin (SAg) gene. **B.** The conditions with tampon usage facilitate growth of the *S aureus* and toxic shock syndrome toxin (TSST-1) SAg production. **C.** The toxin is absorbed from the vagina and circulates. The systemic effects may be due to the direct effect of the toxin or via cytokines released by the superantigen mechanism. The toxin is shown binding directly with the Vβ portion of the T-cell receptor and the class II major histocompatibility complex (MHC) receptor. This Vβ stimulation signals the production of cytokines such as interleukin-1 (IL-1) and tumor necrosis factor (TNF).

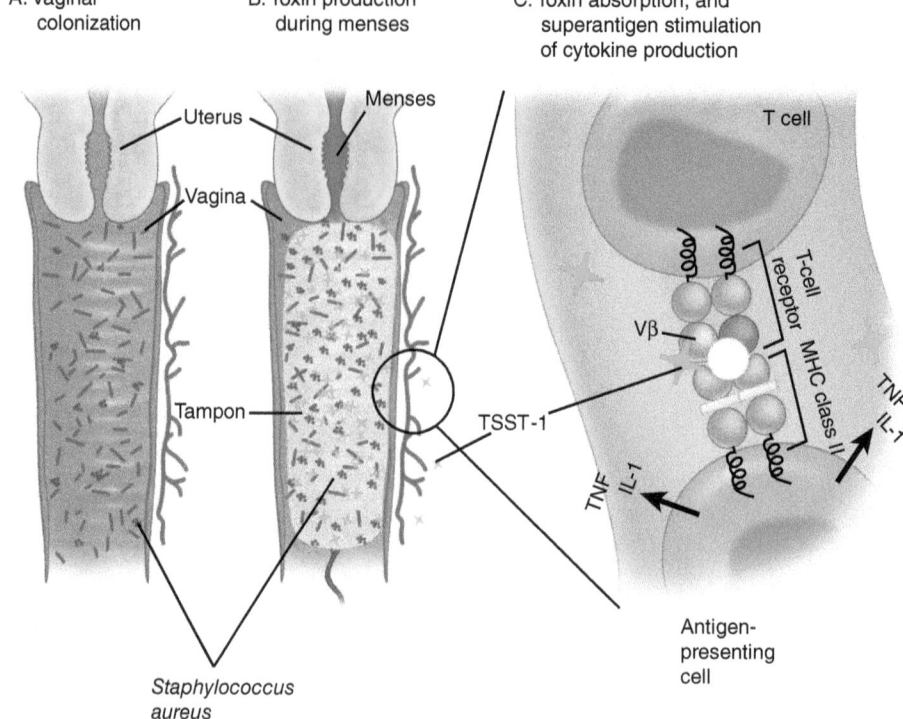

A. Vaginal colonization
B. Toxin production during menses
C. Toxin absorption, and superantigen stimulation of cytokine production

Uterus
Menses
Vagina
T cell
T-cell receptor
MHC class II
Vβ
TNF
IL-1
Tampon
TSST-1
TNF
IL-1
Staphylococcus aureus
Antigen-presenting cell

Nonmenstrual TSS cases may have any SAg strain

Some cases of full-blown staphylococcal TSS are associated with strains that do not produce TSST-1. This is particularly true of nonmenstrual cases. SAgs other than TSST-1 have been detected in these strains and have been shown to produce experimental toxic shock. TSS may be the result of *in vivo* production of a variety of SAgs, with TSST-1 simply the most common offender. The mechanisms by which the pyrogenic exotoxins produce the multiple renal, cutaneous, intestinal, and cardiovascular manifestations of TSS are not known.

IMMUNITY

Relapsing infections show little immunity

The natural history of staphylococcal infections indicates that immunity is of short duration and is incomplete. Chronic furunculosis, for example, can recur over many years. The relative roles of humoral and cellular immune mechanisms are uncertain, and attempts to induce immunity artificially with various staphylococcal products have been disappointing at best.

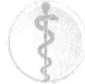 **STAPHYLOCOCCAL INFECTIONS: CLINICAL ASPECTS**

MANIFESTATIONS: PRIMARY INFECTION

◾ Furuncle and Carbuncle

Focal lesions drain spontaneously

✳ Boils develop in hair follicles

Multiple boils become carbuncle

The furuncle or boil (Figure 24–5) is a superficial skin infection that typically develops in a hair follicle, sebaceous gland, or sweat gland. Blockage of the gland duct with inspissation of its contents causes predisposition to infection. Furunculosis is often a complication of acne vulgaris. Infection at the base of the eyelash gives rise to the common stye. The infected patient is often a carrier of the offending *Staphylococcus,* usually in the anterior nares. The course of the infection is usually benign, and the infection resolves upon spontaneous drainage of pus. No surgical or antimicrobial treatment is needed. Infection can spread from a furuncle with the development of one or more abscesses in adjacent subcutaneous tissues. This lesion, known as a carbuncle, occurs most often on the back of the neck (Figure 24–6), but it may involve other skin sites.

◾ Chronic Furunculosis

Some individuals are subject to chronic furunculosis, in which repeated attacks of boils are caused by the same strain of *S aureus*. There is little, if any, evidence of acquired immunity to the disease.

Chronic staphylococcal disease may be associated with factors that depress host immunity, especially in patients with diabetes or congenital defects of polymorphonuclear leukocyte function.

■ Impetigo

S aureus has been long known as a secondary invader in group A streptococcal pustular impetigo (see Chapter 25), but is increasingly seen producing the skin pustules of impetigo on its own. Strains of *S aureus* that produce exfoliatin may cause a characteristic form called **bullous impetigo,** characterized by blisters containing many staphylococci in the superficial layers of the skin.

❋ Produces pustular or bullous impetigo

■ Deep Lesions

S aureus can cause a wide variety of infections of deep tissues by bacteremic spread from a skin lesion that may be unnoticed. These include infections of bones, joints, deep organs, and soft tissues, including surgical wounds. *S aureus* is a common cause of all forms of osteomyelitis and is responsible for a substantial majority of the form of this disease erupting in the long bones of children. Staphylococcal pneumonia is typically secondary to some other insult to the lung, such as influenza, aspiration, or pulmonary edema. A new necrotizing pneumonia has been associated with strains producing the PVL leukocidin. At deep sites, the organism has the same tendency to produce localized, destructive abscesses as it does in the skin. All too often the containment is less effective, and spread with multiple metastatic lesions occurs. Bacteremia and endocarditis can develop. All are serious infections that constitute acute medical emergencies. In all these situations, diabetes, leukocyte defects, or general reduction of host defenses by alcoholism, malignancy, old age, or steroid or cytotoxic therapy can be predisposing factors. Severe *S aureus* infections, including endocarditis, are particularly common in drug abusers using injection methods.

❋ Acute osteomyelitis caused by *S aureus*

Pneumonia, deep tissue lesions highly destructive

Bacteremic spread, endocarditis in drug abusers

MANIFESTATIONS CAUSED BY STAPHYLOCOCCAL TOXINS

■ Scalded Skin Syndrome

Staphylococcal scalded skin syndrome results from the production of exfoliatin in a staphylococcal lesion, which can be minor (eg, conjunctivitis). Erythema and intraepidermal desquamation take place at remote sites from which *S aureus* cannot be isolated (Figure 24–7). The disease is most common in neonates and children less than 5 years of age. The face, axilla, and groin tend to be affected first, but the erythema, bullous formation, and subsequent desquamation of epithelial sheets, can spread to all parts of the body. The disease occasionally occurs in adults, particularly those who are immunocompromised.

Desquamation in neonates caused by exfoliatin-producing strains

■ Toxic Shock Syndrome

TSS was first described in children but came to public attention during the 1980s outbreaks involving hundreds of cases were in young women using intravaginal tampons. The disease is characterized by high fever, vomiting, diarrhea, sore throat, and muscle pain developing within 2 days of the beginning or end of menses. Within 48 hours, it may progress to severe shock with evidence of renal and hepatic damage. A skin rash may develop, later followed by desquamation at a deeper level than in scalded skin syndrome. Blood cultures are usually negative. Nonmenstrual TSS may occur at virtually any body site infected with *S aureus* including surgical wounds. SAgs other than TSST-1 are much more likely to be involved than in the menstrual/tampon-associated cases.

❋ Fever, vomiting, diarrhea, muscle pain early findings

❋ Shock, renal, and hepatic injury may follow

■ Staphylococcal Food Poisoning

Ingestion of staphylococcal enterotoxin-contaminated food results in acute vomiting and diarrhea within 1 to 5 hours. There is prostration, but usually no fever. Recovery is rapid, except sometimes in the elderly and in those with another disease.

Vomiting prominent without fever

DIAGNOSIS

Laboratory procedures to assist in the diagnosis of staphylococcal infections are quite simple. Most acute, untreated lesions contain numerous polymorphonuclear leukocytes and large numbers of Gram-positive cocci in clusters. Staphylococci grow overnight on blood agar incubated aerobically. Catalase and coagulase tests performed directly from colonies on petri dishes are both rapid and simple particularly in separating the more virulent *S aureus* isolates from coagulase-negative isolates. Alternatives designed to correlate with the classical coagulase test include agglutination kits which detect specific *S aureus* antigens. Molecular methods are increasingly used as they become more rapid, less expensive, and offer the prospect of additional information such as the presence of drug-resistance determinants. Routine antibiotic susceptibility tests are indicated because of the emerging resistance to multiple antimicrobials, particularly methicillin-resistant *S aureus* (MRSA). Deep staphylococcal infections such as osteomyelitis and deep abscesses present special diagnostic problems when the lesion cannot be directly aspirated or surgically sampled. Blood cultures are usually positive in conditions such as acute staphylococcal arthritis, osteomyelitis, and endocarditis, but less often in localized infections such as deep abscesses and chronic bone infections.

TREATMENT

Most boils and superficial staphylococcal abscesses resolve spontaneously without antimicrobial therapy. Those that are more extensive, deeper, or in vital organs require a combination of surgical drainage and antimicrobials for optimal outcome. Since the introduction of penicillin the antimicrobial side of this equation has resembled an arms race between the ability of *S aureus* to develop resistance and the ability of drug companies to overcome it with a new antibiotic.

STAPHYLOCOCCAL RESISTANCE

When penicillin was introduced to the general public after World War II, virtually all strains of *S aureus* were highly susceptible due to its disruption of cell wall peptidoglycan synthesis. Since then, the selection of preexisting strains containing a plasmid coding for a penicillinase have compromised its effectiveness. This enzyme opens the β-lactam ring, making the drug unable to bind with its target. The vast majority of clinical isolates are now penicillin resistant. This resistance was overcome by the development of methicillin whose β-lactam ring could not be broken by penicillinase.

Alterations in the β-lactam target, the peptidoglycan transpeptidases (often called penicillin-binding proteins, or PBPs), are the basis for resistance to methicillin. These MRSA strains are also resistant to the newer penicillinase-resistant penicillins such as oxacillin and nafcillin which are now preferred over methicillin. The most common genetic mechanism is the acquisition of a gene (*mecA*) coding for a new bacterial transpeptidase (PBP 2a), which has reduced affinity for β-lactam antibiotics, but is still able to carry out its enzymatic function of cross-linking peptidoglycan.

MRSA

The incidence of MRSA has great geographic variation but rates of 50% or higher are now common.

 Are MRSA strains more virulent than other *S aureus*?

Laboratory susceptibility tests are performed under technical conditions that facilitate detection of what may be a small resistant subpopulation, and the results extrapolated to other relevant agents. For example, oxacillin resistance is considered proof of resistance to nafcillin and all cephalosporins. Methods for direct detection of the *mecA* gene have been developed but face the interpretive dilemma that the gene may be present in phenotypically susceptible isolates. Recent evidence shows that such strains may revert to MRSA during treatment and thus should be considered resistant. Vancomycin is often used to treat serious infections with MRSA. The recent emergence of *S aureus* with decreased susceptibility to vancomycin is still uncommon but of great concern.

MRSA originally associated primarily with hospitals has increasingly emerged in the community (CA-MRSA). At least one clone of CA-MRSA emerging in the United States (USA300) has distinctive pathogenic features beyond methicillin resistance. These strains produce a particularly aggressive necrotizing pneumonia as well as skin and soft tissue infections. This may be due to the almost universal presence of the PVL leucocidin in these *S aureus* isolates.

> Think ▸▸ Apply 24-2: **Virulence and resistance are separate properties unlinked by genetics or pathogenic function. Resistance does give the strain an epidemiologic advantage in spreading but does not enhance disease potential unless some additional virulence factor-like PVL is present.**

Margin notes

* Gram stain, culture primary diagnostic methods

Aspirates, blood cultures for deep infections

Superficial lesions resolve spontaneously

Penicillinase opens the β-lactam ring

MRSAs produce new PBP unaffected by β-lactams

MRSA rates variable but increasing

MRSA testing may include gene detection

Vancomycin use for MRSA threatened

CA-MRSAs produce PVL

ANTIMICROBIAL SELECTION

Although penicillin G is still effective for susceptible strains, it has disappeared from empiric therapy consideration due to the high rate of β-lactamase production as have the penicillinase-resistant penicillins (nafcillin, oxacillin) and cephalosporins (cefazolin, cephalexin) due to the increasing prevalence of MRSA. Once susceptibility testing has been completed the drug selection depends on (1) the presence of MRSA, (2) the severity of the infection, and (3) any patient history of hypersensitivity to β-lactams. The main MRSA alternatives are vancomycin and daptomycin for deep-seated infections (endocarditis, osteomyelitis, bacteremia, pneumonia) with macrolides and tetracyclines restricted to more superficial skin and soft tissue infections.

MRSA, severity, hypersensitivity determine drug selection

PREVENTION

In patients subject to recurrent infection such as chronic furunculosis, preventive measures are aimed at controlling reinfection and, if possible, eliminating the carrier state. Clothes and bedding that may cause reinfection should be dry-cleaned or washed at a sufficiently high temperature (70°C or higher) to destroy staphylococci. In adults, the use of chlorhexidine or hexachlorophene soaps in showering and washing increases the bactericidal activity of the skin. In such individuals, or persons found to be a source of an outbreak, anterior nasal carriage can be reduced and often eliminated by the combination of nasal creams containing topical antimicrobials (eg, mupirocin, neomycin, and bacitracin) and oral therapy with antimicrobials that are concentrated within phagocytes and nasal secretions (eg, rifampin or ciprofloxacin).

Antistaphylococcal soaps block infection

Elimination of nasal carriage difficult

Chemoprophylaxis is effective in surgical procedures such as hip and cardiac valve replacements, in which infection with staphylococci can have devastating consequences. Oxacillin, a cephalosporin, or vancomycin given during and shortly after surgery may reduce the chance for intraoperative infection while minimizing the risk for superinfection associated with longer periods of antibiotic administration.

Chemoprophylaxis during high-risk surgery is effective

COAGULASE-NEGATIVE STAPHYLOCOCCI

In medical practice, the less than 20 species other than *S aureus* that have been isolated from human infections are typically lumped together by a negative characteristic—failure to produce coagulase. These coagulase-negative staphylococci (CoNS) also do not produce α-toxin, exfoliatin, or any of the SAg toxins. They have been shown to have surface adhesins and the ability to produce extracellular polysaccharide biofilms. By far the most common CoNS species isolated from human infections is *S epidermidis*, and *Staphylococcus saprophyticus* is a significant cause of urinary tract infections. Clinical laboratories rarely speciate CoNS isolates, although a simple test (novobiocin resistance) is often used to separate *S saprophyticus* from other urinary isolates.

CoNS DISEASE

S epidermidis and many other species of CoNS are normal commensals of the skin, anterior nares, and ear canals of humans. Their large numbers and ubiquitous distribution result in frequent contamination of specimens collected from or through the skin. In the past, they were rarely the cause of aggressive infections, but with the increasing use of implanted catheters and prosthetic devices, they have emerged as important agents of hospital-acquired infections. Immunosuppressed or neutropenic patients and premature infants have been particularly affected. Other species associated with this kind of disease are *Staphylococcus lugdunensis* and *Staphylococcus haemolyticus* (Table 24-1).

❋ **Common colonizers of the skin**

❋ **Colonize implanted medical devices**

S epidermidis may contaminate prosthetic devices during implantation, seed the device during a subsequent bacteremia, or gain access to the lumina of shunts and catheters when they are temporarily disconnected or manipulated. The outcome of the bacterial contamination is determined by the ability of the microbe to attach to the surface of the foreign body and to multiply there. Central to this process is the ability of some strains to form a viscous extracellular polysaccharide **biofilm.** The biofilm formation begins with attachment to one or more components commonly found in submucosal and deep tissues such as fibrinogen, fibronectin, collagen, and elastin. There is also evidence that many *S epidermidis* strains can bind directly to the plastics increasing found in the same areas due to implantation of medical devices. In this setting production of polysaccharide together with the hydrophobic nature of the synthetic polymers used in medical devices enhances attachment both to the plastic and between CoNS cells. As it expands, this biofilm

***S epidermidis* attaches to medical devices**

❋ **Biofilm mediates attachment to plastics, between CoNS cells**

FIGURE 24-9. Coagulase-negative staphylococcal biofilm. A. *Staphylococcus epidermidis* cocci are shown attached to the surface of a plastic catheter and are starting to produce extracellular polysaccharide biofilm. **B.** After 48 hours, the bacteria are fully embedded in the slime glycocalyx. (Reproduced with permission from Connor DH, Chandler FW, Schwartz DQ, et al: *Pathology of Infectious Diseases.* Stamford CT: Appleton & Lange; 1997.)

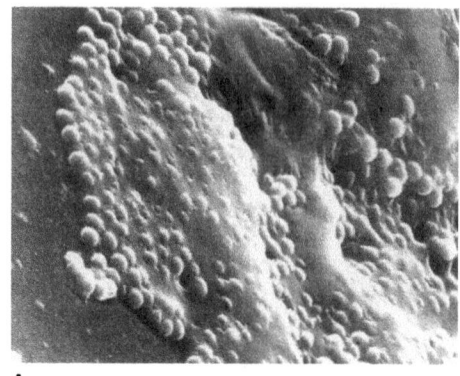

A

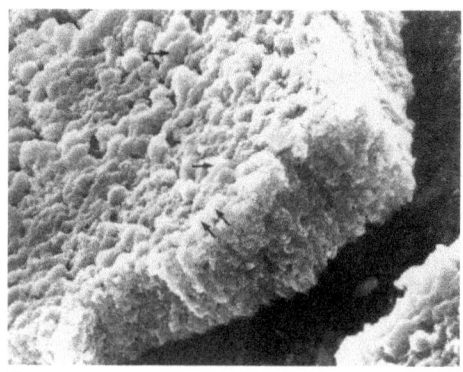

B

provides additional adhesion, encases the entire bacterial population (**Figure 24-9**), and serves as a barrier to antimicrobial agents and host defense mechanisms.

The abovementioned circumstances are found almost exclusively in hospitals and other medical facilities. The most common device colonized is the intravenous catheter, but the same mechanisms apply to any implanted device such as cerebrospinal fluid shunts and artificial heart valves. The ensuing disease is typically low grade with little more than a slowly advancing fever to arouse suspicion. *S aureus* can also produce biofilms, and although a less frequent colonizer of medical devices, it is likely to produce a more aggressive course and metastatic infections. Removal of the contaminated device is the only sure way to avoid these complications.

Catheters, shunts, artificial valves become colonized

The biology of *S saprophyticus* infection is entirely different. Its usual habitat is the gastrointestinal tract, and from that location the organism gains access to the urinary tract. Among sexually active women, *S saprophyticus* is second only to *Escherichia coli* as a cause of acute urinary tract infection. It is rarely found in men. The infection process is aided by surface adhesins to uroepithelial cells and factors aiding survival in urine like the production of a urease. Thus, although other CoNS are causes of infection among compromised patients in hospitals, *S saprophyticus* produces community-acquired infection in women who are otherwise healthy.

❋ *S saprophyticus* causes urinary infections in young women

Most CoNS now encountered are resistant to penicillin, and many are also methicillin-resistant. Resistance to multiple antimicrobials usually active against Gram-positive cocci, including vancomycin, is more common than with *S aureus*. Eradication of CoNS from prosthetic devices and associated tissues with chemotherapy alone is very difficult unless the device is also removed.

Resistance to multiple antimicrobials common

KEY CONCLUSIONS

- *Staphylococcus aureus* (coagulase positive) is by far the most virulent species, launching invasive disease from colonization of the anterior nares.
- Fibronectin-binding proteins mediate surface attachment to skin and mucosal surfaces.
- Coagulase, clumping factor, and protein A disrupt the innate phagocyte response.
- Local production of pore-forming α-toxin destroys cells leading to impetigo, abscesses, pneumonia, osteomyelitis, bacteremia, and endocarditis.
- Exfoliatin production causes blister-like bullous impetigo or, when absorbed by infants, staphylococcal-scalded skin syndrome.
- Strains which produce staphylococcal superantigen toxins (SAgs) cause toxic shock syndrome when absorbed from the vaginal or any other infection.
- SAgs bind directly to the Vβ portion of the T-cell receptors stimulating massive cytokine release.
- Ingestion of preformed SAg enterotoxin causes diarrhea and vomiting within a few hours.
- *S aureus* strains resistant to methicillin (MRSA) have acquired genes for peptidoglycan transpeptidases that do not bind to penicillins.
- CoNS lack the above toxins and cause low-grade disease by producing biofilms adherent to indwelling catheters and other foreign bodies.
- *Staphylococcus saprophyticus* colonizes the intestine and causes urinary tract infections in young women.

Aftermath of a Bicycle Fall

A 14-year-old boy presented with a 3-day history of vomiting, diarrhea, sore throat, headache, weakness, and fever. His temperature was 39.9°C. He had pharyngeal inflammation, and his blood pressure was 60/0 mm Hg while supine and unobtainable when sitting. Initial laboratory findings included white blood cell (WBC) count of 13,600L/mL with a pronounced left shift (ie, many immature forms), blood urea nitrogen (BUN) of 24 mg/dL (normal up to 15 mg/dL), and abnormal urinalysis, with 20 to 30 WBCs and 8 to 10 red blood cells (RBC) per high-power field.

He was treated with large volumes of intravenous fluids and with penicillin; his blood pressure rose, but he had multiple episodes of disorientation, and diffuse erythroderma developed. On admission, a small crusted wound had been noticed on the dorsum of his left foot (the result of a bicycle injury 1 week earlier); 45 hours later the wound became red, warm, and pustular, and a left femoral lymph node became tender and enlarged. A culture of the pustule grew *S aureus* coagulase-positive resistant to penicillin. Several cultures of blood and a throat swab taken before antibiotic therapy was started had been negative. He improved with cephalexin therapy. He had extensive desquamation of the skin of the palms and soles 2 weeks after discharge.

QUESTIONS

1. Which one of the following is most responsible for the nature of the lesion on this boy's foot?
   A. Coagulase
   B. Catalase
   C. Superantigen toxin (StaphSAg)
   D. Exfoliatin
   E. α-Toxin

2. The boy's hypotension and elevated BUN are most probably due to the action of:
   A. α-Toxin
   B. Cytokines
   C. Peptidoglycan
   D. Catalase
   E. Exfoliatin

3. The desquamation of the skin is most probably due to the action of:
   A. Exfoliatin
   B. Coagulase
   C. Superantigen toxin
   D. Penicillin
   E. Fibronectin binding protein

4. The blood culture was negative. What is the best explanation for this?
   A. The penicillin may have caused a false-negative culture.
   B. There must have been a problem with the blood collection.
   C. There must have been an error in the laboratory.
   D. This is typical in staphylococcal toxic shock syndrome. Only the superantigen toxin needs to circulate.

ANSWERS

1. (E)
2. (B)
3. (C)
4. (D)

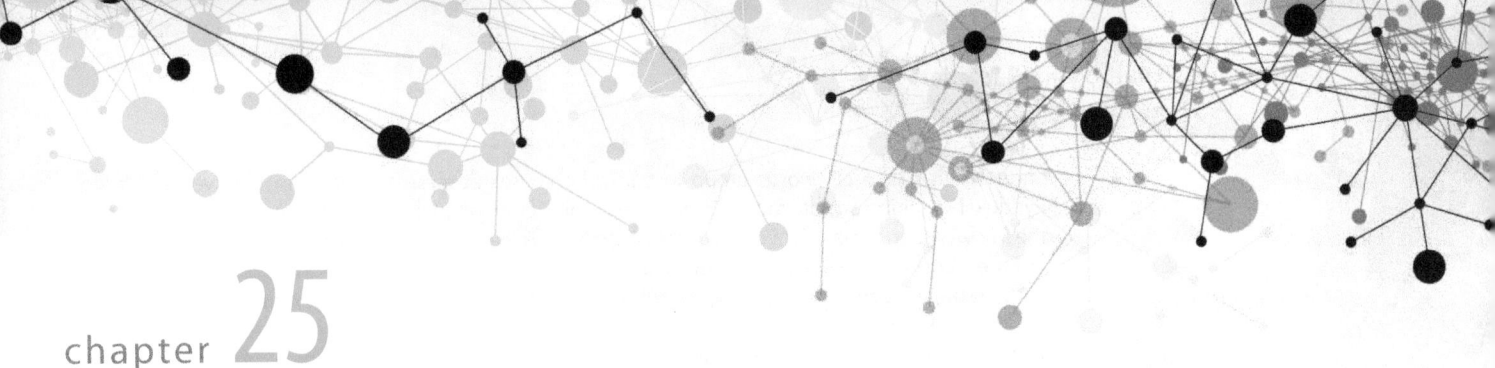

chapter 25

Streptococci and Enterococci

Streptococcus pyogenes (Group A) • *Streptococcus agalactiae* (Group B) • *Streptococcus pneumoniae*

Viridans group streptococci • Enterococci

> *Scarlet fever awes me, and is above my aim. I leave it to the professional and graduated homicides.*
>
> —Sydney Smith, 1833

OVERVIEW

Members of the genus *Streptococcus* and enterococci are all Gram-positive cocci that grow in pairs or short to long chains (**Figure 25–1**) in contrast to the clusters seen with staphylococci. Furthermore, streptococci and enterococci are catalase-negative, whereas staphylococci are catalase-positive. Streptococci and enterococci are classified principally based on their patterns of hemolysis. Streptococci showing β-hemolysis (**Figure 25–2**) are grouped according to the carbohydrate antigens extracted from their cell walls. Groups A and B are the leading pyogenic pathogens of the streptococci having β-hemolysis and cause diverse clinical syndromes. Group A streptococci are the cause of "strep throat," an acute inflammation of the pharynx and tonsils that includes fever and painful swallowing. Skin and soft tissue infections range from the tiny skin pustules called impetigo to a severe toxic and invasive disease that can be fatal in a matter of days. In addition to acute infections, group A streptococci are responsible for inflammatory diseases that are not direct infections but result from an immune response to streptococcal antigens that cause injury to host tissues. Acute rheumatic fever (ARF) is a clinical entity characterized by prolonged febrile inflammation of connective tissues, which can recur after each subsequent attack of streptococcal pharyngitis. Repeated episodes cause permanent scarring of the heart valves. Acute glomerulonephritis is an insidious disease with hypertension, hematuria, proteinuria, and edema due to inflammation of the renal glomerulus.

Group B streptococci (GBS) are harbored in the human gut but may colonize the urethra and vagina. If present in mothers at the time of parturition, their newborns are at risk for severe invasive disease. Insidious initially with fever, lethargy, poor feeding, and respiratory distress, the etiologic diagnosis is disclosed only by isolation of GBS from blood or cerebrospinal fluid.

The α-hemolytic streptococci include *Streptococcus pneumoniae* and the viridans group streptococci. The most common form of infection with *S pneumoniae* is pneumonia, which begins with fever and a shaking chill followed by signs that localize the disease to the lung. These include difficulty breathing and cough with production of purulent sputum, sometimes containing blood. The pneumonia typically fills part or all of a lobe of the lung with inflammatory cells, and the bacteria may spread to the bloodstream and thus to other organs. The most important of the latter is the central nervous system, where seeding with pneumococci leads to acute purulent meningitis. Pneumococci are also a leading cause of otitis media in the early childhood.

Viridans group streptococci are a heterogeneous group of α-hemolytic streptococci that usually are commensal flora of the pharynx and gut but may cause invasive disease such as abscesses or bacterial

(Continued)

endocarditis. The *S anginosus* group in particular causes abscesses, notably in the liver and brain. Pyridoxal-requiring streptococci (*Granulicatella* and *Abiotrophia*) are prone to cause endocarditis as is the *S bovis* group, especially *S gallilyticus* spp. *gallilyticus* that is also highly associated with colon cancer.

Enterococci are usually nonhemolytic (γ) and mostly cause infection in hospitalized patients with trauma, abdominal surgery, or compromised defenses. The primary sites are the urinary tract and soft tissue sites adjacent to the intestinal flora where enterococcal species are resident. The infections themselves are often low grade and have no unique clinical features. A crucial exception is bacteremia caused by *Enterococcus faecalis,* which is an important cause of bacterial endocarditis.

Bacteria of the genus *Streptococcus* are Gram-positive cocci typically arranged in chains of varying length. The genus includes three of the most important pathogens of humans. The group A streptococcus (*S pyogenes*) is the cause of "strep throat," which can lead to scarlet fever, rheumatic fever, and rheumatic heart disease. The ability of some hypervirulent strains of *S pyogenes* to cause catastrophic deep tissue infections led British tabloids to apply the gory label "flesh-eating bacteria." The group B streptococcus (*S agalactiae*) is an important but preventable cause of sepsis in newborns and the pneumococcus (*S pneumoniae*) a leading cause of both pneumonia and meningitis in persons of all ages. Although usually harmless members of the oropharyngeal and gastrointestinal flora, some viridans group streptococci can cause pyogenic infections and others subacute bacterial endocarditis. Similarly, the normally gut dwelling enterococci are an increasingly problematic cause of healthcare-associated infections.

● STREPTOCOCCI

GROUP CHARACTERISTICS

Streptococci stain readily with common dyes, demonstrating that coccal cells are generally smaller and more ovoid in shape than staphylococci. They are usually arranged in chains with oval cells touching end to end, because they divide in one plane and tend to remain attached (Figure 25–1). Length may vary from a single pair to continuous chains of over 30 cells, depending on the species and growth conditions. Medically important streptococci are not acid-fast, do not form spores, and are nonmotile. Some members form capsules composed of polysaccharide complexes or hyaluronic acid.

✳ Oval cells arranged in chains end to end

Streptococci grow best in enriched media under aerobic or anaerobic conditions (facultative). Sheep blood agar is preferred because it satisfies the growth requirements and also serves as an

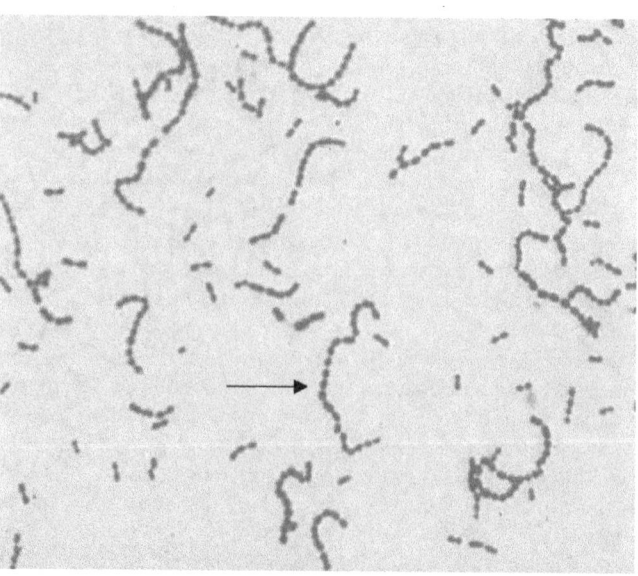

FIGURE 25–1. Group A streptococcus (GAS) Gram stain. Note the oval cocci chaining end-to-end (arrow). (Used with permission from Professor Shirley Lowe, University of California, San Francisco School of Medicine.)

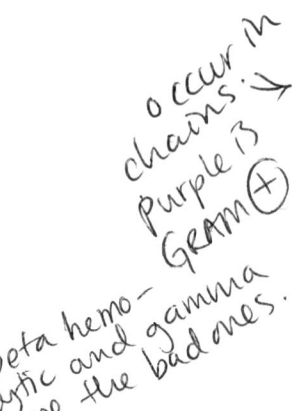

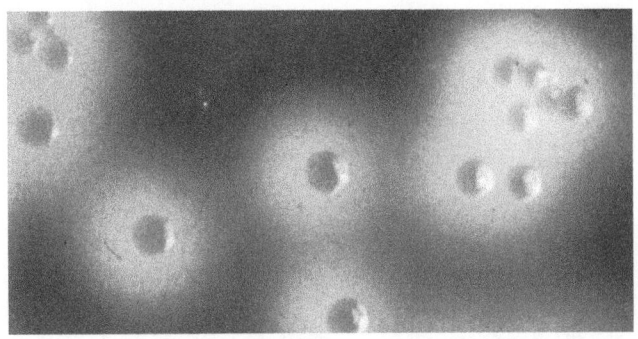

FIGURE 25–2. β-Hemolysis on sheep blood agar plate. Colonies of group A streptococci (GAS) on sheep blood agar plates are surrounded by a zone of complete clearing of the RBCs suspended in the agar. (Reproduced with permission from Nester EW, Anderson DG, Roberts CE Jr, et al: *Microbiology: A Human Perspective,* 6th ed. New York, NY: McGraw Hill; 2008.)

indicator for patterns of hemolysis. The colonies are small, ranging from pinpoint size to 2 mm in diameter, and they may be surrounded by a zone where the erythrocytes suspended in agar have been hemolyzed. When the zone is clear, this state is called **β-hemolysis** (Figure 25–2). When the zone is hazy with a green discoloration of the agar, it is called **α-hemolysis.** Brown discoloration around a colony is termed paradoxically **γ-hemolysis** (nonhemolytic). Streptococci are metabolically active, attacking a variety of carbohydrates, proteins, and amino acids. Glucose fermentation yields mostly lactic acid. In contrast to staphylococci, streptococci are catalase-negative.

* β-Hemolysis is clear

* α-Hemolysis shows greening of blood agar

* Catalase test negative

CLASSIFICATION

At the turn of the 20th century, a classification based on hemolysis and biochemical tests was sufficient to associate some streptococcal species with infections in humans and animals. Rebecca Lancefield, who demonstrated carbohydrate antigens in cell wall extracts of the β-hemolytic streptococci, put this taxonomy on a sounder basis. Her studies formed a classification by serogroups (eg, A, B, C, D, F, and G), each of which is generally correlated with one of the previously established species. Later it was discovered that some nonhemolytic streptococci had the same cell wall antigens. Over the years, it has become clear that possession of one of the Lancefield antigens defines a particularly virulent segment of the streptococcal genus regardless of hemolytic patterns. These are called the **pyogenic streptococci,** and in medical circles they are now better known by their Lancefield letter than the older species name. Pediatricians instantly recognize GBS as an acronym for group B streptococcus, but may be confused by use of the proper name, *Streptococcus agalactiae* (**Table 25–1**).

* Lancefield antigens are cell wall carbohydrates

* Lancefield antigens define the pyogenic streptococci

For practical purposes, the type of hemolysis and certain biochemical reactions remain valuable for the initial recognition and presumptive classification of streptococci, and as an indication of what subsequent taxonomic tests to perform. Thus, β-hemolysis indicates that the strain has one of the Lancefield group antigens, but some Lancefield-positive strains or groups may be α-hemolytic or even nonhemolytic. The streptococci are considered here as follows: (1) pyogenic streptococci (Lancefield groups); (2) pneumococci; and (3) viridans group and other streptococci (Table 25–1).

* Hemolysis a practical guide to classification

* Most pyogenic streptococci β-hemolytic

■ Pyogenic Streptococci χ — *cardiomyocytes*

Of the many Lancefield groups, the ones most frequently isolated from humans are A, B, C, F, and G. Of these, groups A (*S pyogenes*) and B (*S agalactiae*) are the most common causes of serious disease. The group D carbohydrate is found in the *S bovis* group and the genus *Enterococcus,* which used to be classified among the streptococci.

Groups A and B common causes of disease

■ Pneumococci

This category contains a single species, *S pneumoniae*, commonly called the pneumococcus. Its distinctive feature is the presence of a capsule composed of polysaccharide polymers that vary in antigenic specificity. More than 90 capsular immunotypes have been defined. Although the pneumococcal cell wall shares some common antigens with other streptococci, it does not possess any of the Lancefield group antigens. *S pneumoniae* is α-hemolytic.

* Pneumococci have polysaccharide capsule

■ Viridans Group and Other Streptococci

Viridans streptococci are α-hemolytic and lack both the group carbohydrate antigens of the pyogenic streptococci and the capsular polysaccharides of the pneumococcus (Table 25–1). The term

TABLE 25–1   Classification of Streptococci and Enterococci

GROUP/ SPECIES	COMMON TERM	HEMOLYSIS	LANCEFIELD CELL WALL	SURFACE PROTEIN	CAPSULE	VIRULENCE FACTORS	DISEASE
MAJOR ANTIGENS/STRUCTURES							
Streptococci							
Pyogenic							
Streptococcus pyogenes	Group A strep (GAS)	β	A	M protein (100+)	Hyaluronic acid	M protein, lipoteichoic acid, StrepSAgs, streptolysin O, streptokinase	Strep throat, impetigo, pyogenic infections, toxic shock, rheumatic fever, glomerulonephritis
S agalactiae	Group B strep (GBS)	β, –	B	–	Sialic acid (9)	Capsule	Neonatal sepsis, meningitis, pyogenic infections
S dysgalactiae subsp. *equinus*		β	C	–	–	StrepSAg genes	Pyogenic infections
S bovis group *S gallilyticus* subsp. *gallilyticus*		–, α	D	–	–	–	Endocarditis, pyogenic infections, colon cancer association
Pneumococcus							
S pneumoniae	Pneumococcus	α	–	Choline-binding protein	Polysaccharide (90+)	Capsule, pneumolysin, neuraminidase	Pneumonia, meningitis, otitis media, pyogenic infections
Viridans and nonhemolytic							
S sanguis		α	–	–	–	–	Low virulence, endocarditis
S salivarius		α					Low virulence, endocarditis
S mutans		α	–	–			Dental caries
S anginosus group *S constellatus*, *S intermedius*		α, β, –	A, C, F, G	–	–	–	Abscesses, endocarditis
B$_6$-dependent (pyridoxal) streptococci (*Granulicatella*, *Abiotrophia*)		–, α	–				Endocarditis, pyogenic infections
Enterococci							
Enterococcus faecalis	Enterococcus	–, α	D	–	–	–	Urinary tract, pyogenic infections, endocarditis
E faecium	Enterococcus	–, α	D	–	–	–	Urinary tract, pyogenic infections

encompasses several species, including *S sanguis*, *S salivarius*, *S mitis*, and *S mutans*. Viridans streptococci are members of the resident oral microbiota of humans. They rarely demonstrate invasive qualities but can cause endocarditis.

A variety of other streptococci may be encountered, which also lack the features of the pyogenic streptococci or pneumococci. MALDI-TOF mass spectrometry and 16S rRNA sequencing have transformed their identification and taxonomy and have enabled a better understanding of their associations with specific clinical disease entities. Some examples follow. The *S bovis* group (long-known as nonenteroccocal group D streptococci and associated with endocarditis) includes *S gallilyticus* spp. *gallilyticus*, which is now known to be the species most closely linked with endocarditis (90%) and colonic neoplasms (70%) in patients with bacteremia. The *S anginosus* group (includes *S constellatus* and *intermedius*) may be α-, γ-, or β-hemolytic and have A, B, C, or G Lancefield cell wall antigens, but all are pyogenic and associated with abscesses. Lastly, are the nutritionally-variant streptococci (NVS) that require pyridoxal (vitamin B₆), which is lacking in sheep blood, for growth. They are now named *Granulicatella* sp. and *Abiotrophia* sp., and have a striking association with endocarditis.

※ Viridans and nonhemolytic species lack capsules and Lancefield antigens

GROUP A STREPTOCOCCI (*STREPTOCOCCUS PYOGENES*)

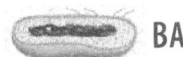 **BACTERIOLOGY**

MORPHOLOGY AND GROWTH

Group A streptococci (GAS) typically appear in purulent lesions or broth cultures as spherical or ovoid cells in chains of short to medium length (4-10 cells). On blood agar plates, colonies are usually compact, small, and surrounded by a 2 to 3 mm zone of β-hemolysis (Figure 25–2), which is easily seen and sharply demarcated. β-Hemolysis is caused by either of two hemolysins, **streptolysin S** and the oxygen-labile **streptolysin O,** both of which are produced by most group A strains. Strains that lack streptolysin S are β-hemolytic only under anaerobic conditions because the remaining streptolysin O is not active in the presence of oxygen. This feature is of practical importance because such strains would be missed in clinical laboratories if cultures were incubated only aerobically.

※ Streptolysins O and S cause β-hemolysis

Aerobically, only streptolysin S active

STRUCTURE

The structure of GAS is illustrated in **Figure 25–3.** The cell wall is built on a peptidoglycan matrix that provides rigidity, as in other Gram-positive bacteria. Within this matrix lies the group carbohydrate antigen, which by definition is present in all GAS. A number of other molecules such as M protein and lipoteichoic acid (LTA) are attached to the cell wall, but extend beyond, often in association with, the hair-like pili. GAS are divided into more than 100 serotypes based on antigenic differences in the M protein.

※ Wall contains group antigen

■ M Protein

The M protein itself is a fibrillar coiled-coil molecule with structural homology to myosin. Its carboxy terminus is rooted in the peptidoglycan of the cell wall, and the amino-terminal regions

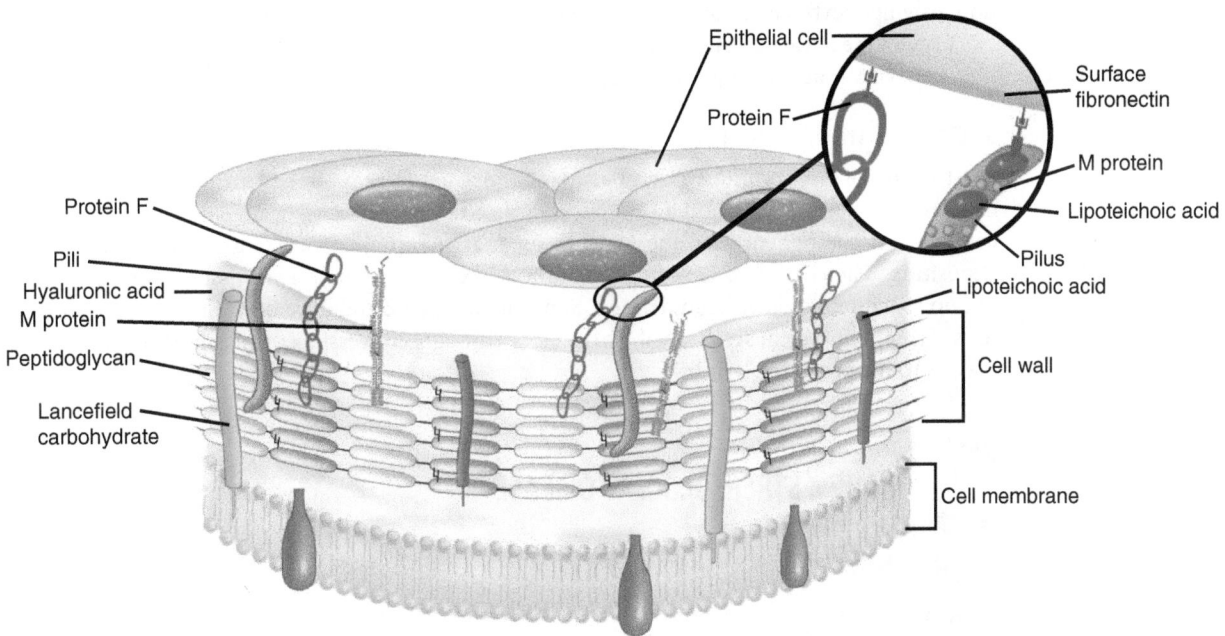

FIGURE 25–3. Antigenic structure of GAS and adhesion to an epithelial cell. The location of peptidoglycan and Lancefield carbohydrate antigens in the cell wall is shown in the diagram. M protein and lipoteichoic acid (LTA) are associated with the cell surface and the pili. LTA and protein F mediate binding to fibronectin on the host surface.

* Coiled-coil structure similar to myosin

* Antigenicity and function differ in domains of the molecule

* 100+ M protein serotypes

extend out from the surface. The specificity of the multiple serotypes of M protein is determined by variations in the amino acid sequences at the amino-terminal portion of the molecule. Because of its exposed location, this part of the M protein is also the most available to immune surveillance (Figure 25–3). The middle part of the molecule is less variable, and some carboxy-terminal regions are conserved across many M types. There is increasing evidence that some of the many known biologic functions of M protein can be assigned to specific domains of the molecule. This includes both antigenicity and the capacity to bind other molecules such as fibrinogen, serum factor H, and immunoglobulins. There are more than 100 immunotypes of M protein, which are the basis of a subtyping system for GAS.

Other Surface Molecules

* Protein F and LTA bind fibronectin

* Hyaluronic acid capsule may be present

A number of surface proteins have been described on the basis of their similarity with M protein or some unique binding capacity. Of these, a fibronectin-binding **protein F** and **LTA** are both exposed on the streptococcal surface (Figure 25–3) and play a role in pathogenesis. An IgG-binding protein has the capacity to bind the Fc portion of antibodies in much the same way as staphylococcal protein A. In principle, this could interfere with opsonization by creating a covering of antibody molecules on the streptococcal surface that are facing the "wrong way." Many GAS have a nonantigenic **hyaluronic acid capsule.** Although this capsule has been shown to be antiphagocytic, its role in disease is clouded by the fact that strains which lack it are still fully virulent.

EXTRACELLULAR PRODUCTS

Streptolysin O

* Streptolysin O is pore-forming and antigenic

Streptolysin O is a pore-forming cytotoxin, lysing leukocytes, tissue cells, and platelets. The toxin inserts directly into the cell membrane of host cells, forming transmembrane pores in a manner similar to complement and staphylococcal α-toxin. Streptolysin O is antigenic, and the quantitation of antibodies against it is the basis of a standard serologic test called antistreptolysin O (ASO).

Streptococcal Superantigen Toxins

* SAgs produced by some strains

* Streptococcal and staphylococcal SAgs are superantigens

Just as with *Staphylococcus aureus*, approximately 10% of GAS produce one of a family of exotoxins whose major biologic effect is through the superantigen (SAg) mechanism (**Figure 22–7**). Over many decades, these toxins have been assigned a number of names linked to their association with **scarlet fever** (erythrogenic toxin) and with streptococcal toxic shock (streptococcal pyrogenic exotoxins [Spe]). As with *S aureus,* there are several antigenically distinct proteins (SpeA, SpeB, and so on). Streptococcal SAgs have multiple effects, including fever, rash (scarlet fever), T-cell proliferation, B-lymphocyte suppression, and heightened sensitivity to endotoxin. Most of these actions are due to cytokine release through the SAg mechanism. At least one streptococcal SAg (SpeB) also has direct enzymatic activity digesting tissue and extracellular matrix proteins.

Other Extracellular Products

* C5a peptidase degrades complement

Most strains of GAS produce a number of other extracellular products including **streptokinase, hyaluronidase,** nucleases, and a **C5a peptidase.** The C5a peptidase is an enzyme that degrades complement component C5a, the main factor that attracts phagocytes to sites of complement deposition. The enzymatic actions of the others likely play some role in tissue injury or spread, but no specific roles have been defined. Some are antigenic and have been the basis of serologic tests. Streptokinase causes lysis of fibrin clots through conversion of plasminogen in normal plasma to the protease plasmin.

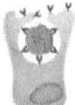

GROUP A STREPTOCOCCAL DISEASE

EPIDEMIOLOGY

Pharyngitis

GAS are the most common bacterial cause of pharyngitis in school-age children 5 to 15 years of age. Transmission is person-to-person from the large droplets produced by infected persons during coughing, sneezing, or even conversation (**Figure 25–4**). This droplet transmission is most

Group A Streptococcus

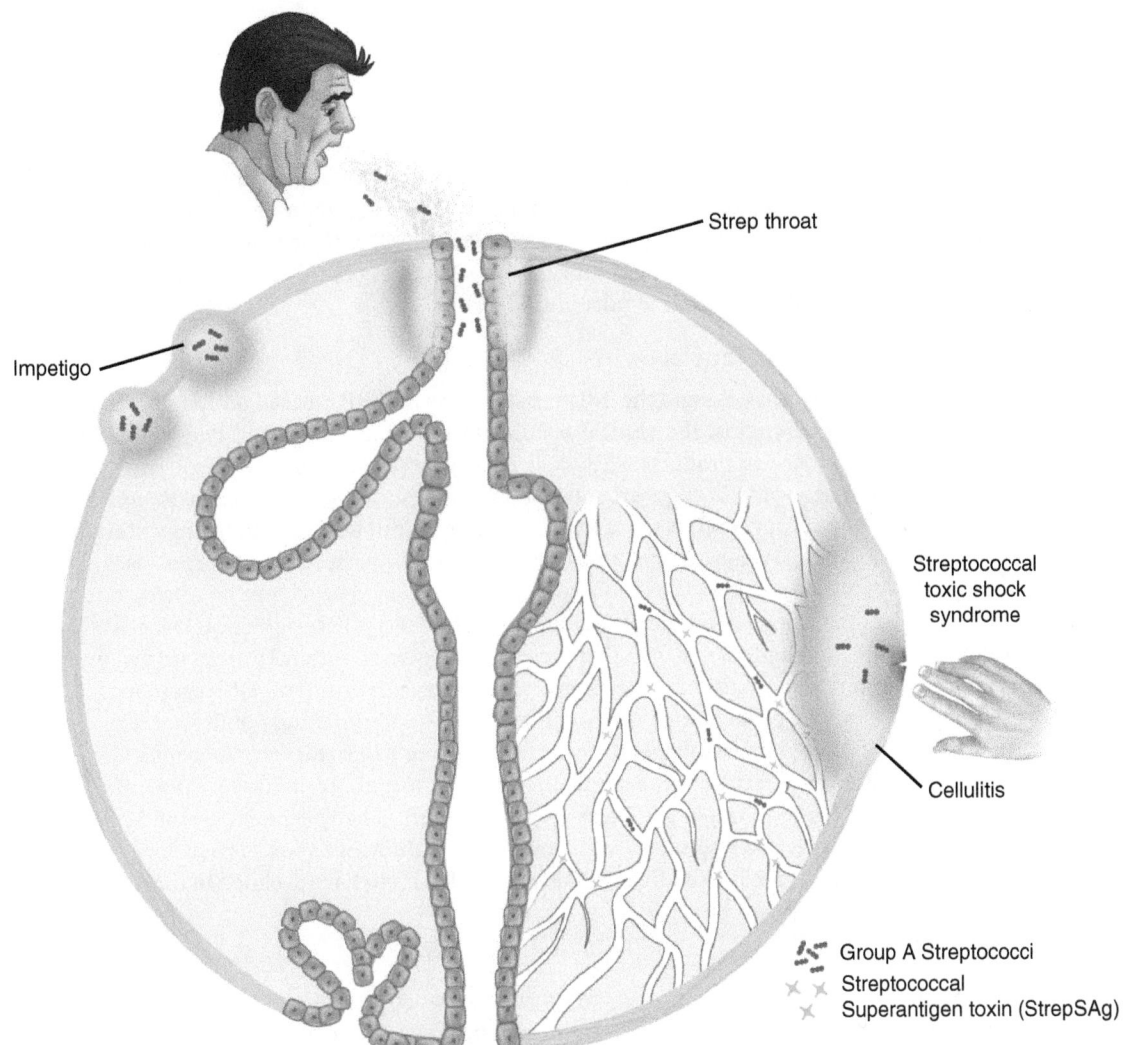

FIGURE 25–4. **GAS disease overview.** The primary sources of infection are respiratory droplets or direct contact with the skin. Impetigo results from minor trauma such as insect bites in skin transiently colonized with GAS. In streptococcal toxic shock, StrepSAgs producing GAS in a superficial lesion spread into the bloodstream. Note both toxin and bacteria are circulating.

efficient at the short distances (2-5 feet) at which social interactions commonly take place in families and schools, particularly in fall and winter months. Asymptomatic carriers (less than 1%) may also be the source of GAS, particularly if colonized in the nose as well as the throat. Although GAS survive for some time in dried secretions, environmental sources and fomites are not important means of spread. Unless the condition is treated, the organisms persist for 1 to 4 weeks after symptoms have disappeared.

※ Most common bacterial cause of sore throat

※ Droplets spread over short distances

■ **Impetigo**

Impetigo occurs when transient skin colonization with GAS is combined with minor trauma such as insect bites. The tiny skin pustules are spread locally by scratching and to others by direct contact or shared fomites such as towels. Impetigo is most common in summer months when insects bite and when the general level of hygiene is low. The M protein types of GAS most commonly associated with impetigo are different from those causing respiratory infection.

※ Skin colonization plus trauma leads to impetigo

■ **Wound and Puerperal Infections**

GAS, once a leading cause of postoperative wound and puerperal infections, retain this potential, but the conditions favoring these diseases are now less common in developed countries. As with staphylococci, transmission from patient to patient is by the hands of physicians or other medical

※ Hospital outbreaks of GAS linked to carriers

attendants who fail to follow recommended handwashing practices. Organisms may be transferred from another patient or may come from the healthcare workers themselves.

■ Streptococcal Toxic Shock Syndrome

Since the late 1980s, a severe invasive form of GAS soft tissue infection appeared with increased frequency worldwide. Rapid progression to death in only a few days has occurred in previously healthy persons. The outstanding features of these infections are their multiorgan involvement, suggesting a toxin and rapid invasiveness with spread to the bloodstream and distant organs. Soft-tissue necrosis and streptococcal gangrenous myositis can rapidly ensue without the trauma associated with clostridial gas gangrene (see **Chapter 29**). The toxic features together with the discovery that almost all the isolates produce streptococcal SAgs have caused this syndrome to be labeled **streptococcal toxic shock syndrome (STSS).**

■ Poststreptococcal Sequelae

The association between GAS and the inflammatory disease ARF is based on epidemiologic studies linking GAS pharyngitis, the clinical features of rheumatic fever, and heightened immune responses to streptococcal products. ARF does not follow skin or other nonrespiratory infection with GAS. Although some M types are more "rheumatogenic," it is not practical to define risk in advance. The general approach is that recurrences of ARF can be triggered by infection with any GAS. Injury to the heart caused by recurrences of ARF leads to **rheumatic heart disease,** a major cause of heart disease worldwide. Although ARF has declined in developed countries, resurgence in the form of small regional outbreaks began in the late 1980s. These outbreaks involved children of a higher socioeconomic status than that previously associated with ARF and a shift in prevalent M types. The underlying basis of the resurgence is unknown. In contrast, ARF is rampant in many developing countries, particularly in Africa, the Middle East, India, and South America.

Poststreptococcal glomerulonephritis may follow either respiratory or cutaneous GAS infection and involves only certain "nephritogenic" strains. It is more common in temperate climates where insect bites lead to impetigo. The average latent period between infection and glomerulonephritis is 10 days from a respiratory infection but generally about 3 weeks from a skin infection. Nephritogenic strains are limited to a few M types and seem to have declined in recent years.

PATHOGENESIS

■ Acute Infections

As with other pathogens, adherence to mucosal surfaces is a crucial step in initiating disease. Along with pili, a dozen specific adhesins have been described that facilitate the ability of the GAS to adhere to epithelial cells of the nasopharynx and/or skin. Of these, the most important are M protein, LTA, and protein F. In the nasopharynx, all three appear to be involved in mediating attachment to the fatty acid-binding sites in the glycoprotein fibronectin covering the epithelial cell surface. The role of M protein in the pharynx is not direct, but it appears to function as an anchor for LTA, which is essential for it to reach its binding site (Figure 25–3).

However, M protein appears to be direct and dominant in binding to the skin through its ability to interact with subcorneal keratinocytes, the most numerous cell type in cutaneous tissue. This adherence takes place at domains of the M protein that bind to receptors on the keratinocyte surface. Protein F is also involved primarily in adherence to antigen-presenting Langerhans cells (Figure 25–3). Expression of M protein and protein F is regulated in response to environmental conditions (O_2, CO_2), which could play a role in establishing the microbe or in relation to the immune response.

Clinical evidence makes it clear that GAS have the capacity to be highly invasive. The events following attachment that trigger invasion are only starting to be understood. It appears that M protein, protein F, and other fibronectin-binding proteins are required for the invasion of nonprofessional phagocytes. There is also evidence that streptococcal SAg genes are linked to invasiveness. The invasion itself involves integrin receptors and is accompanied by cytoskeleton rearrangements, but the molecular events do not yet make a coherent story.

After the initial events of attachment and invasion, the concerted activity of the M protein, immunoglobulin-binding proteins, and the C5a peptidase play the key roles in allowing the streptococcal infection to continue (**Figure 25–5**). M protein plays an essential role in GAS resistance to phagocytosis because of the ability of domains of the molecule to bind serum factor H.

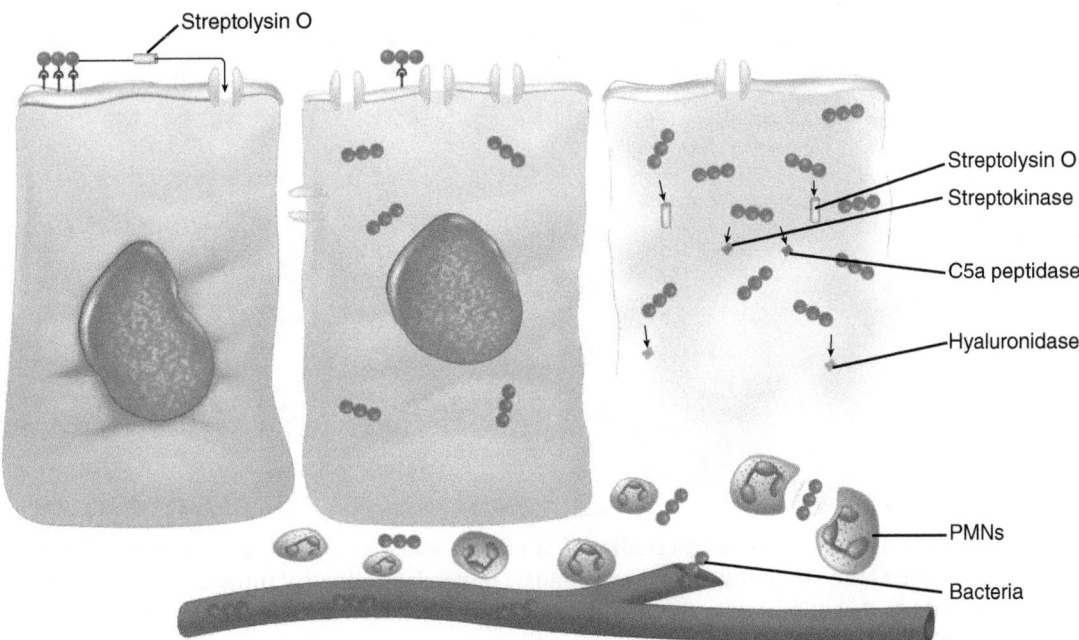

FIGURE 25–5. GAS disease, cellular view. The cellular events are similar to that of *Staphylococcus aureus* (see Figure 24–4). Streptolysin O is a pore-forming toxin, and there are many extracellular products. A difference is that although *S aureus* tends to be localized, GAS tend to spread diffusely, as shown in the cell on the right. This may be due to hyaluronidase (spreading factor) or resistance to phagocytosis. Below the cells, factor H binding is mediating GAS escaping the polymorphonuclear neutrophils (PMNs).

This leads to a diminished availability of alternative pathway-generated complement component C3b for deposition on the streptococcal surface in the same manner as polysaccharide capsules (Figure 22–4). In the presence of M type-specific antibody, classical pathway opsonophagocytosis proceeds, and the streptococci are rapidly killed. As a second antiphagocytic mechanism, the C5a peptidase inactivates C5a and thus blocks chemotaxis of polymorphonuclear neutrophils (PMNs) and other phagocytes to the site of infection.

❋ Surface C3b deposition diminished

❋ C5a peptidase blocks phagocyte chemotaxis

The precise role of other bacterial factors in the pathogenesis of acute infection is uncertain, but the combined effect of streptokinase, DNAase, and hyaluronidase may prevent effective localization of the infection, whereas the streptolysins produce tissue injury and are toxic to phagocytic cells. Antibodies against these components are formed in the course of streptococcal infection but are not known to be protective.

Other virulence factors contribute to spread and injury

In STSS, as with staphylococcal toxic shock syndrome, the findings of shock, renal impairment, coagulopathy, and rash seem to be explained by the massive cytokine release stimulated by the superantigenicity of the streptococcal SAgs. Exotoxin production, however, does not explain the enhanced invasiveness of GAS, which is an added feature of STSS compared to its staphylococcal counterpart. Although the enzymatic activity of some streptococcal SAgs has been linked to invasiveness, the underlying mechanisms are unclear. One theory is that STSS may be due to the horizontal transfer of streptococcal SAg genes to GAS clones with enhanced invasive potential, a deadly combination.

❋ Superantigenicity of SAgs triggers STSS

Invasive component is unexplained

■ **Poststreptococcal Sequelae**

Acute Rheumatic Fever

Of the many theories advanced to explain the role of GAS in ARF, an autoimmune mechanism related to antigenic similarities between streptococci antigens and human tissues has the most experimental support. Streptococcal pharyngitis patients who develop ARF have higher levels of antistreptococcal and autoreactive antibodies than those who do not. Some of these antibodies have been shown to react with both heart tissue and streptococcal antigens.

❋ Autoimmune state induced by GAS

The antigen stimulating these antibodies is most probably M protein, but the group A carbohydrate is also a possibility. There is similarity between the structure of regions of the M protein and myosin, and M protein fragments have been shown to stimulate antibodies that bind to human heart sarcolemma membranes, cardiac myosin, synovium, and articular cartilage. ARF is a prime example of the **molecular mimicry** mechanism of Type II autoimmune hypersensitivity (see

FIGURE 25–6. **Aschoff nodule.** Reacting lymphocytes and large mononuclear cells in myocardium demonstrate a cellular component to the immune reaction in rheumatic fever. (Reproduced with permission from Connor DH, Chandler FW, Schwartz DQ, et al: *Pathology of Infectious Diseases*. Stamford CT: Appleton & Lange; 1997.)

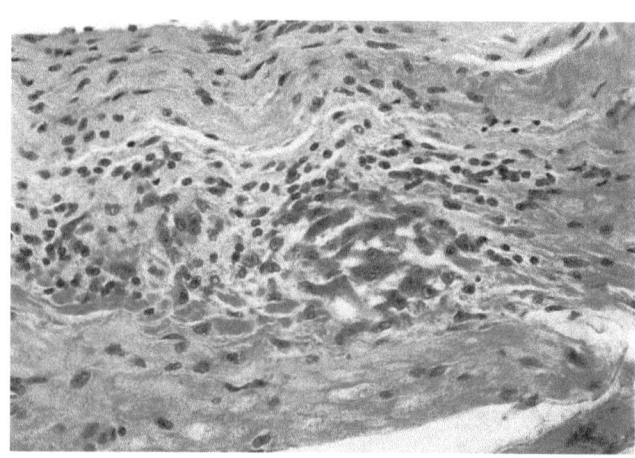

✳ Antibodies react with sarcolemma, myosin, synovium by molecular mimicry

✳ Cross-reactive and protective M protein domains differ

Cell-mediated immunity responses include cytotoxic lymphocytes

Alloantigens associated with hyperreactivity to streptococci

✳ Autoimmune reactions to M protein or streptokinase

✳ Type-specific IgG reverses antiphagocytic effect of M protein

✳ Repeated infections and ARF due to many M types

Chapter 2). Immunochemical studies of M protein are now directed at locating the epitopes in the large M protein molecule, which stimulate protective antibody (anti-factor H binding sites) and those that stimulate antiself antibodies. There is evidence these domains are in different locations in the M protein coiled coil. If they can be separated, there is hope for an M protein-based vaccine that does not cause the very disease (ARF) it is designed to prevent. A further complication with this approach is establishing the consistency of these relationships among the many M types.

Patients with ARF also show enhanced T_H1 responses to streptococcal antigens. Cytotoxic T lymphocytes may be stimulated by M protein, and cytotoxic lymphocytes have been observed in the blood of patients with ARF. A cellular reaction pattern consisting of lymphocytes and macrophages aggregated around fibrinoid deposits is found in human hearts. This lesion, called the Aschoff body (**Figure 25–6**), is considered characteristic of rheumatic carditis.

Genetic factors are probably also important in ARF because only a small percentage of individuals infected with GAS develop the disease. Attack rates have been highest among those of lower socioeconomic status and vary among those of different racial origins. The gene for an alloantigen found on the surface of B lymphocytes occurs four to five times more frequently in patients with rheumatic fever than in the general population. This further suggests a genetic predisposition to hyperreactivity to streptococcal products.

Acute Glomerulonephritis

The renal injury of acute glomerulonephritis is caused by deposition in the glomerulus of antigen-antibody complexes with complement activation and consequent inflammation. This is a type III hypersensitivity (see **Chapter 2**). The M proteins of some nephritogenic strains have been shown to share antigenic determinants with glomeruli, which suggest an autoimmune mechanism similar to rheumatic fever. Streptokinase has also been implicated both through molecular mimicry and through its plasminogen activation capacity.

IMMUNITY

It has long been known that an antibody directed against M protein is protective for subsequent GAS infections. This protection, however, is only for subsequent infection with strains of the same M type. This is called **type-specific immunity.** This protective IgG is directed against factor H-binding epitopes in the amino-terminal regions of the molecule and reverses the antiphagocytic effect of M protein. Streptococci opsonized with type-specific antibody bind complement C3b by the classical pathway, thus facilitating phagocyte recognition. There is evidence that mucosal IgA is also important in blocking adherence, whereas the IgG is able to protect against invasion. Unfortunately, because there are over 100 M types, repeated infections with new M types occur. Eventually, immunity to the common M types is acquired and infections become less common in adults. In ARF patients, it is the hyperreaction seen in each episode that produces the lesions associated with rheumatic heart disease.

GROUP A STREPTOCOCCAL INFECTIONS: CLINICAL ASPECTS

MANIFESTATIONS

Streptococcal Pharyngitis

Although it may occur at any age, streptococcal pharyngitis occurs most frequently between the ages of 5 and 15 years. The illness is characterized by acute sore throat, malaise, fever, and headache. Infection typically involves the tonsillar pillars, uvula, and soft palate, which become red, swollen, and covered with a yellow-white exudate. The cervical lymph nodes that drain this area may also become swollen and tender. This clinical syndrome overlaps with viral pharyngitis taking place at the same age.

GAS pharyngitis is usually self-limiting. Typically, the fever is gone by the third to fifth day, and other manifestations subside within 1 week. Antimicrobial therapy hastens resolution only if begun within a day, but can avert sequelae. Occasionally, the infection spreads locally to produce peritonsillar or retropharyngeal abscesses, otitis media, suppurative cervical adenitis, and acute sinusitis. Rarely, more extensive spread occurs, producing meningitis, pneumonia, or bacteremia with metastatic infection in distant organs. In the preantibiotic era, these suppurative complications were responsible for a mortality rate of 1% to 3% after acute streptococcal pharyngitis. Such complications are much less common now, and fatal infections are rare.

> * Sore throat, fever, and malaise
>
> **Overlaps with viral pharyngitis**
>
> **Spread beyond the pharynx now uncommon**

Impetigo

The primary lesion of streptococcal impetigo is a small (up to 1 cm) vesicle surrounded by an area of erythema. The vesicle enlarges over a period of days, becomes pustular, and eventually breaks to form a yellow crust. The lesions usually appear in 2- to 5-year-old children on exposed body surfaces, typically the face and lower extremities. Multiple lesions may coalesce to form deeper ulcerated areas. Although *S aureus* produces a clinically distinct bullous form of impetigo, it can also cause vesicular lesions resembling streptococcal impetigo. Both pathogens are isolated from some cases.

> * Exposed skin of 2- to 5-year-old children
>
> **Tiny pustules may form ulcers**

Erysipelas

Erysipelas is a distinct form of streptococcal infection of the skin and subcutaneous tissues, primarily affecting the dermis. It is characterized by a spreading area of erythema and edema with rapidly advancing, well-demarcated edges, pain, and systemic manifestations, including fever and lymphadenopathy. Infection usually occurs on the face and a previous history of streptococcal sore throat is common.

> **Spreading dermal erythema**

Puerperal Infection

Infection of the endometrium at or near delivery is a life-threatening form of GAS infection. Now rare in developed countries, sepsis with GAS was a common cause of death in women after childbirth before effective infection control measures (hand sanitation and surgical gloves) were implemented. Other organisms can cause puerperal fever, but this form is the most likely to produce a rapidly progressive infection.

> **GAS causes virulent form of puerperal fever**

Disease Associated With Streptococcal SAg Toxins

Scarlet Fever

Infection with strains that elaborate any of the StrepSAgs may superimpose the signs of scarlet fever on a patient with streptococcal pharyngitis. In scarlet fever, the buccal mucosa, temples, and cheeks are deep red, except for a pale area around the mouth and nose (circumoral pallor). Punctate hemorrhages appear on the hard and soft palates, and the tongue becomes covered with a yellow-white exudate through which the red papillae are prominent (strawberry tongue). A diffuse red "sandpaper" rash appears on the second day of illness, spreading from the upper chest to the trunk and extremities (**Figure 25–7**). Circulating antibody to the toxin neutralizes these effects. For unknown reasons, scarlet fever is both less frequent and less severe than in the early 20th century; however, England is currently experiencing an unprecedented resurgence of scarlet fever owing to a diversity of *emm* types with the highest incidence rates in nearly 50 years. Outbreaks of scarlet fever have also been reported recently from Australia, Hong Kong, and mainland China.

> * Scarlet fever is strep throat with a characteristic rash

FIGURE 25–7. **Scarlet fever.** Rash on the trunk of the adolescent female shown here is characteristic of scarlet fever as are the hyperpigmented linear striations in the antecubital fossa (Pastia lines). (Reproduced with permission from CDC Public Health Image Library.)

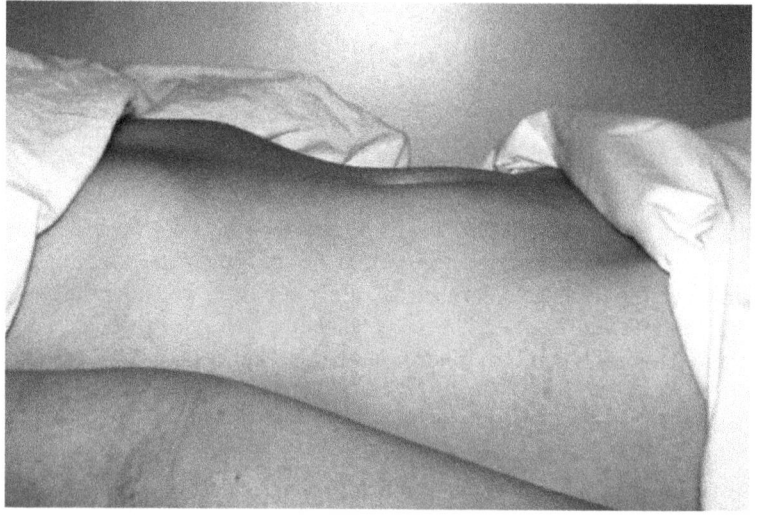

Streptococcal Toxic Shock Syndrome

STSS may begin at the site of any GAS infection even at the site of seemingly minor trauma. The systemic illness starts with vague myalgia, chills, and severe pain at the infected site. Most commonly, this is in the skin and soft tissues and leads to necrotizing fasciitis and myonecrosis. The striking nature of this progression when it involves the extremities is the basis of the label "flesh-eating bacteria." STSS continues with nausea, vomiting, and diarrhea followed by hypotension, shock, and organ failure. The outstanding laboratory findings are a lymphocytosis, impaired renal function (azotemia), and, in over half the cases, bacteremia. Some patients are in irreversible shock by the time they reach a medical facility. Many survivors have been left as multiple amputees as the result of metastatic spread of the streptococci.

STSS is a rapidly progressive multisystem disease

Shock, azotemia, and bacteremia are common

■ Poststreptococcal Sequelae

Acute Rheumatic Fever

ARF is a nonsuppurative inflammatory disease characterized by fever, carditis, subcutaneous nodules, chorea, and migratory polyarthritis. The diagnosis is based on a set of primarily clinical findings (Jones Criteria) recommended by the American Heart Association. Evidence of a previous GAS infection is included in these criteria, but there is no test which is diagnostic of ARF. Cardiac enlargement, valvular murmurs, and effusions are seen clinically and reflect myocardial, endocardial, and epicardial damage, which can lead to heart failure. Attacks typically begin 3 weeks (range 1-5 weeks) after an attack of GAS pharyngitis and, in the absence of antiinflammatory therapy, last 2 to 3 months.

Fever, carditis, nodules, polyarthritis

No single test diagnostic

ARF also has a predilection for recurrence with subsequent streptococcal infections as new M types are encountered. The first attack usually occurs between the ages of 5 and 15 years. The risk of recurrent attacks after subsequent GAS infection continues into adult life and then decreases. Repeated attacks lead to progressive damage to the endocardium and heart valves, with scarring and valvular stenosis or incompetence (rheumatic heart disease).

New M types trigger recurrences

Recurrences lead to rheumatic heart disease

Acute Glomerulonephritis

Poststreptococcal glomerulonephritis is primarily a disease of childhood that begins 1 to 4 weeks after streptococcal pharyngitis and 3 to 6 weeks after skin infection. It is characterized clinically by edema, hypertension, hematuria, proteinuria, and decreased serum complement levels. Pathologically, there are diffuse proliferative lesions of the glomeruli. The clinical course is usually benign, with spontaneous healing over weeks to months. Occasionally, a progressive course leads to renal failure and death.

Children develop a nephritis, which slowly resolves

DIAGNOSIS

Although the clinical features of streptococcal pharyngitis are fairly typical, there is enough overlap with viral pharyngitis that a culture of the posterior pharynx and tonsils is required for diagnosis. A direct Gram-stained smear of the throat is not helpful because of the other streptococci

TABLE 25–2	Usual Hemolytic, Biochemical, and Cultural Reactions of Common Streptococci and Enterococci[a]				
	SUSCEPTIBILITY TO				
	BACITRACIN	OPTOCHIN	BILE SOLUBILITY	BILE/ESCULIN REACTION[b]	PYR
Streptococci					
β-Hemolytic					
Lancefield group A	+	−	−	−	+
Lancefield groups B, C, F, G	−	−	−	−	−
α-Hemolytic					
S pneumoniae	−	+	+	−	−
Viridans group	−	−	−	−	−
Nonhemolytic (usually)					
Enterococci	−	−	−	+	+

PYR, pyrrolidonyl arylamidase test.
[a]All are tests commonly substituted for serologic identification in clinical laboratories.
[b]Tests for the ability to grow in bile and reduce esculin.

in the pharyngeal flora. However, smears from normally sterile sites usually demonstrate streptococci. Sheep blood agar plates incubated anaerobically give the best yield because they favor the demonstration of β-hemolysis (see Streptolysins earlier in the chapter). β-Hemolytic colonies are identified by Lancefield grouping using agglutination methods or polymerase chain reaction (PCR). In smaller laboratories, a surrogate method based on the exquisite susceptibility of GAS to bacitracin (a bacteriocin) and the relative resistance of strains of other groups may be used for presumptive separation of group A strains from the others (**Table 25–2**).

* Throat culture followed by Lancefield grouping

* Bacitracin susceptibility predicts group A

Detection of group A antigen extracted directly from throat swabs is now available in a wide variety of kits marketed for use in physicians' offices. These methods are rapid and specific but are at best only 90% sensitive compared with culture. Given the importance of the detection of GAS in the prevention of ARF (it is the reason physicians culture sore throats), missing 10% or more of cases is not tolerable. Patients with a positive direct antigen test may be treated without culture, but the American Academy of Pediatrics recommends that negative results must be confirmed by culture before withholding treatment.

* GAS antigen test rapid and specific but not sensitive

Several serologic tests have been developed to aid in the diagnosis of poststreptococcal sequelae by providing evidence of a previous GAS infection. They include the ASO, anti-DNAase B, and some tests that combine multiple antigens. High titers of ASO are usually found in sera of patients with rheumatic fever, so that test is used most widely.

ASO antibodies document previous infection

TREATMENT

GAS are highly susceptible to penicillin G, the antimicrobial of choice. Concentrations as low as 0.01 μg/mL have a bactericidal effect, and penicillin resistance is so far unknown. Numerous other antimicrobials are also active, including other β-lactams and macrolides, but not aminoglycosides. Patients allergic to penicillin are usually treated with clindamycin or azithromycin, and impetigo is often treated with clindamycin to cover the prospect of S aureus involvement. Adequate treatment of streptococcal pharyngitis within 10 days of onset prevents rheumatic fever by removing the antigenic stimulus; its effect on the duration of the pharyngitis is not dramatic because of the short course of the natural infection. Treatment of the acute infection may not prevent the development of acute glomerulonephritis.

* GAS remain susceptible to penicillin

* Treatment of GAS pharyngitis for 10 days prevents ARF

PREVENTION

Penicillin prophylaxis with long-acting preparations is used to prevent recurrences of ARF during the most susceptible ages (5-15 years). Patients with a history of rheumatic fever or known rheumatic heart disease may receive antimicrobial prophylaxis while undergoing procedures known

* Prophylactic penicillin prevents ARF recurrences

to cause transient bacteremia, such as dental extraction. Multivalent vaccines using M protein epitopes that are not cross-reactive to self are in clinical trials with encouraging results.

 Why choose M protein for a vaccine? What are the unique problems with widespread use of such a vaccine?

● GROUP B STREPTOCOCCI (*STREPTOCOCCUS AGALACTIAE*)

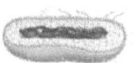 **BACTERIOLOGY**

✻ Nine capsular types contain sialic acid

Group B streptococci (GBS) produce short chains and diplococcal pairs of spherical or ovoid Gram-positive cells. Colonies are larger and β-hemolysis due to a pore-forming cytolysin (β-hemolysin) is less distinct than with GAS and may even be absent. In addition to the Lancefield B antigen, GBS produce polysaccharide capsules of nine antigenic types (Ia, Ib, II–VIII), all of which contain sialic acid in the form of terminal side chain residues. Pili and surface proteins are also present.

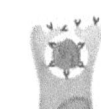 **GROUP B STREPTOCOCCAL DISEASE**

EPIDEMIOLOGY

✻ Neonatal sepsis acquired from mother's vaginal flora

Ruptured membranes, prematurity increase risk

GBS are the leading cause of sepsis and meningitis in the first few days of life. The organism is resident in the gastrointestinal tract, with secondary spread to other sites, the most important of which is the vagina. GBS can be found in the lower gastrointestinal and vaginal flora of 10% to 40% of women. During pregnancy and childbirth, these organisms may gain access to the amniotic fluid or colonize the newborn as it passes through the birth canal (**Figure 25–8**). GBS produce disease in approximately 2% of these encounters. The risk is much higher when factors are present that decrease the infant's innate resistance (prematurity) or increase the chances of transmission such as rupture of the amniotic membranes for 18 hours or more before delivery. Some infants are healthy at birth but develop sepsis 1 to 3 months later. Late-onset cases of GBS sepsis and meningitis have been associated with persistent colonization of mothers and/or their infants with GBS.

PATHOGENESIS

✻ Capsule binds factor H disrupting C3b deposition

✻ Transplacental IgG protective

GBS disease requires the proper combination of organism and host factors. The GBS capsule is the major organism factor. For the initial stages of infection, pili and a number of surface-exposed proteins that attach to fibronectin and extracellular matrix proteins have been identified. The sialic acid moiety of the capsule has been shown to bind serum factor H, which in turn accelerates degradation of C3b before it can be effectively deposited on the surface of the organism. This makes alternative pathway-mediated mechanisms of opsonophagocytosis relatively ineffective (Figure 22–4). Thus, complement-mediated phagocyte recognition requires specific antibody and the classical pathway. Newborns have this antibody only if they receive it from their mother as transplacental IgG. Those who lack the protective antibody specific to the type of GBS they encounter must rely on alternative pathway mechanisms, a situation in which the GBS has an advantage over less virulent organisms. GBS have also been shown to produce a peptidase that inactivates C5a, the major chemoattractant of PMNs. This may correlate with the observation that serious neonatal infections often show a paucity of infiltrating PMNs. The pore-forming cytolysin may contribute to tissue-destructive elements of invasive disease.

Think ▸▸ Apply 25-1: As the antigen on which type-specific immunity is based, M protein is the obvious choice for a vaccine. M protein is also the leading candidate for triggering the immunopathologic events of rheumatic fever. We must avoid causing the disease we are trying to prevent by first analyzing details of the large M protein molecule.

Pneumococcus and GBS

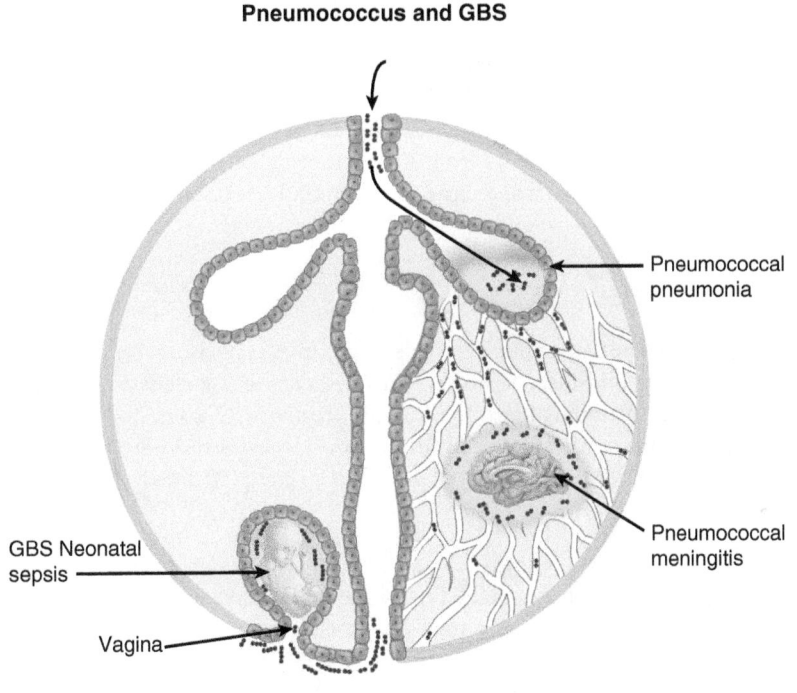

GBS Neonatal sepsis

Vagina

Pneumococcal pneumonia

Pneumococcal meningitis

•• *Streptococcus pneumoniae (pneumococcus)*
•••• Group B streptococcus (GBS)

FIGURE 25–8. **GBS and pneumococcal disease overview.** *Streptococcus pneumoniae* is aspirated from the normal orophyaryngeal flora to the lung where it produces pneumonia. Bacteremic spread can infect other sites particularly the brain where meningitis is produced. GBS vaginal colonization during pregnancy leads to infection of the fetus either in the uterus or during childbirth.

IMMUNITY

Antibody is protective against GBS disease, but as with group A streptococcal M protein, the antibody must be specific to the infecting type of GBS. Fortunately, there are only nine types, and type III is the most common cause of early and late-onset cases. Antibody is acquired by GBS infection, and specific IgG may be transmitted transplacentally to the fetus, providing protection in the perinatal period. In the presence of type-specific antibody, classical pathway C3b deposition, phagocyte recognition, and killing proceed normally.

✳ Type-specific anticapsular antibody protective

 ## GROUP B STREPTOCOCCI: CLINICAL ASPECTS

MANIFESTATIONS

The clinical findings of poor feeding, irritability, lethargy, jaundice, respiratory distress, and hypotension are nonspecific and similar to those found in other serious infections in the neonatal period. Fever is sometimes absent, and infants may even be hypothermic. Pneumonia is common, and meningitis is present in 5% to 10% of cases. Most infections have GBS circulating in the bloodstream without localizing findings. The disease onset is typically in the first few days of life, and signs of infection are present at birth in almost 50% of cases. The late-onset (1-3 months) cases have similar findings but are more likely to have meningitis and focal infections in the bones and joints. Even with increased awareness and improved supportive therapy, the mortality rate for early-onset GBS infection still approaches 10%.

Nonspecific findings evolve to pneumonia and meningitis

Onset is early (1-6 days) or late (1-3 months)

GBS infections in adults are uncommon and fall into two groups. The first group comprises peripartum chorioamnionitis and bacteremia, the mother's side of the neonatal syndrome. Other infections include pneumonia and a variety of skin and soft tissue infections similar to those produced by other pyogenic streptococci. Although adult GBS infections may be serious, they usually are not fatal unless patients are immunocompromised. GBS infections are not associated with rheumatic fever or acute glomerulonephritis.

Maternal and other adult infections can be serious

DIAGNOSIS

✳ Specialized culture to detect vaginal colonization

PCR is sensitive test for GBS detection

The laboratory diagnosis of GBS infection is by culture of blood, cerebrospinal fluid, or other appropriate specimen. Definitive identification involves serologic determination of the Lancefield group by the same methods used for GAS. Maximal detection of vaginal colonization in pregnant women requires obtaining specimens from the rectum as well as vagina. Recovery of GBS by culture necessitates selective media and enrichment broth. PCR is sensitive test for direct detection in intrapartum situations.

TREATMENT

Penicillin is primary antibiotic

GBS are susceptible to the same antimicrobials as group A organisms. Penicillin or ampicillin is the treatment of choice and there is no known resistance to β-lactam agents. However, in the initial stage, neonatal infections are often initially treated with combinations of penicillin (or ampicillin) and an aminoglycoside because of known synergism and the possibility of other bacterial agents. Once GBS is confirmed, therapy can be completed with penicillin alone.

PREVENTION

✳ Intrapartum IV penicillin prophylaxis protective

✳ Third-trimester culture determines risk

Strategies for the prevention of neonatal GBS disease are focused on reducing contact of the newborn with the organism. In colonized women, attempts to eradicate the carrier state have not been successful since GBS reside in the gastrointestinal tract, but intrapartum (during labor) antimicrobial prophylaxis with intravenous penicillin has been shown to reduce transmission and disease. It is now recommended by expert obstetric and perinatology groups that all newborns at risk receive such prophylaxis. Risk is defined by the presence of vaginal or rectal GBS in a culture taken during the third trimester (35-37 weeks). Thus, all expectant mothers must be screened by selective culture or PCR (see Diagnosis) and intrapartum prophylaxis with penicillin (or clindamycin for allergic patients) administered to all found culture-positive or PCR-positive. Although peripartum prophylaxis has reduced early-onset GBS disease in newborns by 60% to 80%, a recent large review of 863 cases from France in 2018 reported a 58% increase in late-onset GBS disease in infants in the same time period.

 Why would peripartum prophylaxis be successful in preventing early-onset GBS disease in newborns but be less effective for late-onset disease?

OTHER PYOGENIC STREPTOCOCCI

Potentially virulent but uncommon

✳ None associated with immunologic sequelae

The other pyogenic streptococci occasionally produce various respiratory, skin, wound, soft tissue, and genital infections, which may resemble those caused by group A and B streptococci. Although a few foodborne outbreaks of pharyngitis have been linked to groups C and G streptococci, their role as a cause of everyday sore throats is not established. These streptococci are susceptible to penicillin, and infections are managed in a manner similar to that with deep tissue infections caused by group A and B strains. None of the non-group A pyogenic streptococci have been associated with poststreptococcal sequelae.

 Think ▶▶ Apply 25-2: Group B streptococci are commensal organisms in the gastrointestinal track and vagina and as such can be temporarily suppressed but not eradicated. The goal of peripartum prophylaxis is to protect the newborn during and immediately after its hazardous journey through the birth canal. That is why cultures for GBS are done at 35-37 weeks' gestation and not earlier. Therapy is not done for eradication of GBS, which has been shown to be futile and been shown to upset the microbiota. Thus, infants remain at risk (albeit reduced as they grow older) for late-onset disease when they or their mothers remain or become colonized with GBS.

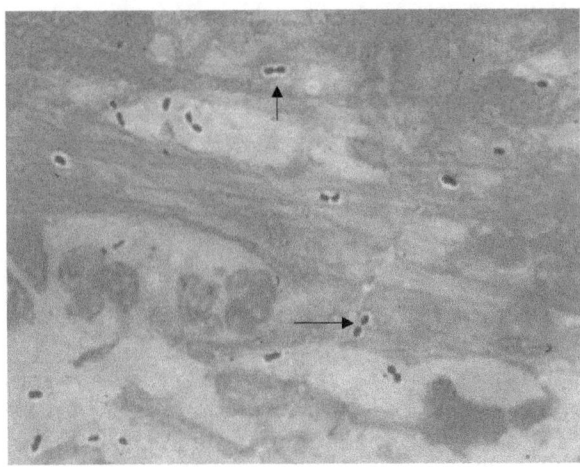

FIGURE 25–9. **Gram stain of sputum in pneumococcal pneumonia.** *Streptococcus pneumoniae* in sputum of patient with pneumonia. Note the marked tendency to form oval diplococci (arrows). The clear halo around the pairs is due to the capsule that does not stain by the Gram method. (Used with permission from Professor Shirley Lowe, University of California, San Francisco School of Medicine.)

STREPTOCOCCUS PNEUMONIAE

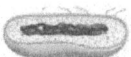 ## BACTERIOLOGY

Streptococcus pneumoniae (pneumococci) are Gram-positive, oval cocci typically arranged end to end in pairs (diplococcus), giving the cells a bullet shape (**Figure 25–9**). On blood agar, pneumococci produce round, glistening 0.5 to 2.0 mm colonies surrounded by a zone of α-hemolysis. Both colonies and broth cultures have a tendency to undergo autolysis because of their susceptibility to peroxides produced during growth and the action of **autolysins,** a family of pneumococcal enzymes that degrade peptidoglycan. Accelerating the autolytic process with bile salts is the basis of the bile solubility test that separates pneumococci from other α-hemolytic streptococci.

Colonies are α-hemolytic

The distinguishing structural feature of the pneumococcus is its capsule (**Figure 25–10**). All virulent strains have surface capsules, composed of high-molecular-weight polysaccharide polymers that are complex mixtures of monosaccharides, oligosaccharides, and sometimes other components. The exact makeup of the polymer is unique and distinctly antigenic for each of more than 90 serotypes. Pneumococcal cell wall structure is similar to that of other streptococci, and a variety of surface proteins are rooted in the peptidoglycan extending outward into the capsule. One group of these, the **choline-binding proteins,** is able to bind to both pneumococcal cell wall cholines and carbohydrates that are present on the surface of epithelial cells.

✻ Capsule has 90+ serotypes

✻ Choline-binding proteins attach to cells

EXTRACELLULAR PRODUCTS

All pneumococci produce **pneumolysin,** which is a member of the family of transmembrane pore-forming toxins that includes staphylococcal α toxin, *S pyogenes* streptolysin O, and others. The pneumococcus does not secrete pneumolysin, but it is released on lysis of the organisms augmented

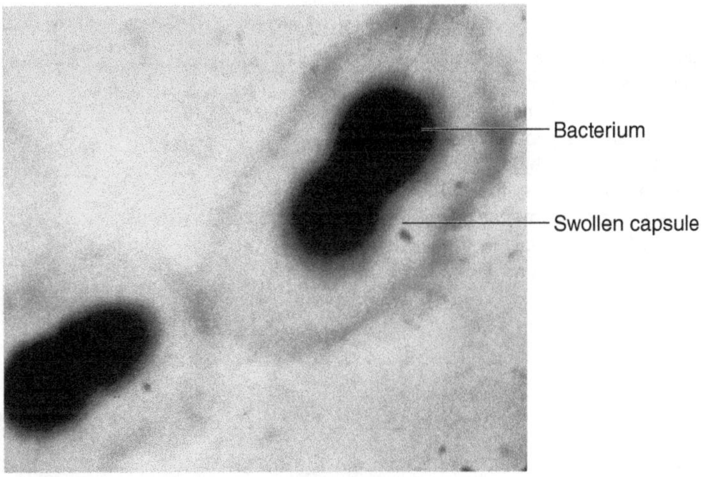

FIGURE 25–10. **Pneumococcal capsule.** In this test, live *Streptococcus pneumoniae* have been mixed with antibody specific to the capsular polysaccharide. The opsonizing antibody defines the capsule, which appears "swollen" when compared with preparations without antibody. (Reproduced with permission from Willey JM: *Prescott, Harley, & Klein's Microbiology,* 7th ed. New York, NY: McGraw Hill; 2008.)

— Bacterium

— Swollen capsule

* Pneumolysin forms pores after release by autolysins

by autolysins. Pneumolysin has a number of other effects, including its ability to stimulate cytokines and disrupt the cilia of human respiratory epithelial cells. Pneumococci also produce a neuraminidase, which cleaves sialic acid that is present in host mucin, glycolipids, and glycoproteins.

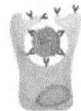 PNEUMOCOCCAL DISEASE

EPIDEMIOLOGY

* Pneumonia common

* Young and old most affected

Streptococcus pneumoniae is a leading cause of pneumonia, acute purulent meningitis, bacteremia, and other invasive infections. In the United States, it is responsible for an estimated 3000 cases of meningitis, 50,000 cases of bacteremia, and 500,000 cases of pneumonia each year. Worldwide, more than 5 million children die every year from pneumococcal disease. *S pneumoniae* is also the most common cause of otitis media, a virtually universal disease of childhood with millions of cases every year. Pneumococcal infections occur throughout life, but are most common in the very young (less than 2 years) and in the elderly (more than 60 years). Alcoholism, diabetes mellitus, chronic renal disease, asplenia, and some malignancies are associated with more frequent and serious pneumococcal infection.

Respiratory colonization is common

Microaerosols transmit person-to-person

Infections are derived from colonization of the nasopharynx, where pneumococci can be found in 5% to 40% of healthy persons depending on age, season, and other factors. The highest rates are among children in the winter. Respiratory secretions containing pneumococci may be transmitted from person to person by direct contact or from the microaerosols created by coughing and sneezing in close quarters. Such conditions are favored by crowded living conditions, particularly when colonized persons are mixed with susceptible ones, as in child care centers, recruitment barracks, and prisons. As with other bacterial pneumonias, viral respiratory infection and underlying chronic disease are important predisposing factors.

Some serotypes are more common

Surveillance data show that just over 20 of the 90 pneumococcal serotypes produce disease more often than the others. There is also a variation among types in the age and geographic distribution of cases. These differences are presumably due to enhanced virulence factors in these types, but the specific reasons are not known. These features do not influence the medical management of individual cases but are important in devising prevention strategies such as immunization (see following text).

PATHOGENESIS

Pneumococcal adherence to nasopharyngeal cells involves multiple factors. The primary relationship is the bridging effect of the choline-binding proteins' attachment to cell wall cholines and carbohydrates covering or exposed on the surface of host epithelial cells. This binding may be aided by the exposure of additional receptors by neuraminidase digestion, viral infection, or pneumolysin-stimulated cytokine activation of host cells. Aspiration of respiratory secretions containing these pneumococci is the initial step leading to pneumonia (**Figure 25–11**). This

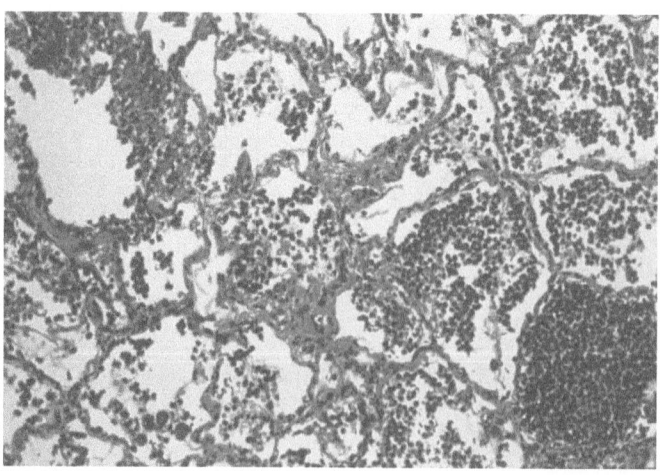

FIGURE 25–11. **Pneumococcal pneumonia.** In this histologic view of infected lung, note that the alveoli are filled with neutrophils but that the alveolar septa are relatively intact despite the high level of cellular infiltrate. The stain used here does not demonstrate the pneumococci, which would be much smaller than the cells at this magnification.

must be a common event. Normally, aspirated organisms are cleared rapidly by the defense mechanisms of the lower respiratory tract, including the cough and epiglottic reflexes; the muco-ciliary "blanket"; and phagocytosis by alveolar macrophages. Host factors that impair the combined efficiency of these defenses allow pneumococci to reach the alveoli and multiply there. These include chronic pulmonary diseases; damage to bronchial epithelium from smoking or air pollution; and respiratory dysfunction from alcoholic intoxication, narcotics, anesthesia, and trauma.

> ❋ Aspiration of colonizing bacteria starts disease process
>
> ❋ Impaired clearance mechanisms enhance susceptibility

When organisms reach the alveolus, pneumococcal virulence factors operate in two stages. The first stage is early in infection, when the capsule and some surface proteins of intact organisms act to block phagocytosis. This allows the organisms to multiply and spread despite an acute inflammatory response. The second stage occurs when organisms begin to disintegrate and release a number of factors either synthesized by the pneumococcus or part of its structure, thus causing injury. These include pneumolysin, autolysin, and components of the cell wall.

> ❋ Capsule interferes with phagocytosis
>
> **Pneumolysin causes injury**

■ Capsule

The polysaccharide capsule of *S pneumoniae* is the major determinant of virulence. Unencapsulated mutants do not produce disease in humans or laboratory animals. Like the GBS capsule, pneumococcal polysaccharide interferes with effective deposition of complement on the organism's surface and thus phagocyte recognition and engulfment. This property is particularly important in the absence of specific antibody, when alternative pathway is the primary means for C3b-mediated opsonization. In addition to the capsule, some of the surface choline-binding proteins may participate in this antiphagocytic effect by binding the serum factor H. When antibody specific to the capsular polysaccharide appears, classical pathway opsonophagocytosis proceeds efficiently.

> ❋ Unencapsulated pneumococci avirulent
>
> ❋ Alternate pathway C3b deposition blocked by capsule

■ Pneumolysin

Some of the clinical features seen in the course of pneumococcal infections are not explainable by the capsule alone. These include the dramatic abrupt onset, toxicity, fulminant course, and disseminated intravascular coagulation seen in some cases. Pneumolysin's toxicity for pulmonary endothelial cells and direct effect on cilia contributes to the disruption of the endothelial barrier and facilitates the access of pneumococci to the alveoli and eventually their spread beyond into the bloodstream. Pneumolysin also has direct effects on phagocytes and suppresses host inflammatory and immune functions. Because pneumolysin is not actively secreted outside the bacterial cell, the action of the autolysins is required to release it.

> ❋ Pneumolysin disrupts cells and cilia
>
> **Lysis required to release from bacterial cell**

The combined effects of pneumococcal and host factors produce a pneumonia, which progresses through a series of stages. Initial alveolar multiplication produces a profuse out-pouring of serous edema fluid, which is then followed by an influx of PMNs and erythrocytes (Figure 25–11). By the second or third day of illness, the lung segment has increased three- to fourfold in weight through accumulation of this cellular, hemorrhagic fluid typically in a single lobe of the lung. In the consolidated alveoli, neutrophils predominate initially, but once actively growing, pneumococci are no longer present, macrophages replace the granulocytes, and resolution of the lesion ensues. A remarkable feature of pneumococcal pneumonia is the lack of structural damage to the lung, which usually leads to complete resolution on recovery.

> ❋ PMNs and red blood cells consolidate alveoli
>
> ❋ Resolves without structural damage

IMMUNITY

Immunity to *S pneumoniae* infection is provided by antibody directed against the specific pneumococcal capsular type. When antibody binds to the capsular surface, C3b is deposited by classical pathway mechanisms, and phagocytosis can proceed. Because the number of serotypes is large, complete immunity through natural experience is not realistic, which is why pneumococcal infections occur throughout life. Infections are most often seen in the very young, when immunologic experience is minimal, and in the elderly, when immunity begins to wane and risk factors are more common. Recently, experience with pneumococcal vaccines has unmasked a phenomenon called **capsule switching** in which the antigenic makeup of the capsule changes. This is felt to be due to *in vivo* transformation and recombination with external DNA. We should not be too surprised at this since the discovery of DNA as the keeper of the genetic code was through experiments transforming pneumococci.

> ❋ Immunity specific to capsular type
>
> ❋ Antibody leads to classical pathway complement deposition
>
> **Capsule switching changes capsule antigenicity**

PNEUMOCOCCAL DISEASE: CLINICAL ASPECTS

MANIFESTATIONS

■ Pneumococcal Pneumonia

Pneumococcal pneumonia begins abruptly with a shaking chill and high fever. Cough with production of sputum pink to rusty in color (indicating the presence of red blood cells) and pleuritic chest pain are common. Physical findings usually indicate pulmonary consolidation. Children and young adults typically demonstrate a lobular or lobar consolidation on chest radiography, whereas older patients may show a less localized bronchial distribution of the infiltrates. Without therapy, sustained fever, pleuritic pain, and productive cough continue until a "crisis" occurs 5 to 10 days after onset of the disease. The crisis involves a sudden decrease in temperature and improvement in the patient's condition. It is associated with effective levels of opsonizing antibody reaching the lesion. Although infection may occur at any age, the incidence and mortality of pneumococcal pneumonia increase sharply after 50 years.

* Shaking chill followed by bloody sputum

* Lung consolidation typically lobar

■ Pneumococcal Meningitis

Streptococcus pneumoniae is one of the three leading causes of acute bacterial meningitis. The signs and symptoms are similar to those produced by other bacteria. Acute purulent meningitis may follow pneumococcal pneumonia or infection at another site or may appear with no apparent antecedent infection. It may also develop after trauma involving the skull. The mortality and frequency of sequelae are higher with pneumococcal meningitis than with other forms of pyogenic meningitis.

Sequelae are higher than with other meningeal pathogens

■ Other Infections

Pneumococci are common causes of sinusitis and otitis media. The latter frequently occurs in children in association with viral infection. Chronic infection of the mastoid or respiratory sinus sometimes extends to the subarachnoid space to cause meningitis. Pneumococci may also cause endocarditis, arthritis, and peritonitis, usually in association with bacteremia. Patients with ascites caused by diseases such as cirrhosis and nephritis may develop spontaneous pneumococcal peritonitis. Pneumococci do not cause pharyngitis or tonsillitis.

* Sinusitis and otitis media common

DIAGNOSIS

Gram smears of material from sputum and other sites of pneumococcal infection typically show Gram-positive, lancet-shaped diplococci (Figure 25–9). Sputum collection may be difficult, however, and specimens contaminated with respiratory flora are useless for diagnosis. Other types of lower respiratory specimens may be needed for diagnosis. *S pneumoniae* grows well overnight on blood agar medium and is usually distinguished from viridans streptococci by susceptibility to the synthetic chemical ethylhydrocupreine (optochin) or by a bile solubility (Table 25–2). Bacteremia is common in pneumococcal pneumonia and meningitis, and blood cultures are valuable supplements to cultures of local fluids or exudates. Detection of pneumococcal antigen in the urine or cerebrospinal fluid (CSF) can be useful, especially when sputum or CSF specimens show no growth owing to prior treatment. This is a simple, rapid card test that detects the C carbohydrate that is found in the cell wall of all pneumococci; it is not based on capsular types. The C antigen is large and is detectable in the urine for weeks to several months after pneumococcal pneumonia.

* Sputum quality complicates diagnosis

* Optochin, bile solubility distinguish from viridans streptococci

Urinary antigen test useful if cultures negative

TREATMENT

For decades pneumococci were uniformly susceptible to penicillin at concentrations of 0.06 µg/mL or less. In the late 1960s, this began to change, and strains with decreased susceptibility to all β-lactams began to emerge that resulted in treatment failures in cases of pneumonia and meningitis. The resistance is not absolute and can be overcome with increased dosage, depending on the minimum inhibitory concentration (MIC) and the site of infection. The mechanism involves alterations in the β-lactam target, the transpeptidase penicillin-binding proteins (PBPs) that crosslink peptidoglycan in cell wall synthesis. Resistant strains have mutations in one or more of

* Altered transpeptidases decrease penicillin susceptibility

these transpeptidases, which cause decreased affinity for penicillin and other β-lactams. Penicillinase is not produced. Resistance rates now exceed 10% in most locales and may be greater than 40% in some areas. Resistance to macrolides is increasing and is more likely with penicillin-resistant strains.

Antibiotic selection differs with the site of the infection and whether it is to be carried out as an outpatient or inpatient. Penicillin is still effective for susceptible strains, but the uncertainty has caused a shift toward azithromycin (outpatient) or ceftriaxone (inpatient) for primary treatment. Patients with meningitis caused by pneumococci with a penicillin MIC of more than 0.06 μg/mL require high doses of ceftriaxone plus vancomycin unless the ceftriaxone MIC is less than or equal to 0.5 μg/mL. The therapeutic response to treatment of pneumococcal pneumonia is often dramatic. Reduction in fever, respiratory rate, and cough can occur in 12 to 24 hours but may occur gradually over several days. Chest radiography may yield normal results only after several weeks.

Resistance criteria differ for meningitis and other sites

PREVENTION

Two pneumococcal vaccines prepared from capsular polysaccharide are now available. The first pneumococcal polysaccharide vaccine (PPV), available since 1977, contains purified polysaccharide extracted from the 23 serotypes of *S pneumoniae* most commonly isolated from invasive disease. It shares the T-cell-independent characteristics of other polysaccharide immunogens and is recommended for use only in those older than 2 years. In 2000, a pneumococcal conjugate vaccine (PCV) was introduced in which polysaccharide was conjugated with protein. This vaccine stimulates T-dependent T_H2 responses and is effective beginning at 2 months of age. In 2010, the original 7-valent vaccine was replaced by a 13-valent (PCV13) conjugate vaccine and is the standard for childhood immunization. Because of its broader coverage, the 23-valent PPV is recommended after age 2 except for immunocompromised children under 5, who should still receive PCV. Adults at age 65 years (or earlier if at special risk) should receive a single dose of PVC13 followed in 6 weeks by a dose of 23-valent PPV. The phenomenon of capsule switching (see Immunity above) is of concern as a mechanism for evading these vaccines. That is, a significant antigenic change in any of the serotypes covered by either vaccine could be the basis of failure to protect.

✴ **23-valent PPV is T-cell independent**

✴ **13-valent PCV stimulates T_H2 in children**

◼ Viridans Group and Nonhemolytic Streptococci

The viridans group comprises all α-hemolytic streptococci that remain after the criteria for defining pyogenic streptococci and pneumococci have been applied. Characteristically, members of the resident flora of the oropharyngeal cavity and gastrointestinal tract, they have the basic bacteriologic features of streptococci but lack the specific antigens, toxins, and virulence factors of the other groups. Although the viridans group includes many species (Table 25–2), they usually are not completely identified in practice because there is little clinical difference among them. The exception is for isolates from blood in patients with visceral or brain abscesses or suspected endocarditis. MALDI-TOF MS has greatly facilitated the identification streptococci within this group that are especially associated with invasive pyogenic infections and endocarditis. Notable examples are members of the *S bovis* group (*S gallilyticus* spp. *gallilyticus*), the *S aginosus* group, and the NVS or pyridoxal-requiring streptococci (*Granulicatella* and *Abiotrophia*). All of these streptococci are important causes of bacterial endocarditis and the S anginosus group (including *S constellatus* and *intermedius*) is also often found in abscesses.

Although their virulence is very low, other viridans group strains can cause disease when they are protected from host defenses. The prime example is subacute bacterial endocarditis. In this disease, viridans streptococci reach previously damaged heart valves as a result of transient bacteremia associated with manipulations, such as tooth extraction, which disturb their usual habitat. Protected by fibrin and platelets, they multiply on the valve, causing local and systemic disease that is fatal if untreated. Extracellular production of glucans, complex polysaccharide polymers, may enhance their attachment to cardiac valves in a manner similar to the pathogenesis of dental caries by *S mutans* (see **Chapter 41**). The clinical course of viridans streptococcal endocarditis is subacute, with slow progression over weeks or months. It is effectively treated with penicillin, but uniformly fatal if untreated. The disease is particularly associated with valves damaged by recurrent rheumatic fever. The decline in the occurrence of rheumatic heart disease has also reduced the incidence of this particular type of endocarditis.

✴ **Low-virulence species may cause endocarditis**

✴ **Glucan production enhances attachment**

Why do NVS (*Granulicatella* and *Abiotrophia*) grow readily in blood cultures but fail to grow when subcultured to sheep blood agar (SBA) plates?

● ENTEROCOCCI

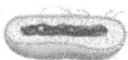

BACTERIOLOGY

* Enterococci have group D antigen

* Intestinal inhabitants resist action of bile salts

Until genomic studies dictated their separation into the genus *Enterococcus*, the enterococci were classified as streptococci. Indeed, the most common enterococcal species share the bacteriologic characteristics previously described for pyogenic streptococci, including presence of the Lancefield group D antigen. The term "enterococcus" derives from their presence in the intestinal tract and the many biochemical and cultural features that reflect that habitat. These include the ability to grow in the presence of high concentrations of bile salts and sodium chloride. Most enterococci produce nonhemolytic or α-hemolytic colonies that are larger than those of most streptococci. A dozen species are recognized based on biochemical and cultural reactions (Table 25–2) of which *Enterococcus faecalis* and *Enterococcus faecium* are the most common. All enterococci are pyrrolidonyl-arylamidase (PYR)-positive.

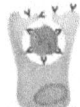

ENTEROCOCCAL DISEASE

EPIDEMIOLOGY

Enterococci are part of the resident intestinal flora. Although they are capable of producing disease in many settings, the hospital environment is where a substantial increase has occurred in the last two decades. Patients with extensive abdominal surgery, transplantation, or indwelling devices or those who are undergoing procedures such as peritoneal dialysis are at greatest risk. Prolonged hospital stays and prior antimicrobial therapy, particularly with fluoroquinolones, cephalosporins, or aminoglycosides, are also risk factors. Most infections are acquired from the endogenous flora but spread between patients has been documented. A substantial number of nosocomial urinary tract, intra-abdominal, and bloodstream infections are due to enterococci.

Endogenous infection is associated with medical procedures

PATHOGENESIS

Enterococci are a significant cause of disease in hospitals and extended-care facilities, but they are not highly virulent. On their own, they do not produce fulminant disease and in wound and soft tissue infections are usually mixed with other members of the intestinal flora. Some have even doubted their significance when isolated together with more virulent members of the Enterobacteriaceae or *Bacteroides fragilis*. *E faecalis* has been shown to form biofilms sticking to medical devices and to possess surface proteins adherent to urinary epithelium. *E faecalis* is also an important cause of bacterial endocarditis. More than anything, enterococci, especially *E faecium*, seem to be very effective at withstanding environmental and antimicrobial agent stresses.

Virulence factors poorly understood

* Persist in healthcare environment

Think ▸▸ Apply 25-3: Human blood has ample pyridoxal (B_6), an essential vitamin for humans, for growth, whereas sheep blood lacks pyridoxal as do SBA plates. Although NVS are not strict anaerobes, they will grow on anaerobic blood agar plates because the base ingredients differ from those in SBAs and include B_6. A simple solution would be to add pyridoxal to SBAs; however, doing so interferes with the quality of β-hemolysis and negates the reason SBAs are preferred. If a paper disk containing pyridoxal is placed on an SBA plate incubated aerobically, growth of colonies around the disk indicates NVS.

⚕ ENTEROCOCCAL DISEASE: CLINICAL ASPECTS

MANIFESTATIONS

Enterococci cause opportunistic urinary tract infections (UTIs) and occasionally wound and soft tissue infections, in much the same fashion as members of the Enterobacteriaceae. Infections are often associated with urinary tract manipulations, malignancies, biliary tract disease, and gastrointestinal disorders. Vascular or peritoneal catheters are often points of entry. Respiratory tract infections are rare. There is sometimes an associated bacteremia, which can result in the development of endocarditis on previously damaged cardiac valves.

※ UTIs and soft tissue infections most common

TREATMENT

The outstanding feature of the enterococci is their high and increasing levels of resistance to antimicrobial agents. Their inherent relative resistance to most β-lactams, complete resistance to all cephalosporins, and high-level resistance to aminoglycosides can be viewed as a kind of virulence factor in the hospital environment where these agents are widely used. Enterococci also have particularly efficient means of acquiring plasmid and transposon resistance genes from themselves and other species. All enterococci require 4 to 16 µg/mL of penicillin for inhibition owing to decreased affinity of their PBPs for all β-lactams. Higher levels of resistance have been increasing, especially in *E faecium*, owing to altered PBPs. Ampicillin remains the most consistently active agent against *E faecalis*.

※ Inherent resistance enhanced by altered PBPs

Enterococci share with streptococci a resistance to aminoglycosides based on failure of the antibiotic to be actively transported into the cell. Despite this, many strains of enterococci are inhibited and rapidly killed by low concentrations of penicillin when combined with an aminoglycoside. Under these conditions, the action of penicillin on the cell wall allows the aminoglycoside to enter the cell, where it can then act at its ribosomal site. Some strains show high-level resistance to aminoglycosides based on mutations at the ribosomal binding site or the presence of aminoglycoside-inactivating enzymes. These strains do not demonstrate synergistic effects with penicillin.

※ Synergy between penicillin and aminoglycosides based on access to ribosomes

Recently, resistance to vancomycin, the antibiotic most often used for ampicillin-resistant strains of enterococci has emerged (almost all are *E faecium* strains) Vancomycin resistance is due to a subtle change in peptidoglycan precursors, which are generated by ligases that modify the terminal amino acids of crosslinking side chains at the point where β-lactams bind. The modifications decrease the binding affinity for penicillins 1000-fold without a detectable loss in peptidoglycan strength. Although hospitals vary, the average rate of resistance in enterococci isolated from intensive care units is around 20%. Enterococci are intrinsically resistant to sulfonamides, clindamycin, and cephalosporins.

※ Vancomycin resistance emerging threat

Ligases modify peptidoglycan side chains

Ampicillin remains the agent of choice for most UTIs and minor soft tissue infections. More severe infections, particularly endocarditis, are usually treated with combinations of a penicillin or ampicillin combined with gentamicin or streptomycin. If susceptible, vancomycin can be used for patients with severe reactions to ampicillin who cannot be desensitized. Linezolid is an alternative if there is no other effective option.

※ Ampicillin or combinations of antimicrobials are used

KEY CONCLUSIONS

- *Streptococcus pyogenes* (Group A) is a preeminent pyogenic pathogen.
- Group A streptococci harbor multiple virulence factors.
- M protein, which is antiphagocytic, is essential in surface attachment and the basis of type-specific immunity.
- Superantigenicity of streptococcal SAgs contributes to invasiveness and STSS.
- Group A streptococci are the foremost cause of bacterial pharyngitis.
- Skin and soft tissue infections are common and may be severe.
- Rheumatic fever and glomerulonephritis are immunopathologic sequelae of GAS infections.
- Group B streptococci (GBS) are important neonatal pathogens due to the presence of a polysaccharide capsule.

- Antimicrobial prophylaxis at delivery for women colonized with GBS is essential.
- *Streptococcus pneumoniae* is also encapsulated and causes pneumonia and meningitis with sequelae.
- *S gallilyticus* subsp. *gallalyticus* is highly associated with endocarditis and colon cancer.
- All enterococci are PYR-positive.
- Enterococci are opportunistic pathogens and often resistant to antimicrobials.
- *Enterococcus faecalis* is an important cause of endocarditis.

CASE STUDY

Sore Throat, Murmur, and Painful Swollen Joints

An 8-year-old boy presented with a 1-day history of fever (39°C), associated with painful swelling of the right wrist and left knee. The patient had a sore throat 2 weeks before the present illness, which was treated with salicylates. No cultures were obtained. The last medical history was essentially negative, and the boy had no history of drug allergy, weight loss, rash, dyspnea, or illness in siblings.

PHYSICAL EXAMINATION: Temperature (39°C), blood pressure 120/80 mm Hg, pulse 110/min, respirations 28/min. The patient was ill-appearing. He avoided movement of the right wrist and left knee, which were swollen, red, hot, and tender. He had a moderately injected oropharynx without exudate and an enlarged right cervical lymph node estimated to be 1 × 1 cm. The precordium was active and, a systolic thrill could be felt. Auscultation of the heart revealed a heart rate of 120/min, normal heart sounds, and a grade III/VI holosystolic murmur over the apex not transmitting toward the axilla. Lungs were clear. No rush or hepatosplenomegaly was present, and the neurologic examination was normal.

LABORATORY DATA:

Hemoglobin 12 g, Hct 37%, WBC 16,500/mm³

Sedimentation rate 90 mm/h

Urinalysis: Normal

Serology: Antistreptolysin O (ASO) titer 666 Todd units (normal <200)

Chest X-ray: Normal (no cardiomegaly)

Throat culture: Negative for group A β-hemolytic streptococci

Blood culture: Negative

Electrocardiogram: Essentially normal except for mild ST depression and nonspecific T-wave changes on V6

Aspirate from left knee: 3 mL of yellow and turbid fluid

WBCs: 3000/mm³ mainly polymorphonuclear leukocytes

Gram stain: Negative

Culture: No growth

QUESTIONS

1. This patient's condition is most probably a case of:
   A. Strep throat
   B. Scarlet fever
   C. Streptococcal toxic shock
   D. Rheumatic fever
   E. Poststreptococcal glomerulonephritis

2. This boy's joint and cardiac findings are due to:
   A. Circulating streptococcal pyrogenic exotoxin
   B. Circulating streptolysin O
   C. Antibody directed against M protein
   D. Antibody directed against streptolysin O (ASO)
   E. Circulating group A streptococci

3. The illness could have been prevented by:
   A. Penicillin treatment of the sore throat
   B. Penicillin treatment at the onset of joint pain
   C. Aspirin at any point
   D. Streptococcal vaccine in infancy
   E. There is no prevention

4. The etiology of the sore throat would have been best determined by:
   A. ASO titer
   B. Throat culture
   C. Throat antigen detection
   D. Exudate on tonsils
   E. Presence of cervical lymphadenopathy

ANSWERS

1. **(D)**

2. **(C)**

3. **(A)**

4. **(B)**

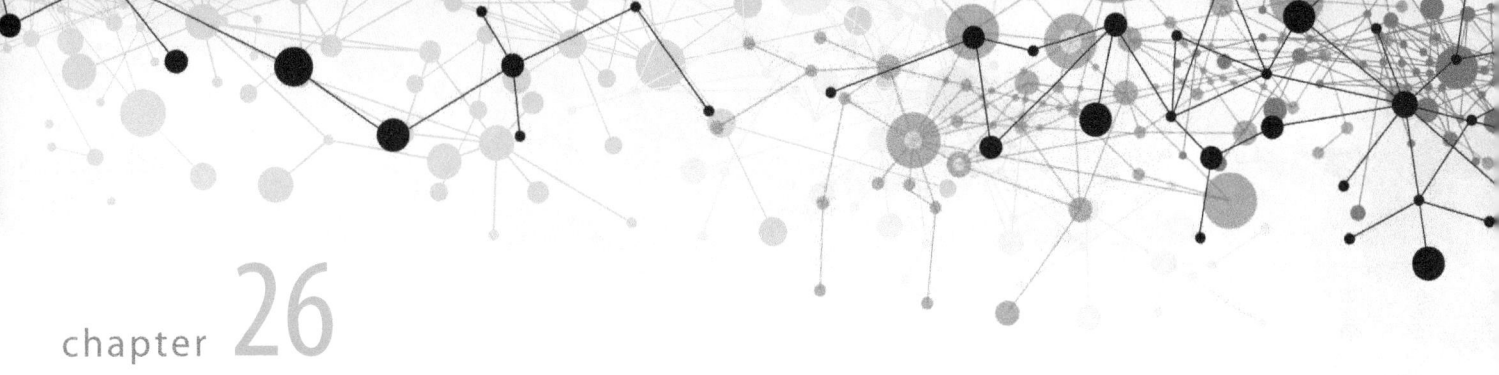

chapter 26

Corynebacterium, Listeria, and Bacillus

Corynebacterium diphtheriae · Listeria monocytogenes · Bacillus anthracis · Bacillus cereus

So Asthma Mark would sit on the corner

And he would play his Diphtheria Blues

—Frank Zappa

OVERVIEW

Corynebacteria are small, pleomorphic Gram-positive rods that include *Corynebacterium diphtheriae*, the foremost pathogen and cause of diphtheria. Other species are common skin flora, rarely cause disease, and often are found as contaminants in blood cultures. Diphtheria is the disease resulting from the local and systemic effects of diphtheria toxin (DT), a potent inhibitor of protein synthesis. The local disease is a severe pharyngitis typically accompanied by a plaque-like pseudomembrane that adheres to and ultimately occludes the throat and trachea. The life-threatening aspects of diphtheria are from suffocation and the consequences of absorption of the DT across the pharyngeal mucosa and its circulation in the bloodstream. Multiple organs are affected, but the most important is the heart, where the toxin produces an acute myocarditis.

Listeria monocytogenes is the only human pathogen in its genus. Importantly, it is catalase positive like corynebacteria, which it resembles morphologically, and unlike catalase-negative Group B streptococci, which it otherwise mimics when isolated on sheep blood agar. *L monocytogenes* causes listeriosis for which pregnant women are at greatest risk. Although insidious in onset, listeriosis can be devastating for the fetus and may result in stillbirth or multiorgan involvement and fulminant sepsis. *Listeria* also causes meningitis in newborns and immunocompromised adults. Although susceptible to ampicillin, *Listeria* are intrinsically resistant to all cephalosporins.

The genus *Bacillus* has hundreds of species of aerobic spore-forming Gram-positive bacilli; only two are human pathogens and of these *Bacillus anthracis* is paramount both for its bioterrorism potential and the severity of disseminated disease owing to its potent tri-component exotoxin (lethal factor, protective antigen, and edema factor). Anthrax occurs in three clinical forms: cutaneous, systemic, and gastrointestinal. When spores are inoculated with trauma to the skin, a localized eschar with surrounding edema ensues (Figure 26–8). When spores are inhaled, lethal hemorrhagic pneumonia, mediastinitis, and meningitis may result. Consumption of meat from infected animals can result in oropharyngeal or gastrointestinal anthrax. *Bacillus cereus* can cause rapidly destructive lesions of the eye following trauma, opportunistic infections, and food poisoning owing to enterotoxin production.

This chapter includes a variety of highly pathogenic Gram-positive rods that are not currently common causes of human disease. Their medical importance lies in the lessons learned when they were more common, and the continued threat their existence poses. *Corynebacterium diphtheriae*, the cause of diphtheria, is a prototype for toxigenic disease. *L monocytogenes* is a sporadic cause of meningitis and other infections in the fetus, newborn, and immunocompromised host. Occurrences in 2001 have served as a painful reminder that *B anthracis*, the cause of anthrax, is still the agent with the most potential for use in bioterrorism. The characteristics of these bacilli are presented in **Table 26–1.**

TABLE 26–1 Features of Aerobic Gram-positive Bacilli

ORGANISM	CAPSULE	ENDOSPORES	MOTILITY	TOXINS	SOURCE	DISEASE
Corynebacterium diphtheriae	–	–	–	DT	Human cases, carriers	Diphtheria
Listeria monocytogenes	–	–	+	LLO	Food, animals	Meningitis, bacteremia
Bacillus						
B anthracis	+	–	–	Exotoxin[a]	Imported animal products	Anthrax
B cereus	–	+	+	Enterotoxin, pyogenic toxin	Ubiquitous	Food poisoning, opportunistic infection
Other species	–	+	+		Ubiquitous	

DT, diphtheria toxin; LLO, listeriolysin O.
[a]Exotoxin contains three components: lethal factor, protective antigen, and edema factor.

● CORYNEBACTERIA

Corynebacteria (from the Greek *koryne*, club) are small and pleomorphic. The genus *Corynebacterium* includes many species of aerobic and facultative Gram-positive rods. The cells tend to have clubbed ends and often remain attached after division, forming "Chinese letter" or palisade arrangements. Spores are not formed. Growth is generally best under aerobic conditions on media enriched with blood or other animal products, but many strains grow anaerobically. Colonies on blood agar are typically small (1-2 mm), and most are nonhemolytic. Catalase is produced, and many strains form acid (usually lactic acid) through carbohydrate fermentation. Surface and cell wall structure is similar to other Gram-positive bacteria. Most corynebacteria are nonpathogenic commensal inhabitants of the pharynx, nasopharynx, distal urethra, and skin; they are collectively referred to as "diphtheroids" and are common contaminants of blood and urine cultures. *Cutibacterium* (*Propionibacterium*) *acnes* grows best anaerobically, is part of the skin microbiota, and usually is a contaminant but rarely can cause infection. Species that have disease associations are included in **Table 26-2**. The foremost exception to the above corynebacteriae is *C diphtheriae* owing to its powerful exotoxin that causes diphtheria.

✳ Pleomorphic club-shaped rods

Corynebacteria called diphtheroids

TABLE 26–2 Other Aerobic and Facultative Gram-positive Bacilli

ORGANISM	FEATURES	EPIDEMIOLOGY	DISEASE
Corynebacterium spp.	Typical club-shape morphology, common contaminant of blood cultures	Normal skin and mucosal flora	Rare cause of bacterial endocarditis
C jeikeium	Multiresistant, often susceptible only to vancomycin	Acquired from skin colonization	Bacteremia, IV catheter colonization
Erysipelothrix rhusiopathiae	Resembles corynebacteria and *Listeria*, intrinsically resistant to vancomycin	Traumatic inoculation from animal and decaying organic matter	Erysipeloid, painful, slow-spreading, erythematous swelling of skin. Occupational disease of fishermen, butchers, and veterinarians
Lactobacillus spp.	Long, slender rods with squared ends, often chain end-to-end	Normal oral, gastrointestinal, and vaginal flora	No human infections *L acidophilus* plays role in pathogenesis of dental caries
Cutibacterium acnes (Propionibacterium)	Resemble corynebacteria, anaerobes, or microaerophiles	Normal skin flora	Rare cause of bacterial endocarditis
Arcanobacterium haemolyticum	Formerly in *Corynebacterium* genus, β-hemolytic	Respiratory flora	Pharyngitis, soft tissue infections

DT, diphtheria toxin; IV, intravenous.

CORYNEBACTERIUM DIPHTHERIAE

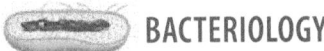 **BACTERIOLOGY**

C diphtheriae (from the Greek *diphthera*, leather) are differentiated from other corynebacteria by the appearance of colonies on the selective media used for its isolation and a variety of biochemical reactions. Strains of *C diphtheriae* may or may not produce **DT.** The gene for DT is contained in the genome of a bacteriophage, which is lysogenic in the *C diphtheriae* chromosome. For strains with the gene, DT production is controlled by a repressor protein (DtxR), which responds to iron concentrations and also regulates other toxin-related functions.

❋ C diphtheriae produces exotoxin

DT gene in lysogenic phage

DT is an A-B toxin that acts in the cytoplasm to inhibit protein synthesis irreversibly in a wide variety of eukaryotic cells. After binding mediated by the B subunit, both the A and B subunits enter the cell in an endocytotic vacuole. In the low pH of the vacuole, the toxin unfolds, exposing sites that facilitate translocation of the A subunit from the phagosome to the cytosol. The target is elongation factor 2 (EF-2), which transfers polypeptidyl-transfer RNA from acceptor to donor sites on the ribosome of the host cell. The specific action of the A subunit is to inactivate EF-2, by **ADP-ribosylation** (ADPR), which shuts off protein synthesis. The details of DT action are illustrated in Chapter 1 (Figure 1–7) as a prototype toxin. *C diphtheriae* itself is unaffected because it uses a protein other than EF-2 for the same steps in protein synthesis.

❋ A subunit enters cytosol from vacuole

❋ EF-2 inactivated by ADPR

❋ tRNA blockage stops protein synthesis

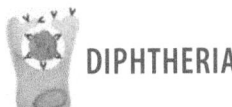 **DIPHTHERIA**

EPIDEMIOLOGY

C diphtheriae is transmitted by droplet spread, by direct contact with cutaneous infections, and, to a lesser extent, by fomites (**Figure 26–1**). Some subjects become convalescent pharyngeal or nasal carriers and continue to harbor the organism for weeks, months, or longer. Diphtheria is rare where immunization is widely practiced. In the United States, for example, fewer than 10 cases are now reported each year. These usually occur as small outbreaks in populations that have not received adequate immunization, such as migrant workers, transients, and those who refuse immunization on religious grounds. It has been more than 25 years since any outbreak exceeded 50 cases.

❋ Transmitted by respiratory droplets

Most cases unimmunized

Diphtheria still occurs in developing countries and in places where public health infrastructure has been disrupted. For example, in the former Soviet Union, where the annual number of diphtheria cases had been below 200, over 47,000 cases and 1700 deaths occurred between 1990 and 1995. This outbreak followed the reintroduction of *C diphtheriae* into a population where the public health systems had broken down as a result of the political situation. Reinstitution of effective immunization brought diphtheria rates back to base levels.

❋ Outbreaks when immunization rates decrease

PATHOGENESIS

C diphtheriae has little invasive capacity, and diphtheria is due to the local and systemic effects of DT, a protein exotoxin with potent cytotoxic features (**Figure 26–2**). It inhibits protein synthesis in cell-free extracts of virtually all eukaryotic cells, from protozoa and yeasts to higher plants and humans. Its toxicity for intact cells varies among mammals and organs, primarily due to differences in toxin binding and uptake. In humans, the B subunit binds to one of a common family of eukaryotic receptors that regulate cell growth and differentiation, thus exploiting a normal cell function.

❋ B subunit binding determines cell susceptibility

The production of DT has both local and systemic effects. Locally, its action on epithelial cells leads to necrosis and inflammation, forming an adherent, leathery pseudomembrane composed of a coagulum of fibrin, leukocytes, and cellular debris. The extent of the pseudomembrane varies from a local plaque to an extensive covering of much of the tracheobronchial tree. Absorption and circulation of DT allow binding throughout the body. Myocardial cells are most affected; eventually, acute myocarditis develops.

❋ Local effects produce pseudomembrane

❋ DT absorption leads to myocarditis

FIGURE 26-1. **Diphtheria overview.** Infection with *Corynebacterium diphtheriae* is acquired by respiratory droplet spread. The throat and upper airways are infected, but there is no invasion. Diphtheria toxin (DT) produced at the primary side is absorbed into the bloodstream and affects multiple organs, particularly the heart where acute myocarditis is produced.

Diphtheria

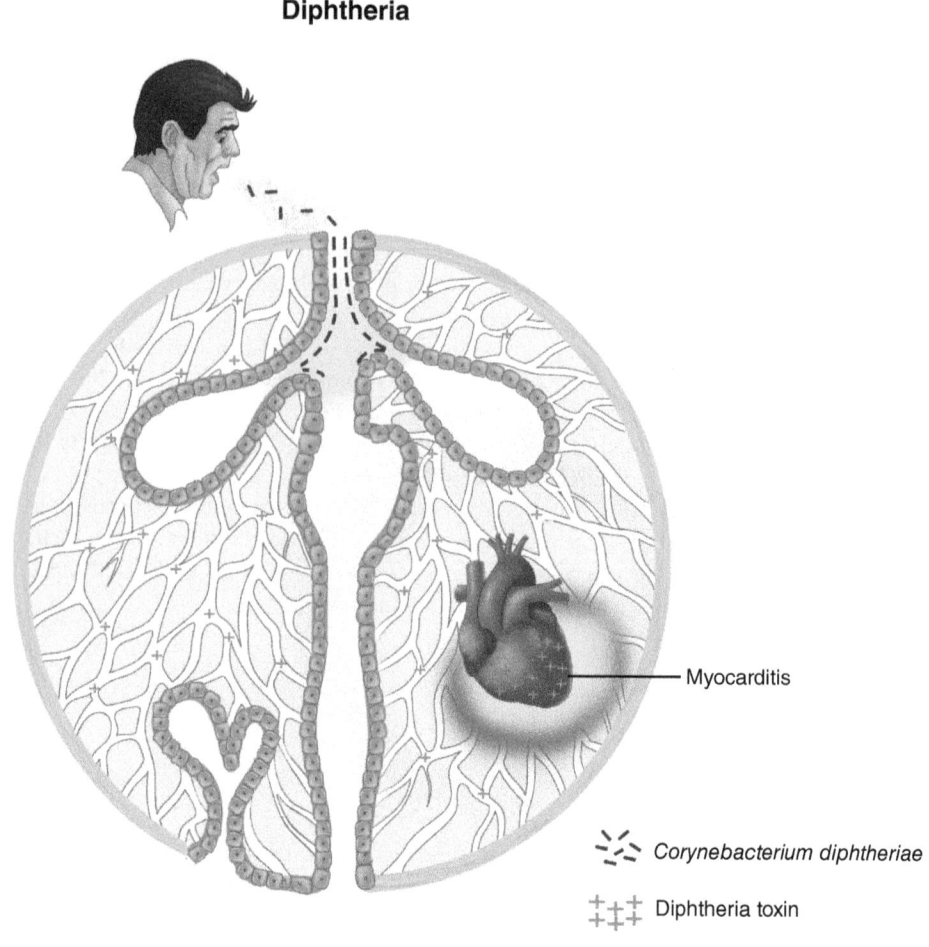

— Myocarditis

Corynebacterium diphtheriae

Diphtheria toxin

IMMUNITY

❋ Antibodies neutralize toxin

❋ Toxoid is inactivated DT

DT is antigenic, stimulating the production of protective antitoxin antibodies during natural infection. Formalin treatment of toxin produces **toxoid,** which retains the antigenicity but not the toxicity of native toxin and is used in immunization against the disease. It is clear that this process functionally inactivates fragment B. Whether it also inactivates fragment A or prevents its ability to dissociate from fragment B is not known. Molecular studies of the A subunit structure and action suggest that another approach to immunization may be by genetic engineering of the A subunit so that it fails to bind EF-2 but retains its antigenicity.

DIPHTHERIA: CLINICAL ASPECTS

MANIFESTATIONS

❋ Severe pharyngitis may have exudate or membrane

After an incubation period of 2 to 4 days, diphtheria usually manifests as pharyngitis or tonsillitis. Typically, malaise, sore throat, and fever occur, and a patch of exudate or membrane develops on the tonsils, uvula, soft palate, or pharyngeal wall. The gray-white pseudomembrane (**Figure 26–3**) adheres to the mucous membrane and may extend from the oropharyngeal area down to the larynx and into the trachea. Associated cervical adenitis is common, and in severe cases cervical adenitis and edema produce a "bull neck" appearance. In uncomplicated cases, the infection gradually resolves, and the membrane is coughed up after 5 to 10 days.

The complications and lethal effects of diphtheria are caused by respiratory obstruction or by the systemic effect of DT absorbed at the site of infection. Mechanical obstruction of the airway produced by the pseudomembrane, edema, and hemorrhage can be sudden and complete and can lead to suffocation, particularly if large sections of the membrane separate from the tracheal or

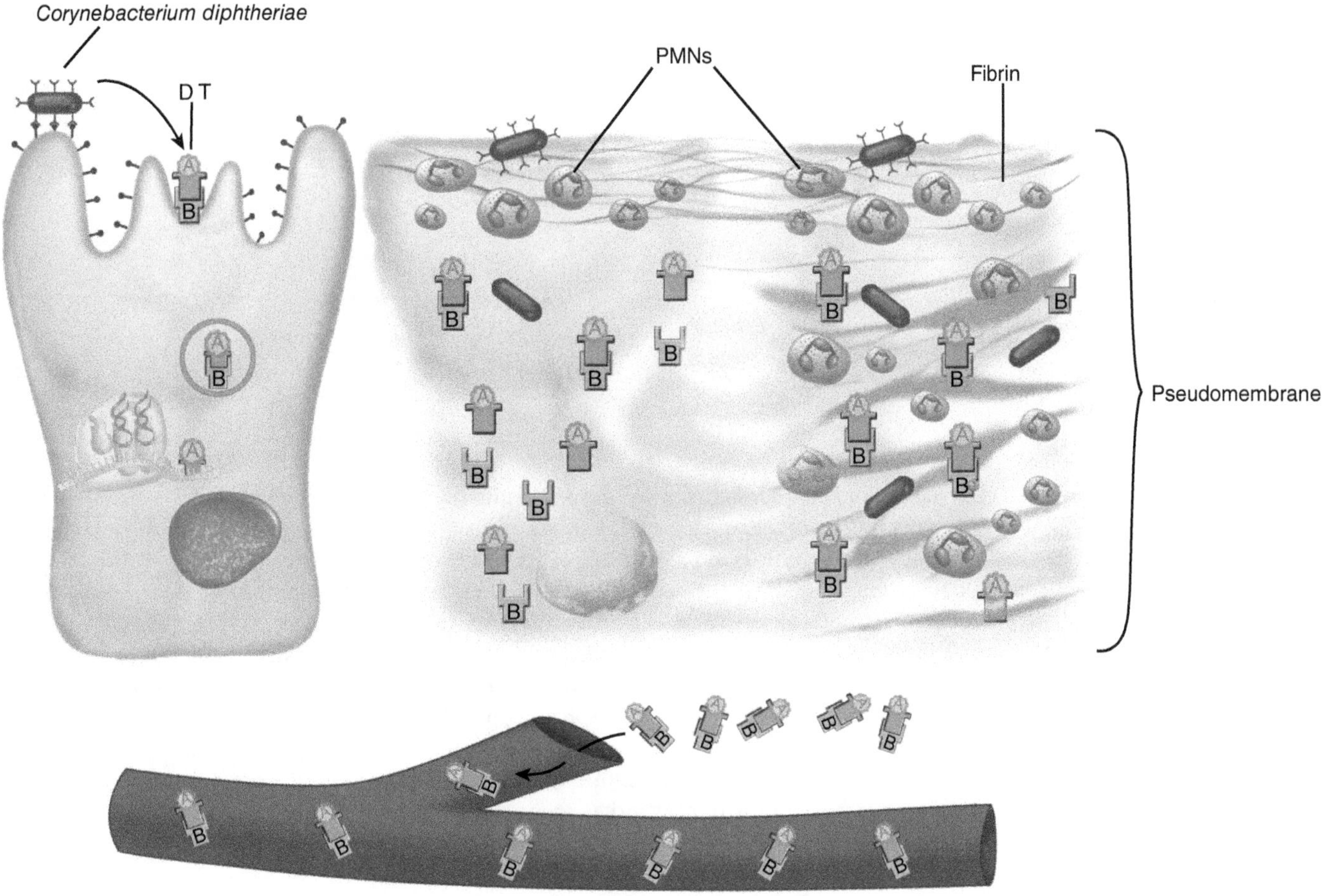

Corynebacterium diphtheriae

D T

PMNs

Fibrin

Pseudomembrane

FIGURE 26-2. Diphtheria cellular view. (*Left*) *Corynebacterium diphtheriae* binds to epithelial cells and secretes diphtheria toxin (DT). The A-B toxin enters the cell, and the A subunit exits the endocytotic vacuole. In the cytoplasm, the A subunit catalyzes the ADP-ribosylation of EF-2, which inhibits protein synthesis at the ribosome (see Figure 1–7). (*Middle*) The cell is dying and superficial inflammation brings polymorphonuclear neutrophils (PMNs) and fibrin. (*Right*) The cell is destroyed and the inflammatory components have coalesced into a pseudomembrane. The bacteria do not invade, but DT enters the bloodstream.

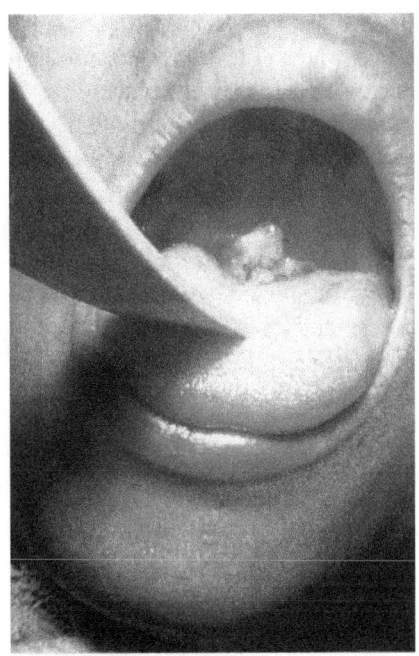

FIGURE 26-3. Diphtheria. Typical appearance of a diphtheritic pseudomembrane adherent to the oropharynx of this child. (Reproduced with permission from Connor DH, Chandler FW, Schwartz DQ, et al: *Pathology of Infectious Diseases.* Stamford CT: Appleton & Lange; 1997.)

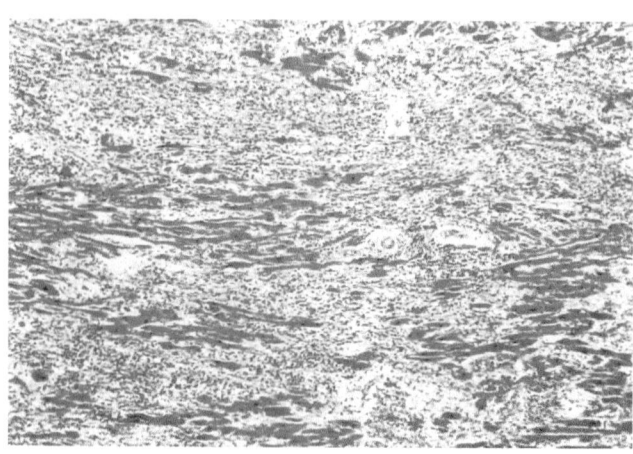

FIGURE 26-4. **Diphtheritic myocarditis.** Necrosis and inflammation are present in this section of myocardium from a fatal case of diphtheria. (Reproduced with permission from Connor DH, Chandler FW, Schwartz DQ, et al: *Pathology of Infectious Diseases.* Stamford CT: Appleton & Lange; 1997.)

laryngeal epithelial surface. The DT absorbed into the circulation causes injury to various organs, most seriously the heart. Diphtheritic myocarditis (**Figure 26–4**) can be detected by electrocardiography in two-thirds of patients and is serious enough to cause cardiac malfunction in up to 25%. It appears during the second or third week and is manifested by cardiac enlargement, arrhythmia, and congestive heart failure with dyspnea. Nervous system involvement appears later in the course of disease, most often involving paralysis of the soft palate, oculomotor (eye) muscles, or select muscle groups. The paralysis is reversible and is generally not serious unless the diaphragm is involved. The disease resolves with the formation of antitoxin antibody.

C diphtheriae may produce nonrespiratory infections, particularly of the skin. The characteristic lesion ranges from a simple pustule to a chronic nonhealing ulcer and is most common in tropical and hot, arid regions. Cardiac and neurologic complications from these infections are infrequent, suggesting that the efficiency of toxin production or absorption is low compared with that in respiratory infections.

* Pseudomembrane can block the airway

* DT myocarditis may lead to congestive heart failure

* Cutaneous ulcerative lesion

DIAGNOSIS

The initial diagnosis of diphtheria is entirely clinical. There are presently no rapid laboratory tests of sufficient value to influence the decision regarding antitoxin administration. Direct smears of infected areas of the throat are not reliable diagnostic tools. Definitive diagnosis is accomplished by isolating and identifying *C diphtheriae* from the infected site and demonstrating its toxigenicity. Isolation is usually achieved with a selective medium containing potassium tellurite (eg, Tinsdale medium).

Although the diagnosis of diphtheria could once be made and confirmed with great confidence, it is now more difficult because experience with the disease is rare. Most physicians have never seen a case of diphtheria, and most laboratories have never isolated the organism and do not even stock the required medium. Because routine throat culture procedures do not detect *C diphtheriae*, the physician must advise the laboratory of the suspicion of diphtheria in advance. Generally, 2 days are required to exclude *C diphtheriae* (no colonies isolated on Tinsdale agar); however, more time is needed to complete identification and toxigenicity testing of a positive culture.

* Primary diagnosis clinical

* Culture requires special medium

Laboratory must be notified of suspicion

TREATMENT

Treatment of diphtheria is directed at neutralization of the toxin with concurrent elimination of the organism. The former is most critical and is accomplished by promptly administering a diphtheria antitoxin, an antiserum produced in horses. It must be administered early because it only neutralizes circulating toxin and has no effect on toxin already fixed to or within cells. *C diphtheriae* is susceptible to multiple antimicrobials, but erythromycin has been the most effective. Penicillin is an alternative. The complications of diphtheria are managed primarily by supportive measures.

* Antitoxin neutralizes free toxin

* Erythromycin effective therapy

PREVENTION

The mainstay of diphtheria prevention is immunization. The vaccine is highly effective. Three to four doses of diphtheria toxoid produce immunity by stimulating antitoxin production. The initial series is begun in the first year of life. Booster immunizations at 10-year intervals maintain immunity. Fully immunized individuals may become infected with *C diphtheriae* because the

* DT toxoid with 10-year boosters

antibodies are directed only against the toxin, but the disease is mild. Serious infection and death occur only in unimmunized or incompletely immunized individuals. Immunization with DT toxoid prevents serious toxin-mediated disease.

KEY CONCLUSIONS

- Corynebacteria are small, pleomorphic catalase-positive rods.
- Pathogenic *C diphtheria* produce potent diphtheria toxin which inhibits protein synthesis.
- Clinical manifestations include pharyngitis, respiratory obstruction, and acute myocarditis. A cutaneous form includes pustule and ulcers.
- Diagnosis is initially clinical; etiologic confirmation requires special media.
- Immunization with inactivated toxin (diphtheria toxoid) is protective.

● LISTERIA MONOCYTOGENES

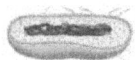 ## BACTERIOLOGY

L monocytogenes is a Gram-positive rod with some bacteriologic features that resemble those of both corynebacteria and streptococci. In stained smears of clinical and laboratory material, the organisms resemble diphtheroids. *Listeria* are not difficult to grow in culture, producing small, β-hemolytic colonies that resemble those of group B streptococci on blood agar. *Listeria* like corynebacteria, however, are catalase positive whereas streptococci are not. An unusual feature for human pathogens is the ability of *L monocytogenes* to grow slowly in the cold, even at temperatures below 0°C. This is due to the action of enzymes (RNA helicases) induced at low temperatures. Growth at refrigerator temperatures turns out to be important in the foodborne transmission of *L monocytogenes* (see epidemiology later). *Listeria* species are catalase positive, which distinguishes them from streptococci, and they produce a characteristic tumbling motility in fluid media at temperatures below 30°C, which distinguishes them from corynebacteria.

L monocytogenes is the only one of six *Listeria* species pathogenic for humans. There are 13 serotypes based on flagellar and surface antigens, but most human cases are limited to only three (1/2a, 1/2b, 4b). The major virulence factors are a group of invasion-associated surface proteins called **internalins** and a pore-forming cytotoxin, **listeriolysin O** (LLO).

＊ Rods resemble corynebacteria

＊ Colonies β-hemolytic

＊ Enzymes allow growth in cold

＊ Internalin, LLO enhance virulence

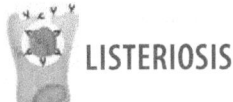 ## LISTERIOSIS

EPIDEMIOLOGY

L monocytogenes is widespread in nature, in soil, ground water, decaying vegetation, and the intestinal tract of animals including those associated with our food supply (eg, fowl and ungulates). The importance of foodborne transmission of listeriosis (**Figure 26–5**) was not recognized until the early 1980s. A widely publicized 1985 California outbreak involved consumption of Mexican-style soft cheese and included 86 cases and 29 deaths; most cases were among mother–infant pairs. The devastating association of listeriosis with pregnancy was dramatically demonstrated in South Africa in 2017 in the largest common source ever reported with 937 cases in which 50% were linked to pregnancy, 87% were in neonates, and 27% died. The culprit was polony (a baloney-like processed meat) processed at a single factory. Dairy product outbreaks have been traced to postpasteurization contamination or deviation from recommended time and temperature guidelines. An important feature of some epidemics has been the ability of *L monocytogenes* to grow at refrigerator temperatures, allowing scant numbers to reach an infectious dose during storage. This persistence is enhanced by its ability to form biofilms, which make surfaces and packages more difficult to decontaminate. Heightened awareness has implicated many other foodstuffs, particularly those prepared from animal products in a ready-to-eat form such as poultry items, sausages, and sliced meats as in the South African catastrophe.

Widespread in nature and animals

＊ Foodborne transmission from animal products

＊ Cold growth, biofilms enhance infectivity

FIGURE 26-5. **Listeriosis overview.** *Listeria monocytogenes* is ingested in dairy and meat products. It invades through the intestinal mucosa producing a bacteremia. The organisms may seed elsewhere particularly the brain (meningitis) or the fetus in pregnancy.

Listeriosis

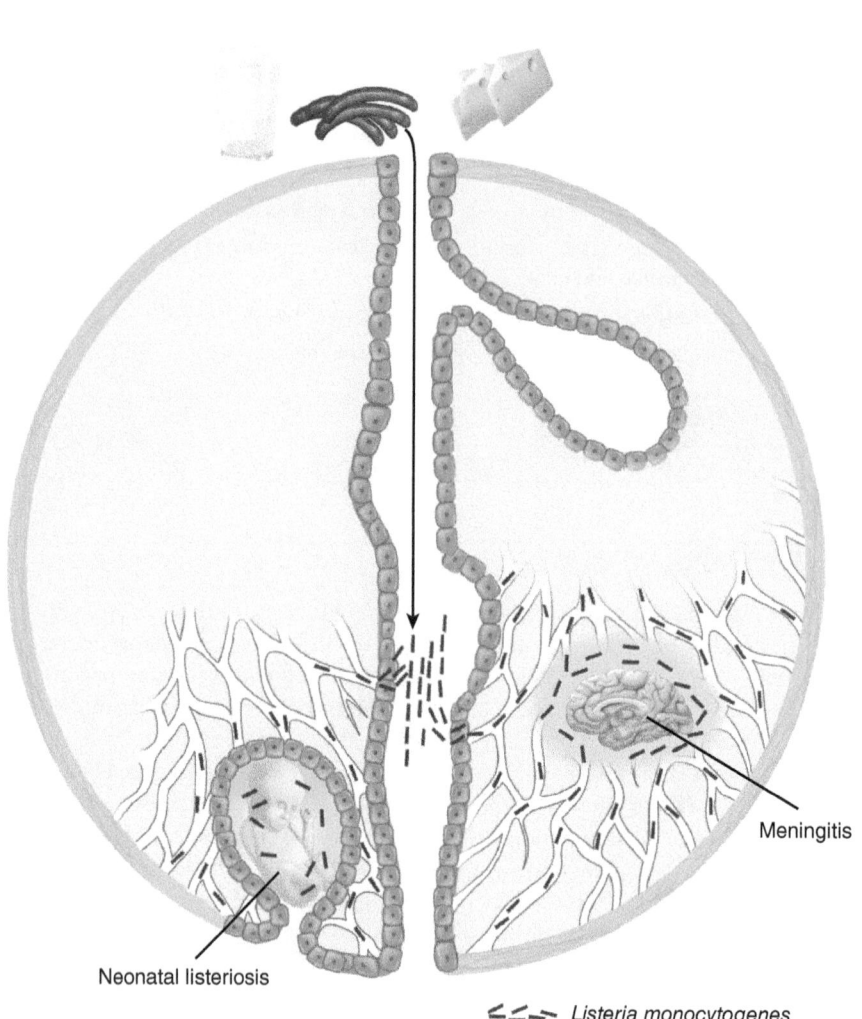

Meningitis

Neonatal listeriosis

⊂⊂⊏ *Listeria monocytogenes*

L monocytogenes may also be transmitted transplacentally to the fetus, presumably following hematogenous dissemination in the mother. It may also be transmitted to newborns in the birth canal in a manner similar to group B streptococci. Listeriosis is still not a reportable disease in the United States, but active surveillance studies indicate that it may account for more than 1000 cases and 200 deaths each year. Most cases occur at the extremes of life (eg, neonates or adults more than 60 years of age).

Transplacental and birth canal transmission can occur

PATHOGENESIS

L monocytogenes animal models have long been used for the study of cell-mediated immunity because of the ability of the organism to grow in nonimmune macrophages and the requirement for activated macrophages to clear the infection. *L monocytogenes* is able to induce its own uptake by nonprofessional and professional phagocytes including enterocytes, fibroblasts, dendritic cells, hepatocytes, endothelial cells, M cells, and macrophages. The first step in this process takes place when various surface proteins bind to fibronectin on the enterocyte surface followed by internalin attaching to its host cell receptor, E-cadherin. The internalin-E-cadherin binding triggers internalization of *L monocytogenes* in an endocytic vacuole. Inside the cell, the organism escapes from the phagosome to the cytosol in a matter of minutes. This escape is mediated by lysing of the vacuole's membrane by the pore-forming LLO and bacterial phospholipases. It takes place so quickly there is no time for lysosomes to fuse with the invading endosome.

Once in the cytosol, *L monocytogenes* continues to move through the cell by disrupting the metabolism of the cell's actin and microtubule infrastructure. This process is mediated by LLO and other proteins, particularly the ones that control actin polymerization (**Figure 26–6**).

✳ Grows in nonimmune macrophages

✳ Surface proteins, internalin start invasion

✳ LLO aids escape from phagosome

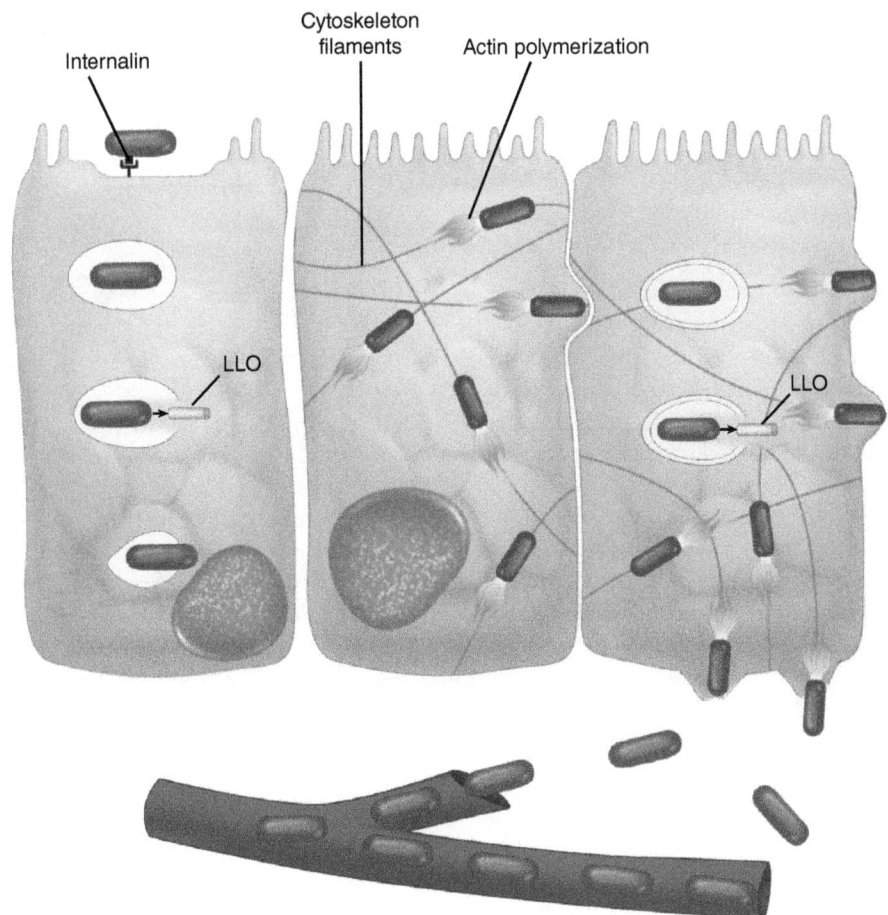

Internalin

Cytoskeleton
filaments

Actin polymerization

LLO

LLO

FIGURE 26-6. Listeriosis, cellular-view. (*Left*) *Listeria monocytogenes* internalin mediates attachment to an enterocyte and enters in an endocytotic vacuole. Listerolysin O (LLO) lyses the vacuole and the organism escapes to the cytoplasm. (*Middle*) The cytoskeleton is modified and the organisms move along fibers by polymerizing actin (comet tail) invading adjacent cells. (*Right*) *Listeria* has entered another cell now in a double vacuole, which LLO again lyses. The process continues with escape to the submucosa and bloodstream invasion.

In this process, actin monomers are sequentially concentrated directly behind the bacterium creating a bacterial "tail" that is connected to the long actin filaments. The addition of new actin units to the tail propels the organisms through the cytosol like a comet through the evening sky. The motile *Listeria* eventually reach the edge of the cell where, rather than stopping, they protrude into the adjacent cell taking the original cell membrane along with them. When these pinch off, the organisms are surrounded by a double set of host cell membranes that are again dissolved by LLO and phospholipases thereby releasing the organisms to restart the cycle in a new cell.

* Actin polymerization propels bacteria through cytoplasm

* Adjacent cells invaded and LLO releases bacteria

This complex strategy allows *L monocytogenes* to survive in macrophages by escaping the phagosome and then to spread from epithelial cell to epithelial cell without exposure to the immune system. How does *Listeria* keep its LLO from destroying the host cell membrane from the inside as the pore-forming toxins of other bacteria do from the outside? It appears that *L monocytogenes* may be able to not only regulate the timely production of LLO but also to trigger its degradation by host cell proteolytic enzymes after it has left the endosome vacuole. LLO is also able to disrupt the response to infection by altering the host cell's posttranslational modification of its own proteins. One of these effects is suppression of antigen-induced T-cell activation. The genes for LLO, actin rearrangement, and several others are part of a virulence regulon contained in a pathogenicity island. The result is a surgically precise deployment of virulence factors.

* Cell-to-cell spread avoids immune system

LLO disrupts protein modification

IMMUNITY

Immunity to *Listeria* infection involves both innate and adaptive immune responses. In addition to neutrophil action, multiple toll-like receptors (TLRs) recognize *Listeria* peptidoglycan, lipoteichoic acid, lipoproteins, and flagellar protein. The adaptive response owes little to humoral and much to T_H1 cell-mediated mechanisms. The generation of antigen-specific CD4+ and CD8+ T-cell subsets is required for the resolution of infection and the establishment of long-lived protection. Cytokine activation and gamma interferon reverse the intracellular growth in macrophages. The importance of cellular immunity is emphasized by the increased frequency of

TLRs recognize peptidoglycan

* *Listeria*-specific T-cell activation protects

listeriosis in immunocompromised patients (eg, advanced age, AIDS, immunosuppressive therapy, or pregnancy.

 ## LISTERIOSIS: CLINICAL ASPECTS

MANIFESTATIONS

Listeriosis usually does not present clinically until there is disseminated infection. In foodborne outbreaks, gastrointestinal manifestations of primary infection such as nausea, abdominal pain, diarrhea, and fever sometimes occur. Disseminated infection in adults is usually occult, involving fever, malaise, and constitutional symptoms without an obvious focus. *L monocytogenes* has a tropism for the central nervous system (CNS), including the brain parenchyma (encephalitis) and brainstem (with cranial nerve deficits), but the meningitis it causes is not clinically distinct from that associated with other leading bacterial pathogens (*Streptococcus pneumoniae* and *Neisseria meningitidis*). *Listeria* meningitis does have a particularly high mortality rate.

Neonatal and puerperal infections appear in settings similar to those of infections with group B streptococci. *L monocytogenes* appears to have a unique ability to infect the placenta (**Figure 26-7**) by taking advantage of the mild impairment of cell-mediated immunity during pregnancy. Intrauterine infection leads to stillbirth or a disseminated infection at or near birth. If the pathogen is acquired in the birth canal, the onset of disease is later. The risk of disease is increased in the elderly and immunocompromised persons as well as in women in late pregnancy. The number of cases in untreated AIDS patients has been estimated at 300 times that of the general population.

DIAGNOSIS

Diagnosis of listeriosis is by culture of blood, cerebrospinal fluid (CSF), or focal lesions. In meningitis, CSF Gram stains are usually positive. The first indication that *Listeria* is involved is often the discovery that the β-hemolytic colonies subcultured from a blood culture bottle are Gram-positive rods rather than cocci and are catalase-positive unlike all streptococci.

TREATMENT AND PREVENTION

L monocytogenes is susceptible to ampicillin and trimethoprim/sulfamethoxazole (TMP/SMX), both of which have been used effectively for treatment, including for meningitis. Ampicillin combined with gentamicin is considered the treatment of choice for fulminant cases and in patients with severe compromise of T-cell function. Intense surveillance to prevent the sale of *Listeria*-contaminated ready-to-eat meat products has led to a marked decrease in the incidence of new infections. Avoidance of unpasteurized dairy products and thorough cooking of animal products are wise measures and mandatory for immunocompromised persons. There is no vaccine available.

* Bacteremia occult

* Meningitis, encephalitis produced

* Puerperal infection leads to stillbirth, dissemination

Increased in AIDS

* Blood, CSF cultures positive

* Ampicillin, TMP/SMX effective

* Resistant to cephalosporins

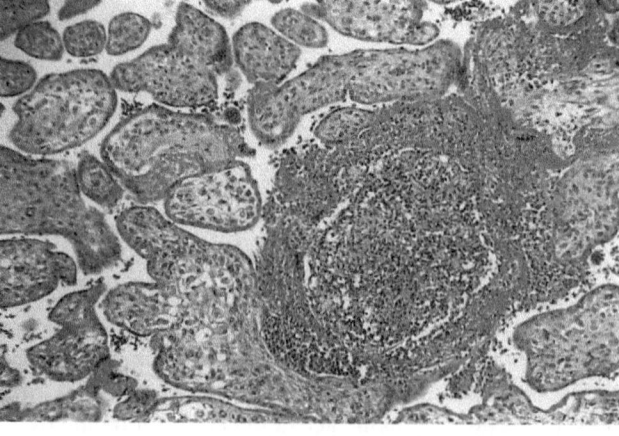

FIGURE 26-7. *Listeria* **placentitis.** This placental villus has been destroyed by a microabscess due to *L monocytogenes*. The infant was stillborn. (Reproduced with permission from Connor DH, Chandler FW, Schwartz DQ, et al: *Pathology of Infectious Diseases.* Stamford CT: Appleton & Lange; 1997.)

How can we tell if cured meat delicacies like Genoa salami are safe?

KEY CONCLUSIONS

- *Listeria* are β-hemolytic, catalase-positive Gram-positive rods.
- Internalin and LLO enhance virulence by enabling survival in macrophages.
- Replication at refrigeration temperatures facilitates foodborne illness.
- Pregnant women and immunocompromised patients are at special risk for listeriosis.
- Clinical presentations include amnionitis, stillbirth, neonatal sepsis, and meningitis.
- Treatment is with ampicillin or TMP/SMX; resistance to cephalosporin is uniform.

● BACILLUS

The genus *Bacillus* includes many species of aerobic or facultative, spore-forming, Gram-positive rods. With the exception of one species, *B anthracis*, they are low-virulence saprophytes widespread in air, soil, water, dust, and animal products. *B anthracis* causes the zoonosis anthrax, a disease of animals that is occasionally transmitted to humans. The genus is made up of rod-shaped organisms that can vary from coccobacillary to rather long-chained filaments. Motile strains have peritrichous flagella. Formation of round or oval spores, which may be central, subterminal, or terminal depending on the species, is characteristic of the genus.

With *Bacillus*, growth is obtained with ordinary media incubated in air and is reduced or absent under anaerobic conditions. The bacteria are catalase positive and metabolically active. The spores survive boiling for varying periods and are sufficiently resistant to heat that those of one species are used as a biologic indicator of autoclave efficiency. Spores of *B anthracis* survive in soil for decades.

Gram-positive spore-forming rods

✳ Aerobic growth

✳ Spores survive boiling

BACILLUS ANTHRACIS

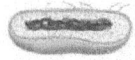 **BACTERIOLOGY**

B anthracis has a tendency to form very long chains of rods and in culture is nonmotile and non-hemolytic; colonies are characterized by a rough, uneven surface with multiple curled extensions at the edge resembling a "Medusa head." *B anthracis* has a polypeptide (poly-d-γ-glutamic acid) capsule of a single antigenic type that has antiphagocytic properties similar to those of bacterial polysaccharide capsules. *Bacillus anthracis* endospores are extremely hardy and have been shown to survive in the environment for decades. The organism also produces a potent exotoxin complex, which consists of two enzymes, edema factor (EF) and lethal factor (LF) together with a receptor-binding protein called protective antigen (PA). When PA binds to either EF or LF it then acts as a translocase forming a pore-like site on the host cell surface. This allows the complexes to enter the cell **(Figure 26–8A)**. Once in the cytosol multiple toxin actions are expressed including adenylate cyclase activity and host protein inactivation. *B anthracis* also produces multiple other proteases that digest tissue components.

✳ Endospores survive in nature

✳ Polypeptide capsule antiphagocytic

✳ Exotoxin complex has multiple components, actions

 Think ▸▸ Apply 26-1: There is no practical way for individuals to detect contamination in advance other than watching for news of outbreaks. Refrigeration is prudent but *Listeria's* cold growth has made even ice-cream a source.

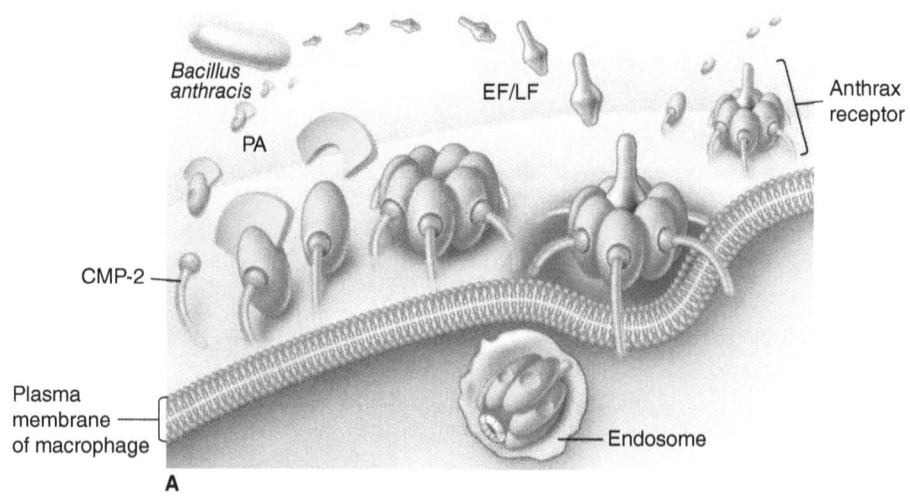

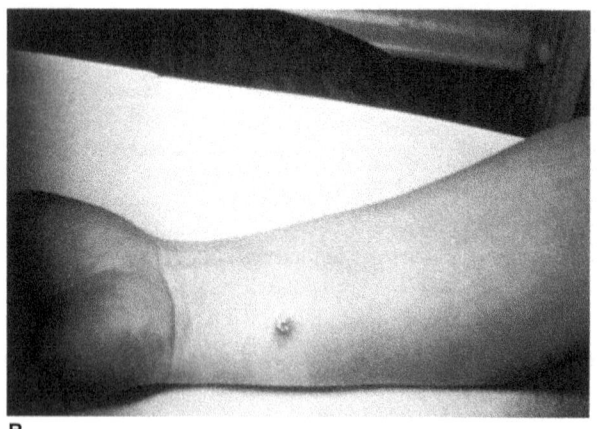

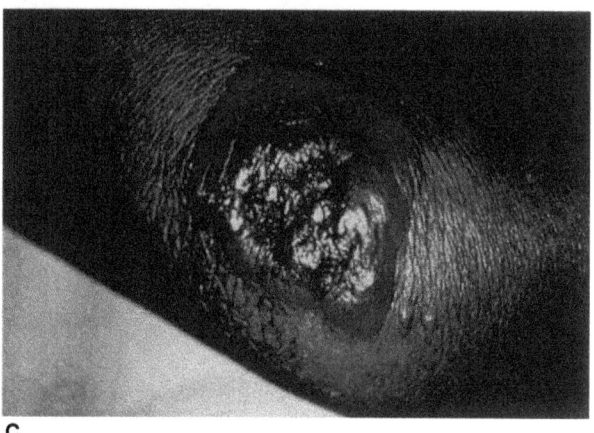

FIGURE 26-8. **Anthrax. A.** A protein called protective antigen (PA) delivers two other proteins, edema factor (EF) and lethal factor (LF), to the capillary morphogenesis protein-2 (CMP-2) receptor on the cell membrane of a target macrophage, where PA, EF, and LF are transported to an endosome. PA then delivers EF and LF from the endosome into the cytoplasm of the macrophage where they exert their toxic effects. **B.** Early anthrax papule that evolves into **C.** The necrotic eschar called the malignant pustule. (Reproduced with permission from Willey JM: *Prescott, Harley, & Klein's Microbiology*, 7th ed. New York, NY: McGraw Hill; 2008.)

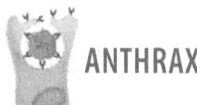 **ANTHRAX**

The isolation of *B anthracis*, the proof of its relationship to anthrax infection, and the demonstration of immunity to the disease are among the most important events in the history of science and medicine. Robert Koch rose to fame in 1877 by growing the organism in artificial culture using pure culture techniques. He defined the stringent criteria needed to prove that the organism caused anthrax (Koch's postulates), then met them experimentally. Louis Pasteur made a convincing field demonstration at Pouilly-le-Fort to show that vaccination of sheep, goats, and cows with an attenuated strain of *B anthracis* prevented anthrax. He was cheered and carried on the shoulders of the grateful farmers of the district in appreciation.

Pasteur animal vaccine attenuated anthrax strain

EPIDEMIOLOGY

Anthrax is primarily a disease of herbivores such as horses, sheep, and cattle, who acquire it from spores of *B anthracis* contaminating their pastures. Humans become infected through contact with these animals or their products in a way that allows the spores to be inoculated through the skin, ingested, or inhaled. In the 1920s, more than 100 cases occurred annually in the United States among farmers, veterinarians, and meat handlers, but the control of animal anthrax in developed countries has made human cases rare. A few endemic foci persist in North America and have been the source of naturally acquired disease. Another source is animal products such

※ Infection through skin injection of spores from herbivores

Anthrax

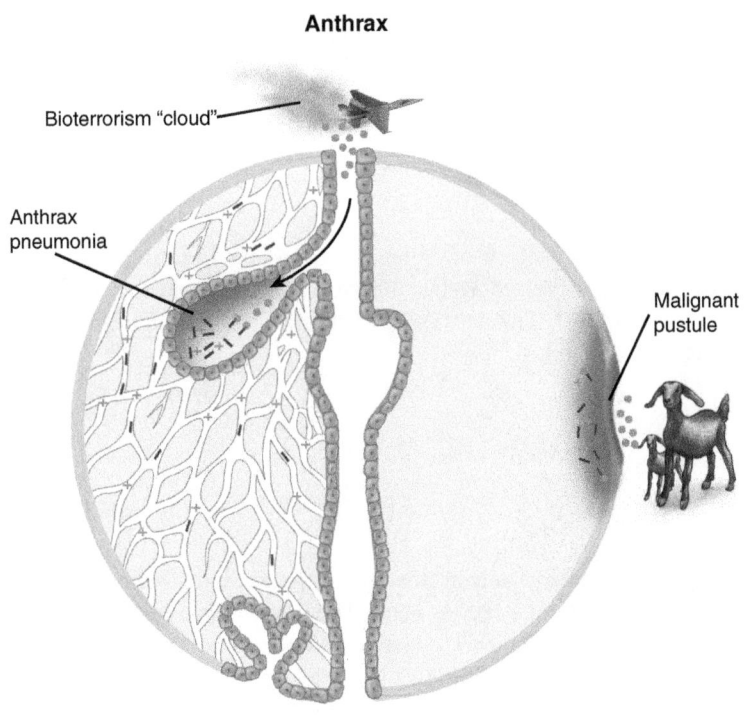

Bioterrorism "cloud"

Anthrax pneumonia

Malignant pustule

 Bacillus anthracis

B anthracis spores

 Anthrax toxin

FIGURE 26-9. **Anthrax overview.** Naturally acquired anthrax (*right*) is from the traumatic inoculation of *Bacillus anthracis* spores derived from animals with anthrax. The lesion is destructive but remains localized. Bioterrorism-acquired anthrax (*left*) would occur by the inhalation of explosive aerosols of *B anthracis* spores. This causes pneumonia with rapid spread to the bloodstream.

as wool, hides, or bone meal fertilizer that have been imported from a country where animal anthrax is endemic. The zoonotic nature of anthrax is highlighted by a 2017 epizootic in Namibia that killed 107 hippopotomuses and 20 Cape buffalo. Eating contaminated meat of infected animals causes gastrointestinal disease; most of these rare cases are in Africa.

* Imported from countries with animal anthrax

The real domestic threat associated with anthrax comes from its use as an agent of biologic warfare or terrorism. The long life, stability, and low mass of the dried spores required make the prospect of someone producing a "cloud of death" leading to massive pulmonary anthrax a chilling reality. Such was the cloud of dust that killed all the Egyptian livestock of an unyielding Pharaoh as recorded in the 9th chapter of *Exodus*. A 1979 episode resulting in more than 60 anthrax deaths in the former Soviet Union was the result of an accidental explosion at a biologic warfare research facility that aerosolized more than 20 lb of anthrax spores. Inhalation anthrax among postal workers after the September 11, 2001 terrorist attacks appears to have been due to the mailing of envelopes containing "weapons-grade" anthrax spores stolen from a biologic warfare research facility. Such spores had been treated to enhance their aerosolization and dissemination. The forms of anthrax are summarized in **Figure 26-9.**

* Biologic warfare continuing threat

* Spread by pulmonary aerosols

* Weapons-grade spores specially treated

What is the most "useful" feature of *B anthracis* as an agent of biology warfare? Are there any deficits?

PATHOGENESIS

When spores of *B anthracis* reach the rich environment of human tissues, they germinate and multiply in the vegetative state. The antiphagocytic properties of the capsule aid in survival, eventually allowing production of enough exotoxin to cause disease. The timing and relative

* Antiphagocytic effect of glutamic acid capsule required for virulence

Think ▶▶ Apply 26-2: The spores of *B anthracis* provide not only hearty survival but also lightweight ideal for creating infectious clouds when launched on warheads. Anthrax does not spread person-to-person, so there is no potential for starting a self-sustaining epidemic as there is with smallpox.

importance of the EF, LF, and PA components are not known. The EF adenylate cyclase activity is believed to correlate with the striking edema seen at infected sites. In pulmonary anthrax the inhaled spores are taken up by alveolar macrophages but apparently do not germinate inside them at least until they drain to the mediastinum via the lymphatics. This most lethal of anthrax forms is manifest in the lung as a mediastinal process and systemically as a virulent bacteremia.

* Edema produced by EF

Pulmonary focus is mediastinum

IMMUNITY

The specific mechanisms of immunity against *B anthracis* are not known. Experimental evidence favors antibody directed against the toxin complex, but the relative role of the components of the toxin is not clear. The capsular glutamic acid is immunogenic, but antibody against it is not protective.

Immune mechanisms are unknown

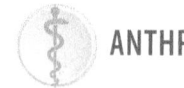 **ANTHRAX: CLINICAL ASPECTS**

MANIFESTATIONS

Cutaneous anthrax usually begins 2 to 5 days after inoculation of spores into an exposed part of the body, typically the forearm or hand. The initial lesion is an erythematous papule, which may be mistaken for an insect bite. This papule usually progresses through vesicular and ulcerative stages in 7 to 10 days to form a black eschar (scab) surrounded by edema (**Figure 26–8B** and **C**). This lesion is known as the "malignant pustule," although it is neither malignant nor a pustule. Associated systemic symptoms are usually mild, and the lesion typically heals very slowly after the eschar separates. Less commonly, the disease progresses with massive local edema, toxemia, and bacteremia.

* Initial papule evolves to malignant pustule

Pulmonary anthrax is contracted by inhalation of spores. Historically, this has occurred when contaminated hides, hair, or wool (wool-sorter disease) are handled in a confined space or after laboratory accidents. Today it is the form we would expect from dissemination of an aerosol of spores in biologic warfare. In the pulmonary syndrome, 1 to 5 days of nonspecific malaise, mild fever, and nonproductive cough lead to progressive respiratory distress and cyanosis. Spread to the bloodstream and CNS follow rapidly. Massive edema and hemorrhage are hallmark features of anthrax meningitis. Mediastinal edema was a prominent finding in the postal workers. If untreated, progression to a fatal outcome is usually very rapid once bacteremia has developed. An intestinal form of anthrax follows ingestion of contaminated food, usually meat. It is characterized by abdominal pain, ascites, and shock.

* Pulmonary anthrax acquired by inhaling spores

* Fever, cough progress to cyanosis and death

* Hemorrhagic mediastinitis and meningitis

DIAGNOSIS

Culture of skin lesions, sputum, blood, and CSF are the primary means of anthrax diagnosis. Given some suspicion on epidemiologic grounds, Gram stains of sputum or other biologic fluids showing large numbers of long Gram-positive bacilli can suggest the diagnosis. In September 2001, diagnosis of the first case in Florida was hastened by an infectious disease specialist who knew such rods were extremely rare in the spinal fluid. Large Gram-positive bacilli are also unusual in sputum. *B anthracis* and other *Bacillus* spp. are not difficult to grow. As common environmental contaminants, however, *Bacillus* saprophytic species are usually β-hemolytic and motile, features not found in *B anthracis*. Blood cultures are positive in most cases of pulmonary anthrax.

Large Gram-positive rods suggestive

* Hemolysis and motility exclude *B anthracis*

* Sputum, blood cultures positive in pneumonia

TREATMENT

Antimicrobial treatment has little effect on the course of cutaneous anthrax but does protect against dissemination. Almost all strains of *B anthracis* are susceptible to penicillin, doxycycline, and ciprofloxacin. Although penicillin has long been the treatment of choice for all forms of anthrax, experience gained during the 2001 outbreak has caused the first-line recommendation to be changed to ciprofloxacin or doxycycline. These antibiotics are also recommended for chemoprophylaxis in the case of known or suspected exposure.

* Ciprofloxacin, doxycycline for treatment and prophylaxis

PREVENTION

The most important preventive measures are those that eradicate animal anthrax and limit imports from endemic areas. Vaccines are also useful. Pasteur's vaccine used a live strain attenuated by repeated subculture that resulted in the loss of a plasmid encoding toxin production.

A similar live vaccine is still effective for animals. The human vaccine licensed in the United States is prepared by extraction from cultures of a nonencapsulated avirulent strain of *B anthracis.* The extract is made up of almost entirely the PA component of the toxin complex. In 2002, the Institute of Medicine issued a detailed analysis of human and animal studies and declared the vaccine both safe and efficacious. Experts also feel that it is very unlikely that the architects of biologic warfare would be able to craft *B anthracis* strains for which this vaccine is not protective. In Russia and China, a live vaccine is used in which spores are inoculated by scarification.

✳ Eradication of animal anthrax important

✳ Live and inactivated vaccines available

OTHER *BACILLUS* SPECIES

Bacillus spores are widespread in the environment, and isolation of one of the more than 20 *Bacillus* species other than *B anthracis* from clinical material usually represents contamination of the specimen. Occasionally *B cereus, B subtilis,* and some other species produce genuine infections, including rapidly destructive infections of the eye, soft tissues, and lung. Infection is usually associated with immunosuppression, trauma, an indwelling catheter, or contamination of complex equipment. The relative resistance of *Bacillus* spores to disinfectants aids their survival in medical devices that cannot be heat sterilized.

✳ Spores enhance survival in medical devices

B cereus deserves special mention. This species is the one most likely to cause opportunistic infection, which suggests a virulence intermediate between that of *B anthracis* and the other species. Genes and plasmids similar to those found in *B anthracis* have been detected as has a destructive pyogenic toxin. Traumatic injuries to the eye can lead to rapid destruction of the globe within hours to days owing to the *B cereus* exotoxin. Treatment is with vancomycin and clindamycin. *B cereus* can also cause food poisoning by means of enterotoxin production.

✳ *B cereus* produces pyogenic toxin and enterotoxin

KEY CONCLUSIONS

- *Bacillus* species survive in the environment by spore formation.
- *Bacillus anthracis* is a demonstrated agent of bioterrorism.
- *B anthracis* evades phagocytosis owing to its polypeptide capsule.
- Anthrax results from a potent tri-component toxin: EF, LF, and PF.
- Inhalation anthrax results in hemorrhagic pneumonia, mediastinitis, and meningitis.
- Postexposure prophylaxis with ciprofloxacin is more effective than treatment.
- *Bacillus cereus* infections of the eye can be rapidly destructive.

CASE STUDY

Sore Throat and Confusion After Summer Camp

A 9-year-old girl developed listlessness and a sore throat on 10 days after arriving at a summer camp operated by a religious group that does not accept immunizations. Four days later, the girl returned home on a camp bus along with other unimmunized children and adults who had also attended the camp. A physician evaluated the patient for a sore throat. A throat culture was taken and oral penicillin was prescribed. The patient was hospitalized for persistent sore throat, diminished fluid intake, and gingival bleeding. Laboratory tests revealed a white blood cell count of 26,500/mm³ with 92% polymorphonuclear cells, blood urea nitrogen of 214 mg/dL, creatinine of 12.4 mg/dL, and a platelet count of 10,000/mm³. The throat culture was reported to contain normal flora, group A β-hemolytic streptococci, and large numbers of diphtheroids. The patient was transferred to a tertiary care children's hospital.

On admission, she was afebrile and had moderate upper airway obstruction, diffuse ecchymoses, bleeding from the nose and gums, prominent cervical adenopathy, and swelling of the jaw and throat. The pharynx revealed severe hemorrhagic and necrotic tonsillitis; no membrane was observed. Treatment with penicillin G, gentamicin, peritoneal dialysis, and platelet transfusions was instituted. The hospital course was complicated by disseminated intravascular coagulation, cardiac conduction abnormalities, and mental confusion. The patient died 2 weeks after the sore throat began. A *Corynebacterium* species isolated from her throat culture was subsequently confirmed to be a toxigenic strain of *C diphtheriae.*

QUESTIONS

1. Attention to what "clue" would have suggested the diagnosis earlier?
   A. Hemorrhagic pharyngitis
   B. Renal failure
   C. Immunization history
   D. Group A strep in throat

2. What treatment might have saved this girl's life?
   A. Intravenous penicillin
   B. Ciprofloxacin
   C. Corticosteroids
   D. Diphtheria toxoid
   E. Diphtheria antitoxin

3. The cardiac conduction abnormalities were probably due to:
   A. Infarction
   B. Inhibition of protein synthesis
   C. Pore-forming toxin
   D. Internalin
   E. Edema factor

ANSWERS

1. **(C)**

2. **(E)**

3. **(B)**

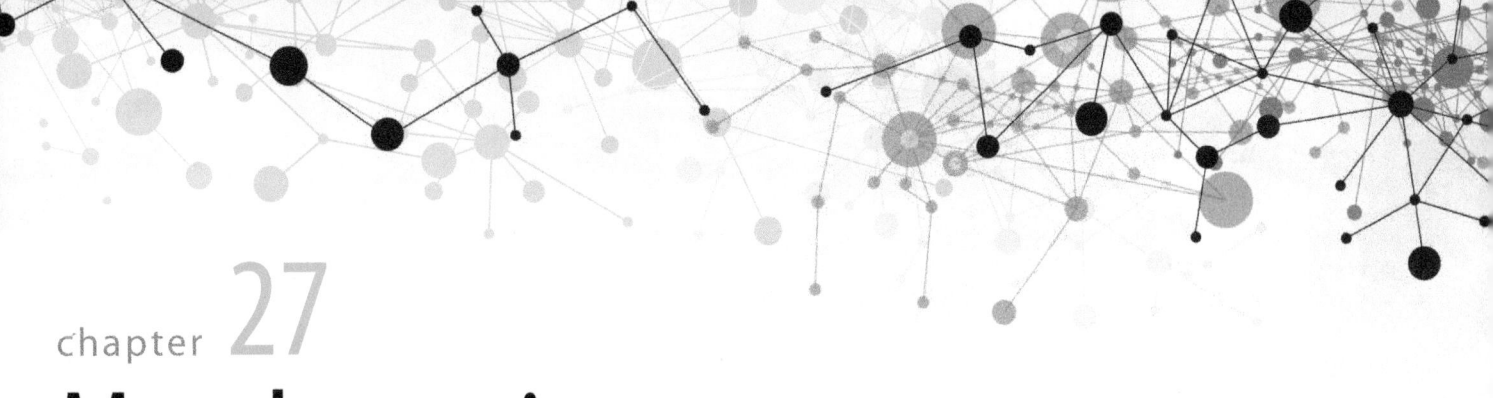

chapter 27

Mycobacteria

Mycobacterium tuberculosis • Mycobacterium leprae • Mycobacterium kansasii • Mycobacterium avium-intracellulare

Mycobacterium scrofulaceum • Mycobacterium fortuitum • Mycobacterium marinum • Mycobacterium ulcerans

A dread disease in which the struggle between soul and body is so gradual, quiet and solemn, and the result so sure that day by day, and grain by grain, the mortal part wastes and withers away. A disease ... which sometimes moves in giant strides and sometimes at a tardy sluggish pace, but, slow or quick, is ever sure and certain.

—Charles Dickens: *Nicholas Nickleby*

*M*ycobacterium is a genus of Gram-positive bacilli which all demonstrate the staining characteristic of acid-fastness. The most important species, *Mycobacterium tuberculosis* (MTB), is the etiologic agent of tuberculosis (TB), the dread disease called consumption in Dickens' time. Mostly out of view in wealthy countries, tuberculosis still infects a third of the world population causing over 10 million new cases and 2 million deaths each year. *Mycobacterium leprae*, is the causative agent of leprosy, an ancient and disfiguring disease. A large number of less pathogenic species are assuming increasing importance as disease agents in immunocompromised patients, particularly those with AIDS.

● *MYCOBACTERIUM*: GENERAL CHARACTERISTICS

 ## BACTERIOLOGY

STRUCTURE

The mycobacteria are slim, poorly staining bacilli, which demonstrate the property of acid-fastness. They are nonmotile, obligate aerobes that do not form spores. The cell wall contains peptidoglycan similar to that of other Gram-positive organisms, to which many branched-chain polysaccharides, proteins, and lipids are attached. Porins and other proteins are found throughout the cell wall. Of particular importance is the presence of long-chain fatty acids called **mycolic acids** (for which the *myco*bacteria are named) and **lipoarabinomannan (LAM)**, a lipid polysaccharide complex extending from the plasma membrane to the surface (**Figure 27–1**). LAM is structurally and functionally analogous to the lipopolysaccharide forming the outer membrane of Gram-negative bacteria. These elements give the mycobacteria a cell wall with unusually high lipid content (greater than 60% of the total cell wall mass). This accounts for many of their biologic characteristics. It can be thought of as a waxy coat that makes them hardy, impenetrable, and hydrophobic. The staining characteristic of acid-fastness is the most frequently observed of these features. The mycobacterial cell wall can be stained only through the use of extreme measures (prolonged staining time, heat, and penetrating agents) but once in, the stain is *fast*. Even the strongest of decolorizing agents (acid and alcohol) do not wash it out (**Figure 27–2**).

Cell wall has high lipid content

* Mycolic acids, LAM form waxy coat

* Acid fastness: once stained, difficult to decolorize

FIGURE 27–1. **Mycobacterial cell wall.** LAM, lipoarabinomannan. (Reproduced with permission from Willey JM: *Prescott, Harley, & Klein's Microbiology*, 7th ed. New York, NY: McGraw Hill; 2008.)

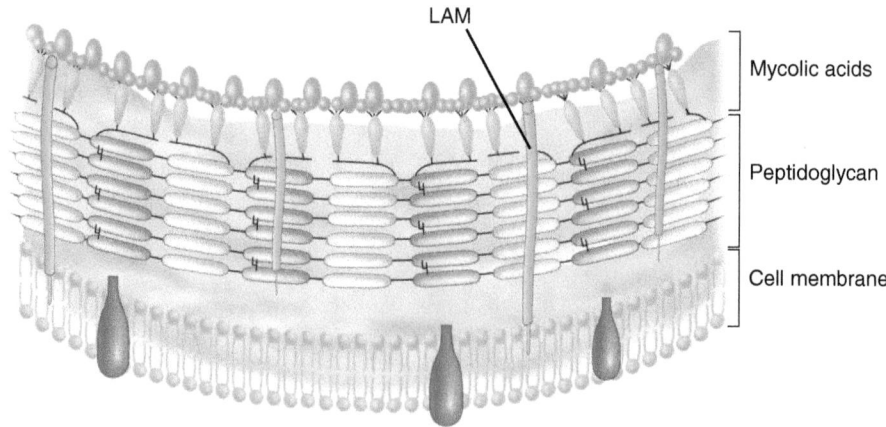

LAM

Mycolic acids

Peptidoglycan

Cell membrane

GROWTH

✳ Strict aerobes, many grow slowly

The most important pathogen, MTB, in the laboratory grows under aerobic conditions enhanced by 10% carbon dioxide and at a relatively low pH (6.5-6.8). Nutritional requirements vary among mycobacterial species and range from the ability of some nonpathogens to multiply on the washers of water faucets to the strict intracellular parasitism of *M leprae*, which does not grow in artificial media or cell culture. Mycobacteria grow more slowly than most pathogenic bacteria because of their hydrophobic cell surface, which causes them to clump and limits permeability of nutrients into the cell.

CLASSIFICATION

Distinguished by cultural features, pathogenicity

Classic mycobacterial classification has been based on a constellation of phenotypic characteristics, including nutritional and temperature requirements, growth rates, pigmentation of colonies grown in light or darkness, key biochemical tests, the cellular constellation of free fatty acids, and the range of pathogenicity in experimental animals. There are now over 120 recognized species, the most important of which are summarized in **Table 27–1**. Increasingly, this classification system is yielding to molecular-based techniques.

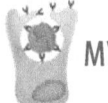 ## MYCOBACTERIAL DISEASE

Mycobacteria include a wide range of species pathogenic for humans and animals. Some, such as MTB, occur exclusively in humans under natural conditions. Others, such as *M intracellulare*, can infect various hosts, including humans, but also exist in a free-living state. Many nonpathogenic

FIGURE 27–2. *Mycobacterium tuberculosis* in sputum stained by the acid-fast technique. The mycobacteria retain the red carbol fuchsin through the decolorization step. The cells, background, and any other organisms stain with the contrasting methylene blue counterstain. (Reproduced with permission from Nester EW, Anderson DG, Roberts CE Jr, et al: *Microbiology: A Human Perspective*, 6th ed. New York, NY: McGraw Hill; 2008.)

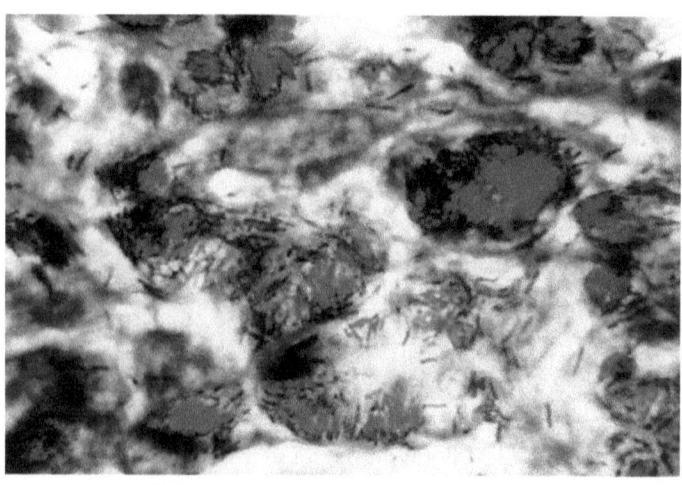

10 µm

TABLE 27–1 Mycobacteria of Major Clinical Importance[a]

SPECIES	RESERVOIR	VIRULENCE FOR HUMANS	DISEASE CAUSED	CHARACTERISTICS						VIRULENCE FOR GUINEA PIGS[d]
				CASE-TO-CASE TRANSMISSION	GROWTH RATE	OPTIMUM GROWTH TEMPERATURE	PIGMENT PRODUCTION[b]	SUBSTANTIAL NIACIN PRODUCTION[c]		
Mycobacterium tuberculosis	Human	+++	Tuberculosis	Yes	S	37	–	+		+
M bovis	Animals	+++	Tuberculosis	Rare	S	37	–	–		+
Bacillus Calmette-Guérin	Artificial culture	±	Local lesion	Very rare	S	37	–	–		–
M kansasii	Environmental	+	Tuberculosis like	No	S	37	Photochromogen	–		–
M scrofulaceum	Environmental	+	Usually lymphadenitis	No	S	37	Scotochromogen	–		–
M avium-intracellulare complex (MAC)[e]	Environmental; birds	+	Tuberculosis like	No	S	37	±	–		–
M fortuitum complex[f]	Environmental	±	Local abscess	No	F	37	±	–		Local abscess
M marinum	Water; fish	±	Skin granuloma	No	S	30	Photochromogen	–		–
M ulcerans	Probably environmental; tropical	+	Severe skin ulceration	No	S	30	–			–
M leprae	Human	+++	Leprosy	Yes	NG	NG	NG	NG		–
M smegmatis	Human, external urethral area	–	None	–	F	37	–	–		–

F, fast (colonies develop in 7 days or less); NG, not grown; S, slow (colonies usually develop in 10 days or more).

[a]Numerous nonpathogenic environmental mycobacteria exist and may contaminate human specimens.

[b]Yellow-orange pigment. Photochromogen is pigment produced in light; scotochromogen is pigment produced in dark or light.

[c]Many other differential biochemical tests used; for example, nitrate reduction, catalase production, Tween 80 hydrolysis.

[d]Disease following subcutaneous injection of light inoculum (eg, 10^2 cells).

[e]Includes M avium, M intracellulare and M chimaera.

[f]Includes M fortuitum, M abscessus, and M chelonae.

Human, animal pathogens

Slowly progressive diseases

species are widely distributed in the environment. Diseases caused by mycobacteria usually develop slowly, follow a chronic course, and elicit a granulomatous response. Infectivity of pathogenic species is high, but virulence for healthy humans is moderate. Clinical disease following infection with MTB is the exception rather than the rule.

MYCOBACTERIUM TUBERCULOSIS (MTB)

Overview

Like other mycobacteria, MTB cells are bacilli with a Gram-positive cell wall structure requiring the acid-fast stain for demonstration. Tuberculosis (TB) is a systemic infection, the most common form of which is a chronic pneumonia with fever, cough, bloody sputum, and weight loss. The natural history follows a course of chronic fever and a wasting to death aptly labeled "consumption" in the 19th century. Disease outside the lung also occurs and is particularly devastating when MTB reaches the central nervous system causing tuberculous meningitis. Most of those infected never develop disease, manifesting infection only by the presence of a skin test or other evidence of an immune response. Although disease may appear immediately following primary infection, in most instances it is delayed following a latent period lasting, months, years, even decades. MTB is not known to produce any classic virulence factors such as toxins. The tissue injury is due to the destructive effects of unremitting delayed-type hypersensitivity in a host whose Th1 cellular immune responses are unable to restrict growth of MTB. Methods for culture diagnosis are sensitive but require specialized expertise. Effective antimicrobial therapy has long been available but multiple drugs are required. The treatment course is prolonged and thus expensive. Together these make TB curable but only in countries that can afford it. TB is the leading infectious cause of premature death in the world.

 ## BACTERIOLOGY

MTB is a slim, strongly acid–alcohol–fast rod. It frequently shows irregular beading in its staining, appearing as connected series of acid-fast granules (Figure 27–2). It grows at 37°C, but not at room temperature, and it requires enriched or complex media for primary growth. The classic medium, Löwenstein-Jensen, contains homogenized egg in nutrient base with dyes to inhibit the growth of nonmycobacterial contaminants. Colonies usually appear after 3 to 6 weeks of incubation. Growth is more rapid in semisynthetic and liquid media. The major phenotypic tests for identification are summarized in Table 27–1. Of particular importance is the ability of MTB to produce large quantities of niacin, which is uncommon in other mycobacteria.

Growth takes weeks

＊ **Niacin test distinguishes MTB**

Because of its hydrophobic lipid surface, MTB is unusually resistant to drying, to most common disinfectants, and to acids and alkalis. Tubercle bacilli are sensitive to heat, including pasteurization, and individual organisms in droplet nuclei are susceptible to inactivation by ultraviolet light. As with other mycobacteria, the MTB cell wall structure is dominated by mycolic acids and LAM. Its antigenic makeup includes many protein and polysaccharide antigens, of which a boiled extract called **tuberculin** is the most studied. It consists of heat-stable proteins liberated into liquid culture media creating the **purified protein derivative (PPD)** of tuberculin used for skin testing. It is standardized in tuberculin skin test (TST) units according to activity.

Resistance to drying and disinfectants

＊ **PPD mix of MTB proteins**

 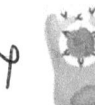 ## TUBERCULOSIS

EPIDEMIOLOGY

A recognized disease of antiquity, tuberculosis reached epidemic proportions in the Western world during the 18th and 19th centuries. Associated with urbanization and crowding, consumption accounted for 20% to 30% of all deaths in cities, winning tuberculosis the appellation "the captain of all the men of death." The disease has had major sociologic impacts, flourishing with ignorance, poverty, and poor hygiene, particularly during the social disruptions of war and

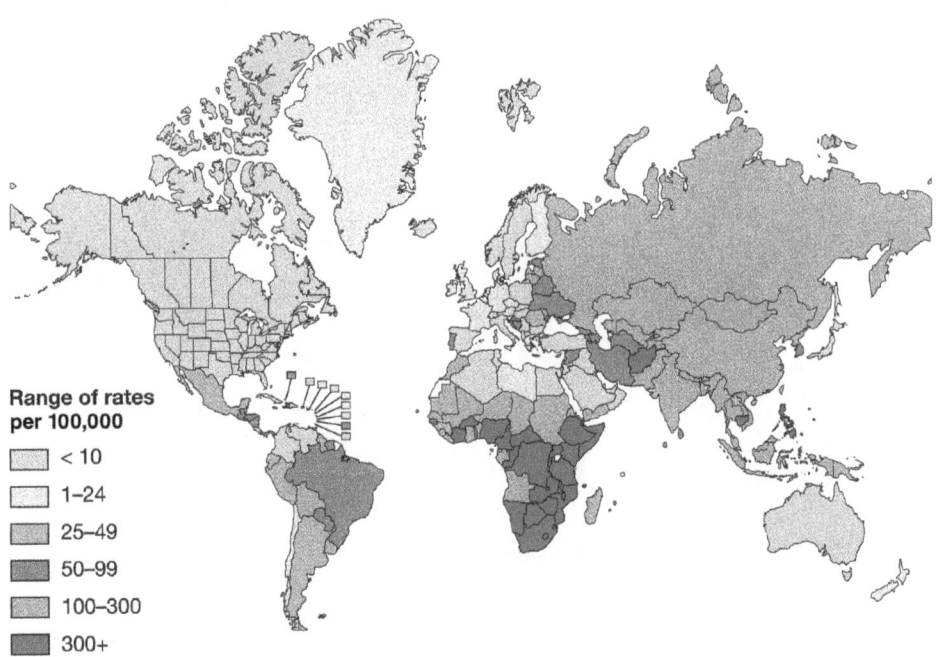

FIGURE 27–3. The worldwide incidence and distribution of tuberculosis. (Reproduced with permission from Willey JM: *Prescott, Harley, & Klein's Microbiology*, 7th ed. New York, NY: McGraw Hill; 2008.)

Range of rates per 100,000

	< 10
	1–24
	25–49
	50–99
	100–300
	300+

economic depression. The poor are the major victims, but all sectors of society are at risk. Chopin, Paganini, Rousseau, Goethe, Chekhov, Thoreau, Keats, and the Brontës, to name but a few, were all lost to TB in their prime. Over the past two centuries, more people have died from TB than from plague, cholera, malaria, influenza, smallpox, and HIV/AIDS combined.

With knowledge of the cause and transmission of the disease and the development of effective antimicrobial agents, tuberculosis was increasingly brought under control in developed countries. Unfortunately, morbidity and mortality remain at 19th-century levels in many developing countries. Worldwide, TB is the leading cause of death from a single infectious agent. A third of the world population is infected, 30 million have active disease, with over 10 million new cases every year. There are more than 30 thousand TB **deaths** *every week*. In the United States, the TB mortality rate has decreased over the last 25 years from 10.5 to 2.8 cases per 100,000 population. The majority of these are concentrated in ethnic and racial minorities and medically underserved populations. As shown in **Figure 27–3** the global distribution is unequal largely due to the relative availability of the public health and medical resources necessary to control TB. Twenty-two high-burden countries account for 80% of active cases.

The majority of TB infections are contracted by inhalation of droplet nuclei carrying the causative organism (**Figure 27–4**). Humans may also be infected through the gastrointestinal tract after ingestion of milk from tuberculous cows (now uncommon because of pasteurization) or, rarely, through abraded skin. Although a number of animals may become infected, humans are the primary reservoir for MTB. It has been estimated that a single cough can generate as many as 3000 infected droplet nuclei which dry while airborne and remain suspended for long periods. The likelihood of spreading infection thus relates to the numbers of organisms in the sputum of an open case of the disease, the frequency and efficiency of the coughs, the closeness of contact, and the adequacy of ventilation in the contact area. Epidemiologic data indicate that large doses or prolonged exposure to smaller infecting doses is usually needed to initiate infection. In some closed environments, such as a submarine or a crowded nursing home, a single open case of pulmonary TB can infect the majority of nonimmune individuals sharing sleeping accommodations. Most infections are acquired in places outside the home like workplaces, schools, churches, and bars. It is estimated that a room previously occupied by an active TB patient may remain infectious for 30 minutes or more. Infection outdoors is less likely due to greater ventilation and the susceptibility of MTB to ultraviolet light.

The AIDS pandemic and the spread of MTB strains resistant to multiple drugs have added to the TB burden. It is estimated that patients with latent TB increase their risk of reactivation disease by a factor 200 to 300 times with the development of HIV coinfection. HIV-infected persons are also at particularly high risk for primary infection even in their first year when CD4+ T cell counts are still high. TB is the leading cause of death in HIV patients. With this dark synergy, TB and AIDS have been leading causes of premature death in the world for decades.

Peak in 18th and 19th centuries

Attack rates relate to health resources

❋ Infection by respiratory droplets

❋ Coughing generates infectious dose

Poor ventilation increases risk

❋ AIDS, drug resistance enhance spread

FIGURE 27–4. Tuberculosis. A. Primary tuberculosis. *Mycobacterium tuberculosis* is inhaled in droplet nuclei from an active case of tuberculosis. Initial multiplication is in the alveoli with spread through lymphatic drainage to the hilar lymph nodes. After further lymphatic drainage to the bloodstream, the organisms are spread throughout the body. **B. Alveolar macrophage.** The two-stage battle being carried out between A and C is shown. Ingested bacteria multiply in the nonactivated macrophage. (1) Th1 cellular immune responses attempt to activate the macrophage by secreting cytokines (interferon-gamma [IFN-γ]). If successful, the disease is arrested. (2) Inflammatory elements of delayed-type hypersensitivity (DTH) are attracted and cause destruction. If activation is not successful, DTH injury and disease continue. **C. Reactivation tuberculosis.** Reactivation typically starts in the upper lobes of the lung with granuloma formation. DTH-mediated destruction can form a cavity, which allows the organisms to be coughed up to infect another person.

✳ In alveoli AMs initial site of infection

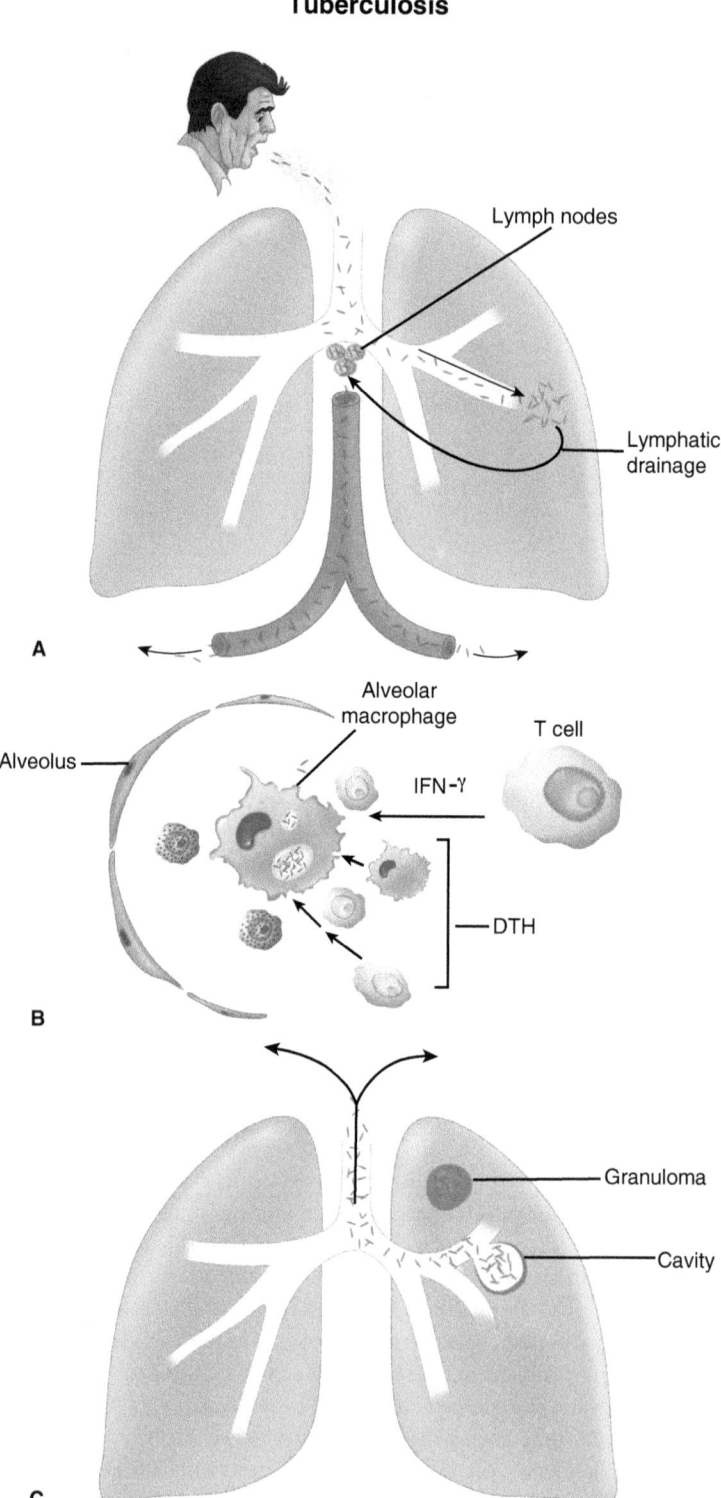

Tuberculosis

PATHOGENESIS

■ Primary Tuberculosis

MTB is a facultative intracellular pathogen whose success depends on avoiding the killing mechanisms of professional phagocytes. Primary TB is the initial infection in which inhaled droplet nuclei containing tubercle bacilli are deposited in the peripheral respiratory alveoli, most frequently those of the well-ventilated midlung zones of the middle and lower lobes. At the earliest stages surface proteins may facilitate binding to laminin in the basement membrane of alveolar epithelial cells. In the alveoli the bacteria are recognized by alveolar macrophages (AMs) and phagocytosed. This inaugurates a two-stage battle within the AM, which may be resolved in weeks or last for decades.

The first stage is MTB's interference with AM phagosome/lysosome fusion and its ability to interfere with the acidification required for maximal efficiency of lysosomal enzymes. These actions allow the bacteria to multiply freely in a phagosome within the nonactivated macrophage (Figure 27–4). MTB cells escaping AMs are trafficked by dendritic cells from the alveoli to regional lymph nodes in the interstitial space under the direction of a specialized secretion system (EXS-1). From there, a low-level bacteremia disseminates the bacteria to a number of sites, including the liver, spleen, kidney, bone, brain, meninges, and apices of the lung. Although enlarged hilar lymph nodes can be detected radiologically, the distant sites usually have no findings. In fact, the primary evidence for their existence is reactivation TB appearing at nonpulmonary sites later in life. TB meningitis, universally fatal in the preantibiotic era, is the most serious of these.

The second stage is the triggering of MTB-specific Th1 immune responses, beginning with digestion, antigen-presenting cell presentation of MTB components to naïve T cells, and ending with cytokine activation of the macrophages. The short- and long-term outcomes of the infection depend on the ability of the macrophage activation process to reverse the intracellular edge that MTB has as a result of its ability to block bactericidal mechanisms inside the AM. This is accomplished as macrophages and dendritic cells release cytokines particularly interferon-gamma (IFN-γ) and interleukin (IL)-12 which attract T cells and other inflammatory cells to the site. The recruited CD4+ T cells initiate the Th1 immune response over the following 3 to 9 weeks in which IFN-γ is the primary activator of macrophages. This includes CD8+ cytotoxic T cells which recognize and destroy MTB-infected macrophages. From the beginning of primary infection, MTB multiplication also generates mycobacterial proteins which trigger a delayed-type hypersensitivity (DTH) response with its phagocytes generating fluid, and release of digestive enzymes. This adds a destructive component to the process and is the sole known source of injury in tuberculosis. The magnitude of the DTH is directly related to the size of the MTB population at its local tissue destruction sites. If the Th1immune process is effective, the antigenic source of DTH stimulation wanes and the disease resolves. Stimulation of the DTH component of this response is the basis of the TST (see Diagnosis).

The mixture of the Th1 immune and DTH responses is manifest in a microscopic structure called a **granuloma,** which is composed of lymphocytes, macrophages, epithelioid cells (activated macrophages), fibroblasts, and multinucleated giant cells (fused macrophages) all in an organized pattern (**Figure 27–5**). As the granuloma grows, the destructive nature of the hypersensitivity component leads to necrosis usually in the center of the lesion. This is termed **caseous necrosis** because of the cheesy, semisolid character of material at the center of large gross lesions, but the term fits the smooth glassy appearance of microscopic granulomas as well. Foamy macrophages

* MTB multiplies in AMs

* Acidification of phagosome blocked

* Spread to lymph nodes, bloodstream

* Cytokines attract T cells, Th1 immune response

* Primary cytokine is IFN-γ

* Triggers DTH and injury

* Granuloma includes macrophages, lymphocytes

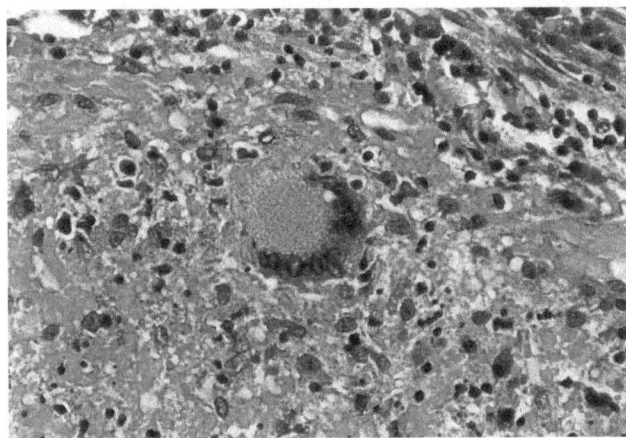
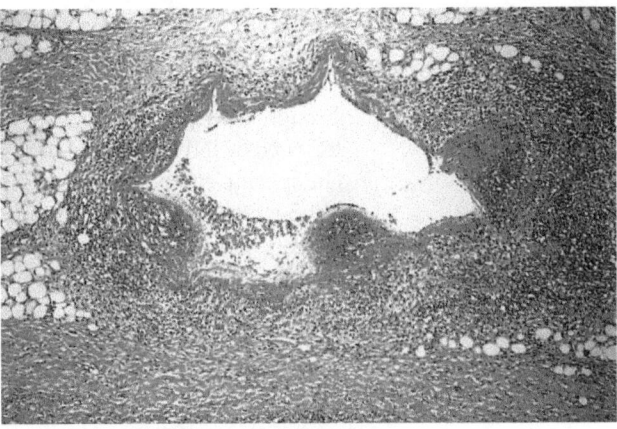

A   B

FIGURE 27–5. **Tuberculous granulomas. A.** Early granuloma with lymphocytes, epithelioid cells, and fibroblasts organizing around a central focus. The multinucleate giant cell in the center is typical of granulomas but not exclusive to *Mycobacterium tuberculosis.* **B. Multiple granulomas** surround and invade a vein near the lung hilum. Central degeneration is starting to appear and will eventually become caseous necrosis. (Reproduced with permission from Connor DH, Chandler FW, Schwartz DQ, et al: *Pathology of Infectious Diseases.* Stamford CT: Appleton & Lange; 1997.)

* Caseous necrosis due to DTH

seen on the interlayers of the granuloma are due to lipid droplets felt to provide nutrition to the inflammatory cells.

■ Latent Tuberculosis

* Primary lesions heal

* Some MTB enter latent state

Hypoxia triggers latency

Primary infections are handled well once the Th1 immune response halts the intracellular growth of MTB. Bacterial multiplication ceases, the lesions heal by fibrosis, and the organisms appear to slowly die. This sequence occurs in infections with multiple other infectious agents for which it is the end of the story. However, when faced with oxygen and nutrient deprivation, MTB is able to deploy regulators integrating nitrogen metabolism and hypoxia. This may allow at least some cell populations to enter a prolonged dormant state called latency instead of dying. Some view the arrival of MTB specific T cells 3 to 4 weeks after infection as the start of containment rather than cure. Specific factors facilitating survival are not known but the waxy nature of the MTB cell wall must be of aid as it is in the environment. It has long been assumed that these latent bacilli are primarily in healed granulomas in the lung, but we now know they are widely distributed with or without evidence of local granulomatous inflammation. This surviving MTB subpopulation in the lung and elsewhere lies waiting for reactivation months, years, or decades later. For the vast majority (90%) of persons who undergo a primary infection this never happens, either because of the complete killing of the original population or the variability of the factors favoring latency or reactivation to materialize. We do not know which.

■ Reactivation (Adult) Tuberculosis

* Latent reactivation at aerobic sites

* DTH destruction forms pulmonary cavities

Of the 10% of infected (TST-positive) persons who will reactivate disease, 3% to 4% take place during the year following skin test conversion. Most of the rest take place within 2 years but the risk continues into old age. Although mycobacterial factors have been identified (resuscitation-promoting factor), little is known of the mechanisms of reactivation of these latent foci. It has generally been attributed to some selective waning of immunity. The new foci are usually located in body areas of relatively high oxygen tension that would favor growth of the aerobe MTB. The apex of the lung is the most common of these, with spreading, coalescing granulomas, and large areas of caseous necrosis. Necrosis often involves the wall of a small bronchus from which the necrotic material is discharged, resulting in a pulmonary cavity and bronchial spread. Small blood vessels are also eroded. The destructive nature of these lesions cannot be directly attributed to any products or structural components of MTB. It is due to the failure of the host to control growth of MTB and thus the rising load of mycobacterial proteins, which stimulate the autodestructive DTH response.

IMMUNITY

Innate immunity high

Humans have a high innate immunity to the development of disease. This was tragically illustrated in the Lübeck disaster of 1926, in which infants were administered wild-type MTB instead of an intended vaccine strain. Despite the large dose, only 76 of 249 died. As stated earlier, over 90% of immunocompetent persons infected with MTB never develop active disease. There is epidemiologic and historic evidence for differences in the immunity in certain population groups and between identical and nonidentical twins.

* Th1 immunity most important

* CD8+ lymphocytes participate

Adaptive immunity to TB is primarily related to the development of reactions mediated through CD4+ T lymphocytes via Th1 pathways. Intracellular killing of MTB by macrophages activated by INF-γ and the CD8+ mediated killing of infected macrophages are the essential steps. The specific components of MTB that are important in initiating these reactions are not known. Although antibodies to MTB are formed in the course of disease, there is no evidence they play any role in immunity.

TUBERCULOSIS: CLINICAL ASPECTS

MANIFESTATIONS

■ Primary Tuberculosis

* Mid-lung infiltrates, adenopathy

Primary TB is either asymptomatic or manifests only by fever and malaise. Radiographs may show infiltrates in the mid-zones of the lung (Ghon focus) and later enlarged draining lymph nodes in the area around the hilum. When these lymph nodes fibrose and sometimes calcify, they produce a characteristic radiologic picture (Ghon complex). In less than 5% of patients, the primary disease is not controlled and merges into the reactivation type of tuberculosis, or disseminates to many organs. The latter may also result from a necrotic tubercle eroding into a small blood vessel.

Primary may progress to reactivation or dissemination

■ Reactivation Tuberculosis

The times of life when persons infected with MTB are most likely to develop clinical disease are infancy (primary), young adult (primary or reactivation), or old age (reactivation). In Western countries, reactivation of previous quiescent lesions occurs most often after age 50 and is more common in men. Reactivation is associated with a period of immunosuppression precipitated by malnutrition, alcoholism, diabetes, old age, or a dramatic change in the individual's life, such as loss of a spouse. In areas in which tuberculosis is most prevalent, reactivation is more frequently seen in young adults experiencing the immunosuppression that accompanies puberty and pregnancy. Recently, reactivation and progressive primary TB among younger adults have increased as a complication of AIDS.

✳ Factors include underlying disease, life events, AIDS

 How can it take this long for disease to develop?

Cough is the universal symptom of TB. It is initially dry, but as the disease progresses sputum is produced, which even later is mixed with blood (hemoptysis). Fever, malaise, fatigue, sweating, and weight loss all progress with continuing disease. Radiographically, infiltrates appearing in the apices of the lung coalesce to form cavities with progressive destruction of lung tissue. Less commonly, reactivation TB can also occur in other organs, such as the kidneys, bones, lymph nodes, brain, meninges, bone marrow, and bowel. Disease at these sites ranges from a localized tumor-like granuloma (tuberculoma) to a chronic meningitis due to rupture of a subependymal lesion into the subarachnoid space. Untreated, the progressive cough, fever, and weight loss of pulmonary TB create an internally consuming fire that usually takes 2 to 5 years to cause death. The course in AIDS and other T-cell–compromised patients is more rapid.

✳ Cough universal

✳ Cavities in lung apices

DIAGNOSIS

■ Tuberculin Test

The TST (**Figure 27–6**) measures DTH to an international reference tuberculoprotein preparation called PPD. The TST involves an intradermal injection that is read 48 to 72 hours later. An area of induration of 15 mm or more accompanied by erythema constitutes a positive reaction, and no induration indicates a negative reaction. A positive PPD test indicates that the individual

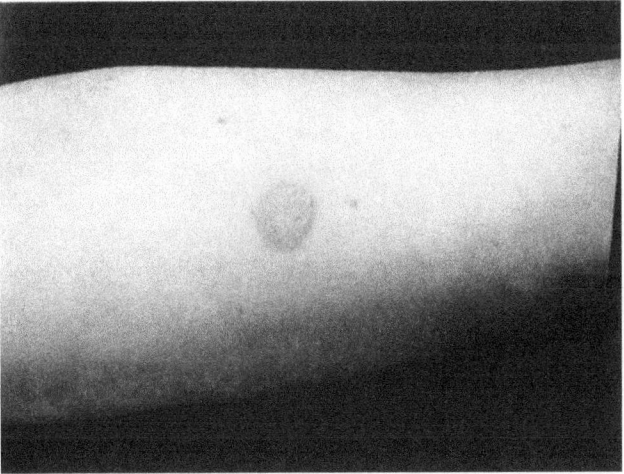

FIGURE 27–6. **Tuberculin skin test.** The purified protein derivative tuberculoprotein was injected intradermally at this site 48 hours previously. The erythema and induration (>15 mm) that are present indicate the development of delayed-type (type IV) hypersensitivity. (Reproduced with permission from Nester EW, Anderson DG, Roberts CE Jr, et al: *Microbiology: A Human Perspective,* 6th ed. New York, NY: McGraw Hill; 2008.)

 Think ▸▸ Apply 27-1: **This is due to the long survival of the cells that enter the state of latency. The MTB have been inert but "alive" all this time.**

✳ PPD indicates past or current
infection

✳ Other mycobacteria, BCG
immunization intermediate

✳ TST interpretation depends
on prevalence, BCG status

✳ IFN-γ tests specific for MTB

✳ AFB detected in 65% of
culture-positive sputum

Resident flora chemically
treated

Mucolytic agents concentrate
sputum

✳ Classic culture takes
3+ weeks

Colorimetric indicators speed
detection

✳ NAA detects MTB, rifampin
resistance

has developed DTH through infection at some time with MTB, but carries no implication as to whether the disease is active. Persons who have been infected with another mycobacterial species or immunized with the bacillus Calmette-Guérin (BCG) vaccine may also be reactive, but the induration is usually in the 5 to 10 mm range. Patients with severe disseminated disease, those on immunosuppressive drugs, or those with immunosuppressive diseases such as AIDS, may fail to react or produce 5 to 10 mm reactions due to anergy. A positive TST should not be attributed to BCG unless the vaccination was recent.

The predictive value of the TST depends on the prevalence of tuberculosis and other mycobacterial diseases in the population and public health practices, particularly the use of BCG immunization. In the United States, where BCG is not used and the disease prevalence is low, a positive test is very strong evidence of previous MTB infection. In countries that use BCG, the skin test can only be used selectively. A new group of tests detect the release of IFN-γ from T cells stimulated with MTB-only proteins in whole blood. These IFN-γ release assays (IGRA) are not positive in persons immunized with BCG or infected with other mycobacteria but are no better indicator of active tuberculosis than the TST. IGRA tests are more expensive but this expense is often offset by their value in immigrant populations and in facilitating clinical decision making such as hospital isolation.

■ Laboratory Diagnosis

Acid-fast Smears

MTB can be detected microscopically in smears of clinical specimens using one of the acid-fast staining procedures discussed in Chapter 4. Because the number of bacteria present is often small, specimens such as sputum and cerebrospinal fluid are concentrated by centrifugation before staining to improve the sensitivity of detection. In one of the acid-fast procedures, the stain is fluorescent, which enhances the chances that a microscopist will be able to find the few that may be present in an entire acid-fast bacilli (AFB) smear. Even with the best of concentration and staining methods, little more than half (~65%) of culture-positive sputum samples yield positive AFB smears. The yield from other sites is even lower, particularly cerebrospinal fluid. The presence of AFB is not specific for MTB because other mycobacteria may have a similar morphology.

Culture

Whether the AFB smear is positive or not, culture of the organism is essential for confirmation and for antimicrobial susceptibility testing. Specimens from sites, such as cerebrospinal fluid, bone marrow, and pleural fluid, can be seeded directly to culture media used for MTB isolation. Samples from sites inevitably contaminated with resident microbiota, such as sputum, gastric aspirations (cultured when sputum is not produced), and voided urine, are chemically treated (alkali, acid, and detergents) using concentrations, experience has shown to kill the bulk of contaminating flora but not mycobacteria. Sputum specimens also require the use of agents to dissolve mucus so the specimen can be concentrated by centrifugation or filtration before inoculation onto the culture media just described.

Cultures on solid media usually take 3 weeks or longer to show visible colonies. Growth is more rapid in liquid media in which detection time may be further decreased by radiometric, fluorometric, and colorimetric growth indicator systems. These systems may also be automated and have become the standard for all that can afford them. Identification of the isolated mycobacterium is achieved with a number of cultural and biochemical tests, including those shown in Table 27–1, but this process takes weeks more. Nucleic acid amplification (NAA) procedures targeting both DNA and ribosomal RNA sequences in clinical specimens have been developed and applied worldwide with increasing success. A rapid commercial system shows high specificity for MTB and sensitivities for sputum specimens from patients with positive AFB smears which approach that of culture. The system also detects sequences associated with resistance to rifampin, a first-line drug (see treatment). Even with improved sensitivity, direct NAA methods cannot yet completely substitute for culture due to the need for live bacteria to carry out comprehensive antimicrobial susceptibility testing. Rifampin is not only a first-line agent for TB treatment but is considered a surrogate marker for resistance to multiple drugs. Automated systems able to detect both MTB and drug resistance markers directly in sputum samples are now available.

TABLE 27–2	Antimicrobics Commonly Used in Treatment of Tuberculosis
FIRST-LINE DRUG	**SECOND-LINE DRUG**[a]
Isoniazid	*para*-Aminosalicylic acid
Ethambutol	Ethionamide
Rifampin	Cycloserine
Pyrazinamide	Fluoroquinolones

[a]Second-line drugs added to combinations if resistance or toxicity contraindicates first-line agent.

TREATMENT

Before effective antimycobacterial drugs became available over half the patients with active pulmonary TB died of their disease, most within 2 years. The development of effective drugs is complicated by the need for them to pass the unusually impermeable lipid-rich mycobacterial cell wall. However, several antimicrobial agents have been shown to be effective in the treatment of MTB infection (**Table 27–2**). The term **first-line** is used to describe the primary drugs of choice (isoniazid, ethambutol, rifampin, and pyrazinamide) that have long clinical experience to back up their efficacy and to manage their side effects. **Second-line** agents are less preferred and reserved for use when there is resistance to the first-line agents.

The approach with new cases is to start the patient on multiple first-line drugs (often all four) while waiting for the results of susceptibility tests. When these results are available, the regimen is adjusted to two or three agents proven by susceptibility testing to be active against the patient's isolate. Isoniazid and rifampin are active against both intra- and extracellular organisms, and pyrazinamide acts at the acidic pH found within cells. The use of streptomycin, the first antibiotic active against MTB, is now limited by resistance, toxicity, and the requirement for parenteral administration. MTB is also susceptible to other drugs that may be used to replace those of the primary group due to resistance or drug toxicity. The fluoroquinolones, such as ciprofloxacin and ofloxacin, are active against MTB and penetrate well into infected cells. Their role in the treatment of tuberculosis is promising but they require further clinical evaluation. Isoniazid and ethambutol act on the mycolic acid (isoniazid) and LAM (ethambutol) elements of mycobacterial cell wall synthesis. The molecular targets of the other agents have yet to be defined except for the general antibacterial agents (rifampin, streptomycin, and fluoroquinolones) discussed in Chapter 23.

Because of the high bacterial load and long duration of anti-MTB therapy, the emergence of resistance during treatment is of greater concern than with more acute bacterial infections. This is the reason the use of multiple drugs each with a different mode of action is the norm. Expression of resistance would then theoretically require a double mutant, a very low probability when the frequency of single mutants is 10^{-7} to 10^{-10}. The percentage of new infections with strains resistant to first-line drugs varies between 5% and 15%, but it is increasing, particularly among those who have been treated previously. Of particular concern is the emergence in the last two decades of multidrug-resistant tuberculosis (MDR-TB) strains, defined as resistance to isoniazid and rifampin, the mainstays of primary treatment. MDR-TBs now represent 1% of United States cases but up to 6% of worldwide cases. Over half of these are concentrated in China, India, and the countries of the former Russian federation. MDR-TB resistance can be either primary or emerge after antituberculosis therapy. Strains that add resistance to one or more second-line drugs like fluoroquinolones are called extensively drug-resistant (XDR-TB). Although still uncommon such strains are increasingly being seen.

Why doesn't the mutant lead to a new subpopulation of resistant MTB?

These therapeutic advances make curing tuberculosis a realistic goal for all with active disease. Effective treatment renders the patient noninfectious within 1 or 2 weeks, which has shifted the care of tuberculous patients from isolation hospitals and sanatoriums to home or a general hospital. The duration of therapy varies, based on some clinical factors but is usually 6 to 9 months. In patients whose organisms display resistance to one or more of these drugs, and in those with HIV infection, a more intensive and prolonged treatment course is used. Chemotherapy for tuberculosis is among

* Must penetrate lipid-rich cell wall

* Resistance requires second-line drugs

Antimicrobials act intra- and extracellularly

Resistance, toxicity limit some agents

* Multidrug therapy decreases resistance expression

* MDR-TB resistant to isoniazid and rifampin

* Treatment 6 to 9 months

* Compliance a major problem

the most successful and cost-effective of all health interventions. Failure is most often due to lack of adherence to the regimen by the patient, the presence of resistant organisms, or both.

PREVENTION

There are a number of situations in which persons are felt to be at increased risk for TB even though they have no clinical evidence of disease (healthy + negative chest X-ray). The most common of these situations are close exposure to an open case (particularly a child) and/or conversion of the TST from negative to positive. In these instances, prophylactic chemotherapy with isoniazid (alone) is administered for 6 to 9 months. In the exposed person, the goal is to prevent a primary infection. The TST-positive person has already had a primary infection; therefore, the goal is to reduce the chance of reactivation TB by killing all MTB in the body before they enter the nonreplicating latent state. This chemoprophylaxis has clear value for recently exposed persons demonstrating skin test conversion. It is less certain for those whose time of conversion is unknown and could have been many years ago. Isoniazid may cause a form of hepatitis in adults, so its administration carries some risk.

Exposure, PPD conversion warrant isoniazid prophylaxis

Goal is eradication prior to latency

BCG is a live vaccine derived originally from a strain of *M bovis* that was attenuated by repeated subculture. It is administered intradermally to tuberculin-negative subjects and leads to self-limiting local multiplication of the organism with development of tuberculin DTH. The latter negates the TST as a diagnostic and epidemiologic tool. BCG has been used for the prevention of TB in various countries since 1923, but its overall efficacy remains controversial. Its ability to prevent disseminated disease in newborns and children is generally acknowledged, but prevention of chronic pulmonary disease in adults is not. TB would not be the world leading killer if BCG was effective in preventing pulmonary reactivation disease. The use of BCG in any country is a matter of public health policy balancing the potential protection against the loss of case tracking through the skin test. BCG is not used in the United States, but is used in many other counties, particularly those that lack the infrastructure for case tracking. BCG is contraindicated for individuals in whom T-cell–mediated immune mechanisms are compromised, such as those infected with HIV. Current TB vaccine strategies are focused on genomic manipulations of BCG which has a long experience of safety in diverse populations. Strategies include the insertion or modification of genes for proteins for which there is evidence of immunizing potential.

BCG vaccine stimulates DTH

Effectiveness in adults variable

Modified BCG basis for future vaccines

KEY CONCLUSIONS

- High-lipid mycobacterial cell wall contains mycolic acids and lipoarabinomannan (LAM) which are responsible for the staining property called acid-fastness.
- Infection is by inhalation of respiratory droplets coughed up by human cases.
- Primary pulmonary infection leads to systemic spread of *Mycobacterium tuberculosis* (MTB).
- MTB interferes with killing mechanisms of alveolar macrophages.
- MTB-specific macrophage activation by IFN-γ leads to resolution in most infected persons.
- Incomplete macrophage activation leads to progressive disease (tuberculosis).
- Delayed-type hypersensitivity (DTH) is the sole known cause of injury.
- Entry of MTB into inactive latent state creates risk of reactivation disease in the lung or other sites (much less often) years to decades later.
- DTH response to tuberculin skin test (TST) indicates previous infection but not active disease.
- Definitive diagnosis is by acid-fast bacilli (AFB) smear, culture, or nucleic acid amplification (NAA) procedures on sputum or other tissues.
- Bacillus Calmette-Guérin (BCG) vaccine offers childhood protection but does not prevent reactivation. It also causes a DTH response to TST.
- Antimicrobial chemotherapy of tuberculosis is effective, but few agents able to penetrate the MTB cell wall are available. Cost and compliance limit worldwide effectiveness.
- Up to four drugs are used simultaneously to prevent expression of resistant mutants.

Think ▸▸ Apply 27-2: The mutant cell cannot replicate because it is still susceptible to the action (at a different molecular site) of at least one of the other drugs in the regimen. Expression would require two or three independent mutations in the genome of a single cell, an unlikely event.

Overview

Mycobacterium leprae is a mycobacterial species yet to be grown in culture. Its disease, leprosy, is a chronic granulomatous inflammation of the peripheral nerves and superficial tissues, which is particularly distinctive in the nasal mucosa. The extent of disease depends on the effectiveness of Th1 immune responses and ranges from slowly resolving anesthetic skin lesions to the disfiguring facial lesions responsible for the social stigma and ostracism of the individuals with leprosy (lepers). Effective chemotherapy produces cures and is responsible for closing of the infamous leper colonies.

BACTERIOLOGY

Mycobacterium leprae, the cause of leprosy (Hanson disease), is an AFB that has not been grown in artificial media or tissue culture beyond a few generations. However, it will grow slowly (doubling time 14 days) in some animals (mice, armadillos). Although lack of *in vitro* growth severely limits study of the organism, the structure and cell wall components appear to be similar to those of other mycobacteria. One mycoside (phenolic glycolipid I [PGL-1]) is synthesized in large amounts and found only in *M leprae*.

❋ Has not been grown in artificial culture

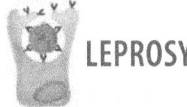

LEPROSY

EPIDEMIOLOGY

The exact mode of transmission is unknown but appears to be by generation of small droplets from the nasal secretions from cases of florid leprosy. Traumatic inoculation through minor skin lesions or tattoos is also possible. The central reservoir is infected humans, but infection may be acquired from environmental sources. The incubation period as estimated from clinical observations is generally 2 to 7 years, but sometimes up to four decades. The infectivity of *M leprae* is low. Most new cases have had prolonged close contact with an infected person. Biting insects may also be involved. The introduction of effective chemotherapy in 1981 reduced the incidence of new cases worldwide from over 5 million to less than 200 thousand by 2017. Now virtually absent from North America and Europe, India; Brazil and Indonesia account for the most disease. Nine-banded armadillos found in South America and the southern United States are known to carry *M leprae* and have been associated with cases in persons who have never left the United States.

❋ Nasal droplets transmit infection

Rare in North America

PATHOGENESIS

M leprae is an obligate intracellular pathogen that must multiply in host cells to persist. In humans, the target is Schwann cells, the glial cells of the peripheral nervous system. PGL-1 and a laminin-binding protein facilitate both invasion of Schwann cells and binding to basal lamina of the peripheral nerve axon units. This leads to cell injury and demyelination of peripheral nerves, which precede but is enhanced by the DTH immune response to *M leprae*. This invasion and demyelination of peripheral sensory nerves cause local anesthesia and other changes in the skin depending on the location and degree of immune response. Individual variability in the extent of immune response is responsible for two major forms of leprosy with a spectrum of illness in between. In the **tuberculoid** form, few *M leprae* are seen in lesions with well-formed granulomas, abundant CD4+ T cells, extensive epithelioid cells, giant cells, and lymphocytic infiltration. In **lepromatous** leprosy there is a lack of CD4+ T cells, numerous CD8+ T cells, foamy macrophages, and dense infiltration with leprosy bacilli.

❋ Schwann cells are target

❋ Peripheral nerves demyelinated

❋ Tuberculoid and lepromatous vary in CD4+ T-cell response

IMMUNITY

Immunity to *M leprae* is T-cell–mediated. Tuberculoid cases have minimal disease and evidence of Th1 immune responses including production of typical cytokines (IL-2, IFN-γ). Lepromatous cases have progressive disease and lack Th1 mediators. In the past, this range of disease also correlated with DTH responsiveness to lepromin, a skin test antigen no longer available.

❋ Th1 immunity determines extent of disease

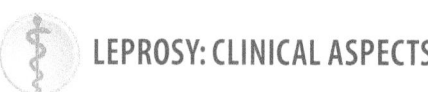

LEPROSY: CLINICAL ASPECTS

MANIFESTATIONS

■ Tuberculoid Leprosy

Tuberculoid leprosy involves the development of macules or large, flattened plaques on the face, trunk, and limbs, with raised erythematous edges and dry, pale, hairless centers. When the bacterium has invaded peripheral nerves, the lesions are anesthetic. The disease is indolent, with simultaneous evidence of slow progression and healing. Because of the small number of organisms present, this form of the disease is usually noncontagious.

■ Lepromatous Leprosy

In lepromatous leprosy, skin lesions are infiltrative, extensive, symmetric, and diffuse, particularly on the face, with thickening of the looser skin of the lips, forehead, and ears (**Figure 27–7**). Damage may be severe, with loss of nasal bones and septum, sometimes of digits, and testicular atrophy in men. Peripheral neuropathies may produce deformities or nonhealing painless ulcers. The organism may spread systemically, with involvement of the reticuloendothelial system.

DIAGNOSIS

Leprosy is primarily a clinical diagnosis confirmed by demonstration of AFB in stained scrapings of infected tissue, particularly nasal mucosa or ear lobes. Because *M leprae* is more sensitive to decolorization than MTB, a variant of the standard acid-fast procedure (Fite stain) must be employed to avoid false-negative results. AFB demonstration is readily achieved in lepromatous leprosy because of the typically large numbers of bacteria present. Tuberculoid leprosy is confirmed by the histologic appearance of full-thickness skin biopsies and hopefully a few AFB.

TREATMENT AND PREVENTION

Treatment has been revolutionized by the development of sulfones, such as dapsone, which blocks *para*-aminobenzoic acid metabolism in *M leprae*. Treatment regimens are different for patients with multiple AFB smear-positive skin lesions (multibacillary) and those in which AFB are difficult to detect (paucibacillary). For multibacillary disease, dapsone and clofazimine are combined with monthly rifampin doses for a year. For paucibacillary leprosy dapsone combined with monthly rifampin usually cures disease when given for 6 months. Prevention of leprosy involves recognition and treatment of infectious patients and early diagnosis of the disease in close contacts.

* Skin, nerve involvement

* Anesthetic lesions

* Lesions infiltrative and diffuse

* Modified AFB smears, biopsies

* Sulfones, clofazimine combined with rifampin

AFBs in skin lesions determine drug combinations and duration

FIGURE 27–7. **Lepromatous leprosy.** Note the cutaneous plaques, infiltrates, and loss of eyebrows. Scrapings of the ear lobes would reveal numerous acid-fast bacilli. This advanced case will still respond to appropriate chemotherapy. (Reproduced with permission from Connor DH, Chandler FW, Schwartz DQ, et al: *Pathology of Infectious Diseases.* Stamford CT: Appleton & Lange; 1997.)

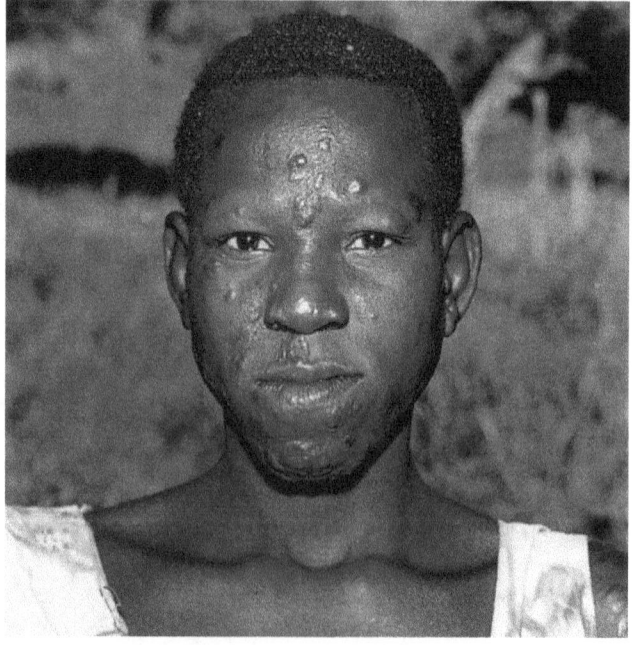

A possible diagnosis of leprosy elicits fear and distress in patients and friends out of proportion to its risks. Few clinicians in the United States have the experience to make such a diagnosis, and expert help should be sought from public health authorities before reaching this conclusion or indicating its possibility to the patient.

● MYCOBACTERIA CAUSING TUBERCULOSIS-LIKE DISEASES

Mycobacteria causing diseases that often resemble tuberculosis are listed in Table 27–1. With the exception of *M bovis*, mycobacteria have become relatively more prominent in developed countries as the incidence of tuberculosis has declined. All have known or suspected environmental reservoirs, and all the infections they cause appear to be acquired from these sources. Immunocompromised individuals or those with chronic pulmonary conditions or malignancies are more likely to develop disease. There is no evidence of case-to-case transmission. Environmental mycobacteria that cause tuberculosis-like infections are usually more resistant than *M tuberculosis* to the antimicrobials used in the treatment of mycobacterial diseases, and susceptibility testing is essential as a guide to therapy.

✳ Environmental source

✳ No human transmission

Resistance common

■ *Mycobacterium avium–intracellulare* Complex

The *Mycobacterium avium–intracellulare* complex (MAC) includes three closely related mycobacteria, *M avium*, *M intracellulare*, and *M chimaera* that grow only slightly faster than *M tuberculosis*. Among them are organisms that cause tuberculosis in birds (and sometimes swine), but rarely lead to disease in humans. Others may produce disease in mammals, including humans, but not in birds. They are found worldwide in soil and water and in infected animals.

✳ Associated with birds, mammals

Second AFB cause in developed countries

The most common infection in humans is cavitary pulmonary disease, often superimposed on chronic bronchitis and emphysema. Most individuals infected are white men of 50 years of age or more. Cervical lymphadenitis, chronic osteomyelitis, and renal and skin infections also occur. The organisms in this group are substantially more resistant to antituberculosis drugs than most other species, and treatment with the three or four agents found to be most active often requires supplementation with surgery. About 20% of patients suffer relapse within 5 years of treatment.

Wide disease range; most pulmonary

Resistance to antituberculosis drugs

Disseminated MAC infections, once considered rare, are now a common systemic bacterial superinfection in patients with AIDS. They usually develop when the patient's general clinical condition and CD4+ T cell concentrations are declining. Clinically, the patient experiences progressive weight loss and intermittent fever, chills, night sweats, and diarrhea. Histologically, granuloma formation is muted, and there are aggregates of foamy macrophages containing numerous intracellular AFB. The diagnosis is most readily made by blood culture, using a variety of specialized cultural techniques. Response to chemotherapeutic agents is marginal, and the prognosis is grave. *M chimaera* infections are similar but generally less virulent.

✳ Common AIDS coinfection

✳ Isolated from blood

■ *Mycobacterium kansasii*

Mycobacterium kansasii is a species that forms pigmented colonies after about 2 weeks of incubation. In the United States, infection tends to affect urban residents; it is uncommon in the Southeast. There is no evidence of case-to-case transmission, but the reservoir has yet to be identified. It causes about 3% of non-MTB mycobacterial disease in the United States. *M kansasii* infections resemble TB and tend to be slowly progressive without treatment. Cavitary pulmonary disease, cervical lymphadenitis, and skin infections are most common, but disseminated infections also occur. They are an important cause of disease in patients with HIV infection and CD4+ T lymphocyte counts of less than 200 cells/μL; clinical features closely resemble TB in patients with AIDS. Hypersensitivity to proteins of *M kansasii* develops and cross-reacts almost completely with that caused by TB. Positive TST tests may thus result from clinical or subclinical *M kansasii* infection. Prolonged combined chemotherapy with isoniazid, rifampin, and ethambutol is usually effective.

Mycobacterium scrofulaceum

Mycobacterium scrofulaceum occurs in the environment under moist conditions. It forms yellow colonies in the dark or light within 2 weeks, and it shares several features with MAC. *M scrofulaceum* is now one of the more common causes of granulomatous cervical lymphadenitis in young children. The infection manifests as an indolent enlargement of one or more lymph nodes with little, if any, pain or constitutional signs. It may ulcerate or form a draining sinus to the surface. It does not cause TST conversion. Treatment usually involves surgical excision.

● MYCOBACTERIA CAUSING SOFT TISSUE INFECTIONS

Mycobacterium fortuitum Complex

In addition to *Mycobacterium fortuitum* this complex includes *M abscessus* and *M chelonae*. All are free-living, rapidly growing AFB, which produce colonies within 3 days. Human infections are rare. Abscesses at injection sites in drug abusers are probably the most common lesions. Occasional secondary pulmonary infections develop. Some cases have been associated with implantation of foreign material (eg, breast prostheses, artificial heart valves). Except in the case of endocarditis, infections usually resolve spontaneously with removal of the prosthetic device.

Mycobacterium marinum

Mycobacterium marinum causes disease in fish. It is widely present in fresh and salt waters, and grows at 30°C but not at 37°C. It occurs in considerable numbers in the slime that forms on rocks or on rough walls of swimming pools and thrives in tropical fish aquariums. It can cause skin lesions in humans. Classically, a swimmer who abrades elbows or forearms climbing out of a pool develops a superficial granulomatous lesion that finally ulcerates. It usually heals spontaneously after a few weeks, but is sometimes chronic. The organism may be sensitive to tetracyclines as well as to some antituberculosis drugs. A recent outbreak was associated with fish handlers in a New York City Chinatown market.

Mycobacterium ulcerans

Mycobacterium ulcerans is serious cause of superficial infection. Like *M marinum*, *M ulcerans* grows at 30°C but not at 37°C [see Table 27–1]). Cases usually occur in the tropics, most often in parts of Africa, New Guinea, and northern Australia, but have been seen elsewhere sporadically. Children are most often affected. The source of infection and mode of transmission are unknown. Infected individuals develop severe ulceration involving the skin and subcutaneous tissue that is often progressive unless treated effectively. Surgical excision and grafting are usually needed. Antimicrobial treatment is often unsuccessful.

Marginal notes

* Resembles TB
* Infection may cause TST conversion

* Granulomatous cervical lymphadenitis in children

* Cause abscesses, infections of prostheses

* Cause of fish-associated tuberculosis

Occurs in tropical areas

Progressive ulcerations require surgical removal

CASE STUDY

Jail, HIV, and AFB

A 55-year-old man with a 2-month history of fevers, night sweats, increased cough with bloody sputum production, and a 25-lb weight loss was seen in the emergency room. He reported no intravenous drug use or homosexual activity but had multiple sexual encounters in the previous year. He "sips" a pint of gin a day and was jailed 2 years ago in New York City related to a fight with gunshot and stab wounds. His physical examination revealed bilateral anterior cervical and axillary adenopathy and a temperature of 39.4°C. His chest radiograph showed peritracheal adenopathy and bilateral interstitial infiltrates. His laboratory findings showed a positive HIV serology and a low absolute CD4 lymphocyte count. An acid-fast organism grew from the sputum and bronchoalveolar lavage (BAL) fluid from the right middle lobe.

QUESTIONS

1. The most likely etiologic agent(s) for this patient's infection are:
   A. *Mycobacterium tuberculosis*
   B. *Mycobacterium avium–intracellulare*
   C. *Mycobacterium leprae*
   D. A and B
   E. B and C

2. All of the following factors increase this man's risk of developing active tuberculosis *except*:
   A. Homosexual relations
   B. Jail
   C. HIV
   D. Alcoholism

3. If the acid-fact bacterium isolated from the man's sputum is identified as *Mycobacterium tuberculosis* and he is placed on a two-drug antituberculous regimen, the resolution of his disease depends primarily on:
   A. Antibody to LAM
   B. Lifestyle changes
   C. Th1 immune responses
   D. Th2 immune responses
   E. Active DTH

ANSWERS

1. (D)

2. (A)

3. (C)

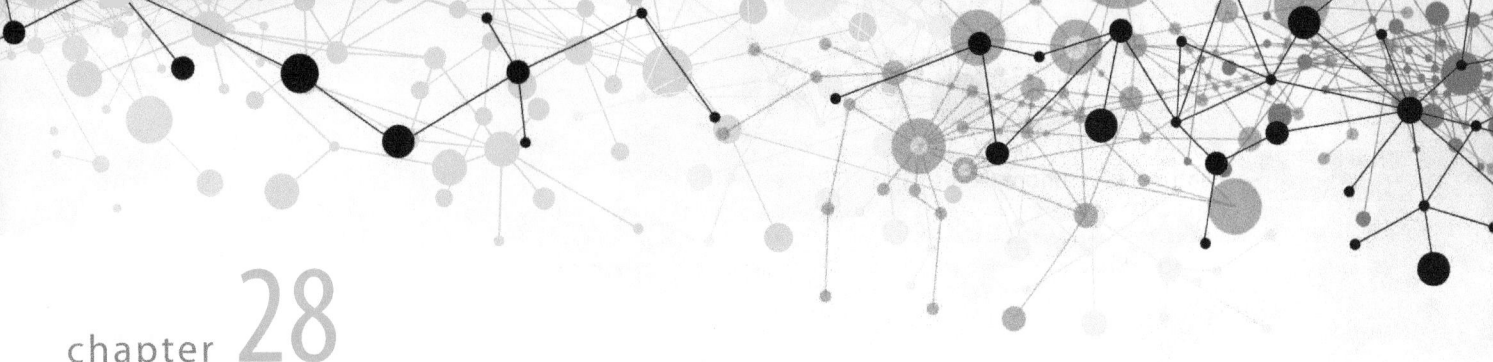

chapter 28

Actinomyces and *Nocardia*

Actinomyces israelii • *Nocardia asteroids* • *Nocardia brasiliensis* • *Rhodococcus equi*

Actinomyces and *Nocardia* are Gram-positive rods characterized by filamentous, tree-like branching growth, which has caused them to be confused with fungi in the past. They are opportunists that can sometimes produce indolent, slowly progressive diseases. A related genus, *Streptomyces*, is of medical importance as a producer of many antibiotics, but it rarely causes infections. Important differential features of these groups and of the mycobacteria to which they are related are shown in **Table 28–1**.

● ACTINOMYCES

OVERVIEW

Actinomycosis is a chronic inflammatory condition originating in the tissues adjacent to mucosal surfaces caused by anaerobic Gram-positive branching bacilli of the genus Actinomyces that are present in the microbiota of the alimentary tract. Disease occurs when minor trauma displaces these bacteria below the mucosal barrier. The lesions follow a slow burrowing course with considerable induration and draining sinuses, eventually opening through the skin. The exact nature depends on the organs and structures involved.

 ## BACTERIOLOGY

Actinomyces are typically elongated Gram-positive rods that branch at acute angles (**Figure 28–1**). They are Gram-positive bacilli that grow slowly (4-10 days) under microaerophilic or strictly anaerobic conditions. In pus and tissues, the most characteristic form is the sulfur granule (**Figure 28–2**). This yellow-orange granule, named for its gross resemblance to a grain of sulfur, is a microcolony of intertwined branching *Actinomyces* filaments solidified with elements of tissue exudate.

⁎ Anaerobic branching Gram-positive rods

Species of *Actinomyces* are distinguished on the basis of biochemical reactions, cultural features, and cell wall composition. Most human actinomycosis is caused by *Actinomyces israelii*, but other species have been isolated from typical actinomycotic lesions. Another group of *Actinomyces* species have been associated with dental and periodontal infections (see Chapter 41).

⁎ Most infections *A israelii*

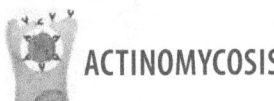 ## ACTINOMYCOSIS

Actinomyces are normal inhabitants of some areas of the gastrointestinal tract of humans and animals from the oropharynx to the lower bowel. These species are highly adapted to mucosal surfaces and do not produce disease unless they transgress the epithelial barrier under conditions

TABLE 28-1	Features of Actinomycetes				
GENUS	**MORPHOLOGY**	**ACID-FASTNESS**	**GROWTH**	**SOURCE**	**DISEASE**
Actinomyces	Branching bacilli	None	Anaerobic	Oral, intestinal endogenous flora	Chronic cellulitis, draining sinuses
Nocardia	Branching bacilli	Weak[a,b]	Aerobic	Soil	Pneumonia, skin pustules, brain abscess
Rhodococcus	Cocci to bacilli	Variable (weak[a])	Aerobic	Soil, horses[c]	Pneumonia
Streptomyces	Branching bacilli	None	Aerobic	Soil	Extremely rare[d]

[a]Modified stain, fast only to weak decolorizer (1% H_2SO_4).
[b]*N asteroides* and *N brasiliensis;* other species variable.
[c]*R equi.*
[d]Nonpathogen, but important producer of antibiotics.

* Microbiota in gastrointestinal tract

* Displacement into tissues

Sinus tracts with sulfur granules

Little evidence of immunity

* Linked to poor dental hygiene

Surgery, trauma, intrauterine devices provide access

that produce a sufficiently low oxygen tension for their multiplication (**Figure 28-3**). Such conditions usually involve mechanical disruption of the mucosa with necrosis of deeper, normally sterile tissues (eg, following tooth extraction). Once initiated, growth occurs in microcolonies in the tissues and extends without regard to anatomic boundaries. The lesion is composed of inflammatory sinuses, which ultimately discharge to the surface. As the lesion enlarges, it becomes firm and indurated. Sulfur granules are present within the pus but are not numerous. Free *Actinomyces* or small branching units are rarely seen, although contaminating Gram-negative rods are common. As with other anaerobic infections, most cases are polymicrobial involving other flora from the mucosal site of origin including other *Actinomyces* species.

Human cases of actinomycosis provide little evidence of immunity to *Actinomyces*. Once established, infections typically become chronic and resolve only with the aid of antimicrobial therapy. Antibodies can be detected in the course of infection, but seem to reflect the antigenic stimulation of the ongoing infection rather than immunity. Infections with *Actinomyces* are endogenous, and case-to-case transmission does not appear to occur.

ACTINOMYCOSIS: CLINICAL ASPECTS

MANIFESTATIONS

Actinomycosis exists in several forms that differ according to the original site and circumstances of tissue invasion. Infection of the cervicofacial area, the most common site of actinomycosis (**Figure 28-4**), is usually related to poor dental hygiene, tooth extraction, or some other trauma to the mouth or jaw. Lesions in the submandibular region and the angle of the jaw give the face a swollen, indurated appearance.

Thoracic and abdominal actinomycosis are rare and follow aspiration or traumatic (including surgical) introduction of infected material leading to erosion through the pleura, chest, or abdominal wall. Diagnosis is usually delayed because only vague or nonspecific symptoms are produced until a vital organ is eroded or obstructed. The firm, fibrous masses are often initially mistaken for a malignancy. Pelvic involvement as an extension from other sites also occurs occasionally.

FIGURE 28-1. **Actinomyces.** Note the angular branching of the Gram-positive bacilli. (Reproduced with permission from Willey JM: *Prescott, Harley, & Klein's Microbiology,* 7th ed. New York, NY: McGraw Hill; 2008.)

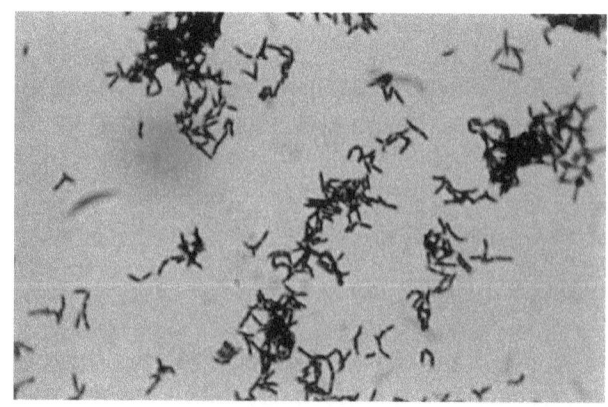

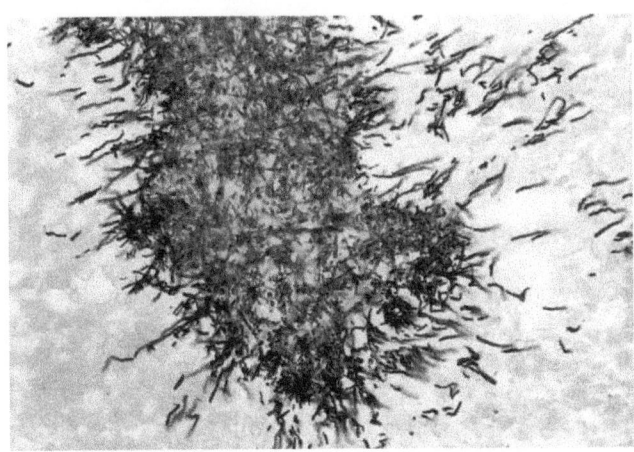

FIGURE 28-2. **Sulfur granule.** The mass is a microcolony of bacteria Gram-positive bacteria and tissue elements. The branching is clearly seen only at the edge. (Reproduced with permission from Connor DH, Chandler FW, Schwartz DQ, et al: *Pathology of Infectious Diseases*. Stamford CT: Appleton & Lange; 1997.)

It is particularly difficult to distinguish from other inflammatory conditions or malignancies. A more localized chronic endometritis, due to *Actinomyces*, is associated with the use of intrauterine contraceptive devices.

DIAGNOSIS

A clinical diagnosis of actinomycosis is based on the nature of the lesion, the slowly progressive course, and a history of trauma or of a condition predisposing to mucosal invasion by *Actinomyces*. The etiologic diagnosis can be difficult to establish with certainty. Although the lesions may be extensive, the organisms in pus may be few and concentrated in sulfur granule microcolonies deep in the indurated tissue. The diagnosis is further complicated by heavy colonization of the moist draining sinuses with other bacteria, usually Gram-negative rods. This contamination not only causes confusion regarding the etiology but interferes with isolation of the slow-growing anaerobic *Actinomyces*. Material for direct smear and culture should include as much pus as possible to increase the chance of collecting the diagnostic sulfur granules.

Sinus drainage contains few Actinomyces

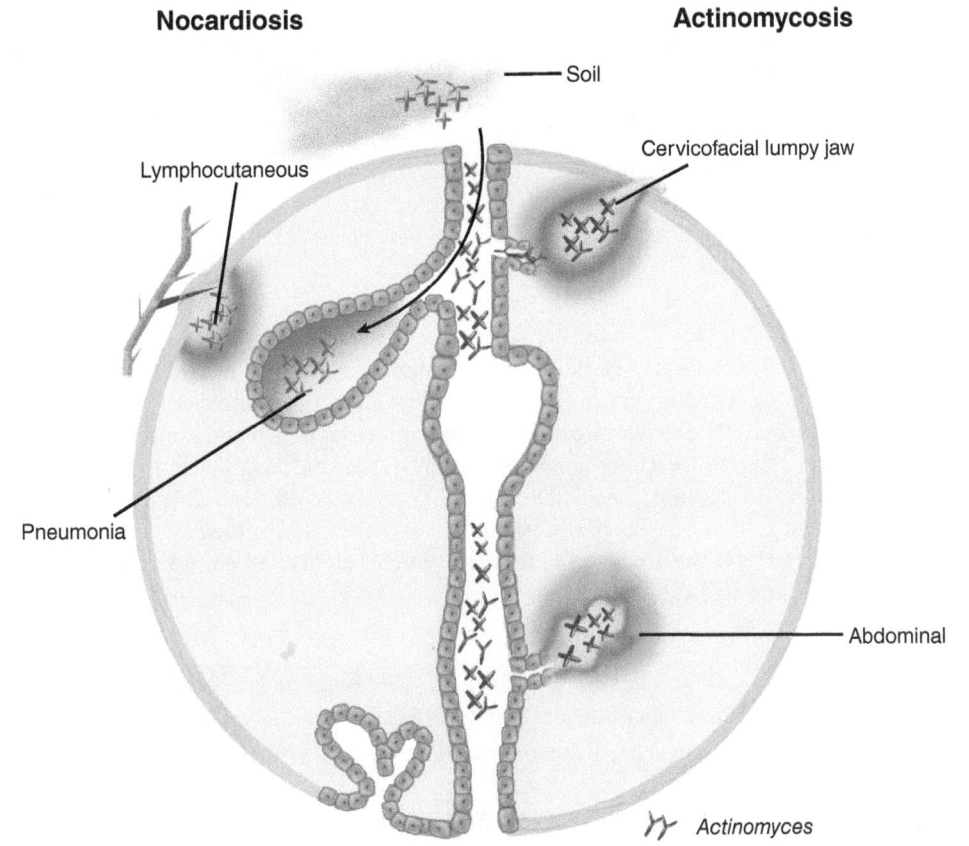

FIGURE 28-3. **Actinomycosis and Nocardiosis.** (*Right*) *Actinomyces* are members of the normal flora throughout the alimentary tract. Minor trauma allows access to tissues where they create burrowing abscesses that may break through to the surface. (*Left*) *Nocardia* is present in the soil, where it may be either inhaled to produce a pneumonia or traumatically injected to produce cutaneous pustules and lymphadenitis.

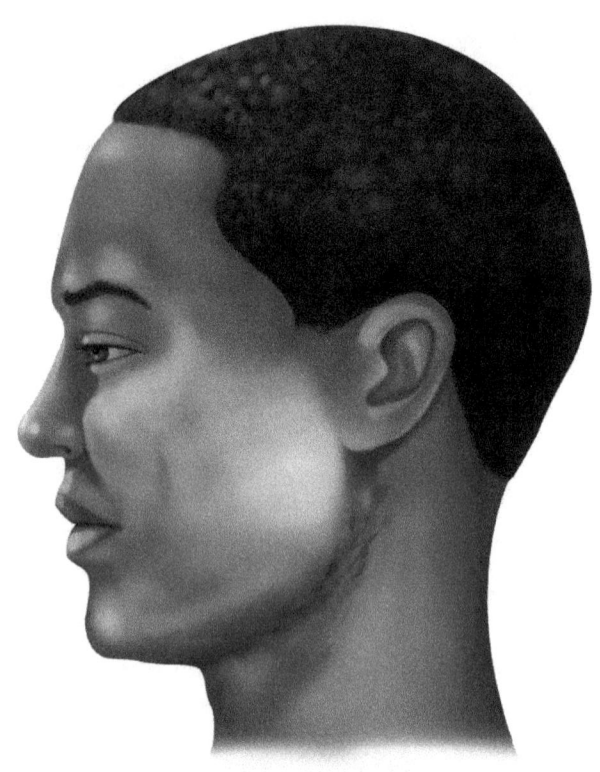

FIGURE 28–4. Cervicofacial actinomycosis. The classic "lumpy jaw" is shown with draining sinuses at the angle of the jaw. The lesion would be very firm on palpation. (Reproduced with permission from Connor DH, Chandler FW, Schwartz DQ, et al: *Pathology of Infectious Diseases.* Stamford CT: Appleton & Lange; 1997.)

✳ Gram stains show branching rods

Anaerobic culture required

Biopsy shows clubbed lesions

Penicillin is effective

Sulfur granules crushed and stained show a dense, Gram-positive center with individual branching rods at the periphery (Figure 28–2). Granules should also be selected for culture, because material randomly taken from a draining sinus usually grows only superficial contaminants. Culture media and techniques are the same as those used for other anaerobes. Incubation must be prolonged because some strains require 7 days or more to appear. Identification requires a variety of biochemical tests to differentiate *Actinomyces* from *Propionibacteria*, which may show a tendency to form short branches.

Biopsies for culture and histopathology are useful, but it may be necessary to examine many sections and pieces of tissue before sulfur granule colonies of *Actinomyces* are found. The morphology of the sulfur granule in tissue is quite characteristic with routine hematoxylin and eosin (H&E) or histologic Gram staining. With the histologic H&E stain, the edge of the granule shows amorphous eosinophilic "clubs" formed from the tissue elements and containing the branching actinomycotic filaments.

TREATMENT

Penicillin G is the treatment of choice for actinomycosis, although a number of other antimicrobics (ampicillin, doxycycline, erythromycin, and clindamycin) are active *in vitro* and have shown clinical effectiveness. Metronidazole is not active. High doses of penicillin must be used and therapy prolonged for up to 6 weeks or longer before any response is seen. The initial treatment course is usually followed with an oral penicillin for 6 to 12 months. Although slow, response to therapy is often striking given the degree of fibrosis and deformity caused by the infection. Because detection of the causative organism is difficult, many patients are treated empirically as a therapeutic trial based on clinical findings alone.

KEY CONCLUSIONS

- Anaerobic branching Gram-positive rods grow in microcolonies called sulfur granules.
- Displacement from microbiota habitat across oropharyngeal or intestinal mucosa leads to burrowing lesions.
- Culture diagnosis from draining sinuses complicated by contaminating bacteria.
- Penicillin and other β-lactams are effective treatment.

● *NOCARDIA*

OVERVIEW

Nocardia species are aerobic Gram-positive rods which typically demonstrate acid-fastness. They are present in soil and other environmental sites. Nocardiosis occurs in two major forms. The pulmonary form is an acute bronchopneumonia with dyspnea, cough, and sputum production. A cutaneous form produces localized pustules in areas of traumatic inoculation, usually the exposed areas of the skin.

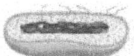

BACTERIOLOGY

Nocardia species are Gram-positive, rod-shaped bacteria related to mycobacteria and like them abundant mycolic acids are present in their cell wall. They show true branching both in culture and in stains from clinical lesions. The microscopic morphology is similar to that of *Actinomyces*, although *Nocardia* tend to fragment more readily and are found as shorter branched units throughout the lesion rather than concentrated in a few colonies or granules. Many strains of *Nocardia* take the Gram stain poorly, appearing "beaded" with alternating Gram-positive and Gram-negative sections of the same filament (**Figure 28–5A and B**). The species most common in human infection are *Nocardia abscessus* (formerly *N asteroides*) and *Nocardia brasiliensis*, which are weakly acid-fast.

In contrast to *Actinomyces*, *Nocardia* species are strict aerobes. Growth typically appears on ordinary laboratory medium (blood agar) after 2 to 3 days incubation in air. Colonies initially have a dry, wrinkled, chalk-like appearance, are adherent to the agar, and eventually develop white to orange pigment. Speciation involves uncommon tests such as the decomposition of amino acids and casein.

✳ Beaded, branching Gram-positive rods, weakly acid-fast

Grow on blood agar in 2 to 3 days

NOCARDIOSIS

EPIDEMIOLOGY

Nocardia species are ubiquitous in the environment, particularly in soil. In fact, fully developed colonies of *Nocardia* give off the aroma of wet dirt. The organisms have been isolated in small numbers from the respiratory tract of healthy persons, but are not considered members of the microbiota. The pulmonary form of disease follows inhalation of aerosolized bacteria, and the cutaneous form follows injection by a thorn prick or similar accident (Figure 28–3). Most

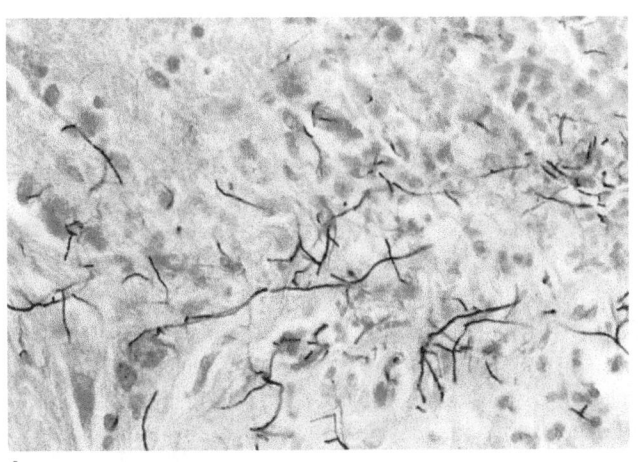 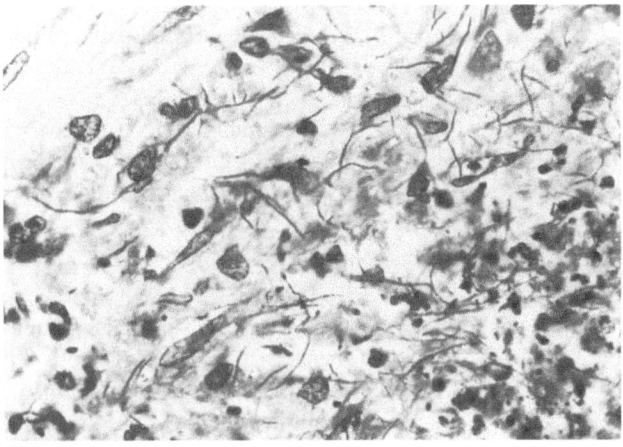

A   **B**

FIGURE 28–5. *Nocardia* in sputum. A. Note the filamentous bacteria forming tree-like branches among the neutrophils. The beaded appearance of the rods is typical. **B.** The same sputum stain with the modified (weaker) acid-fast method. Note the red filaments with the same branching pattern as in A. (Reproduced with permission from Connor DH, Chandler FW, Schwartz DQ, et al: *Pathology of Infectious Diseases.* Stamford CT: Appleton & Lange; 1997.)

* Primary source is soil

pulmonary cases occur in patients with compromised immune systems due to underlying disease or the use of immunosuppressive therapy. Transplant patients have been a prominent representative of the latter group. There is no case-to-case transmission.

PATHOGENESIS

* Survive in phagocytes

CNS invasion produces brain abscesses

Factors leading to disease after inhalation of *Nocardia* are poorly understood. Neutrophils are prominent in nocardial lesions, but appear to be relatively ineffective. The bacteria have the ability to resist the microbicidal actions of phagocytes and may be related to the disruption of phagosome acidification or resistance to the oxidative burst. No specific virulence factors are known. The primary lesions in the lung show acute inflammation, with suppuration and destruction of parenchyma. Multiple, confluent abscesses may occur. Unlike *Actinomyces* infections, there is little tendency toward fibrosis and localization. Dissemination to distant organs, particularly the brain, may occur. In the central nervous system (CNS), multifocal abscesses are often produced.

* Cutaneous infections follow
  minor trauma

Skin infections follow direct inoculation of *Nocardia*. This mechanism is usually associated with some kind of outdoor activity and with relatively minor trauma. The species is usually *N brasiliensis*, which produces a superficial pustule at the site of inoculation. If *Nocardia* gain access to the subcutaneous tissues, lesions resembling actinomycosis may be produced, complete with draining sinuses and sulfur granules.

IMMUNITY

* CMI mechanisms dominant

There is evidence that effective T-cell–mediated immunity is dominant in host defense against *Nocardia* infection. Increased resistance to experimental *Nocardia* infection in animals has been mediated by cytokine-activated macrophages, and activated macrophages have enhanced capacity to kill *Nocardia* that they have engulfed. Patients with impaired cell-mediated immune responses are at greatest risk for nocardiosis. There is little evidence for effective humoral immune responses.

 NOCARDIOSIS: CLINICAL ASPECTS

MANIFESTATIONS

Pulmonary infection is usually a confluent bronchopneumonia that may be acute, chronic, or relapsing. Production of cavities and extension to the pleura are common. Symptoms are those of any bronchopneumonia, including cough, dyspnea, and fever. The clinical signs of brain abscess depend on its exact location and size; the neurologic picture can be particularly confusing when multiple lesions are present.

 How would Nocardia get to the brain?

* Bronchopneumonia and
  cerebral abscess

The combination of current or recent pneumonia and focal CNS signs is suggestive of *Nocardia* infection. The cutaneous syndrome typically involves a pustule, fever, and tender lymphadenitis in the regional lymph nodes.

DIAGNOSIS

The diagnosis of *Nocardia* infection is much easier than that of actinomycosis because the organisms are present in greater numbers and distributed more evenly throughout the lesions. Filaments of Gram-positive rods with primary and secondary branches can usually be found in sputum and are readily demonstrated in direct aspirates from skin or other purulent sites. Demonstration of acid-fastness, when combined with other observations, is diagnostic of *Nocardia*

 Think ►► Apply 28-1: Presumably by inhalation from soil into the lung followed by hematogenous dissemination to the central nervous system.

(Figure 28–5). The acid-fastness of *Nocardia* species is not as strong as that of mycobacteria. Like *Mycobacterium leprae*, the staining method (Kinyoun technique) uses a decolorizing agent weaker than that used for the classic AFB stains. Culture of *Nocardia* is not difficult because the organisms grow on blood agar. It is still important to alert the laboratory to the possibility of nocardiosis, because the slow growth of *Nocardia* could cause it to be overgrown by the respiratory flora commonly found in sputum specimens. Due to competition from local microbiota the yield from respiratory specimens may be improved by the use of selective media. Specific identification can take weeks due to the unconventional tests involved. Nucleic acid amplification methods have been developed but are not widely available.

Gram-positive

* Weak acid fastness

Blood agar culture

TREATMENT

For decades, Nocardia infection has been one of the few indications for systemic use of sulfonamides alone or combined with trimethoprim. Recent surveys indicate an increase in resistance to sulfonamides including the trimethoprim–sulfamethoxazole combination. Technical difficulties in susceptibility testing have hampered the rational selection and study of other antimicrobials. Although most *Nocardia* strains are relatively resistant to penicillin, some of the newer β-lactams (imipenem, meropenem, cefotaxime) have been effective, as have minocycline, doxycycline, erythromycin, and amikacin. Antituberculous agents and antifungal agents such as amphotericin B have no activity against *Nocardia*.

* Sulfonamides + trimethoprim active but increased resistance

KEY CONCLUSIONS

- Aerobic Gram-positive branching rods are weakly acid-fast.
- Nocardia are common in dirt and other environmental sites.
- Inhalation of *N asteroides* leads to pneumonia particularly in immunocompromised.
- Traumatic inoculation (typically *N brasiliensis*) leads to localized pustules.
- Culture requires 3 to 5 days.
- Sulfamethoxazole/trimethoprim and some newer β-lactams may be effective but susceptibility is variable.

RHODOCOCCUS

Rhodococcus is a genus of aerobic actinomycetes with characteristics similar to those of *Nocardia*. Morphologically the rods vary from cocci to long, curved, clubbed forms. Some strains are acid-fast. *Rhodococcus* has recently been recognized as an opportunistic pathogen causing an aggressive pneumonia in severely immunocompromised patients, particularly those with AIDS. The organisms are found in the soil. One species, *Rhodococcus equi*, has an association with horses where it also causes pneumonia in foals. This species is a facultative intracellular pathogen of macrophages with features somewhat similar to those of *Legionella* and *Listeria*. Optimal treatment is unknown, although combinations of a macrolide, rifampin, and fluoroquinolones show *in vitro* activity.

Vary from cocci to acid-fast rods

Pneumonia associated with horses

CASE STUDY

Lung Lesions and a Brain Abscess

The patient was a 34-year-old man with a history of tobacco and alcohol abuse (12 cans of beer per day). Two months before admission, he was seen at a hospital, where radiographs revealed a necrotic lesion in his right upper lobe. He was PPD-negative and three sputum cultures analyzed for *Mycobacterium* were negative. He had no risk factors for HIV infection. Four weeks later, he presented with fever, productive cough, night sweats, chills, and a 10 lb (4.5 kg) weight loss.

He was treated with ampicillin for 14 days. Fever, chills, and night sweats decreased. On admission, he presented with a firm right chest wall mass (4 × 4 cm), which was aspirated. The aspirated material was dark green and extremely viscous. Two days later, the nurses found him urinating on the wall of his room. Because of this behavior, it was decided to perform a CT scan of the head; the scan revealed multiple, ring-enhancing lesions. The patient was taken to surgery and the central nervous system lesions were drained. A Gram stain of the organism recovered from the brain aspirate showed a branching, beaded Gram-positive rod. The laboratory noted that it was also acid-fast.

QUESTIONS

1. The material in the brain aspirate most likely contains which of the following?
   A. *Actinomyces*
   B. *Nocardia*
   C. *Mycobacterium tuberculosis*
   D. Another *Mycobacterium*
   E. *Rhodococcus*

2. What risk factor is likely to have contributed the most to this patient's infection?
   A. Occupation
   B. Alcoholism
   C. HIV
   D. Smoking

3. The infection was most likely acquired from which of the following?
   A. Family member
   B. Pet
   C. Wild animal
   D. Soil
   E. Water

ANSWERS

1. **(B)**

2. **(B)**

3. **(D)**

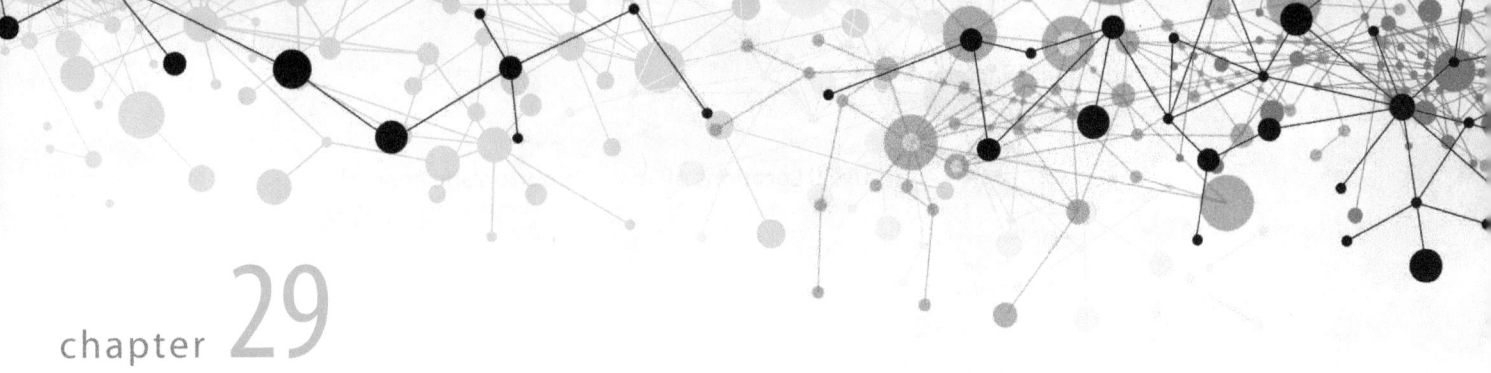

chapter 29

Clostridium, Bacteroides, and Other Anaerobes

Clostridium perfringens · *Clostridium botulinum* · *Clostridium tetani* · *Clostridium difficile* · *Bacteroides fragilis*

Can you watch placidly the horrible struggles of lock-jaw? ... If you can, you had better leave the profession: cast your diploma into the fire; you are not worthy to hold it.

—Jacob M. Da Costa (1833-1900): *College and Clinical Record*

The bacteria discussed in this chapter are united by a common requirement for anaerobic conditions for growth. Organisms from multiple genera and all Gram-stain categories are included. Most of them produce endogenous infections adjacent to the mucosal surfaces, especially when they are members of the indigenous microbiota. The clostridia form spores that allow them to produce diseases such as tetanus and botulism after environmental contamination of tissues or foods. Another anaerobic genus of bacteria, *Actinomyces*, is discussed in Chapter 28.

● ANAEROBES AND ANAEROBIC INFECTION: GROUP CHARACTERISTICS

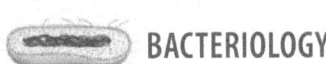 ## BACTERIOLOGY

THE NATURE OF ANAEROBIOSIS

Anaerobes not only survive under anaerobic conditions but they also require an oxygen-depleted environment to initiate and sustain growth. By definition, anaerobes fail to grow in the presence of 10% oxygen, but some are sensitive to oxygen concentrations as low as 0.5%, and can be killed by even brief exposures to air. However, **oxygen tolerance** is variable, and many organisms can survive briefly in the presence of 2% to 8% oxygen, including most of the species pathogenic for humans. The mechanisms involved are incompletely understood, but clearly represent a continuum from species described as **aerotolerant** to those so susceptible to oxidation that growing them in culture requires the use of media prepared and stored under anaerobic conditions.

✻ Anaerobes require low oxygen to initiate growth

Oxygen tolerance is a continuum

Anaerobes lack the cytochromes required to use oxygen as a terminal electron acceptor in energy-yielding reactions and thus generate energy solely by fermentation (see Chapter 21). Some anaerobes do not grow unless the oxidation–reduction potential is extremely low (–300 mV); because critical enzymes must be in the reduced state to be active; indeed, aerobic conditions create a metabolic block.

✻ Low redox potential is required

Another element of anaerobiosis is the direct susceptibility of anaerobic bacteria to molecular oxygen. For most aerobic and facultative bacteria, **catalase** and/or **superoxide dismutase** neutralize the toxicity of the oxygen products **hydrogen peroxide** and **superoxide.** Most anaerobes lack these enzymes and are injured when these oxygen products are formed in their

Antioxidant defense typically lacking

TABLE 29–1	Usual Locations of Some Opportunistic Anaerobes				
ORGANISM	GRAM STAIN	MOUTH OR PHARYNX	INTESTINE	UROGENITAL TRACT	SKIN
Peptoniphilus	Positive cocci	+	+	+	–
Propionibacterium	Positive rods	–	–	–	+
Clostridium	Positive rods (large)	–	+	–	–
Veillonella	Negative cocci	–	+	–	–
Bacteroides fragilis group	Negative rods (coccobacillary)	–	+	–	–
Fusobacterium	Negative rods (elongated)	+	+	–	–
Prevotella	Negative rods	+		+	–
Porphyromonas	Negative rods	+		+	

Pathogens often produce catalase and superoxide dismutase

microenvironment. However, and as discussed in the following text, many of the more virulent anaerobic pathogens are able to produce antioxidant enzymes like catalase or superoxide dismutase.

CLASSIFICATION

The anaerobes indigenous to humans include almost every morphotype and hundreds of species. Typically, biochemical and culture-based tests are used for classification, although this is difficult because the growth requirements of each anaerobic species must be satisfied. Characterization of cellular fatty acids and metabolic products by chromatography (or more recently, mass spectrometry) has been useful for many anaerobic groups. Nucleic acid base composition and homology have been used extensively to rename older taxonomy. The genera most commonly associated with disease are shown in **Table 29–1** and discussed later.

Biochemical, cultural, and molecular criteria define many species

■ Anaerobic Cocci

The medically important species of anaerobic Gram-positive cocci include species of the genus, *Peptoniphilus, Aerococcus,* and others. With Gram staining, these bacteria are most often seen as long chains of tiny cocci. On the Gram-negative side, *Veillonella* deserves mention because of its potential for confusion with *Neisseria* (other genera such as *Megasphera* and *Anaeroglobus* may also be confused with the neisseriae).

Gram (+) *in long chains*

Veillonella *may resemble* Neisseria

■ Clostridia

The clostridia are large, spore-forming, Gram-positive bacilli. Like their aerobic counterpart, *Bacillus*, clostridia can form spores that are resistant to heat, desiccation, and disinfectants. They are able to survive for decades in the environment and return to the vegetative form when exposed to a favorable milieu. The shape of the vegetative cell and location of the spore vary with the species. For some clostridial genera, the spores themselves (**Figure 29–1**) may be rarely seen in clinical specimens.

The medically important clostridia are potent producers of one or more protein exotoxins. The histotoxic group including *Clostridium perfringens* and five other species (**Table 29–2**) produces hemolysins at the site of acute infections; these have lytic effects on a wide variety of cells. The neurotoxic group including *Clostridium tetani* and *Clostridium botulinum* produces neurotoxins that exert their effect at neural sites remote from bacterial entry points. *Clostridioides difficile* produces enterotoxins and disease in the intestinal tract. Many of the more than 80 other nontoxigenic clostridial species are also associated with disease.

Spores vary in shape and location

Hemolysin, neurotoxin, and enterotoxin production cause disease

■ Nonsporulating Gram-positive Bacilli

Propionibacterium is a genus of small pleomorphic bacilli sometimes called anaerobic diphtheroids because of its morphologic resemblance to corynebacteria. They are among the most common bacteria in the resident microbiota of the skin. *Eubacterium* is a genus that includes long slender bacilli commonly found in the colonic flora. These organisms are occasionally isolated

Low-virulence members of skin, oral, and intestinal flora

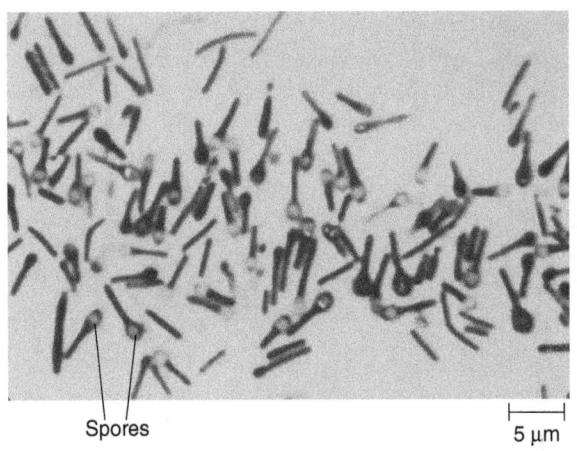

FIGURE 29–1. *Clostridium tetani.* Many of these bacilli show the typical terminal "tennis racquet" spores typical of this species. (© Arthur Siegelman/Visuals Unlimited)

Spores

5 μm

from infections in combination with other anaerobes, but they rarely produce disease on their own. Other anaerobic Gram-positive bacilli play roles in dental caries (see Chapter 41).

■ Gram-negative Bacilli

Gram-negative, non–spore-forming bacilli are the most common bacteria isolated from anaerobic infections. In the past, most species were consolidated into the genus *Bacteroides,* which still exists along with five other genera. Of these, *Fusobacterium, Porphyromonas,* and *Prevotella* are medically the most important. The *Bacteroides fragilis* group contains *B fragilis* and 10 similar

Bacteroides and other genera are medically important

TABLE 29–2	Features of Pathogenic Anaerobes			
ORGANISM	**BACTERIOLOGIC FEATURES**	**EXOTOXINS**	**SOURCE**	**DISEASE**
Gram-positive Cocci				
Peptoniphilus			Mouth, intestine	Oropharyngeal infections, brain abscess
Gram-negative Cocci				
Veillonella			Intestine	Rare opportunist
Gram-positive Bacilli				
Clostridium perfringens	Spores	α-Toxin, θ-toxin, enterotoxin	Intestine, environment, food	Cellulitis, gas gangrene, enterocolitis
Histotoxic species similar to *C perfringens*[a]	Spores		Intestine, environment	Cellulitis, gas gangrene
C tetani	Spores	Tetanospasmin	Environment	Tetanus
C botulinum	Spores	Botulinum	Environment	Botulism
C difficile	Spores	A enterotoxin, B cytotoxin	Intestine, environment (nosocomial)	Antibiotic-associated diarrhea, enterocolitis
Propionibacterium			Skin	Rare opportunist
Eubacterium			Intestine	Rare opportunist
Gram-negative Bacilli				
Bacteroides fragilis[b]	Polysaccharide capsule	Enterotoxin	Intestine	Opportunist, abdominal abscess
Bacteroides species			Intestine	Opportunist
Fusobacterium			Mouth, intestine	Opportunist
Prevotella	Black pigment		Mouth, urogenital	Opportunist
Porphyromonas			Mouth, urogenital	Opportunist

[a]*C histolyticum, C noyyi, C septicum, C bifermentans,* and *C sordellii.*
[b]The *Bacteroides fragilis* group includes *B fragilis, B distasonis, B ovatus, B vulgatus,* and *B thetaiotaomicron.*

species noted for their virulence, production of β-lactamases, and in some strains, production of an enterotoxin (species outside this group generally lack these features and are more similar to the other anaerobic Gram-negative bacilli). *Bacteroides fragilis* is a relatively short Gram-negative bacillus with rounded ends sometimes giving a coccobacillary appearance. Almost all *B fragilis* strains have a polysaccharide capsule and are particularly oxygen-tolerant. *Prevotella, Porphyromonas,* and *Fusobacterium* are distinguished by biochemical and other taxonomic features. *Prevotella melaninogenica* forms a black pigment in culture, and *Fusobacterium,* as its name suggests, is typically elongated and has tapered ends.

B fragilis group is oxygen tolerant and produces β-lactamase

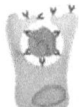

ANAEROBIC INFECTIONS

EPIDEMIOLOGY

Despite our constant immersion in air, anaerobes are able to colonize the many oxygen-deficient or oxygen-free microenvironments of the body. These conditions are created by the presence of resident microbiota whose growth reduces oxygen and decreases the local oxidation–reduction potential. Such sites include the sebaceous glands of the skin, the gingival crevices of the gums, the lymphoid tissue of the throat, and the lumina of the intestinal and urogenital tracts. Except for infections with some environmental clostridia, anaerobic infections are almost always endogenous with the infective agent(s) derived from the patient's own microbiota. The specific anaerobes involved are linked to their prevalence in the flora of the relevant sites as shown in Table 29–1. However, spores of some anaerobes (eg, Clostridia) that are normally resident in the lower intestinal tract of humans and animals may also be widely distributed in the environment, particularly in soil exposed to animal excreta. The spores may contaminate any wound caused by a nonsterile object (eg, splinter, nail) or exposed directly to soil.

Low redox microbiota sites are the origin of most infections

Spore-forming clostridia also come from the environment

PATHOGENESIS

The anaerobic microbiota normally lives in a harmless commensal relationship with the host. However, when displaced from their niche on the mucosal surface into normally sterile tissues, these organisms may cause life-threatening infections. This can occur as the result of trauma (gunshot, surgery), disease (diverticulosis, cancer), or isolated events (aspiration). Host factors such as malignancy or impaired blood supply increase the probability that the dislodged flora will eventually produce an infection. The anaerobes most often causing infection are those both present in the microbiota at the adjacent mucosal site and which possess other features enhancing their virulence. For example, *B fragilis* represents a small percent of the normal colonic flora but is the bacterial species most frequently isolated from intraabdominal abscesses.

Anaerobes displaced from normal flora to deeper sites may cause disease

＊ **Trauma and host factors create the opportunity for infection**

The relation between the microbiota and site of infection may be indirect. For example, aspiration pneumonia, lung abscess, and empyema typically involve anaerobes found in the oropharyngeal flora. The brain is not a particularly anaerobic environment, but brain abscess is most often caused by these same oropharyngeal anaerobes. This presumably occurs by extension across the cribriform plate to the temporal lobe, the typical location of brain abscess. In contaminated open wounds, clostridia can come from the intestinal flora or from spores surviving in the environment.

Flora may be aspirated or displaced at a distance

＊ **Brain abscess typically involves anaerobic bacteria**

Although gaining access to tissue sites provides the opportunity, additional virulence factors are needed for anaerobes to produce infection. Some anaerobic pathogens produce disease even when present as a minor part of the displaced resident flora, and other common members of the microbiota rarely cause disease. Classic virulence factors such as toxins and capsules are known only for the toxigenic clostridia and *B fragilis,* but a feature such as the ability to survive brief exposures to oxygenated environments can also be viewed as a virulence factor. Anaerobes found in human infections are far more likely to produce catalase and superoxide dismutase than their more docile counterparts of the microbiota. Exquisitely oxygen-sensitive anaerobes are seldom involved, probably because they are injured by even the small amounts of oxygen dissolved in tissue fluids.

Capsules and toxins are known for some anaerobes

Survival in oxidized conditions can be a virulence factor

A related feature is the ability of the bacteria to create and control a reduced microenvironment, often with the apparent help of other bacteria. Most anaerobic infections are mixed; that is, two or more anaerobes are present, often in combination with facultative bacteria such as *Escherichia coli.* In some cases, the components of these mixtures are believed to synergize each other's growth either by providing growth factors or by lowering the local oxidation–reduction potential. These conditions may have other advantages such as the inhibition of oxygen-dependent leukocyte bactericidal functions under the anaerobic conditions in the lesion. Anaerobes that produce specific toxins have a pathogenesis on their own, which are discussed in the sections devoted to individual species.

Mixed infections may facilitate an anaerobic microenvironment

 ## ANAEROBIC INFECTIONS: CLINICAL ASPECTS

MANIFESTATIONS

Bacteroides, Fusobacterium, and anaerobic cocci, alone or together with other facultative or obligate anaerobes, are responsible for the overwhelming majority of localized abscesses within the cranium, thorax, peritoneum, liver, and female genital tract. As indicated earlier, the species involved relate to the pathogens present in the microbiota of the adjacent mucosal surface. Those derived from the oral flora also include dental infections and infections of human bites.

Abscesses are caused by *Bacteroides, Fusobacterium,* or anaerobic cocci

In addition, anaerobes play causal roles in chronic sinusitis, chronic otitis media, aspiration pneumonia, bronchiectasis, cholecystitis, septic arthritis, chronic osteomyelitis, decubitus ulcers, and soft tissue infections of patients with diabetes mellitus. Dissection of infection along fascial planes (necrotizing fasciitis) and thrombophlebitis are common complications. Foul-smelling pus and crepitation (gas in tissues) are signs associated with, but by no means exclusive to, anaerobic infections. As with other bacterial infections, they may spread beyond the local site and enter the bloodstream. The mortality rate of anaerobic bacteremias arising from nongenital sources is equivalent to the rates with bacteremias due to staphylococci or Enterobacteriaceae.

Foul-smelling pus suggests anaerobic infection

DIAGNOSIS

The key to detection of anaerobes is a high-quality specimen, preferably pus or fluid taken directly from the infected site. The specimen needs to be taken quickly to the microbiology laboratory and protected from oxygen exposure while on the way. Special anaerobic transport tubes may be used, or by expression of any air from the syringe in which the specimen was collected. A generous collection of pus serves as its own best transport medium unless transport is delayed for hours.

Specimens must be direct and protected from oxygen

A direct Gram-stained smear of clinical material demonstrating Gram-negative and/or Gram-positive bacteria of various morphologies is highly suggestive, often even diagnostic of anaerobic infection. Because of the typically slow and complicated nature of anaerobic culture, the Gram stain often provides the most useful information for clinical decision making. Isolation of the bacteria requires the use of an anaerobic incubation atmosphere and special media protected from oxygen exposure. Although elaborate systems are available for this purpose, the simple anaerobic jar is sufficient for isolation of the clinically significant anaerobes. The use of media that contain reducing agents (cysteine, thioglycollate) and growth factors needed by some species further facilitates isolation of anaerobes. The polymicrobial nature of most anaerobic infections requires the use of selective media to protect the slow-growing anaerobes from being overgrown by hardier facultative bacteria, particularly members of the Enterobacteriaceae. Antibiotics, particularly aminoglycosides (and sometimes cephalosporins) to which all anaerobes are resistant, are frequently incorporated in culture media. Once the bacteria are isolated, identification procedures include morphology, biochemical characterization, and metabolic end-product detection by gas chromatography or mass spectrometry.

Gram staining is particularly useful

Anaerobic incubation jar provides atmosphere

Selective media inhibit facultative bacteria

TREATMENT

As with most abscesses, drainage of the purulent material is the primary treatment, in association with appropriate chemotherapy. Antimicrobial agents alone may be ineffective because of failure to penetrate the site of infection. Their selection is empiric to a large degree because such infections typically involve mixed species. Culture-based diagnosis is delayed by the slow growth and the time required to distinguish multiple species. In addition, antimicrobial susceptibility testing methods are slow and not generally available for anaerobic bacteria. The usual approach involves selection of antimicrobials based on the expected susceptibility of the anaerobes known to produce infection at the site in question. For example, anaerobic organisms derived from the oral flora are often susceptible to penicillin, but infections below the diaphragm are caused by

Mixed infections and slow growth dictate empiric therapy

Abdominal infections require β-lactamase-resistant antimicrobials

fecal anaerobes including *B fragilis* which is resistant to many β-lactams. These latter infections are most likely to respond to metronidazole, imipenem, or cefotaxime, a cephalosporin not inactivated by the β-lactamases produced by anaerobes.

● *CLOSTRIDIUM* PERFRINGENS

OVERVIEW

Clostridium perfringens is a spore-forming Gram-positive rod commonly found in the intestine and environment. It produces a wide range of wound and soft tissue infections, many of which are no different from those caused by other opportunistic bacteria. The most dreaded of these, gas gangrene, begins as a wound infection but progresses to shock and death in a matter of hours. Another form of *C perfringens*-caused disease, food poisoning, is characterized by diarrhea without fever or vomiting.

 ## BACTERIOLOGY

Hemolysis and gas production are characteristic

C perfringens is a large, Gram-positive, nonmotile rod with square ends. It grows overnight under anaerobic conditions, producing hemolytic colonies on blood agar. In the broth containing fermentable carbohydrate, growth of *C perfringens* is accompanied by the production of large amounts of hydrogen and carbon dioxide gas, which can also be produced in necrotic tissues; hence the term gas gangrene.

Typing system is based on toxins

C perfringens produces multiple exotoxins that have different pathogenic significance in different animal species and serve as the basis for classification of the five types (A-E). Type A is by far the most important in humans and is found consistently in the colon and often in soil. The most important exotoxin is the **α-toxin,** a phospholipase that hydrolyzes lecithin and sphingomyelin, thus disrupting the cell membranes of various host cells, including erythrocytes, leukocytes, and muscle cells. The **θ-toxin** alters capillary permeability and is toxic to heart muscle. This toxin also has pore-forming activity similar to streptolysin O. A minority of strains (less than 5%) produce an **enterotoxin,** which inserts into enterocyte membranes to form pores leading to alterations in intracellular calcium, membrane permeability, and the integrity of cell-to-cell tight junctions. This leads to loss of cellular fluid and macromolecules.

✻ Phospholipase α-toxin lyses RBCs and other cells

✻ Pore-forming θ-toxin and enterotoxin disrupt cells

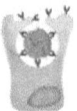 ## *CLOSTRIDIUM PERFRINGENS* DISEASE

EPIDEMIOLOGY

■ Gas Gangrene

Spores from the host or environment contaminate wounds

Delays allow multiplication

Gas gangrene (clostridial myonecrosis) develops in traumatic wounds with significant avascular muscle necrosis when they are contaminated with dirt, clothing, or other foreign material containing *C perfringens* or another species of histotoxic clostridia (see Table 29–2). The clostridia can come from the patient's own intestinal flora or spores in the environment. Compound fractures, bullet wounds, or the kind of trauma seen in wartime are prototypes for this infection. A significant delay (many hours) between the injury and definitive surgical management is required for bacterial multiplication and toxin production to develop. In peacetime these conditions are more likely to be satisfied in a remote hiking accident than in an automobile collision. The difference is the time between injury and medical intervention.

■ Clostridial Food Poisoning

Bacteria multiply in meat dishes

C perfringens can cause food poisoning if spores of an enterotoxin-producing strain contaminate food. Outbreaks usually involve rich meat dishes such as stews, soups, or gravies that have been kept warm for a number of hours before consumption. This allows time for the infecting dose to be reached by conversion of spores to vegetative bacteria, which then multiply in the food. Clostridial food poisoning is common in developed countries and is second among foodborne illnesses in the United States with over a million cases per year.

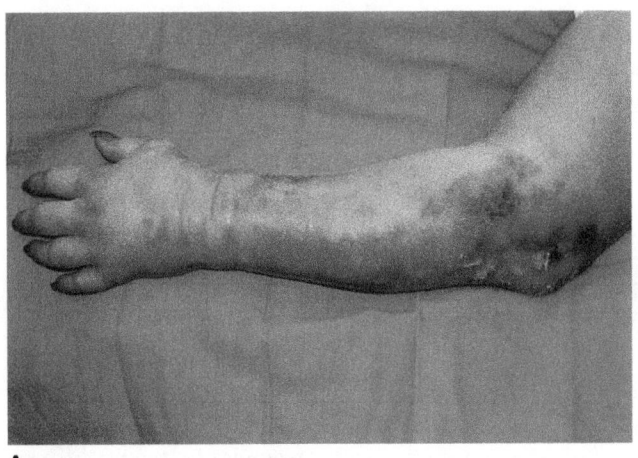
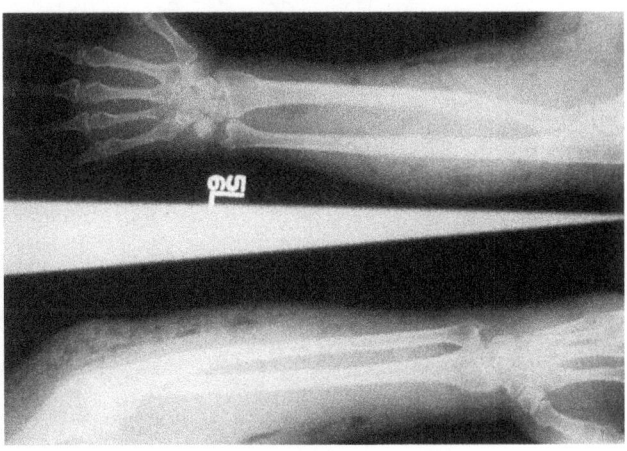

FIGURE 29–2. Gas gangrene. A. Arm of a drug abuser with ulcers and swelling traced to needle tracks. **B.** Radiographs from the same patient demonstrating gas (clear spaces) in the tissues. (Reproduced with permission from Connor DH, Chandler FW, Schwartz DQ, et al: *Pathology of Infectious Diseases.* Stamford CT: Appleton & Lange; 1997.)

PATHOGENESIS

Gas Gangrene

If the oxidation–reduction potential in a wound is sufficiently low, *C perfringens* spores can germinate and then multiply, elaborating α-toxin. The process passes along the muscle bundles, producing rapidly spreading edema and necrosis as well as conditions that are favorable for growth of the anaerobes. Very few leukocytes are present in the myonecrotic tissue (**Figure 29–2**). As the disease progresses, increased vascular permeability and systemic absorption of the toxin lead to shock. α-Toxin is the major cause of both local destruction and shock. θ-Toxin and oxygen deprivation due to the metabolic activities of *C perfringens* are probable contributors. The basis for the profound systemic effects is not known, but α-toxin absorption and circulation seems probable because fatal cases occur without bacteremia.

Low redox favors multiplication and α-toxin production

✳ *α-Toxin circulation leads to shock*

Clostridial Food Poisoning

The spores of some *C perfringens* strains are often particularly heat-resistant and can withstand temperatures of 100°C for an hour or more. Thus, spores that survive initial cooking can convert to the vegetative form and multiply when food is not refrigerated or is rewarmed. After ingestion, the enterotoxin is released into the upper gastrointestinal tract, causing a fluid outpouring in which the ileum is most severely involved.

Spores survive cooking

✳ *Vegetative cells produce enterotoxin*

 CLOSTRIDIUM PERFRINGENS: CLINICAL ASPECTS

MANIFESTATIONS

Gas Gangrene

Gas gangrene usually begins 1 to 4 days after the injury but may start within 10 hours. The earliest reported finding is severe pain at the site of the wound accompanied by a sense of heaviness or pressure. The disease then progresses rapidly with edema, tenderness, and pallor, followed by discoloration and hemorrhagic bullae. The gas is apparent as crepitance in the tissue, but this is a late sign. Systemic findings are those of shock with intravascular hemolysis, hypotension, and renal failure leading to coma and death. Patients are often remarkably alert until the terminal stages.

✳ *Wound pain evolves to edema and shock*

Anaerobic Cellulitis

Anaerobic cellulitis is a clostridial infection of wounds and surrounding subcutaneous tissue in which there is marked gas formation (more than in gas gangrene), but in which the pain, swelling, and toxicity of gas gangrene are absent. This condition is much less serious and can be controlled with antimicrobial therapy.

Gas is more likely than in gas gangrene

■ Endometritis

If *C perfringens* gains access to necrotic products of conception retained in the uterus, it may multiply and infect the endometrium. Necrosis of uterine tissue and bacteremia with massive intravascular hemolysis due to α-toxin may then follow. Clostridial uterine infection is particularly common after an incomplete abortion with inadequately sterilized instruments.

■ Food Poisoning

The particularly short incubation period of 8 to 24 hours is followed by nausea, abdominal pain, and diarrhea. There is no fever, and vomiting is rare. Spontaneous recovery usually occurs within 24 hours.

DIAGNOSIS

Diagnosis is based substantially on clinical observations. Bacteriologic studies are adjunctive. *C perfringens* is readily isolated in anaerobic cultures, which are routine for all wound cultures. It is common, for example, to isolate *C perfringens* from contaminated wounds of patients who have no evidence of clostridial disease. The organism can also be isolated from the postpartum uterine cervix of healthy women or from those with only mild fever. In clostridial food poisoning, isolation of high numbers of *C perfringens* in the ingested food in the absence of any other cause is usually sufficient to confirm an etiology of a characteristic food poisoning outbreak.

TREATMENT AND PREVENTION

Treatment of gas gangrene and endometritis must be initiated immediately because these conditions are almost always fatal if untreated. Excision of all devitalized tissue is of paramount importance because it denies the organism the anaerobic conditions required for further multiplication and toxin production. This often entails wide resection of muscle groups, hysterectomy, and even amputation of limbs. Administration of massive doses of penicillin is an important adjunctive procedure. Because nonclostridial anaerobes and members of Enterobacteriaceae frequently contaminate injury sites, broad-spectrum cephalosporins are often added to the antibiotic regimen. Placement of patients in a hyperbaric oxygen chamber, which increases the tissue level of dissolved oxygen, has been shown to slow the spread of disease, probably by inhibiting bacterial growth and toxin production and by neutralizing the activity of θ-toxin.

The most effective method of prevention of gas gangrene is the surgical debridement of traumatic injuries as soon as possible. Wound cleansing, removal of dead tissue and foreign bodies, and drainage of hematomas limit organism multiplication and toxin production.

 What if I am in a remote area, suspect gas gangrene but am not a surgeon?

Antimicrobial prophylaxis is indicated but cannot replace surgical debridement, because the antimicrobial agents may fail to reach the organism in devascularized tissues.

Prevention of food poisoning involves good cooking hygiene and adequate refrigeration. There is growing evidence that enterotoxin-producing strains of *C perfringens* may also be responsible for some cases of antimicrobial agent-induced diarrhea in a setting similar to that of *C difficile* (see the following discussion).

KEY CONCLUSIONS

- *Clostridium perfringens* α-toxin, a phospholipase, causes hemolysis, tissue destruction, and shock.
- Gas gangrene requires traumatic avascular muscle necrosis.
- Surgery is essential to remove dead tissue and restore circulation.
- Endometritis follows nonsterile abortion.
- Enterotoxin-producing strains cause short incubation food poisoning.

 Think ▸▸ Apply 29-1: If this is truly gas gangrene the patient may die within hours unless the infected dead tissue is removed and circulation restored. You must arrange an airlift or other transport to a facility where there is a surgeon.

CLOSTRIDIUM BOTULINUM

OVERVIEW

Botulism is caused by ingestion of botulinum toxin preformed by *C botulinum* contaminating foods inadequately sterilized and stored unrefrigerated for long periods. The toxin acts at the neuromuscular junction blocking acetylcholine release leading to flaccid paralysis. The disease begins with cranial nerve palsies and develops into descending symmetric motor paralysis, which may involve the respiratory muscles. No fever or other signs of infection occur. A slower moving form of the disease occurs when the toxin is produced endogenously in the intestinal tract or a wound.

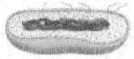 ### BACTERIOLOGY

C botulinum is a large Gram-positive rod much like the rest of the clostridia. Its spores resist boiling for long periods, and moist heat at 121°C is required for certain destruction. Germination of spores and growth of *C botulinum* can occur in a variety of alkaline or neutral foodstuffs when conditions are sufficiently anaerobic.

The major characteristic of medical importance is that when *C botulinum* grows under these anaerobic conditions, it elaborates a family of neurotoxins of extraordinary toxicity. **Botulinum toxin** is among the most potent toxins known in nature, with an estimated lethal dose of less than 1 μg for humans. Botulinum toxin is an enzyme (metalloproteinase) that acts at neuromuscular junctions (**Figure 29–3**). Once bound, it cleaves attachment protein receptors (SNARE proteins), which effectively block the release of the neurotransmitter acetylcholine from vesicles at the presynaptic membrane of the synapse. Because acetylcholine mediates activation of motor neurons, the blockage of its release causes flaccid paralysis of the motor system.

C botulinum is classified into multiple types (A-G) based on the antigenic specificity of the neurotoxins. All the toxins are heat-labile and destroyed rapidly at 100°C, but are resistant to the

❋ Cells germinating from spores produce neurotoxin in food

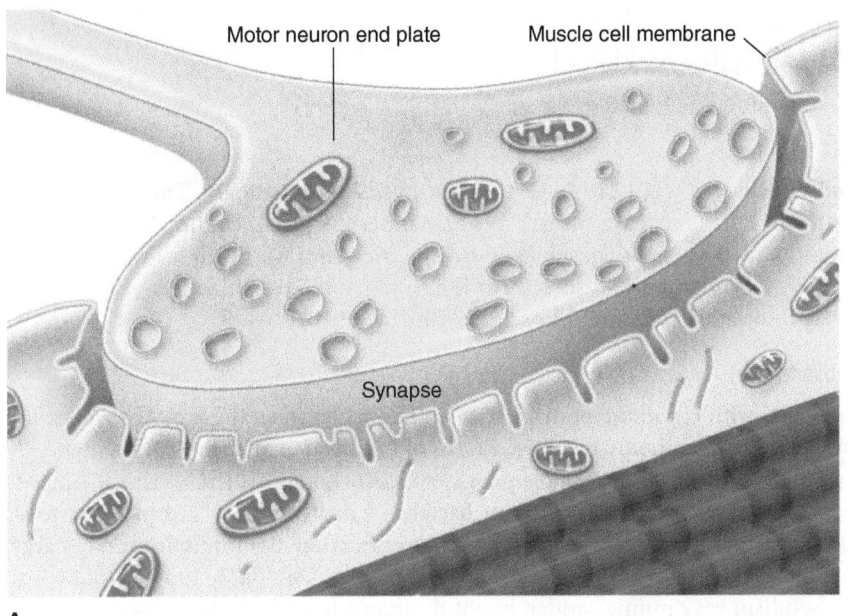
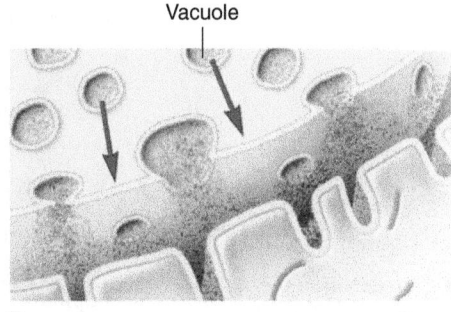
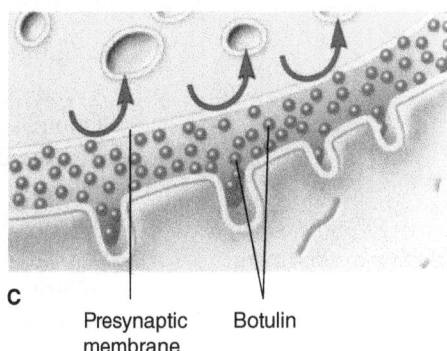

FIGURE 29–3. Clostridial tetanus and botulinum neurotoxins. A. The motor neuron endplate, synapse, and neuromuscular junction are shown. For tetanus toxin, the neurons have an inhibitory function; for botulinum, they are active motor neurons. **B.** Vesicles releasing neurotransmitters across the synapse to the muscle cell membrane are shown. **C.** In the presence of toxin, the release of neurotransmitter vesicles into the synapse is blocked. For botulinum toxin, the neurotransmitter is acetylcholine, and motor neurons are blocked giving flaccid paralysis. For tetanus toxin, release of neurotransmitters activating inhibitory neurons is blocked resulting in spasmodic contractions. (Reproduced with permission from Willey JM: *Prescott, Harley, & Klein's Microbiology,* 7th ed. New York, NY: McGraw Hill; 2008.)

enzymes of the gastrointestinal tract. If unheated toxin is ingested, it is readily absorbed and distributed in the bloodstream.

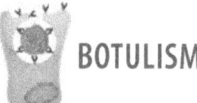 BOTULISM

EPIDEMIOLOGY

Spores of *C botulinum* are found in soil, pond, and lake sediments in all parts of the world. If spores contaminate food, they may convert to the vegetative state, multiply, and produce toxin in storage under certain conditions. This may occur with no change in food taste, color, or odor. The alkaline conditions provided by vegetables, such as green beans, and mushrooms and fish particularly support the growth of *C botulinum*. Botulism most often occurs after ingestion of home-canned products that have not been heated at temperatures sufficient to kill *C botulinum* spores, although inadequately sterilized commercial fish products have also been implicated. Because the toxin is heat-labile, in order to produce disease the food must be ingested uncooked or after insufficient cooking. Botulism often occurs in small family outbreaks in the case of home-prepared foods or less often as isolated cases connected to commercial products. Infant and wound botulism result when the toxin is produced endogenously, beginning with spores that are either ingested in difficult to sterilize foods (honey) or contaminate wounds.

PATHOGENESIS

Foodborne botulism is an intoxication not an infection. The ingested preformed toxin is absorbed in the intestinal tract and reaches its neuromuscular junction target via the bloodstream. Once bound there, its inhibition of acetylcholine release causes paralysis due to lack of neuromuscular transmission. The specific disease manifestations depend on the specific nerves to which the circulating toxin binds. Cardiac arrhythmias and blood pressure instability are believed to be due to effects of the toxin on the autonomic nervous system. The damage to the synapse once the toxin has bound is permanent, and recovery requires growth of presynaptic axons and formation of new synapses.

 BOTULISM: CLINICAL ASPECTS

MANIFESTATIONS

Foodborne botulism usually starts 12 to 36 hours after ingestion of the toxin. The first signs are nausea, dry mouth, and, in some cases, diarrhea. Cranial nerve signs, including blurred vision, pupillary dilatation, and nystagmus, occur later. Symmetric paralysis begins with the ocular, laryngeal, and respiratory muscles and spreads to the trunk and extremities. The most serious finding is complete respiratory paralysis. Mortality is 10% to 20%.

■ Infant Botulism

A syndrome associated with *C botulinum* that occurs in infants between the ages of 3 weeks and 8 months is now the most commonly diagnosed form of botulism. The organism is apparently introduced on weaning or with dietary supplements, especially honey, which is virtually impossible to sterilize. Ingested spores yield vegetative bacteria, which multiply and produce small amounts of toxin in the infant's colon. The infant shows constipation, poor muscle tone, lethargy, and feeding problems and may have ophthalmic and other paralyses similar to those in foodborne botulism. Infant botulism may mimic sudden infant death syndrome. The benefits of antitoxin and antimicrobial agents have not been clearly established.

■ Wound Botulism

Very rarely, wounds infected with other organisms may allow *C botulinum* to grow. Wound botulism in parenteral users of cocaine and maxillary sinus botulism in intranasal users of cocaine has been reported. Disease similar to that from food poisoning may develop, or it may begin with weakness localized to the injured extremity. Botulism without an obvious food or wound source is occasionally reported in individuals beyond infancy. It is possible that some such cases result

---

Margin notes (left column):

✳ Blockage of synaptic acetylcholine release causes paralysis

Toxin is destroyed by boiling

Spores are widely distributed

Alkaline foods favor toxin production

✳ Inadequately heated home-canned foods most common source

Preformed toxin is readily absorbed

✳ Acetylcholine block leads to paralysis

✳ Blurred vision progresses to symmetrical paralysis

✳ Nonsterile honey introduces spores to intestine

Lethargy, poor feeding occur in addition to adult signs

Contaminated wounds of drug users are sites of toxin production

from ingestion of spores of *C botulinum* with subsequent *in vivo* production of toxin in a manner similar to that in infant botulism.

DIAGNOSIS

The toxin can be demonstrated in blood, intestinal contents, or remaining food by immunoassay or nucleic acid amplification (NAA) methods, but these tests are available only in reference laboratories. *C botulinum* may also be isolated from stool or from foodstuffs suspected of responsibility for botulism.

❋ Toxin detected by EIA, NAA

TREATMENT AND PREVENTION

The availability of intensive supportive measures, particularly mechanical ventilation, is the single most important determinant of clinical outcome. With proper ventilatory support, mortality rate should be less than 10%. The administration of large doses of horse *C botulinum* antitoxin is thought to be useful in neutralizing free toxin. Frequent hypersensitivity reactions related to the equine origin of this preparation make it unsuitable for use in infants. Antimicrobial agents are given only to patients with wound botulism.

Adequate pressure cooking or autoclaving in the canning process kills spores, and heating food at 100°C for 10 minutes before eating destroys the toxin. Food from damaged cans or those that present evidence of positive inside pressure should not even be tasted because of the extreme toxicity of the *C botulinum* toxin.

In an interesting twist, botulinum toxin as Botox has itself become a therapeutic agent. Originally licensed as a treatment of spasmotic neuromuscular conditions by direct injection into muscle, it has found a far larger use for cosmetic applications. For those that can afford it, a temporary respite from the wrinkles of aging can be gained from Botox injections administered by dermatologists and plastic surgeons.

Supportive measures and antitoxin allow survival

❋ Cooking food inactivates toxin

Botox relieves wrinkles

● *CLOSTRIDIUM TETANI*

OVERVIEW

Tetanus follows production of a neurotoxin in a wound infected by *C tetani*. Like botulinum tetanospasmin toxin acts at the neuromuscular junction. It blocks postsynaptic inhibition thus enhancing muscular contraction. The striking feature of tetanus is severe muscle spasms (or "lock-jaw" when the jaw muscles are involved). This occurs despite minimal or no inflammation at the primary site of infection, which may be unnoticed even though the outcome is fatal. The disease is caused by *in vivo* production of a neurotoxin that acts centrally, not locally. Immunization with inactivated toxin prevents tetanus.

BACTERIOLOGY

C tetani is a slim, Gram-positive rod, which forms spores readily in nature and in culture, yielding a round terminal spore that gives the organism a drumstick-like appearance (Figure 29–1). *C tetani* requires strict anaerobic conditions. Its identity is suggested by culture-based as well as biochemical characteristics, but definite identification depends on demonstrating the neurotoxic exotoxin. *C tetani* spores remain viable in soil for many years and are resistant to most disinfectants and to boiling for several minutes.

Gram-positive rods with drumstick-like spore

The most important product of *C tetani* is its neurotoxic exotoxin, **tetanospasmin** or tetanus toxin, a metalloproteinase that has structural and pharmacologic features similar to those of botulinum toxin. Tetanus toxin degrades a protein required for neurotransmitter release from vesicles at the appropriate site on presynaptic membranes (Figure 29–3). The most important difference from botulinum toxin is that the neurotransmitters in this case (glycine and γ-aminobutyric acid [GABA]) are the ones that affect inhibitory neurons. The result is unopposed firing of the active motor neurons, generating spasms, and spastic paralysis, which are the opposite of the botulinum flaccid paralysis. The toxin is heat-labile, antigenic, readily neutralized by antitoxin, and rapidly destroyed by intestinal proteases. Treatment with formaldehyde yields a nontoxic product or **toxoid** that retains the antigenicity of toxin and thus stimulates the production of antitoxin.

❋ Toxin blocks release of glycine, GABA

❋ Formaldehyde treatment removes toxicity but retains antigenicity

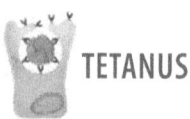 TETANUS

EPIDEMIOLOGY

✴ Spores from environment germinate in wounds

Nonsterile technique can lead to tetanus

The spores of *C tetani* exist in many soils, especially those that have been treated with manure, and the organism is sometimes found in the lower intestinal tract of humans and animals. The spores are introduced into wounds contaminated with soil or foreign bodies. The wounds are often small (eg, a puncture wound with a splinter). In many developing countries, the majority of tetanus cases occur in recently delivered infants when the umbilical cord is severed or bandaged in a nonsterile manner. Similarly, tetanus may follow an unskilled abortion, scarification rituals, female circumcision, and even surgery performed with nonsterile instruments or dressings.

PATHOGENESIS

Trauma provides growth conditions

✴ Tetanospasmin produced at the local site ascends through nerves to anterior horn

✴ Blockage of reflex inhibition causes spasmodic contractions

The usual predisposing factor for tetanus is an area of very low oxidation–reduction potential in which tetanus spores can germinate, such as a large splinter, an area of necrosis from introduction of soil, or necrosis after injection of contaminated illicit drugs. Infection with facultative or other anaerobic organisms can contribute to the development of an appropriate anaerobic nidus for spore germination. Tetanus bacilli multiply locally and neither damage nor invade adjacent tissues. Tetanospasmin is produced at the site of infection and enters the presynaptic terminals of lower motor neurons, reaching the central nervous system (CNS) mainly by exploiting the retrograde axonal transport system in the nerves. In the spinal cord, it acts at the level of the anterior horn cells, where its blockage of postsynaptic inhibition of spinal motor reflexes produces spasmodic contractions of both protagonist and antagonist muscles. This process takes place initially in the area of the causative lesion, but may extend up and down the spinal cord. Minor stimuli, such as a sound or a draft, can provoke generalized spasms.

 TETANUS: CLINICAL ASPECTS

MANIFESTATIONS

The incubation period of tetanus is from 4 days to several weeks. The shorter incubation period is usually associated with wounds in areas supplied by the cranial motor nerves, probably because of a shorter transmission route for the toxin to the CNS. In general, shorter incubation periods are associated with more severe disease.

Incubation period varies with distance to CNS

✴ Masseter muscle contraction causes lock-jaw

The diagnosis is clinical; neither culture nor toxin testing is useful. Although tetanus may be localized to muscles innervated by nerves in the region of the infection, it is usually more generalized. The masseter muscles are often the first to be affected, resulting in inability to open the mouth properly (**trismus**); this effect accounts for the term **lock-jaw.** As other muscles become affected, intermittent spasms can become generalized to include muscles of respiration and swallowing. In extreme cases, massive contractions of the back muscles (opisthotonos) develop (**Figure 29–4**).

FIGURE 29–4. **Tetanus.** Opisthotonic posturing caused by involvement of the spinal musculature in a child with generalized tetanus. (Reproduced with permission from Connor DH, Chandler FW, Schwartz DQ, et al: *Pathology of Infectious Diseases.* Stamford CT: Appleton & Lange; 1997.)

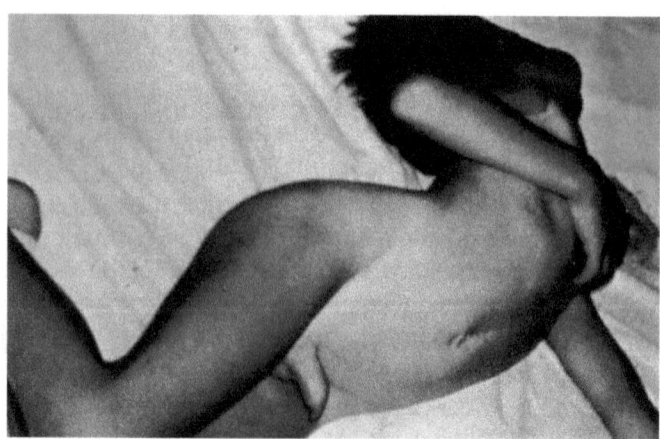

Untreated patients with tetanus retain consciousness and are aware of their plight, in which small stimuli can trigger massive contractions. In fatal cases, death results from exhaustion and respiratory failure. Untreated, the mortality rate caused by the generalized disease varies from 15% to more than 60%, according to the lesion, incubation period, and age of the patient. Mortality is highest in neonates and in elderly patients.

✳ Respiratory failure leads to death

TREATMENT

Specific treatment of tetanus involves neutralization of any unbound toxin with large doses of human tetanus immune globulin (HTIG), which is derived from the blood of volunteers hyperimmunized with toxoid. Most important in treatment are nonspecific supportive measures, including maintenance of a quiet dark environment, sedation, and provision of an adequate airway. Benzodiazepines are also used to indirectly antagonize the effects of the toxin. The value of antimicrobials is not clear. Because toxin binding is irreversible, recovery requires the generation of new axonal terminals.

✳ HTIG neutralizes unbound toxin

Supportive treatment required until axons regenerate

PREVENTION

Routine active immunization with tetanus toxoid, combined with diphtheria toxoid and pertussis vaccine (DTaP) for primary immunization in childhood and DT for adults, can completely prevent tetanus. It has reduced the incidence of tetanus in the United States to less than 50 reported cases per year. Five doses of DT are recommended, to be given at the ages of 2, 4, 6, and 18 months, and once again between the ages of 4 and 6 years. Thereafter, a booster of adult-type tetanus diphtheria toxoid should be given every 10 years. Unfortunately, routine childhood immunization is not administratively and economically feasible in many less well-developed countries, where as many as 1 million cases of tetanus occur annually. In such settings, immunization efforts have been focused on pregnant women, because transplacental transfer of antibodies to the fetus also prevents the highly lethal neonatal tetanus.

✳ Childhood toxoid immunization prevents disease

Unimmunized subjects with tetanus-prone wounds should be given passive immunity with a prophylactic dose of HTIG as soon as possible. This immunization provides immediate protection. Those who have had a full primary series of immunizations and appropriate boosters are given toxoid for tetanus-prone wounds if they have not been immunized within the previous 10 years in the case of clean minor wounds or 5 years for more contaminated wounds. If immunization is incomplete or the wound has been neglected and poses a serious risk of disease, HTIG is also appropriate. Penicillin therapy is a prophylactic adjunct in serious or neglected wounds, but in no way alters the need for specific prophylaxis.

Childhood toxoid immunization prevents disease

Boosters required every 10 years

✳ Passive immunization for unimmunized

KEY CONCLUSIONS

- Vegetative cells germinating in wounds contaminated with *C tetani* spores produce tetanospasmin, a neurotoxin at the local site.
- Tetanospasmin migrates through the axonal transport system to CNS neuromuscular junctions.
- The toxin blocks the release of neurotransmitters affecting inhibitory neurons causing unrestrained muscular contraction.
- Hypercontraction of muscle groups leads to lockjaw (masseter muscles) and opisthotonus (back muscles).
- Immunization with tetanus toxoid prevents disease.

● *CLOSTRIDIOIDES DIFFICILE*

OVERVIEW

Clostridioides difficile spores are either resident in the intestinal microbiota or ingested from the environment. When other members of the microbiota are suppressed by antibiotics these spores germinate and the vegetative cells produce powerful toxins. *C difficile* infection (CDI) is the most common and deadly cause of diarrhea that develops in association with the use of antimicrobial agents. The diarrhea ranges from a few days of intestinal fluid loss to life-threatening toxic megacolon and pseudomembranous colitis (PMC). PMC is associated with intense inflammation and the formation of a pseudomembrane composed of inflammatory debris on the mucosal surface.

 **BACTERIOLOGY**

* A and B toxins disrupt cytoskeleton signal transduction

Enterocytes show altered enterocyte secretion and inflammation

CDT inhibits actin polymerization

Clostridioides difficile (formerly *Clostridium difficile*) is a Gram-positive rod that readily forms spores both in the environment and *in vivo*. Under circumstances described as follows, spores present in the intestinal microbiota may germinate to the metabolically active vegetative form. The *C difficile* germination mechanism differs from that of most other spore-forming bacteria in that it is triggered by bile salts. In the vegetative form *C difficile* has a most important medical feature: its ability to produce toxins. In this species, two distinct large polypeptide toxins, Toxin A (TcdA) and Toxin B (TcdB), with similar structure (45% homology) are released during late growth phases, perhaps at the time of cell lysis. Both toxins are glucosyltransferases and act in the cytoplasm by inactivating signal transduction proteins (Rho GTPases), particularly those that control the actin cytoskeleton. This results in the disruption of intercellular tight junctions followed by altered membrane permeability and fluid secretion. Within hours of contact with enterocytes, cell rounding and neutrophilic infiltration also appear. In recent years, a third toxin, *C difficile* Binary toxin (CDT), has been discovered, which exerts an ADP-ribosylating action which inhibits actin cytoskeleton polymerization within the enterocyte.

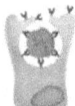 *CLOSTRIDIOIDES DIFFICILE* **INFECTION (CDI)**

EPIDEMIOLOGY

* Source is endogenous or environmental

C difficile is present in the stool of 2% to 15% of the general population, sometimes at higher rates among hospitalized persons and infants. Infants largely remain asymptomatic; the molecular basis for this is not known. More than two decades of the antibiotic era had elapsed before the medical importance of *C difficile* was recognized through its association with antibiotic-associated diarrhea (AAD). Although CDI is endogenous in most cases, hospital outbreaks have clearly established that the environment can be the source as well. CDI is clearly on the rise worldwide and is now the leading cause of death due to an acute diarrheal illness. New strains combining more potent A and B toxins, along with the CDT toxin, have been particularly virulent.

C difficile is not the only cause of AAD, but it is the most common identifiable cause. In simple diarrhea following antimicrobial administration, this organism is responsible for approximately 30% of cases. As the disease is colitis, the association is stronger, rising to 90% if pseudomembranous colitis (PMC) is present.

 Is antibiotic resistance an essential component of AAD?

Most frequent cause of AAD

Major cause of PMC

* Environmental spores cause hospital outbreaks

* Antimicrobial effect on microbiota selects for *C difficile*

* Spore germination triggered by bile salts

Although CDI is primarily an endogenous infection, the generation of spores from excretions provides the prospect for person-to-person spread. This is the basis of the hospital outbreaks but can occur in any situation where *C difficile* spores lurk in a closed space.

PATHOGENESIS

When *C difficile* becomes established in the colon of individuals with normal gut microbiota, few, if any, direct consequences result, probably because its numbers are dwarfed by the other flora. Alteration of the colonic flora with antimicrobials (particularly ampicillin, cephalosporins, and clindamycin) favors *C difficile* in two ways. First, strains resistant to the antimicrobial agent can grow in its presence and assume a larger if not dominant position in the flora. Second, in an antimicrobial milieu, the readiness with which *C difficile* forms spores may favor its survival over

 Think ▶▶ Apply 29-2: No. Resistance may hasten the emergence of *C difficile* strains, but it is the inert spore that allows its survival. Fully susceptible strains cause CDI usually just after the antibiotic is discontinued.

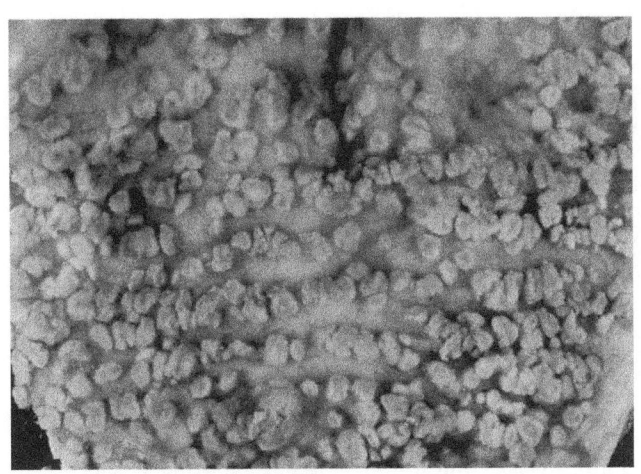
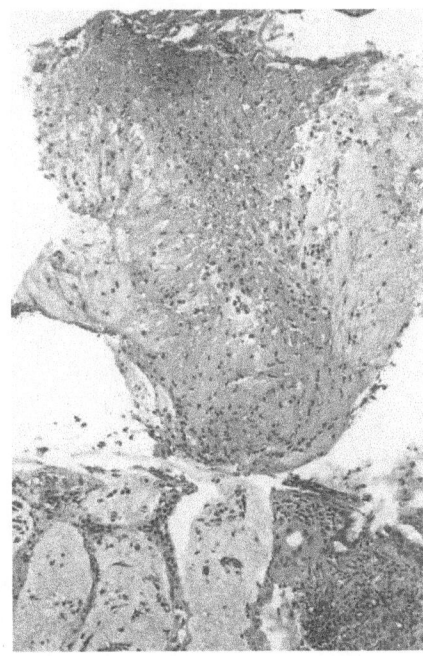

A   B

FIGURE 29–5. ***Clostridium difficile* pseudomembranous colitis. A.** Colon with discrete plaques of pseudomembrane. **B.** Histopathology demonstrates the pseudomembrane above the mucosa. It is "pseudo" because
it is composed of only fibrin and inflammatory cells. (Reproduced with permission from Connor DH, Chandler FW,
Schwartz DQ, et al: *Pathology of Infectious Diseases*. Stamford CT: Appleton & Lange; 1997.)

non–spore-forming bacteria. A distinctive feature of *C difficile* spores is that their germination is
triggered by taurocholate, a bile salt, through a receptor in the spore itself. Thus, in the situation of
general suppression of intestinal flora by antimicrobial agents, *C difficile* has a double advantage.
Its spores are specifically triggered to germinate by normal intestinal secretions, and the resultant
vegetative cells have less competition for nutrients. Eventually, the minor niche of the species is
improved to the point where the effect of its toxins on the colonic mucosa becomes significant.

Increased numbers increase toxin injury

Although most strains produce both toxins, the relative contribution of TcdA and TcdB has
been much debated. The toxins have similar actions and it seems both are important. Recently
emerged strains may produce high levels of both toxins, including a variant of TcdB, and also
secrete the new CDT. This combination has been responsible for more cases and more deaths.
In PMC, the colonic mucosa is studded with inflammatory plaques, which may coalesce into
an overlying "pseudomembrane" composed of fibrin, leukocytes, and necrotic colonic cells
(**Figure 29–5**).

Hypervirulent strains produce three toxins

IMMUNITY

Antibody against the TcdA and TcdB have been associated with resolution of disease in experimental animals. This is a long way from concluding that humoral antitoxin immunity is protective when we know serial relapses with toxin production are common.

 CLOSTRIDIOIDES DIFFICILE DIARRHEA: CLINICAL ASPECTS

MANIFESTATIONS

Diarrhea is a common side effect of antimicrobial treatment. In *C difficile*-caused diarrhea, the
onset is usually 5 to 10 days into the antibiotic treatment, but the range is from the first day to weeks
after cessation. The diarrhea may be mild and watery or bloody and accompanied by abdominal
cramping, leukocytosis, and fever. In PMC, it progresses to a severe, occasionally lethal inflammation of the colon that can be demonstrated by endoscopic examination. Systemic signs of inflammation are common and WBC counts of more than 15,000 per cubic millimeter are considered
ominous. Toxic megacolon is the most serious complication leading to colectomy or death.

✱ Diarrhea ranges from mild to toxic megacolon

DIAGNOSIS

Although selective media have been developed for isolation of *C difficile*, direct detection of toxins in the stool has largely replaced culture for diagnostic purposes. *C difficile* is the only pathogen for which detection of its toxin has become routine. The original cell culture toxicity assays were replaced by immunoassays, which reveal TcdA and/or TcdB in the stool. These tests are now being superseded by NAA as well as mass spectrometric methods with improved sensitivity and specificity.

TREATMENT

In AAD discontinuing the implicated antimicrobial often results in the resolution of clinical symptoms. Once *C difficile* toxins are detected in the stools, treatment with metronidazole, vancomycin, or fidaxomicin is indicated. Vancomycin is not absorbed orally which is an advantage in this situation because the toxin production is taking place in the bowel lumen. Metronidazole is only used for mild to moderate CDI. Fidaxomicin is a narrower-spectrum antimicrobial, so is employed when intestinal dysbiosis control is expediently required. *C difficile* is susceptible to penicillins and cephalosporins *in vitro*, but these drugs are ineffective because of access in the intestinal lumen and the hazard of destruction by β-lactamases produced by other bacteria. With all antimicrobial regimens, relapses are common and often multiple episodes occur (more than 20), presumably due to the survival of the inert spores following a treatment course. The relapse rate appears to be less with fidaxomicin a newer drug. Other treatment strategies include the use of intravenous monoclonal antibody-based passive immunization; however, this is limited to hospital patients with severe (or recurrent) disease. Treatments under investigation include probiotics, and molecules that bind the toxin(s) or its intestinal toxin receptor. These approaches are usually combined with antimicrobial therapy. The emergence of PMC with toxic megacolon requires a high-risk colectomy.

PREVENTION

Strategies to prevent recurrences of CDI have generated some highly creative approaches. In pulsed-treatment, a single dose of vancomycin is given once every few days rather than multiple times a day as in standard treatment. The idea is to allow time for the vegetative bacteria to emerge from the inert spore and then block their cell wall synthesis as they start to multiply. After multiple "hits," this approach has ended long sequences of relapses. The most recent and sensational approach has been the infusion of donor feces into the intestine in an effort to reestablish an effective competitive flora. This "fecal microbiota transplant" (FMT) has now moved from anecdotal relapse cures to greater than 90% success in controlled trials including the use of standardized preparations in capsules. The elements of the microbiota included in these capsules are a matter of great debate. Finally, another strategy is aimed at preventing germination of *C difficile* spores by administration of competitive inhibitors of the bile salts known to trigger germination. If successful, this could be applied to any situation where CDI was a risk.

● *BACTEROIDES FRAGILIS*

OVERVIEW

Bacteroides fragilis, a minor component of the intestinal microbiota, is a leading cause of intraabdominal abscess. When displaced beyond mucosal barriers, oxygen tolerance and a polysaccharide capsule allow this anaerobic Gram-negative rod to cause local injury. Deep pain and tenderness anywhere below the diaphragm are typical of the onset of *B fragilis* infection. Depending on the extent and spread of the intraabdominal abscess, fever and widespread findings of an acute abdomen may also be seen. Production of β-lactamases, unusual for anaerobes, complicates treatment.

BACTERIOLOGY

The *B fragilis* group constitutes the most common opportunistic pathogens of the genus *Bacteroides*. These slim, pale-staining, capsulated, Gram-negative rods form colonies overnight on blood agar medium incubated anaerobically. The implication of fragility in the name is misleading, because they are actually among the hardier and more easily grown anaerobes. Most strains produce superoxide dismutase and are relatively tolerant to atmospheric oxygen. *B fragilis* has adhesive surface pili and a capsule composed of a polymer of two polysaccharides. The LPS endotoxin in the *B fragilis* outer membrane is less toxic than that of most other Gram-negative bacteria, possibly owing to modification or absence of the lipid A portion.

✳ Polysaccharide capsule present

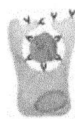

BACTEROIDES FRAGILIS DISEASE

EPIDEMIOLOGY

Like the other Gram-negative anaerobes, *B fragilis* infections are endogenous, originating in the patient's own intestinal microbiota. Given the mass and diversity of intestinal anaerobes, the frequent presence of *B fragilis* in clinically significant infections is striking. It is typically mixed with other anaerobes and facultative bacteria. Human-to-human transmission is not known and seems unlikely.

✳ Endogenous infection mixed with other intestinal bacteria

PATHOGENESIS

The relative oxygen tolerance of *B fragilis* probably plays a role in its virulence by aiding its survival in oxygenated tissues in the period between its displacement from the intestinal flora and the establishment of a reduced local microenvironment. *B fragilis* cells can withstand up to 3 days of exposure to atmospheric levels of oxygen due to activation of an oxidative stress response which deploys detoxifying enzymes like catalase and superoxide dismutase.

Oxygen tolerance mediated by oxidative stress response

The polysaccharide capsule confers resistance to phagocytosis, inhibits macrophage migration, and mediates binding to the peritoneum. The capsule is also involved in the most distinguishing pathogenic feature of *B fragilis*, its ability to cause abscess formation. Experimentally, the *B fragilis* capsular polysaccharide stimulates abscess formation, even in the absence of live cells, a property not found in the capsules of bacteria like *Streptococcus pneumonia* or *Neisseria meningitidis*. Within the bowel, *B fragilis* polysaccharides have immunomodulatory effects which may influence the presence and course of inflammatory bowel disease. That the same polysaccharides cause abscesses outside their usual habitat may involve their triggering of Toll-like receptors. *B fragilis* and other *Bacteroides* species produce a number of extracellular enzymes (collagenase, fibrinolysin, heparinase, hyaluronidase) that may also contribute to the formation of the abscess.

✳ Capsule directly causes abscess formation

Immunomodulatory effects may influence inflammatory bowel disease

Some strains of *B fragilis* produce an enterotoxin that causes enteric disease in animals, and in some studies they have been associated with a self-limited, watery diarrhea in children. Because these enterotoxin-producing strains are found in up to 10% of healthy individuals, their pathogenic importance is still undetermined.

Diarrheal enterotoxin causes diarrhea

IMMUNITY

Although it has been demonstrated that antibody to capsular polysaccharide facilitates classical complement pathway killing, there is no evidence that this confers immunity to reinfection. In contrast, there is some evidence that cell-mediated immunity may be protective.

Cell-mediated immunity may be protective

BACTEROIDES FRAGILIS: CLINICAL ASPECTS

MANIFESTATIONS

Some event that displaces *B fragilis* along with other members of the intestinal flora is required to initiate infection; there is no evidence the organism is invasive on its own. This mucosal break may be the result of trauma or other disease states such as diverticulitis.

The local effects of the developing abscess include abdominal pain and tenderness, often with a low-grade fever. The subsequent course depends on whether the abscess remains localized or ruptures through to other sites such as the peritoneal cavity. This may cause several other abscesses or peritonitis. The course of illness is strongly influenced by the other bacteria in the abscess, particularly members of the Enterobacteriaceae. Spread to the bloodstream is more common with *B fragilis* than any other anaerobe.

Abdominal pain, fever evolve to peritonitis

Abscesses combined with anaerobes and Enterobacteriaceae

TREATMENT

Drainage of abscesses and debridement of necrotic tissue are the mainstays of the treatment of *B fragilis* infections, as with anaerobic infections in general. The accompanying antimicrobial therapy is complicated by the fact that abdominal *B fragilis* isolates almost always produce a β-lactamase, which not only inactivates penicillin but other β-lactams, including many cephalosporins. Resistance to tetracycline is also common, but most strains are susceptible to clindamycin, and metronidazole. Among the β-lactams, aztreonam, imipenem, and cefotaxime have been used effectively, as have combinations of a β-lactamase inhibitor (cilastatin, tazobactam) and a β-lactam (imipenem, piperacillin).

❋ β-lactamase action includes some cephalosporins

KEY CONCLUSIONS

- *Bacteroides fragilis* is a leading cause of intraabdominal abscesses often in combination with other intestinal bacteria.
- Superoxide dismutase mediated oxygen tolerance and a polysaccharide capsule causing abscess production act as virulence factors.
- Production of β-lactamase limits the use of antimicrobials active against other anaerobes.

CASE STUDY
Compound Fracture and a Sense of Doom

A 24-year-old man, an automobile accident victim, was brought to the hospital with a compound fracture of the distal left tibia and fibula. Within 6 hours of the accident, the patient was taken to surgery where the wound was debrided, the leg was immobilized, and therapy was begun (cephalothin sodium IV, 1 g/4 h). The patient was afebrile. The hematocrit reading was 41%, the WBC count 10,900/mm³, and blood pressure and pulse rate within normal limits. He did well until the fourth postoperative day when he was noted to have a temperature of 38.3°C orally, a tachycardia rate of 120 bpm, a painful left leg, and a sense of impending doom.

The cast was opened and the entire lower leg was found to be swollen and reddish-brown, and was exuding a serosanguineous foul-smelling discharge. Crepitations were palpable over the anterior tibial and entire gastrocnemius areas. His blood pressure became unstable and then dropped to 70/20 mm Hg. A Gram stain of an aspirate from the gastrocnemius demonstrated both Gram-negative and Gram-positive rods, but no spores were seen. At this time, the hematocrit reading had decreased to 35%, and WBC count was 12,000/mm³, with 85% polymorphonuclear leukocytes.

Therapy was begun with IV penicillin G aqueous, 5 million units every 6 hours. The man was taken to surgery, where an above-knee amputation was performed. While the patient was receiving cephalothin, cultures of the necrotic muscle grew *E coli* and *C perfringens*. Within 3 hours after amputation, the patient had a sense of well-being, and complete recovery followed.

QUESTIONS

1. The crepitations in the wound are most likely due to:
   A. Production of CO_2 by *Clostridium perfringens*
   B. Bowel leakage into the tissue
   C. Foreign bodies from the accident
   D. Surgical introduction of air
   E. Local hematoma

2. The clostridia in the wound most likely came from:
   A. Intestinal flora
   B. Skin flora
   C. Soil
   D. Insect bite
   E. Water

3. The injury in the tissue is produced by which of the following?
    A. ADP-ribosylating toxin
    B. Lecithinase α-toxin
    C. Pore-forming θ-toxin
    D. Enterotoxin
    E. Spores

4. The most important treatment for this condition is:
    A. Antimicrobials
    B. Antitoxin
    C. Hyperbaric oxygen
    D. Surgery
    E. Bed rest

ANSWERS

1. **(A)**

2. **(C)**

3. **(B)**

4. **(D)**

chapter 30

Neisseria

Neisseria meningitidis • *Neisseria gonorrhoeae*

> *Like all real heroes, Charley had a fatal flaw. He refused to believe that he had gonorrhea, whereas the truth was that he did.*
>
> —Kurt Vonnegut, *God Bless You, Mr. Rosewater*

The genus *Neisseria* contains the two Gram-negative cocci which are established human pathogens. The genus also contains many commensal species, most of which are harmless inhabitants of the upper respiratory and alimentary tracts. The pathogenic species are *Neisseria meningitidis* (meningococcus), a major cause of meningitis and bacteremia, and *Neisseria gonorrhoeae* (gonococcus), the cause of gonorrhea.

● *NEISSERIA:* GENERAL FEATURES

Neisseria typically appear in pairs (diplococcic) with the opposing sides flattened, imparting a "kidney bean" appearance (**Figure 30–1**). They are nonmotile, non–spore-forming, and non–acid-fast. Their cell walls are typical of Gram-negative bacteria, with a peptidoglycan layer and an outer membrane containing polysaccharides complexed with lipid and protein. The structural elements of *N meningitidis* and *N gonorrhoeae* are the same, except that the meningococcus has a polysaccharide capsule external to the cell wall.

Diplococci bean shaped

Gonococci and meningococci require an aerobic atmosphere with added carbon dioxide and enriched medium for optimal growth. Gonococci grow more slowly and are more fastidious than meningococci, which can grow on routine blood agar. All *Neisseria* are oxidase-positive. Species are defined by growth characteristics and patterns of carbohydrate fermentation. Procedures are also available to distinguish *N gonorrhoeae* and *N meningitidis* from the other *Neisseria* by immunoassay and nucleic acid amplification (NAA).

Gonococci more fastidious

＊ All oxidase-positive

Both pathogenic species possess pili and outer membrane proteins (OMPs), which vary in their function and antigenic composition. In the study of these meningococcal and gonococcal proteins, investigators have assigned names for molecules which appear to have similar functions in pathogenesis. **Table 30–1** is an attempt to show similarities and differences. It should be understood that the assignment of the same name (eg, PorA) to a protein found in both species does not mean they are identical. It does suggest that they have similar structure and function.

Pili, OMPs, similar

The outer membrane of the two pathogenic *Neisseria* contains a lipopolysaccharide (LPS) variant which differs from that of most other Gram-negative bacteria. The major difference is that the polysaccharide side chains are shorter, lacking the variable O-antigen units of most other Gram-negative bacteria. This short-chain neisserial polymer is called lipooligosaccharide (LOS). The lipid A and core oligosaccharide are structurally and functionally similar to the LPS of other Gram-negative bacteria and LOS has the same endotoxic power of LPS. The pili, OMPs, and LOS are antigenic and have been used in typing schemes.

LOS has short side chains

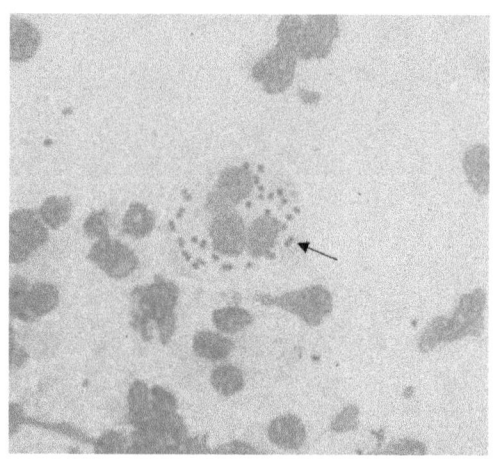

FIGURE 30–1. *Neisseria gonorrhoeae.* Gram stain of urethral exudate. Note the many pairs of Gram-negative bean-shaped diplococci (arrow) collected in polymorphonuclear neutrophils (PMNs) and free in the purulent material. The morphology of *N meningitidis* and other *Neisseria* is identical. (Used with permission from Professor Shirley Lowe, University of California, San Francisco School of Medicine.)

● *NEISSERIA MENINGITIDIS*

OVERVIEW

Meningococci are aerobic Gram-negative diplococci which are irregular but usually quiescent members of the nasopharyngeal flora. Under conditions poorly understood they may invade producing fulminant infection of the bloodstream and/or the central nervous system (CNS). There is little warning; localized infections that precede systemic spread are rarely recognized. The major disease is an acute purulent meningitis with fever, headache, seizures, and mental signs secondary to inflammation and increased intracranial pressure. Even when the CNS is not involved, *N meningitidis* infections have a marked tendency to be accompanied by rash, purpura, thrombocytopenia, and other manifestations associated with endotoxemia. This bacterium causes one of the few infections in which patients may progress from normal health to death in less than a day. It can also spread quickly in family, school, and even national outbreaks.

TABLE 30–1   Bacteriologic and Pathogenic Features of *Neisseria*, Other Gram-negative cocci

| | GROWTH | | ANTIGENIC STRUCTURE | | | | | | |
| | | | | OUTER MEMBRANE PROTEINS | | | | | |
ORGANISM	BLOOD AGAR	ML AGAR[a]	CAPSULE	PILI	ADHERENCE ASSOCIATED	PORINS	BLOCKING AB ASSOCIATED[b]	TRANSMISSION	DISEASE
N meningitidis	+	+	Polysac-charide (12 sero-groups)[c]	Class I,[d] II Anti-genically diverse	Class 5 (4 variants)	PorA, PorB[e]	Class 4	Inhalation of respiratory droplets	Meningitis, septic shock
N gonorrhoeae	–	+	None[f]	Anti-genically diverse[d]	Protein II or Opa (12 variants)	Por1BA, Por1BB	Protein III	Sexual contact of mucosal surfaces	Urethritis, cervicitis, PID
N lactamica, Moraxella	+	–	None	Present	Unknown	Unknown	Absent	Respiratory microbiota	None

PID, pelvic inflammatory disease.
[a]Martin-Lewis or similar selective medium.
[b]Bind IgG in a way that interferes with bactericidal activity of antibodies directed at other antigens.
[c]A, B, C, H, I, K, L, X, Y, Z, 29E, W-135.
[d]Gonococcal and meningococcal class I are similar to each other and members of a class of bacterial pili with amino-terminal *N*-methylphenylalanine residues (*Bacteroides, Moraxella, Pseudomonas aeruginosa*).
[e]Two antigenic classes.
[f]Lipooligosaccharide sialylation has some of the effects of a capsule (see text).

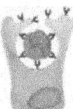 BACTERIOLOGY

Meningococci produce medium-sized smooth colonies on blood agar plates after overnight incubation. Carbon dioxide enhances growth, but is not required. Thirteen serogroups have been defined based on the antigenic specificity of their polysaccharide capsule. The most important disease-producing serogroups are A, B, C, W-135, and Y. In addition to the group polysaccharides, individual *N meningitidis* strains may contain distinct classes of pili and OMPs including porins and adherence proteins, some of which have structural and functional similarities to those found in gonococci. Outer membrane porins mediate cellular interactions. Of these, PorA is a target of new meningococcal group B (MenB) vaccines as are factor H binding proteins (FHbp).

* Serogroups based on polysaccharide capsule

OMPs similar to gonococci

MENINGOCOCCAL DISEASE

EPIDEMIOLOGY

The combination of rapidly progressive disease and obvious person-to-person spread has long made meningococcal disease one of the most feared of all infections. In fact, meningococci are found in the nasopharyngeal flora of 3% to 25% of healthy individuals. Transmission occurs by inhalation of aerosolized respiratory droplets. Close, prolonged contact such as occurs in families and closed populations promotes transmission. The estimated attack rate among family members residing with an index case is 1000 times higher than in the general population; this fact is evidence of the contagious nature of meningococcal infection. Other factors that foster transmission are contact with a virulent strain and host susceptibility (lack of protective antibody). Typical settings of larger outbreaks are schools, dormitories, and camps for military recruits. In these close living circumstances, *N meningitidis* spreads readily among newly exposed individuals, but disease develops only in those who lack group-specific antibody.

* NP colonization common

* Spread by respiratory droplets

The incidence of invasive meningococcal infection varies widely depending on age, geographic locale, and serogroup. In the United States, attack rates vary between 0.5 and 1.5 cases per 100,000 population, but in some countries rates as high as 25 per 100,000 have been sustained for some time. Most disease occurs in children 6 months to 5 years old with a second peak at 18 to 25 years of age (Figure 30–4). Most cases are sporadic or in small family or closed-population (school, day care center) outbreaks. B, C, Y, and W-135 are the most common serogroups in developed countries. Serogroup A strains tend to emerge every 10 to 15 years in large epidemics largely confined to China, Russia, the Middle East, and Africa.

* Groups B, C, Y, W-135 most common

* Group A causes epidemics

PATHOGENESIS

The meningococcus is an exclusively human parasite; it can either exist as an apparently harmless member of the resident microbiota or produce acute disease. For most individuals, the carrier state is an immunizing process associated with acquisition of protective antibodies, but for some, spread from the nasopharynx to produce bacteremia, endotoxemia, and meningitis takes place too quickly for immunity to develop. Meningococcal pili (type IV) protruding through the capsule are the primary mediators of initial attachment to surface proteins (CD46) on nonciliated cells in the nasopharyngeal epithelium. This is a prelude to invasion. In this process, the pili aggregate the bacteria into microcolonies which move as a unit (twitching motility) on the epithelial cell surface. These units bind to microvilli and enter these cells in membrane-bound vesicles. Once inside, meningococci quickly pass through the cytoplasm, exiting into the submucosa and eventually the bloodstream (**Figure 30–2**). In the process, they damage the ciliated cells, possibly by direct release of endotoxin.

Mobile microcolonies

Attachment to microvilli precedes invasion

Once meningococci gain access to the submucosa, their ability to produce disease is enhanced by factors that allow them to scavenge essential nutrients like iron and evade the host immune response. As with other encapsulated bacteria, the polysaccharide capsule enables meningococci to resist complement-mediated bactericidal activity by binding serum factor H to their surface (see Chapter 22). Meningococci also have surface proteins which bind this down-regulator of C3b deposition. In addition, the LOS side chains are able to incorporate sialic acid, another factor H binder, from host substrates.

Proteins scavenge iron

* Capsule, proteins bind factor H

* LOS + sialic acid interferes with C3b deposition

FIGURE 30-2. **Gonococcus and meningococcus, cellular view.** *Neisseria gonorrhoeae* and *Neisseria meningitidis* differ in that *N meningitidis* has a capsule. (*Left*) Both attach to microvillus cells by outer membrane proteins (OMP) and pili. They are endocytosed in vacuoles. (*Middle*) Both multiply freely in the cytoplasm. (*Right*) Both escape to the submucosa, but the gonococcus is actively phagocytosed and remains localized. The meningococcal capsule allows it to evade phagocytosis and it enters the bloodstream. PMNs, polymorphonuclear neutrophils.

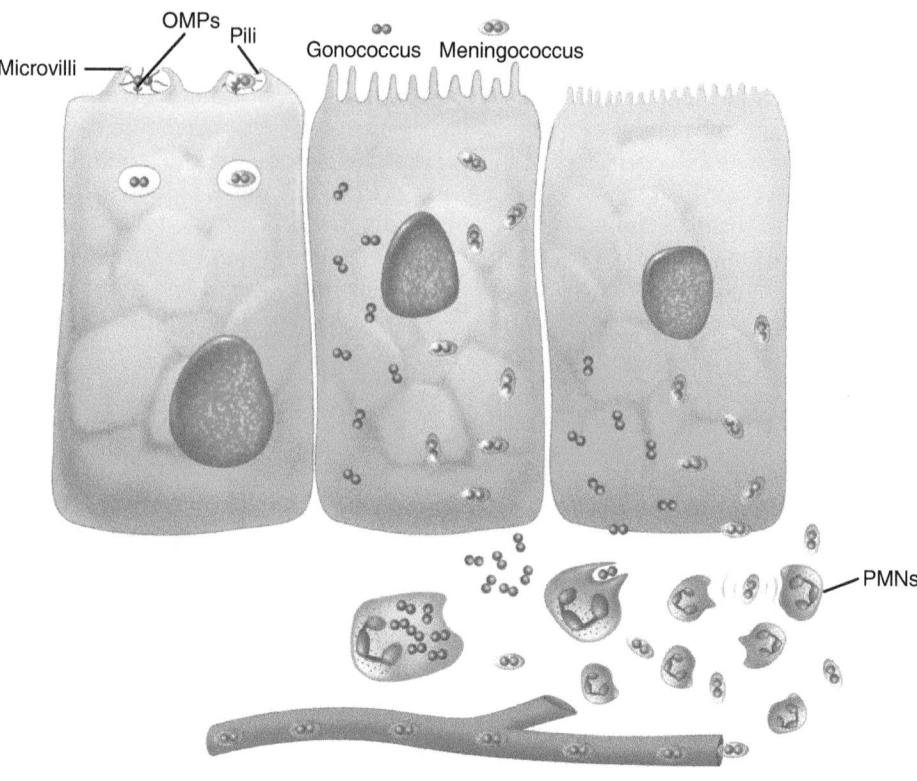

* Spread produces systemic endotoxemia

* LOS, peptidoglycan trigger cytokines

* Outer membrane blebs contain endotoxin

The most serious manifestations of meningococcal disease are related to its spread to the bloodstream and, its namesake, the meninges. The exact mechanism of CNS invasion is unclear but is probably related to the level of the bacteremia. It occurs in the choroid plexus with its exceptionally high rate of blood flow. After CNS invasion, an intense subarachnoid space inflammatory response is induced by the release of cell wall peptidoglycan fragments, LOS, and possibly other virulence factors. This causes the release of inflammatory cytokines. A prominent feature of meningococcal disease with or without CNS invasion is systemic endotoxin activity (see Manifestations). When grown in culture, *N meningitidis* readily releases endotoxin-containing blebs of its outer membrane from the cell surface as shown in **Figure 30–3.** It is not known whether this occurs *in vivo*, but the model of the meningococcus as a hyperproducer of endotoxin certainly fits with its most serious disease manifestations.

IMMUNITY

* Group-specific antibody protective

Immunity to meningococcal infections is related to group-specific antipolysaccharide antibody, which is bactericidal and facilitates phagocytosis. The bactericidal activity is due to complement-mediated cell lysis via the classical complement pathway. Individuals with deficiencies in the

FIGURE 30-3. *Neisseria meningitidis.* Cell wall is shown shedding multiple "blebs" (*arrows*) containing lipopolysaccharide–endotoxin. Note the typical trilamellar Gram-negative cell wall structure in the wall and the blebs. (Reproduced with permission from Devoe IW, Gilcrist JE: Release of endotoxin in the form of cell wall blebs during in vitro growth of Neisseria meningitides, *J Exp Med* 1973; Nov 1;138(5):1156-1167.)

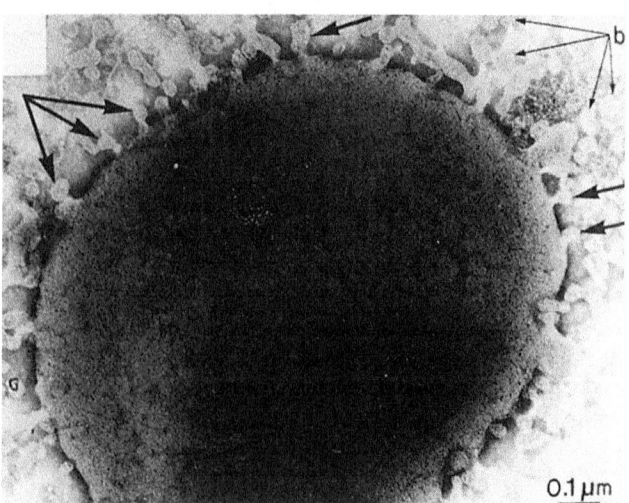

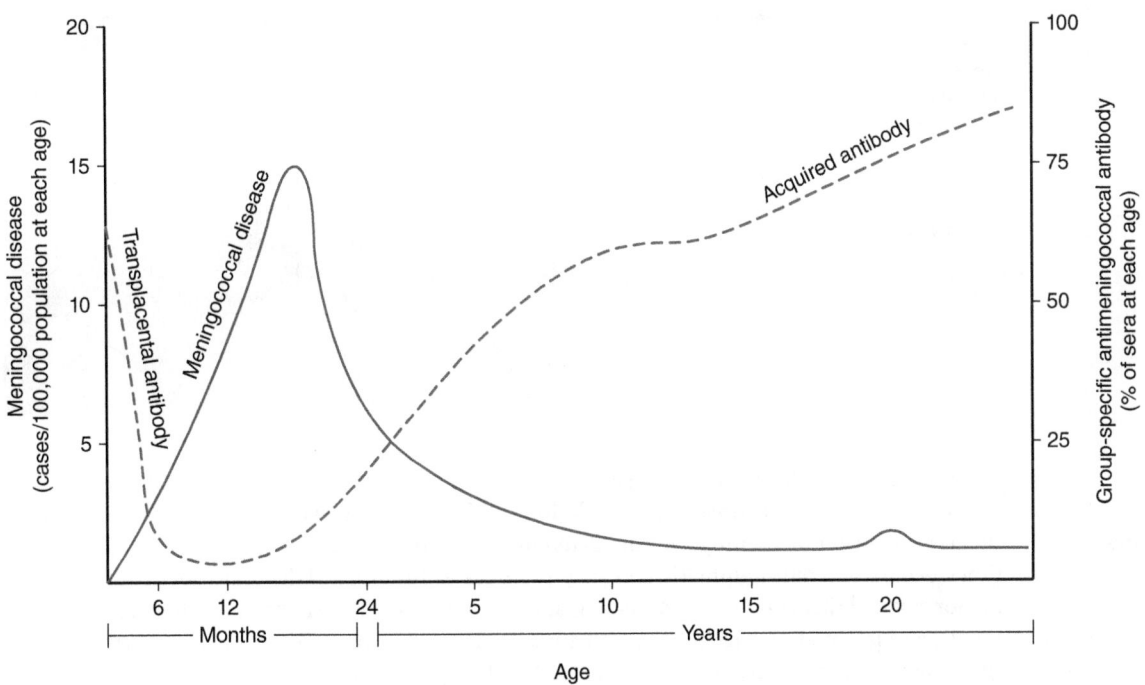

FIGURE 30–4. **Immunity to the meningococcus.** The inverse relationship between bactericidal meningococcal anti-body and meningococcal disease is demonstrated. The "blip" in the disease curve around age 20 is attributable in part to military and other closed-population outbreaks. (Adapted with permission from Goldschneider I, Gotschlich EC, Liu TY, et al: Human immunity to the meningococcus I. The role of humoral antibodies, *J Exp Med* 1969; Jun 1;129(6):1307–26.)

terminal complement components have an enhanced risk for meningococcal disease but not for other polysaccharide capsule pathogens, such as *Haemophilus influenzae* type b.

Through the first 12 years of life, the incidence of meningococcal meningitis is inversely proportional to the percentage of the population with bactericidal antibody (**Figure 30–4**). The peak incidence of disease occurs between 6 months and 2 years of age. This corresponds to the nadir in the prevalence of bactericidal antibody in the general population. This is the time gap between loss of maternal transplacental antibody and the appearance of naturally acquired antibody. By adult life, serum antibody to one or more meningococcal serogroups is usually present, but an immune deficit remains for the serogroups not encountered in the local community. Infections appear when populations carrying virulent strains mix (college, summer camp, military barracks) allowing susceptible individuals encounter strains of serogroups for which they have no immunologic experience.

Protective antibody is stimulated by infection and through the carrier state, which produces immunity within a few weeks. The natural immunization shown in Figure 30–4 may not require colonization with every serogroup or even with *N meningitidis*, because antibody may be produced in response to cross-reactive polysaccharides possessed by other *Neisseria* or even other genera. For example, *Escherichia coli* strains of a particular serotype (K1) have a polysaccharide capsule identical to that of the group B meningococcus.

Purified capsular polysaccharides are immunogenic, generating T-cell–independent immune responses. As with other polysaccharide immunogens, these responses are not strong, lack memory, and mature slowly. In particular they may not yet be mature in early childhood when the risk of meningococcal disease is greatest. The group B polysaccharide differs from that of the other groups in failing to stimulate bactericidal antibody at all. This is believed to be due to the similarity of its sialic acid polymer to human neural cell adhesion molecules. That is, it is recognized as self.

Common age 6 to 24 months

✳ Antibody lack = susceptibility

Carrier state, other polysaccharides stimulate antibody

✳ T-cell–independent mechanisms weak

✳ Group B not immunogenic

MENINGOCOCCAL DISEASE: CLINICAL ASPECTS

MANIFESTATIONS

The most common form of meningococcal infection is acute purulent meningitis, with clinical and laboratory features similar to those of meningitis from other causes. A prominent feature of meningococcal meningitis is the appearance of scattered skin petechiae, which may evolve into

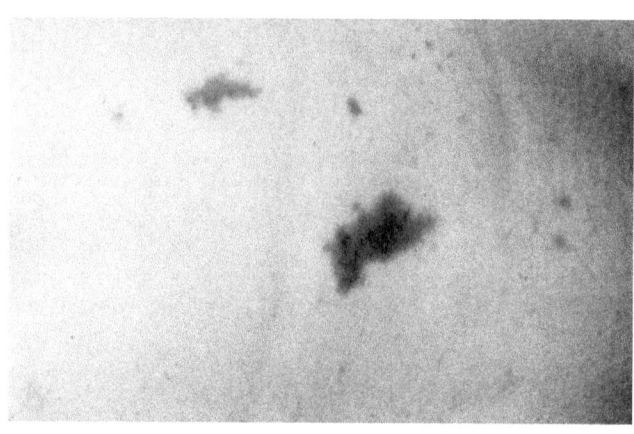

FIGURE 30–5. **Meningococcemia.** Small and large coalesced petechiae are shown in the skin of a patient with meningococci circulating in the blood. (Reproduced with permission from Nester EW, Anderson DG, Roberts CE Jr, et al: *Microbiology: A Human Perspective*, 6th ed. New York, NY: McGraw Hill; 2008.)

ecchymoses or a diffuse petechial rash (**Figure 30–5**). These cutaneous manifestations are signs of the disseminated intravascular coagulation (DIC) syndrome, which is part of the endotoxic shock brought on by meningococcal bacteremia (meningococcemia). Meningococcemia sometimes occurs without meningitis and may progress to fulminant DIC and shock with bilateral hemorrhagic destruction of the adrenal glands (Waterhouse-Friderichsen syndrome). However, the disease is not always fulminant, and some patients have only low-grade fever, arthritis, and skin lesions that develop slowly over a period of days to weeks. Meningococci are a rare cause of other infections such as pneumonia, but it is striking that localized infections are almost never recognized in advance of systemic disease.

Meningitis most common

✳ Meningococcemia, rash progress to DIC

✳ Resemble endotoxic shock

DIAGNOSIS

Direct Gram smears of cerebrospinal fluid (CSF) in meningitis usually demonstrate the typical bean-shaped, Gram-negative diplococci (Figure 30–1). Definitive diagnosis is by culture of CSF, blood, or skin lesions. Although *N meningitidis* is reputed to be somewhat fragile, it requires no special laboratory handling for isolation from presumptively sterile sites such as blood and CSF. Growth is good on blood or chocolate agar after 18 hours of incubation. Serogrouping has no immediate clinical importance.

Gram smears diagnostic

✳ Culture on blood agar

TREATMENT

Penicillin resistance mediated by both β-lactamase and altered penicillin-binding proteins (PBPs) is over 10%. Third-generation cephalosporins such as ceftriaxone and cefotaxime are now the treatments of choice for acute meningitis. For those with β-lactam hypersensitivity, moxifloxacin and chloramphenicol are alternatives.

✳ Cephalosporins replace penicillin

PREVENTION

Until the development and spread of sulfonamide resistance in the 1960s, chemoprophylaxis with these agents was the primary means of preventing spread of meningococcal infections. Rifampin, ceftriaxone, ciprofloxacin, or azithromycin are now the primary chemoprophylactic agents. In the absence of resistance, penicillin is still not effective for prophylaxis, probably due to inadequate penetration into the uninflamed nasopharyngeal mucosa. Selection of cases to receive prophylaxis is based on epidemiologic assessment. Risk is highest for siblings of the index case and declines with increasing age. The closeness and duration of contact with the index case are also important. For example, an infant sibling sharing a room with a person with meningococcal disease would be at the highest risk. Typically, family members are given prophylaxis, but other adults are not. Common-sense exceptions, such as playmates and healthcare workers with very close contact (eg, mouth-to-mouth resuscitation), are made at the discretion of the physician or epidemiologist. The presence or absence of nasopharyngeal carriage of *N meningitidis* plays no role in this decision because it does not accurately predict risk of disease.

Rifampin, ceftriaxone, ciprofloxacin, azithromycin for chemoprophylaxis

Close contact is indication

The first purified polysaccharide vaccines were shown to stimulate group-specific antibody and to prevent disease in military and adult civilian populations. A vaccine containing A, C, Y, and W-135 polysaccharides was licensed in the United States but proved poorly immunogenic for infants and children under 2 years of age. This was a huge disappointment because young children are the largest group at risk (Figure 30–4). We now know the reason. Purified polysaccharide vaccines only stimulate T-cell–independent responses and these become fully developed only after 2 years of age. As with pneumococcal and *H influenzae* polysaccharide vaccines, this problem was overcome by conjugating the polysaccharide to a protein carrier (diphtheria toxoid). This quadrivalent meningococcal Conjugate Vaccine (MenACWY) stimulates T-cell–dependent responses, which are both stronger and present at an earlier age. Its use now is licensed and universally recommended beginning at age 11 with boosters at 16 years.

 11 years! Why not start at 6 months like other vaccines?

MenACWY is also recommended down to the age of 9 months for anyone at high risk for meningococcal disease (complement deficiency, asplenia, HIV infection). Hopefully, further experience and solution of the group B (MenB) problem (see later) will push universal application of this protection down to infants and toddlers as is done with the highly successful *H influenzae* Hib vaccine (see Chapter 31).

The protein conjugate approach faces a unique difficulty with the meningococcus—the failure of the MenB polysaccharide to be immunogenic at all. This appears to be due to its similarity to a human neural cell adhesion molecule. This means that even if the lack of antigenicity was overcome by protein conjugation, the risk of the new vaccine stimulating an autoimmune reaction would be unacceptable. MenB causes up to one-third of all disease, so no vaccine that omits it is likely to be completely successful. For this reason, discarding the group polysaccharide entirely in favor of other approaches particularly the use of surface proteins as immunogens has been pursued. Of the two new licensed MenB vaccines one uses two serum factor H binding proteins (FHbp) and the other an FHbp plus a well-known meningococcal surface protein, PorA. Both vaccines have been shown to be immunogenic and safe, as well as appearing to control a number of college campus outbreaks. These vaccines are recommended for immunization of young adults 16 to 18 years old or earlier if the any of the predisposing conditions discussed above for MenACWY are present.

* Polysaccharides only stimulate T-cell–independent immunity

* MenACWY stimulates T-cell–dependent immunity

* MenB vaccines now available

* FHbp, PorA proteins are immunogens

KEY CONCLUSIONS

- The *N meningitidis* polysaccharide comes in multiple antigenic groups of which 5 (A, B, C, W-135, Y) are common causes of disease.
- Disease may be endogenous (respiratory microbiota) or transmitted from a case by respiratory droplets.
- Pili and OMPs mediate attachment and invasion of respiratory epithelial cells.
- Hyperproduction of endotoxin causes fulminant sepsis and/or meningitis without a preceding local infection.
- MenACWY polysaccharide/conjugate vaccine includes groups A, C, W-135, and Y.
- Group B polysaccharide is recognized as self and thus not immunogenic. New MenB vaccines use surface FHbp and PorA proteins as immunogens.

● *NEISSERIA GONORRHOEAE*

OVERVIEW

Bacteriologically, gonococci are similar to meningococci except they are more fragile and lack a capsule. The contrast in disease is considerable. Gonorrhea (*gonos* [semen], *rhoia* [to flow]) is primarily localized to mucosal surfaces with relatively infrequent spread to the bloodstream or deep tissues. Infection is sexually acquired by direct genital contact, and the primary manifestation is pain and purulent discharge at the infected site. In men, this is typically the urethra, and in women, the uterine cervix. Direct extension of the infection up the fallopian tubes produces fever and lower abdominal pain, a syndrome called pelvic inflammatory disease (PID). For women, sterility or ectopic pregnancy can be long-term consequences of gonorrhea.

 Think ▸▸ Apply 30-1: **There is less experience with these protein-conjugate vaccines and the "hole" created by absence of a group B component could have epidemic potential. In practice the age is being slowly and cautiously dropped down.**

BACTERIOLOGY

Chocolate agar for growth

✳ Pili, LOS, and OMPs in outer membrane

✳ Opas mediate adherence

N gonorrheae grows well only on chocolate agar and other specialized media enriched to ensure its growth. It requires carbon dioxide supplementation. Small, smooth, nonpigmented colonies appear after 18 to 24 hours and are well developed (2-4 mm) after 48 hours. Gonococci possess numerous pili (type IV) which are structurally similar to those of meningococci and extend beyond the outer membrane (**Figure 30–6**) (Table 30–1). In addition to intergonoccocal and epithelial cell adherence, these fibers contract causing "twitching" motility of entire microcolonies. They also facilitate direct uptake of DNA (transformation) by gonococci. The gonococcal outer membrane is composed of phospholipids, LOS, and several distinct OMPs. The OMPs include porins (Por1BA and Por1BB) and adherence proteins known as Opa.

ANTIGENIC VARIATION

Pili, OMPs, LOS vary antigenically

✳ Pilin subunit genes undergo recombination

✳ Outcome nonfunctional or antigenically altered pili

✳ Opa genes "on" or "off"

N gonorrhoeae and *N meningitidis* are among several microorganisms whose surface structures are known to change antigenically from generation to generation during growth of a single strain. The mechanisms involved have been more extensively studied in gonococci but appear to be similar in both species. The major gonococcal structures known to undergo antigenic variation are pili, Opa proteins, and LOS. The genetic mechanisms are discussed in the following discussion and illustrated in Figure 22–5.

Gonococcal pili are antigenically variable to an extraordinary extent. There are multiple genetic mechanisms, but the most important is recombinational exchange between the multiple pilin genes present in the chromosome of every strain. Some of these genes are complete and able to express pilin (*pilE*). Others are not, due to lack of an effective promoter and are thus silent (*pilS*). When recombination between expression and silent loci results in the donation of new sequences to an expression locus, the result can be expression of a pilin with changes in its amino acid composition and thus its antigenicity. The recombination could also involve exogenous DNA from another cell or strain, because gonococci naturally take up species-specific DNA by transformation. The numerous possible outcomes include no pilin subunits, pilin subunits unable to assemble, mature pili with altered functional characteristics, and fully functional pili with a new antigenic makeup.

The multiple gonococcal Opa proteins are each encoded by separate genes scattered around the genome. Various combinations of these genes may be either "on" or "off" at any one time. The

FIGURE 30–6. *Neisseria gonorrhoeae* **pili.** This view is a cross-section of the microcolony of gonococci on the surface of an epithelial cell originally shown in Figure 22–2 (inset). Pili are actively attaching to the epithelial cell surface and using a contractile force (twitching motility) to move and modify the surface. (Used with permission from Dustin L. Higashi and Magdalene So.)

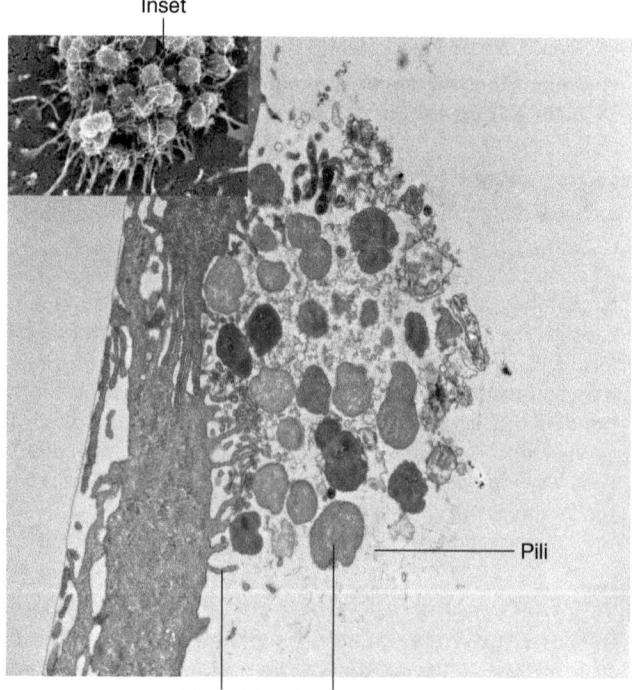

Inset

Pili

Microvilli   Gonococci

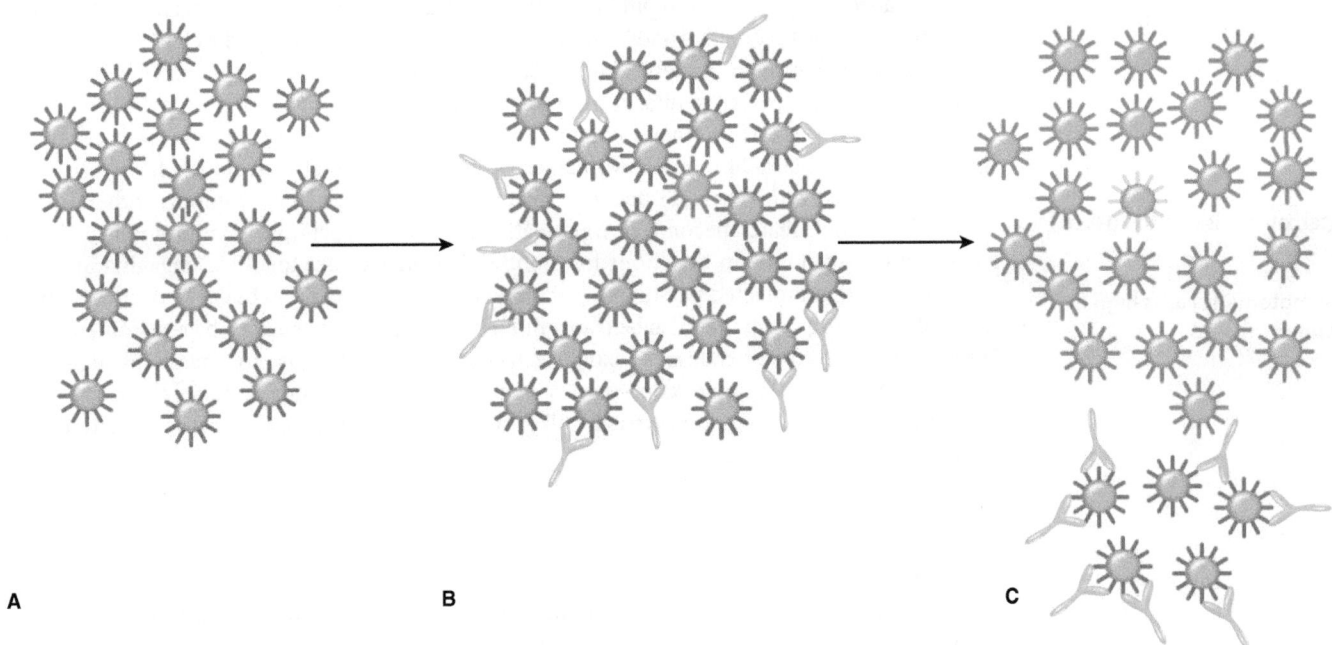

A   B   C

FIGURE 30–7. **Gonococcal antigenic variation. A.** A population of gonococci is shown with surface pili. There are two antigenic types of pili in the population, one of which is dominant. **B.** IgG against the dominant blue pilin type is introduced and binds all the cells with that pilin type on the surface. **C.** Later, the bound gonococci with their pili are clumped at the bottom. The minor (red) pilin type present in A now predominates, and a new one (green) has appeared but is still a minority member of the population. Antibody directed against the now dominant member would allow the new green one to take over. The same kind of population change occurs based on antigenic variation of outer membrane proteins. The genetic mechanisms involved in generating multiple antigenic types are illustrated in Figure 22–5.

switch is set during the transcription of each Opa gene for the next cell generation. As a result of a process called replicative slippage, the number of repeats of particular gene sequence can vary. When the time comes for translation, the number of repeats determines whether the gene will be in or out of frame to translate its Opa protein. If it is in frame, the gene is "on"; if not, the switch is "off." Variation in gonococcal LOS has been observed in volunteer subjects challenged with intraurethral *N gonorrhoeae*, but the genetic mechanism is unknown.

⁎ Frame shift controls Opa switch

LOS varies antigenically

These changes in the gonococcal surface are random events which may or may not have survival value. During the early stages of infection, there could be positive selection for the expression of pili and Opas that mediate adherence. If the host has antibodies against one or more of these proteins, they would be removed and the infecting population would shift to cells expressing pili or Opas to which there is no immunologic experience. An example of how these antigenic variants could be selected is shown in **Figure 30–7**. Taken together, these multifactorial, antigenic variations of the gonococcal surface may serve the dual purposes of escape from immune surveillance and timely provision of the ligands required to bind to human cell receptors.

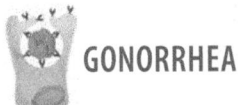 GONORRHEA

EPIDEMIOLOGY

Gonorrhea is one of our greatest public health problems. The hundreds of thousands of cases reported in the United States each year are felt to represent less than 50% of the true number and the rates for adolescents are alarmingly high and increasing by 10% a year. The highest rates are in women between the ages of 15 and 19 years and in men between the ages of 20 and 24 years. No truly effective means of control is yet in sight. Our ability to stem the tide of changed sexual mores continues to be hampered by lack of an effective means to detect asymptomatic cases, resistance of *N gonorrhoeae* to antibiotics (see Treatment), and, to some extent, lack of appreciation of the importance of this disease. The latter is evidenced by failure of patients to seek medical care

Rates among adolescents are high and increasing

and reluctance to report cases to public health authorities due to privacy concerns. In the minds of too many, syphilis is dreaded and "unclean," whereas gonorrhea is only "the clap" ("clap" is from the archaic French *clapoir*, "a rabbit warren"; later, "a brothel").

Gonorrhea is acquired by genital contact with an infected person. The major reservoir for continued spread is the asymptomatic patient. Screening programs and case contact studies have shown that almost 50% of infected women are asymptomatic or at least do not have symptoms usually associated with venereal infection. Most men (95%) have acute symptoms with infection. Many who are not treated become asymptomatic but remain infectious. Asymptomatic male and female patients can remain infectious for months. The attack rates for those engaging in sexual intercourse with an infected person are estimated to be 20% (female to male) to over 50% (male to female). The organism may also be transmitted by oral–genital contact or by rectal intercourse. When all these factors operate in a sexually active population, it is easy to explain the high prevalence of gonorrhea. Although gonococci can survive for brief periods on toilet seats, nonsexual transmission is extremely rare. Virtually all gonococci isolated from children can be traced to sexual abuse by an infected adult.

Intercourse risk up to 20% to 50%

Asymptomatic cases high in women

PATHOGENESIS

■ Attachment and Invasion

Gonococci are not normal inhabitants of the respiratory or genital microbiota. When introduced onto a mucosal surface by sexual contact with an infected individual, adherence ligands such as pili and Opa proteins allow initial attachment of the bacteria to receptors (CD46, CD66, integrins) on nonciliated epithelial cells (Figure 30–2). Initial attachment by the pili is mediated by the active force they generate in movement of their microcolonies across the cell surface (Figure 30–6). This is followed by a tighter attachment owing to Opa proteins. This close binding provides an opportunity for other OMPs (Por1BA) to trigger signaling cascades activating multiple enzymatic systems within the host cell. These reactions lead to induction of phagocytosis of the gonococci in a process involving microfilaments and microtubules of the invaded cell. The microvilli surround the bacteria and appear to draw them into the host cell in the same manner as meningococci. Thus, after initial attachment the gonococcus induces the host cell to actively take it inside (Figure 30–2). Once inside, the bacteria transcytose the cell and exit through the basal membrane to enter the submucosa.

Pili, Opa attach to nonciliated epithelium

Induce phagocytosis

Pass to submucosa

■ Survival in the Submucosa

Once in the submucosa, the bacteria must survive and resist innate host defenses as well as adaptive immune responses acquired from a previous infection. Although gonococci lack the polysaccharide capsule of the meningococcus, they still have multiple mechanisms that protect them against serum complement and antibody. One of these is LOS sialylation in which the gonococcus is able to incorporate host sialic acid onto its own surface. This provides a mechanism for blocking surface C3b deposition by direct LOS/sialic acid binding of factor H or by facilitating its binding to surface porins.

Even when phagocytes do encounter gonococci, surface factors such as pili and Opa proteins interfere with effective phagocytosis. The organisms are also able to defend against oxidative killing inside the phagocyte by upregulation of catalase production and an efficient antioxidant defense system. Taken together, these factors provide ample evidence that killing by neutrophils is sufficiently retarded to allow prolonged survival of gonococci in mucosal and submucosal locations.

Phagocytosed gonococci resist PMN killing

■ Spread and Dissemination

In contrast to meningococci, *N gonorrhoeae* bacteria tend to remain localized to genital structures, causing inflammation and local injury, which no doubt facilitates their continued venereal transmission. Purulent exudates containing "sticky" clusters of gonococci held together by Opa proteins could be the primary infectious unit. Infection may spread to deeper structures by progressive extension to adjacent mucosal and glandular epithelial cells. These include the prostate and epididymis in men and the paracervical glands and fallopian tubes in women (**Figure 30–8**). Spread to the fallopian tubes is facilitated by pilus-mediated twitching motility, attachment to sperm, and finally to the microvilli of nonciliated fallopian tube cells. Injury to the fallopian epithelium is mediated by the local effect of outer membrane LOS. Gonococci are also known to turn over their peptidoglycan rapidly during growth, releasing peptidoglycan fragments which are toxic to the ciliated epithelium of the fallopian tube.

In a small proportion of infections, organisms reach the bloodstream to produce disseminated gonococcal infection (DGI). When this happens, the systemic findings have their own pattern (see Manifestations) and seldom take on the endotoxic shock picture of meningococcemia. Although differences have been noted between *N gonorrhoeae* strains that remain localized and those that produce DGI, their connection to pathogenesis is unknown. Both DGI and salpingitis tend to begin during or shortly after completion of menses. This may relate to changes in the cervical mucus and reflux into the fallopian tubes during menses.

✳ LOS, peptidoglycan shedding causes injury

DGI differs from endotoxic shock

✳ Reflux during menses facilitates spread

■ Genetic Regulation of Virulence

Through all the stages of gonorrhea, gonococci are able to use a particularly rich variety of genetic mechanisms in deployment of the virulence factors previously described at the right time. Some are regulatory responses to environmental cues, such as iron in relation to iron-binding proteins, whereas others involve changes in the genome. Antigenic changes in both pili and Opa proteins have been demonstrated in human infection, including the isolation of antigenic variants from different sites in the same patient. These presumably take place by the recombinational and translational mechanisms described above (see Antigenic Variation) as the organisms replicate in the patient.

Regulation, recombination, translation of virulence factors

IMMUNITY

The apparent lack of immunity to gonococcal infection has long been frustrating. Among sexually active persons with multiple partners, repeated infections are the rule rather than the exception.

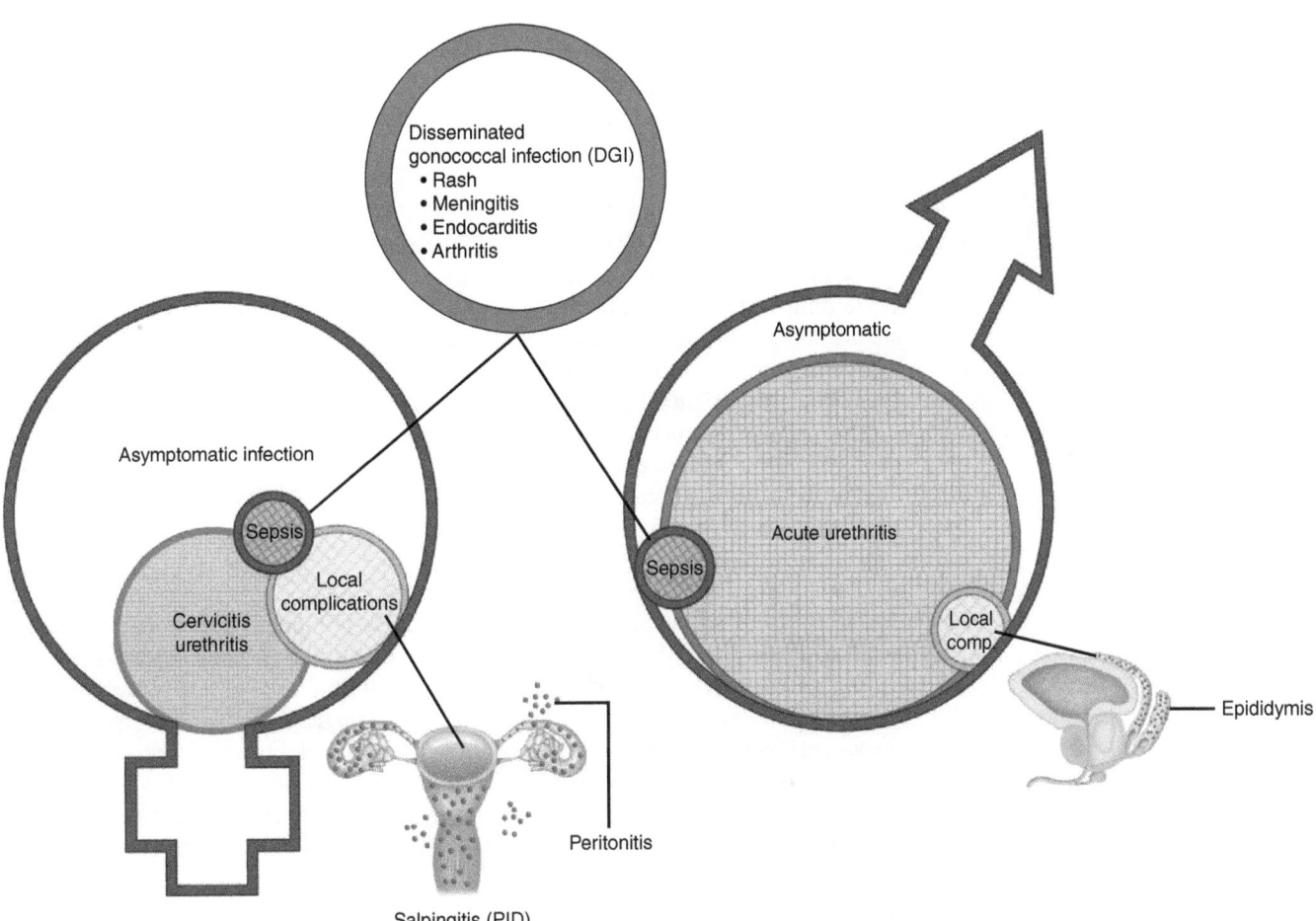

FIGURE 30–8. Gonorrhea in men and women. The majority of cases in women are asymptomatic. Local extension up the fallopian tubes causes salpingitis. The majority of men have acute urethritis, and only a small percentage have local extension to the epididymis. A very small part of either spectrum results in bacteremia and disseminated gonococcal infection.

How can there be so little immunity to an infectious agent that produces such intense acute inflammation?

Both serum and secretory antibodies are generated during natural infection, but the levels are generally low, even after repeated infections. Another aspect is that even when antibodies are formed, antigenic variation defeats their effectiveness and allows the gonococcus to escape immune surveillance. Antigenic variation of pili, Opa proteins, and LOS is particularly likely to be important. Outbreaks have been traced to a single strain that demonstrated multiple pilin variations and Opa types in repeated isolates from the same individual or from sexual partners. In experimental models, passive administration of antibody directed against one pilin type has been followed by emergence of new pilin variants presumably through the sequence illustrated in Figure 30–7. It appears that although some immunity to gonococcal infection is present, its effectiveness is compromised by the ability of the organism to change key structures during the course of infection.

Antibody response weak

✱ Antigenic variation evades immune surveillance

 ## GONORRHEA: CLINICAL ASPECTS

MANIFESTATIONS

■ Genital Gonorrhea

The clinical spectrum of gonorrhea differs substantially in men and women (Figure 30–8). In men, the primary site of infection is the urethra. Symptoms begin 2 to 7 days after infection and consist primarily of purulent urethral discharge and dysuria. Although uncommon, local extension can lead to epididymitis or prostatitis. The endocervix is the primary site in women, in whom symptoms include increased vaginal discharge, urinary frequency, dysuria, abdominal pain, and menstrual abnormalities. As mentioned previously, symptoms may be mild or absent in either sex, particularly women.

Urethritis and endocervicitis in primary infections

■ Other Local Infections

Rectal gonorrhea occurs after rectal intercourse or, in women, after contamination with infected vaginal secretions. This condition is generally asymptomatic, but may cause tenesmus, discharge, and rectal bleeding. Pharyngeal gonorrhea is transmitted by oral–genital sex and, again, may be asymptomatic. Sore throat and cervical adenitis may occur. Infection of other structures near primary infection sites, such as Bartholin glands in women, may lead to abscess formation.

Inoculation of gonococci into the conjunctiva produces a severe, acute, purulent conjunctivitis. Although this infection may occur at any age, the most serious form is gonococcal ophthalmia neonatorum, a disease acquired during childbirth by a newborn from an infected mother. The disease was formerly a common cause of blindness, which is now prevented by the administration of prophylactic topical eye drops or ointment (erythromycin or tetracycline) at birth.

Rectal, pharyngeal infections relate to sexual practices

Transmission at birth causes ophthalmia neonatorum

■ Pelvic Inflammatory Disease

The clinical syndrome of pelvic inflammatory disease (PID) develops in 10% to 20% of women with gonorrhea. The findings include fever, lower abdominal pain (usually bilateral), adnexal tenderness, and leukocytosis with or without signs of local infection. These features are caused by spread of organisms along the fallopian tubes to produce salpingitis and into the pelvic cavity to produce pelvic peritonitis and abscesses (**Figure 30–9**). PID is also known to develop when other genital pathogens ascend by the same route. These organisms include anaerobes and *Chlamydia trachomatis*, which may appear alone or mixed with gonococci. The most serious complications of PID are infertility and ectopic pregnancy secondary to scarring of the fallopian tubes.

✱ Salpingitis, peritonitis cause scarring, infertility

 Think ▸▸ Apply 30-2: The primary culprit is antigenic variation of the primary virulence factors. Whatever immune response is mounted finds a changed pathogen even during the course of a single infection. Any effective vaccine would have to use a highly conserved pilin or OMP epitope.

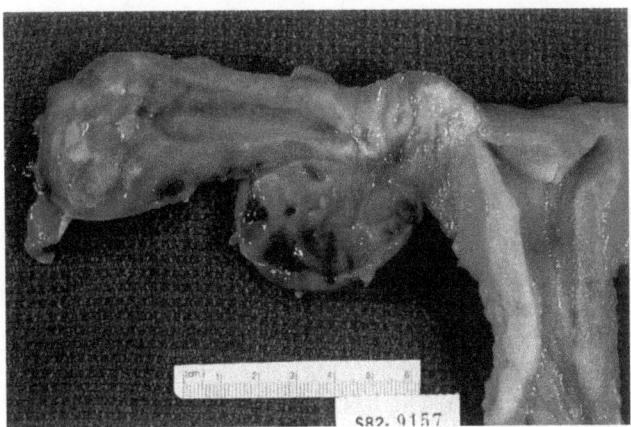

FIGURE 30–9. Tubo-ovarian abscess. This large abscess in the fallopian tube is part of the spectrum of pelvic inflammatory disease (PID) of which *Neisseria gonorrhoeae* is a major cause. (Reproduced with permission from Connor DH, Chandler FW, Schwartz DQ, et al: *Pathology of Infectious Diseases*. Stamford CT: Appleton & Lange; 1997.)

■ Disseminated Gonococcal Infection

Any of the local forms of gonorrhea or their extensions such as PID may lead to bacteremia. In the bacteremic DGI phase, the primary features are fever, migratory polyarthralgia, and a petechial, maculopapular, or pustular rash. Some of these features may be immunologically mediated. Gonococci are infrequently isolated from the skin or joints at this stage despite their presence in the blood. The bacteremia may lead to metastatic infections such as endocarditis and meningitis, but the most common is purulent arthritis. The arthritis typically follows the bacteremia and involves large joints such as elbows and knees. Gonococci are readily cultured from the pus.

Skin rash, arthralgia, and arthritis with bacteremia

Purulent arthritis in large joints

DIAGNOSIS

■ Gram Smear

The presence of multiple pairs of bean-shaped, Gram-negative diplococci within a neutrophil is highly characteristic of gonorrhea when the smear is from a genital site (Figure 30–1). The direct Gram smear is more than 95% sensitive and specific in symptomatic men. Unfortunately, it is only 50% to 70% sensitive in women, and its specificity is complicated by the presence of other bacteria in the female genital flora that have similar morphology. A positive Gram smear is generally accepted as diagnostic in men. It should not be used as the sole source for diagnosis in women or when the findings have social (divorce) or legal (rape, child abuse) implications.

✻ Smear diagnostic in men

■ Culture

Attention to detail is necessary for isolation of the gonococcus because it is a fragile organism that is often mixed with hardier members of the genital flora. In men, the best specimen is urethral exudate or urethral scrapings (obtained with a loop or special swab). In women, cervical swabs are preferred over urethral or vaginal specimens. Rectal cultures in men and throat cultures are needed only when indicated by sexual practices. The selective medium (eg, Martin-Lewis agar) is an enriched selective chocolate agar with antibiotics active against Gram-positive bacteria (vancomycin), Gram-negative bacteria (colistin, trimethoprim), and fungi (nystatin).

Urethra, cervix preferred culture sites

ML agar inhibits competing flora

■ Direct Detection

Much effort has been directed at developing immunoassay and NAA methods that detect gonococci in genital and urine specimens without culture. Such methods have particular importance for screening populations in which culture is impractical. After a series of improvements NAA methods are now considered the diagnostic standard. NAA results are considered diagnostic from genital sites (including urine) but may need to be confirmed by culture from other sites. The cost/benefit ratio of NAA tests has been improved by combining them with *Chlamydia* detection (see Chapter 39), which targets the same clinical population.

NAA methods sensitive and specific

Gonococci and *Chlamydia* combined

TREATMENT

Penicillin, which once was active against all known gonococci at extremely low concentrations (less than 0.1 μg/mL), is no longer used due to the development of multiple mechanisms of resistance. Third-generation cephalosporins resistant to the β-lactamases prevalent in gonococci are

GC and Chlamydia treated together

IM ceftriaxone

now the standard. In addition, it is now recommended that all patients treated for gonorrhea also be treated for *Chlamydia* infection. For gonorrhea, ceftriaxone is given in a single intramuscular injection. Until late 2020, oral azithromycin, which is also effective against *Chlamydia*, was added to follow the ceftriaxone dose but has now been dropped in favor of a higher dose of ceftriaxone. Resistance rates up to 25% have taken fluoroquinolones out of the picture.

PREVENTION

Condoms block transmission

Condoms provide a high degree of protection against both infection with *N gonorrhoeae* and transmission to a sexual partner. Spermicides and other vaginal foams and douches are not reliable protection. The classic public health methods of case–contact tracing and treatment are important but difficult because of the size of the infected population. The availability of a good serologic test would greatly aid control, as it has for syphilis. Although candidate immunogens continue to be studied, the development of a vaccine is a high but distant goal.

KEY CONCLUSIONS

- *Neisseria gonorrhoeae* is more fastidious than *N meningitis* and lacks a capsule.
- Gonorrhea is sexually transmitted.
- Pili and outer membrane proteins (OMPs) mediate attachment and invasion of urethral and cervical epithelial cells.
- Intense inflammation typically extends only locally (fallopian tubes, epididymis) not systemically.
- Pelvic inflammatory disease (PID), ectopic pregnancy and sterility are consequences in women.
- Antigenic variation of pili and OMPs confounds lasting immunity, vaccine strategies.
- Nucleic acid amplification methods have replaced culture for definitive diagnosis.
- Emergence of β-lactamase-mediated resistance requires treatment with ceftriaxone.

CASE STUDY

Recruit with Fever, Backache, and Rash

A 20-year-old man presented to the emergency room because of fever and backache. A basic trainee on leave from a naval training station, he was perfectly well until the day of admission when he awakened with fever, malaise, and lumbar backache, all of which gradually worsened over the ensuing 6 hours.

Examination revealed an acutely ill man with blood pressure of 105/65 mm Hg, pulse rate 120/min, and temperature 104°F. A few small petechiae were on the volar surfaces of each forearm. The muscles of the back, arms, and legs were tender to palpation. The remainder of the examination was normal. A lumbar puncture showed 1500 white blood cells/mL, 95% of which were PMNs. CSF cultures were obtained.

QUESTIONS

1. Which factor would most influence the likely etiologic agents?
   A. Height of fever
   B. Number of PMNs in CSF
   C. Immunization status
   D. Extent of petechiae
   E. Prior antibiotics

2. What is the primary cause of the patient's petechiae?
   A. Superantigen production
   B. Pore-forming toxin
   C. Endotoxin
   D. Pili
   E. OMPs

3. In addition to culture of the CSF, culture of what other site would be most valuable?
    A. Throat
    B. Sputum
    C. Petechiae
    D. Blood

4. If the CSF cultures are positive for *N meningitidis*, is any preventive action appropriate for the man's contacts?
    A. Conjugate vaccine for family
    B. Conjugate vaccine for healthcare workers
    C. Chemoprophylaxis for family
    D. Chemoprophylaxis for healthcare workers
    E. No action required

ANSWERS

1. (C)

2. (C)

3. (D)

4. (C)

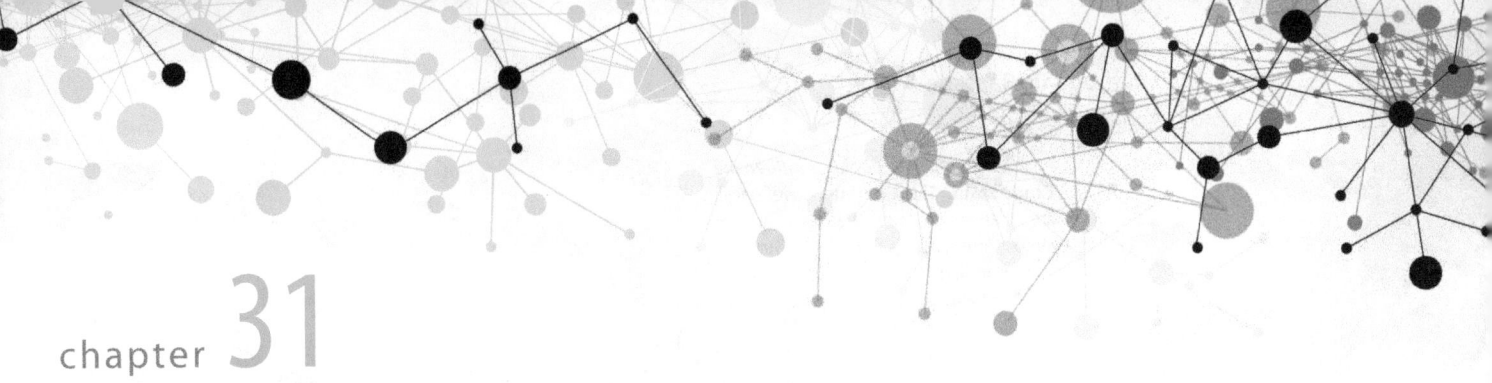

chapter 31

Haemophilus and *Bordetella*

Haemophilus influenzae · *Haemophilus ducreyi* · *Bordetella pertussis*

> *Whooping cough—why, he nearly whooped himself to death.*
>
> —Rosa Nouchette Carey: *Uncle Max* (1887)

OVERVIEW

Haemophilus and *Bordetella* are small, Gram-negative rods that tend to assume a coccobacillary shape. Members of both genera contain species exclusively found in humans and cause respiratory tract infections. The major species are *Haemophilus influenzae*, the cause of acute purulent meningitis, and *Bordetella pertussis*, the cause of whooping cough. *H influenzae* type b (Hib) produces acute, life-threatening infections of the central nervous system, epiglottis, and soft tissues, primarily in children. Disease begins with fever and lethargy, and in the case of acute meningitis, can progress to coma and death in less than 1 day. In affluent countries, Hib disease has been controlled by immunization. *H influenzae* also produces common but less fulminant infections of the bronchi, respiratory sinuses, and middle ear; the latter are usually associated with nonencapsulated strains. Pertussis is a prolonged illness caused by toxins produced by *Bordetella pertussis* bacteria attached to the cilia of respiratory epithelial cells. It progresses in stages over many weeks, beginning with rhinorrhea (runny nose), and evolving into a persistent paroxysmal cough lasting weeks more. The term "whooping cough" comes the inspiratory "whoop" made by children after an exhausting series of retching coughs. Pertussis vaccine has reduced disease incidence in developed countries, but vaccine modifications to reduce febrile seizures have led to important reductions in effectiveness.

HAEMOPHILUS

Haemophilus are among the smallest of bacteria. The curved ends of the short (1.0-1.5 μm) bacilli make many appear nearly round; hence the term coccobacilli (**Figure 31–1**). The cell wall has a structure similar to that of other Gram-negative bacteria. The most virulent strains of *H influenzae* have a polysaccharide capsule, but other species of *Haemophilus* are not encapsulated.

Cultivation of *Haemophilus* (Greek *haema*, blood, and *philos*, loving) species requires the use of culture media enriched with blood or blood products for optimal growth. This requirement reflects bacterial need for exogenous hematin and/or nicotinamide adenine dinucleotide (NAD). These growth factors, also termed X factor (hematin) and V factor (NAD), are present in erythrocytes. In culture media, optimal concentrations are not available unless the red blood

Tiny Gram-negative coccobacilli

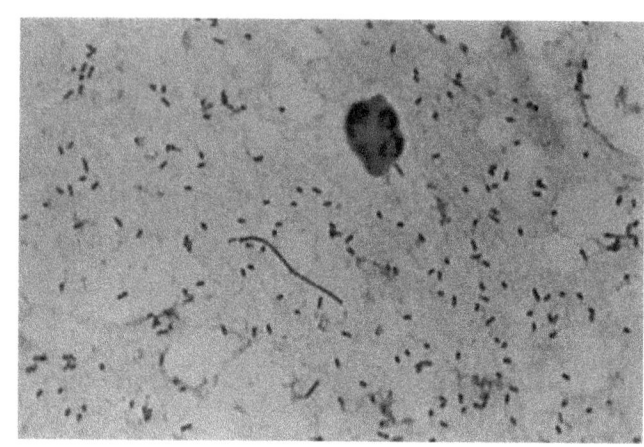

FIGURE 31-1. *Haemophilus influenzae* **Gram stain.** The Gram-negative bacilli are small and so short that some appear almost round. This is the basis of the term coccobacilli. The morphology of *Bordetella pertussis* is the same. (Reproduced with permission from Connor DH, Chandler FW, Schwartz DQ, et al: *Pathology of Infectious Diseases.* Stamford CT: Appleton & Lange; 1997.)

✳ Require hematin and/or NAD

Staphylococcus aureus may provide NAD

Non-*influenzae Haemophilus* species similar to nonencapsulated *H influenzae*

cells are lysed by gentle heat (chocolate agar) or added separately as a supplement. Although erythrocytes are the only convenient source of hematin, sufficient amounts of NAD may be provided by certain other bacteria and yeasts. This is responsible for the "satellite phenomenon," in which colonies of *Haemophilus* have been observed to grow only in the vicinity of a colony of *Staphylococcus aureus.* The several species of *Haemophilus* are defined by their requirement for hematin and/or NAD, dependence on CO_2, and other growth-related characteristics (**Table 31–1**). Species of *Haemophilus* other than *H influenzae* (eg, *H parainfluenzae*, associated with some cases of endocarditis) have the same biology described below for the nonencapsulated strains of *H influenzae.*

TABLE 31–1	Features of *Haemophilus* and *Bordetella*						
SPECIES	**TYPE**	**GROWTH REQUIREMENT**	**CAPSULE**	**ADHERENCE FACTORS**	**TOXINS**	**EPIDEMIOLOGY**	**DISEASE**
Haemophilus							
H influenzae	a–f	Hematin and NAD	Polysaccharide	Pili, HMW	—	Microbiota, respiratory droplet spread	Meningitis, epiglottitis, arthritis, sepsis, otitis media
H influenzae	—	Hematin and NAD	—	Pili, HMW	—	Microbiota, respiratory droplet spread	Otitis media, bronchitis, sinusitis
H ducreyi	—	Hematin	—	Pili	Cytolethal distending toxin	Sexual contact	Chancroid
Other species[a]	—	Hematin or NAD	—	—	—	Microbiota	Bronchitis, endocarditis
Bordetella							
B pertussis	—	Nicotinamide[b]	—	Pili, FHA, PT, pertactin	PT, AC, TCT	Strict pathogen, respiratory droplet spread	Whooping cough
B bronchiseptica	—	Nicotinamide	—	Pili, FHA	AC, TCT	Dogs, rabbits, swine	Kennel cough, rhinitis
B parapertussis	—	Nicotinamide	—	Pili, FHA	AC, TCT	Minor cause of pertussis	Whooping cough (mild)

HMW, high-molecular-weight proteins (HMW1, HMW2); FHA, filamentous hemagglutinin; PT, pertussis toxin; AC, adenylate cyclase; TCT, tracheal cytotoxin
[a]*H parainfluenzae, H aphrophilus, H hemolyticus.*
[b]Also requires additives such as charcoal to neutralize toxicity in standard media.

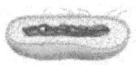

● *HAEMOPHILUS INFLUENZAE*

BACTERIOLOGY

Haemophilus that meets the species requirements for *H influenzae* may or may not have a capsule. Those that do are divided into six serotypes, a through f, based on the capsular polysaccharide antigen. The type b capsule comprises a polymer of ribose, ribitol, and phosphate, called **polyribitol phosphate (PRP)**. These surface polysaccharides are strongly associated with virulence, particularly in *H influenzae* type b (**Hib**). The surface of *H influenzae* features pili and an outer membrane similar to the structure of other Gram-negative bacteria. The outer membrane includes high molecular weight proteins (HMW1, HMW2), lipopolysaccharide (LPS), and lipooligosaccharides (LOS). The nonencapsulated, and thus nontypable, *H influenzae* (NTHi) can be classified by various typing schemes based on outer membrane proteins (OMPs) and other factors. *H influenzae* produces no known exotoxins.

Six serotypes based on capsular polysaccharide

❋ *Hib capsule is PRP*

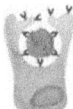

HAEMOPHILUS INFLUENZAE DISEASE

EPIDEMIOLOGY

H influenzae is a strictly human pathogen and has no known animal or environmental sources. It can be found in the nasopharyngeal flora of 20% to 80% of healthy persons, depending on age, season, and other factors. Most of these are NTHi, but encapsulated strains (including Hib) are not rare. Spread is by respiratory droplets, as with streptococci. Before the introduction of effective vaccines, approximately 1 in every 200 children developed invasive disease by the age of 5 years; meningitis was the most common invasive form and most often attacked those under 2 years of age. Cases of epiglottitis and pneumonia tended to peak in the 2- to 5-year age group. More than 90% of these cases were due to a single serotype, Hib.

❋ *Nasopharyngeal colonization common*

❋ *Meningitis in children under 2 years*

The introduction of universal immunization with the Hib protein conjugate vaccine (see Prevention) has reduced invasive disease rates by 99%. Most of the cases in immunized populations are now caused either by serotypes other than b or nonencapsulated strains. Evidence suggests a steady increase in infections worldwide due to nonencapsulated strains, primarily targeting perinatal infants, young children, and the elderly. And as before, in countries and populations unable to afford the vaccine, Hib disease continues.

❋ *Immunization (where implemented) has dramatically reduced disease*

At one point in time, *H influenzae* that caused meningitis were believed to be isolated, endogenous infections, but reports of outbreaks in closed populations and careful epidemiologic studies of secondary spread in families have changed this view. The risk of serious infection for unimmunized children younger than 4 years of age living with an index case is more than 500-fold than for unexposed children. This risk indicates a need for protection of susceptible contacts with postexposure antibiotic prophylaxis (see Prevention).

Prophylaxis limits person-to-person spread

PATHOGENESIS

■ Invasive Disease

For unknown reasons, *H influenzae* strains commonly found in the microbiota of the nasopharynx occasionally invade deeper tissues. Bacteremia then enables spread to the central nervous system and metastatic infections at distant sites, such as bones and joints (**Figure 31–2**). These events seem to take place within a short period (<3 days) after an encounter with a new virulent strain. Systemic spread is typical only for encapsulated *H influenzae* strains, and more than 90% of invasive strains exhibit type b capsule. Even among Hib strains there are distinct clones, which account for approximately 80% of all invasive disease worldwide.

❋ *Encapsulated strains more invasive*

Certain clones account for most disease

Attachment to respiratory epithelial cells is mediated by pili and OMPs. Evidence suggests that this depends on a complex regulatory cascade, coordinating capsular biosynthesis and adherence factors that act cooperatively in establishing the microbe within susceptible hosts. *H influenzae* can be seen to invade between the cells of the respiratory epithelium (**Figure 31–3**), and for a time resides between and below them. Once past the mucosal barrier, the antiphagocytic capsule confers resistance to C3b deposition in the same manner as it does for other encapsulated bacteria.

❋ *Capsule prevents phagocytosis*

Pili, other adhesins bind to epithelial cells

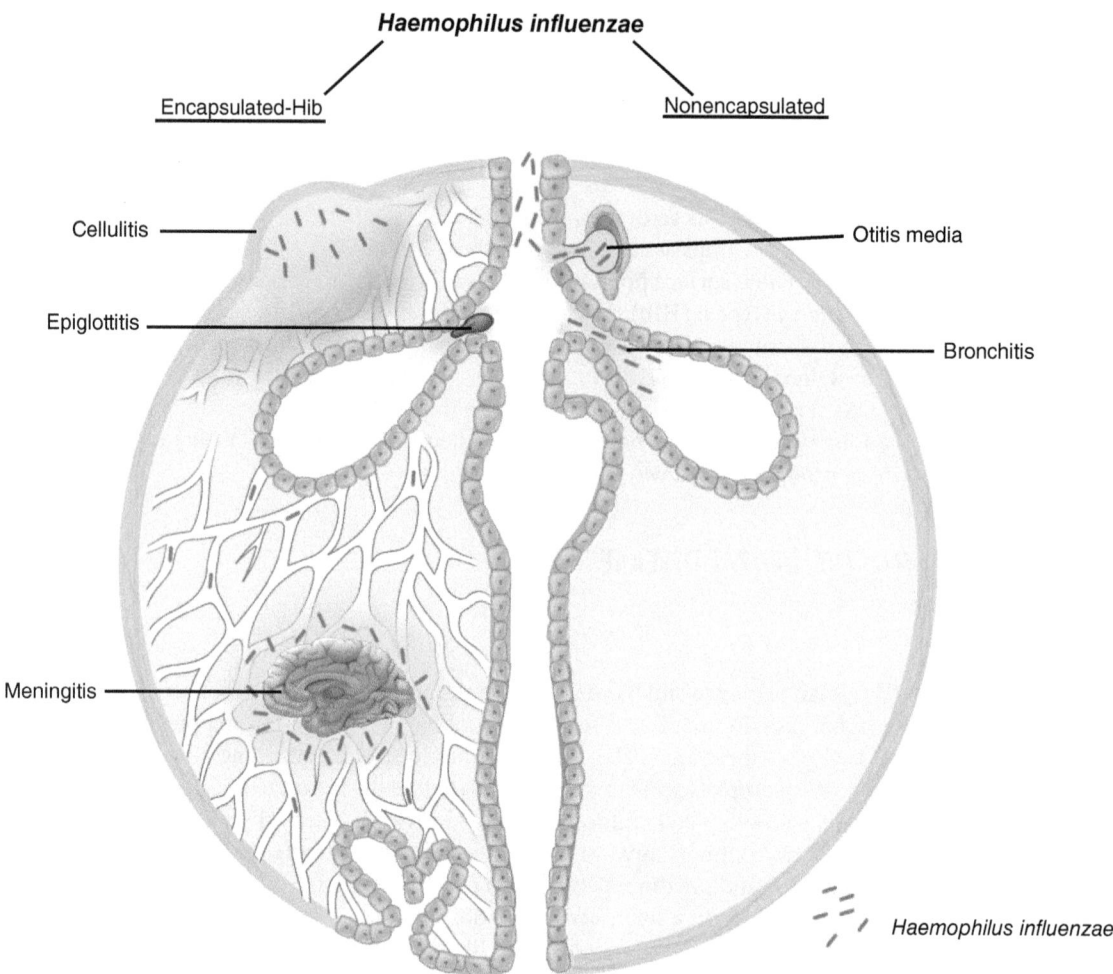

FIGURE 31–2. *Haemophilus* **disease overview.** (*Left*) Invasive disease is caused by encapsulated strains, mostly type b (Hib). From a nasopharyngeal colonization site, the organisms invade locally to produce cellulitis or epiglottitis. Invasion of the blood occurs in all Hib diseases and can lead to meningitis. (*Right*) Localized disease is produced when nonencapsulated strains from the nasopharynx are trapped in the middle ear, paranasal sinuses or compromised bronchi.

FIGURE 31–3. *Haemophilus influenzae* **disease, cellular view.** Organisms attach to epithelial cells using pili and outer membrane proteins (OMP). Invasion takes place between cells by disruption of cell–cell adhesion molecules. In the submucosa, the capsule allows the bacteria to evade phagocytosis and enter the bloodstream. PMNs, polymorphonuclear neutrophils.

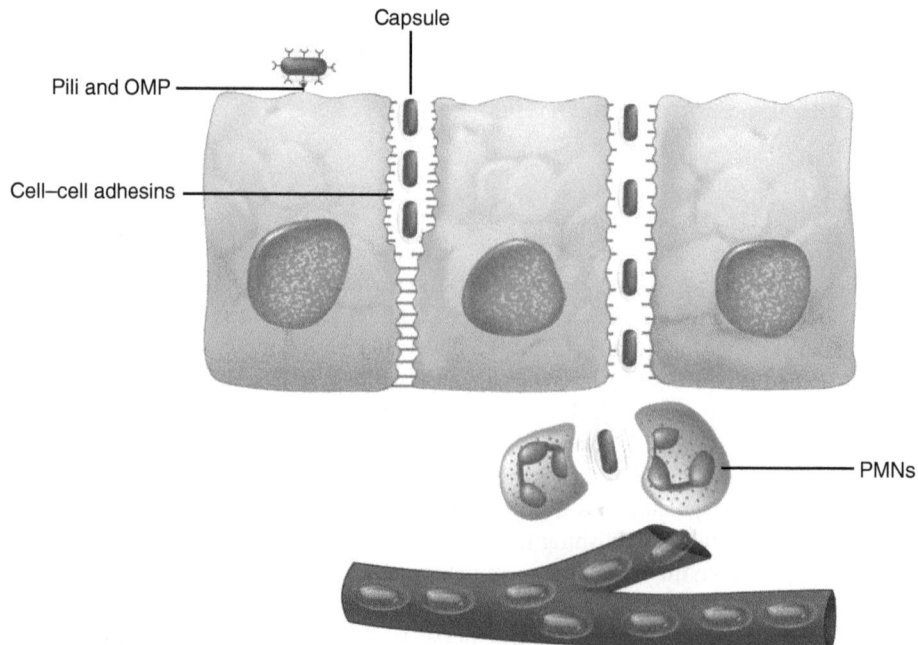

As with pathogenic *Neisseria*, there is evidence that *H influenzae* LOS may provide an antiphago-cytic effect by binding host components such as sialic acid. Outer membrane LOS is toxic to ciliated respiratory cells, and when circulating in the bloodstream, produces all the features of endotoxemia.

Invasion goes between cells

■ Localized Disease

NTHi produce disease under circumstances in which they are entrapped at a luminal site adjacent to the respiratory microbiota, such as the middle ear, sinuses, or bronchi (Figure 31–2), usually when normal clearing mechanisms have been disrupted, for example by a viral infection or struc-tural damage. NTHi attach to bronchial epithelial cells and laminin using pili, OMPs, and other proteins. Consistent with their relative prevalence in the respiratory tract, NTHi account for more than 90% of localized *H influenzae* disease, particularly otitis media, sinusitis, and exacerbations of chronic bronchitis.

NTHi trapped in middle ear, sinuses, bronchi produce localized infections

Adherence by pili, OMPs, other proteins

IMMUNITY

Immunity to Hib infections has long been associated with the presence of anticapsular (PRP) antibodies, which are bactericidal in the presence of complement. The infant is usually protected by passively acquired maternal antibody for the first few months of life. Thereafter, actively acquired antibody increases with age; it is present in the serum of most children by 10 years of age. The peak incidence of Hib infections in unimmunized populations occurs at 6 to 18 months of age, when serum antibody is least likely to be present. This inverse relationship between infec-tion and serum antibody is similar to that for *Neisseria meningitidis* (see Figure 30–4). The major difference is that substantial immune protection is provided by antibody directed against a single serotype (Hib) rather than the multiple types of other encapsulated bacteria, such as *N meningitidis* and *S pneumoniae*. Thus, systemic *H influenzae* infections (meningitis, epiglottitis, cellulitis) are rare in adults, but where such infections develop, the immunologic deficit is typically the same as that with meningococci—lack of type-specific circulating antibody.

✳ **Anticapsular antibody is bactericidal and protective**

✳ **Hib infections occur at ages when antibody is absent**

Like other polysaccharides, Hib PRP behaves as a T-cell–independent antigen. Antibody responses to immunization are poor in children younger than 18 months of age, and boosters do not elicit significant secondary responses. The conjugation of PRP to protein dramatically improved immunogenicity by eliciting T-cell–dependent responses while preserving the specific-ity for PRP, and this maneuver represented a significant breakthrough in vaccine immunology in the 1980s.

✳ **T-cell–independent PRP response poor at less than 18 months**

✳ **Protein conjugate vaccines elicit protective T-cell responses**

HAEMOPHILUS INFLUENZAE DISEASE: CLINICAL ASPECTS

MANIFESTATIONS

Of the major acute Hib infections, meningitis accounts for just over 50% of cases; the remaining cases involve pneumonia, epiglottitis, septicemia, cellulitis, and septic arthritis. Localized infec-tions can be caused by encapsulated strains including Hib, but most are caused by NTHi.

■ Meningitis

Hib meningitis follows the same pattern as other causes of acute purulent bacterial meningitis. The initial signs and symptoms may be those of an upper respiratory infection, such as pharyn-gitis, sinusitis, or otitis media; whether these represent a predisposing viral infection or early invasion by the organism is not known. Just as often, meningitis is preceded by vague malaise, lethargy, irritability, and fever. Mortality is 3% to 6% despite appropriate therapy, and roughly one-third of all survivors have significant neurologic sequelae.

Acute purulent meningitis follows sinusitis, otitis media

Mortality, neurologic sequelae significant

■ Acute Epiglottitis

Acute epiglottitis is a dramatic infection in which the inflamed epiglottis and surrounding tissues obstruct the airway; Hib is one of several causes. Onset is sudden, with fever, sore throat, hoarse-ness, an often muffled cough, and rapid progression to severe prostration within 24 hours. Affected children have air hunger, inspiratory stridor, and retraction of the soft tissues of the chest with each inspiration. The hallmark of the disease is an inflamed, swollen, cherry-red epiglottis

FIGURE 31-4. The swollen epiglottis characteristic of *Haemophilus influenzae* acute epiglottitis. (Reproduced with permission from Connor DH, Chandler FW, Schwartz DQ, et al: *Pathology of Infectious Diseases*. Stamford CT: Appleton & Lange; 1997.)

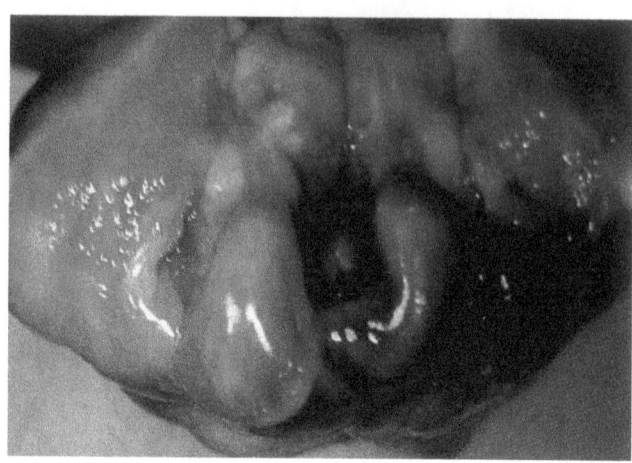

* Cherry-red, swollen epiglottis and stridor are hallmarks

* Attention to airway maintenance critical

that protrudes into the airway (**Figure 31-4**) and can be visualized on lateral X-rays. As with meningitis, this infection must be treated as a medical emergency, with primary emphasis on maintenance of a patent airway (by tracheostomy or endotracheal intubation) and antimicrobial therapy. Clinical maneuvers such as direct examination or attempting to take a throat swab may trigger acute obstruction and fatal laryngospasm.

Cellulitis and Arthritis

* Cellulitis is usually facial

Arthritis involves large joints

A tender, reddish-blue swelling in the cheek or periorbital areas is the usual presentation of Hib cellulitis. This picture may follow an upper respiratory infection or otitis media; fever and a moderately toxic state are usually present. Joint infection begins with fever, irritability, and local signs of inflammation, often in a single large joint. *Haemophilus* arthritis is occasionally the cause of a more subtle set of findings in which fever occurs without clear clinical evidence of joint involvement. Bacteremia is often present in both cellulitis and arthritis.

Other Infections

* Nonencapsulated strains are common in otitis media, sinusitis, and bronchitis

Pneumonia may arise in damaged airways

Haemophilus influenzae is an important cause of conjunctivitis, otitis media, and acute and chronic sinusitis. It is also one of several common respiratory organisms that can cause and exacerbate chronic bronchitis. Most of these infections are caused by NTHi strains and remain localized without bacteremia. Disease may be acute or chronic, depending on the anatomic site and underlying pathology. For example, otitis media is acute and painful because of the small, closed space involved, but after antimicrobial therapy and reopening of the eustachian tube, the condition usually clears without sequelae. The association of *H influenzae* with chronic bronchitis is more complex. There is evidence to suggest that *H influenzae* and other bacteria play a role in inflammatory exacerbations, but a direct cause-and-effect relationship has been difficult to prove. The underlying cause of the bronchitis is usually related to chronic damage resulting from factors such as smoking. *Haemophilus* pneumonia may be caused by either encapsulated or non-encapsulated organisms. Encapsulated strains have been observed to produce a disease much like pneumococcal pneumonia; however, NTHi strains may also produce pneumonia, particularly in patients with chronic bronchitis. The closely related *H parainfluenzae* belongs to the so-called HACEK group of fastidious Gram-negative bacteria (*Haemophilus, Aggregatibacter, Cardiobacterium, Eikenella, Kingella kingae*) that are known to produce up to 3% of all infective endocarditis cases, typically in patients with prosthetic valves or underlying heart disease.

 Is *Haemophilus* otitis media the event preceding systemic infections like meningitis?

DIAGNOSIS

The combination of clinical findings and a typical Gram smear may be sufficient to make a presumptive diagnosis of *Haemophilus* infection. The tiny cells are usually of uniform shape except in cerebrospinal fluid, where some may be elongated to several times their usual length (Figure 31-1). The diagnosis is usually confirmed by isolation of the organism from the site of infection or from the blood. Blood cultures are particularly useful in systemic *H influenzae* infections because it is often difficult to obtain an adequate specimen directly from the site of infection. Bacteriologically, small coccobacillary Gram-negative rods that grow on chocolate agar but not blood agar strongly suggest *Haemophilus*. Confirmation and speciation depend on demonstration of the requirement for hematin (X factor) and/or NAD (V factor) and/or biochemical tests. Serotyping is unnecessary for clinical purposes, but important in epidemiologic and vaccine studies.

* X and V factor requirements distinguish species

Blood cultures useful in systemic infections

TREATMENT

All forms of *H influenzae* disease were effectively treated with ampicillin until the 1970s, when resistance emerged, in a pattern similar to that of *Neisseria gonorrhoeae*. The major mechanism was production of a β-lactamase identical to that found in *Escherichia coli*. The frequency of β-lactamase–producing strains varies between 5% and 50% in different geographic areas, with rates of 20% to 30% appearing in recent North American isolate collections. More recently, ampicillin resistance has emerged in β-lactamase–negative strains due to alterations in the transpeptidase site of the penicillin-binding protein, PBP3. Current practice is to start empiric therapy with a third-generation cephalosporin (eg, ceftriaxone), which can be narrowed to ampicillin if laboratory testing indicates that the infecting strain is susceptible.

* β-lactamase-producing strains ampicillin-resistant

* Third-generation cephalosporin treatment

PREVENTION

Purified PRP vaccines became available in 1985; however, owing to the typically poor immune response of infants to polysaccharide antigens, their use was limited to children 24 months of age and older. Because immunization at this age failed to protect those most susceptible to Hib invasive disease, a new vaccine strategy was needed to evoke the improved stimulation of T-cell–dependent immune responses in infants. To achieve this, the first protein conjugate vaccines were developed by linking PRP to proteins derived from bacteria (diphtheria toxoid, *N meningitidis* OMP). The first PRP–protein conjugate vaccines were licensed in 1989; by late 1990, they were recommended for universal immunization in children, beginning at 2 months of age. As illustrated in **Figure 31–5,** the impact has been dramatic. This 99% reduction in what was once one of the most feared diseases of childhood is one of the greatest achievements in medical history. Fortunately, the decline in Hib has not been accompanied by compensatory rise in the numbers of non-b cases or in the other causes of acute purulent meningitis. An unexpected concomitant finding has been a dramatic drop in *H influenzae* colonization rates in immunized populations. Under the direction of the World Health Organization, government and philanthropic efforts like those of the Gates Foundation continue to implement Hib immunization in children across the globe.

* PRP vaccine missed peak age of disease

* Vaccines conjugating PRP to bacterial proteins stimulate T cells

* Dramatic reductions in Hib disease have been sustained

As with *N meningitidis*, rifampin chemoprophylaxis is indicated for unimmunized close contacts of cases for children and adults alike.

Rifampin prophylaxis indicated

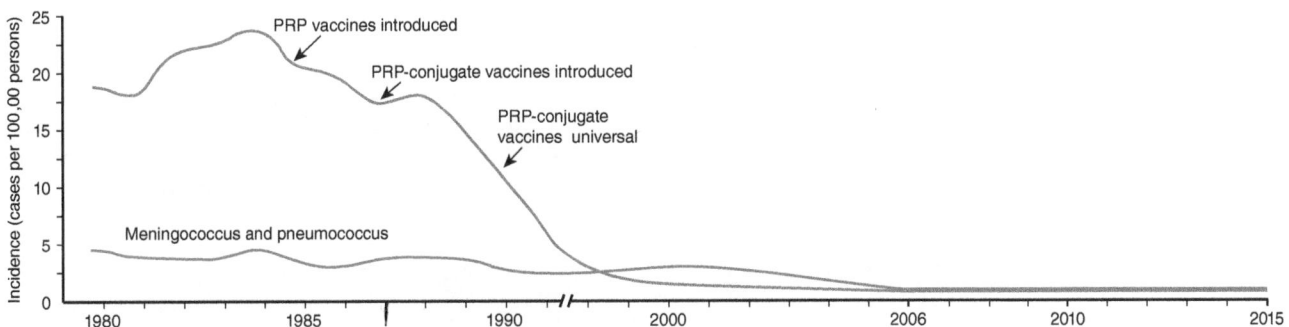

FIGURE 31–5. The decline in *Haemophilus influenzae* type b (Hib) meningitis in association with the introduction of new vaccines is shown. Note also the steady state of the other major causes of childhood meningitis; they did not increase to "fill in the gap" nor did *H influenzae* invasive disease caused by other serotypes.

 Think ▸▸ Apply 31-1: **If so, this would only happen with encapsulated strains, which are the minority in OM. Although probable because of the high prevalence of OM, the specific epidemiologic evidence is lacking for this connection.**

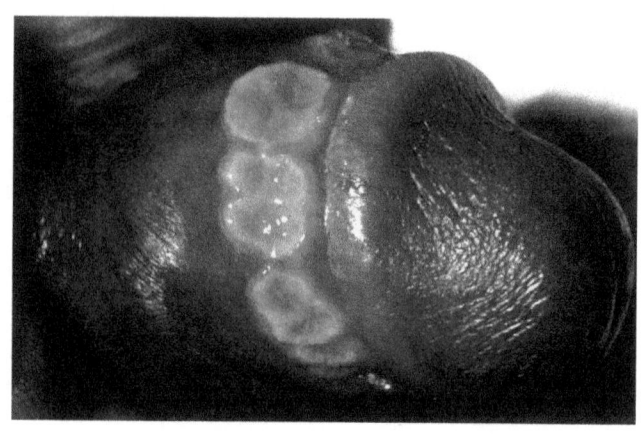

FIGURE 31–6. **Chancroid.** These penile ulcers are caused by *Haemophilus ducreyi*. In contrast to the ulcers of syphilis, they are soft and painful. (Reproduced with permission from Nester EW, Anderson DG, Roberts CE Jr, et al: *Microbiology: A Human Perspective,* 6th ed. New York, NY: McGraw Hill; 2008.)

● HAEMOPHILUS DUCREYI

Haemophilus ducreyi causes chancroid, a common cause of genital ulcer that has been found in Africa, Southeast Asia, India, and Latin America. Occasional outbreaks in North America have most often been associated with the exchange of sex for drugs or money. The typical lesion is a tender papule on the genitalia that develops into a painful ulcer with sharp margins (**Figure 31–6**). Satellite lesions may develop by autoinfection, and regional lymphadenitis is common. The incubation period is usually short (2-5 days). The lack of induration around the ulcer has caused the primary lesion to be called "soft chancre" to distinguish it from the primary syphilitic chancre, which is typically indurated and painless. The presence of open genital sores due to *H ducreyi* greatly enhances the risk of transmission of HIV by providing a portal of entry and/or by the recruitment of CD4+ cells to the site. This may contribute to the heterosexual spread of HIV on the African continent, where chancroid is common. However, determination of the true global incidence of chancroid has been obviated by widespread practice of syndromic management for bacterial genital ulcer disease—that is, empiric treatment with agents effective against both syphilis and chancroid. *H ducreyi* has also recently been identified as a causative agent of nongenital cutaneous ulcers in children in tropical regions where yaws is endemic (eg, Papua New Guinea, the Solomon Islands).

Candidate *H ducreyi* virulence factors include pili and an OMP (DsrA) which mediates attachment to epithelial cells and resistance to complement-mediated killing. In the lesion, *H ducreyi* localizes with neutrophils and macrophages but remains extracellular. There is evidence to suggest that the organism may gain an advantage by secreting antiphagocytic proteins and by resisting antimicrobial peptides that are part of the innate immune response. Host immunity may be dampened by the action of cytolethal distending toxin on T cells.

The specific diagnosis of *H ducreyi* infection is difficult. Although the organism grows on chocolate agar, it does so slowly, and other organisms in the genital flora are apt to over-grow the plates. Incorporating antibiotics (usually vancomycin) in the agar overcomes this problem, but few laboratory suppliers in the United States produce this selective medium. Preferred treatments for chancroid include single doses of either azithromycin or ceftriaxone; alternative agents include multiple-dose regimens of ciprofloxacin or erythromycin. Condoms are effective in blocking transmission.

● BORDETELLA

The genus *Bordetella* contains seven species; *Bordetella pertussis* is by far the most important because it is the cause of classic pertussis (whooping cough). Nucleic acid homology and other analyses indicate that *Bordetella parapertussis* and *B bronchiseptica* are almost similar enough to *B pertussis* to be considered variants of the same species. *B parapertussis* occasionally causes a disease similar to, but milder than, pertussis and has appeared together with *B pertussis* in outbreaks. This mild phenotype is probably due to its lack of pertussis toxin (PT) production, even though a silent copy of the toxin gene is present. The remainder of this section focuses on *B pertussis*.

✳ Soft chancre: a nonindurated genital ulcer with satellite lesions

May contribute to spread of HIV in Africa

✳ Culture requires selective medium

✳ Species similar to *B pertussis* may cause mild whooping cough

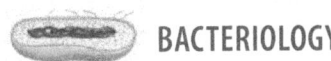
BORDETELLA PERTUSSIS

BACTERIOLOGY

GROWTH AND STRUCTURE

Bordetella pertussis is a tiny (0.5-1.0 μm), Gram-negative coccobacillus morphologically similar to *Haemophilus*. Growth requires a special medium with nutritional supplements (nicotinamide), additives (charcoal) to neutralize the inhibitory effect of compounds in standard bacteriologic media, and antibiotics to inhibit other respiratory flora. Under the best conditions, growth is still slow, requiring 3 to 7 days for isolation. The organism is also very susceptible to environmental changes and survives only briefly outside the human respiratory tract.

The cell wall of *B pertussis* has the structure typical of Gram-negative bacteria, although the outer membrane lipopolysaccharide differs significantly in structure and biologic activity from that of the Enterobacteriaceae. The surface exhibits a rod-like protein called the **filamentous hemagglutinin (FHA)** because of its ability to bind to and agglutinate erythrocytes. FHA has strong adherence qualities, based on domains in its structure that interact with an amino acid sequence present in host integrins, epithelial cells, and macrophages. FHA also stimulates cytokine release and interferes with T_H1 immune responses. The organism surface also contains other adhesive structures including **pili** and an OMP called **pertactin.**

> **Morphologically similar to** *Haemophilus*
>
> ✳ Growth slow, requires nicotinamide
>
> ✳ FHA binds amino acid sequences found on host cells
>
> ✳ Pili and pertactin are adhesins

EXTRACELLULAR PRODUCTS

■ Pertussis Toxin

PT is the major virulence factor of *B pertussis*. It is an A-B toxin produced from a single operon as an enzymatic subunit and five binding subunits that are assembled into the complete toxin on the bacterial surface. The binding subunits mediate attachment of the toxin to carbohydrate moieties on the host cell surface. The enzymatic subunit is then internalized and ADP-ribosylates a G protein that affects adenylate cyclase (AC) activity. Unlike cholera toxin, which keeps cyclase activity switched on, PT freezes the opposite side of the regulatory circuit and cripples the capacity of the host cell to inactivate cyclase activity. Multiple intracellular signaling pathways are disrupted by this G protein modification. Among the results of this action are lymphocytosis, insulinemia, and histamine sensitization.

> ✳ A-B toxin ADP-ribosylates G protein
>
> ✳ Adenylate cyclase and cell regulation are disrupted

■ Other Toxins

Another potent toxin, a pore-forming **adenylate cyclase**, enters host cells and catalyzes the conversion of host cell ATP to cyclic AMP at levels far above what can be achieved by normal mechanisms. This activity interferes with cellular signaling, chemotaxis, superoxide generation, and function of immune effector cells, including PMNs, lymphocytes, macrophages, and dendritic cells. AC can also induce programmed cell death (apoptosis). **Tracheal cytotoxin (TCT)** is a monomer of *B pertussis* peptidoglycan generated during cell wall synthesis. The fragments are released into the environment by multiplying bacterial cells because *B pertussis* lacks mechanisms present in other bacteria for recycling these monomers. TCT is directly toxic to ciliated tracheal epithelial cells, causing their extrusion from the mucosa and eventual death; there is little or no effect on the nonciliated cells.

> ✳ Toxin adenylate cyclase disrupts immune cell function
>
> ✳ Peptidoglycan fragments injure ciliated tracheal cells

PERTUSSIS (WHOOPING COUGH)

EPIDEMIOLOGY

Pertussis is a major health problem worldwide, with an estimated 50 million cases and 300,000 deaths annually. More than 90% of the cases are in developing nations and most of the deaths are among infants. *Bordetella pertussis* is spread by airborne droplet nuclei and remains localized to the tracheobronchial tree. It is highly contagious, infecting more than 90% of exposed susceptible persons. Secondary spread in families, schools, and hospitals is rapid. Sporadic epidemics occur, but there is no strong seasonal pattern. *B pertussis* is a strictly human pathogen. It is not

※ Highly contagious, spread by airborne droplet nuclei

※ Immunization reduces disease but outbreaks continue

found in animals and survives poorly in the environment. Asymptomatic carriers are rare except in outbreak situations. The introduction of immunization in the 1940s produced a dramatic reduction in disease, but outbreaks persisted in 3- to 5-year cycles. Large outbreaks have occurred in populations where the immunization rates fell, for example, as a result of concerns about febrile reactions to the original pertussis vaccine.

※ Undiagnosed adult disease facilitates spread

※ Infants have high mortality

※ Waning immunity needs boosting

Immunization also produced a change in the age distribution of the residual cases. Previously a disease of toddlers and young children, pertussis began to appear in infants and—due to the relatively short duration (10-12 years) of immunity—adults, beginning in late adolescence. Upon exposure, susceptible adults usually have a milder form of the disease, which is often not recognized as pertussis. These unwitting adults then are the major source for outbreaks in highly susceptible populations, such as infants. In the preimmunization era, newborns were usually protected by maternal transplacental IgG stimulated by the almost universal exposure to *B pertussis* in the general population. In an immunized population with waning immunity, this antibody has frequently dropped below protective levels by the childbearing years. In a cruel twist, infants have the most severe form of the disease; more than 70% of fatal cases occur in children younger than 1 year of age. These problems appear to have worsened with the switch to an acellular vaccine whose protection is of even shorter duration. (See Prevention)

PATHOGENESIS

When introduced into the respiratory tract, *B pertussis* has a remarkable tropism for ciliated bronchial epithelium, attaching to the cilia themselves. This adherence is mediated by FHA, pili, pertactin, and the binding subunits of PT. Once attached, the bacteria immobilize the cilia and begin a sequence in which the ciliated cells are progressively destroyed and extruded from the epithelial border (**Figures 31–7** and **31–8**). This local injury is caused primarily by the action of TCT. This toxicity eventually produces an epithelium devoid of the ciliary blanket, needed to move foreign matter away from the lower airways. Persistent coughing is the clinical correlate of this ciliary defect. Although considerable local inflammation and exudate are produced in the bronchi, *B pertussis* does not directly invade the cells of the respiratory tract or spread to deeper tissue sites.

※ Attachment to cilia provides site for toxin production

※ Mucosa becomes devoid of ciliated cells

■ Virulence Factors

In addition to the local effects on bronchial epithelium, other virulence factors of *B pertussis* contribute to the disease in diverse ways. The combined action of PT and AC on neutrophils, macrophages, and lymphocytes creates paralysis and even death of these crucial effector cells of the immune system. Many of the systemic manifestations of the disease, such as lymphocytosis, histamine sensitization, and insulin secretion, are due to the action of circulating PT absorbed at the primary infection site. The specific biologic effect depends on how disruption of G-protein regulation by PT is manifested by the host cell type that the toxin reaches. Pertussis is the result of a well-orchestrated delivery by *B pertussis* of toxic and adhesive factors to host cells at local and distant sites to produce a disease that persists for many weeks.

PT and AC attack immune cells

Absorbed PT acts on multiple cell types

■ Genetic Regulation of Pathogenicity

How *B pertussis* deploys its repertoire of virulence genes is a model for the regulation of bacterial pathogenicity. *B pertussis* regulates the synthesis of PT, AC, FHA, pili, and many other genes through genetic loci that control the expression of at least 20 unlinked chromosomal genes at the transcriptional level. Expression is modulated in a two-component system by changes in specific environmental parameters, including temperature. The induction of virulence factors in *B pertussis* is sequential, with expression of adhesins (FHA and pili) preceding expression of factors involved in tissue injury (PT, AC). The finely honed responses of *B pertussis* virulence factors to changes in temperature and ionic conditions presumably play a role in the pathogenesis of infection and help the organism adapt in a stepwise fashion to the diverse local conditions throughout the human respiratory tract. Details of the genetic mechanisms involved are discussed in Chapter 22 and illustrated in Figure 22–8.

Multiple virulence genes respond to temperature, ionic changes

Virulence genes regulated in two-component model

Adherence factors precede injury products

IMMUNITY

Although IgG antibodies are produced to PT, pili, and pertactin during the course of natural infection and by immunization, they are not long-lasting, and their role in immunity is not well understood. Although naturally acquired immunity is not lifelong, second attacks (when recognized) tend to be mild.

※ Immunity is not lifelong

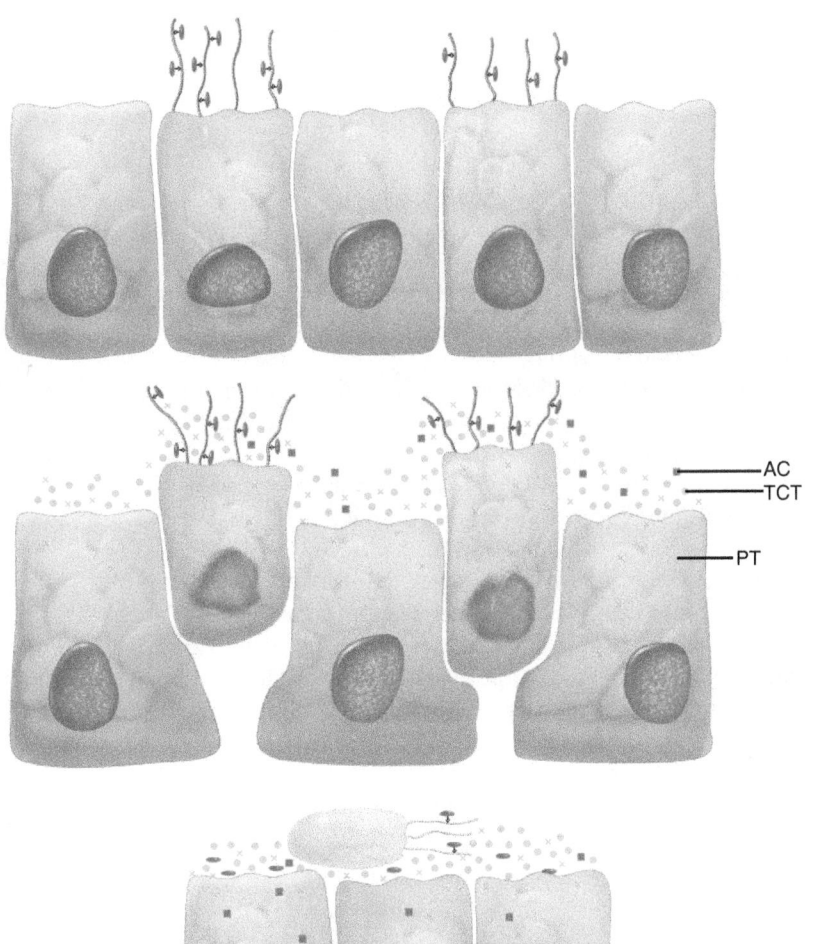

FIGURE 31–7. **Whooping cough, cellular view.** (*Top*) *Bordetella pertussis* attaches to the cilia of cells in the respiratory epithelium. Attachment is mediated by pili, filamentous hemagglutinin, and pertactin. (*Middle*) Regulatory systems initiate production of pertussis toxin (PT) and adenylate cyclase (AC), which injure the cells and they begin to be extruded. Additional injury is from the peptidoglycan fragments of tracheal cytotoxin (TCT). (*Bottom*) The ciliated cells are destroyed, leaving a denuded mucosa without protective cilia. PT is absorbed into the bloodstream to act throughout the body.

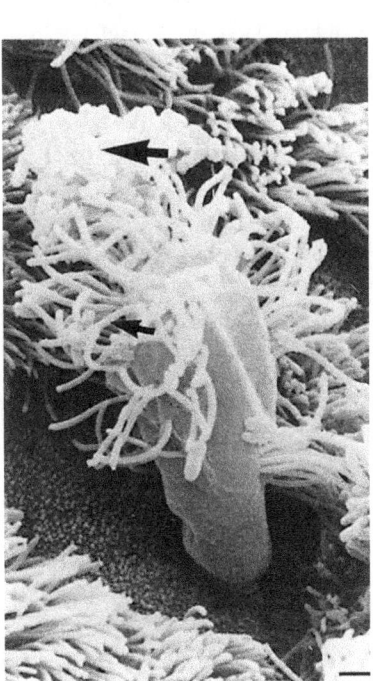

FIGURE 31–8. A tracheal organ culture 72 hours after infection with *Bordetella pertussis*. The organisms have attached to the cilia of some cells and killed them. These balloon-like cells with attached bacteria are extruded from the epithelium. The large arrow shows the *Bordetella,* and the small arrow shows cilia. Note the background of uninfected ciliated cells and denuded epithelium where nonciliated cells remain. (Reproduced with permission from Muse KE, Collier AM, Baseman JB: Scanning electron microscopic study of hamster tracheal organ cultures infected with Bordetella pertussis, *J Infect Dis* Dec;136(6):768-777.)

PERTUSSIS: CLINICAL ASPECTS

MANIFESTATIONS

After an incubation period of 7-10 days, pertussis follows a prolonged course consisting of three overlapping stages: (1) catarrhal, (2) paroxysmal, and (3) convalescent. In the catarrhal stage, the primary feature is profuse mucoid rhinorrhea, which persists for 1 to 2 weeks. Nonspecific findings such as fever, malaise, sneezing, and anorexia may also be present. The disease is most communicable at this stage because large numbers of organisms are present in the nasopharynx and the mucoid secretions.

The appearance of a persistent cough marks the transition from the catarrhal to the paroxysmal coughing stage. At this time, episodes of paroxysmal coughing occur up to 50 times a day for 2 to 4 weeks. The characteristic inspiratory whoop follows a series of coughs as air is rapidly drawn in through the narrowed glottis; vomiting may follow the whoop. The combination of mucoid secretions, whooping cough, and vomiting produces a miserable, exhausted child barely able to breathe. Apnea may follow such episodes, particularly in infants. Marked lymphocytosis reaches its peak at this time, with absolute lymphocyte counts of up to 40,000/mm^3.

During the 3- to 4-week convalescent stage, the frequency and severity of paroxysmal coughing and other features of the disease gradually fade. Partially immune persons and infants younger than 6 months of age may not show all the typical features of pertussis. Some evolution through the three stages is usually seen, but paroxysmal coughing and lymphocytosis may be absent.

The most common complication of pertussis is pneumonia caused by a superinfecting organism such as *Streptococcus pneumoniae*. Atelectasis is also common but may be recognized only by radiologic examination. Other complications, including convulsions and subconjunctival— or even intracerebral—bleeding, are related to the venous pressure effects of the paroxysmal coughing and the anoxia produced by inadequate ventilation and apneic spells.

DIAGNOSIS

A clinical diagnosis of pertussis is best confirmed by detection of *B pertussis* in nasopharyngeal secretions or swabs. Throat swabs are not suitable because the cilia to which the organism attaches are not found there. Specimens collected early in the course of disease (during the catarrhal or early paroxysmal stage) provide the greatest chance of successful isolation. Unfortunately, the diagnosis is frequently not considered until paroxysmal coughing has been present for some time, by which point the number of organisms has decreased significantly. Usually, the nasopharyngeal specimens are plated onto a special charcoal blood agar medium made selective by the addition of a cephalosporin; this allows the slow-growing *B pertussis* to be isolated in the presence of more rapidly growing members of the normal upper respiratory flora. The characteristic colonies appear after 3 to 7 days of incubation and look like tiny drops of mercury. Immunologic methods (agglutination, immunofluorescence) are required for specific identification.

A direct immunofluorescent antibody (DFA) technique has been successfully applied to nasopharyngeal smears for rapid diagnosis of pertussis. DFA is particularly helpful in pertussis because of the many days required for culture results. Nucleic acid amplification tests are now replacing both culture and DFA as they have proven to be more timely and sensitive than the classic methods. However, culture confirmation should be considered before declaring an epidemic. Serologic tests are widely used for epidemiologic studies but not diagnosis of individual clinical cases.

TREATMENT

Once the paroxysmal coughing stage has been reached, the treatment of pertussis is primarily supportive. Antimicrobial therapy is useful at earlier stages and for limiting the spread to other susceptible individuals. Of a number of antimicrobial agents active *in vitro* against *B pertussis*, macrolides are preferred for both treatment and prophylaxis. Erythromycin has the greatest clinical experience, but azithromycin and clarithromycin are equally effective.

Marginal notes:

* Catarrhal phase most communicable

* Paroxysmal coughing lasts for weeks

* Inspiratory whoop, coughing may lead to apnea

* Marked lymphocytosis

* Convalescent phase a gradual fading

Atelectasis and superinfection are major complications

* Nasopharyngeal swab is plated on charcoal blood agar

Organisms are often gone by later paroxysmal phase

* DFA and/or PCR allow rapid diagnosis

* Macrolide antibiotics most effective in catarrhal phase

PREVENTION

Active immunization is the primary method of preventing pertussis. The original vaccine, which produced a dramatic reduction in disease (Figure 31–9), was prepared from inactivated whole cell suspensions and given together with diphtheria and tetanus toxoids as DTP. The undoubted efficacy of this vaccine was colored by a high rate of side effects due to the crude nature of the whole cell preparation. These included local inflammation, fever and, rarely, febrile seizures. Although permanent neurologic sequelae were never convincingly linked to pertussis immunization, some argued that the vaccine was worse than the disease. This led to the development of acellular vaccines containing virulence factors purified from inactivated whole cell preparations.

The multiple acellular vaccine products have different combinations of virulence factors. All contain PT and FHA, and some add pertactin or pili (vaccine manufacturers use the term fimbriae). In combination with diphtheria and tetanus toxoids, the acellular vaccine has now replaced the whole cell DTP as DTaP ("a" for acellular). This vaccine is now recommended for the full primary immunization series (at 2, 4, and 6 months) and boosters (at 15-18 months, 4-6 years). The safety and efficacy of these vaccines have now been extensively evaluated. All have dramatically less frequent side effects compared with the whole cell preparations, but their efficacy is increasingly in question. In the United States, major pertussis outbreaks in 2005, 2010, and 2012 have been traced to vaccine failures in fully immunized adolescents and even preadolescent children. Clearly, the acellular vaccine does not provide immunity for as long as the product it replaced. The concern for transmission to newborns (Figure 31–10) has led to a strategy called cocooning, in which all family members are newly immunized or boosted before the baby comes home. There appears to be no going back to the whole cell vaccine, but adjustments in booster schedules and vaccine formulation are ahead.

* Whole cell vaccine effective but had side effects

* Acellular vaccines are purified

* Vaccines include PT, FHA, and other virulence factors

* DTaP has replaced DTP

* Duration of immunity from acellular vaccine in question

 Do we need a new vaccine?

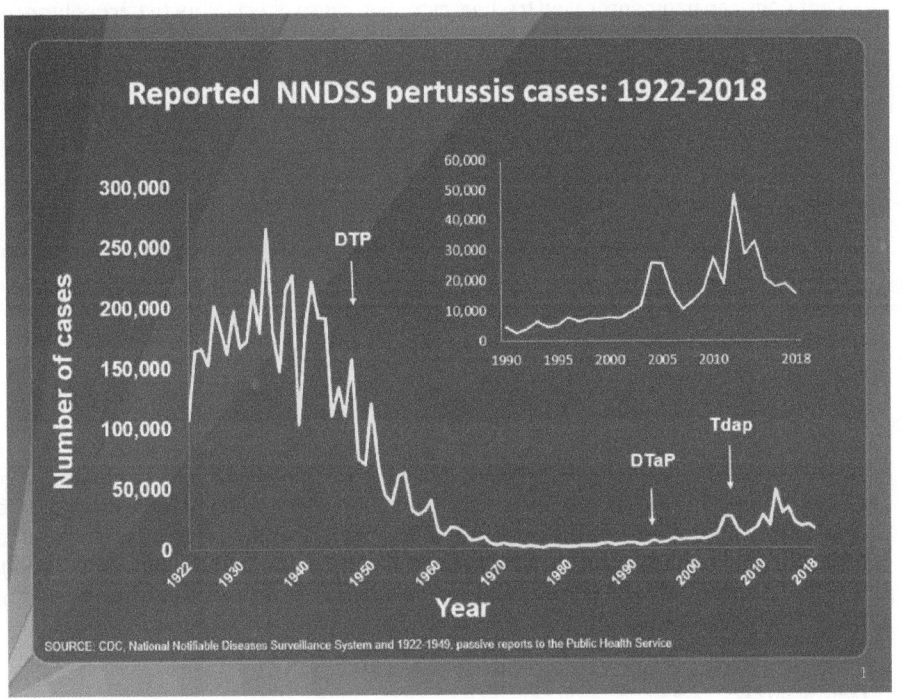

FIGURE 31–9. **Impact of pertussis vaccines 1922-2018.** The changes in pertussis incidence produced by diphtheria/tetanus/pertussis (DTP [whole cell]) and the acellular (DTaP, Tdap) vaccines are shown. (Reproduced with permission from Centers for Disease Control and Prevention. U.S. Department of Health & Human Services. Pertussis [Whooping Cough]. December, 2019.)

 Think ▸▸ Apply 31-2: **It looks more and more like this is the case, but there are big problems. The scientific evidence for new immunogens is lacking and activities of antivaccine groups discourage commercial development.**

FIGURE 31–10. Impact of acellular pertussis vaccines by age group 1990-2018. Note the predominance of cases in infants less than 1 year of age. (Reproduced with permission from Centers for Disease Control and Prevention. U.S. Department of Health & Human Services. Pertussis [Whooping Cough]. December, 2019.)

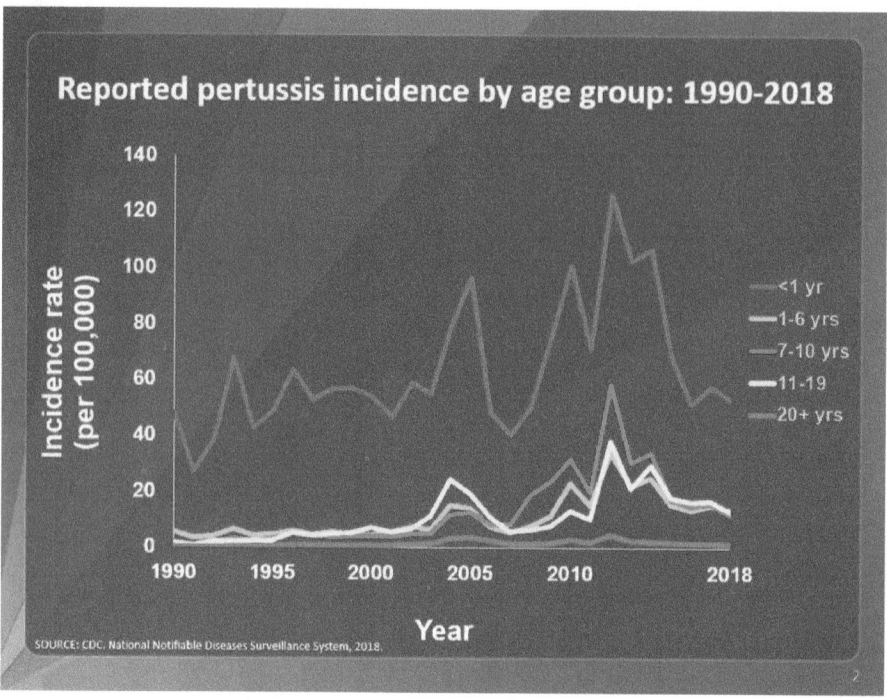

KEY CONCLUSIONS

- *Bordetella pertussis* is slow growing and requires a special selective medium for growth.
- *B pertussis* pili and filamentous hemagglutinin attach directly to respiratory cilia. The organism does not invade tissues.
- Pertussis toxin stimulates regulatory G-proteins disrupting cell functions locally and systemically.
- Peptidoglycan fragments called tracheal cytotoxin cause direct injury to tracheobronchial epithelium.
- High infectivity and waning immunity have shifted pertussis incidence to highly vulnerable infants.
- Absolute lymphocytosis is a unique diagnostic finding.
- Nucleic acid amplification methods provide the most rapid and specific means of laboratory diagnosis.
- The new acellular vaccine is less toxic but has a shorter duration of protection than the old whole cell vaccine.

✳ Vaccines include PT, FHA, and other virulence factors

✳ DTaP has replaced DTP

✳ Duration of immunity from acellular vaccine in question

CASE STUDY

A Choking, Coughing Infant

A male infant born prematurely was still in the pediatric intensive care unit at 12 days old. On the eighth day, he began to exhibit repetitive coughing, which progressed to his turning red, choking, and gasping for breath. The episodes were sometimes followed by vomiting. On the tenth day, he suffered apnea and then required ventilatory assistance. His physical examination was significant for a pulse of 160 bpm and respiratory rate of 72/min (both highly elevated). The child's chest radiograph was clear. There was no evidence of tracheal abnormalities. The infant's white cell count was 15,500/mm³ with 70% lymphocytes.

QUESTIONS

1. Which of this patient's findings are most unique for pertussis?
    - A. Cough
    - B. Choking
    - C. Vomiting
    - D. Leukocytosis
    - E. Lymphocytosis

2. Which of the following would yield the most rapid confirmation of a whooping cough diagnosis?
    A. Throat culture
    B. Nasopharyngeal culture
    C. Nasopharyngeal direct fluorescent antibody smear
    D. Throat direct fluorescent antibody smear
    E. *B pertussis* serology

3. What is the most likely source of this child's infection?
    A. Sibling
    B. Parent
    C. Delivery room environment
    D. Healthcare worker carrier
    E. Healthcare worker with disease

ANSWERS

1. **(E)**

2. **(C)**

3. **(E)**

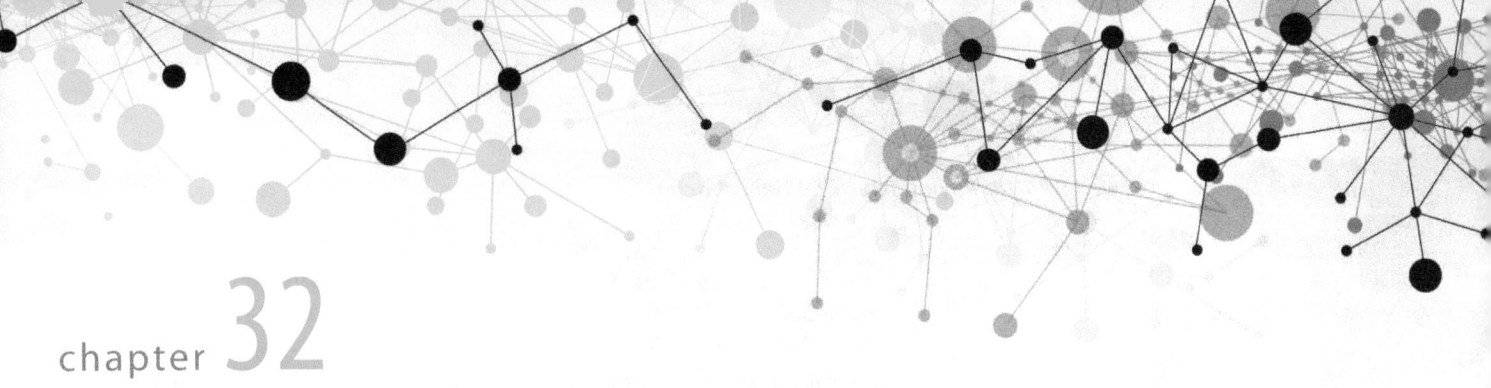

chapter 32

Vibrio, Campylobacter, and Helicobacter

Vibrio cholerae • Campylobacter jejuni • Helicobacter pylori

I am poured out like water, and all my bones are out of joint: my heart is like wax; it is melted in the midst of my bowels.

—The Bible: *Psalms* 22:14

OVERVIEW

Vibrio cholerae is a motile (flagellated), comma-shaped oxidase-positive Gram-negative rod that grows best on specialized media. Although many infections are asymptomatic, epidemic cholera produces the most dramatic watery diarrhea known. Intestinal fluids pour out in voluminous bowel movements, which untreated rapidly leads to dehydration and electrolyte imbalance. The pathogenesis is solely due to the action of cholera enterotoxin secreted by *V cholerae* in the bowel lumen. Despite the profound physiologic effects, there is no fever, inflammation, or direct injury to the bowel mucosa.

Campylobacter jejuni is the most common of the pathogenic *Campylobacter* species all of which are curved, motile Gram-negative rods. Clinical disease with *C jejuni* typically begins with lower abdominal pain, which evolves into diarrhea over a matter of hours. The diarrhea may be watery or dysenteric, with blood and pus in the stool. Most patients are febrile. The illness resolves spontaneously after a few days to 1 week.

Helicobacter pylori is also a curved, flagellated, small Gram-negative rod that is distinguished by being catalase, oxidase, and urease positive. Infections are limited to the mucosa of the stomach in which urease production enables survival in the acid milieu. Most are asymptomatic even after many years. Burning pain in the upper abdomen, accompanied by nausea and sometimes vomiting, is a symptom of gastritis, but peptic gastric or duodenal ulcers may ensue with additional symptoms and complications including bleeding and perforation.

This group of curved Gram-negative rods includes *Vibrio cholerae*, the cause of cholera and one of the first proven infectious diseases, along with *Campylobacter jejuni* and *Helicobacter pylori*, which were incriminated as pathogens late in the 20th century (Table 32–1). Cholera has undergone resurgence in recent decades and has now spread from its historic roots in South Asia to Africa and the Americas, including the coastline of the United States. *C jejuni* is one of the most common causes of diarrhea in virtually every country of the world. The peptic ulcer disease now known to be caused by *H pylori* had been long accepted to be due to stress and disturbed gastric acid secretion.

● VIBRIO

Vibrios are curved, Gram-negative rods commonly found in saltwater. Cells may be linked end to end, forming S shapes and spirals. They are highly motile with a single polar flagellum, non–spore-forming, and oxidase-positive, and they can grow under aerobic or anaerobic conditions. The cell envelope structure is similar to that of other Gram-negative bacteria. *V cholerae* is the prototype cause of a water-loss diarrhea called **cholera.** Other species causing diarrhea, wound infections, and, rarely, systemic infection are listed in **Table 32–2.**

✳ Motile curved rods found in seawater

TABLE 32–1	Features of *Vibrio, Campylobacter, and Helicobacter*[a]					
	BACTERIOLOGY			PATHOGENESIS		
ORGANISM	GROWTH	UREASE	EPIDEMIOLOGY	ADHERENCE	TOXINS	DISEASE
Vibrio cholerae	Facultative	–	Fecal–oral, water-borne, pandemics	Surface protein[b], pili	CT[c]	Watery diarrhea (cholera)
Campylobacter jejuni	Microaerophilic	–	Animals, unpasteurized milk	Unknown	Unknown	Dysentery, watery diarrhea
Helicobacter pylori	Microaerophilic	+	Human, gastric secretions	OMPs[d]	Urease,[e] VacA,[f] Cag[g]	Chronic gastritis, ulcers, adenocarcinoma, lymphoma

[a]All are curved Gram-negative rods with similar morphology.
[b]Surface protein able to bind to chitin and human intestine.
[c]Cholera toxin.
[d]OMPs, outer membrane proteins (especially BabA, which binds to Lewis b blood group antigen)
[e]Urease enables survival in acid milieu of stomach by producing ammonia.
[f]Vacuolating cytotoxin (VacA).
[g]Cytotoxin associated gene A (CagA) is strongly associated with virulence.

● *VIBRIO CHOLERAE*

BACTERIOLOGY

GROWTH AND STRUCTURE

V cholerae has a low tolerance for acid, but grows readily under alkaline (pH 8.0-9.5) conditions that inhibit many other Gram-negative bacteria. It is distinguished from other vibrios by biochemical reactions, lipopolysaccharide (LPS) O antigenic structure, and production of cholera toxin (CT). There are over 200 O antigen serotypes, only two of which (O1 and O139) cause cholera. *V cholerae* biogroup El Tor, an O1 variant, is a biotype of the classic strain. The O139

TABLE 32–2	Features of Less Common *Vibrio* and *Campylobacter* Species		
ORGANISM	FEATURES	EPIDEMIOLOGY	DISEASE
Vibrio			
V mimicus	Closely related to *V cholerae*, cholera-like enterotoxin, sucrose-negative	Ingestion of raw seafood	Watery diarrhea
V parahaemolyticus	Produces two enterotoxins, sucrose-negative	Coastal seawater; ingesting raw seafood; outbreaks on cruise ships; common in Japan	Watery diarrhea, occasionally dysentery
V vulnificus	Siderophores scavenge iron from host transferrin and lactoferrin; two cytotoxins include pore-forming activity	Coastal seawater, particularly when water temperatures rise; ingesting raw seafood or contamination of wound with seawater	Fulminant bacteremia following ingestion, cellulitis from wound contamination, high fatality rate in those with iron-storage disease or cirrhosis
V alginolyticus		Wounds contaminated by seawater	Cellulitis
Campylobacter			
C fetus	Fails to grow on selective medium used for *C jejuni*	Cause of abortion in cattle and sheep	Bacteremia, thrombophlebitis
C upsaliensis	Fails to grow on selective medium used for *C jejuni*	Associated with dogs and cats	Diarrhea similar to *C jejuni*
C hyointestinalis		Enteritis in swine	Diarrhea in immunocompromised and homosexual men
C lari		Associated with birds	Diarrhea, bacteremia in immunocompromised

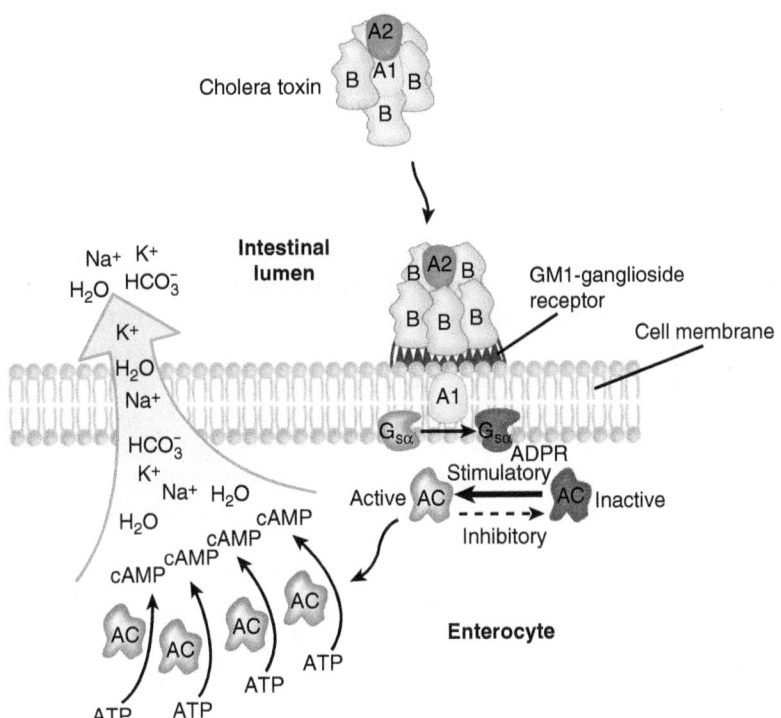

FIGURE 32–1. **The action of cholera toxin.** The complete toxin is shown binding to the GM1-ganglioside receptor on the cell membrane via the binding (B) subunits. The active portion (A1) of the A subunit catalyzes the ADP-ribosylation (ADPR) of the G_s (stimulatory) regulatory protein, "locking" it in the active state. Because the G_s protein acts to return adenylate cyclase from its inactive to active form, the net effect is persistent activation of adenylate cyclase. The increased adenylate cyclase (AC) activity results in accumulation of cyclic adenosine 3′,5′-monophosphate (cAMP) along the cell membrane. The cAMP causes the active secretion of sodium (Na^+), chloride (Cl^-), potassium (K^+), bicarbonate (HCO_3^-), and water out of the cell into the intestinal lumen.

strains phenotypically resemble O1 El Tor strains but also produce a polysaccharide capsule. *V cholerae* possess long filamentous pili that form bundles on the bacterial surface and belong to a family of pili whose chemical structure is similar to those of the gonococcus and a number of other bacterial pathogens. All strains capable of causing cholera produce a colonizing factor known as the toxin-coregulated pilus (TCP) because its expression is regulated together with CT. In aquatic environments, *V cholerae* produces polysaccharide biofilms, which contain carbohydrate moieties mediating cell–cell adhesion and attachment to surfaces.

✳ Grow in alkaline conditions

✳ Cholera limited to O1, O139 serotypes

✳ Biofilm produced in environment

CHOLERA TOXIN

The structure and mechanism of action of CT have been studied extensively (**Figure 32–1**). CT is an A–B type ADP-ribosylating (ADPR) toxin. Its molecule is an aggregate of multiple polypeptide chains organized into two toxic subunits (A1, A2) and five binding (B) units. The B units bind to a GM1-ganglioside receptor found on the surface of many types of cells. Once bound, the A1 subunit is released from the toxin molecule by reduction of the disulfide bond that binds it to the A2 subunit, and it enters the cell by translocation. In the cell, it exerts its effect on the membrane-associated adenylate cyclase system at the basolateral membrane surface. The target of the toxic A1 subunit is a guanine nucleotide (G) protein, Gsα, which regulates activation of the adenylate cyclase system. CT catalyzes the ADPR (Figure 21–16) of the G-protein, rendering it unable to dissociate from the active adenylate cyclase complex. This causes persistent activation of intracellular adenylate cyclase, which in turn stimulates the conversion of adenosine triphosphate to cyclic adenosine 3′,5′-monophosphate (cAMP). The net effect is excessive accumulation of cAMP at the cell membrane, which causes hypersecretion of chloride, potassium, bicarbonate, and associated water molecules out of the cell. Strains of *V cholerae* other than the two epidemic serotypes may or may not produce CT.

✳ B subunit receptor surface ganglioside

✳ A1 ADPRs G-protein

✳ Adenylate cyclase locked in active state

✳ cAMP accumulation causes water, electrolyte hypersecretion

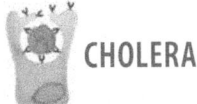

CHOLERA

EPIDEMIOLOGY

Epidemic cholera is spread primarily by contaminated water under conditions of poor sanitation, particularly where sewage treatment is absent or defective. Even though convalescent human carriage is brief, if the numerous vibrios purged from the intestines of those infected with cholera are able to reach the primary water supply, the conditions for spread are established. The short incubation period (2 days) ensures that organisms ingested by others quickly enter the epidemic cycle. Even so, modern travel makes imported cases of cholera possible. For instance, one man developed diarrhea in Florida after eating ceviche (marinated uncooked fish) just before departure from an airport in Ecuador.

Cholera is endemic in the Indian subcontinent and now in Africa. Over the last two centuries, cholera has periodically spread beyond its historic locale to other parts of Asia, Indonesia, and even Europe in the 1800s during successive pandemics, each lasting 5 to 25 years. The current pandemic has brought cholera to the Western Hemisphere for the first time since 1911. Sporadic cases of cholera in the United States first appeared in the early 1970s and were traced to inadequately cooked crabs and shrimp caught off the Gulf Coast of Louisiana and Texas. In 1991, Latin America was hit with epidemic cholera with cases reported from 21 countries from Peru to northern Mexico. A massive epidemic of cholera followed the devastating earthquake of 2010 in Haiti. *V cholerae* O1, biotype El Tor was reintroduced into East Africa between 2015 and 2016 and is now endemic with tens of thousands of cases and thousands of deaths being reported. Currently, war-torn Yemen is experiencing the largest outbreak in recent history of O1, biotype El Tor cholera with over a million cases as a consequence of disrupted sanitation and water supplies.

The dominant strain of the 20th century was the El Tor biotype, first isolated from pilgrims to Mecca at the El Tor quarantine camp in Egypt in 1905 by Koch. This strain survives slightly longer in nature and is more likely to produce subclinical cases of cholera, both of which facilitate its spread. In 1992, the first cases of cholera due to a serotype other than O1 were detected in India and Bangladesh. The new serotype (O139 Bengal) is fully virulent with the additional threat of enhanced ability to produce disease in persons whose immunity is due to exposure to the old serotype. Genomic analysis of the clonal Haitian epidemic strains showed them to be nearly identical to variant *V cholera* El Tor O1 strains isolated from Bangladesh in 2002 and 2008, likely introduced into Haiti by asymptomatic UN peacekeepers from South Asia, and quite different from earlier Peruvian isolates. These realities illustrate the potential for the global spread of cholera and the challenges for the vaccine strategies designed to prevent it.

 Cholera was unknown in Haiti before 2010. How could an earthquake cause an epidemic there?

The epidemic potential of *V cholerae* depends on its ability to survive in both aquatic environments and human hosts. In the environment, it persists in a dormant state in association with shellfish and plankton by attaching to their chitinous exoskeleton in the biofilms formed in the dormant seawater state but not during infection. This dual life is facilitated by a surface protein able to bind a constituent of chitin as well as glycoproteins and lipids on the intestinal epithelium. Satellite tracking has linked periodic climate changes (warming seawater), plankton blooms, and cholera epidemics along the coast of South America. Otherwise, the organism is fragile, surviving only a few days in the environment outside its human or crustacean hosts.

PATHOGENESIS

To produce cholera, *V cholerae* must reach the small intestine, swim to the intestinal crypts, multiply, and produce virulence factors. In healthy people, ingestion of large numbers of bacteria is required to offset the acid barrier of the stomach. Colonization of the entire intestinal tract from the jejunum to the colon by *V cholerae* requires adherence to the epithelial surface by the abovementioned protein and surface pili. Bacteria recently passed from cholera cases are hyperinfectious by virtue of chemotactic motility facilitating colonization of the small intestine. The

Margin notes (left column):

* Transmission through untreated water

* Incubation period 2 days

* Endemic on Indian subcontinent, East Africa

* Pandemics span decades

* Gulf Coast cases from undercooked shellfish

* Latin American epidemics widespread

* *V cholerae* O1, biotype El Tor dominated 20th century

* New O139 serotype spreading

* Survival in shellfish and plankton facilitates epidemics

* Large doses pass stomach acid barrier

* Pili, proteins mediate adherence

 Think ▶▶ Apply 32-1: The sanitary infrastructure disruptions caused by earthquakes can contribute to epidemics but only if the pathogen is already present. Ironically, in this case, it was the aid workers flown in to help who brought the *V cholerae* with them. The absent immunity in the Haitian population accelerated spread and heightened morbidity.

outstanding feature of *V cholerae* pathogenicity is the ability of virulent strains to secrete CT, which is responsible for the disease cholera. The water and electrolyte shift from the cell to the intestinal lumen is the fundamental cause of the watery diarrhea of cholera. Non-O1, non-O139 strains have been sporadically isolated from cases of gastroenteritis but do not produce CT, and thus not the disease cholera.

❋ CT-stimulated hypersecretion causes diarrhea

The fluid loss that results from the adenylate cyclase stimulation of cells depends on the balance between the amount of bacterial growth, toxin production, fluid secretion, and fluid absorption in the entire gastrointestinal tract. The outpouring of fluid and electrolytes is greatest in the small intestine, where the secretory capacity is high and absorptive capacity is low. The diarrheal fluid can amount to many liters per day, with approximately the same NaCl content as plasma, but also significant potassium and bicarbonate. The result is dehydration (isotonic fluid loss), hypokalemia (potassium loss), and metabolic acidosis (bicarbonate loss). The intestinal mucosa remains unaltered except for some hyperemia because *V cholerae* does not invade or otherwise injure the enterocyte.

❋ Small intestine loses fluid

❋ K⁺ plus bicarbonate loss causes hypokalemia, acidosis

■ Genetic Regulation of Virulence

The expression of the multiple virulence factors of *V cholerae* is controlled in a coordinated two-component systems involving environmental sensors and as many as 20 chromosomal genes divided between a pathogenicity island (PAI) containing CT and one containing TCP. The chief regulator is a transmembrane protein (ToxR) that "senses" environmental changes in pH, osmolarity, and temperature, which convert it to an active form. In the active state, ToxR can directly turn on CT genes as well as activate transcription of a second regulatory protein, ToxT. ToxT, whose natural effector may be bile, then activates transcription of virulence genes in both PAIs, including TCP and CT. Another set of environmental sensors switch *V cholerae* from free-swimming forms to the sessile, biofilm-forming state associated with environmental persistence in crustaceans. Quorum-sensing systems deploy expression of these virulence genes at a time when a critical mass of *V cholerae* is present to sustain it.

❋ ToxR controls CT and TCP genes

❋ Biofilm formation expressed in environmental crustaceans

IMMUNITY

Nonspecific defenses such as gastric acidity, gut motility, and intestinal mucus are important in preventing colonization with *V cholerae*. For example, in persons who lack gastric acidity (gastrectomy or achlorhydria from malnutrition), the attack rate of clinical cholera is higher. The immune state has been most strongly associated with sIgA directed against O-antigen LPS, CT (B subunit), and TCP. The precise protective mechanisms remain to be established.

❋ Rate higher with achlorhydria

❋ sIgA associated

CHOLERA: CLINICAL ASPECTS

MANIFESTATIONS

Typical cholera has a rapid onset, beginning with abdominal fullness and discomfort, rushes of peristalsis, and loose stools. Vomiting may also occur. The stools quickly become watery, voluminous, almost odorless, and contain mucus flecks, giving it an appearance called **rice-water stools.** Neither white blood cells nor blood are in the stools, and the patient is afebrile. Clinical features of cholera result from the extensive fluid loss and electrolyte imbalance, which can lead to extreme dehydration, hypotension, and death within hours if untreated. No other disease produces dehydration as rapidly as cholera.

❋ Watery diarrhea causes large fluid loss

❋ Dehydration and electrolyte imbalance

DIAGNOSIS

The initial suspicion of cholera depends on recognition of the typical clinical features in an appropriate epidemiologic setting. A bacteriologic diagnosis is accomplished by isolation of *V cholerae* from the stool. The organism grows on common clinical laboratory media such as blood agar and MacConkey agar, but its isolation is enhanced with a selective medium that contains thiosulfate–citrate–bile salt–sucrose (TCBS agar). Once isolated, *V cholerae* (sucrose-fermenting yellow colonies on green background) is readily identified by biochemical reactions. Outside cholera-endemic areas, the TCBS agar is not routinely used for stool cultures, so clinical laboratories must be alerted to the suspicion of cholera.

Stool culture uses TCBS selective agar

TREATMENT

The outcome of cholera depends on balancing the diarrheal fluid and ionic losses with adequate fluid and electrolyte replacement. This is accomplished by oral and/or intravenous administration of solutions of glucose with near physiologic concentrations of sodium and chloride and higher than physiologic concentrations of potassium and bicarbonate. Exact formulas are available as dried packets to which a given volume of water is added. Oral replacement, particularly if begun early, is sufficient for all but the most severe cases and has substantially reduced the mortality from cholera. Antimicrobial therapy plays a secondary role in fluid replacement by shortening the duration of diarrhea and magnitude of fluid loss. A single dose of azithromycin provides optimal antimicrobial therapy, but doxycycline, a fluoroquinolone, or trimethoprim-sulfamethoxazole also are effective agents.

✳ Oral or IV fluid and electrolyte replacement

✳ Antimicrobials reduce duration, severity

PREVENTION

Epidemic cholera, a disease of poor sanitation, does not persist where treatment and disposal of human waste are adequate. Because good sanitary conditions do not exist in much of the world, secondary local measures such as boiling and chlorination of water during epidemics are required. Cholera associated with ingestion of crabs and shrimp can be prevented by adequate cooking (10 minutes) and avoidance of recontamination from containers and surfaces. Vaccines prepared from whole cells, lipopolysaccharide, and CT B subunit have been disappointing providing protection that is not long-lasting. Live attenuated strains of *V cholerae* have garnered the most research interest because of their potential to stimulate a sIgA immune response in the gut. In 2016, the FDA first approved such a vaccine, for use in adults 18 through 64 years of age traveling to cholera-affected areas, based on challenge studies in nonimmune individuals of whom 91% seroconverted with a fourfold rise in serum vibriocidal antibody. The active component of this vaccine is lyophilized *V cholerae* CVD 103-HgR. There are caveats: efficacy has not been established in persons with any preexisting immunity due to exposure to *V cholerae* (as in endemic or epidemic areas) or receipt of a cholera vaccine and it has not been shown to protect against V cholera serogroup O139 or other non-O1 serogroups.

✳ Water sanitation, cooking shellfish

Killed vaccines disappointing

✳ Live oral vaccine approved

OTHER *VIBRIOS*

Species of *Vibrio* other than *V cholerae* may still produce disease, but are uncommon and typically restricted to seacoast locales. *Vibrio parahaemolyticus* produces a diarrheal illness after ingestion of raw or inadequately cooked seafood due to the production of a pair of its own enterotoxins. For virulence *Vibrio vulnificus* stands out because it can produce a rapidly progressive cellulitis in wounds sustained in seawater as well as a fatal bacteremic infection after ingestion of raw seafood. The latter has been common enough in Florida to threaten the local oyster trade. Cases were also seen in the area devastated by hurricane Katrina. *V vulnificus* is also a spectacular scavenger of host iron stores and produces particularly fulminant disease in persons with iron-overload states (eg, thalassemia and hemochromatosis) and those with cirrhosis of the liver. Features of these and other less common vibrios are shown in Table 32–2.

✳ *V parahaemolyticus* diarrhea from undercooked seafood

***V vulnificus* sepsis, wound infections linked to raw oysters, iron overload**

KEY CONCLUSIONS

- *Vibrio cholerae* produces an enterotoxin that activates the adenylate cyclase system.
- Cholera reemerges when public health infrastructure breaks down.
- *V cholerae* survives and persists in saltwater plankton and crustaceans.
- Accumulations of cAMP in enterocytes result in massive outpouring of intestinal fluid.
- Voluminous diarrhea leads to dehydration, acidosis, and death swiftly unless replaced.
- Effective therapy (single dose of azithromycin) halts toxin production and thereby shortens duration.
- *Vibrio parahaemolyticus* causes diarrhea after seafood ingestion.
- *Vibrio vulnificus* and other halophilic species cause soft tissue infections and sepsis in patients with cirrhosis or iron overload.

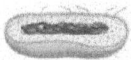

• CAMPYLOBACTER

Campylobacters are motile, curved, oxidase-positive, Gram-negative rods similar in morphology to vibrios. The cells have polar flagella and are often attached at their ends giving pairs "S" shapes or a "seagull" appearance. More than a dozen *Campylobacter* species have been associated with human disease. Of these, *C jejuni* is by far the most common and is discussed here as the prototype for intestinal disease. The features of other species are summarized in Table 32–2.

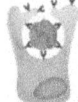

BACTERIOLOGY: *CAMPYLOBACTER JEJUNI*

Before 1973, *C jejuni* was not recognized as a cause of human disease. Not until selective methods for its isolation were developed was it recognized as one of the most common causes of infectious diarrhea. Like other campylobacters, *C jejuni* grows well only on enriched media at 42°C under microaerophilic conditions. That is, it requires oxygen at reduced tension (5-10%), presumably because of the vulnerability of some of its enzyme systems to superoxides. Growth usually requires 2 to 4 days, sometimes as much as 1 week. *C jejuni* has the structural components found in other Gram-negative bacteria (eg, outer membrane, LPS, and LOS). The cells are actively motile through the action of a polar flagellum. In contrast to the vibrios, *C jejuni* does not break down carbohydrates but uses amino acids and metabolic intermediates for energy. It is one of a number of pathogens that produce a membrane-bound protein called cytolethal-distending toxin (CDT). CDT has an A/B toxin structure in which the A subunit is able to cause cell cycle arrest.

* Microaerophilic atmosphere for growth

* CDT is cytotoxin

CAMPYLOBACTER ENTERITIS

EPIDEMIOLOGY

It is humbling to consider how a pathogen as common as *C jejuni* could have been missed for decades. Rates of campylobacteriosis vary widely around the world but at 4% to 30% of diarrheal stools, it is the leading cause of gastrointestinal infection in developed countries. Over 2 million cases occur each year in the United States at a rate roughly double that of *Salmonella*, the second most common bacterial enteric pathogen. This high rate of disease is facilitated by the low infecting dose of *C jejuni*—only a few hundred cells.

The primary reservoir is in animals, and the bacteria are transmitted to humans by ingestion of contaminated food or by direct contact with pets. Campylobacters are commonly found in the normal gastrointestinal and genitourinary flora of warm-blooded animals, including sheep, cattle, chickens, wild birds, and many others. The most common source of human infection is undercooked poultry, but outbreaks have been caused by contaminated rural water supplies and unpasteurized milk often consumed as a "natural" food. Sometimes a direct association can be made with a household pet, particularly a new puppy just brought home from a kennel.

* Diarrhea worldwide

* Infecting dose low

* Reservoir in animals

* Undercooked poultry, unpasteurized milk major sources

PATHOGENESIS

Infection is established by oral ingestion, followed by colonization of the intestinal mucosa. Adherence to enterocytes is facilitated by action of the flagellum followed by entrance into cells in endocytotic vacuoles. Once inside, they move in association with the cell's microtubule structure, rather than the actin microfilaments associated with some other invasive bacteria. Candidate injury mechanisms include the cytotoxic CDT and the action of lipooligosaccharides (LOS) released in outer membrane vesicles. The intestinal pathology is that of an invasive pathogen with acute inflammation, crypt abscesses, and occasional seeding of the bloodstream.

There is an association between *C jejuni* infection and **Guillain-Barré syndrome (GBS),** an acute demyelinating neuropathy that is frequently preceded by an infection. Although *C jejuni* is not the only antecedent to this syndrome, it is the most common of identifiable causes. Up to 40% of patients have culture or serologic evidence of *Campylobacter* infection at the time the neurologic symptoms occur. The mechanism is a type II hypersensitivity involving antibody elicited by epitopes in the *C jejuni* outer membrane LOS that cross-react with host peripheral nerve

Intracellular microtubule movement

* Invasion, CDT, LOS vesicles cause injury

* GBS may follow infection

* Anti-LOS antibodies cross-react with neural gangliosides

myelin gangliosides. These antiganglioside antibodies are found in the serum of patients with GBS motor neuropathies. This molecular mimicry is similar to the mechanism of group A streptococcal rheumatic fever. Reactive arthritis may also occur following infection.

IMMUNITY

✴ Immune mechanisms unclear

Acquired immunity after natural infection with *C jejuni* has been demonstrated in volunteer studies, but the mechanisms involved are unknown. Secretory and serum IgA are formed in the weeks after infection but decline thereafter. The high rate of *Campylobacter* infection in patients with AIDS suggests the importance of cellular immune mechanisms.

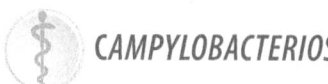 *CAMPYLOBACTERIOSIS:* CLINICAL ASPECTS

MANIFESTATIONS AND DIAGNOSIS

Abdominal pain and dysentery

Culture on selective medium in microaerophilic atmosphere

The illness typically begins 1 to 7 days after ingestion, with fever and lower abdominal pain that may be severe enough to mimic acute appendicitis. These are followed within hours by dysenteric stools that usually contain blood and pus. The illness is typically self-limiting after 3 to 5 days but may last 1 to 2 weeks. The diagnosis is confirmed by isolation of the organism from the stool. This requires a special medium made selective for *Campylobacter* by inclusion of antimicrobials that inhibit the normal facultative microbiota of the bowel. Plates must be incubated in a microaerophilic atmosphere, which can now be conveniently generated in a sealed jar by hydration of commercial packs similar to those used for anaerobes.

TREATMENT

✴ Azithromycin drug of choice

Since less than 50% of patients clearly benefit from antimicrobial therapy, cases of *Campylobacter* infection are usually not treated unless the disease is severe or prolonged (lasting longer than 1 week). *Campylobacter jejuni* is typically susceptible to macrolides and fluoroquinolones but resistant to β-lactams. Azithromycin is the therapy of choice but must be given early for maximal effect; erythromycin is an alternative. Fluoroquinolones are also effective, but resistance is becoming more common, especially in patients with HIV infection who have difficulty clearing the organism despite treatment.

KEY CONCLUSIONS

- *Campylobacter jejuni* causes diarrhea by invasion and cytotoxin production.
- Found in the intestine of many animals, especially poultry, it is a foodborne pathogen.
- The disease is self-limited, but excretion and transmission are halted by macrolide therapy.
- Carriage after infection is transient except in HIV-infected patients.
- Guillian-Barré syndrome can follow infection by virtue of molecular mimicry.

● *HELICOBACTER*

Almost everything we once knew about ulcers was wrong

In 1983 an Australian internist and pathologist (Warren and Marshall) postulated that gastritis and peptic ulcers were infectious diseases. Subsequently, they fulfilled Koch's postulates by self-experimentation with Warren's ingestion of a broth slurry of *H pylori*, his development of gastritis, and the recovery of *H pylori* in pure culture from his gastric mucosa. Later the 2005 Nobel Prize in Medicine was awarded to the pair for their scientific contradiction of long-held beliefs. Ironically, the 10th edition of *Harrison's Principles of Internal Medicine* published in 1983 described peptic ulcers as due to an unfavorable balance between gastric acid–pepsin secretion and gastric or duodenal mucosal resistance. Underlying causes cited included genetic and lifestyle (smoking) as well as psychologic factors (anxiety, stress). Treatment with bismuth salts, antacids, and inhibitors of acid secretion gave relief but not cure. Relapsing patients (50-80%) were subjected to surgical treatments (vagotomy, partial gastrectomy), which had their own set of complications (reflux, afferent loop, and dumping syndromes). All of this seemed logical and supported by clinical observations and research studies but was simply incorrect. The bacteria now called *Helicobacter* had been observed but dismissed because they were so common and their urease was once considered a secretory product of the stomach itself. The Nobel Prize-winning studies that stimulated the reversal of this dogma have led to cures with antibacterial agents and new ideas linking *Helicobacter* infection to cancer. This experience has also left us with a sense that we can never be smug about what we "know" in medicine.

 ## BACTERIOLOGY: *HELICOBACTER PYLORI*

H pylori has morphologic and growth similarities to the campylobacters, with which they were originally classified. The cells are slender, curved rods with polar flagella. The cell wall structure is typical of other Gram-negative bacteria. Growth requires a microaerophilic atmosphere and is slow (3-5 days). The cells are rapidly motile due to the action of multiple polar flagella.

※ Similar to Campylobacter

A number of unique bacteriologic features have been found in *H pylori*. The most distinctive is a **urease** whose action allows the organism to persist in low pH environments by the generation of ammonia. The urease is produced in amounts so great (6% of bacterial protein) that its action can be demonstrated within minutes of placing *H pylori* in the presence of urea. Another secreted protein called the **vacuolating cytotoxin** (VacA) causes apoptosis in eukaryotic cells it enters generating multiple large cytoplasmic vacuoles (**Figure 32–2**). The vacuoles are felt to be

※ Urease raises pH

※ VacA injures lysosomal, endosomal membranes

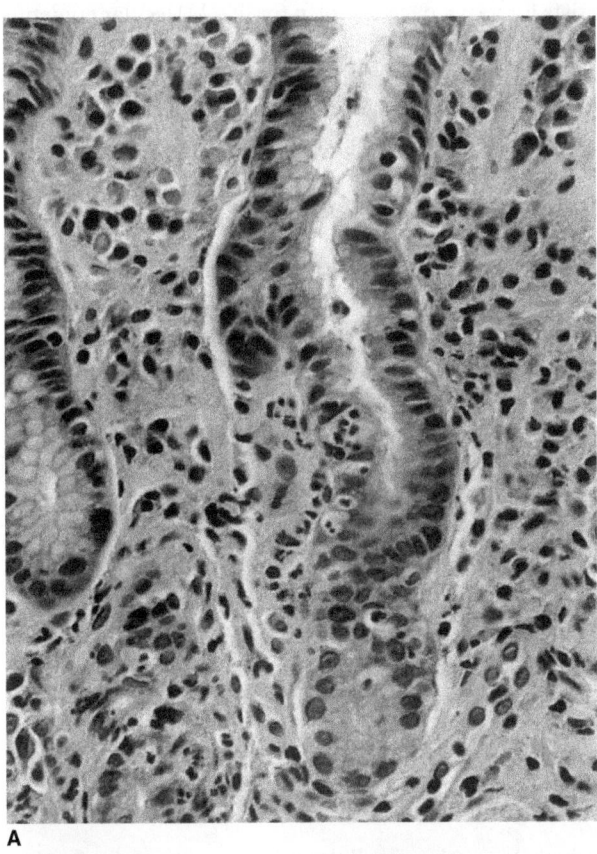

FIGURE 32–2. *Helicobacter* **gastritis.** High magnification shows curved bacilli and vacuolization of some cells. (Reproduced with permission from Connor DH, Chandler FW, Schwartz DQ, et al: *Pathology of Infectious Diseases.* Stamford CT: Appleton & Lange; 1997.)

A

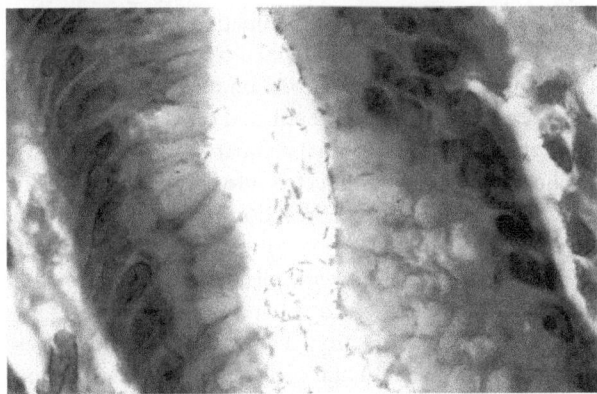

B

generated by the toxin's formation of channels in lysosomal and endosomal membranes. Another protein, CagA, induces changes in multiple cellular proteins and has a strong association with virulence. Both VacA and CagA are delivered to cells by injection secretion systems (type IV). The genes for CagA and the components of its secretion system are located in a large PAI.

* CagA induces multiple changes

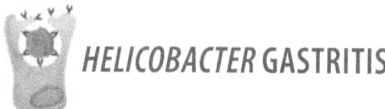 *HELICOBACTER* GASTRITIS

EPIDEMIOLOGY

* Transmitted by human fecal, gastric secretions

* Gastric colonization prevalent worldwide

Infection with *H pylori* causes what is perhaps the most prevalent disease in the world. The organism is found in the stomachs of 30% to 50% of adults in developed countries, and it is almost universal in developing countries. The exact mode of transmission is not known, but is presumed to be person to person by the fecal–oral route or by contact with gastric secretions in some way. Colonization increases progressively with age, and children are believed to be the major amplifiers of *H pylori* in human populations. A declining prevalence in developed countries may be due to decreased transmission because of less crowding and frequent exposure to antimicrobial agents.

* Colonization persists

* Ethnic links strong

Once established, the same strain persists for years, decades, even for life. Molecular epidemiologic analysis indicates the strains themselves have strong linkages to ethnic origins that can be traced back to the earliest known patterns of human migration. *H pylori* has been called an "accidental tourist," which was established in the stomachs of humans thousands of years ago and remained bound to the original population as it dispersed from continent to continent.

* Sole nondrug cause of gastritis, ulcers

* Adenocarcinoma, lymphoma preceded by infection

H pylori is the most common precursor of gastritis, gastric ulcer, and duodenal ulcer cases which are not due to drugs. In addition, *Helicobacter* gastritis caused by Cag+ strains is acknowledged to be an antecedent of gastric adenocarcinoma, one of the most common causes of cancer death in the world. It is also linked to a gastric mucosa-associated lymphoid tissue (MALT) lymphoma, which is less common but shows the striking property of regressing with antimicrobial therapy. *H pylori* gained the dubious distinction of being the first bacterium declared a class I carcinogen by the World Health Organization.

Other helicobacters in animals

H pylori is exclusive to humans, but other species have been found in the stomachs of a wide range of animals, where they are also associated with gastritis. It is difficult to imagine the old "stress ulcer" theories surviving the discovery of a cheetah with *Helicobacter* gastritis. Speculation that domestic animals may serve as a reservoir for human infection has not been confirmed.

PATHOGENESIS

* Urease neutralizes gastric acid

* Motility facilitates microenvironment survival

To persist in the hostile environs of the stomach, *H pylori* uses many mechanisms to adhere to the gastric mucosa and survive the acid milieu of the stomach (**Figure 32–3**). Motility provided by the flagella allows the organisms to swim to the less acidic locale beneath the gastric mucus, where the urease further creates a more neutral microenvironment by ammonia production. Urease production is regulated in response to changes in the gastric acidity such as rises to a pH as high as 6.0 following the buffering effect of meals. At the mucosa, adherence is mediated by multiple outer membrane proteins which bind to the surface of gastric epithelial cells and certain erythrocyte antigens (Lewis b).

Multiple inflammation factors

* VacA induces cellular changes, death

* CagA alters cytoskeleton

H pylori colonization is almost always accompanied by a cellular infiltrate ranging from minimal mononuclear infiltration of the lamina propria to extensive inflammation with neutrophils, lymphocytes, and microabscess formation. Both gastritis and duodenal ulcers are most strongly associated with colonization of the antrum area of the stomach. The inflammation may be due to toxic effects of the urease or the VacA transported into the gastric epithelial cells by the secretion system. Inside the cell, VacA causes vacuolization of the endosomal compartment and has other effects including altered T-cell function. The CagA protein is injected into the gastric epithelial cell by the secretion system, where it triggers multiple enzymatic reactions including those that cause reorganization of the actin cytoskeleton and stimulation of cytokines. Variations in the genes contained in the PAI generate a mixed population of *H pylori* cells particularly in relation to the multiple properties of CagA. Added together urease, CagA, and VacA provide ample explanation for the gastritis that is universal in *H pylori* infection. This prolonged and aggressive inflammatory response could lead to epithelial cell death and ulcers. The progression from

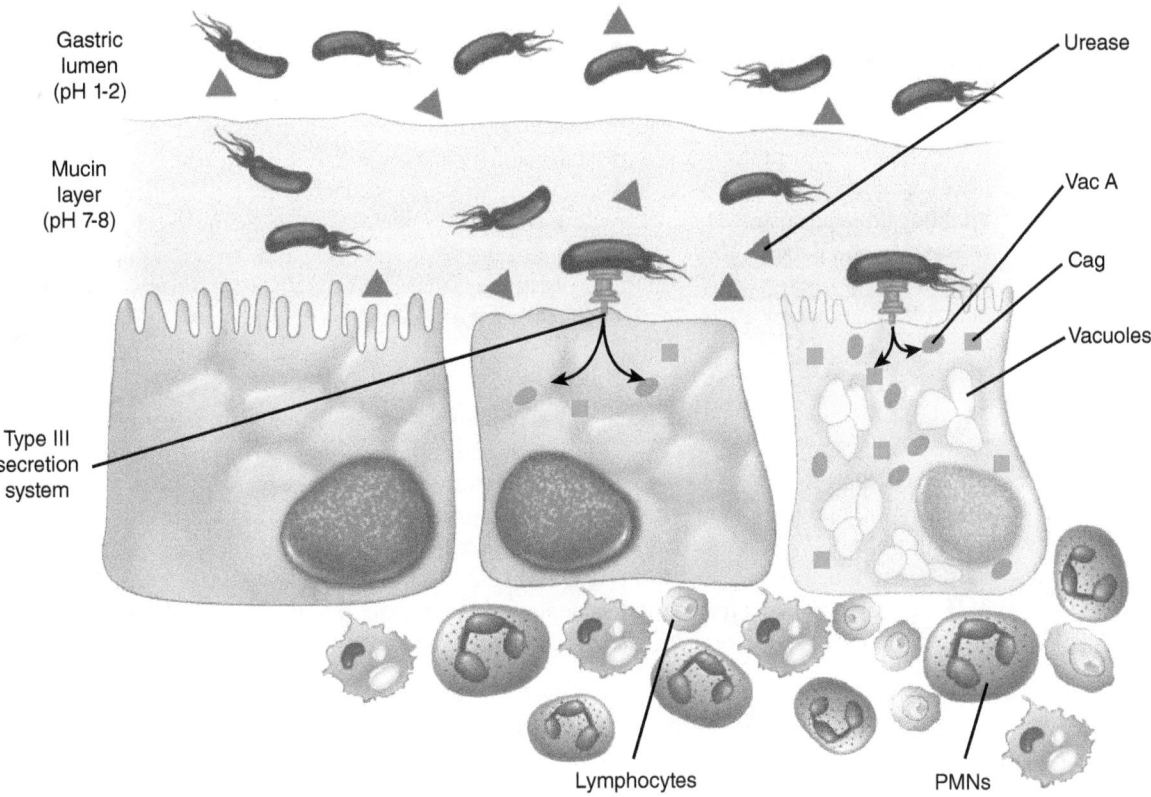

FIGURE 32–3. *Helicobacter* gastritis, cellular view. From the low pH gastric lumen *H pylori* swims beneath the mucus layer, produces urease, and persists in a more physiologic environment. A type III secretion system injects the vacuolating cytotoxin (VacA), and Cag, into the gastric cells. Acute and chronic inflammatory cells gather in the submucosa. PMNs, polymorphonuclear neutrophils.

gastritis to ulcer remains to be explained although a duodenal ulcer-promoting gene has been identified.

That decades of inflammation and assault by the virulence factors just described could cause metaplasia, and eventually cancer seems logical, but the specific mechanisms of carcinogenesis have only recently been explored. CagA, for example, has been shown to trigger a cascade of interactions leading to growth-promoting oncogenic signals. The gastric lymphomas may represent neoplastic transformation of B-lymphocyte clones proliferating in response to chronic antigenic stimulation. The discovery that *H pylori* colonization may affect hormones involved in glucose homeostasis has led to other hypotheses involving type 2 diabetes.

✳ Chronic inflammation leads to metaplasia

✳ CagA triggers oncogenic signals

IMMUNITY

There is obviously little evidence of natural immunity in an infection that typically lasts for decades. The immunosuppressive effect of virulence factors such as VacA may be responsible in combination with yet to be discovered mechanisms.

 HELICOBACTER DISEASE: CLINICAL ASPECTS

MANIFESTATIONS

Primary infection with *H pylori* is either silent or causes an illness with nausea and upper abdominal pain lasting up to 2 weeks. Years later, the findings of gastritis and peptic ulcer disease include nausea, anorexia, vomiting, epigastric pain, and even less specific symptoms such as belching. Many patients are asymptomatic for decades, even up to perforation of an ulcer. Perforation can lead to extensive bleeding and peritonitis due to the leakage of gastric contents into the peritoneal cavity.

✳ Epigastric pain, nausea signs of gastritis

DIAGNOSIS

The most sensitive means of diagnosis is endoscopic examination, with biopsy and culture of the gastric mucosa. The *H pylori* urease is so potent that its activity can be directly demonstrated in biopsies in less than an hour. Noninvasive methods include serology and a urea breath test. For the breath test, the patient ingests ^{13}C- or ^{14}C-labeled urea, from which the urease in the stomach produces products that appear as labeled CO_2 in the breath. A number of methods for the detection of antibody directed against *H pylori* are now available. Because IgG or IgA remains elevated as long as the infection persists, these tests are valuable both for screening and for evaluation of therapy. The advantage of direct detection of the organism is that culture is the most sensitive indicator of cure following therapy. A stool antigen detection test is also a sensitive indicator of colonization.

* Culture, urease, or antigen detection

* Serology demonstrates chronic infection

TREATMENT AND PREVENTION

H pylori is susceptible to a wide variety of antimicrobial agents. Bismuth subsalicylate (eg, Pepto-Bismol), which in the past was believed to act by coating the stomach, also has antimicrobial activity. Cure rates approaching 90% have been achieved with a quadruple regimen (14 days) of bismuth subsalicylate, a protein pump inhibitor (PPI) (omeprazole), tetracycline, and metronidazole. Triple therapy with a PPI, clarithromycin, and amoxicillin is less effective. These combination regimens must be continued for at least 2 weeks and may be difficult for some patients to tolerate. Prevention of *H pylori* disease awaits further understanding of transmission and immune mechanisms. Prophylactic treatment of asymptomatic persons colonized with *H pylori* is not yet recommended.

* Combination therapies achieve cures

* Regimen difficult to tolerate

 Should everyone be screened for *H pylori* colonization?

KEY CONCLUSIONS

- *Helicobacter pylori* is found worldwide as a common inhabitant of the stomach.
- *H pylori* is also the sole nondrug cause of gastritis and gastric and duodenal ulcers.
- Its toxins VacA and CagA cause chronic inflammation that can lead to gastric adenocarcinoma.
- Diagnosis of active disease is done by endoscopic biopsy, the breath test for urease, or stool antigen detection.
- Quadruple therapy with bismuth, omeprazole, tetracycline, and metronidazole is optimal.

CASE STUDY

Raw Oysters in Rifle

On August 17, 1988, a 42-year-old man was treated for profuse, watery diarrhea, vomiting, and dehydration at an emergency room in Rifle, Colorado. On August 15, he had eaten approximately 12 raw oysters from a new oyster-processing plant in Rifle. Approximately 36 hours after eating the oysters, he had sudden onset of symptoms and passed 20 stools during the day before seeking medical attention. Stool culture subsequently yielded toxigenic *Vibrio cholerae* O1, El Tor biotype. The patient had no underlying illness, was not taking medications, and had not traveled outside the region during the month before onset.

The oysters had been harvested on August 8, 1988, in a bay off the coast of Louisiana. Approximately 1000 bushels (200,000 oysters) arrived by refrigerator truck at the plant in Rifle on August 11. The patient purchased three dozen of these oysters on August 15. During a 6-day period, eight other persons shared the oysters purchased by the patient. None became ill. Although one of seven tested had a vibriocidal antibody titer of 1:640, none had elevated antitoxic antibody titers, and none had *V cholerae* isolated from stool. Physicians and local health departments were asked to notify the Colorado Department of Health about similar cases, but no cases were reported.

 Think ▸▸ Apply 32-2: **Widespread screening to prevent ulcers remains controversial in asymptomatic persons. In parts of the world with high *H pylori* prevalence and gastric adenocarcinoma rates, screening followed by treatment of positives is under study as a means of cancer prevention. The diversity of regimes used worldwide and the paucity of controlled trials with adequate follow-up, however, have hampered definitive conclusions.**

QUESTIONS

1. What is the probable source of this patient's *V cholerae* infection?
    A. Oyster bar employee
    B. An imported case from Asia
    C. Gulf of Mexico
    D. Rifle groundwater
    E. South America

2. What would you expect a biopsy of this patient's small intestine to show?
    A. Hyperemia
    B. Pseudomembrane
    C. Flask-shaped ulcers
    D. Enterocyte necrosis
    E. Focal hemorrhage

3. Which of the following measures would be the *least effective* in preventing a recurrence of this outbreak?
    A. Disinfecting the plant
    B. A new source for oysters
    C. Prophylactic rifampin
    D. Cooking the oysters

ANSWERS

1. (C)

2. (A)

3. (C)

chapter *33*

Enterobacteriaceae

Escherichia coli • Shigella species • Salmonella enterica • Yersinia • Klebsiella • Enterobacter • Serratia • Proteus • Morganella • Providencia

> *She died of a fever / And no one could save her / And that was the end of sweet Molly Malone / But her ghost wheels her barrow / Through streets broad and narrow / Crying cockles and mussels alive, alive o!*
>
> —James Yorkston: Irish Ballad

OVERVIEW

The Enterobacteriaceae are a large and diverse family of Gram-negative rods, members of which are both free-living and part of the indigenous flora of humans and animals; a few are adapted strictly to humans. The Enterobacteriaceae grow rapidly under aerobic or anaerobic conditions and are metabolically active. They are by far the most common cause of urinary tract infections (UTIs), and a limited number of species are also important etiologic agents of diarrhea. Entry into the bloodstream may cause Gram-negative endotoxin shock, a dreaded and often fatal complication. Historically, dying "of a fever" usually meant typhoid fever (*Salmonella* ser. Typhi), which because of its prolonged course and lack of localizing signs, caused unfortunates like Molly Malone to appear to be dying of fever alone. The term UTI encompasses a range of infections from simple cystitis involving the bladder to full-blown infection of the entire urinary tract, including the renal pelvis and kidney (pyelonephritis). The primary feature of cystitis is frequent urination, which often has a painful burning quality. In pyelonephritis, symptoms include fever, general malaise, and flank pain in addition to frequent urination. Cystitis is usually self-limiting, but infection of the upper urinary tract carries a risk of spread to the bloodstream. It is the leading cause of Gram-negative sepsis and septic shock. Diarrhea is the universal finding with *Escherichia coli* strains that are able to cause intestinal disease; the nature of the diarrhea varies depending on the pathogenic mechanism. Enterotoxigenic and enteropathogenic strains produce a watery diarrhea, the enterohemorrhagic strains produce a bloody diarrhea, and the enteroinvasive strains may cause dysentery with blood and pus in the stool. The diarrhea is usually self-limiting after only 1-3 days. The enterohemorrhagic *E coli* are an exception, with life-threatening manifestations outside the gastrointestinal tract due to Shiga toxin production. *Shigella* is the classic cause of dysentery, which is typically spread person to person under poor sanitary conditions. The illness begins as a watery diarrhea but evolves into an intense colitis with fever and frequent small-volume stools that contain blood and pus. Despite the invasive properties of the causal organism, the infection usually does not spread outside the intestinal tract. Typhoid fever has a slow, insidious onset and, if untreated, lasts for weeks. The primary symptom is a slowly rising fever, often accompanied by abdominal pain but little else. It ends either by gradual resolution or in death due to complications (eg, rupture of the intestine or spleen). Family members may note only the extended fever, although physicians may observe a subtle rash or feel an enlarged spleen. Diarrhea may occur sporadically during the course but is not a consistent feature.

● GENERAL CHARACTERISTICS

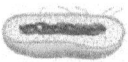 **BACTERIOLOGY**

Rods are large

The Enterobacteriaceae are among the largest bacteria, measuring 2 to 4 μm in length with parallel sides and rounded ends. Forms range from large coccobacilli to elongated, filamentous rods. The organisms do not form spores or demonstrate acid-fastness.

O = LPS

H = flagellar protein

K = polysaccharide capsule

The cell wall, cell membrane, and internal structures are morphologically similar for all Enterobacteriaceae, and follow the cell plan described in Chapter 21 for Gram-negative bacteria. Components of the cell wall and surface, which are antigenic, have been extensively studied in some genera and form the basis of systems dividing species into serotypes. The outer membrane lipopolysaccharide (LPS) is called the **O antigen.** Its antigenic specificity is determined by variation in the sugars that form the long terminal polysaccharide side chains linked to the core polysaccharide and lipid A. Cell surface polysaccharides may form a well-defined capsule or an amorphous slime layer and are termed the **K antigen** (from the Danish *kapsel*, capsule). Motile strains have protein peritrichous flagella, which extend well beyond the cell wall and are called the **H antigen.** Many Enterobacteriaceae have adhesive surface pili (fimbriae), which are antigenic proteins, but not part of traditional typing systems.

Facultative growth is rapid

Enterobacteriaceae grow readily on simple media, often with only a single carbon energy source. Growth is rapid under both aerobic and anaerobic conditions, producing 2 to 5 mm colonies on agar media and diffuse turbidity in broth after 12 to 18 hours of incubation. All Enterobacteriaceae ferment glucose, reduce nitrates to nitrites, and are oxidase-negative.

CLASSIFICATION

Genus and species designations are based on phenotypic characteristics such as patterns of carbohydrate fermentation and amino acid breakdown. The O, K, and H antigens are used to further divide some species into multiple **serotypes**. These types are expressed with letter and number of the specific antigen, such as *Escherichia coli* O157:H7, the cause of numerous foodborne outbreaks. These antigenic designations have been established only for the most important species and are limited to known antigenic structures. For example, many species lack capsules and/or flagella. In recent years, DNA and rRNA homology comparisons have been used to validate these relationships and establish new ones. The genera containing the species most virulent for humans are *Escherichia, Shigella, Salmonella, Klebsiella,* and *Yersinia.* Other less common but medically important genera are *Enterobacter, Serratia, Proteus, Morganella,* and *Providencia.* Multiple locus sequence typing (MLST) schemes have been developed in order to facilitate identification of and communication about important clones within these key pathogenic species.

✳ Biochemical characteristics establish species

✳ Antigenic features define serotypes within species

TOXINS

All have LPS

Cytotoxins kill host cells

Enterotoxins cause secretion and diarrhea

In addition to the **LPS endotoxin** common to all Gram-negative bacteria, some Enterobacteriaceae also produce **protein exotoxins,** which act on host cells by damaging membranes, inhibiting protein synthesis, or altering metabolic pathways. The end result of these actions may be cell death (cytotoxins) or a physiologic alteration, the net effect of which depends on the function of the affected cell. For example, enterotoxins act on intestinal enterocytes, causing the net secretion of water and electrolytes into the gut to produce diarrhea. Although these toxins are most strongly associated with *E coli, Shigella,* and *Yersinia,* others with the same or very similar actions have now been discovered in other species. Toxins found in another species may differ slightly in protein structure and genetic regulation, but still have the same biologic action on host cells. Details of these toxins are discussed later in this chapter in relation to their prototype species.

 DISEASES CAUSED BY ENTEROBACTERIACEAE

EPIDEMIOLOGY

Most Enterobacteriaceae are primarily colonizers of the lower gastrointestinal tract of humans and animals. Many species survive readily in nature and live freely anywhere that water and minimal energy sources are available. In humans, they are the major facultative components of the

Enterobacteriaceae

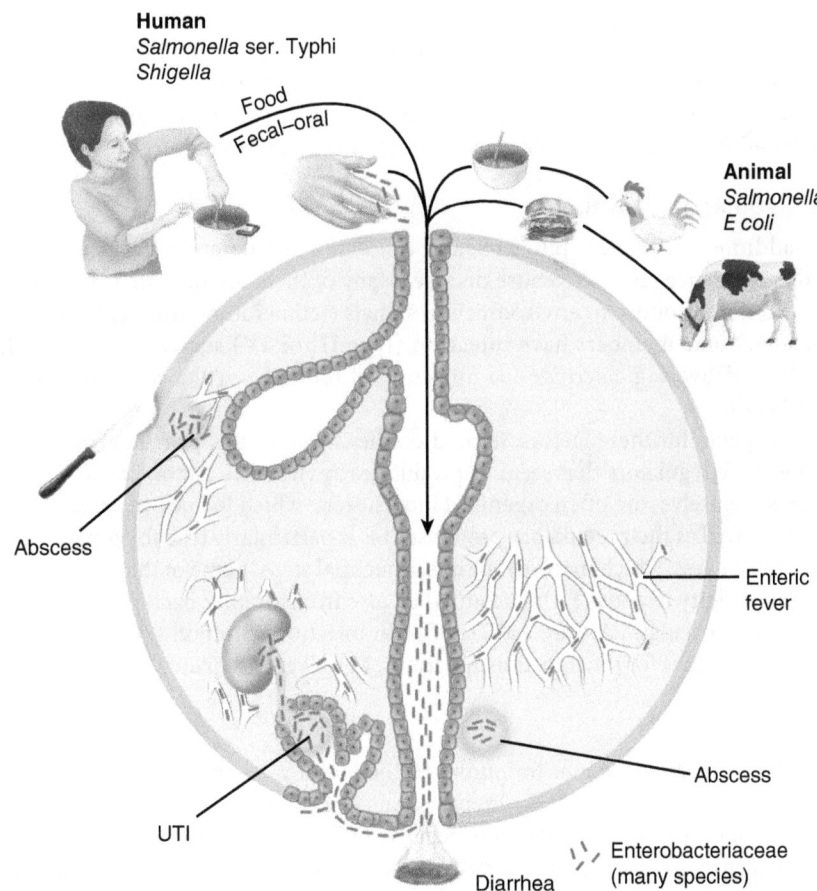

Human
Salmonella ser. Typhi
Shigella

Food

Fecal–oral

Animal
Salmonella
E coli

Abscess

Enteric
fever

Abscess

UTI

Diarrhea

Enterobacteriaceae
(many species)

FIGURE 33–1. **Enterobacteriaceae disease overview.** The external sources of infection are frequently animal sources, but some pathogens are strictly human (*Shigella*, *Salmonella* ser. Typhi). Endogenous flora are the source of opportunistic infection, particularly urinary tract infection (UTI). Bacteria of any source entering the blood may cause endotoxic shock.

colonic bacterial flora but are also found in the female genital tract and as transient colonizers of the skin. Enterobacteriaceae are scant in the respiratory tract of healthy individuals; however, their numbers may increase in hospitalized patients with intensive antibiotic exposure. *E coli* is the most common species of Enterobacteriaceae found among the indigenous flora, followed by *Klebsiella*, *Proteus*, and *Enterobacter* species. *Salmonella* and *Shigella* species are not considered members of the resident microbiota, although carrier states can exist. *Shigella* and *Salmonella* serovar Typhi are strict human pathogens with no animal reservoir. An overview of these infections is illustrated in **Figure 33–1**.

Present in nature and the intestinal tract

✳ *Shigella* and *S* Typhi are found only in humans

PATHOGENESIS

■ Opportunistic Infections

Enterobacteriaceae are often poised to take advantage of their presence in the environment and among human microbiota to produce disease whenever they gain access to normally sterile body sites. Surface structures such as pili have been proven to aid this process for some species, and likely do so for many others as well. Once in deeper tissues, bacteria may persist and cause injury using strategies that, with the exception of LPS endotoxin and production of exotoxins or capsules, are still not well understood. The prototype infectious syndrome is the UTI, in which Enterobacteriaceae gain access to the urinary bladder due to minor trauma or instrumentation. Strains able to adhere to uroepithelial cells can persist and multiply in the nutrient-rich urine, sometimes ascending by way of the ureters to the renal pelvis and kidney, producing pyelonephritis. Likewise, mucosal or skin trauma can allow access to underlying soft tissue, and aspiration can provide access to the lung when the relevant sites are colonized with Enterobacteriaceae.

✳ Colonization presents opportunity when defense barriers open

✳ Access and adherence to bladder mucosa may lead to UTI

■ Intestinal Infections

Salmonella, *Shigella*, *Yersinia enterocolitica*, and certain strains of *E coli* are able to produce disease in the intestinal tract. These intestinal pathogens have invasive properties or virulence factors

* Cell destruction causes dysentery

* Enterotoxins cause watery diarrhea

* Enteric fever is a systemic illness

* Secretion systems inject virulence factors

Virulence genes are organized into gene clusters

PAIs contain multiple genes

* Expression stimulated by environmental cues

travel on plasmids.

* Immunity is short-lived

* UTI and acute diarrhea are most common

* MacConkey agar demonstrates lactose fermentation

* Selective media required for *Salmonella* and *Shigella* in stools

Gene probes allow direct detection

such as cytotoxins and enterotoxins, which correlate with the type of diarrhea they produce. In general, the invasive and cytotoxic strains produce an inflammatory diarrhea called **dysentery** with white blood cells (WBCs) and/or blood in the stool. The enterotoxin-producing strains cause a **watery diarrhea** in which fluid loss is the primary pathophysiologic feature. For a few species, the intestinal tract may be the original portal of entry, but the disease ultimately becomes systemic as a result of spread of bacteria to multiple organs. **Enteric (typhoid) fever** caused by *Salmonella enterica* ser. Typhi is the prototype of this form of infection.

■ Regulation of Virulence

In addition to adhesive pili, LPS, and exotoxins, the Enterobacteriaceae produce a myriad of other virulence factors to cause disease. Many of them are deployed in complex and sequential fashion, in response to environmental signals (temperature, iron, calcium) or as-yet unknown factors. Some members have **injection (type III or IV) secretion systems** that target human cells by delivering a syringe-like injection of multiple virulence factors into the cytoplasm of host cells.

The genes for these factors, located on the chromosome, plasmids, or both, are controlled by interactive regulators that seem to produce each virulence factor exactly when it is needed. The genes themselves are often organized into clusters, which include the genes for the effector molecules as well as their regulatory proteins. This is particularly true for complex characteristics such as invasiveness, which involve multiple sequential steps. Some of these gene clusters reside within **pathogenicity islands (PAIs)** acquired *en bloc* from another bacterium in the genetically distant past. In particular, PAIs are associated with injection secretion systems, where they contain the structural genes for the injection apparatus, as well as the virulence factors injected.

IMMUNITY

Little is understood about immunity to the broad range of opportunistic infections caused by Enterobacteriaceae. Antibody directed against an LPS core antigen has been shown to provide a degree of protection against Gram-negative endotoxemia, but the diversity of antigens and virulence factors among the Enterobacteriaceae is too great to expect broad immunity in any given host. Immunity to intestinal infection is generally short-lived and will be discussed where relevant to specific intestinal pathogens.

ENTEROBACTERIACEAE: CLINICAL ASPECTS

MANIFESTATIONS

The Enterobacteriaceae produce the widest variety of infections of any group of microbial agents, including two of the most common infectious states, UTI and acute diarrhea. Urinary tract infections are manifested by dysuria and urinary frequency when infection is limited to the bladder, with the addition of fever and flank pain when the infection spreads to the kidney. Enterobacteriaceae are by far the most common cause of UTIs, and the most common species involved is *E coli*.

DIAGNOSIS

Culture is the primary method of diagnosis; all Enterobacteriaceae are readily isolated on routine media under almost any incubation conditions. Special indicator media such as MacConkey agar are commonly used in primary isolation to promote rapid identification of the pathogen from many possible species. For example, the common pathogens *E coli* and *Klebsiella* typically ferment lactose rapidly, producing acid (pink) colonies on MacConkey agar, whereas the intestinal pathogens *Salmonella* and *Shigella* do not. Separation of the intestinal pathogens from all the other Enterobacteriaceae in stool requires highly selective media designed solely for this purpose. (These are discussed as they relate to individual pathogens.) Improved understanding of the genetic and molecular basis for virulence has led to the development of direct nucleic acid and immunodiagnostic techniques for direct detection of toxin, adhesin, and invasin proteins or their genes in clinical materials, such as stool. Once too expensive for use in clinical laboratories, these methods are emerging as primary diagnostic tools.

TREATMENT

Antimicrobial therapy is crucial to the outcome of certain infections caused by Enterobacteriaceae. Unfortunately, combinations of chromosomal and plasmid-determined resistance render them the most variable of all bacteria in susceptibility to antimicrobial agents. They are intrinsically resistant to penicillin G, erythromycin, and clindamycin, but may be susceptible to the extended-spectrum β-lactams, carbapenems, aminoglycosides, tetracyclines, chloramphenicol, sulfonamides, quinolones, nitrofurantoin, and the polypeptide antibiotics. The emergence and spread of multidrug resistance plasmids featuring hydrolytic enzymes such as extended-spectrum cephalosporinases or carbapenemases have fundamentally altered the empiric treatment of Gram-negative infections. Because the probability of resistance varies among genera and in different epidemiologic settings, the susceptibility of any individual strain must be determined by antimicrobial susceptibility tests. Typical patterns of resistance for some of the more common Enterobacteriaceae appear in **Appendix 23–1**.

✳ Susceptibility to antimicrobials is highly variable

● *ESCHERICHIA COLI*

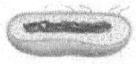 ## BACTERIOLOGY

Most strains of *E coli* ferment lactose rapidly and produce indole. These and other biochemical reactions are sufficient to separate it from the other pathogenic Enterobacteriaceae. There are over 150 distinct O antigens and a large number of K and H antigens, all of which are designated by number. The antigenic formula for serotypes is described by linking the letter (O, K, or H) and the assigned number of the antigen(s) present (eg, O18:K1:H7). In the sequencing era, the emergence of multidrug-resistant clones has led to the use of alternative nomenclature (eg, *E coli* Sequence Type 131, *Klebsiella pneumoniae* Sequence Type 258).

✳ Serotypes use O, K, H antigens

PILI

Pili play a role in virulence as mediators of attachment to human epithelial surfaces. They show marked tropism for different epithelial cell types, which is determined by the availability of their specific receptor on the host cell surface. Most *E coli* express **type 1**, or common, **pili**. Type 1 pili bind to the D-mannose residues commonly present on epithelial cell surfaces and thus mediate binding to a wide variety of cell types. More specialized pili are found in select clones of *E coli*. **P pili** bind to digalactoside (Gal–Gal) moieties particularly common on kidney cells and erythrocytes of the P blood group. Pili that mediate binding to enterocytes are found among the diarrhea-causing *E coli* and are specific to the pathogenic type, as shown in **Figure 33–2** and listed in **Table 33–1**. *E coli* also causes diarrhea in animals, and different sets of pili exist with host-specific

Type 1 pili bind mannose

P pili bind kidney cells

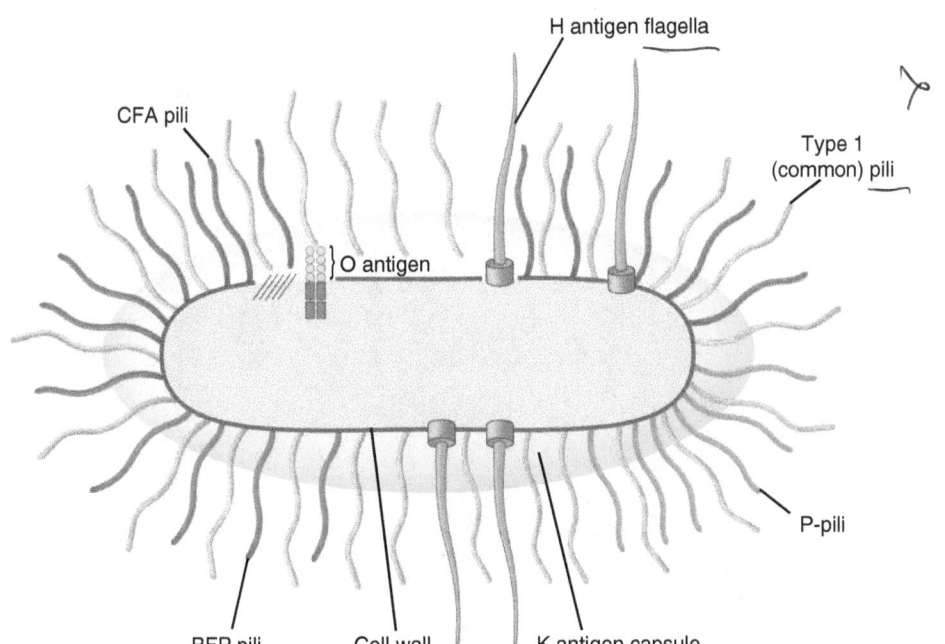

FIGURE 33–2. **Antigenic structure of *Escherichia coli*.** The O antigen is contained in the repeating polysaccharide units of the lipopolysaccharide (LPS) in the outer membrane of the cell wall. The H antigen is the flagellar protein. The K antigen is the polysaccharide capsule present in some strains. Most *E coli* have type 1 (common) hair-like pili extending from the surface. Some *E coli* have specialized P pili, colonization factor antigens (CFAs), or bundle-forming pili (Bfp), as well as type 1 pili.

TABLE 33–1 Characteristics of Pathogenic Enterobacteriaceae

	DIAGNOSTIC ANTIGENS O, H, K	PILI	ADHESIN OR CAPSULE	EXOTOXIN	PATHOGENIC LESIONS	SECRETED PROTEINS[a]	GENETICS	TRANSMISSION	DISEASE
Escherichia coli									
Newborn meningitic (NMEC)	O18:K1:H7, O1:K1, O2:K1	Type 1[b]	K1 polysaccharide	α-Hemolysin	Inflammation		PAI	Intestinal flora	Opportunistic, newborn meningitis
Uropathogenic (UPEC)		Type 1[b], P (Gal–Gal)		α-Hemolysin	Inflammation		PAI	Fecal flora, ascending	UTI
Enterotoxigenic (ETEC)		CFs		LT, ST	Hypersecretion		Plasmid (CF, LT, ST)	Fecal–oral	Watery diarrhea (travelers)
Enteropathogenic (EPEC)		Bfp	Intimin		A/E, small intestine	Esps	PAI	Fecal–oral	Watery diarrhea
Enteroinvasive (EIEC)			Ipas		Invasion, inflammation, ulcers	Ipas	Large plasmid, PAI	Fecal–oral	Dysentery
Enterohemorrhagic (EHEC)	O157:H7	Lpf	Intimin	Stx	A/E, colon, hemorrhage	Esps	Prophage, PAI	Fecal–oral direct, low dose, cattle	Bloody diarrhea, HUS
Enteroaggregative (EAEC)		AAFs		Stx[d]	Adherent biofilm				Watery diarrhea; bloody diarrhea and HUS[d]
Shigella	**O serogroups**								
S dysenteriae	A (10 types)		Ipas	Stx (serotype AI most potent)	Invasion, inflammation, colonic ulcers	Ipas	Large plasmid, PAI	Fecal–oral, direct, low dose	Dysentery (severe), HUS
S flexneri	B (6 types)		Ipas	Stx (variable)	Invasion, inflammation, colonic ulcers	Ipas	Large plasmid, PAI	Fecal–oral, direct, low dose	Dysentery, HUS
S boydii	C (15 types)		Ipas	Stx (variable)	Invasion, inflammation, colonic ulcers	Ipas	Large plasmid, PAI	Fecal–oral, direct, low dose	Dysentery, HUS
S sonnei	D		Ipas	Stx (variable)	Invasion, inflammation, colonic ulcers	Ipas	Large plasmid, PAI	Fecal–oral, direct, low dose	Dysentery, HUS

Salmonella enterica	O, H_1, H_2 K								
Serotypes	>2000 serovars	Type 1[b]			Ruffles, invasion, inflammation	Inv, Spa, others	PAI	Fecal–oral, animals and humans	Gastroenteritis, sepsis
Typhi	O group D	Type 1[b]	Vi polysaccharide		Macrophage survival, RES growth	As in serotypes[c]	PAI	Fecal–oral, moderate dose, humans only	Enteric (typhoid) fever
Yersinia	O, H								
Y pestis			Invasin	Protease, fibrinolysin	RES growth, bacteremia, pneumonia	Yops	PAI	Rats, flea bite, aerosol (human)	Plague
Y pseudotuberculosis	10 types		Invasin		RES growth, microabscesses	Yops	PAI	Fecal–oral, animal	Mesenteric adenitis
Y enterocolitica	>50 types		Invasin		RES growth, microabscesses	Yops	PAI	Fecal–oral, animals	Mesenteric adenitis, enteric fever
Klebsiella	70 capsular types	Pili	Polysaccharide					Intestinal flora	Opportunistic, pneumonia, UTI
K pneumoniae		Pili	K1, K2 polysaccharide		Abscesses			Intestinal flora	Liver abscess, endophthalmitis
Enterobacter, Serratia, Citrobacter								Intestinal flora	Opportunistic, UTI
Proteus						Urease		Intestinal flora	UTI

A/E, attaching and effacing lesion; Bfp, bundle-forming pili; CFs, colonizing factor antigens; Esps, *E coli*-secreted proteins; HUS, hemolytic uremic syndrome; Ipas, invasion protein antigens; LT, labile toxin; Lpf, long polar fimbrae; PAI, pathogenicity island; RES, reticuloendothelial system; ST, stable toxin; UTI, urinary tract infection; Yops, *Yersinia* outer membrane proteins.

[a]Delivered by injection (type III) secretion system.

[b]Bind to mannose.

[c]No animal model, presumed to be similar to *S enterica* serotypes.

[d]Major outbreak in 2011 due to EAEC serotype O104:H4 that acquired shiga toxin stx_2.

Pili of diarrhea strains bind
enterocytes

tropism for their enterocytes. The receptor(s) for the enteric pili are not known in detail but include glycolipids and glycoproteins on the enterocyte surface.

The genetics of pilin expression are complex. The genes are organized into multicistronic clusters that encode structural pilin subunits and regulatory functions. Pili of different types may coexist on the same bacterium, and their expression may vary under different environmental conditions. Type 1 pilin expression can be turned on or off by inversion of a chromosomal DNA sequence containing the promoter responsible for initiating transcription of the pilin gene. Other genes control the orientation of this switch.

Type 1 has on–off switch

TOXINS

As a single species, *E coli* can produce every kind of protein exotoxin found among the Enterobacteriaceae. These include a pore-forming cytotoxin, inhibitors of protein synthesis, and a number of toxins that alter messenger pathways in host cells. The **α-hemolysin** is a pore-forming cytotoxin that inserts into the plasma membrane of a wide range of host cells in a manner similar to streptolysin O (Chapter 25) and *Staphylococcus aureus* α-toxin (Chapter 24). The toxin causes leakage of cytoplasmic contents and eventually cell death. The more recently discovered **cytotoxic necrotizing factor (CNF)** is often produced in concert with α-hemolysin. CNF is an A-B toxin that disrupts G proteins regulating signaling pathways in the cell cytoplasm with multiple effects including cytoskeleton rearrangement and apoptosis.

α-Hemolysin is pore-forming
cytotoxin

CNF disrupts intracellular
signaling

Shiga toxin (Stx) is named for the microbiologist who discovered *Shigella dysenteriae*, and this toxin was once believed to be limited to that species. It is now recognized to exist in at least two molecular forms released upon bacterial lysis by multiple *E coli* and *Shigella* strains. In the years after the discovery of this toxin, the term Shiga toxin was reserved for the original toxin, while others were called Shiga-like. In this book, the term Stx is used for all molecular variants that have the same mode of action regardless of the species under consideration. Stx is an A–B type toxin. The B unit directs binding to a specific glycolipid receptor (Gb$_3$) present on eukaryotic cells and leads to internalization by an endocytotic vacuole. Inside the cell, the A subunit crosses the vacuolar membrane in the trans-Golgi network, exits to the cytoplasm, and enzymatically modifies the ribosome site (28S-RNA of 60S subunit) where amino-acyl tRNA binds. This alteration blocks protein synthesis, leading to cell death (**Figure 33–3**). This action is very similar to the plant toxin ricin.

✳ Shiga toxin is produced by
Shigella and *E coli*

✳ Inhibits protein synthesis by
ribosomal modification

Labile toxin (LT) is also an A–B toxin. Its name relates to the physical property of heat lability, which was important in its discovery, and contrasts with the heat-stable toxin (ST) also produced by *E coli*. The B subunit binds to the cell membrane, and the A subunit catalyzes the ADP-ribosylation of a regulatory G protein located in the membrane of the intestinal epithelial cell. This inactivation of part of the G protein complex causes permanent activation of the membrane-associated adenylate cyclase system and a cascade of events, the net effect of which depends on the biologic function of the stimulated cell. If the cell is an enterocyte, the result is the stimulation of chloride secretion out of the cell and the blockage of NaCl absorption; the net effect is the secretion of water and electrolytes into the bowel lumen. The structure and action of LT are nearly identical with that already described for cholera toxin (CT), but LT is less potent than CT.

✳ LT ADP-ribosylates G protein

✳ Adenylate cyclase
stimulation similar to cholera

Stable toxin is a small peptide that binds to a glycoprotein receptor, resulting in the activation of a membrane-bound guanylate cyclase. The subsequent increase in cyclic GMP concentration causes an LT-like net secretion of fluid and electrolytes into the bowel lumen.

✳ ST stimulates guanylate
cyclase

E COLI EXTRAINTESTINAL INFECTIONS

URINARY TRACT INFECTION

■ Epidemiology

E coli accounts for more than 90% of the more than 7 million cases of cystitis and 250,000 of pyelonephritis estimated to occur in otherwise healthy individuals every year in the United States. Urinary tract infections are much more common in women, 40% of whom have an episode in their lifetime, usually when they are sexually active. The reservoir for these infections is the patient's own intestinal *E coli* flora, which colonize the perineal and urethral area. In individuals with urinary tract obstruction or instrumentation, exogenous sources assume greater importance.

Perineal flora is reservoir of
common cystitis

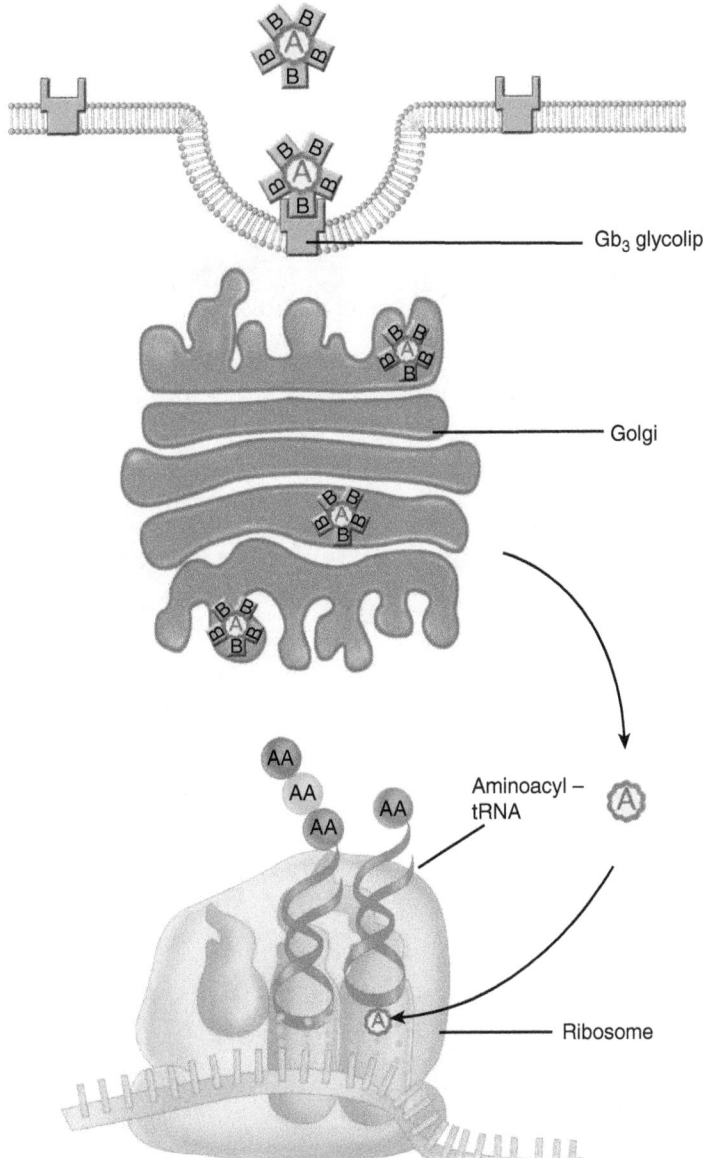

FIGURE 33-3. **Stx (Shiga) toxin.** The A-B toxin binds to the cytoplasmic membrane, enters in an endocytotic vacuole, and enters the Golgi network. Exiting to the cytoplasm, it combines at ribosome sites involved with tRNA binding. The result is interference with protein synthesis.

Gb₃ glycolipid

Golgi

Aminoacyl – tRNA

Ribosome

■ Pathogenesis

Relatively minor trauma or mechanical disruptions can allow bacteria colonizing the periurethral area brief access to the urinary bladder. These bacteria originally derived from the intestinal flora are frequently present in the bladder of women immediately after sexual intercourse. In most instances, they are purged by the flushing action of voiding, but may persist to cause a UTI, depending on host and bacterial factors. Although most UTIs occur in otherwise healthy women, host situations that violate bladder integrity (urinary catheters) or that obstruct urine outflow (in men, enlarged prostate) may allow the bacteria more time to attach, multiply, and cause injury. Here, bacterial virulence factors are important, and *E coli* is the prototype UTI pathogen. Fewer than 10 *E coli* clones (whether characterized as serotypes or sequence types) account for the majority of UTI cases, and these UTI clones are not the most common ones in the fecal flora. These *E coli* with enhanced potential to produce UTI are called **uropathogenic** *E coli* (**UPEC**).

The ability of UPEC to produce UTI begins with type 1 pili, which are the most important for both periurethral and bladder colonization. The tips of such pili attach to mannose moieties presented by membrane proteins (uroplakins) in the transitional epithelium of the bladder. Other pili such as P pili may add to the strength of this attachment; however, because their cognate Gal–Gal receptor is most abundant in the renal pelvis and kidney, P pili are more important for upper urinary tract disease. Strains possessing P pili are a minor percentage of fecal *E coli* (<20%), but the proportion of P⁺ strains progressively rises with the severity of UTI, reaching 70%

Minor trauma admits *E coli* to the bladder

UPEC cause most UTIs

FIGURE 33–4. **Urinary tract infection due to *Escherichia coli*.** Features of the lower female urinary tract, including the bladder, perineal mucosa, and urethra, are shown. *E coli* from the nearby rectal flora have colonized the perineum, utilizing binding by type 1 (common) pili. Also present are *E coli* with P pili, though these adhesins are of no use at this site. **A.** A few *E coli* have gained access to the bladder owing to mechanical disruptions, such as sexual intercourse or instrumentation (catheters). Note that receptors for the P pili, absent on the perineal mucosa, are found on the surface of bladder mucosal cells. **B.** During voiding, the bladder has expelled the *E coli*, which have only type 1 pili. The P pili-containing bacteria remain behind due to the strong binding to the P (Gal–Gal) receptor. **C.** The remaining *E coli* have multiplied and are causing a UTI (cystitis) with inflammation and hemorrhage. In some cases, the bacteria ascend the ureter to cause pyelonephritis in the kidney, where the P (Gal–Gal) receptor is most abundant. WBCs, white blood cells.

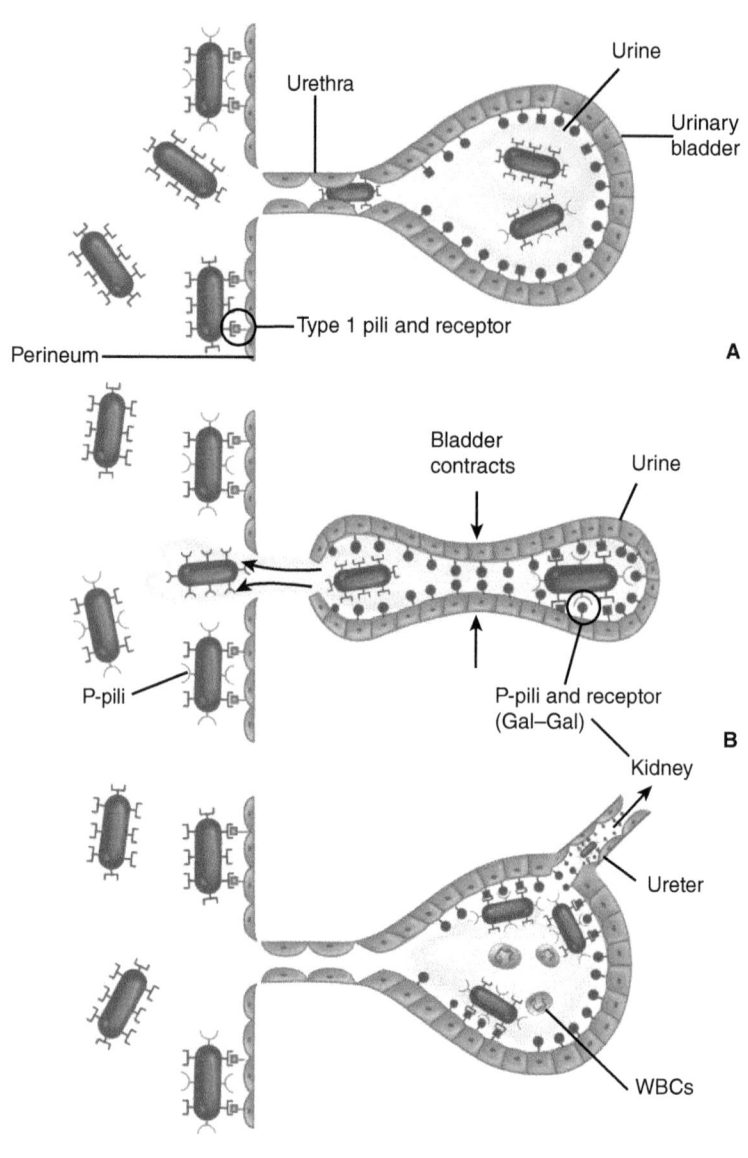

✳ Type 1 pili adhere to periurethral and bladder cells

P pili prominent in pyelonephritis

among pyelonephritis isolates. Motility driven by flagellar motors also plays a role both in access to the bladder and swimming up the ureter to the kidney. Because adherence and motility operate at cross purposes, UPEC reciprocally regulate these features with on/off switching of fimbrial expression. But even with type 1 fimbriae switched on, UPEC can alternate between swimming and adherent phases due to the catch-bond properties of the tip adhesin. Another pathogenic feature of UPEC is the ability to invade superficial epithelial cells. The raft-like clusters formed by this maneuver have been proposed to aid persistence against the periodic flushing of the bladder. Once bacteria are established, LPS and the production of other virulence factors such as α-hemolysin and CNF cause injury. Spread to the bloodstream leads to LPS-induced septic shock. The adherence aspects of UPEC are illustrated in **Figure 33–4**.

OTHER EXTRAINTESTINAL INFECTIONS

■ Meningitis

E coli is one of the most common causes of neonatal meningitis, producing many features similar to group B streptococcal disease. The pathogenesis involves colonization of the infant with maternal *E coli* via ruptured amniotic membranes or during childbirth. Failure of protective maternal IgM antibodies to cross the placenta and the immunologic immaturity of newborns surely play a role. Fully 75% of cases of newborn meningitis are caused by strains possessing the sialic

✳ From vaginal flora-like group B strep

acid-containing K1 capsular polysaccharide, which is structurally identical to the group B poly-saccharide of *Neisseria meningitidis*, another cause of meningitis.

With the exception of UTIs, extraintestinal *E coli* infections are uncommon unless there is a significant breach in host defenses. Opportunistic infection may follow mechanical damage, such as trauma or a ruptured intestinal diverticulum, or involve a generalized impairment of immune function. The virulence factors involved are likely the same as with UTI (eg, pili, α-hemolysin), but have been less specifically studied. Host failure to control local infection can lead to spread and eventually Gram-negative septic shock. A significant proportion of blood isolates have the K1 surface polysaccharide. The particular diseases that result depend on the sites involved.

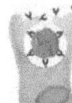 ## *E COLI* INTESTINAL INFECTIONS

Diarrheal illnesses continue to produce a tremendous mortality burden worldwide, particularly in children under 5 years of age, with the largest numbers of deaths occurring in sub-Saharan Africa and South Asia. *E coli* and *Shigella* (which are specialized *E coli*) are among the top causes of moderate-to-severe diarrhea among children in these areas. Diarrhea-causing *E coli* are classi-fied according to their virulence properties as **enterotoxigenic (ETEC), enteropathogenic (EPEC), enteroinvasive (EIEC), enterohemorrhagic (EHEC),** or **enteroaggregative (EAEC).** Each group causes disease by a different mechanism, and the resulting syndromes usually differ clinically and epidemiologically. For example, ETEC and EIEC strains infect only humans. Food and water contaminated with human waste and person-to-person contact are the principal means of infection. A summary of the pathogenesis of infection, clinical syndromes, and epidemiology of infection for each enteropathogen is shown in Table 33–1.

ENTEROTOXIGENIC *E COLI*

■ Epidemiology

Enterotoxigenic *E coli* (ETEC) produce diarrhea in infants in developing countries, where they are a leading cause of morbidity and mortality during the first 2 years of life. ETEC is also the most important cause of traveler's diarrhea in visitors to these countries. Repeated bouts of diar-rhea caused by ETEC and other infectious agents are an important cause of growth retardation, malnutrition, and developmental delay in developing countries where ETEC are endemic. ETEC disease is rare in industrialized nations, although recent outbreaks suggest that it may be underestimated.

Transmission is by consumption of food and water contaminated by infected human or conva-lescent carriers. Uncooked foods such as salads or marinated meats and vegetables are associated with the greatest risk. Direct person-to-person transmission is unusual because the infecting dose is high. Animals are not involved in ETEC disease.

■ Pathogenesis

ETEC diarrhea is caused by strains of *E coli* that produce LT and/or ST enterotoxins in the proxi-mal small intestine. ST seems to be more potent than LT, and strains that elaborate both cause the most severe illness. Adherence to surface microvilli, mediated by multiple variants of colonizing factor (CF) pili, is essential for the efficient delivery of toxin to the target enterocytes. The genes encoding the ST, LT, and the CF pili are borne on plasmids; a single plasmid can carry all three sets of genes. The bacteria remain on the epithelial surface, where the adenylate cyclase-stimulating action of the toxin(s) creates the flow of water and electrolytes from the enterocyte into the intes-tinal lumen. The mucosa becomes hyperemic but is not injured in the process. There is no inva-sion or inflammation.

■ Immunity

Although infections with ETEC do stimulate immunity, individuals may experience more than one episode of ETEC diarrhea. Travelers from industrialized nations have a much higher attack rate than adults living in the endemic area. This natural immunity is presumably mediated by sIgA specific for LT and CFs; the small ST peptides are nonimmunogenic. The disease is of very low incidence in breastfed infants, underscoring the protective effect of maternal antibody and the importance of transmission by contaminated food and water.

* K1 capsule identical to meningococcus

* Non-UTI infections require breach of defenses

* Several pathogenic mechanisms have distinctive epidemiologic and clinical features

* Traveler's diarrhea affects children in developing countries

High dose in uncooked foods required

* LT and/or ST cause fluid outpouring in small intestine

CF pili are required

sIgA to LT and CFs may provide some protection

ENTEROPATHOGENIC *E COLI*

■ Epidemiology

Enteropathogenic *E coli* (EPEC) strains were first identified as the cause of explosive outbreaks of diarrhea in hospital nurseries in the United States and Great Britain during the 1950s. The link to *E coli* was established on epidemiologic grounds alone, using serotyping of stool isolates—no small task. In 1987, the World Health Organization recognized a group of 12 EPEC serotypes that remain of epidemiologic significance. The disease seems to have disappeared in industrialized nations, although it may be underestimated because of the diagnostic challenges. In developing countries throughout the world, EPEC account for up to 20% of diarrheal illnesses in bottle-fed infants younger than 1 year of age. The reservoir is infant cases and adult carriers, with transmission by the fecal–oral route. Nursery outbreaks demonstrate the importance of spread by fomites, suggesting that the infecting dose for infants is low. Adult cases are felt to require a very high infecting dose (10^8 to 10^{10} bacteria).

Nursery outbreaks and endemic diarrheas in developing world

■ Pathogenesis

Enteropathogenic *E coli* initially attach to small intestine enterocytes using **bundle-forming pili (Bfp)** to form clustered microcolonies on the enterocyte cell surface. The lesion then progresses with localized degeneration of the brush border, loss of the microvilli, and changes in the cell morphology including the production of dramatic "pedestals" with the EPEC bacterium at their apex. These actions in combination result in the **attachment and effacing (A/E)** lesion (**Figure 33–5**). The many steps involved in the formation of the A/E lesion are genetically controlled in a PAI, which includes the genes for the major EPEC attachment protein, **intimin,** and an injection (type III) secretion system. The secretion system injects over 30 *E coli* **secretion proteins (Esps)** into the host cell cytoplasm, including—remarkably—the surface receptor (Tir) for intimin, which migrates to the surface after its injection. The other *E coli* secretion proteins perturb intracellular signal transduction pathways, one effect of which is the induction of modifications in enterocyte cytoskeleton proteins actin and talin. The cytoskeleton accumulates beneath the attached bacteria to form the pedestals and complete the actin-rich A/E lesion (**Figure 33–6**). The Esps cause a host of other intracellular disruptions, including mitochondrial injury and induction of apoptosis. The link between the morphologic changes of the A/E lesion and diarrhea is not known, but the injected Esps have been shown to change electrolyte transport across the luminal membrane.

✳ Intimin receptor and Esps are injected

✳ Cytoskeleton modification produces A/E lesion

■ Immunity

In endemic areas, EPEC can be isolated often from the stool of asymptomatic adults, but unlike ETEC, these strains do not seem to cause traveler's diarrhea in individuals new to the area. This observation obscures whether adults have acquired immunity or resistance based on physiologic factors.

Little evidence for immunity

FIGURE   33–5. **Enteropathogenic** *Escherichia coli* **(EPEC) attachment to epithelial cells.** The EPEC are attaching to and effacing the microvilli on the epithelial cell surface. The cell's filamentous actin is rearranged at the attachment point. Note the pedestal below the EPEC cell.

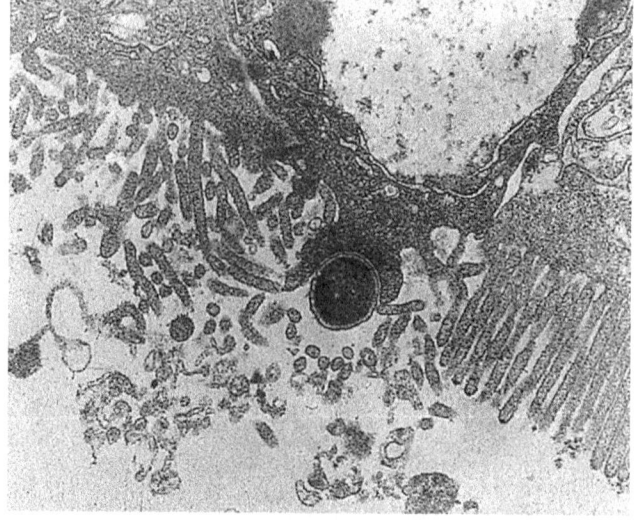

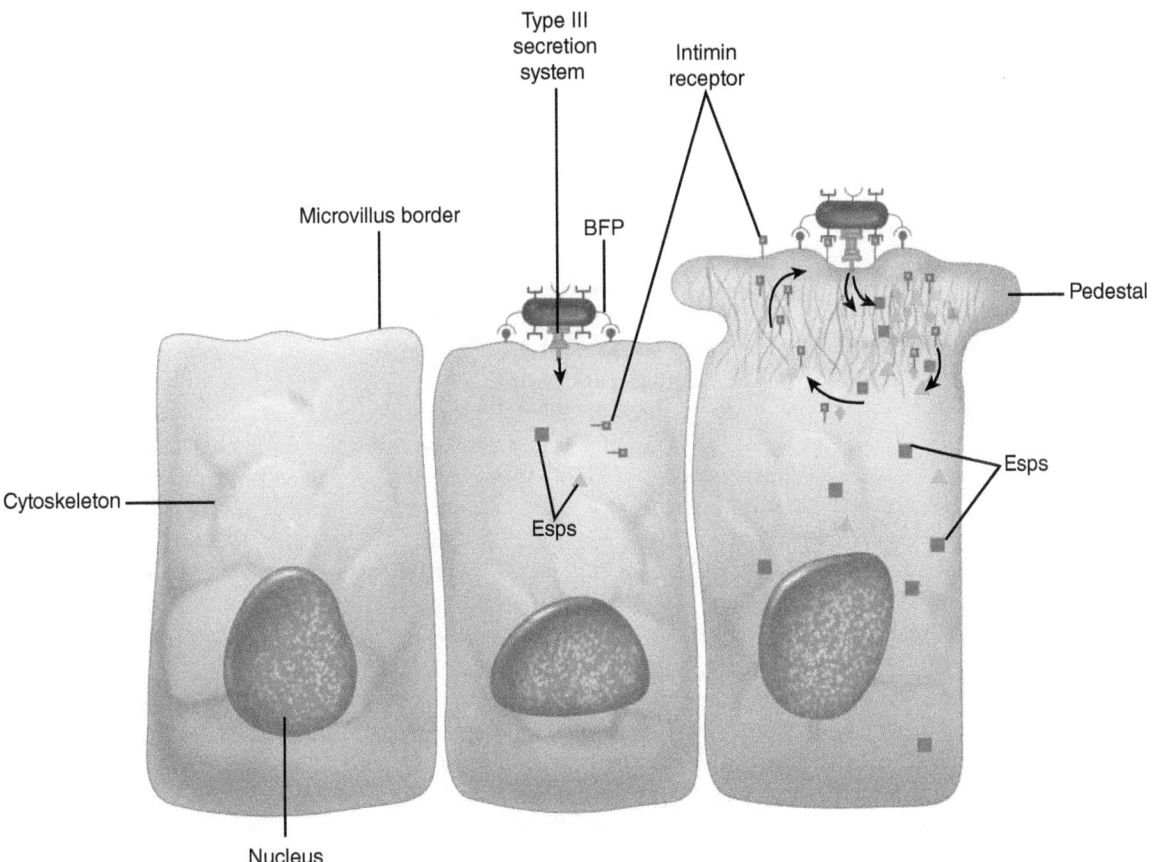

FIGURE 33–6. Enteropathogenic *Escherichia coli* (EPEC) contact secretion system. (*Left*) An enterocyte is shown with a microvillus border and a delicate supporting cytoskeleton. (*Middle*) An EPEC has attached to the cell surface by binding of the bundle-forming pili to receptors on the host cell surface. A type III secretion system apparatus has been inserted into the cell and is exporting secretion proteins (Esps) into the cytoplasm. One of these is the receptor for intimin. (*Right*) The intimin receptor has been inserted below the host cell membrane and is now mediating tight binding to the surface. The other Esps have disrupted multiple cellular functions, including the structure of the cytoskeleton. Cytoskeleton elements have been concentrated to form a pedestal cradling the EPEC (Figure 33–5). Bfp, bundle-forming pili.

ENTEROHEMORRHAGIC *E COLI*

■ Epidemiology

Enterohemorrhagic *E coli* (EHEC) disease and the associated **hemolytic uremic syndrome (HUS)** result from the consumption of products from animals colonized with EHEC strains. It is also clear from secondary cases in families during outbreaks that person-to-person transmission also occurs. This disease occurs more in developed than developing countries.

EHEC was first recognized when outbreaks of HUS (hemolytic anemia, renal failure, and thrombocytopenia) were linked to a single *E coli* serotype, O157:H7. Since then, EHEC disease has emerged as an important cause of **bloody diarrhea** in industrialized nations and retained a remarkable, though not exclusive, relationship with the O157:H7 serotype. Regional and national outbreaks associated with ground beef, unpasteurized juices, and fresh vegetables often catch the attention of the public, the press, and the government, and at times bring renewed scrutiny to food safety policies and practices in public and private sectors.

The emergence of EHEC is related to its virulence, low infecting dose, common reservoir (cattle), and changes in the modern food processing industry that provide fresher meat (and bacteria) over wider distribution networks. The infecting dose, estimated to be as low as 100 organisms, is particularly important. This is a level at which food need not come directly from the infected animal, but only be contaminated by it. For example, large modern meat-processing plants can mix EHEC from colonized cattle at one ranch into beef from hundreds of other farms and quickly ship it all over the country. Therefore, the worst outbreaks have been seen in

Consumption of contaminated animal products the main source

✴ Bloody diarrhea and HUS linked to O157:H7

✴ Low infecting dose facilitates transmission

countries with the most advanced food production and distribution systems. If the organisms are ground into hamburger meat, an infecting dose of EHEC may remain even after cooking if the meat is left rare in the middle. Unpasteurized milk carries an obvious risk, but fruits and vegetables have also been the source for EHEC infection. In these instances, the EHEC from the manure of cattle grazing nearby has contaminated fruit in the field. The bacterial dose from a few "drop" apples (those picked up from the ground) included in a batch of cider has been enough to cause disease.

■ Pathogenesis

EHEC strains cause the A/E lesions previously described for EPEC, but also produce the Stx toxin. The EHEC pathotype, which was first described in O157:H7 strains in 1982, is proposed to have evolved by an EPEC acquiring the genes for Stx via prophage. Apparently, the injection secretion system which creates the A/E pedestals also facilitates delivery of Stx to the enterocyte. Stx secretion is regulated through a quorum-sensing system which awaits a critical EHEC population to activate. The interaction of EHEC with enterocytes is much the same as that of EPEC, except that EHEC strains do not form localized microcolonies on the mucosa and have their own adhesive pili (long polar fimbriae [Lpf]), which mediate attachment in the colon rather than the small intestine. The outer membrane protein intimin mediates tight adherence, and the injection secretion system introduces the *E coli* secretion proteins, which cause alterations in the host cytoskeleton. The genes for these properties are also found in a PAI. The multiple extraintestinal features such as HUS are the result of circulating Stx.

The A/E features alone are sufficient to cause nonbloody diarrhea. On top of this, Stx production causes capillary thrombosis and inflammation of the colonic mucosa, leading to a hemorrhagic colitis. (The distinctive association between shiga toxin and bloody diarrhea has given rise to the term STEC, or shiga toxin-producing *E coli*, as an alternate pathotype descriptor for EHEC.) Although it has not been detected in the blood of human cases, Stx is presumed to be absorbed across denuded intestinal mucosa. Circulating Stx binds to renal tissue, where its glycoprotein receptor globotriaosylceramide (Gb3) is particularly abundant, causing glomerular swelling and the deposition of fibrin and platelets in the microvasculature. How Stx causes hemolysis is less clear; perhaps the erythrocytes are simply damaged as they attempt to traverse the occluded capillaries. Cases and outbreaks caused by Stx-producing *E coli* of other serotypes are common in many countries.

ENTEROINVASIVE *E COLI*

The biochemistry, genetics, and pathogenesis of enteroinvasive *E coli* (EIEC) strains are so close to those of *Shigella* that our understanding of EIEC disease is generally extrapolated from that genus—EIEC disease is essentially a mild version of shigellosis. Epidemiologically, EIEC infections are primarily seen in children younger than 5 years living in developing countries. The occasional documented outbreaks in industrialized nations are usually linked to contaminated food or water. There is a lower incidence of person-to-person transmission of EIEC, which correlates with the observation that the infecting dose is higher than it is for *Shigella*. Humans are the only known reservoir.

ENTEROAGGREGATIVE *E COLI*

Enteroaggregative *E coli* (EAEC) is associated with a protracted (>14 days) watery diarrhea that occasionally features blood and mucus. First recognized in infants and children in developing countries, EAEC is increasingly diagnosed in a variety of community settings. EAEC strains are identified by the "stacked brick" pattern the bacteria make when adhering to cultured mammalian cells. The EAEC pili (aggregative adherence fimbriae [AAF]) mediate tight adherence to the intestinal mucosa, but the A/E lesions of the EPEC and EHEC are not present. The pathogenesis of diarrhea involves formation of a thick mucus–bacteria biofilm on the intestinal surface.

This view of EAEC was dramatically altered by a 2011 German outbreak of serotype O104:H4 initially thought to be caused by EHEC based on clinical features. There were a thousand cases of bloody diarrhea and 53 deaths due to HUS, but the rate of HUS development was twice that typical for EHEC disease. It turned out that the responsible strain had all the essential features of EAEC, but with the addition of Stx genes. There was no injection secretion system or A/E lesions.

---

* Modern meat processing facilitates outbreaks

* Unpasteurized beverages another risk

* Produce both A/E lesions and Stx

* Quorum-sensing regulates Stx

Lesions are in colon

* Stx causes capillary thrombosis and inflammation

* Circulating Stx leads to HUS

* EIEC closely resemble *Shigella*

Adherence and biofilm cause diarrhea

Apparently, the tight adherence of EAEC provided a particularly effective mechanism for delivery of Stx to the intestinal mucosa.

✳ Outbreak strain acquired Stx genes

E COLI INFECTIONS: CLINICAL ASPECTS

MANIFESTATIONS

■ Extraintestinal Infections

The most common symptoms of *E coli* UTI are dysuria and urinary frequency – as they are for UTI produced by the other, less common Gram-negative urinary pathogens. If the infecting bacteria ascend the ureters to produce pyelonephritis, fever and flank pain are common and bacteremia may develop. Although *E coli* may have enhanced virulence in the production of pneumonia as well as soft tissue and other infections, no clinical features distinguish these cases from those caused by other members of the Enterobacteriaceae.

✳ Dysuria and frequency are features of UTIs

 If the EHEC diarrhea is bloody, why would fever not be more prominent?

■ Intestinal Infections

Infection caused by any *E coli* intestinal pathotype usually begins with a mild watery diarrhea starting 2 to 4 days after ingestion of an infectious dose. In most instances, the duration of diarrhea is limited to a few days, with the exception of EAEC diarrhea, which can last for weeks. With ETEC and EPEC, the diarrhea remains watery, but with EIEC and EHEC, a dysenteric illness follows. Some EPEC cases may also become chronic. EHEC disease begins like the others but often also includes vomiting; in 90% of cases, this is followed in 1 to 2 days by intense abdominal pain and bloody diarrhea, but fever is not prominent. Some EHEC cases develop into a dysentery illness that is less severe than that seen in shigellosis. Colonoscopy reveals edema, hemorrhage, and pseudomembrane formation. Resolution usually takes place over a 3- to 10-day period, with few residual effects on the bowel mucosa.

✳ ETEC and EPEC diarrhea is watery

✳ EIEC and EHEC diarrhea is bloody

HUS develops as a complication in 5% to 10% of cases of EHEC hemorrhagic colitis, primarily in children under 10 years of age. The disease begins with decreased urine output, edema, and pallor, progressing to the triad of microangiopathic hemolytic anemia, thrombocytopenia, and renal failure. The systemic effects are often life-threatening, requiring transfusion and hemodialysis for survival. The mortality rate is 5%, and up to 30% of those who survive suffer sequelae such as renal impairment or hypertension.

✳ HUS begins as oliguria and may progress to renal failure

DIAGNOSIS

Like the rest of the Enterobacteriaceae, *E coli* is readily isolated in culture. In UTIs, the bacteria typically reach high numbers (>10⁵/mL), which makes them readily detectable by Gram stain even in an unspun urine specimen (**Figure 33–7**). For the diagnosis of intestinal disease, separating the virulent types discussed previously from the numerous other *E coli* strains universally found in stool presents a special problem. A myriad of immunoassay and nucleic acid amplification methods have been described that are able to detect the toxins (LT, ST, Stx) or genes associated with virulence. These methods work but their clinical use is hampered by limited positive predictive value—healthy persons may also have positive test results with these methods—and high cost, especially in developing countries where ETEC, EIEC, EPEC, and EAEC are prevalent. A screening test for EHEC takes advantage of the observation that the O157:H7 serotype typically fails to ferment sorbitol. Incorporating sorbitol in place of lactose in MacConkey agar provides an

Bacterial counts in urine are high

Diarrhea requires immunoassay or gene probe

 Think ▸▸ Apply 33-1: The blood in the stool in EHEC is due to the action of Stx and not due to destruction of enterocytes. It usually takes cellular destruction to cause inflammation and thus fever. This is a feature of shigellosis (see below).

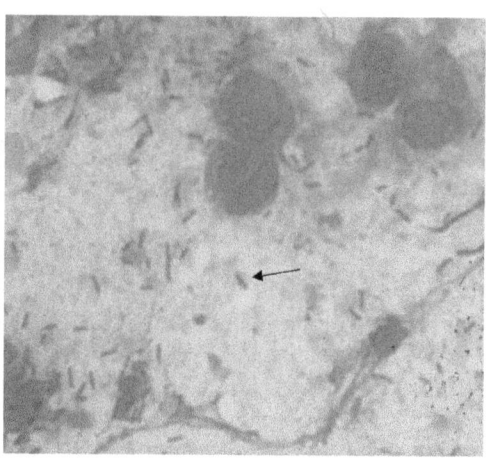

FIGURE 33–7. *Escherichia coli* **urinary tract infection.** The ready observation of the large Gram-negative bacilli (such as that indicated by the arrow) and WBCs in a drop of unspun urine indicates the number of bacteria in the urine is high. (Used with permission from Professor Shirley Lowe, University of California, San Francisco School of Medicine.)

✳ Sorbitol agar screens for O157:H7

indicator medium from which suspect (colorless) colonies can be selected and then confirmed with O157 antisera. This procedure has become routine in areas where EHEC is endemic but does not detect the non-O157 EHEC strains.

TREATMENT

Acute uncomplicated UTIs are often treated empirically. Because of widespread resistance to earlier agents like ampicillin, use of trimethoprim/sulfamethoxazole (TMP-SMX) and fluoroquinolones for this purpose rose steadily. In turn, use of these agents set the stage for the rise of international multidrug-resistant clones like *E coli* Sequence Type 131, which wields chromosome-encoded fluoroquinolone resistance and plasmid-borne resistance to TMP-SMX, gentamicin and, not infrequently, extended-spectrum cephalosporins. Thus, in many clinical settings domestically and abroad, *E coli* resistance to these latter agents has now exceeded the 20% level used to indicate the suitability of antibiotics for empiric use. In cases of empiric treatment failure, selection of other antimicrobials must be guided by antimicrobial susceptibility testing of the patient's isolate.

Resistance patterns influence antimicrobial selection

Antibiotics may shorten symptoms for ETEC, EIEC, and EPEC

✳ Antibiotics may increase risk of HUS in EHEC

Because most *E coli* diarrheas are mild and self-limiting, treatment is usually not required. When it is, rehydration and supportive measures are the mainstays of therapy, regardless of the causative agent. In the case of EHEC with hemorrhagic colitis and HUS, heroic supportive measures such as hemodialysis or plasmapheresis may be required. Treatment with TMP-SMX or fluoroquinolones reduces the duration of diarrhea in ETEC, EIEC, and EPEC infection. However, because the risk of HUS may be increased by the use of antimicrobial agents, their use is contraindicated when EHEC is even suspected. Antimotility agents are not helpful and are contraindicated when EIEC or EHEC could be the etiologic agent.

PREVENTION

✳ Avoid uncooked foods

✳ Chemoprophylaxis works for defined periods

Traveler's diarrhea is usually little more than an inconvenience. Because the infecting dose is high, the incidence of the disease can be greatly reduced by eating only cooked foods and peeled fruits and drinking hot or carbonated beverages. Avoiding nonbottled water, ice, salads, and raw vegetables is a wise precaution when traveling in developing countries. High-priced hotel accommodations have no protective effect. Chemoprophylaxis against traveler's diarrhea is not routinely recommended, and in fact may increase risk of intestinal colonization with multidrug-resistant Enterobacteriaceae encountered abroad. Short courses of TMP-SMX or ciprofloxacin (<2 weeks) have been recommended for those at high risk for disease resulting from such chronic conditions as achlorhydria, gastric resection, prolonged use of H_2 blockers or antacids, and underlying immunosuppressive diseases.

✳ Rare hamburgers carry risk for EHEC

These public health measures apply equally to EHEC, but here prevention is more difficult because the infecting dose is so low. Cooking hamburgers all the way through is sensible, but abstinence from salads at home has only been recommended in defined outbreak scenarios associated with romaine lettuce. Recent U.S. recommendations for the irradiation of meats and the extension of pasteurization requirements to fruit juices are designed largely to stem the spread of EHEC.

● SHIGELLA

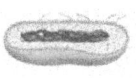

BACTERIOLOGY

Shigella species may be considered specialized *E coli*. Their antigenic makeup has been character-ized in a manner similar to that of *E coli*, with the exception that they lack flagella (and thus H antigens). All *Shigella* species are nonmotile. The genus is divided into four species, which are defined by biochemical reactions and specific O antigens organized into serogroups. The species are *Shigella dysenteriae* (serogroup A), *Shigella flexneri* (serogroup B), *Shigella boydii* (serogroup C), and *Shigella sonnei* (serogroup D). All but *S sonnei* are further subdivided, producing a total of 38 indi-vidual O antigen serotypes specified by numbers. *Shigella* is the prototype invasive bacterial patho-gen. All species are able to invade and multiply inside a wide variety of epithelial cells, including their natural target, the enterocyte. *Shigella dysenteriae* type 1, the Shiga bacillus, is the most potent producer of Stx. Other *Shigella* species produce various molecular forms and quantities of Stx.

✳ O antigens and biochemicals define four species

✳ Invasiveness and Stx production are virulence factors

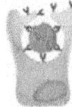

SHIGELLOSIS ⚕

EPIDEMIOLOGY

Shigellosis is a strictly human disease with no animal reservoirs. Worldwide, it is consistently one of the most common causes of infectious diarrhea, with over 150 million cases and 600,000 deaths per year. As with almost all infectious diarrheas, the incidence is related to general levels of sani-tation, but *Shigella* disease remains important in both developed and developing countries. This high prevalence despite lack of a nonhuman reservoir is primarily due to highly efficient trans-mission by the fecal–oral route. This spread by person-to-person contact is so effective because the infecting dose is extremely low, as few as 10 organisms in some studies. The secondary attack rates among family members are as high as 40%. *Shigella* is also spread by food or water contam-inated by human waste products.

✳ Strictly human disease

✳ Low infecting dose facilitates fecal–oral spread

The incidence and spread of shigellosis are directly related to individual- and community-level behaviors and practices. In developed countries, shigellosis has often been seen as a pediatric disease producing daycare-associated outbreaks, as well as an adult syndrome in men who have sex with men. In countries where the sanitary infrastructure is inadequate and in institutions plagued by crowding and poor hygienic conditions, the disease may be more widespread; war-time and natural disasters create similar circumstances. The most common species are *S flexneri* and *S sonnei*, with *S dysenteriae* largely limited to underdeveloped tropical areas. *S dysenteriae* type 1 produces the most severe disease, historically known as "bacillary dysentery." This condi-tion slowed the march of many an army; it was the leading cause of death in the notorious Ander-sonville prison camp during the American Civil War.

✳ Individual behaviors or community sanitary practices determine incidence

✳ Wars and disasters enable outbreaks

PATHOGENESIS

Shigella, unlike *Vibrio cholerae* and most *Salmonella* species, is acid-resistant and survives passage through the stomach to reach the intestine. Once there, the fundamental pathogenic event is invasion and destruction of the human colonic mucosa. This triggers an intense acute inflamma-tory response with mucosal ulceration and abscess formation. The steps involved in this process constitute one of the richest tales in bacterial pathogenesis (**Figure 33–8**). Most pathogenesis research has been done with *S flexneri*, but there is no reason to believe it does not apply equally to the three other species and to EIEC.

✳ *Shigella* pass stomach acid and invade colon

Shigella initially cross the mucosal membrane by entering the follicle-associated M cells of the intestine, which lack the highly organized brush borders of absorptive enterocytes. *Shigella* adhere selectively to M cells, enter, and then transcytose through them into the underlying collection of macrophages. Inside macrophages, the organisms escape from the phagosome to the cytoplasm and activate programmed cell death (apoptosis) in the macrophage. Bacteria released from the dead macrophage contact the basolateral side of enterocytes and initiate a multistep invasion process mediated by a set of **invasion plasmid antigens** (IpaA–IpaD). On contact with the enterocyte, these proteins are injected by an injection (type III)

✳ Transcytose M cells to macrophages

Invade enterocytes from dead macrophages

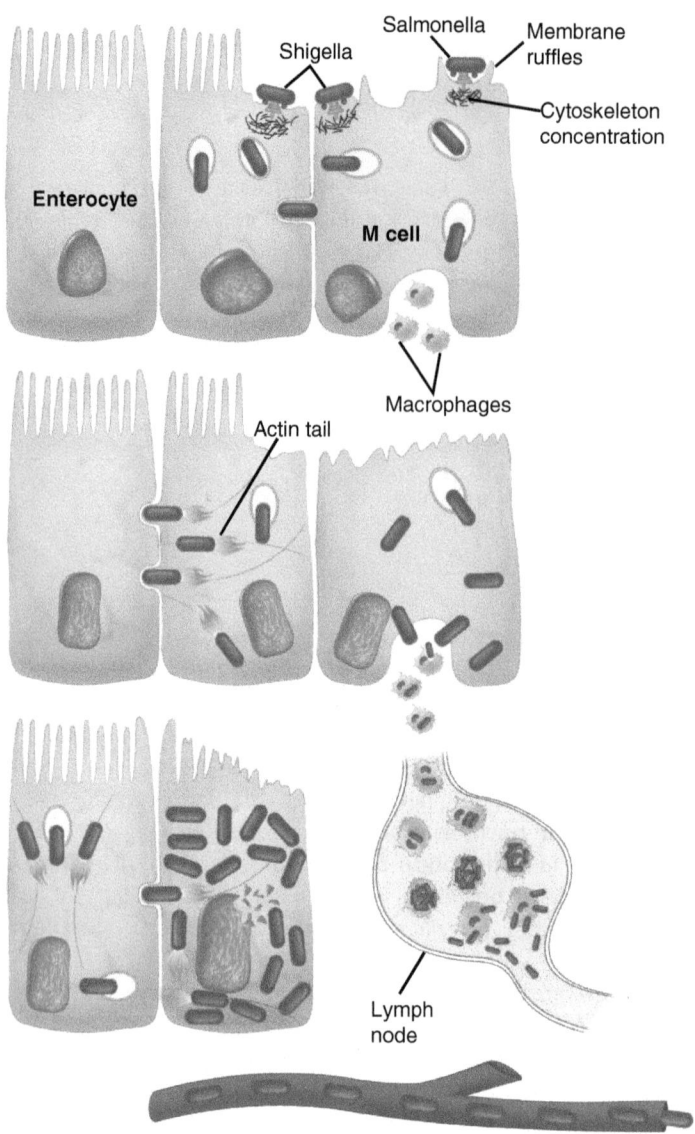

…E 33-8. Invasion by _Shig-a flexneri_ and _Salmonella_ serotype Typhi. _Shigella_ and _Salmonella_ are shown invading the intestinal M cells but taking different paths after escaping the endocytotic vacuole. The _Shigella_ multiplies in the cell and propels itself through the cytoplasm to invade adjacent cells, and the _Salmonella_ passes through the cell to the submucosa, where it is taken up by macrophages. Serovar Typhi is able to multiply in the macrophages in the lymph node and other reticuloendothelial sites. Both organisms induce apoptosis in their host cells. In the case of _Shigella_, this produces a mucosal ulcer; in the case of Typhi, it leads to seeding of the bloodstream and typhoid fever.

Injected Ipa proteins induce endocytosis

❋ Escape phagosome to cytoplasm

❋ Polymerization of cytoskeletal actin propels bacteria

Microtubules are digested

Adjacent enterocytes are invaded directly

Double-membrane lysis restarts process

secretion system and induce cytoskeleton reorganization, actin polymerization, and other changes, particularly at the cell surface. Rather than create the A/E lesions of the EPEC and EHEC, this cytoskeleton modification process induces engulfment and internalization of _Shigella_ into the host cell by endocytosis.

Shigella are highly adapted to the intracellular environment and make unique use of it to continue the infection. Although initially the bacteria are surrounded by a phagocytic vacuole, they quickly escape and enter the cytoplasmic compartment of the host cell. Almost immediately, they orient in parallel with the filaments of the cell's actin cytoskeleton and initiate a process in which they control polymerization of the monomers that make up the actin fibrils. This process creates an actin "tail" at one end of the microbe, which appears to propel it through the cytoplasm like a comet. This exploitation of the cytoskeletal apparatus allows nonmotile _Shigella_ to not only replicate in the cell but to move efficiently through it. Apparently, the cell's microtubule network is an obstruction, so the bacteria produce an enzyme that digests this. One microbiologist called this strategy "bushwhacking through a microtubule jungle."

Eventually, the bacteria encounter the host cell membrane, much of which is adjacent to the neighboring enterocytes. At this point, some _Shigella_ rebound but others push the membrane as much as 20 μm into the adjacent cell; this invasion of the neighboring enterocyte forms finger-like projections, which eventually pinch off, placing the bacterium within a new cell but surrounded by a double membrane. The organisms then lyse both membranes and are released into the cytoplasm, free to begin their relentless invasion anew.

The cell-by-cell extension of this process radially destroys enterocytes and creates focal ulcers in the mucosa, particularly in the colon. The ulcers add a hemorrhagic component and allow *Shigella* to reach the lamina propria, where they evoke an intense acute inflammatory response. Extension of the infection beyond the lamina (for example, to the bloodstream) is unusual in healthy individuals. The diarrhea created by this process is almost purely inflammatory, consisting of small-volume stools containing WBCs, RBCs, bacteria, and little else—this is classic dysentery.

⁑ **Enterocyte invasion creates ulcers**

⁑ **Diarrhea + WBCs + RBCs = dysentery**

Some *Shigella* also produce Stx, which is not essential for disease but does contribute to the severity of the illness. The original and most potent producer of Stx, *S dysenteriae* type 1, is the only *Shigella* with a significant mortality rate in previously healthy individuals. This is probably due to systemic effects of the toxin, which can be the same as previously described for the EHEC, including HUS. The role, if any, of Stx in enterocyte injury and diarrhea is uncertain.

⁑ **Stx increases severity of disease**

All virulent *Shigella* and EIEC carry a very large plasmid that has several genes essential for the attachment and entry process, including the Ipa genes. The characteristics of *Shigella* entry and interaction with cellular elements are very similar to those observed with *Listeria monocytogenes*, which is Gram-positive and motile and prefers livestock to humans. Finding that such dissimilar bacteria use such similar tactics to infect their preferred host suggests commonality among the selective pressures on a microbe to become a "successful" enteric pathogen (convergent evolution).

⁑ **Large plasmid containing Ipa genes required for virulence**

IMMUNITY

Episodes of *Shigella* infection produce modest immunologic protection against infection by homologous serotypes, but do not significantly protect against other serotypes. Recently, large-scale epidemiologic studies have elucidated the predominant *Shigella* serogroups responsible for the major burden of disease, invigorating the prospects for design of a multivalent vaccine.

Immunity is brief

 ## SHIGELLOSIS: CLINICAL ASPECTS

MANIFESTATIONS

Shigella organisms cause an acute inflammatory colitis and bloody diarrhea, which in the most characteristic state presents as a dysentery syndrome—a clinical triad consisting of cramps, painful straining to pass stools (tenesmus), and a frequent, small-volume, bloody, mucoid fecal discharge. However, most clinical shigellosis due to *S sonnei* is a watery diarrhea that is often indistinguishable from that of other bacterial or viral diarrheal illness. The disease usually begins with fever and systemic manifestations of malaise, anorexia, and sometimes myalgia. These nondescript symptoms are followed by the onset of watery diarrhea containing the large numbers of leukocytes detectable by light microscopy. The diarrhea may turn bloody with or without the other classic signs of dysentery. The manifestations may be more severe when *S flexneri*, the species that predominates in the developing world, is involved and most severe with *S dysenteriae* type 1 (Shiga bacillus). Although most cases of shigellosis resolve spontaneously after 2 to 5 days, the mortality rate in Shiga epidemics in Asia, Latin America, and Africa has been as high as 20%.

⁑ **Watery diarrhea followed by fever, bloody mucoid stools, and cramping**

⁑ **Mortality significant with *S dysenteriae* type 1**

⁑ **Most infections self-limiting**

 Why is *Shigella* so potent in producing epidemics in conditions of poor sanitation or natural disaster?

DIAGNOSIS

All *Shigella* species are readily isolated using selective media (eg, Hektoen enteric agar) that are part of the routine stool culture protocol in all clinical laboratories. These media contain chemical

 Think ▸▸ Apply 33-2: Epidemics with most enteric pathogens require widespread distribution in food (*Listeria*, EHEC). This also occurs with *Shigella,* but in addition, its resistance to gastric acid and low infecting dose facilitates human-to-human transmission by direct contact. This is magnified when basic sanitation is compromised (war, natural disaster) or nonexistent.

additives shown to inhibit facultative flora (eg, *E coli*, *Klebsiella*) with relatively little effect on *Shigella* (or *Salmonella*). They also contain indicator systems that use typical biochemical reactions to mark suspect *Shigella* colonies among the other flora. Isolates are identified with further biochemical tests. Slide agglutination tests using O group-specific antisera (A, B, C, D) confirm both the species and the *Shigella* genus.

TREATMENT

Though hydration and maintenance or restoration of electrolyte balance remain the cornerstones of management, various antimicrobial agents have been used in the treatment of shigellosis over time. Because the disease is usually self-limiting, the beneficial effect of treatment is in shortening the duration of the illness and the period of excretion of organisms. Ampicillin was once the treatment of choice, but resistance rates as high as 50% have caused a shift to other agents; in recent years, increasing rates of nonsusceptibility to ciprofloxacin, ceftriaxone, and azithromycin have raised grave concerns about the continued effectiveness of these agents. Antispasmodic agents may aggravate the condition and are contraindicated in shigellosis and other invasive diarrheas.

PREVENTION

Standard sanitation practices such as sewage disposal and water chlorination are important in preventing the spread of shigellosis. In certain circumstances, insect control may also be important, because flies can serve as passive vectors when open sewage is present. Good individual sanitary practices, such as handwashing and proper cooking of food, are highly protective. Parenteral vaccines have proved disappointing thus far, particularly in infants. Ongoing efforts encompass development and testing of a wide range of formulations, including live attenuated, formalin-killed whole cell, glycoconjugate, subunit and novel antigen (such as Type III secretion systems and outer membrane protein) vaccines.

● *SALMONELLA*

 ### BACTERIOLOGY

More than any other genus, *Salmonella* has been a favorite of those who love to subdivide and name biologic entities. At one time, there were over 2000 names for various members of this genus, many colorfully reflecting aspects of place or circumstances of the original isolation (eg, *S budapest*, *S seminole*, *S tamale*, *S oysterbeds*). This rich nomenclature has now been streamlined to a single species—*S enterica*—with the previous species names relegated to the status of serovars. Adding to this robust picture is a large number of lipopolysaccharide O antigens, a few capsular K antigens, and flagellar H antigens that undergo phase variation (thus doubling the possible H antigenic states for each strain). As in *Shigella*, the specific O antigens are organized into serogroups (eg, A, B, K, and so on), to which the two H and K (if present) antigen designations are appended to achieve the full antigenic formula. It is not difficult to understand why microbiologists—confronted by a salmonella with the antigenic formula O:group B [1,4,12] H:I;1,2—still prefer to call it *Salmonella typhimurium*. The proper name for this organism is *S enterica* serovar Typhimurium, but indulging in the convenience of elevating the serotype to species status is still common.

Another feature distinguishing *Salmonella* serotypes is their host range. Some are highly adapted to particular mammals or amphibians while others infect a broad range of hosts. Of interest for medical microbiology are those strictly adapted to humans and those that infect humans and other animals. *S enterica* serovar Typhi is the prototype for the former, and *S enterica* serovar Typhimurium the prototype for the latter. In the following discussions, the Typhi descriptor is used for the strictly human species that produce enteric (typhoid) fever. Unless otherwise specified, *S enterica* is used for serotypes such as Typhimurium, which are able to infect animals or humans and typically cause gastroenteritis in the latter.

Salmonellae possess multiple types of pili, one of which is morphologically and functionally similar to *E coli* type 1 pili and binds D-mannose receptors on various eukaryotic cell types. Most strains are motile through the action of their flagella. *S* Typhi has a surface polysaccharide called the Vi antigen, but capsules have not been as important in the other *Salmonella*.

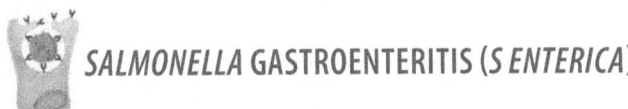 *SALMONELLA* GASTROENTERITIS (*S ENTERICA*)

CLINICAL CAPSULE

The typical example of *Salmonella* "food poisoning" is the community picnic, in which participants prepare poultry, salads, and other potential culture media to be eaten later in the day. Because the refrigerators are filled with beer and soda, the food is left out in covered pans. A near-physiologic incubation temperature is provided by the still-warm contents and the afternoon sun. This allows the organisms to enter logarithmic growth during the softball game. The bacteria usually produce no noticeable change in the food. One to two days after the feast, a significant proportion of the revelers develop abdominal pain, nausea, vomiting, and diarrhea lasting for 3 or 4 days. An investigation points to a particular food, such as potato salad or turkey dressing, exposure to which correlates with both attack rate and severity of illness.

EPIDEMIOLOGY

S enterica gastroenteritis is predominantly a disease of industrialized societies and improper food handling, which allows the transmission from the animal reservoir to humans. The infecting dose of *S enterica* infection varies widely with serotype (from 200 to 10^6 bacteria) but is generally considerably higher than *Shigella*. This makes human-to-human transmission by direct contact unlikely, so these infections are transmitted under conditions in which the bacteria increase their numbers by growth in contaminated foods before ingestion. Achlorhydric individuals or those taking antacids can be infected with smaller inocula. Consistently, salmonellae are a leading cause of foodborne intestinal infection in circumstances like those described in the preceding capsule.

Poultry products, including eggs (infected transovarially), are most often implicated as the vehicle of infection of *Salmonella* gastroenteritis. Food storage and preparation practices that permit growth of bacteria to an infecting dose before ingestion are commonly involved. The incidence in the United States is estimated at 1.35 million illnesses annually (compared to 450,000 illnesses due to *Shigella*), leading to 26,500 hospitalizations and over 400 deaths each year. The number of cases varies seasonally, with peak incidence in summer and fall.

The highest rates of infection are in children under 5 years of age, persons aged 20 to 30, and those older than 70. If one household member becomes infected, the probability that another will become infected approaches 60%. Nearly one-third of all *Salmonella* epidemics occur in nursing homes, hospitals, mental health facilities, and other institutional settings. Increases in the popularity of raw milk have been associated with outbreaks of *Salmonella* (and *Campylobacter*) infection. Exotic pets, including turtles, bearded dragons, and hedgehogs, have also been the source of infection. Humans can also be the source of disease: fully 5% of patients recovering from gastroenteritis still shed the organisms 20 weeks later. Chronic carriers who are food handlers are an important reservoir in the epidemiology of foodborne disease.

In recent years, the number of multistate outbreaks has increased, often through the contamination of foodstuffs during large-scale production at a single plant, as in a 2009 U.S. outbreak involving peanut products and encompassing over 700 cases in 48 states. Efficient interstate and international distribution systems that deliver large amounts of the contaminated food over a wide area facilitate spread, as with a 2013 U.S. outbreak involving chicken products that infected over 600 persons across 29 states and Puerto Rico. Under these conditions, an attack rate as low as 0.5% can still produce many infections because of the large number of persons at risk. It is of concern that relatively small numbers of cases sprinkled over a massive area will be missed by local surveillance systems hampered by chronic budgetary cutbacks.

PATHOGENESIS

Ingested *S enterica* cells that surmount the stomach acid and swim through the intestinal mucous layer eventually reach the small bowel, where they must compete with indigenous host flora and evade enteric defenses. Though it is not clear whether the initial host cell contact there may be

❋ Infecting dose is higher than Shigella

❋ Poultry products are common source

❋ Outbreaks in institutions common

❋ Human carriers a source

❋ Modern food production and delivery systems can spread disease efficiently

FIGURE 33–9. **Salmonella ruffles.** *S* serovar Typhimurium is shown inducing wave-like ruffles on an intestinal M cell. This leads to induction of uptake of the bacteria by the M cell. (Reproduced with permission from Nester EW, Anderson DG, Roberts CE Jr, et al: Microbiology: *A Human Perspective*, 6th ed. New York, NY: McGraw Hill; 2008.)

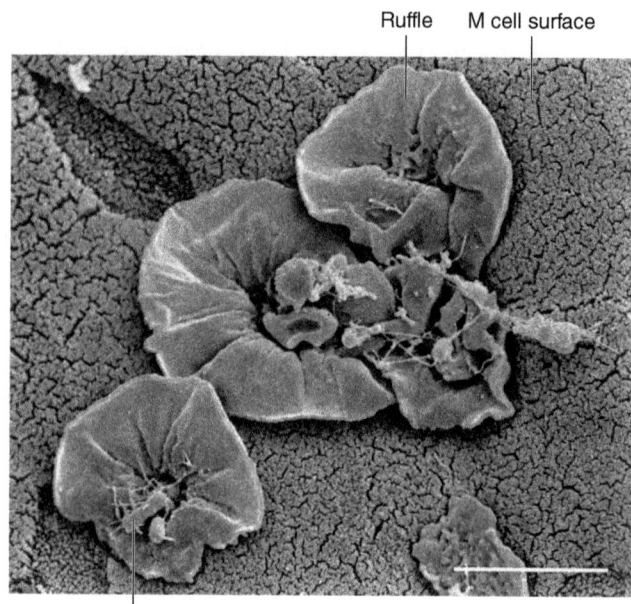

Ruffle   M cell surface

Bacterial cell

* Adherence triggers surface ruffles

* Secretion system genes are in PAIs

with M (microfold) cells, enterocytes, or columnar epithelial cells, the initial adherence is probably mediated by pili. Upon engagement of *S enterica* injection (type III) secretion systems, formation of membrane "ruffles" dramatically alters the normal host cell architecture within minutes (**Figure 33–9**). These ruffles are specialized plasma membrane sites of filamentous actin cytoskeletal rearrangement, normally induced by physiologic molecules such as growth factors. The bacterial secretion systems inject multiple other effectors coded by genes located within PAIs in the *Salmonella* genome; the virulence factors coded by PAI genes are either components of the injection system apparatus itself or the effector proteins it injects.

* Ruffles induce endocytosis

* Macrophage apoptosis aids survival

Persisters may lead to relapse

The ruffles seem to engulf the organism in an endocytic vacuole, permitting it to transcytose from the apical surface to the basolateral membrane. Once in the cell, *S enterica* multiplies in the vacuole and continues on through the cell, entering the lamina propria; there the bacteria typically induce a profound inflammatory response and are phagocytosed by neutrophils and macrophages. Then, by deploying a second injection secretion system from inside the host macrophage, bacteria induce apoptosis, killing the macrophages and thus persisting in the lamina propria. This process contrasts with *Shigella*, which escapes the endocytic vacuole (and double vacuole) to the cytoplasm and prefers to invade adjacent enterocytes rather than move through to the submucosa. Alternatively, *Salmonella* may become nonreplicating persisters within host cells, enacting survival programs induced by vacuolar acidification and nutritional deprivation; subsequent resumption of intracellular growth by these persisters may be the basis for relapsing infection.

* Invasion and inflammation cause diarrhea

Enterotoxin role is unclear

The joint impact of invasion and transcytosis of enterocytes, together with the associated increased vascular permeability and inflammatory response, may account in aggregate for diarrhea. The release of prostaglandins and chemotactic factors may trigger inflammation and biochemical changes in enterocytes. Although the process remains localized to the mucosa and submucosa with most *S enterica* strains, some invade more deeply, reaching the bloodstream and distant organs; some serotypes (eg, *S* ser. Choleraesuis) invade so rapidly that they produce minimal diarrhea and are isolated more frequently from the blood than stool. Although various enterotoxins have been described in *Salmonella*, their role in diarrhea is unclear.

IMMUNITY

Evidence that both humoral and cell-mediated immune responses are stimulated by infection with *S enterica* is ample. *Salmonella* pathogens are also able to exploit some of these responses to compete successfully with resident microbiota and promote their own survival within the host. While several of these host-pathogen interactions have been characterized in great detail, the key determinants in the outcome of infectious episodes (resolution, dissemination, chronic infection) remain to be determined.

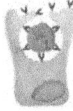 # ENTERIC (TYPHOID) FEVER (*SALMONELLA* SEROVAR TYPHI)

EPIDEMIOLOGY

Typhoid fever is a strictly human disease; chronic carriers of *S* Typhi are the primary reservoir. Some patients become carriers for years (witness the infamous "Typhoid Mary" Mallon), usually because of chronic infection of a biliary tract where gallstones are present. All cases can and should be traced back to their human source; if a patient with typhoid has not traveled to an endemic area, the source must be a visitor or someone else who prepared food. The pathogen can be transmitted in the water supply in endemic areas or anywhere that structural defects allow sewage from carriers to contaminate drinking water. Transmission is by the fecal–oral route. The infecting dose of 10^5 to 10^6 bacteria is intermediate between *Shigella* and most *S enterica*, and Typhi's Vi capsule may further reduce the number of organisms needed to infect. Three serotypes called Paratyphi (A, B, C) have features similar to *S* Typhi, including the production of an enteric fever syndrome; cases are likewise traceable to a human source.

✳ Fecal–oral transmission requires moderate dose

Typhoid fever is still an important cause of morbidity and mortality worldwide, producing 16 million cases and 600,000 deaths a year. In developed countries, it is mostly seen in travelers returning from endemic areas in Latin America, Asia, and India. Visitors from these areas who are carriers are often the source of isolated cases. The decline in disease in industrialized nations largely reflects the availability of clean water supplies and improved disposal of human waste.

✳ Prevalence is linked to sanitation infrastructure

PATHOGENESIS

There is no animal model for the strictly human *S* Typhi. The details of the cellular events are inferred from studies of Typhimurium, which in mice produces a disease similar to typhoid (thus the name). The invasion and killing of intestinal M cells and macrophages are presumed to follow the same pattern as that of *S enterica*, with two key differences: the Vi surface polysaccharide and the extensive multiplication of Typhi in macrophages. In the submucosa, Vi (for virulence) blocks neutrophil phagocytosis by interfering with complement deposition in a manner similar to that of other bacterial surface polysaccharides. This may favor uptake by macrophages, where at least some Typhi cells establish a privileged niche, and the Vi⁺ phenotype in turn favors intracellular multiplication. Like other serotypes of *Salmonella*, Typhi remains within a membrane-bound vacuole, but unlike them, it enters a stage of extended replication rather than killing the macrophage.

✳ Typhi invades M cells and macrophages

✳ Vi polysaccharide limits PMN (neutrophil) phagocytosis

The primary feature distinguishing Typhi from the other serotypes—the prolonged intracellular survival in macrophages—is due to Typhi's ability to inhibit the oxidative metabolic burst and thus continue to multiply. As they proliferate in macrophages, Typhi bacteria are carried through the lymphatic circulation to the mesenteric nodes, spleen, liver, and bone marrow, all elements of the reticuloendothelial system (RES). At the RES sites, Typhi continue to multiply, infecting new host macrophages. Rather than the acute inflammatory response seen with *S enterica*, *S* Typhi generates a mononuclear response so mild as to spare the host from diarrhea; this may be due to the down-regulation of innate toll-like receptor responses in the intestinal mucosa by the Vi antigen.

✳ Macrophage oxidative burst inhibited

✳ Infection spreads through RES

Eventually, the burgeoning bacterial population begins to reach the bloodstream (Figure 33–8). The entry of Gram-negative bacteria and their LPS endotoxin into the blood triggers fever that increases slowly. Continued seeding of *S* Typhi into the blood feeds the fever and sometimes leads to metastatic infection of other organs including the urinary tract and the biliary tree; the latter may ultimately cause reinfection of the bowel. This cycle, beginning and ending in the small intestine, takes approximately 2 weeks to complete.

✳ RES sites seed the bloodstream and other organs

✳ Endotoxin produces the fever

IMMUNITY

Natural infection with *S* Typhi confers immunity; reinfection is rare unless the course was short-ened by early administration of antimicrobials. The immune response is both T_H1- and T_H2-mediated. In nonfatal cases, antibody and activated macrophages eventually subdue untreated infection over a period of about 3 weeks. Which antigens stimulate this immunity is not clearly understood; the Vi antigen is usually credited, but various surface proteins are also candidates.

✳ Immunity follows natural infection

SALMONELLOSIS: CLINICAL ASPECTS

MANIFESTATIONS

The clinical patterns of salmonellosis can be divided into gastroenteritis, bacteremia with or without focal extraintestinal infection, enteric fever, and the asymptomatic carrier state. In principle any *Salmonella* serotype may cause any of these clinical manifestations under appropriate conditions, but in practice the *S enterica* serotypes are mainly associated with gastroenteritis, and Typhi and related serotypes (Paratyphi) cause enteric fever.

■ Gastroenteritis

Typically, the episode begins 24 to 48 hours after ingestion, with nausea and vomiting followed by, or concomitant with, abdominal cramps and diarrhea. Diarrhea persists as the predominant symptom for 3 to 4 days and usually resolves spontaneously within 7 days. Fever (39°C) is present in about 50% of the patients. The spectrum of disease ranges from a few loose stools to a severe dysentery-like syndrome.

■ Bacteremia and Metastatic Infection

The acute gastroenteritis caused by *S enterica* can be associated with transient or persistent bacteremia. Frank sepsis is uncommon, except in those with compromised cell-mediated immunity; *Salmonella* infection in patients with acquired immunodeficiency syndrome (AIDS) is common and often severe. Bacteremia occurs in 70% of these patients and can cause septic shock and death. Despite adequate antimicrobial coverage, relapses are common. Patients with T-cell defects, such as lymphoproliferative diseases, or those receiving immune-suppressive agents after organ transplant are also highly susceptible to disseminated salmonellosis. Metastatic spread by salmonellae is a significant risk when bacteremia occurs. These organisms have a unique ability to colonize sites of preexisting structural abnormality, including atherosclerotic plaques, sites of malignancy, and the meninges (especially in infants). *Salmonella* infection of the bone typically involves the long bones; in particular, sites of trauma, sickle cell injury, and skeletal prosthetics are at risk.

■ Enteric Fever

Enteric fever is a multiorgan *Salmonella* infection characterized by prolonged fever, sustained bacteremia, and profound involvement of the mesenteric lymph nodes, liver, and spleen. The manifestations of typhoid (**Figure 33–10**) have been well documented in human volunteer studies conducted during vaccine trials. The mean incubation period is 13 days, and the first sign of disease is fever associated with a headache. The fever rises in stepwise fashion over the next 72 hours; a slow

---

⁎ *S enterica* = gastroenteritis

⁎ Typhi = enteric fever

⁎ Diarrhea, vomiting, and cramps are common

⁎ Bacteremia is most common and severe in the immunocompromised

⁎ Metastatic sites linked to previous injury, particularly sickle cell anemia

⁎ Slowly increasing fever lasts for weeks

FIGURE 33–10. **Natural history of enteric (typhoid) fever.** The course of disease without antimicrobial therapy. Fever chart shows time course for typical patient. Culture and agglutinating antibody show timing and probability of positive results in a group of typhoid fever patients.

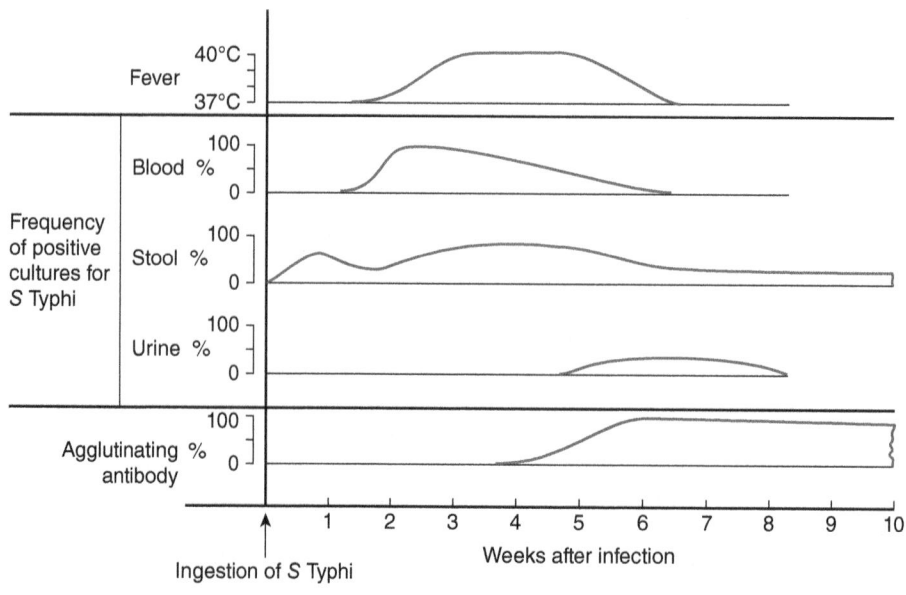

pulse, rather than the quickened pulse typical of fever, is pathognomonic for typhoid fever. In untreated patients, elevated temperature persists for weeks. Many patients are constipated, but up to one-third of patients have mild diarrhea; as untreated disease progresses, diarrhea may become more prominent. A faint rash (rose spots) appears during the first few days on the abdomen and chest; few in number, these spots may be missed by clinicians on the skin of people of color.

※ Diarrhea is intermittent or absent

 Why does it take so long? Why is there no diarrhea?

Obviously, prolonged infection of the bloodstream is serious, and the effects of endotoxin can lead to myocarditis, encephalopathy, or disseminated intravascular coagulation. Moreover, the persistent bacteremia can lead to infection at other sites. Of particular importance is the biliary tree, with reinfection of the intestinal tract and diarrhea late in the disease. Urinary tract infection and metastatic lesions in bone, joint, liver, and meninges may also occur. However, the most important complication of typhoid fever is intestinal perforation (through the wall of the terminal ileum or proximal colon at the site of necrotic Peyer patches) and hemorrhage; these occur in patients whose disease has been progressing for 2 weeks or more.

※ Biliary tree infection reseeds intestine

※ Urinary tract, bone, and joints are metastatic sites

DIAGNOSIS

Culture of *Salmonella* from the blood or stool is the primary diagnostic method. Early in the course of enteric fever, blood is far more likely to give a positive culture result than culture from any other site. The media used for stool culture are the same as those used for *Shigella*. Failure to ferment lactose and the production of hydrogen sulfides from sulfur-containing amino acids are characteristic features used to identify suspect colonies on the selective isolation media. Characteristic results of biochemical tests are used to identify the genus, though an isolate may also be subjected to O serogroup antisera for confirmation in larger laboratories. Typhi has a pattern of biochemical reactions distinctive enough to permit identification without reliance on serotype. All isolates should be referred to public health laboratories for confirmation and epidemiologic tracing; whole genome sequencing and other molecular typing methods have continued to gain prominence in these settings.

※ Stool and blood culture are routine

※ Typhi has characteristic features

TREATMENT

The primary therapeutic approach to *Salmonella* gastroenteritis consists of fluid and electrolyte replacement and the control of nausea and vomiting. Antibiotic therapy is not indicated in most cases because it may promote and prolong the carrier state. When used to eradicate the carrier state, antibiotics produce only erratic success and may fail altogether in the presence of biliary tract disease. Therefore, the use of antimicrobial agents in *S enterica* gastroenteritis is restricted to those with severe infections or underlying risk factors (such as immunosuppressive illnesses or therapies) and to infants less than 3 months old; in these instances, antimicrobial use is intended to prevent systemic spread.

※ Antimicrobials are of limited use in gastroenteritis

In typhoid fever, antimicrobial therapy is clearly indicated. Chloramphenicol (no longer in use) and then ampicillin were the first antibiotics used and reduced the mortality rate from 20% to less than 2%. Use of ampicillin is now limited by widespread resistance, leaving the extended-spectrum cephalosporins (ceftriaxone, cefixime) and ciprofloxacin as preferred first-line agents. As seen in other pathogenic enteric species (*E coli, K pneumoniae*), global patterns of antimicrobial resistance in *S* Typhi have been reshaped by the recent emergence of a single multidrug resistant clone. Nonetheless, with effective antimicrobial therapy, patients feel better in 24 to 48 hours, their temperature returns to normal in 3 to 5 days, and they are generally well in 10 to 14 days.

Antibiotics effective but multidrug resistance is increasing

 Think ►► Apply 33-3: **In the 2 weeks before the onset of fever, *S* Typhi is multiplying in macrophages and spreading to lymph nodes, spleen, and other elements of the RES. There may be a transient diarrhea but too mild for most to seek medical attention and have a culture taken. The disease is due to circulating LPS, not enterocyte dysfunction or destruction.**

PREVENTION

Killed whole bacterial vaccines have been available for typhoid since the late 19th century, with protection in the range of 50% to 70%. Newer vaccines—one that uses a live attenuated Typhi strain, the other a polysaccharide vaccine containing the Vi antigen—give slightly higher protection, but none lasting more than a few years. The newest vaccine contains Vi antigen conjugated to a bacterial protein in the manner of Hib, meningococcal, and pneumococcal vaccines. It shows promise for both higher efficacy and use in children less than 5 years of age. No human vaccine is available for the other *Salmonella* serotypes. When all is said and done, the provision of clean water supplies and the treatment of carriers would still go a long way toward eradicating typhoid. The importance of carriers and sanitation was emphasized by a 1973 typhoid outbreak among migrant workers in Florida; the source was traced to leakage of sewage into the water supply, failure of chlorination, and a chronic carrier. All three are required to sustain an outbreak when adequate sanitary infrastructure is in place.

✳ Typhoid vaccines are only moderately effective

✳ Sanitation and public health measures can eliminate Typhi

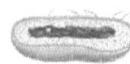

● YERSINIA

BACTERIOLOGY

Morphologically, *Yersinia* tend to be coccobacillary and to retain staining at the ends of the cells (bipolar staining). Growth and metabolic characteristics are the same as those of other Enterobacteriaceae, although some strains grow more slowly or have optimal growth temperatures lower than 37°C. The genus includes 11 species, of which *Yersinia pestis, Yersinia pseudotuberculosis,* and *Yersinia enterocolitica* are pathogenic for humans. *Yersinia pestis* is antigenically homogenous, but *Y pseudotuberculosis* and *Y enterocolitica* have multiple O and H antigen serotypes. *Yersinia* are primarily animal pathogens, with occasional transmission to humans through direct or indirect contact. *Yersinia pestis,* the cause of plague, is discussed in Chapter 36, although features of its pathogenesis common to other *Yersinia* are included below.

✳ Coccobacillary and grow at variable temperatures

✳ Human pathogens linked to animals

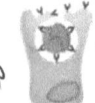

YERSINIA DISEASES (*Y PSEUDOTUBERCULOSIS* AND *Y ENTEROCOLITICA*)

EPIDEMIOLOGY

In animals, *Y pseudotuberculosis* causes pseudotuberculosis, a disease characterized by local necrosis and granulomatous inflammation in the lymph nodes, spleen, and liver. In humans, the portal of entry is the gastrointestinal tract, presumably by consumption of contaminated food or water; farm animals and wild rodents are among the most likely source of infection. Rates of *Y enterocolitica* infection vary markedly by geographic region, with the highest rates reported in Scandinavian and other European countries, and much lower rates in the United Kingdom and the United States. However, *Y enterocolitica* infection may be underdiagnosed due to lack of routine testing by many laboratories.

✳ Transmitted by ingestion from animal source

Geographic variation is great

PATHOGENESIS

Enteropathogenic *Yersinia* enter the human host in contaminated food and invade the M cells of the Peyer patch. The invasive process and its effects on the host cell are driven by a large array of virulence factors that are deployed under complex genetic and environmental regulation. These proteins include **invasin,** which binds to integrins on the surface of host cells, and the major effector proteins called Yersinia outer membrane proteins (**Yops**). The Yops are delivered by yet another injection (type III) secretion system; when injected into the host cell, they trigger cytotoxic events, including disruption of biochemical pathways (dephosphorylation, serine kinase), sensor functions, and the actin cytoskeleton.

Some of the virulence factors produced by *Yersinia* are regulated in response to either temperature or free calcium (Ca^{2+}) concentration. The physiologic temperature in a mammalian host is different from that in an insect or the environment, and the intracellular calcium concentration is markedly different from that of extracellular fluids; by sensing the environment, *Yersinia* are able

✳ Intestinal M cells are invaded

✳ Secreted Yops disrupt cellular function

Ca^{2+} and temperature regulate virulence factor expression

to express or suppress virulence factors at different stages of the pathogenic process. The results seem timed to support the pathogenic strategy of *Yersinia*, which is to paralyze the phagocytic activity of defending macrophages and neutrophils and thus nullify the host cellular immune response. The virulence determinants are encoded both on the bacterial chromosome and on a plasmid that contains genes for the secretion apparatus as well as the Yops. Another genetic component is a PAI, which is found only in the three pathogenic species and not other *Yersinia*.

The biological outcome of this extraordinary multifactorial process is the enhanced capacity of the pathogenic *Yersinia* to enter and replicate within the RES and to delay the cellular immune response. This leads to the formation of microabscesses and destruction of the cytoarchitecture of Peyer patches and the mesenteric lymph nodes. The systemic symptoms seen with dissemination can largely be attributed to the effects of endotoxin.

Yersinia pestis is a specialized variant closely related to *Y pseudotuberculosis*. Instead of entering the intestinal tract, *Y pestis* reaches the dermal lymphatics by the bite of an infected flea. It has its own invasin-like adhesin as well as two plasmids not found in the enteropathogenic *Yersinia*. Unique virulence factors for *Y pestis* include a capsular protein antigen with antiphagocytic properties, a plasminogen activator protease that promotes adherence to basement membranes, and a fibrinolysin that may play a survival role in the flea.

> **Plasmid and PAI contain virulence genes**
>
> ✻ Spread leads to microabscesses in lymph nodes
>
> ✻ *Y pestis* has capsule, plasminogen activator, and fibrinolysin

 ## *YERSINIA* INFECTIONS: CLINICAL ASPECTS

Both *Y enterocolitica* and *Y pseudotuberculosis* cause acute mesenteric lymphadenitis, a syndrome involving fever and abdominal pain that often mimics acute appendicitis. *Y enterocolitica* produces a wider variety of manifestations as well. The most common of these is enterocolitis, which usually occurs in children and is characterized by fever, diarrhea, and abdominal pain. *Y enterocolitica* also causes enteric fever, terminal ileitis, and an immune-mediated polyarthritic syndrome occurring after acute infection. Few laboratories in the United States routinely screen stools for *Yersinia* because yield has been low and good selective media are not available.

The role of antimicrobial therapy in enteric *Yersinia* infections is uncertain as the episodes are usually self-limiting. *Y pseudotuberculosis* is susceptible to ampicillin, cephalosporins, aminoglycosides, and tetracyclines, but *Y enterocolitica* is usually resistant to penicillins and cephalosporins through the production of β-lactamases.

> ✻ Mesenteric lymphadenitis creates abdominal pain
>
> **Not routinely sought in stools**
>
> **Antimicrobials not needed for self-limited disease**
>
> **Resistance patterns vary by species**

● OTHER ENTEROBACTERIACEAE

All Enterobacteriaceae described here are capable of producing opportunistic infections of the type discussed under *E coli*; none is considered a primary cause of enteric disease in the normal host. The genera isolated in at least moderate frequency are discussed briefly below. There are many other less common species.

KLEBSIELLA

The most distinctive bacteriologic features of the genus *Klebsiella* are the absence of motility and the presence of a polysaccharide capsule; the latter gives colonies a glistening, mucoid character and forms the basis of a serotyping system. Over 70 capsular types have been defined, including some that cross-react with those of other encapsulated pathogens, such as *Streptococcus pneumoniae* and *Haemophilus influenzae*. Limited studies suggest that the capsule interferes with complement activation as it does in other encapsulated pathogens. *Klebsiella* also express several types of pili on the cell surface which probably aid in adherence to respiratory and urinary epithelium.

Klebsiella pneumoniae, the most common species, is able to cause classic lobar pneumonia, a characteristic of other encapsulated bacteria; most *Klebsiella* pneumonias are indistinguishable from those produced by other members of the Enterobacteriaceae. Highly mucoid *K pneumoniae* bearing K1 or K2 capsule have been associated with distinctive clinical syndromes featuring liver abscess and endophthalmitis, particularly in Southeast Asian countries. Of all the Enterobacteriaceae, *Klebsiella* species are now among the most resistant to antimicrobial agents. In the early 2000s, a single *K pneumoniae* clone (Sequence Type 258), now notorious for its near pan-resistant

> ✻ Polysaccharide capsule blocks complement deposition

properties, emerged as a devastating cause of hospital-acquired infection (bloodstream, respiratory tract, urinary tract) in the northeastern United States and spread rapidly around the globe. The rise and spread of this and other highly resistant "superbugs" have led to concerns about a postantibiotic era.

ENTEROBACTER

Enterobacter species generally ferment lactose promptly and produce colonies similar to those of *Klebsiella*, though not as mucoid. A differential feature is motility by peritrichous flagella, which are generally present in *Enterobacter* species but uniformly absent in *Klebsiella*. *Enterobacter* species, which are generally less virulent than *Klebsiella*, have attracted increasing attention as a cause of infections acquired in the hospital, where their intrinsic antibiotic resistance properties undoubtedly confer a selective advantage. In addition to ampicillin, most isolates are resistant to first-generation cephalosporins. Though *Enterobacter* may appear susceptible to later-generation cephalosporins, resistance to these agents may emerge during treatment via derepression of β-lactamase production in patients with inadequate source control, such as those with incompletely drained abscesses or devitalized/necrotic tissue where bacteria may persist.

SERRATIA

Serratia strains ferment lactose slowly (3-4 days), if at all. Some produce distinctive brick-red colonies. Although less common, this genus produces the same range of opportunistic infections seen with other Enterobacteriaceae. *Serratia* strains show consistent intrinsic resistance to ampicillin and cephalothin/cefazolin, and like Enterobacter, may become further resistant to later generation cephalosporins during treatment. Circulating hospital strains may acquire plasmids conferring resistance to other antimicrobial classes including the aminoglycosides. Sporadic infections and nosocomial outbreaks with multiresistant strains have often been difficult to control.

CITROBACTER

Though biochemically and serologically similar to *Salmonella*, the genus *Citrobacter* is an uncommon cause of opportunistic infection. Like many other Enterobacteriaceae, *Citrobacter* strains may be present in the intestinal microbiota and cause opportunistic infections. Despite reports of association with diarrheal disease, present evidence does not indicate that *Citrobacter* should be considered an enteric pathogen of humans. *Citrobacter freundii* has been associated with neonatal meningitis and brain abscess.

PROTEUS, PROVIDENCIA, AND MORGANELLA

Proteus, *Morganella*, and *Providencia* are also opportunistic pathogens found with varying frequencies in the intestinal microbiota. *Proteus mirabilis*, the most commonly isolated member of the group, is one of the most susceptible of the Enterobacteriaceae to the penicillins. Other Proteae (typically, indole-positive species like *P vulgaris*) are intrinsically resistant to ampicillin and the cephalosporins. *Proteus mirabilis* and *P vulgaris* share the ability to swarm over the surface of microbiologic media, rather than remaining confined to discrete colonies; this characteristic makes them readily recognizable in the laboratory—often to the microbiologist's dismay, as this spreading growth covers other organisms in the culture and thus delays their isolation. Swarming coupled with motility could facilitate the production of UTI by propelling *Proteus* up urinary catheters. *Proteus* and *Morganella* differ from other Enterobacteriaceae in the production of a very potent **urease**, which allows for their rapid identification; it also contributes to the formation of urinary stones and produces alkalinity and an ammoniac odor to the urine. *Providencia* species do not produce urease, are the least frequently isolated, and are generally the most resistant of the group to antimicrobials.

Margin notes

* Often multidrug resistant

* Resistance can emerge during treatment

Modest virulence but are linked to hospital acquisition

* Red pigment and multidrug resistance are characteristic

* Opportunistic infection and brain abscess are uncommon

* Swarming is a feature of some species

* Urease production is linked to urinary stones

CASE STUDY

Hamburgers and Hemorrhage

A 24-year-old woman was seen in a hospital emergency department with a history of nausea, vomiting, and nonbloody diarrhea, which progressed to bloody diarrhea. Four days earlier, she had eaten a hamburger at a fast-food restaurant. To replace fluid lost from diarrhea, she was given 2 liters of IV fluid. She felt better and was sent home with antinausea medication.

After 2 days, the vomiting, nausea, and bloody diarrhea persisted, along with abdominal cramps and orthostatic dizziness. She returned to the emergency department, was admitted, again given IV fluids, and discharged after 2 days of hospitalization. A stool sample was taken for culture.

Three days later, the patient awoke with vomiting and contacted her private physician. Laboratory tests were done with the following results: blood urea nitrogen 67.0 mg/dL (ref. 7-19); white blood cells 13 100/mL; hemoglobin 7.0 g/dL (ref. 11.5-15.5); platelet count 75 000/µL (ref. >150 000). The stool culture taken earlier was positive for *E coli* O157:H7.

The patient was transferred to the ICU the same day and was described as severely ill. She was fatigued, very dehydrated, with abdominal tenderness and back pain but no neurologic problems. Steroids were the only additional medication given in addition to plasmapheresis, which was done five times during her hospitalization. She gradually recovered and was discharged.

QUESTIONS

1. Which of the following is probably the source of this patient's infection?
   A. Colonized cow
   B. Colonized restaurant worker
   C. Contaminated restaurant water
   D. Family member
   E. Restaurant air

2. What bacterial product was primarily responsible for the hemorrhage and renal injury?
   A. Endotoxin
   B. α-Toxin
   C. Labile toxin (LT)
   D. Stable toxin (ST)
   E. Shiga toxin (Stx)

3. If hamburger is the source, this infection could have been prevented by which of the following?
   A. Screening the restaurant workers
   B. Handwashing
   C. Disinfectants
   D. Complete cooking
   E. Antibiotic prophylaxis

ANSWERS

1. (A)

2. (E)

3. (D)

chapter 34

Legionella and *Coxiella*

Legionella pneumophila • *Coxiella burnetii*

The death toll in the outbreak of the mysterious respiratory disease in Philadelphia rose by two to 25 as medical detectives accelerated efforts today to seek a chemical or poison as the possible cause.

—*The New York Times*, August 7, 1976

OVERVIEW

Legionella are thin, pleomorphic, long, Gram-negative rods that stain poorly and require special media for isolation. They are ubiquitous and persistent in the environment, especially in water and soil. When inhaled into the lung, *Legionella* enter alveolar macrophages, escape host defenses, and produce a destructive pneumonia marked by headache, fever, chills, dry cough, and chest pain. There may be multiple foci in both lungs and extension to the pleura, but spread outside the respiratory tract is very rare.

Coxiella (agent of Q fever) are tiny Gram-negative coccobacilli that when inhaled from animal and soil environmental sources cause pneumonia. In addition to the lung, *Coxiella* also have a tropism for the liver where they reside in macrophages and cause granulomatous hepatitis. Less commonly, *Coxiella* causes infective endocarditis not detected by culturing blood.

*L*egionella is a genus of Gram-negative bacilli that takes its name from the outbreak at the American Legion convention where it was first discovered. The name of the type species, *Legionella pneumophila*, reflects its propensity to cause the necrotizing pneumonia known as Legionnaires disease. *Legionella* species are now known to be widespread in the environment in ponds, amoebas, and the plumbing of large buildings. *Coxiella*, a cause of pneumonia known long before *Legionella*, shares many pathogenic, epidemiologic, and clinical features with it.

● *LEGIONELLA*

 ## BACTERIOLOGY

STRUCTURE

L pneumophila is a thin, pleomorphic, Gram-negative rod that may show elongated, filamentous forms up to 20 μm long. In clinical specimens, the organism stains poorly or not at all by Gram stain or the usual histologic stains; however, it can be demonstrated by silver impregnation methods (Dieterle stain). Polar, subpolar, and lateral flagella may be present and most species of *Legionella* are motile. Spores are not found.

Structurally, *L pneumophila* has features similar to those of Gram-negative bacteria with a typical outer membrane, thin peptidoglycan layer, and cytoplasmic membrane. The toxicity of *L pneumophila* lipopolysaccharide (LPS) is significantly less than that of other Gram-negative bacteria such as *Neisseria* and the Enterobacteriaceae. This has been attributed to chemical makeup of the LPS side chains that renders the cell surface highly hydrophobic, a property which may promote distribution in aerosols.

✳ Gram negative rods stain with difficulty

✳ LPS less toxic than other Gram negatives

Side chains hydrophobic

METABOLISM

* Intracellular parasite of protozoa

* Biofilms in water systems

* Requires L-cysteine, ferric ions, low pH

Legionella is a facultative intracellular pathogen multiplying to high numbers inside free-living amoebas, other protozoa, and macrophages. In human-made water systems the organisms persist in a low metabolic state imbedded in biofilms. *In vitro L pneumophila* fails to grow on common enriched bacteriologic media such as blood agar due to requirements for certain amino acids (L-cysteine), ferric ions, and slightly acidic conditions (optimal pH 6.9). Even when these requirements are met, growth under aerobic conditions is slow, requiring 2 to 5 days to produce colonies that have a distinctive surface resembling ground glass. Although a few enzymatic actions (catalase, oxidase, β-lactamase) are demonstrable, the classification of *Legionella* depends largely on antigenic features, chemical analysis, and nucleic acid homology comparisons. The closest relative among pathogenic bacteria is *Coxiella burnettii* (see later).

Multiple serogroups, other species

L pneumophila has multiple serogroups (16) and there are over 50 other *Legionella* species (eg, *Legionella longbeachae*, *Legionella bozemanii*, *Legionella dumoffii*, *Legionella micdadei*). The original Philadelphia strain (serogroup 1) is still the most common, and a limited number of *L pneumophila* serogroups account for 80% to 90% of cases. This suggests enhanced virulence for humans, since the frequency of *L pneumophila* among species found in the environment is below 30%. Less than half of the non–*L pneumophila* species have been isolated from human infections.

 ## LEGIONNAIRES DISEASE

EPIDEMIOLOGY

1976 outbreak led to discovery

Earlier outbreaks solved

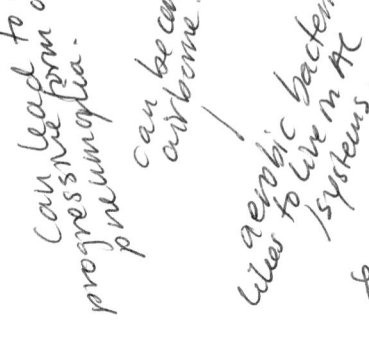
[handwritten margin notes: Can lead to a progressive form of pneumonia. Can become airborne. Uses aerobic bacteria that likes to live in AC systems.]

The widely publicized outbreak of pneumonia among attendees of the 1976 American Legion convention in Philadelphia led to the isolation of a previously unrecognized infectious agent, *L pneumophila*. The event was unique in medical history. For months, the American public entertained theories of its cause that ranged from chemical sabotage to viroids and fears that something like Michael Crichton's 1969 novel *The Andromeda Strain* was ahead. It was almost a letdown to find that a Gram-negative rod that could not be stained or grown by the common methods was responsible. The Centers for Disease Control investigation was an outstanding example of the benefits of pursuing sound epidemiologic evidence until it is explained by equally sound microbiologic findings. We now know the disease had occurred for many years. Specific antibodies and organisms have been detected in material preserved from the 1950s, and a mysterious hospital outbreak in 1965 has been solved retrospectively by examination of preserved specimens. Today, most cases of Legionnaires disease in the United States are caused by just a few *L pneumophila* serogroups, including the original Philadelphia strain, but there is considerable variation worldwide. In Australia, New Zealand, and Japan *L longbeachae* and *L pneumophila* are found with similar frequency.

* Freshwater amoebas are reservoir

* Aerosols distributed by humidifying and cooling systems

In nature, *Legionella* species are ubiquitous in freshwater lakes, streams, and subterrestrial groundwater sediments. They are also found in moist potting soil, mud, and riverbanks. In these sites, they also exist as parasites of protozoa including numerous species of amoebas, which appear to be the environmental reservoir. Transmission to humans occurs when aerosols are created in manmade water supplies that harbor *Legionella*. Most outbreaks have occurred in or around large buildings such as hotels, factories, and hospitals with cooling towers or some other part of an air-conditioning system as the dispersal mechanism. Some hospital outbreaks have implicated respiratory devices and potable water coming from parts of the hot water system such as faucets and showerheads. Even the mists used in supermarkets to make the vegetables look fresh have been the source of outbreaks. *Legionella* can persist in a water supply despite standard disinfection procedures, particularly when the water is warm and the pipes contain scale or low-flow areas that compromise the effectiveness of chlorine compounds.

* Person-to-person transmission, carriers unknown

* Disease rate low

It is difficult to ascertain the overall incidence of *Legionella* infections because most information has been from outbreaks that constitute only a small part of the total cases. Estimates based on seroconversions suggest approximately 25,000 cases in the United States each year. The attack rate among those exposed is estimated at less than 5% and serious cases are generally limited to immunocompromised persons. Person-to-person transmission has not been documented, and the organisms have not been isolated from healthy individuals. Growth in free-living amoebas produces *Legionella* cells that are more resistant to environmental stress (acid, heat, osmotic) and have enhanced infectivity.

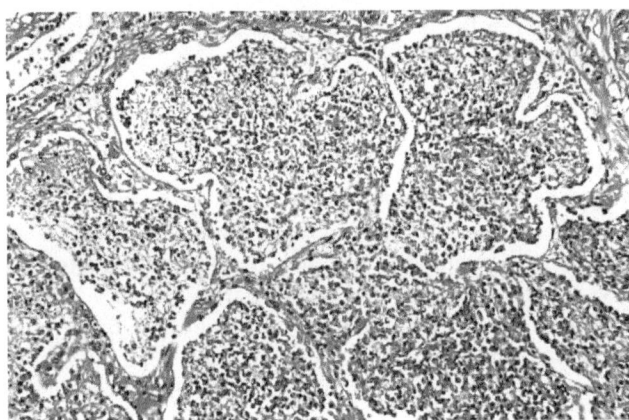

FIGURE 34-1. *Legionella pneumonia.* Note the filling of alveoli with exudate. Some of the alveolar septa are starting to degenerate. (Reproduced with permission from Connor DH, Chandler FW, Schwartz DQ, et al: *Pathology of Infectious Diseases.* Stamford CT: Appleton & Lange; 1997.)

PATHOGENESIS

L pneumophila is striking in its propensity to attack the lung, producing a necrotizing multifocal pneumonia. Microscopically, the process involves the alveoli and terminal bronchioles, with relative sparing of the larger bronchioles and bronchi (**Figure 34–1**). The inflammatory exudate contains fibrin, neutrophils, macrophages, and erythrocytes. A striking feature is the preponderance of bacteria within phagocytes and the lytic destruction of inflammatory cells.

Inhaled *Legionella* bacteria reach the alveoli, where they attach to their pathogenic target the alveolar macrophage. In this process, they are aided by flagella, pili, and a variety of other proteins. Following attachment the bacteria enter the macrophage in an endocytic vacuole. Inside the cell *L pneumophila* initiates a process which prevents fusion with the lysosome and instead recruits ribosomes, mitochondria, and elements of the host cell endoplasmic reticulum (ER) into its own phagosome called the Legionella-containing vacuole (LCV). In the LCV niche protected from lysosomal digestion, the organisms multiply to high numbers (**Figure 34-2**). They eventually kill the macrophage releasing new cells to repeat the cycle. The multiple enzymes released in this process lead to inflammation, destructive lesions in the lung, and a systemic toxicity that may be related to cytokine release.

L pneumophila accomplishes this control of the phagocyte through the complex deployment of over 200 proteins. Only a few of these proteins have functions which are known or have been inferred by genomic analysis. It is known that the majority of these proteins are produced by an injection secretion system (type IV) which in contrast to those described in other Gram-negative pathogens operates from *inside* the unfortunate macrophage. As the intracellular population grows, the virulence protein deployment shifts to products facilitating egress from the LCV and macrophage with some causing pore-forming membrane lysis. The entire process in environmental protozoa is similar to that in the macrophage. In both amoebas and humans this rapid growth takes place under nutrient-rich conditions. Similar to other intracellular bacterial pathogens (*Chlamydia, Chlamydophila,* and *Coxiella*), *L pneumophila* also has a nutrient-restricted phase in which elements that mediate resistance to environmental stress and facilitate future infectivity

* Tropism for lung

* Pneumonia with intracellular bacteria

* Invades alveolar macrophages

* Lysosomal fusion blocked

* Host ER incorporated into LCV

Protein secretion system inside host cell

* Macrophage, amoeba replication similar

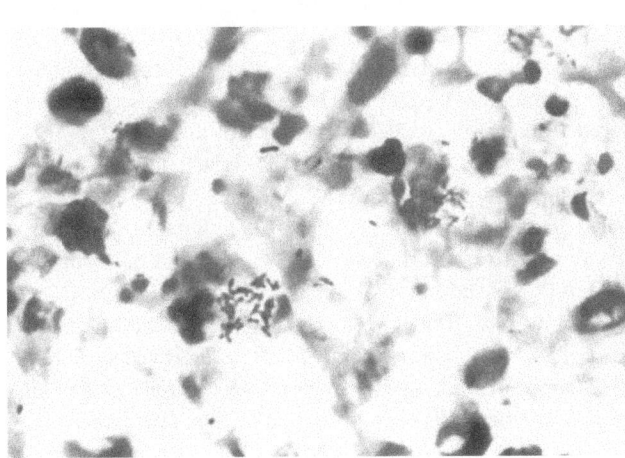

FIGURE 34-2. **Legionnaires disease.** Imprint smear of lung shows *L pneumophila* (*stained red*) mostly inside alveolar macrophages. (Reproduced with permission from Connor DH, Chandler FW, Schwartz DQ, et al: *Pathology of Infectious Diseases.* Stamford CT: Appleton & Lange; 1997.)

are produced. This appears to be the situation in the low metabolic state of biofilm-imbedded cells, which lurk in the pipes of human-constructed water systems.

IMMUNITY

Just as intracellular multiplication is the key to *L pneumophila* virulence, its arrest by innate and adaptive mechanisms is the most important aspect of immunity. The high level of innate immunity to *Legionella* infection in most persons is related to brisk pattern recognition responses triggered by toll-like receptors (TLRs) in macrophages and dendritic cells that recognize *Legionella* LPS. The activation of the T_H1 adaptive immune response and its associated cytokines (IFN-γ, IL-12, IL-18) completes the process of macrophage activation and intracellular killing of the invading *Legionella*. Failure of this aspect of the immune response is the primary reason for most cases of progressive Legionnaires disease in the immunocompromised. Antibodies formed in the course of *Legionella* infection are useful for diagnosis, but do not appear to be important in immunity. It is unknown whether humans who have had Legionnaires disease are immune to reinfection and disease.

Innate defenses triggered by TLRs

✳ Cytokine-activated macrophages limit intracellular growth

Antibody less important

LEGIONNAIRES DISEASE: CLINICAL ASPECTS

MANIFESTATIONS

Legionnaires disease is a severe toxic pneumonia that begins with myalgia and headache, followed by a rapidly rising fever. A dry cough may develop and later become productive, but sputum production is not a prominent feature. Chills, pleuritic chest pain, vomiting, diarrhea, confusion, and delirium may all be seen. Radiologically, patchy or interstitial infiltrates with a tendency to progress toward nodular consolidation are present unilaterally or bilaterally. Liver function tests often indicate some hepatic dysfunction. In the more serious cases, the patient becomes progressively ill and toxic over the first 3 to 6 days, and the disease terminates in shock, respiratory failure, or both. The overall mortality rate is about 15%, but it has been higher than 50% in some hospital outbreaks. Mortality is particularly high in patients with serious underlying disease or suppression of cell-mediated immunity.

A less common form of disease called **Pontiac fever** (named for a 1968 Michigan outbreak), is a nonpneumonic illness that resembles influenza with fever, myalgia, dry cough, and a short incubation period (6-48 hours). Pontiac fever is a self-limiting illness and may represent a reaction to endotoxin or hypersensitivity to components of the *Legionella* or their protozoan hosts.

✳ Toxic pneumonia in 5% of exposed

✳ Mortality high in immunocompromised

DIAGNOSIS

The diagnosis of *Legionella* pneumonia requires a high-quality specimen. Lung aspirates, bronchoalveolar lavage, or biopsies are preferred, because the organism may not be found in sputum. Typically, the Gram smear fails to show bacteria owing to poor staining, but organisms may be seen by DFA based on *L pneumophila*-specific conjugates. Non-*L pneumophila* species are not detected and DFA yields a positive result in only 25% to 50% of culture-proved cases. Multiplex PCR platforms for *L pneumophila* are increasingly being used for diagnosis; however, non-*L pneumophila* species require culture.

Cultures must be made on buffered charcoal yeast extract (BCYE) agar medium that includes supplements (amino acids, vitamins, L-cysteine, ferric pyrophosphate), which meets the growth requirements of *Legionella*. It is buffered to meet the acidic conditions—optimal for *Legionella* growth. The isolation of large Gram-negative rods on BCYE after 2 to 5 days that have failed to grow on routine media (blood agar, chocolate agar) is presumptive evidence for *Legionella*. The BCYE also allows isolation of species of *Legionella* species other than *L pneumophila*.

The difficulty and slow speed of culture together with the low sensitivity of DFA have spurred searches for other methods. This has led to the development of nucleic acid amplification (NAA) procedures for use in respiratory specimens and immunoassay methods for the detection of antigen in urine. NAA methods such as the polymerase chain reaction (PCR) have proved to be rapid and much more sensitive than DFA. A simple card-based antigenuria detection test has also proved to be sensitive for the common *L pneumophila* serogroup 1 but does not detect other

✳ Lung specimens needed

✳ DFA only 50% sensitive

✳ Culture on BCYE

Other species isolated

serogroups or other *Legionella* species. The primary barrier to making these methods more widely used is that Legionnaires disease is uncommon except in immunocompromised populations. This tends to limit their availability to reference laboratories and hospitals serving immunocompromised patients. Demonstrating a significant rise in serum antibody is used primarily for retrospective diagnosis and in epidemiologic studies.

PCR rapid and sensitive

✳ Antigenuria detects serogroup 1

TREATMENT

The best information on antimicrobial therapy is still provided by the original Philadelphia outbreak. Because the cause of Legionnaires disease was completely obscure at the time, the cases were treated with many different regimens. Patients treated with erythromycin clearly did better than those given the penicillins, cephalosporins, or aminoglycosides. Subsequently, it was shown that most *Legionella* produce β-lactamases. Currently, therapy with levofloxacin (or moxifloxacin) or azithromycin is preferred.

Fluoroquinolone, azithromycin treatments of choice

PREVENTION

The prevention of legionellosis involves minimizing production of aerosols in public places from water that may be contaminated with *Legionella*. Prevention is complicated by the fact that, compared with other environmental bacteria, *Legionella* bacteria are relatively resistant to chlorine and heat. The bacteria have been isolated from hot water tanks held at over 50°C. Methods for decontaminating water systems are still under evaluation. Some outbreaks have been terminated by hyperchlorination, by correcting malfunctions in water systems, or by temporarily elevating the system temperature above 70°C. The installation of silver and copper ionization systems similar to those used in large swimming pools has been effective as a last resort in hospitals plagued with recurrent nosocomial legionellosis. An outbreak reported from a neonatal intensive care unit in Cyprus was traced to free-standing humidifiers which had been filled with tap water. This underscores both the ubiquity of *Legionella* and the need to at least start with sterile water wherever possible.

✳ Preventing aerosols primary goal

✳ Heat, hyperchlorination, metal ions in institutional water systems

● *COXIELLA*

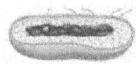

BACTERIOLOGY

C burnetii is a Gram-negative bacillus and the cause of **Q fever.** Its intracellular growth has caused it to be discussed with the rickettsiae; however, it is now known to be most closely related to *Legionella*. Previously thought to be an obligate intracellular parasite, *C burnetii* does not suffer the metabolic deficits of the *Rickettsia* and has now been grown in a cell-free environment. The primary growth niche of *C burnetii* in humans is the alveolar macrophage where it deploys the same secretion system (type IV) used by *L pneumophila*. *C burnetii* continues to multiply even following phagosome/lysosome fusion, because it is adapted to growth at low pH and resists lysosomal enzymes. In its growth cycle *Coxiella* includes a form that is resistant to drying and other environmental conditions much like a bacterial spore. These forms do not have the chemical composition of *Bacillus* or *Clostridium* spores but do survive prolonged periods in the environment. It is felt that this accounts for the ability of *C burnetii* to produce infection by aerosol inhalation, often at considerable distance from the presumed source.

✳ Multiplies in alveolar macrophage

✳ Resists acid and enzymes of phagolysosome

✳ Spore-like forms survive in environment

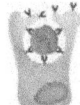

COXIELLA INFECTION: Q FEVER

Q fever is primarily a zoonosis transmitted from animals to humans by inhalation rather than by arthropod bite. Its distribution is worldwide among a wide range of mammals, of which cattle, sheep, and goats are most associated with transmission to humans. *C burnetii* grows particularly well in placental tissue, attaining huge numbers (less than 10^{10} per gram), which at the time of parturition contaminate the soil and fomites, where it may survive for years. Q fever occurs in those who are exposed to infected animals or their products, particularly farmers, veterinarians, and workers involved in slaughtering. Another high-risk environment is animal research facilities

✴ Transmission by inhalation; occasionally ingestion

✴ Exposure in abattoirs, research facilities

that have not provided adequate protection for personnel. Infection in all of these circumstances is believed to result from inhalation, which may be at some distance from the site of generation of the infectious aerosols. Infection can also occur from ingestion of animal products such as unpasteurized milk.

 ## Q FEVER: CLINICAL ASPECTS

✴ Systemic infection without rash

✴ Pneumonia and endocarditis

C burnetii has an affinity for the reticuloendothelial system, but little is known of the pathology, because fatal cases are rare. As in livestock, most human infections are unapparent. When clinically evident, Q fever usually begins at an average of 20 days after inhalation, with abrupt onset of fever, chills, and headache. A mild, dry, hacking cough and patchy interstitial pneumonia may or may not be present. There is no rash. Hepatosplenomegaly and abnormal liver function tests are common. Complications such as myocarditis, pericarditis, and encephalitis are rare. Chronic infection is also rare, but particularly important when it takes the form of endocarditis. There is evidence that the strains associated with endocarditis constitute an antigenic subgroup of *C burnetii*.

Diagnosis serologic or PCR

Diagnosis of Q fever is usually made by demonstrating high or rising titers of antibody to Q fever antigen by complement fixation, IFA, or enzyme immunoassay procedures or by PCR. Although most infections resolve spontaneously, doxycycline therapy is believed to shorten the duration of fever and reduce the risk of chronic infection. Vaccines have been shown to stimulate antibodies, and some studies have suggested a protective effect for heavily exposed workers.

KEY CONCLUSIONS

- *Legionella pneumophila* is acquired by inhalation and multiplies within pulmonary alveolar macrophages.
- *Legionella* are found widely in the environment persisting in amoebas in standing water. Biofilm formation and dormancy facilitate survival in the pipes of large buildings.
- *L pneumophila* serogroup 1 can be diagnosed with a specific urinary antigen test. Other diagnostics include immunofluorescent staining, specialized culture, and NAA methods.
- Levofloxacin or azithromycin are preferred for treatment.
- *Coxiella burnetii* causes Q fever after inhalation of aerosols from animal or soil sources.
- *Coxiella* survives in macrophages and causes pneumonia and granulomatous hepatitis.
- Q fever is underrecognized as cause of culture-negative endocarditis

CASE STUDY

Fatal Pneumonia with Mystery Gram-Negative Bacillus

A 54-year-old man with multiple myeloma was admitted with a 2-day history of fever, nausea, and diarrhea. His lungs were initially clear, but during the first 3 days of his hospitalization he developed a progressive right lower lobe pneumonia and pleural effusion. Initial antibiotic therapy included cephalothin, tobramycin, and ticarcillin. On day 3, intravenous erythromycin was added.

Initial cultures of blood, sputum, urine, cerebrospinal fluid, and stool failed to reveal an etiologic agent. A transtracheal aspirate was also obtained with negative results, including a *Legionella* DFA. There was no resolution of the pneumonia, and spiking fevers continued. On day 13, his respiratory difficulties increased, with frank bleeding from the upper respiratory tract, and he died.

At autopsy, the most prominent findings were bronchopneumonia with focal organization and hemorrhage in the right lung. Stains of the lung tissue were negative by Gram, methenamine silver, and acid-fast methods, but Dieterle silver stains revealed short bacilli. Lung cultures yielded Gram-negative bacilli, which grew aerobically on buffered charcoal–yeast extract, but not on blood or chocolate agar. The organisms resembled *Legionella*, but failed to stain with immunofluorescence conjugates for *Legionella pneumophila* and multiple other species (*L micdadei, L longbeachae, L gormanii, L dumoffii,* and *L bozemanae*). The organism was sent to the Centers for Disease Control and Prevention, where it was eventually identified as a new species of *Legionella*.

QUESTIONS

1. What is the most probable source of this man's infection?
    A. Family member
    B. Water
    C. Food
    D. Insect
    E. Bioterrorism

2. What cell type did the organism initially infect in this patient?
    A. Ciliated epithelial cell
    B. Squamous epithelial
    C. Microvillous cell
    D. M cell
    E. Alveolar macrophage

3. Which of the following contributes most to the ability of *Legionella* to multiply in host phagocytes?
    A. Pore-forming toxin
    B. Superantigen action
    C. Cytokine stimulation
    D. Inhibition of lysosome fusion
    E. Inhibition of protein synthesis

ANSWERS

1. **(B)**

2. **(E)**

3. **(D)**

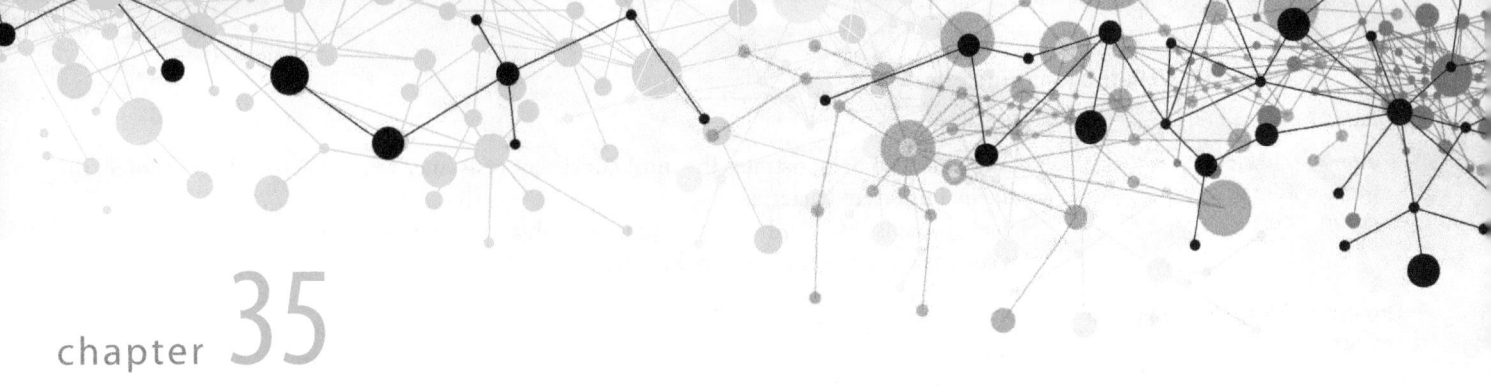

chapter 35

Pseudomonas and Other Opportunistic Gram-negative Bacilli

Pseudomonas aeruginosa · Burkholderia pseudomallei · Burkholderia cepacia · Acinetobacter

Moraxella · Aeromonas and *Plesiomonas*

OVERVIEW

A number of opportunistic Gram-negative rods of several genera not considered in other chapters are included here. With the exception of *Pseudomonas aeruginosa*, they rarely cause true disease, and all are frequently encountered as superficial colonizers or contaminants; the significance of their isolation from clinical material thus depends on the circumstance and site of culture and on the clinical situation of the patient. *P aeruginosa* produces infection at a wide range of pulmonary, urinary, and soft tissue sites, much like the Enterobacteriaceae. The clinical manifestations of these infections reflect the organ system involved and are not unique for *Pseudomonas*. However, once established, infections are particularly virulent and difficult to treat, likely because affected patients almost always have some form of debilitation or compromise of immune defenses and the bacteria themselves may be highly resistant to antibiotics.

● PSEUDOMONAS

There is a large number of *Pseudomonas* species, the most important of which is *Pseudomonas aeruginosa*. *Pseudomonas* species are most frequently seen as colonizers and contaminants but are able to cause opportunistic infections; however, the number of human infections produced by the other species together is far lower than that produced by *P aeruginosa* alone. The assignment of species names has little clinical importance beyond differentiation from *P aeruginosa*. Reports vary regarding the frequency of their isolation from cases of bacteremia, arthritis, abscesses, wounds, conjunctivitis, and urinary tract infections. In general, unless isolated in pure culture from a high-quality (direct) specimen, particularly from a normally sterile site, it is difficult to attach pathogenic significance to any of the miscellaneous *Pseudomonas* species.

❋ *P aeruginosa* most important pathogen

❋ Other *Pseudomonas* species cause opportunistic infection

PSEUDOMONAS AERUGINOSA

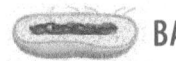 BACTERIOLOGY

P aeruginosa is an aerobic, motile, Gram-negative rod that is slimmer and more pale-staining than members of the Enterobacteriaceae. Its most striking bacteriologic feature is the production of vivid and colorful water-soluble pigments. Of all the medically important bacteria,

* Pigment-producing rod resistant to many antimicrobials

Grows aerobically with minimal requirements

* Colonies are oxidase-positive

* Blue pyocyanin produced only by *P aeruginosa*

* Yellow fluorescein and pyocyanin combine for green color

* Outer membrane porins are relatively impermeable

* Secreted alginate forms a slime layer

* Overproduction due to regulatory mutations

* Multiple extracellular enzymes produced

* ExoA action same as diphtheria toxin

* ExoS or ExoU injected by secretion system

* Primary habitat environmental

* Occasionally colonizes humans

* Multiplies in humidifiers, solutions, medications

* Risk highest for immunocompromised persons

(handwritten margin notes: Psephalosporins are naturally choice. associated w. pneumonia and (gas gangrene))

P aeruginosa also demonstrates the most consistent resistance to antimicrobial agents of all the medically important bacteria.

P aeruginosa is sufficiently versatile in its growth and energy requirements to use simple molecules such as ammonia and carbon dioxide as sole nitrogen and carbon sources. Thus, it does not require enriched media for growth and can survive and multiply over a wide temperature range (20–42°C) in almost any environment, including those with high salt content. The organism uses oxidative energy-producing mechanisms and has high levels of cytochrome oxidase ("oxidase-positive"). Although an aerobic atmosphere is necessary for optimal growth and metabolism, most strains multiply slowly in an anaerobic environment if nitrate is present as an electron acceptor.

Growth on all common isolation media is luxurious, and colonies have a delicate, fringed edge. Confluent growth often has a characteristic metallic sheen and emits an intense fruity odor. Hemolysis is usually produced on blood agar. The positive oxidase reaction of *P aeruginosa* differentiates it from the Enterobacteriaceae, and its production of blue, yellow, or rust-colored pigments differentiates it from most other Gram-negative bacteria. The blue pigment, **pyocyanin,** is produced only by *P aeruginosa*. **Fluorescein,** a yellow pigment that fluoresces under ultraviolet light, is produced by *P aeruginosa* and other free-living, less pathogenic *Pseudomonas* species. Pyocyanin and fluorescein combined to produce a bright green color that diffuses throughout the medium.

Lipopolysaccharide (LPS) is present in the outer membrane, as are porin proteins, which differ from those of the Enterobacteriaceae family in offering much less permeability to molecules including antibiotics. Pili composed of repeating monomers of the pilin structural subunit extend from the cell surface. A single polar flagellum rapidly propels the organism and assists in binding to host tissues.

A mucoid exopolysaccharide slime layer is present outside the cell wall in some strains. This layer is created by secretion of **alginate,** a copolymer of D-mannuronic and L-guluronic acids. It is created by the action of several enzymes that effectively channel carbohydrate intermediates into the alginate polymer. All *P aeruginosa* produce moderate amounts of alginate, but those with mutations in regulatory genes overproduce the polymer; such mutants appear as striking mucoid colonies in cultures from the respiratory tract of patients with cystic fibrosis (CF).

Most strains of *P aeruginosa* produce multiple extracellular products, including **exotoxin A (ExoA)** and other enzymes with phospholipase, collagenase, adenylate cyclase, or elastase activity. ExoA is a secreted protein that inactivates eukaryotic elongation factor 2 (EF-2) by ADP ribosylation (ADPr). This arrests translation, leading to shutdown of protein synthesis and cell death. Although this action is the same as diphtheria toxin, the two toxins are otherwise unrelated. The **elastase** acts on a variety of biologically important substrates, including elastin, human IgA and IgG, complement components, and some collagens. Then, the vast majority of *P aeruginosa* strains encode a type III secretion system (T3SS) that injects virulent effector proteins— exoenzymes T (**ExoT**), along with either **ExoS** for most strains or **ExoU** for a small minority— directly into host cells. Inside the cell, ExoT and ExoS disrupt formation of reactive oxygen species and promote apoptosis, while the phospholipase ExoU functions as a cytotoxin.

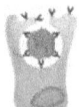 *P AERUGINOSA* DISEASE ρ

EPIDEMIOLOGY

The primary habitat of *P aeruginosa* is the environment; it is found in water, soil, and various types of vegetation throughout the world. *P aeruginosa* has been isolated from the throat and stool of 2% to 10% of healthy persons, but colonization rates are quite likely higher in hospitalized patients. *P aeruginosa* rarely infects previously healthy persons, but represents one of the most dreaded causes of invasive infection in hospitalized patients with serious underlying disease, such as leukemia, CF, and extensive burns (**Figure 35–1**).

The ability of *P aeruginosa* to survive and proliferate in water with minimal nutrients can lead to heavy contamination of any nonsterile fluid, such as that in the humidifiers of ventilator circuits. Inhalation of aerosols from such sources can bypass the normal respiratory defense mechanisms and initiate pulmonary infection. Infections have resulted from the growth of *Pseudomonas* in medications, contact lens solutions, and even some disinfectants. Sinks and faucet aerators may be heavily contaminated and serve as the environmental source for contamination of other items. The presence

Pseudomonas

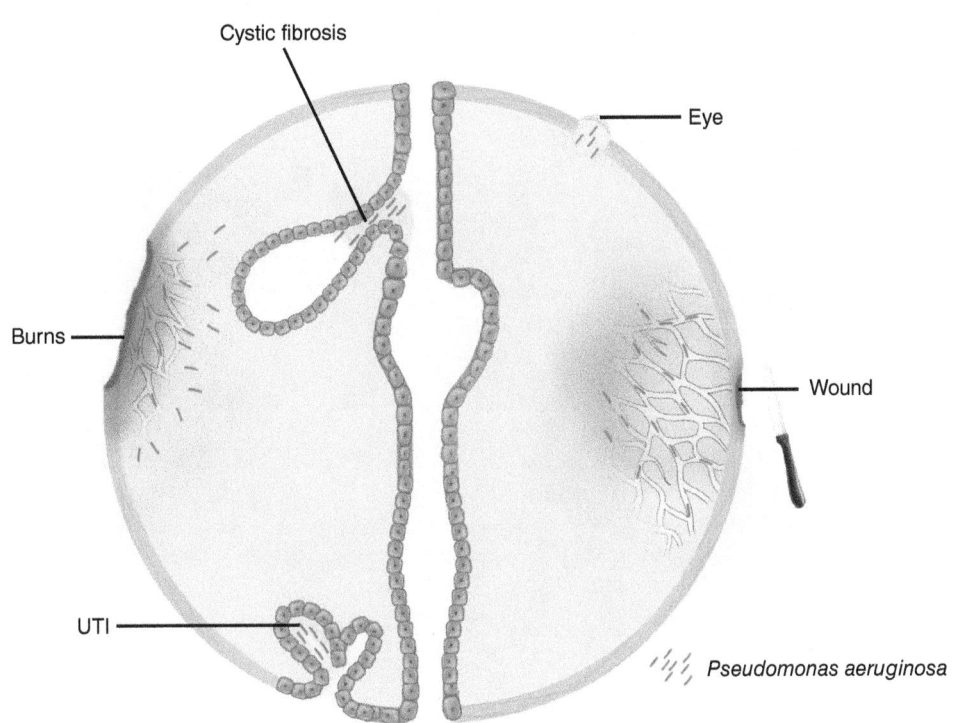

FIGURE 35–1. *Pseudomonas* disease overview. *P aeruginosa* is a leading cause of opportunistic infection in the eye (contact lenses), wounds, urinary tract, and burns. In a special case, it colonizes the respiratory tract of persons with cystic fibrosis by formation of a biofilm (see Figure 35–4). UTI, urinary tract infection.

of *P aeruginosa* in drinking water or food is not a cause for alarm; the risk lies in the access of materials susceptible to contamination to portals of entry in persons uniquely predisposed to infection.

    P aeruginosa is now the most common bacterial pathogen to complicate the management of patients with CF, an inherited defect in chloride ion transport that leads to a buildup of thick mucus in ducts and the tracheobronchial tree. In a high percentage of patients, the respiratory tract eventually becomes colonized with *P aeruginosa*; once established, the organism may evolve in complex ways but remains essentially impossible to eradicate. This infection is a leading cause of morbidity and eventual death of these patients.

※ **Respiratory colonization of CF patients becomes chronic**

PATHOGENESIS ℗

Although *P aeruginosa* is an opportunistic pathogen, it is one of particular virulence. The organism usually requires a significant break in first-line defenses (such as a wound) or a route past them (such as a contaminated solution or endotracheal tube) to initiate infection. Attachment to epithelial cells is the first step in infection and is likely mediated by pili, flagella, and the extracellular polysaccharide slime. The receptors include sialic acid and *N*-acetyl glucosamine borne by cell surface glycolipids. Attachment is favored by loss of surface fibronectin, which may in part explain the propensity for debilitated persons.

※ **Needs break in first-line defenses**

Pili, flagella, and slime mediate adherence

    Given the proper susceptible host, the virulence of *P aeruginosa* is not unexpected, given its myriad enzymes and other factors (**Figure 35–2**). The importance of ExoA is supported by studies in humans and animals, which correlate its presence with a fatal outcome and antibody against it with survival. The effect of ExoA is not immediate, since it is one of a number of virulence factors activated through a gene-regulating system called **quorum sensing.** Under these conditions, lactones and/or quinolones secreted by *P aeruginosa* signal their presence to the other bacterial cells. The system is quantitative so when the *Pseudomonas* cell population reaches a certain threshold, the signals direct the cytotoxin gene to be transcribed, and the toxin is then produced by the entire population at once. No diphtheria-like systemic effect of ExoA has been demonstrated, but its action correlates with the primarily invasive and locally destructive lesions seen in *P aeruginosa* infections.

※ **ExoA secretion triggered by quorum sensing**

※ **ExoA correlates with invasion, destruction**

    Elastase and phospholipase degrade proteins and lipids, respectively, allowing the organism to acquire nutrients from the host and disseminate from the local site. The many biologically important substrates of **elastase**—particularly its namesake, elastin—argue for its importance. Elastin is

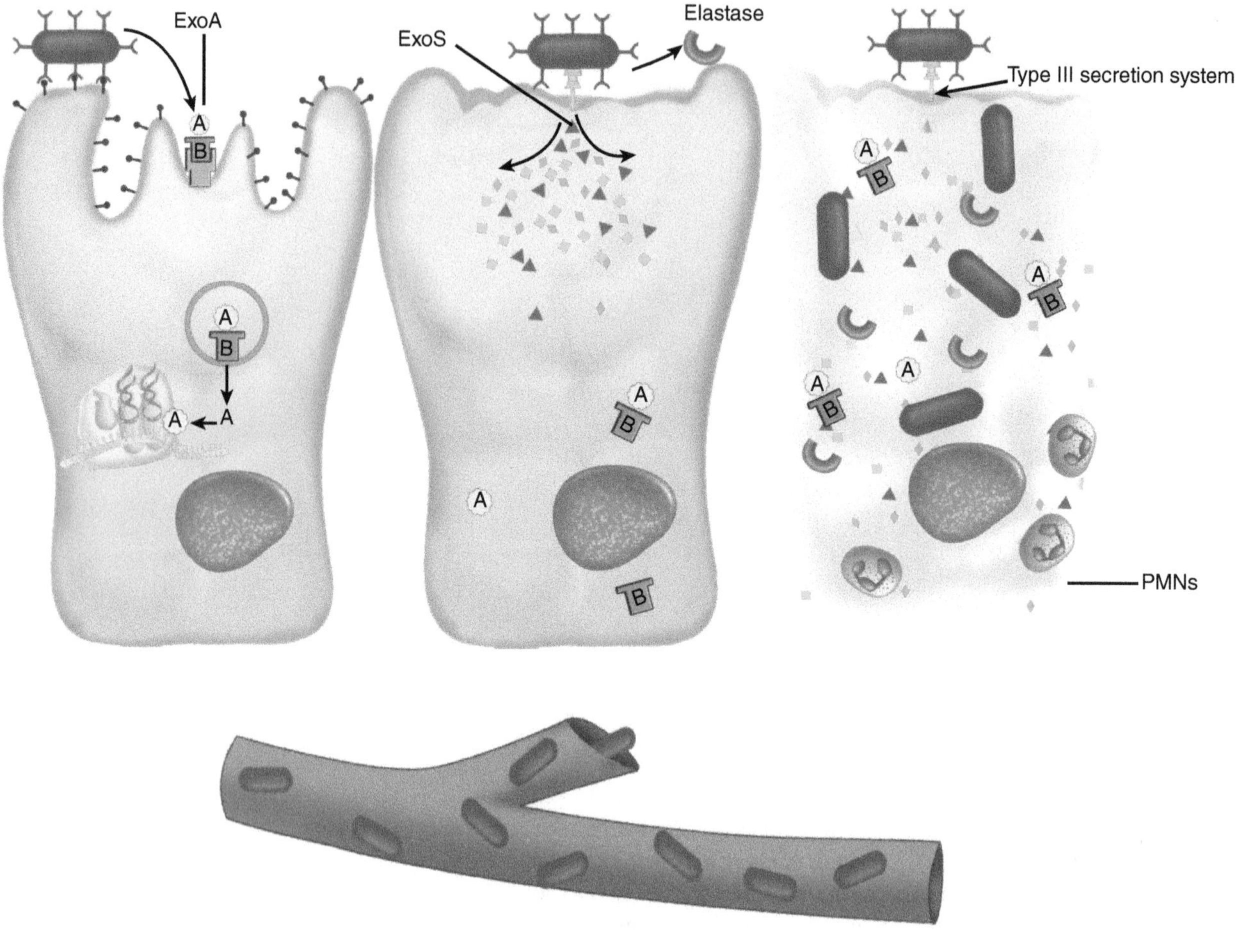

ExoA

ExoS

Elastase

Type III secretion system

PMNs

A B

A B

A ← A

A B

A

B

A B

A B

A B

A

A

FIGURE 35–2. *Pseudomonas* **disease, cellular view.** (*Left*) *P aeruginosa* binds and secretes the A–B exotoxin A (ExoA), which acts on protein synthesis by the same mechanism as diphtheria toxin. (*Middle*) A type III injection secretion system delivers exoenzyme S (ExoS) to the cell cytoplasm. Elastase is secreted extracellularly. (*Right*) All toxins act to destroy the cell and the bacteria may enter the blood.

found at some sites that *P aeruginosa* preferentially attacks, such as the lung and blood vessels. Elastase-mediated hemorrhagic destruction, including the walls of blood vessels (**Figure 35–3**), is the histologic hallmark of *Pseudomonas* infection. The intracellular dysfunction caused by ExoS and other factors injected by the secretion system begin immediately upon contact with the host cell. ExoS is associated with dissemination from burn wounds and with actions destructive to cells, including its action on the cytoskeleton. The blue pigment pyocyanin has been detected in human lesions and shown to have a toxic effect on respiratory ciliary function.

✳ Elastase attacks lung and blood vessels

✳ Injected ExoS disrupts cells

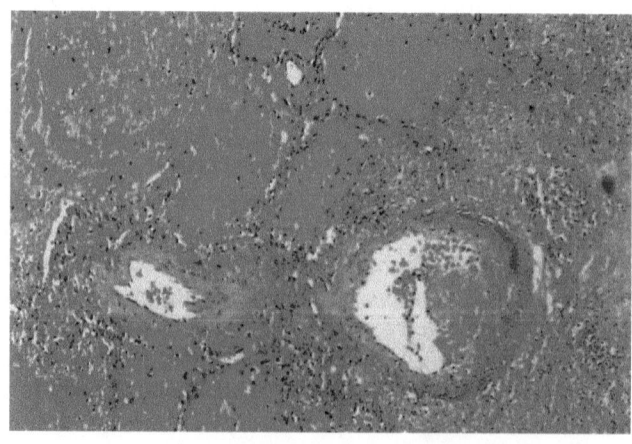

FIGURE 35–3. *Pseudomonas aeruginosa* **pneumonia.** This blood vessel in the lung of a fatal case is infected with *P aeruginosa* and is undergoing destruction. A thrombus is forming in the lumen as well. (Reproduced with permission from Connor DH, Chandler FW, Schwartz DQ, et al: *Pathology of Infectious Diseases.* Stamford CT: Appleton & Lange; 1997.)

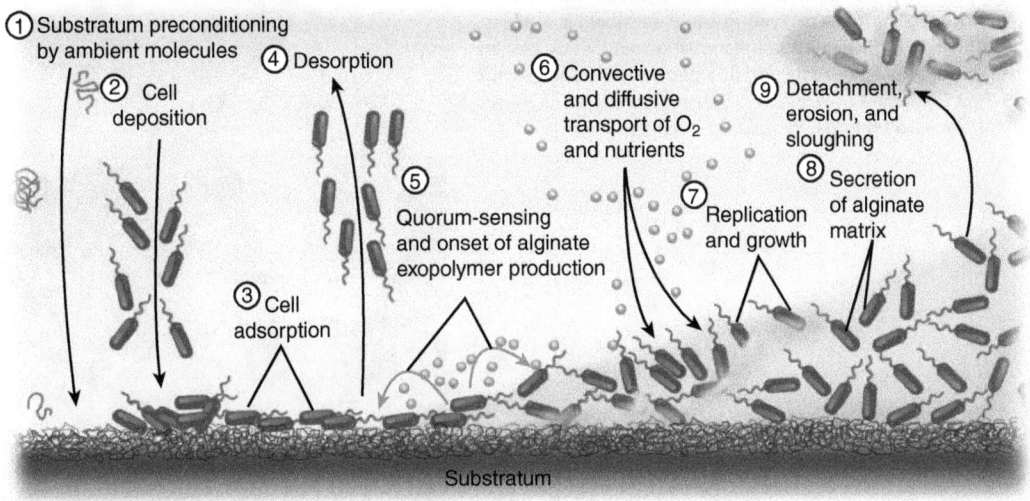

FIGURE 35–4. *Pseudomonas aeruginosa* alginate biofilm in cystic fibrosis. (Reproduced with permission from Willey JM: *Prescott, Harley, & Klein's Microbiology*, 7th ed. New York, NY: McGraw Hill; 2008.)

■ *Pseudomonas aeruginosa* and Cystic Fibrosis

P aeruginosa is the most persistent of the infectious agents that complicate the course of CF. Initial colonization may be aided by the fact that cells from CF patients are less highly sialylated than normal epithelial cells, providing improved access to receptors suitable for *P aeruginosa* attachment; defects in the epithelia of CF patients may also impede bacterial clearance by desquamation. The most striking feature of this host-pathogen relationship is the appearance of strains with multiple mutations in regulatory genes, causing overproduction of the thick alginate polymer. The colonization of the bronchi then becomes a **biofilm** with microcolonies of bacteria and debris embedded in the alginate (**Figure 35–4**). The high osmolarity of characteristically thick CF secretions facilitates expression of these alginate-hyperproducing mutants. For *P aeruginosa*, biofilm confers highly advantageous protection from the immune system (complement, antibody, phagocytes) and antimicrobial agents. The global regulatory networks responsible for quorum sensing, and their effects on alginate production and other virulence-related behaviors, remain a central focus in the search for novel therapeutics.

* Mutants overproduce alginate polymer

* Biofilm protects bacteria

IMMUNITY

Human immunity to *Pseudomonas* infection is not well understood. Inferences from animal studies and clinical observations suggest that both cell-mediated and humoral immunity are important. The strong propensity of *P aeruginosa* to infect those with defective cell-mediated immunity indicates that these responses are important, while provocative studies on the **host interleukin IL-17** have highlighted the humoral response. The versatile IL-17 cytokine recruits inflammatory cells to sites of infection and promotes release of neutrophilic cytokines at epithelial surfaces. While this cytokine appears critical to prevention of chronic infection, experimental deficiency has also been protective against an acute lethal response; in aggregate, these findings demonstrate the delicate balance that the immune system must strike between harmful and beneficial responses.

* Humoral and cellular immune responses both important

Immune system balance between benefit and harm

 ## *P AERUGINOSA* DISEASE: CLINICAL ASPECTS

MANIFESTATIONS

P aeruginosa can produce any of the opportunistic extraintestinal infections caused by members of the Enterobacteriaceae. Burn, wound, urinary tract, skin, eye, ear, and respiratory infections all occur and may give rise to bacteremia. *P aeruginosa* is also one of the most common causes of infection in environmentally contaminated wounds (eg, osteomyelitis after compound fractures or nail puncture wounds of the foot).

* Infects burns and environmentally contaminated wounds

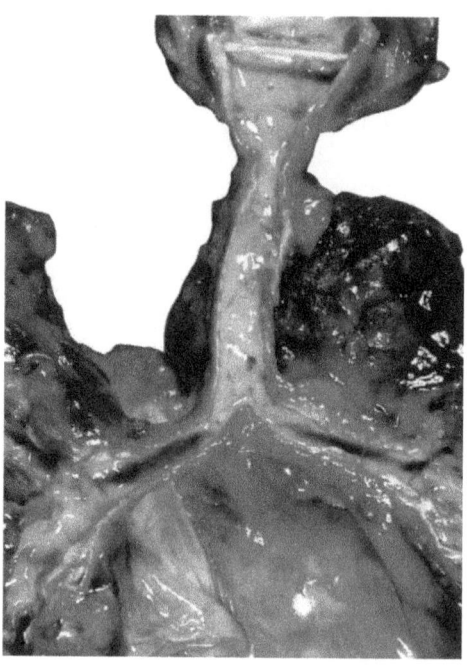

FIGURE 35–5. *Pseudomonas aeruginosa* and cystic fibrosis. The lungs of a young adult are shown at autopsy. There is both extensive inflammation and thick biofilm throughout. (Reproduced with permission from Connor DH, Chandler FW, Schwartz DQ, et al: *Pathology of Infectious Diseases*. Stamford CT: Appleton & Lange; 1997.)

* Pneumonia aggressive in immunocompromised, chronic in CF

Particularly in patients with neutropenia, *P aeruginosa* pneumonia is a rapid, destructive infection associated with alveolar necrosis, vascular invasion, infarcts, and bacteremia. Pulmonary infection in CF patients is different; it is a chronic infection that alternates between a state of colonization and more overt bronchitis or pneumonia (**Figure 35–5**). Although the more aggressive features of *Pseudomonas* infection in the immunocompromised are not common in CF, the infection is still serious enough to be a leading cause of death in CF patients.

* Common cause of otitis externa

* Contact lens contamination leads to keratitis

* Bacteremia may cause ecthyma gangrenosum

P aeruginosa is also a common cause of otitis externa, including "swimmer's ear" and a rare but life-threatening **malignant otitis externa** seen in patients with diabetes. Folliculitis of the skin may follow soaking in hot tubs that have become heavily contaminated with the organism. *P aeruginosa* can cause conjunctivitis, keratitis, or endophthalmitis when introduced into the eye by trauma or contaminated medication or contact lens solution. Keratitis can progress rapidly and destroy the cornea within 24 to 48 hours. In some cases of *P aeruginosa* bacteremia, cutaneous papules develop which progress to black, necrotic ulcers—a condition called **ecthyma gangrenosum**. The lesions are the result of direct invasion and destruction of blood vessel walls by the organism.

DIAGNOSIS

* Pigments produced in culture

P aeruginosa is readily grown in culture. The combination of characteristic oxidase-positive colonies, pyocyanin production (**Figure 35–6**), and the ability to grow at 42°C is sufficient to distinguish *P aeruginosa* from other *Pseudomonas* species. Although biochemical tests can identify other species, such tests are usually not done unless the clinical evidence for infection is very strong.

TREATMENT

* Multidrug resistance due to restricted permeability

Of the pathogenic bacteria, *P aeruginosa* is the organism most consistently resistant to many antimicrobials. Inherent resistance is due to the porins that restrict entry of antibiotic compounds to the periplasmic space. *P aeruginosa* strains are uniformly resistant to penicillin, ampicillin, cephalothin, tetracycline, chloramphenicol, sulfonamides, and the earlier aminoglycosides (streptomycin, kanamycin). Much effort has been directed toward the development of antimicrobials with anti-*Pseudomonas* activity. All treatment must be guided by antimicrobial susceptibility testing as resistance patterns are highly variable. The aminoglycosides in current use—gentamicin, tobramycin, and amikacin—all are still active against most strains. Among β-lactams, clinicians have relied on the anti-pseudomonal workhorses (piperacillin/tazobactam, cefepime, ceftazidime,

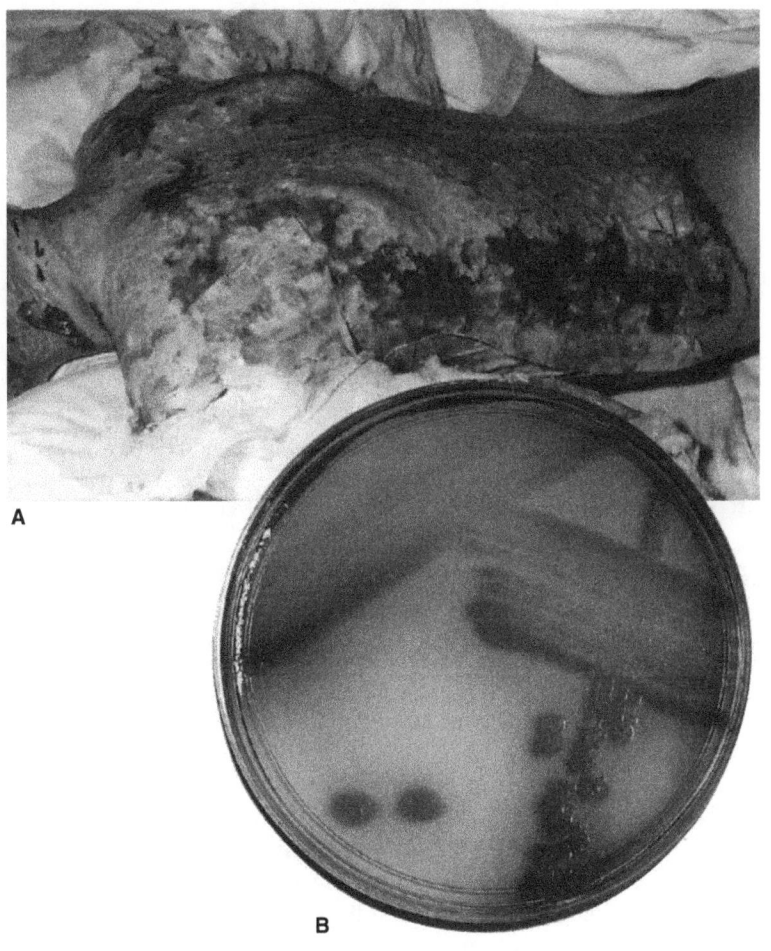

FIGURE 35–6. ***Pseudomonas aeruginosa* pigment production.** The blue color of pyocyanin when mixed with yellow tissue or media components typically produces a green discoloration. This is sometimes seen in clinical cases **A.** and regularly seen on culture plates **B.** (Reproduced with permission from Nester EW, Anderson DG, Roberts CE Jr, et al: *Microbiology: A Human Perspective*, 6th ed. New York, NY: McGraw Hill; 2008.)

imipenem/cilastatin, meropenem, doripenem), but may have additional options with more recently developed β-lactam/β-lactam inhibitor combinations. In general, urinary infections may be treated with a single drug, but more serious systemic *P aeruginosa* infections are initially treated with a combination of an anti-pseudomonal β-lactam and an aminoglycoside, particularly in neutropenic patients; fluoroquinolones may also be used as monotherapy or in combination against susceptible strains. Long simmering interest in phage therapy has risen in recent years, with sporadic reports of experimental use for treatment of extensively resistant *P aeruginosa* infections, but remains under study.

* Resistance to penicillins and aminoglycosides is common

* Ceftazidime and cefepime (third- and fourth-generation cephalosporins) often active

The treatment for *P aeruginosa* infection in CF presents special problems because most of the effective antimicrobials are only given intravenously. To avoid hospitalization, oral agents are often used to manage mild exacerbations. Patients that have persistent or progressive symptoms will then be admitted for "cleanout" with multiple intravenous antibiotics. The chronic nature of *P aeruginosa* colonization leads to progressive development of resistance over the course of patients' disease. Aerosolized tobramycin has been used in many CF patients, with evidence of clinical effectiveness in improving pulmonary function and decreasing risk of hospitalization.

* Effective oral agents scarce

* Inhaled tobramycin provides benefit

PREVENTION

Vaccines incorporating somatic antigens from multiple *P aeruginosa* serotypes have been developed and proved immunogenic in humans. The primary candidates for such preparations are patients with burn injuries, CF, or immunosuppression. Although some protection has been demonstrated, these preparations have generally proven disappointing.

Vaccines are experimental

  Why would aerosolized tobramycin be used in this situation?

BURKHOLDERIA

Burkholderia pseudomallei is a saprophyte in soil, ponds, rice paddies, and vegetables found in Southeast Asia, the Philippines, Indonesia, and other tropical areas. Infection is acquired by direct inoculation or by inhalation of aerosols or dust containing the bacteria. The resultant disease, **melioidosis,** is usually an acute pneumonia; however, it is sufficiently variable that subacute, chronic, and even relapsing infections may follow systemic spread. Some American soldiers relapsed years after their return from Vietnam. The clinical and radiologic features may resemble tuberculosis. In fulminant cases of melioidosis, rapid respiratory failure may ensue and metastatic abscesses develop in the skin or other sites. Though intrinsically resistant to a wide range of antibacterials, *B pseudomallei* may be susceptible to tetracycline, sulfonamides, and trimethoprim-sulfamethoxazole (as well as chloramphenicol, though its toxicity precludes its use in many developed countries). *Burkholderia cepacia* complex is a group of opportunistic species that has been found to contaminate laboratory reagents, disinfectants, and medical devices in much the same manner as *P aeruginosa*. They have also complicated the course of CF, even producing a life-threatening necrotizing pneumonia ("cepacia syndrome"), but do not produce the mucoid polymer seen with *P aeruginosa*.

✳ Melioidosis is a tropical pneumonia that relapses

✳ *B cepacia* infects CF patients and hospitalized patients

ACINETOBACTER

The genus *Acinetobacter* comprises Gram-negative coccobacilli that occasionally appear sufficiently round on Gram smears to be confused with *Neisseria*. On primary isolation, they closely resemble Enterobacteriaceae in growth pattern and colonial morphology but are distinguished by their failure to ferment carbohydrates or reduce nitrates. As with most of the organisms discussed in this chapter, the isolation of *Acinetobacter* from specimens other than normally sterile sites (blood, bronchoalveolar lavage fluid) does not define infection because these bacteria appear frequently as skin and respiratory colonizers. They are most frequently found as contaminants of almost anything wet, including soaps and some disinfectant solutions. Pneumonia is the most common infection, followed by urinary tract and soft tissue infections. Nosocomial respiratory infections have been traced to contaminated inhalation therapy equipment, and bacteremia to infected intravenous catheters. While treatment is frequently complicated by resistance to penicillins, cephalosporins, and occasionally aminoglycosides, virtually pan-resistant *Acinetobacter* isolates have produced outbreaks in intensive care units and military hospitals abroad.

✳ Respiratory and urinary infections come from soil and water

MORAXELLA

Moraxella is another genus of Gram-negative organisms that are usually paired end-to-end. Though many *Moraxella* species exhibit coccobacillary morphology, *Moraxella catarrhalis* isolates appear as diplococci; indeed, the morphology, fastidious growth (some species require enriched media, such as blood or chocolate agar), and positive oxidase reaction of *Moraxella* species can result in confusion with *Neisseria* in the laboratory. *M catarrhalis* is found in the normal oropharyngeal flora, and it is an occasional cause of lower respiratory tract infection and otitis media. In otitis media cases, *M catarrhalis* has been detected in mixed culture with pathogens like *Haemophilus influenzae* and *Streptococcus pneumoniae*; because *M catarrhalis* frequently produces β-lactamase, it has been blamed for "protecting" the other pathogens when β-lactam treatment fails.

✳ Bronchitis and otitis arise from respiratory flora

✳ *M catarrhalis* diplococci may be confused with *Neisseria*

AEROMONAS AND *PLESIOMONAS*

The genera *Aeromonas* and *Plesiomonas* have bacteriologic features similar to those of the Enterobacteriaceae, *Vibrio*, and *Pseudomonas*. They are aerobic and facultatively anaerobic, attack carbohydrates fermentatively, and demonstrate various other biochemical reactions. *Aeromonas* colonies are typically β-hemolytic. The resemblance of *Aeromonas* and *Plesiomonas*

 Think ▸▸ Apply 35-1: There is no oral form of tobramycin. CF patients infected with *P aeruginosa* infected alginate biofilms need to be treated outside the hospital often for long periods. Aerosolization provides this safety and convenience and may also enhance delivery of the drug directly to biofilms at effective concentrations.

TABLE 35-1   *Pseudomonas* and Other Opportunistic Gram-negative Rods

| SPECIES | BACTERIOLOGIC FEATURES | | PIGMENTS | ADHERENCE | VIRULENCE FACTORS | EPIDEMIOLOGY | DISEASE |
	MACCONKEY GROWTH	CO_2 REQUIRED					
Pseudomonas							
P aeruginosa	+	–	Pyocyanin, fluorescein	Pili, flagella, alginate slime	Exotoxin A, exoenzyme S, elastase, alginate slime	Environmental, normal flora, mucosal breaks, nosocomial	Wounds, pneumonia, burns, otitis externa, cystic fibrosis
P fluorescens	+	–	Fluorescein			Environmental	Opportunistic
Other species	+	–	Fluorescein			Environmental	Opportunistic
Stenotrophomonas maltophilia	+	–	–		Protease	Environmental, mucosal breaks, water, nosocomial	Pneumonia, bacteremia
Acinetobacter	+	–	–		Capsule	Environmental, skin colonization, water, nosocomial	Respiratory, urinary catheter bacteremia
Burkholderia							
B mallei	+	–	–			Contact with horses	Glanders
B pseudomallei	+	–	–		Facultative intracellular growth	Environmental in Southeast Asia and tropical regions	Melioidosis
B cepacia	+	–	–	Pili	Invasion, elastase, biofilm	Environmental, mucosal breaks, water, nosocomial	Wounds, pneumonia, cystic fibrosis
Aeromonas	+	–	–		Enterotoxin, cytotoxin	Environmental, fresh and salt water, leeches, intestinal flora	Wounds, diarrhea
Plesiomonas	+	–	–		Enterotoxin	Water, seafood, soil	Diarrhea
Aggregatibacter[a]	+	+	–			Respiratory flora	Endocarditis, periodontal disease
Cardiobacterium[a]	+	+	–			Nasopharyngeal, intestinal flora	Endocarditis
Eikenella[a]	+	+	–			Periodontal flora	Endocarditis, oropharyngeal abscess, draining sinuses
Alcaligenes	+	–	–			Respiratory, intestinal flora	Blood, urine, wounds
Chromobacterium	+	+	Violet			Water, soil (tropical)	Cellulitis, bacteremia
Flavobacterium	+	+	Yellow			Environmental, nosocomial	Meningitis
Moraxella	+	+		Pili		Respiratory flora	Bronchitis, pneumonia

[a]Along with *Haemophilus* and *Kingella* species, these species constitute the HACEK group of pathogens that produce endocarditis of insidious onset.

Resemble other enteric bacteria

to *Pseudomonas* arises from their shared oxidase positivity and polar flagella. Their habitat is basically environmental (water and soil), but they can occasionally be found in the human intestinal tract.

Acquired in fresh or salt water, *Aeromonas* is an uncommon but highly virulent cause of wound infections. The onset can be as rapid as 8 hours after the injury, and the cellulitis can progress rapidly to fasciitis, myonecrosis, and bacteremia in less than a day. *Aeromonas* is also the leading cause of infections associated with the medical use of leeches, owing to its regular presence in the leech foregut. In addition to opportunistic infection, some evidence suggests an occasional role for *Aeromonas* in gastroenteritis through production of toxins with enterotoxic and cytotoxic properties. *Plesiomonas* is also associated with an enterotoxic diarrhea. These associations have not been strong enough to warrant routine efforts to isolate *Aeromonas* and *Plesiomonas* from diarrheal stools, but newer molecular tests may raise clinical awareness of their prevalence in the community. Resistance to penicillins and first-generation cephalosporins is typical. Most strains show susceptibility to fluoroquinolones and tetracyclines, with variable susceptibility to aminoglycosides, including gentamicin.

✳ Rapid cellulitis follows injury in water

✳ Diarrheal illnesses relate to enterotoxin production

"HACEK" GROUP

The HACEK acronym denotes species from the genera *Haemophilus*, *Aggregatibacter*, *Cardiobacterium*, *Eikenella*, and *Kingella* that have been implicated in up to 3% of all cases of infective endocarditis. These pathogens typically produce infection in individuals with prosthetic heart valves or other underlying heart disease. These species are part of the microbiota of the oral cavity and upper respiratory tract in humans and tend to produce syndromes that are insidious in onset and challenging to diagnose. Treatment with third-generation cephalosporins produces a favorable outcome in 80% to 90% of cases.

OTHER GRAM-NEGATIVE RODS

There are many other Gram-negative rods that rarely cause disease in humans. Some are members of the microbiota, and others come from the environment. Because many of these do not ferment carbohydrates or react in many of the tests routinely used to characterize bacteria, their identification is frequently delayed while additional tests are performed or the organism is sent to a reference laboratory. The clinical significance of all these organisms is essentially the same: the clinician usually receives report of a "non-fermenter" (or other descriptive term) and a susceptibility test result, and the significance of the isolate must then be determined on clinical grounds. The major characteristics of some of these organisms are shown in **Table 35-1**. The types of infection listed represent the most common among scattered case reports and should not be interpreted as typical for each organism.

✳ Rare species interpreted based on their clinical setting

Some Gram-negative bacilli fail to conform to any of the species currently recognized. If clinically important, such strains are sent to reference centers, such as the Centers for Disease Control and Prevention (CDC) in Atlanta, Georgia. Eventually, some are given designations such as "CDC group IIF," which may appear in clinical reports. Much later, a new genus and/or species name may be issued if agreement among taxonomists is sufficient.

Some bacteria remain unnamed for years

CASE STUDY

Leukemia and Black Skin Ulcers

An 8-year-old boy with recently diagnosed acute leukemia was treated with potent cytotoxic drugs in an effort to induce remission. Within 5 days of starting chemotherapy, his total white blood cell count had fallen from 60,000/mm³ pretreatment to 300/mm³, with no granulocytes present. On the sixth day, the boy developed a high fever (40.1°C) with no focal findings except for the appearance of several faintly erythematous nodules on the thighs.

Over the next 2 days, his skin lesions became purple, then black, and necrotic, eventually forming multiple deep ulcers. Chest radiographs taken at the onset of fever were clear, but the following day showed diffuse infiltrates in both lungs. All blood cultures taken on day 6 were positive for an oxidase-positive, Gram-negative rod that produced blue-green discoloration of the culture plates.

QUESTIONS

1. This infection is most likely due to which of the following:
   A. *Pseudomonas aeruginosa*
   B. *Burkholderia pseudomallei*
   C. *Burkholderia cepacia*
   D. *Aeromonas*
   E. *Acinetobacter*

2. Which is the most important predisposing feature for this infection?
   A. Hospital environment
   B. Antibiotic treatment
   C. Neutropenia
   D. Age

3. The skin lesions are most likely due to the action of:
   A. Alginate
   B. Pyocyanin
   C. Oxidase
   D. Elastase
   E. Flagella

ANSWERS

1. **(A)**

2. **(C)**

3. **(D)**

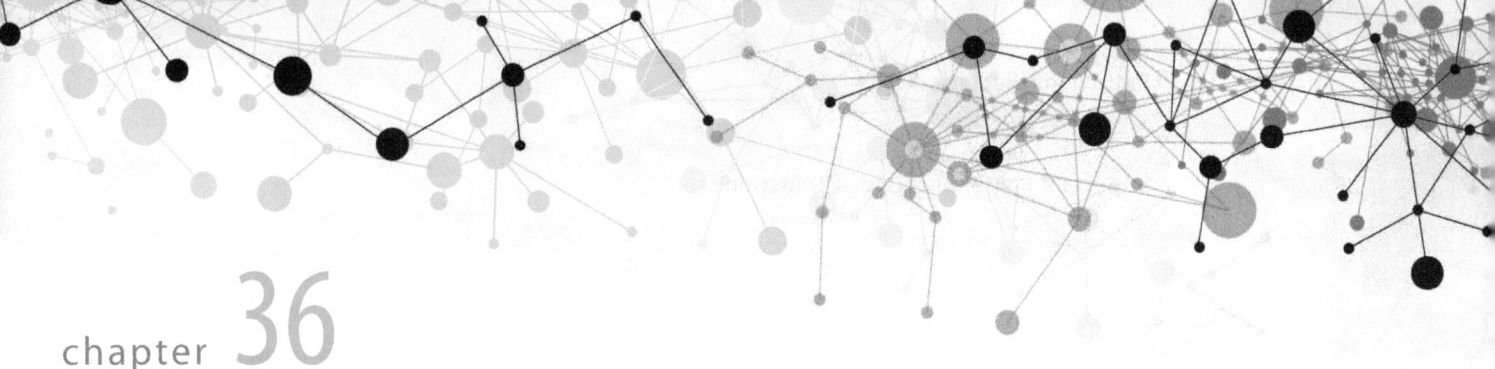

Plague and Other Bacterial Zoonotic Diseases

Brucella abortus · Yersinia pestis · Francisella tularensis · Pasteurella multocida

> *Dr. Rieux resolved to compile this chronicle…to state quite simply what we learn in a time of pestilence: that there are more things to admire in men than to despise.*
>
> —Albert Camus: *The Plague*

OVERVIEW

Zoonoses are infections in humans acquired by direct or indirect contact with animals. There are many zoonoses and more are being recognized (**Table 36–1**), but those covered herein are of great importance historically and still occur. The three principle species/variants of *Brucella* and their associated animals are *abortus* (cattle), *melitensis* (sheep and goats), and *suis* (pigs) in whom they cause genitourinary tract disease. Humans such as farmers, slaughterhouse workers, and veterinarians become infected directly by occupational contact or indirectly by consumption of contaminated animal products such as milk. In humans *Brucella* evade toll-like receptors (TLRs) and innate immunity, survive in macrophages by inhibiting myeloperoxidase and lysosome fusion, and produce a chronic illness characterized by fever, night sweats, and weight loss lasting weeks to months. Because the infection is localized in reticuloendothelial organs, there are few physical findings unless the liver or spleen becomes enlarged. When patients develop a cycling pattern of nocturnal fevers, the disease has been called undulant fever. The diagnosis is made by culturing blood or retrospectively by serology.

Yersinia pestis causes plague, an infection of rodents that is transmitted to humans by the bite of infected fleas and is the most explosively virulent disease known owing to its complex array of mechanisms to avoid host defenses. Most cases begin with a painful swollen lymph node (bubo) from which the bacteria rapidly spread to the bloodstream. Pneumonic plague (Black Death) is produced by pulmonary seeding from the bloodstream or is acquired directly from another patient with hemorrhagic pneumonia. All forms cause a toxic picture with shock and death within a few days. No other disease regularly kills previously healthy persons so rapidly. *Y pestis* is readily recovered on media used for other Enterobacteriaceae from aspirates of lymph nodes, blood cultures, and sputum in patients with pneumonia.

Tularemia is a disease of wild mammals caused by *Francisella tularensis*. Humans usually become infected by direct contact with infected animals or through the bite of a vector (tick or deer fly). Contact with water contaminated by ill animals has also been well documented. The illness is characterized by a local ulcer with high fever and severe constitutional symptoms. Typhoid-like illness with systemic symptoms only has been described. The epidemiology of tularemia and many features of the clinical infection are similar to those of plague.

Pasteurella multocida is found normally in the respiratory tract of many companion and other domestic and wild animals. When humans sustain a penetrating bite or scratch, most often by a cat, a rapidly destructive local soft tissue infection results.

TABLE 36–1	Some Important Bacterial Zoonotic Infections					
DISEASE	ETIOLOGIC AGENT	USUAL RESERVOIR	USUAL MODE OF TRANSMISSION TO HUMANS	TRANSMISSION BETWEEN HUMANS	MODE OF TRANSMISSION BETWEEN HUMANS	SPECIAL CHARACTERISTICS
Anthrax	*Bacillus anthracis*	Cattle, sheep, goats	Infected animals or products	No		Resistant spores
Bovine tuberculosis	*Mycobacterium bovis*	Cattle	Milk	No		
Brucellosis	*Brucella abortus*	Cattle, swine, goats	Milk, infected carcasses	No		
Campylobacter infection	*Campylobacter jejuni*	Wild mammals, cattle, sheep, pets	Contaminated food and water	Yes	Fecal–oral	
Leptospirosis	*Leptospira* spp.	Cattle, rodents	Water contaminated with urine	No		
Lyme disease	*Borrelia burgdorferi*	Deer, rodents	Ticks, transplacentally	No		Late sequelae
Pasteurellosis	*Pasteurella multocida*	Animal oral cavities	Bites, scratches	No		
Plague	*Yersinia pestis*	Rodents	Fleas	Yes	Droplet (pneumonic) spread	Great epidemic potential
Other *Yersinia* infections	*Y enterocolitica, Y pseudotuberculosis*	Wild mammals, pigs, cattle, pets	Fecal–oral	Yes	Fecal–oral	
Relapsing fever	*Borrelia* spp.	Rodents, ticks	Ticks	No	Tick	
Salmonellosis	*Salmonella* serotypes	Poultry, livestock	Contaminated food	Yes	Fecal contamination of food	
Rickettsial spotted fevers	*Rickettsia rickettsii*[a]	Rodents, ticks, mites	Ticks, mites	No		
Epidemic typhus	*R prowazeki*	Humans	Body louse	Yes	Body louse	Epidemic potential
Murine typhus	*Rickettsia typhi*	Rodents	Fleas	No		
Q fever	*Coxiella burnetii*	Cattle, sheep, goats	Contaminated dust and aerosols	No		

[a]One of several etiologic agents.

Many bacterial, rickettsial, and viral diseases are classified as zoonoses, because they are acquired by humans either directly or indirectly from animals. This chapter considers bacteria that cause four zoonotic infections not covered in other chapters. All four etiologic agents, *Brucella abortus, Yersinia pestis, Francisella tularensis,* and *Pasteurella multocida,* are Gram-negative bacilli that are primarily animal pathogens. The diseases they cause, brucellosis, plague, tularemia, and pasteurellosis, are now mostly rare in humans and develop only after unique animal contact. The full range of zoonoses considered in this and other chapters is shown in Table 36–1.

● *BRUCELLA*

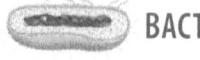 ## BACTERIOLOGY

Brucella species are small, coccobacillary, Gram-negative rods that morphologically resemble *Haemophilus* and *Bordetella.* They are nonmotile, non–acid-fast, and non–spore-forming. The cells have a typical Gram-negative structure, and the outer membrane contains proteins. The genus *Brucella* contains nine closely related variants that differ primarily in their preferred terrestrial or marine hosts. Taxonomists vacillate as to whether they should be called species or something else. The three most commonly infecting humans, *B abortus* (cattle), *B melitensis* (sheep, goats), and *B suis* (swine), will all be referred to here as *B abortus* or simply *Brucella*. Their growth is relatively slow, requiring at least 2 to 3 days of aerobic incubation in enriched broth or on blood agar. They produce catalase, oxidase, and urease, but do not ferment carbohydrates. The lipid composition of the *Brucella* envelope is unusual in that the dominant phospholipid component (phosphatidylcholine) is more typical of eukaryotic than bacterial cells.

Coccobacilli resemble *Haemophilus*

✳ Variants infect cattle, sheep, goats, swine

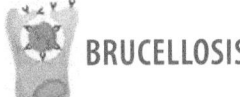

BRUCELLOSIS

EPIDEMIOLOGY

Brucellosis, a chronic infection that persists for life in animals, is an important cause of abortion, sterility, and decreased milk production in cattle, goats, and hogs. It spreads among animals by direct contact with infected tissues and ingestion of contaminated feed. It causes chronic infection of the mammary glands, uterus, placenta, seminal vesicles, and epididymis.

Abortion in cattle, goats, pigs

Humans acquire brucellosis by occupational exposure or consumption of unpasteurized dairy products. The bacteria may gain access through cuts in the skin, contact with mucous membranes, inhalation, or ingestion. In the United States, the number of cases has dropped steadily from a maximum of more than 6000 per year in the 1940s to the current level of fewer than 100 per year. Of these cases, 50% to 60% are in abattoir employees, government meat inspectors, veterinarians, and others who handle livestock or meat products. Consumption of unpasteurized dairy products, which accounts for 8% to 10% of infections, is the leading source in persons who have no connection with the meat-processing or livestock industries. The distribution of human cases of brucellosis in the United States includes virtually every state, but is concentrated in states with large livestock industries or the populous states bordering Mexico (California, Arizona, Texas). An outbreak in Texas was traced to unpasteurized goat cheese brought in from Mexico.

✳ Occupational disease for veterinarians

✳ Unpasteurized dairy products a risk

PATHOGENESIS

All *Brucella* are facultative intracellular parasites of epithelial cells and professional phagocytes. After they penetrate the skin or mucous membranes, they are able to evade aspects of the innate immune system, particularly Toll-like receptors (TLRs). This may be due to the more eukaryotic than prokaryotic nature of their outer membrane lipids. Once past the epithelial and innate immune barriers they enter and multiply in macrophages in the liver sinusoids, spleen, bone marrow, and other components of the reticuloendothelial system and eventually form granulomas (**Figure 36–1**). Intracellular survival is facilitated by inhibition of both the myeloperoxidase

✳ Evades TLRs, multiplies in macrophages

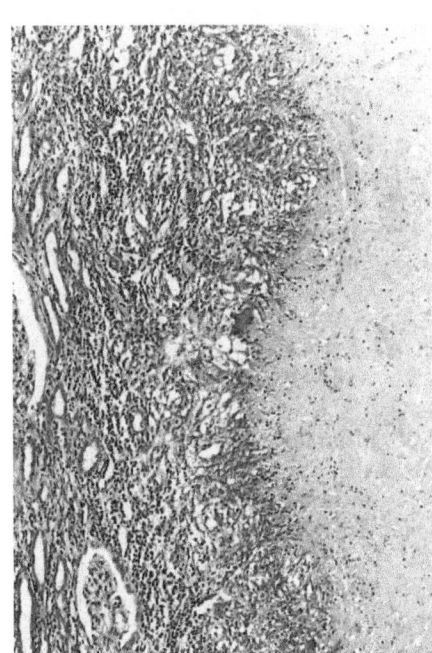

FIGURE 36–1. **Brucellosis.** Caseating granuloma in the kidney of a midwestern cattle farmer. The giant and epithelioid cells are pallisaded around the caseating area on the right. Glomeruli are compressed on the left. (Reproduced with permission from Connor DH, Chandler FW, Schwartz DQ, et al: *Pathology of Infectious Diseases.* Stamford CT: Appleton & Lange; 1997.)

system and of phagosome–lysosome fusion. This is accompanied by multiplication in their own replicative compartment in association with the endoplasmic reticulum (ER). This intracellular strategy includes a contact secretion system (type IV) and is similar to that of *Legionella pneumophila* (see Chapter 34). *Brucella* is also able to inhibit apoptosis, thus prolonging the life of the host cell where it is replicating. In cows, sheep, pigs, and goats, erythritol, a four-carbon alcohol present in chorionic tissue, markedly stimulates growth of *Brucella*. This stimulation probably accounts for the tendency of the organism to locate in these sites. The human placenta does not contain erythritol.

If not controlled locally, infection progresses with the formation of small granulomas in the reticuloendothelial sites of bacterial multiplication and with release of bacteria back into the systemic circulation. These bacteremic episodes are largely responsible for the recurrent chills and fever of the clinical illness. These events resemble the pathogenesis of typhoid fever (see Chapter 33).

IMMUNITY

Although antibodies are formed in the course of brucellosis, there is little evidence that they are protective. Control of disease is due to T-cell–mediated cellular immune responses. Development of T_H1-type responses with the production of cytokines (tumor necrosis factors [TNF-α, TNF-γ, IL-1] and interleukin [IL-12]) are associated with the elimination of *Brucella* from macrophages.

BRUCELLOSIS: CLINICAL ASPECTS

MANIFESTATIONS

Brucellosis starts with malaise, chills, and fever 7 to 21 days after infection. Drenching sweats in the late afternoon or evening are common, as are temperatures in the range of 39.4°C to 40°C. The pattern of periodic nocturnal fever (undulant fever) typically continues for weeks, months, or even 1 to 2 years. Patients become chronically ill with associated body aches, headache, and anorexia. Weight loss of up to 20 kg may occur during prolonged illness. Despite these dramatic effects, physical findings and localizing signs are few. Less than 25% of patients show detectable enlargement of the fixed macrophage or reticuloendothelial organs, the primary site of infection. Of such findings, splenomegaly is most common, followed by lymphadenopathy and hepatomegaly. Occasionally, localized infection develops in the lung, bone, brain, heart, or genitourinary system. These cases usually lack the pronounced systemic symptoms of the typical illness.

DIAGNOSIS

Definitive diagnosis of brucellosis requires isolation of *Brucella* from the blood or from biopsy specimens of the liver, bone marrow, or lymph nodes. The slower growth of *Brucella* may require longer incubation of agar plates than for most bacteria; however, blood cultures are positive in 2 to 5 days with newer automated systems and improved media. The diagnosis is often made serologically, but is subject to the same interpretive constraints as are all serologic tests. Antibodies that agglutinate suspensions of heat-killed organisms typically reach titers of 1:640 or more in acute disease. Lower titers may reflect previous disease or cross-reacting antibodies. Titers return to the normal range within 1 year of successful therapy.

TREATMENT AND PREVENTION

Doxycycline in combination with rifampin or gentamicin is the primary treatment for brucellosis. Ciprofloxacin, and trimethoprim-sulfamethoxazole are also used in combinations. Although β-lactams may be active *in vitro*, clinical response is poor, probably as a result of failure to penetrate the intracellular location of the bacteria. The therapeutic response is not rapid; 2 to 7 days may pass before patients become afebrile. Up to 10% of patients have relapses in the first 3 months after therapy. Prevention is primarily by measures that minimize occupational exposure and by the pasteurization of dairy products. Control of brucellosis in animals involves a combination of immunization with an attenuated strain of *B abortus* and eradication of infected stock. No human vaccine is in use.

Margin notes

✳ Inhibits myeloperoxidase, lysosome fusion, apoptosis

Animal placental erythritol stimulates growth

✳ Macrophage killing requires T_H1 responses

✳ Recurrent bacteremia from reticuloendothelial sites

✳ Night sweats, periodic fevers without a focus

✳ Blood culture primary

✳ Serologic tests may be useful

✳ Doxycycline plus rifampin

✳ Pasteurization primary prevention

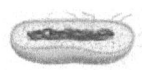 *YERSINIA PESTIS*

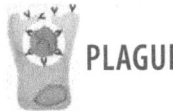 ## BACTERIOLOGY

Y pestis is a nonmotile, non–spore-forming, Gram-negative bacillus with a tendency toward pleomorphism and bipolar staining. It is a member of the Enterobacteriaceae family (see Chapter 33) and shares features of the other *Yersinia* pathogenic for humans (*Y pseudotuberculosis, Y enterocolitica*), such as virulence plasmids and multiple *Yersinia* outer membrane proteins (Yops). In addition, *Y pestis* has two virulence plasmids, which code for a glycoprotein gel-like capsule called the F1 antigen and enzymes with phospholipase, protease, fibrinolytic, and plasminogen-activating activity. *Y pestis* also has its own adhesin similar to the invasins of the other *Yersinia*.

Member of Enterobacteriaceae

✳ Yops, glycoprotein capsule, multiple enzymes

PLAGUE

EPIDEMIOLOGY

The term **plague** is often used generically to describe any explosive pandemic disease with high mortality. Medically, it refers only to infection caused by *Y pestis*, and this appellation was justly earned because *Y pestis* was the cause of the most virulent epidemic plague of recorded human history, the Black Death of the Middle Ages. In the 14th century, the estimated population of Europe was 105 million; between 1346 and 1350, 25 million died of plague. Pandemics continued through the end of the 19th century and the early 20th century despite elaborate quarantine measures developed in response to the obvious communicability of the disease. Yersin isolated the etiologic agent in China in 1894 and named it after his mentor, Pasteur (*Pasteurella pestis*). The name was later changed to honor Yersin (*Yersinia pestis*).

Black Death into 20th century

Plague is a disease of rodents transmitted by the bite of rat fleas (*Xenopsylla cheopis*) that colonize them. It exists in two interrelated epidemiologic cycles, the **sylvatic** and the **urban** (**Figure 36–2**). Endemic transmission among wild rodents in the sylvatic (Latin *sylvaticus*, belonging to or found in the woods) is the primary reservoir of plague. When infected rats enter a city, circumstances for the urban cycle are created. Humans can enter the cycle from the bite of the flea in either environment. However, chances are greater in the urban setting, particularly with crowding and poor sanitation.

✳ Sylvatic transmission among rodents Is primary reservoir

The plagues of the Middle Ages are examples of the urban cycle involving rats and humans. When food is scarce in the countryside, rats migrate to cities. This facilitates rat-to-rat transmission and brings the primary reservoir into closer contact with humans. When the number of nonimmune rats is sufficient, epizootic plague develops among them, with bacteremia and high mortality. Fleas feeding on the rats become infected, and the bacteria multiply in their intestinal tract eventually blocking the proventriculus, a valve-like organ connecting the esophagus to the midgut. When the rat dies, the fleas seek a new host, which is usually another rat but may be a nearby human. Because of the intestinal blockage, the infected flea regurgitates *Y pestis* into the new bite wound. Therefore, the probability of transmission to humans is greatest when both rat population and rat mortality are high.

✳ Rat migration to cities increases human risk

✳ Fleas regurgitate into bite wounds

✳ Bubo initial lesion

✳ Pneumonia is contagious

The bite of the flea is the first event in the development of a case of **bubonic plague,** which, even if serious enough to kill the patient, is not contagious to other humans. However, some patients with bubonic plague develop a secondary pneumonia by bacteremic spread to the lungs. This **pneumonic plague** is highly contagious person to person by the respiratory droplet route. It is not difficult to understand how rapid spread proceeds in conjunction with crowded unsanitary conditions and continued flea-to-human transmission. A 20th century urban plague epidemic is vividly described through the eyes of a physician in Albert Camus' novel, *The Plague*.

Although urban plague epidemics have been essentially eliminated by rat control and other public health measures, sylvatic transmission cycles persist in many parts of the world, including North America. These cycles involve nonurban mammals such as prairie dogs, deer mice, rabbits, and wood rats. Transmission between them involves fleas. Coyotes or wolves may be infected by the same fleas or by ingestion of infected rodents. By their nature, the reservoir animals rarely come in contact with humans; when they do, however, the infected fleas they carry can transmit *Y pestis*. The

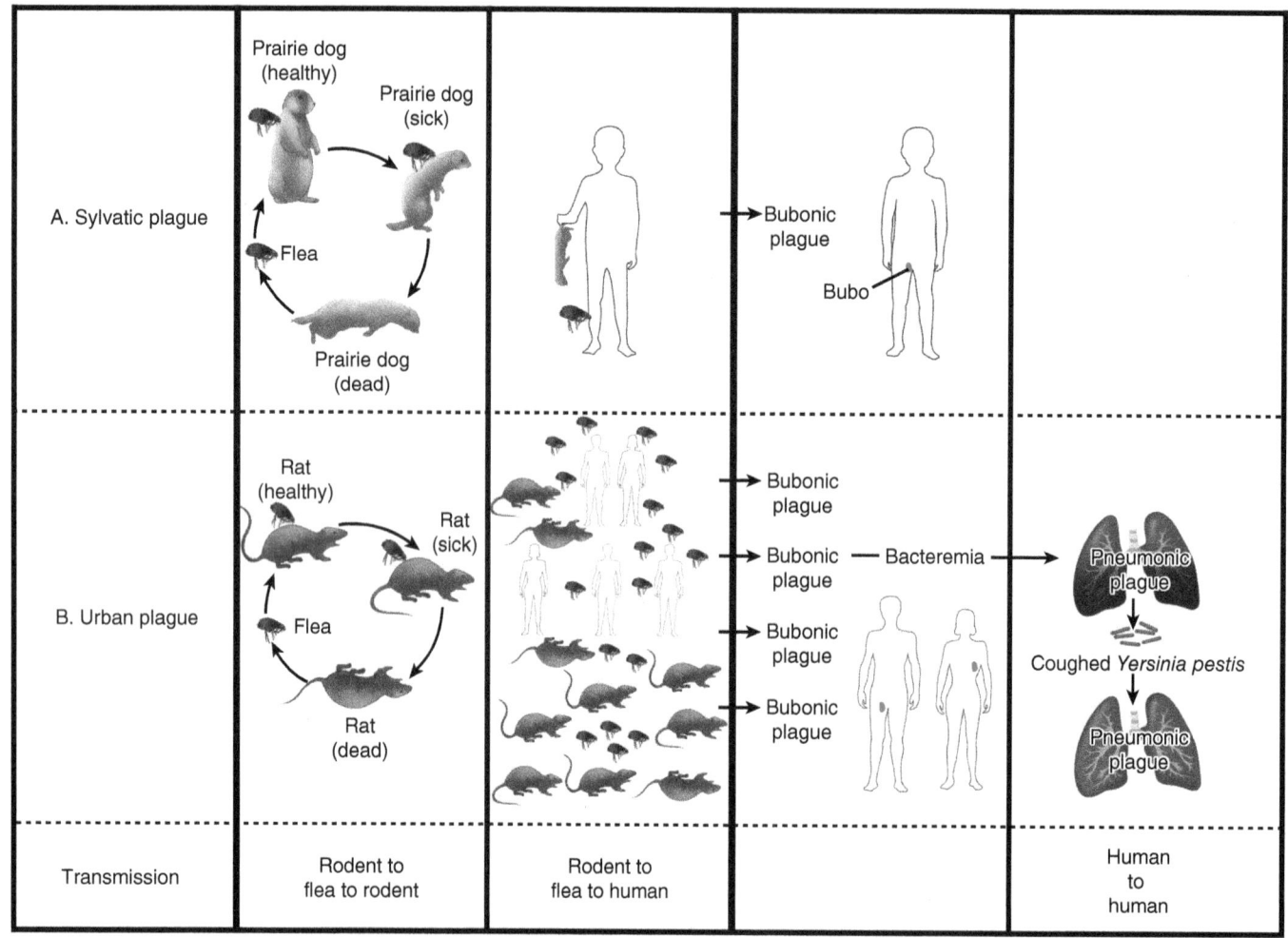

FIGURE 36–2. The epidemiology of plague. A. In the sylvatic cycle, fleas leaving infected rodents, such as mice and prairie dogs, pass the infection to others in the population. Humans rarely contact these rodents but when they do, the flea bite transmits plague. **B.** In the urban cycle, masses of rats are in closer contact with humans, and bites from infected fleas transmit the infection to many. In both cycles, initial transmissions result in bubonic plague. Bacteremia with *Y pestis* may infect the lungs to cause pneumonic plague. Pneumonic plague is transmitted human to human by the respiratory route without the involvement of fleas.

✻ Nonepidemic disease due to wild animal contact

most common circumstance is a child who is exploring the outdoors, comes across a dead or dying prairie dog, and pokes, carries, or touches it long enough to be bitten by the fleas leaving the animal. The result is a sporadic case of bubonic plague, which occasionally becomes pneumonic.

Sylvatic plague is found in Africa, North and South America, and Asia; however, 95% of human cases currently occur in Africa and Madagascar accounts for nearly half of those. In the United States, the primary enzootic areas are the semiarid plains of the western states. Infected animals and fleas have been detected from the Mexican border to the arid eastern half of Washington State. The geographic focus of human plague in the United States is in the "four corners" area, where Arizona, New Mexico, Colorado, and Utah meet, but cases have occurred in California, west Texas, Idaho, and Montana. Most years, as many as 15 cases of plague are reported, although this number rose to 30 to 40 in the mid-1980s. These variations are strongly related to changes in the size of the sylvatic reservoir.

✻ Most U.S. cases in arid western states

PATHOGENESIS

Multiplication in flea foregut aided by low temperature, virulence factors

It should not be surprising that the molecular pathogenesis of plague is quite complex, given its extremely high virulence in both insect and mammalian environments. Of more than 20 known virulence factors, some are deployed primarily in the flea, whereas others are produced only in the rodent or human victim. *Y pestis* has regulatory systems that sense temperature, calcium, and

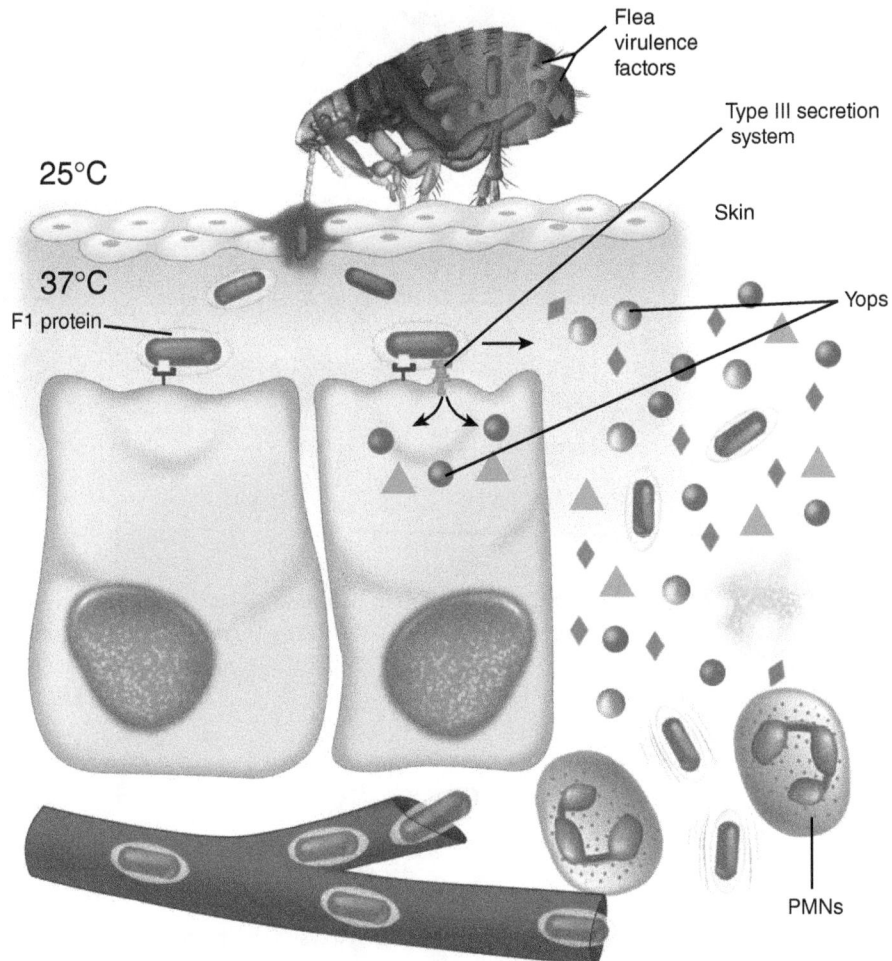

25°C

37°C

F1 protein

Flea virulence factors

Type III secretion system

Skin

Yops

PMNs

FIGURE 36–3. **Plague, cellular view.** (*Top*) *Yersinia pestis* is growing in the flea and producing virulence factors unique to that environment. Bacteria are regurgitated as part of the flea's feeding on human skin and reach the subepithelial tissues. Here, triggered by environmental cues such as a new warmer temperature (37°C), they start to produce a new set of virulence factors unique to mammalian victims such as the F1 protein capsule. (*Left*) *Yersinia pestis* attaches to an epithelial cell. (*Middle*) *Yersinia* outer membrane proteins (Yops) begin to be produced. Some are injected by a type III secretion system, others are secreted on the surface. (*Right*) The cell is destroyed and the organisms evade phagocytosis to enter the bloodstream. PMNs, polymorphonuclear neutrophils.

surely other environmental triggers to turn the production of appropriate virulence factors on or off. At ambient temperature (20–28°C) in the flea, factors that facilitate multiplication of the organism (fibrinolysin, phospholipase) and blockage of the proventriculus (coagulase, polysaccharide biofilm) are produced. The flea, sensing starvation, feeds voraciously but due to the intestinal blockage repeatedly regurgitates blood and bacteria into the bite wound. In this wound (rat or human), *Y pestis* is suddenly moved into a new environment.

In a new warm-blooded (35-37°C) host, *Y pestis* produces a second set of virulence factors including the F1 capsule, a plasminogen activator (Pla), and the Yops (**Figure 36–3**). At this temperature it also synthesizes a form of lipopolysaccharide (LPS) that is not recognized by the TLRs that respond to Gram-negative bacteria. The F1 protein forms a gel-like capsule with antiphagocytic properties that allow the bacteria to persist and multiply. Pla facilitates metastatic spread through enzymatic activity and adhesion to extracellular matrix proteins. The Yops, though named as a protein family (YopA, YopB, and so on), have diverse biologic activities that fall into two categories. The first is direct destructive enzymatic activity directed at host cells. The other set of actions disrupt intracellular function and are mediated through injection secretion systems (type III). Once inside host cells, including professional phagocytes, these secreted proteins disrupt signaling pathways, destroy cytoskeleton structure, trigger apoptosis, and inhibit cytokine production and acidification of phagosomes.

The organisms eventually reach the regional lymph nodes through the lymphatics, where they multiply rapidly and produce a hemorrhagic suppurative lymphadenitis known clinically as the **bubo.** Spread to the bloodstream quickly follows. The extreme systemic toxicity that develops with bacteremia appears to be due to LPS endotoxin combined with the many actions of Yops, proteases, and other extracellular products. The bacteremia causes seeding of other organs, most notably the lungs, and produces a necrotizing hemorrhagic pneumonia known as pneumonic plague.

✳ Flea regurgitates bacteria into bite wound

✳ F1 protein capsule antiphagocytic

✳ Pla, Yops produced at 37°C

✳ Yops destroy and disrupt

✳ Bubo progresses to bacteremia

✳ LPS, other products produce shock

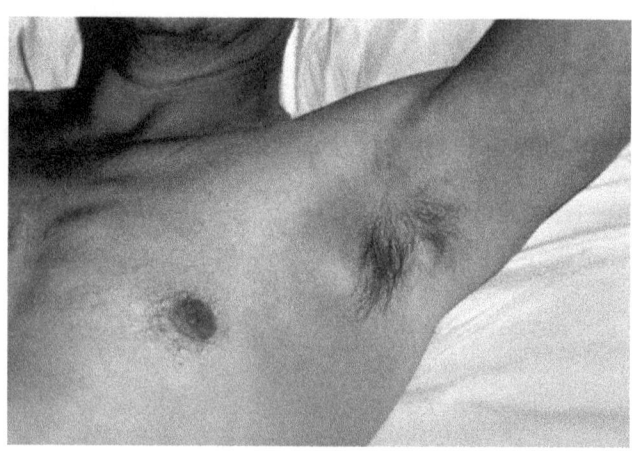

FIGURE 36–4. Bubonic plague. A swollen bubo is seen in the axilla of this man. (Reproduced with permission from Public Health Image Library [PHIL]. Centers for Disease Control and Prevention. Photo contributor Dr. Karl F. Meyer, ID #2061.)

IMMUNITY

Anticapsular antibody may be protective

Recovery from bubonic plague appears to confer lasting immunity, but for obvious reasons the mechanisms in humans have not been extensively studied by modern immunologic methods. Animal studies suggest that antibody against the F1 capsular glycoprotein is protective by enhancing phagocytosis, but cell-mediated mechanisms are required for intracellular killing.

 PLAGUE: CLINICAL ASPECTS

MANIFESTATIONS

✳ **Bubonic plague mortality up to 75%**

✳ **Pneumonic plague fatal if untreated**

Terminal cyanosis = Black Death

The incubation period for bubonic plague is 2 to 7 days after the flea bite. Onset is marked by fever and a painful bubo, usually in the groin (bubo is from the Greek *boubon* for "groin") or, less often, in the axilla (**Figure 36-4**). Without treatment, 50% to 75% of patients progress to bacteremia and die in Gram-negative septic shock within hours or days of development of the bubo. About 5% of victims develop pneumonic plague with mucoid, then bloody sputum. Primary pneumonic plague has a shorter incubation period (2-3 days) and begins only with fever, malaise, and a feeling of tightness in the chest. Cough, production of sputum, dyspnea, and cyanosis develop later in the course. Death on the second or third day of illness is common, and there are no survivors without antibiotic therapy. A terminal cyanosis seen with pneumonic plague is responsible for the term Black Death. Even today, plague pneumonia is almost always fatal if appropriate treatment is delayed more than a day from the onset.

DIAGNOSIS

Immunofluorescent staining, PCR available

Cultures grow on routine media

Gram-stained smears of aspirates from the bubo typically show bipolar-staining Gram-negative bacilli. RT-PCR for the *Y pestis*-specific *pla* gene and detection of F1 antigen by immunofluorescence are available in public health laboratories in endemic areas for immediate identification of smears or cultures. *Y pestis* is readily isolated on the media used for other members of the Enterobacteriaceae (blood agar, MacConkey agar), although growth may require more than 24 hours of incubation. The appropriate specimens are bubo aspirate, blood, and sputum. Laboratories must be notified of the suspicion of plague to avoid delay in the bacteriologic diagnosis and to guard against laboratory infection.

TREATMENT

✳ **Gentamicin/streptomycin +/– doxycycline**

Gentamicin or streptomycin with or without doxycycline is the treatment of choice for both bubonic and pneumonic plague. Ciprofloxacin or chloramphenicol (if meningitis is present) are alternatives. Timely treatment reduces the mortality of bubonic plague to less than 10%, but the mortality rate of human cases of plague reported in developed countries is still around 20% because of delays in initiation of appropriate therapy.

PREVENTION

Urban plague has been prevented by rat control and general public health measures such as use of insecticides. Sylvatic plague is virtually impossible to eliminate because of the size and dispersion of the multiple rodent reservoirs. Disease can be prevented by avoidance of sick or dead rodents and rabbits. Eradication of fleas on domestic pets, which have been known to transport infected fleas from wild rodents to humans, is recommended in endemic areas. The continued presence of fully virulent plague in its sylvatic cycle poses a risk of extension to the urban cycle and epidemic disease in the event of major disaster or social breakdown. Chemoprophylaxis with doxycycline or ciprofloxacin is recommended for those who have had close contact with a case of pneumonic plague. It is also used for the household contacts of a person with bubonic plague because they may have had the same flea contact.

✳ Avoid sick or dead wild rodents

✳ Chemoprophylaxis for respiratory exposure

● *FRANCISELLA*

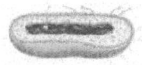 ## BACTERIOLOGY

F tularensis is a small, facultative, coccobacillary, Gram-negative rod with much the same morphology as *Brucella*. Virulent strains possess a lipid-rich capsule. *F tularensis* is one of the bacterial species of medical importance that does not grow well on routine media used for wound cultures in most clinical laboratories, but it will grow on chocolate agar. *F tularensis* has a special requirement for sulfhydryl compounds, and growth occurs best on a cysteine–glucose blood agar medium after 2 to 10 days of incubation. *Francisella* has the general structure of other Gram-negative bacilli but its outer membrane LPS is unusual in that it fails to stimulate innate immune responses but does induce specific protective antibodies.

✳ Growth requirement for –SH compounds

LPS does not stimulate protective antibodies

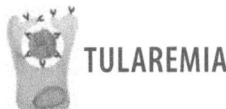 ## TULAREMIA

EPIDEMIOLOGY

Humans most often acquire *F tularensis* by contact with an infected mammal or a blood-feeding arthropod. Because the infecting dose is very low (less than 100 organisms), many routes of infection are possible. A tick bite or direct contact with an infected animal via a minor skin abrasion is the most common mechanism of infection. About 10% of cases have been linked to contaminated water by contact or ingestion, especially in Europe. Many wild mammals can be infected, including squirrels, muskrats, beavers, and deer. A common history is that of skinning wild rabbits on a hunting trip. Inhalation may also lead to disease. In an outbreak of pulmonary tularemia on Cape Cod, experts believed that lawn mowing and brush cutting facilitated inhalation. Occasionally, the bite or scratch of a domestic dog or cat has been implicated when the animal has ingested or mouthed an infected wild mammal. Infected animals may not show signs of infection, because the organism is well adapted to its natural host. The usual vectors in animals are ticks and deer flies. Ticks may also serve as a reservoir of the organism by transovarial transmission to their offspring.

✳ Infecting dose low

✳ Acquired by tick bites or directly from wild mammals

Tularemia is distributed throughout the Northern Hemisphere, although there are wide variations in specific regions. The highly virulent tick/rabbit-associated strains are common only in North America and cases have declined steadily since World War II. In the United States, 100 to 200 cases are reported each year, half of which are in the lower midwestern states (Arkansas, Missouri, Oklahoma). Tularemia is not found in the British Isles, Africa, South America, or Australia.

✳ Distribution throughout Northern Hemisphere

PATHOGENESIS

Initial entry of *Francisella* is through a cut, insect bite, or inhalation of airborne bacteria. As with *Brucella* and *Y pestis* the lipid components of its LPS are not recognized by innate TLRs so growth is unimpeded until phagocytes are encountered. Once ingested by macrophages, *Francisella*

✳ Entry by trauma, insect, or airborne

resides in a phagosome for a time but resists lysosome fusion and escapes to the host cell cytoplasm. These are the general properties of a facultative intracellular pathogen and indeed the virulence of F tularensis has been linked to its ability to multiply within many cell types, including hepatocytes, kidney, and alveolar epithelial cells. A lesion often develops at the site of infection, which becomes ulcerated. The organism then infects the reticuloendothelial organs, often forming granulomas. Early bacteremic spread probably occurs, although it is rarely detected.

IMMUNITY

Naturally acquired infection appears to confer long-lasting immunity. Antibody titers remain elevated for many years, but cellular immunity plays the major role in resistance to reinfection. T-cell–dependent reactions involving either CD4+ or CD8+ cell are detectable even before antibody responses.

 ## TULAREMIA: CLINICAL ASPECTS

MANIFESTATIONS

After an incubation period of 2 to 5 days, tularemia may follow a number of courses, depending on the site of inoculation and extent of spread. All begin with the acute onset of fever, chills, and malaise. In the ulceroglandular form, a local papule at the inoculation site becomes necrotic and ulcerative (**Figure 36–5**). Regional lymph nodes become swollen and painful. The oculoglandular form, which follows conjunctival inoculation, is similar except that the local lesion is a painful purulent conjunctivitis. Ingestion of large numbers of F tularensis (more than 10^8) leads to typhoidal tularemia, with abdominal manifestations and a prolonged febrile course that is similar to that of typhoid fever. Oral contamination results in the oropharyngeal form with mucosal ulcers and painful swollen cervical lymph nodes. Inhalation of the organisms can result in pneumonic tularemia or a more generalized infection resembling typhoid. As with plague pneumonia, tularemic pneumonia may also develop through seeding of the lungs by bacteremic spread from any of the other forms. All forms of tularemia may progress to a systemic infection with lesions in multiple organs.

Without treatment, mortality rate ranges from 5% to 30%, depending on the type of infection. Ulceroglandular tularemia, the most common form, generally carries the lowest risk of a fatal outcome estimated at 2%.

DIAGNOSIS

Because tularemia is uncommon and F tularensis has unique growth requirements, the diagnosis is easily overlooked. Although most strains grow on chocolate agar, laboratories must be alerted to the suspicion of tularemia so that specialized media supplemented with cysteine can

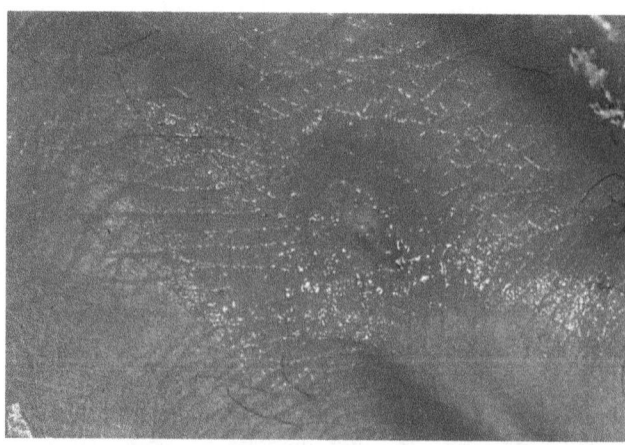

FIGURE 36–5. **Tularemia.** Ulcer on the hand of a trapper is infected with F tularensis. (Reproduced with permission from Connor DH, Chandler FW, Schwartz DQ, et al: Pathology of Infectious Diseases. Stamford CT: Appleton & Lange; 1997.)

be prepared and precautions taken against the considerable risk of laboratory infection. Where available, PCR-based based assays are useful for samples from humans, animals, and the environment. An immunofluorescent reagent is available in reference laboratories for use directly on smears from clinical material. Because of the difficulty and risk of cultural techniques, many cases of tularemia are diagnosed by serologic tests. Agglutinating antibodies are usually present in titers of 1:40 by the second week of illness, increasing to 1:320 or greater after 3 to 4 weeks. Unless previous exposure is known, single high antibody titers are considered diagnostic.

* Special media for culture

* Serodiagnosis common

* PCR useful

TREATMENT AND PREVENTION

Gentamicin or streptomycin is the treatment of choice in all forms of tularemia. Doxycycline or ciprofloxacin have also been effective, but relapses are more common than with an aminoglycoside and doxycycline combination. Prevention mainly involves the use of rubber gloves and eye protection when handling potentially infected wild mammals. Prompt removal of ticks is also important. A live attenuated vaccine exists, but it is used only in laboratory workers and those who cannot avoid contact with infected animals.

* Streptomycin or gentamicin effective

● *PASTEURELLA MULTOCIDA*

P multocida, one of many species of *Pasteurella* in the respiratory flora of animals, is a cause of respiratory infection in some. This small, coccobacillary, Gram-negative organism grows readily on blood agar but not on MacConkey agar. It is oxidase-positive and ferments a variety of carbohydrates. Unlike most Gram-negative rods, *P multocida* is susceptible to penicillin. Humans are usually infected by the bite or scratch of a domestic dog or cat. Infection develops at the site of the lesion, often within 24 hours. The typical infection is a diffuse cellulitis with a well-defined erythematous border. The diagnosis is made by culture of an aspirate of pus expressed from the lesion. Frequently, too few organisms are present to be seen on a direct Gram smear. *P multocida* is by far the most common cause of an infected dog or cat bite. *P multocida* is occasionally isolated from the sputum of patients with bronchiectasis and has been traced to contamination of home inhalation equipment by cats. Infections are treated with penicillin, but amoxicillin-clavulanate is often used empirically because animal bite wounds initially may be polymicrobial.

* Penicillin-susceptible, Gram-negative rods

* Most common cause of infected animal bites or scratches

KEY CONCLUSIONS

- *Brucella, Yersinia pestis,* and *F tularensis* all share the ability to evade TLRs and innate immunity and survive in macrophages by inhibiting lysosome fusion.
- *Brucella* thrives in the placental tissue of host animals owing to presence of erythritol; human placentas lack erythritol.
- *Brucella* causes genitourinary tract infections in animals; in humans it causes a chronic systemic illness with recurrent fever, headache, and arthralgia.
- Diagnosis of brucellosis is made by culturing blood or retrospectively by serology.
- *Y pestis* has a plethora of virulence factors (over 20 known) and is often lethal.
- Most plague in humans is bubonic and results from the bites of fleas who feed on infected rodents. Bacteremic spread to the lungs produces pneumonic plague.
- Human to human transmission of pneumonic plague is by direct inhalation of lung secretions.
- Gentamicin therapy with or without doxycycline can be life saving.
- Infections with *F tularensis* are acquired primarily through inhalation, inoculation, or the bite of ticks or deerflies.
- Tularemia has ulceroglandular, oculoglandular, typhoidal, and pneumonic forms.
- Streptomycin or gentamicin is the primary tularemia treatment and doxycycline is an alternative.
- *Pasteurella multocida* causes soft tissue infections most often after a cat bite or scratch; penicillin is effective but amoxicillin-clavulanate is used empirically.

CASE STUDY

Downhill to Death Following Cat Exposure

A 31-year-old man had just returned from visiting a friend in Chaffee County, Colorado. While there, he helped remove an obviously ill domestic cat from the crawl space under a friend's cabin. They also noticed a number of dead chipmunks in a nearby arroyo. Two days after returning to his home in Tucson, the man began to have abdominal cramps. The next day, he had the onset of fever, nausea, vomiting, severe diarrhea, and cough. On the third day, he consulted a physician because of diarrhea and vomiting. On examination, he was febrile (104°F) and dehydrated; no abnormal chest sounds were heard, and he had no lymphadenopathy. The man was treated for gastroenteritis with clindamycin and given oral ciprofloxacin to be taken the following day. The next day, he was hospitalized with cyanosis and septic shock. Chest radiographs revealed a right upper lobar pneumonia. A Gram stain of a sputum sample obtained at hospital admission showed numerous Gram-negative rods. Antibiotic therapy with ceftazidime, erythromycin, and one dose each of penicillin and gentamicin was initiated for treatment of overwhelming sepsis and pneumonia. He died 24 hours after admission.

Investigation by Chaffee County public health officials indicated that the cat, reported to have submandibular abscesses and oral lesions consistent with feline plague, died on August 19 before being evaluated by a veterinarian. The cat was cremated without diagnostic studies. A dead chipmunk found in the area where the cat lived was culture-positive for *Y pestis*.

QUESTIONS

1. This man most probably had which disease?
    A. Brucellosis
    B. Bubonic plague
    C. Pneumonic plague
    D. Typhoidal tularemia
    E. Pneumonic tularemia

2. By which of the following was his infection likely transmitted?
    A. Flea
    B. Cat
    C. Chipmunk
    D. Rat
    E. Human

3. Which of the following contributed to his death?
    A. Yops
    B. Biofilm
    C. Erythritol
    D. Adenylate cyclase
    E. ADP-ribosylation

ANSWERS

1. (C)

2. (A)

3. (A)

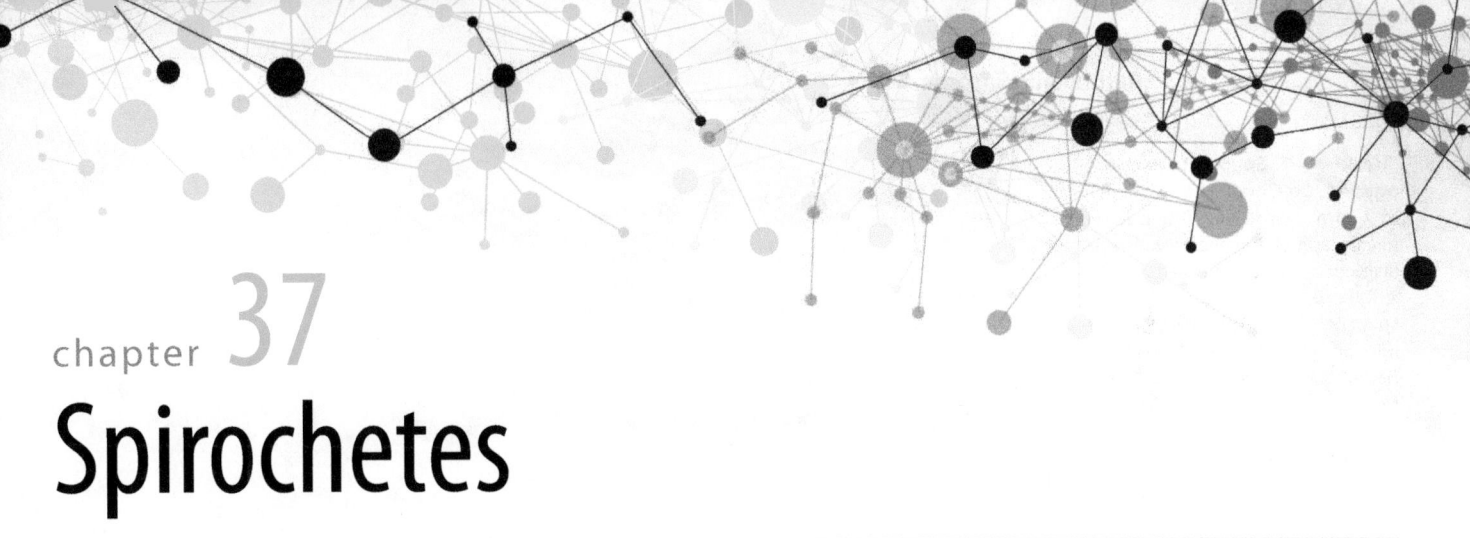

chapter 37

Spirochetes

Treponema pallidum · Leptospira interrogans · Borrelia recurrentis · Borrelia hermsii · Borrelia burgdorferi

> *The French disease, for it was that, remained in me more than four months dormant before it showed itself, and then it broke out over my whole body at one instant…with certain blisters, of the size of six-pence, and rose colored.*
>
> —Benvenuto Cellini (1500-1571): *The Life of Benvenuto Cellini*

Spirochetes are bacteria with a spiral morphology ranging from loose coils to a rigid corkscrew shape. The three medically important genera include the cause of syphilis, the ancient scourge of sexual indiscretion, and Lyme disease, a more recently discovered consequence of an innocent walk in the woods.

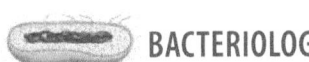 BACTERIOLOGY

MORPHOLOGY AND STRUCTURE

The spiral morphology of spirochetes (**Figure 37–1**) is produced by a flexible, peptidoglycan cell wall around which several axial fibrils are wound. The cell wall and axial fibrils are completely covered by an outer bilayered membrane similar to the outer membrane of other Gram-negative bacteria. In some species, a hyaluronic acid slime layer forms around the exterior of the organism and may contribute to its virulence. Spirochetes are motile, exhibiting rotation and flexion; this motility is believed to result from movement of the axial filaments, although the mechanism is not clear.

Spiral structure around axial filaments

Motil rotation and flexion

Many spirochetes are difficult to see by routine microscopy. Although they are Gram negative, many either take stains poorly or are too thin to fall within the resolving power of the light microscope. Only darkfield microscopy (**Figure 37–2**), immunofluorescence, or special staining techniques can demonstrate these spirochetes. Other spirochetes such as *Borrelia* are wider and readily visible in stained preparations, even routine blood smears.

Take stains poorly

Darkfield demonstrates

GROWTH AND CLASSIFICATION

Parasitic spirochetes grow more slowly *in vitro* than most other disease-causing bacteria. Some species, including the causative agent of syphilis, have not been grown beyond a few generations in cell culture. Some are strict anaerobes, others require low concentrations of oxygen, and still others are aerobic. Compared with other bacterial groups, the taxonomy of the spirochetes is underdeveloped. Because spirochetes are difficult to grow and study; thus, there are relatively few phenotypic properties on which to base a classification. The medically important genera *Treponema*, *Leptospira*, and *Borrelia* have been distinguished primarily by morphologic characters such as the nature of their spiral shape and the arrangement of flagella.

Some not isolated in culture

Aerobic or anaerobic

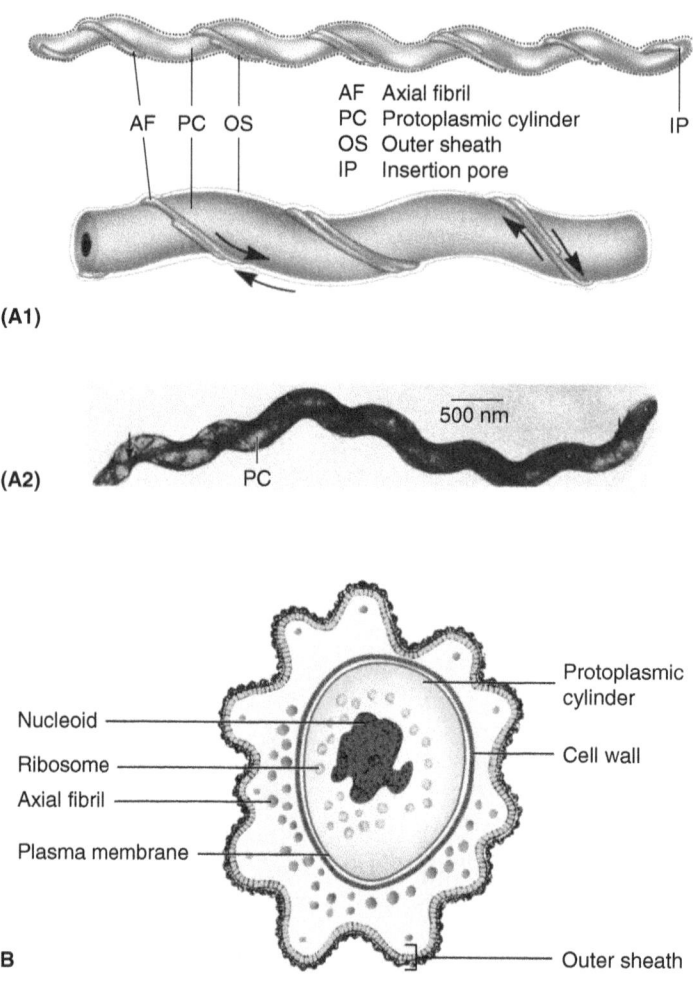

AF   Axial fibril
PC   Protoplasmic cylinder
OS   Outer sheath
IP   Insertion pore

(A1)

(A2)

B

Nucleoid

Ribosome

Axial fibril

Plasma membrane

Protoplasmic cylinder

Cell wall

Outer sheath

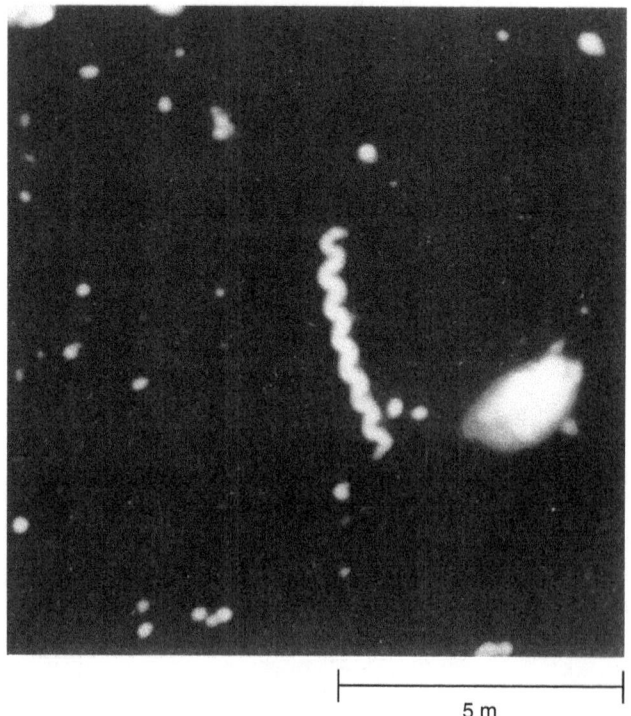

5 m

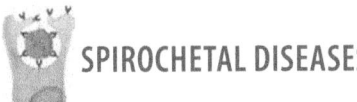

SPIROCHETAL DISEASES

Some spirochetes are free living; some are members of the microbiota of humans and animals. The oral cavity, particularly the dental crevice, harbors a number of nonpathogenic species of *Treponema* and *Borrelia* as part of its microbiome (**Table 37–1**). Under unusual conditions, these spirochetes, together with anaerobes in the flora, can cause necrotizing, ulcerative infection of the gums, oral cavity, or pharynx (Vincent infection, trench mouth).

Part of oropharyngeal flora

The major spirochetal diseases are caused by selected species of three genera that are not found in the microbiota, *Treponema* (*T pallidum*), *Leptospira* (*L interrogans*), and *Borrelia* (***Borrelia recurrentis*, *B hermsii*, and *B burgdorferi*). Most *Borrelia* and *Leptospira* infections are zoonoses transmitted from wild and domestic animals. *Treponema pallidum* is a strict human pathogen transmitted by sexual contact. Some rare nonvenereal treponemal diseases are summarized in **Appendix 37–1**.

Diseases are zoonoses or venereal

● *TREPONEMA PALLIDUM*

OVERVIEW

Treponema pallidum is a highly motile corkscrew-shaped spirochete containing a minimum of proteins and no lipopolysaccharide (LPS). It has not been isolated in culture. Its disease, syphilis, is typically acquired by the direct contact of mucous membranes during sexual intercourse. The disease begins with a lesion at the point of entry, usually a genital ulcer. After healing of the ulcer, the organisms spread systemically, and the disease may return weeks later as a generalized maculopapular rash called secondary syphilis. The disease may then enter a second eclipse phase called latency. The latent infection may be cleared by the immune system or reappear as tertiary syphilis years to decades later. Tertiary syphilis is characterized by focal lesions whose locale determines the injury. Isolated foci in bone or liver may be unnoticed, but infection of the cardiovascular or nervous systems can be devastating. Progressive dementia or a ruptured aortic aneurysm are two of many fatal outcomes of untreated syphilis.

TABLE 37–1	Features of Spirochetal Diseases						
					DIAGNOSIS		
ORGANISM	**MORPHOLOGY**	**TRANSMISSION**	**RESERVOIR**	**MICROSCOPY**	**CULTURE**	**SEROLOGY**	**DISEASE**
Treponema pallidum	Corkscrew spirals	Sexual, transplacental, transfusion	Humans	Darkfield of chancre or secondary lesions	None	VDRL, RPR, FTA-ABS, MHA-TP	Syphilis
Leptospira interrogans	Close spirals, hooked ends	Ingestion of contaminated water	Rodents, cattle, dogs	Not recommended[a]	Rarely performed[b]	MAT	Fever, meningitis, hepatitis
Borrelia recurrentis	Loose spirals	Lice	Humans	Giemsa or Wright stain of blood smear	Rarely performed[c]	None	Relapsing fever
Borrelia hermsii	Loose spirals	Ticks[d]	Rodents	Giemsa or Wright stain of blood smear	Rarely performed[c]	None	Relapsing fever
Borrelia burgdorferi	Loose spirals	Ticks[e]	White-footed mice, other rodents (deer)[f]	Not recommended[a]	Rarely performed[c]	EIA + Immunoblot	Lyme disease

EIA, enzyme immunoassay; FTA-ABS, fluorescent treponemal antibody; MAT, microagglutination test; MHA-TP, microhemagglutination test for *T pallidum*; RPR, rapid plasma reagin; VDRL, Venereal Disease Research Laboratory.

[a]Organisms are small in number and rarely seen in clinical lesions.

[b]Culture of blood or urine in semisolid Fletcher medium takes 1 to many weeks and is generally not available.

[c]Culture of blood in liquid Barbour-Stoener-Kelly medium takes 1 to many weeks and is generally not available.

[d]*Ornithodoros hermsii*, p. 9.

[e]*Ixodes scapularis* in the eastern and central United States, *I pacificus* in the western United States.

[f]Transmitting ticks mature on deer that are not actually a reservoir.

T pallidum is the causative agent of syphilis, a venereal disease first recognized in the 16th century as the "great pox," which rapidly spread through Europe in association with urbanization and military campaigns. Its extended course and the protean, often dramatic nature of its findings (genital ulcer, ataxia, dementia, ruptured aorta) are due to a state of balanced parasitism that spans decades. The cause of syphilis is actually a subspecies (*T pallidum* subsp. *pallidum*) closely related to other agents that cause rare nonvenereal treponematoses (Appendix 37-1). *T pallidum* is used here to indicate the *pallidum* subspecies.

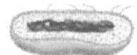 ## BACTERIOLOGY

Corkscrew spirals spin

Heat, drying, disinfectants kill

T pallidum is a slim spirochete 5 to 15 μm long with regular spirals whose wavelength and amplitude resemble a corkscrew (Figure 37–2). The organism is readily seen only by immunofluorescence, darkfield microscopy, or silver impregnation histologic techniques. Live cells show characteristic rotating motility with sudden 90-degree angle flexions, which suggest a gentleman quickly bowing at the waist. *T pallidum* is extremely susceptible to any deviation from physiologic conditions. It dies rapidly on drying and is readily killed by a wide range of detergents and disinfectants.

Beyond these observations, the study of the biology and pathogenesis of *T pallidum* is severely impeded by our inability to grow the organism in culture. It multiplies for only a few generations in cell cultures and is difficult to subculture. Sustained growth is achieved only in animals (rabbit testes), which are the sole source of bacteria for diagnostic reagents and scientific study. The *T pallidum* genome is amenable to study, and much of what follows is based on extrapolations comparing genomic sequences found there with those in other pathogenic bacteria. The picture of the syphilis spirochete is that of a minimalist pathogen, growing very slowly and producing few definitive structures or products.

✻ **Growth only in animals**

The sluggish growth (mean generation time more than 30 hours) of *T pallidum* is felt to be due to lack of enzymes that detoxify reactive oxygen species (catalase, oxidase) and the absence of efficient energy (ATP)-producing pathways such as the tricarboxylic acid cycle and electron transport chain. *T pallidum* shares the Gram-negative structural style of other spirochetes, but its outer membrane lacks LPS and contains few proteins.

No LPS, few proteins in outer membrane

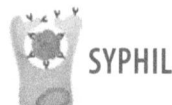 ## SYPHILIS ৸

EPIDEMIOLOGY

T pallidum is an exclusively human pathogen under natural conditions. In most cases, infection is acquired from direct sexual contact with a person who has an active primary or secondary syphilitic lesion (**Figure 37–3**). Partner notification studies suggest transmission occurs in over 50% of sexual contacts in which a lesion is present. Less commonly, the disease may be spread by nongenital contact with a lesion (eg, of the lip), sharing of needles by intravenous drug users, or transplacental transmission to a fetus within the first 3 years of the maternal infection. Late disease is not infectious. Modern screening procedures have essentially eliminated blood transfusion as a source of the disease. The incidence of new cases of primary and secondary syphilis in developed countries declined to an all time low at the end of the 20th century, but since then has risen more than 10%. Worldwide, syphilis remains a major public health problem, with an estimated six million new cases annually. There is evidence that syphilitic lesions are a portal for HIV transmission.

✻ **Transmission via mucosal surfaces, blood**

✻ **Congenital transplacental infection**

Tertiary syphilis not infectious

PATHOGENESIS

The spirochete reaches the subepithelial tissues through unapparent breaks in the skin or possibly by passage between the epithelial cells of mucous membranes aided by at least one adhesin that binds to fibronectin and elements of the extracellular matrix. Beyond a few candidate adherence or digestive proteins there is little to explain the organism's invasiveness beyond the propulsive motility generated from its corkscrew structure. In the submucosa, it multiplies slowly stimulating little initial tissue reaction. This is probably due to the relative paucity of antigens in the *T pallidum* outer membrane that could be exposed to the immune system. As lesions develop, the basic

Mucosal spread to blood

✻ **Multiplication produces endarteritis, granulomas**

Syphilis

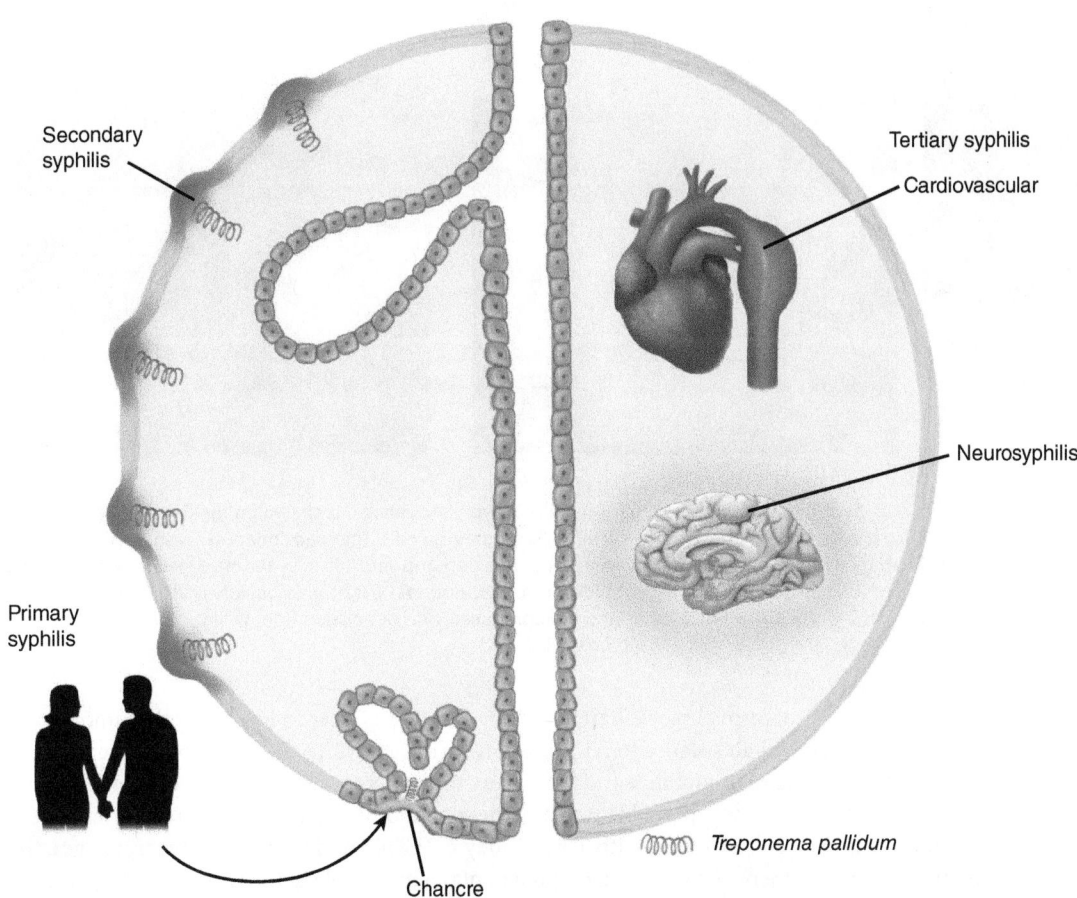

Secondary
syphilis

Tertiary syphilis

Cardiovascular

Neurosyphilis

Primary
syphilis

Chancre

Treponema pallidum

FIGURE 37–3. Syphilis overview. Infection is acquired by sexual contact, and the primary lesion is an ulcer on the genitalia called the chancre. The major feature of secondary syphilis is a maculopapular rash that is teeming with spirochetes. Tertiary syphilis (*right*) involves multiple organ systems. Shown are an aortic aneurysm as part of cardiovascular syphilis and inflammation of the brain in neurosyphilis.

pathologic finding is an endarteritis. The small arterioles show swelling and proliferation of their endothelial cells. This reduces or obstructs local blood supply, probably accounting for the necrotic ulceration of the primary lesion and subsequent destruction at other sites (**Figure 37–4A–C**). There is no evidence that this injury is due to any toxins or other classic virulence factors produced by *T pallidum*. Although the primary lesion heals spontaneously, the bacteria have already disseminated to other organs by way of local lymph nodes and the bloodstream.

* Ulcer heals but spirochetes disseminate

The disease is clinically silent until the disseminated secondary stage develops and then is silent again with entry into latency. Although evasion of host defenses is clearly taking place, the mechanisms involved are unknown. *T pallidum* strains found in secondary lesions have not been demonstrated to differ antigenically from those in the primary chancre. It may be that the combination of the low antigen content of its outer membrane combined with the extremely slow multiplication rate allows the organism to stay below whatever critical antigenic mass is required to trigger an effective immune response.

Minimal triggers for immune response

IMMUNITY

Clinical observations suggest an immune response in syphilis that is slow and imperfect. Immunity to reinfection does not appear until early latency, and for at least one-third of those infected the subsequent host response is successful in clearing most but not all of the treponemes.

Immunity slow, incomplete

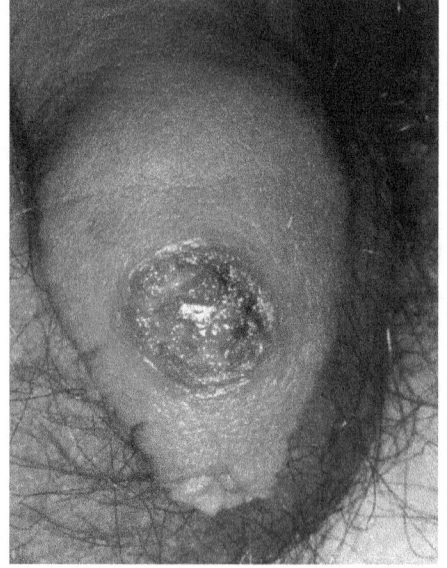
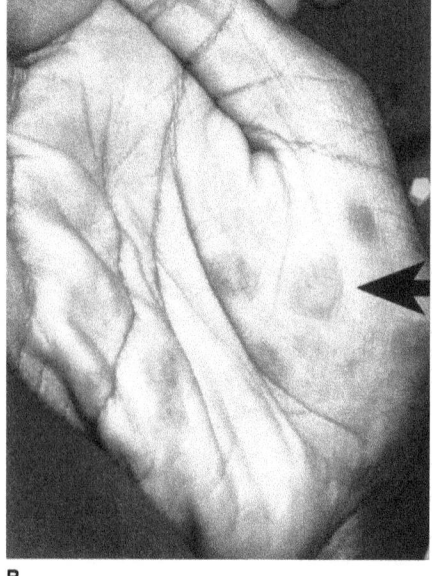
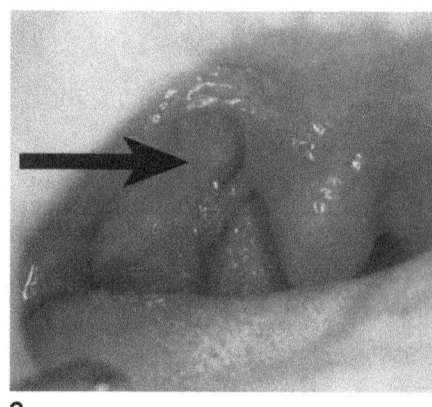

(handwritten, top margin): ←broad dissemination also transmissable from saliva·

A

B

C

(handwritten, left margin): painless chancers ↑ ↑ primary syphilis ↑ usually self-limiting

FIGURE 37–4. Syphilitic lesions. A. Primary syphilis. A syphilitic chancre is shown on the foreskin of the penis. Note the sharp edge and raw base of the ulcer. **B.** Secondary syphilis. The maculopapular rash appears on the palm. **C.** Tertiary syphilis. A ruptured gumma appears as a lump and ulcer in the hard palate of the mouth. (A, Reproduced with permission from Nester EW, Anderson DG, Roberts CE Jr, et al: *Microbiology: A Human Perspective*, 6th ed. New York, NY: McGraw Hill; 2008. B and C, Reproduced with permission from Willey JM: *Prescott, Harley, & Klein's Microbiology*, 7th ed. New York, NY: McGraw Hill; 2008.)

OMP antibodies with reinfection resistance

T-lymphocyte suppression may link stages

The immune mechanisms involved are far from clear, but appear to involve both humoral and cell-mediated responses. Resistance to reinfection is correlated with appearance of antitreponemal antibody, which is able to immobilize and kill the organism. Exposed treponemal outer membrane proteins (OMPs) are the most probable target of these antibodies. Cell-mediated responses appear to be dominant in syphilitic lesions with T lymphocytes (CD4+ and CD8+) and macrophages, the primary cell types, present. Activated macrophages play a major role in the clearance of *T pallidum* from early syphilitic lesions. The relapsing course of primary and secondary syphilis may reflect shifts in the balance between developing cellular immunity and suppression of T lymphocytes. Syphilis in immunocompromised patients such as those with acquired immunodeficiency syndrome (AIDS) may present with unusually aggressive or atypical manifestations.

SYPHILIS: CLINICAL ASPECTS

MANIFESTATIONS

■ Primary Syphilis

✶ Painless, indurated chancre

Heals after weeks

The primary syphilitic lesion is a papule that evolves to an ulcer at the site of infection. This is usually the external genitalia or cervix but could be in the anal or oral area depending on the nature of sexual contact. The lesion becomes indurated and ulcerates but remains painless, though slightly sensitive to touch. The fully developed ulcer with a firm base and raised margins is called the **chancre** (Figure 37–4A). Firm, nonsuppurative, painless enlargement of the regional lymph nodes usually develops within 1 week of the primary lesion and may persist for months. The median incubation period from contact until appearance of the primary lesion is about 3 weeks (range 3-90 days). It heals spontaneously after 4 to 6 weeks.

■ Secondary Syphilis

✶ Generalized lymphadenopathy, maculopapular rash

Secondary or disseminated syphilis develops 2 to 8 weeks after the appearance of the chancre in about a third of primary patients. The primary lesion has usually healed but may still be present. This most florid form of syphilis is characterized by a symmetric mucocutaneous maculopapular rash and generalized nontender lymph node enlargement with fever, malaise, and other manifestations of systemic infection. Skin lesions are distributed on the trunk and extremities, often including the palms (Figure 37–4B), soles, and face, and can mimic a variety of infectious and noninfectious skin eruptions. Some patients develop painless mucosal warty erosions called **condylomata lata.** These erosions usually develop in warm, moist sites such as the genitals and perineum. All the lesions of secondary syphilis are teeming with spirochetes and are highly infectious. They resolve spontaneously after a few days to many weeks, but the infection itself has resolved in only one-third of patients. In the remaining two-thirds, the illness enters the latent state.

✳ Spirochetes abundant

Disease continues in one-third

■ Latent Syphilis

Latent syphilis is by definition a stage in which no clinical manifestations are present, but continuing infection is evidenced by serologic tests. In the first few years, latency may be interrupted by progressively less severe relapses of secondary syphilis. In late latent syphilis (>4 years), relapses cease, and patients become resistant to reinfection. Transmission to others is possible from relapsing secondary lesions and by transfusion or other contact with blood products. Mothers may transmit *T pallidum* to their fetus throughout latency. About one-third of untreated cases do not have any manifestation of disease beyond this stage.

Relapses interrupt latency

Bloodborne transmission risk

■ Tertiary Syphilis — goes to CNS, destroys brain → dementia → death within 15 yrs.

Another one-third of patients with untreated secondary syphilis develop tertiary syphilis. The manifestations may appear as early as 5 years after infection but characteristically occur after 15 to 20 years. The manifestations depend on the body sites involved, the most important of which are the nervous and cardiovascular systems.

Neurosyphilis is due to the damage produced by a mixture of meningovasculitis and degenerative parenchymal changes in virtually any part of the nervous system. The most common entity is a chronic meningitis with fever, headache, focal neurologic findings, and increased cells and protein in the cerebrospinal fluid (CSF). Cortical degeneration of the brain causes mental changes ranging from decreased memory to hallucinations or frank psychosis. In the spinal cord, demyelination of the posterior columns, dorsal roots, and dorsal root ganglia produces a syndrome called **tabes dorsalis (Figure 37–5),** which includes ataxia, wide-based gait, foot slap, and loss of sensation. The most advanced central nervous system (CNS) findings include a combination of neurologic deficits and behavioral disturbances called **paresis,** which is also a mnemonic (**p**ersonality, **a**ffect, **r**eflexes, **e**yes, **s**ensorium, **i**ntellect, **s**peech) for the myriad of changes seen.

✳ Meningitis, degenerative changes, psychosis

✳ Demyelination causes neuropathies

Paresis has many signs

Cardiovascular syphilis is due to arteritis involving the vasa vasorum of the aorta and causing a medial necrosis and loss of elastic fibers. The usual result is dilatation of the aorta and aortic valve ring. This in turn leads to aneurysms of the ascending and transverse segments of the aorta and/or aortic valve incompetence. The expanding aneurysm can produce pressure necrosis of adjacent structures or even rupture. In **gummatous syphilis** a localized, granulomatous reaction to *T pallidum* infection called a **gumma** (Figure 37–4C) may be found in skin, bones, joints, or other organs. Any clinical manifestations are related to the nature of the mass and local destruction as with other mass-producing lesions like tumors.

✳ Aortitis leads to aneurysm

✳ Gummas localized granulomas

■ Congenital Syphilis

Fetuses are susceptible to syphilis only after the fourth month of gestation and adequate treatment of infected mothers before that time prevents fetal damage. Because active syphilitic infection is devastating to infants, routine serologic testing is performed in early pregnancy and should be repeated in the last trimester in women at high risk for acquiring syphilis. Untreated maternal infection may result in fetal loss or congenital syphilis, which is analogous to secondary syphilis in the adult. Although there may be no physical findings, the most common are rhinitis and a

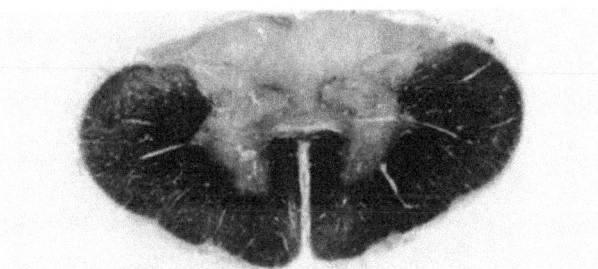

FIGURE 37–5. **Tabes dorsalis.** Loss of axons and myelin is evident in the posterior columns of the spinal cord (Woelke stain). (Reproduced with permission from Connor DH, Chandler FW, Schwartz DQ, et al: *Pathology of Infectious Diseases.* Stamford CT: Appleton & Lange; 1997.)

* Rhinitis, rash, bone changes

Congenital syphilis increasing

maculopapular rash. Bone involvement produces characteristic changes in the architecture of the entire skeletal system (saddle nose, saber shins). Anemia, thrombocytopenia, and liver failure are terminal events. The incidence of congenital syphilis in the United States more than doubled between 2013 and 2017 reaching 918 cases, the most in 20 years.

DIAGNOSIS

■ Microscopy

T pallidum can be seen by darkfield microscopy in primary and secondary lesions, but the execution of this procedure requires experience and attention to detail. The microscopist must observe the corkscrew morphology and characteristic motility to make a diagnosis (Figure 37–2). A negative result from examination does not exclude syphilis; to be readily seen, the fluid must contain thousands of treponemes per milliliter. Darkfield microscopy of oral and anal lesions is not recommended because of the risk of misinterpretation of other spirochetes present in the resident flora.

Darkfield requires fluid deep in lesion

* Negative if small numbers

 Would a darkfield exam work during secondary syphilis?

Direct fluorescent antibody methods have been developed but are available only in certain centers.

■ Serologic Tests

Most cases of syphilis are diagnosed using serologic tests that detect antibodies directed at either lipid or specific treponemal antigens. The former, called nontreponemal tests are positive only in active syphilis at the expense of a small proportion of false positives. The latter, called treponemal tests, detect antibody directed at *T pallidum* antigens. Treponemal tests are thus more specific than the nontreponemal, but do not distinguish between active and long past, even successfully treated syphilis. Their complementary deployment in the screening, diagnosis, and therapeutic evaluation of syphilis is described below.

■ Nontreponemal Tests

Nontreponemal tests measure antibody directed against **cardiolipin,** a lipid complex so called because one component was originally extracted from beef heart. Anticardiolipin antibody is called **reagin,** and the tests that detect it depend on immune flocculation of cardiolipin in the presence of other lipids. The most common nontreponemal tests are the rapid plasma reagin (RPR) and the Venereal Disease Research Laboratory (VDRL). The results become positive in the early stages of the primary lesion and, with the possible exception of some patients with advanced HIV infection, are uniformly positive during the secondary stage. They slowly wane in the later stages of the disease. In neurosyphilis, VDRL test results on CSF may be positive when the serum VDRL has reverted to negative. Nontreponemal tests are nonspecific; they may be falsely positive in a variety of autoimmune diseases or in diseases involving substantial tissue or liver destruction, such as lupus erythematosus, viral hepatitis, infectious mononucleosis, and malaria. False-positive results can also occur occasionally in pregnancy and in patients with HIV infection.

* Reagin is antibody to a lipid complex

Levels peak in secondary syphilis

* Nonspecific reactions in autoimmune diseases

* Titer used to follow therapy

Sensitivity and low cost make nontreponemal tests preferred for screening, but positive results must be confirmed by one of the more specific treponemal tests described in the following text. The tests are also valuable for monitoring treatment because the height of the antibody titer is directly related to activity of disease. With successful antibiotic therapy, positive nontreponemal serologies slowly revert to negative.

■ Treponemal Tests

Treponemal tests detect antibody specific to *T pallidum*. The microhemagglutination test for *T pallidum* (MHA-TP), uses antigens attached to the surface of erythrocytes, which then agglutinate in the presence of specific antibody. A variety of enzyme immunoassay (EIA) procedures also detect specific antibody.

* *T pallidum* is the antigen

 Think ▶▶ Apply 37-1: **Although it is not so easy to get specimens from skin papules a darkfield should be positive because the rash lesions are teeming with *T pallidum* spirochetes. The serologic tests are all positive too.**

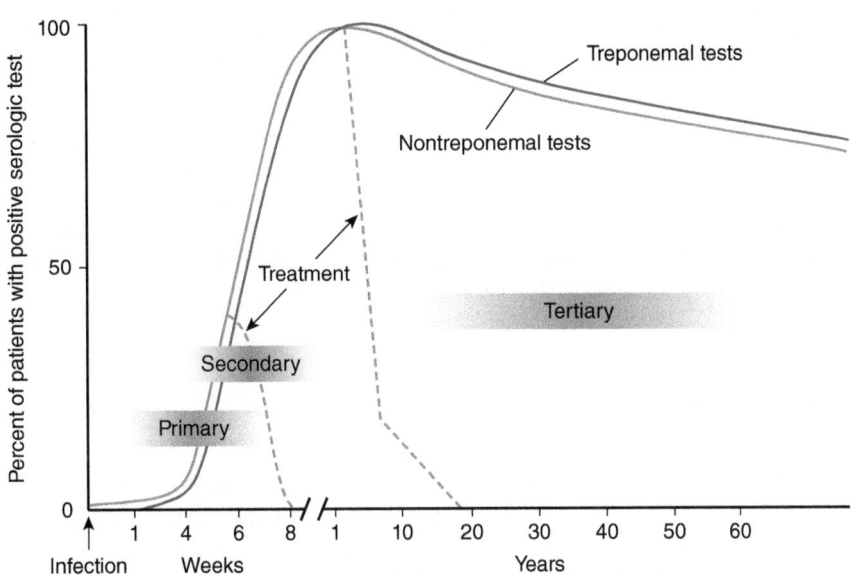

FIGURE 37–6. **Syphilis serology.** The time course of treponemal and nontreponemal tests in treated and untreated syphilis is shown. The non-treponemal test results (VDRL, RPR) rise during primary syphilis and reach their peak in secondary syphilis. They slowly decline with advancing age. With treatment, they revert to normal over a few weeks. The treponemal tests (FTA-ABS, MHA-TP) follow the same course but remain elevated even after successful treatment. FTA-ABS, fluorescent treponemal antibody; MHA-TP, microhemagglutination test for *T pallidum*; RPR, rapid plasma reagin; VDRL, Venereal Disease Research Laboratory.

Treponemal tests are considerably more specific than the cardiolipin-based nontreponemal tests. Their primary role in diagnosis is to confirm positive RPR and VDRL results obtained in the evaluation of a patient suspected of having syphilis or in screening programs. These tests are less useful for screening or after therapy because, once positive, they usually remain so for life except for the immunocompromised. The traditional approach is a two-step process. Initial screening is done with a nontreponemal test, and if positive, the result is confirmed with a treponemal test. In recent years, a "reverse algorithm" has become increasing popular with the availability of automated treponemal methods. Here the treponemal test is done first followed by the nontreponemal if positive. For persons with symptoms the added cost of this approach may be offset by improved efficiency of emergency room and hospital isolation decision-making. The time course of serologic tests in the various stages of syphilis is illustrated in **Figure 37–6**.

> ✳ Treponemal positive confirms RPR, VDRL

Reverse algorithm increasing

The use of serologic tests in the diagnosis of congenital syphilis is complicated by the presence of IgG antibodies in infants, who acquire it transplacentally from their mothers. If available, treponemal IgM tests are useful in establishing the presence of an acute infection in infants.

IgM for congenital syphilis

TREATMENT AND PREVENTION

T pallidum remains exquisitely sensitive to penicillin, which is the preferred treatment in all stages. In primary, secondary, or latent syphilis, persons hypersensitive to penicillin may be treated with doxycycline or tetracycline. The efficacy of agents other than penicillin has not been established in tertiary or congenital syphilis. It is recommended that penicillin-hypersensitive patients with neurosyphilis or congenital syphilis be desensitized rather than use an alternate antimicrobial. The Jarisch-Herxheimer reaction is a bacterial sepsis like reaction beginning in the first 8 hours after penicillin administration. It is prevented or treated with antiinflammatory agents like asprin.

> ✳ Penicillin is preferred

KEY CONCLUSIONS

- The corkscrew morphology of *Treponema pallidum* can be seen by darkfield microscopy but the organism has not been grown in culture.
- *T pallidum* has minimal structural proteins, no LPS and a very small genome. It persists by failing to trigger an effective immune response while slowly causing an endarteritis at multiple times and locations.
- Syphilis occurs in three stages. Primary syphilis includes the chancre (ulcer) and systemic dissemination. Secondary syphilis is manifest by a diffuse maculopapular rash. Tertiary syphilis includes destructive cardiovascular, nervous system, and tissue lesions.
- A latent phase between secondary and tertiary syphilis may last for decades.
- Diagnosis of syphilis is by darkfield microscopy together with treponemal and nontreponemal serologic tests.
- Penicillin treatment stops the disease process at any stage.

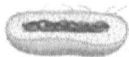 **LEPTOSPIRA INTERROGANS**

OVERVIEW

Leptospira interrogans may be seen by darkfield microscopy or grown in culture but is primarily detected by serologic testing. Leptospirosis is a systemic flu-like illness associated with water contaminated by animal urine. It begins with fever, nausea, vomiting, headache, abdominal pain, and severe myalgia. In severe cases, a second phase is characterized by impaired hepatic and renal function with jaundice, prostration, and circulatory collapse. The CNS is often involved, with stiff neck and inflammatory changes in the CSF.

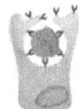 **BACTERIOLOGY**

Loose spirals seen in darkfield

L interrogans is a member of the genus *Leptospira* that is pathogenic to humans and animals. There are other free-living species of *Leptospira*. This species is a slim spirochete 5 to 15 μm long, with a single axial filament; fine, closely wound spirals; and hooked ends (**Figure 37–7**). It is not visualized with the usual staining procedures, and detection is best accomplished using darkfield microscopy. The outer membrane contains LPS and OMPs with adhesive or factor H-binding properties.

✳ **Survives in water**

L interrogans has over 200 serotypes which are of epidemiologic and epizoologic importance but have no clinical significance. *L interrogans* can survive days or weeks in some waters in the environment at a pH above 7.0. Acidic conditions, such as those that may be found in urine, rapidly kill the organism. It is highly sensitive to drying and to a wide range of disinfectants.

LEPTOSPIROSIS

EPIDEMIOLOGY

Leptospirosis is a worldwide disease of a variety of wild and domestic animals, particularly rodents, cattle, and dogs. It is usually transmitted to humans directly or indirectly through water contaminated with animal urine. Secondary human-to-human transmission occurs rarely. Individuals who are exposed to animals (eg, farmers, veterinarians, slaughterhouse employees) are at increased risk, although most clinical cases are now associated with recreational exposure to contaminated water (eg, irrigation ditches or other bodies of water receiving farmland drainage).

✳ **Animals transmit via water**

FIGURE 37–7. *Leptospira interrogans.* Note the tight primary coiling, loose loops, and hooked ends of the spirochete. (Reproduced with permission from Nester EW, Anderson DG, Roberts CE Jr, et al: *Microbiology: A Human Perspective*, 6th ed. New York, NY: McGraw Hill; 2008.)

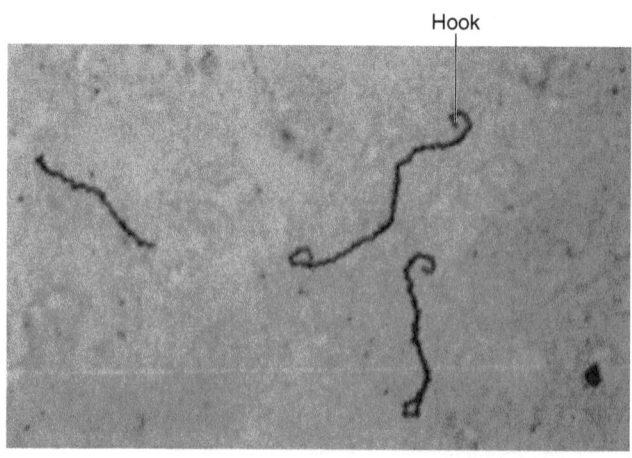

Hook

5 m

PATHOGENESIS AND IMMUNITY

The organism gains entrance to the tissues through small skin breaks, the conjunctiva, or, most commonly, ingestion through the upper alimentary tract mucosa. The active motility of the hooked ends driven by periplasmic flagella may allow the organism to burrow into tissues. A few OMPs mediate adherence and one with serum factor H-binding properties interferes with complement-mediated killing. The organisms spread widely through the bloodstream to all parts of the body including the CSF. The kidney is a target organ in human disease, causing tubular infection and interstitial nephritis.

Clearing of the bacteremia is associated with the appearance of circulating antibody but little else is known of immune mechanisms. Antibody is also rising during the second phase of the disease, which suggests an immunologic component to its pathogenesis. This is supported by the absence of response to antimicrobials when given at this stage and the typical failure to recover the organism from the CSF in cases of leptospiral meningitis.

* Enters through mucosal breaks

* Blood and CNS spread

Antibody may be part of disease

 ## LEPTOSPIROSIS: CLINICAL ASPECTS

MANIFESTATIONS

Most infections are subclinical and detectable only serologically. After an incubation period of 7 to 13 days, an influenza-like febrile illness with fever, chills, headache, conjunctival suffusion, and muscle pain develops in persons who become ill. This disease phase is associated with bacteremia. Leptospires are also found in the CSF at this stage, but without clinical or cytologic evidence of meningitis. The fever often subsides after about a week coincident with the disappearance of the organisms from the blood, but it may recur with a variety of clinical manifestations depending partly on the serogroup involved. This second phase of the disease usually lasts 3 or more weeks and may manifest as an aseptic meningitis resembling viral meningitis or as a more generalized illness with muscle aches, headache, rash, pretibial erythematous lesions, biochemical evidence of hepatic and renal involvement, or all of these. In its most severe form (Weil disease), there is extensive vasculitis, jaundice, renal damage, and sometimes a hemorrhagic rash. The mortality rate in such cases may be as high as 10%.

Initial disease flu-like

* Meningitis, muscle aches

DIAGNOSIS

The diagnosis of leptospirosis is primarily serologic. Although the spirochetes can theoretically be detected, darkfield examination of body fluids is not recommended. The yield is very low and the chance for confusion with fibrin and debris is significant. Likewise, leptospires can be isolated from the blood, CSF, or urine, but culture is rarely attempted because the organisms take weeks to grow in a special medium that few laboratories bother to stock. The standard serologic test the microscopic agglutination test (MAT) is limited to reference laboratories. There are two FDA-approved serologic test kits that may be available in locales where the disease is common.

Primary diagnosis serologic

TREATMENT AND PREVENTION

Penicillin is the primary treatment for all forms of leptospirosis. Doxycycline and ceftriaxone are alternatives. Doxycycline is recommended as chemoprophylaxis for individuals engaging in high-risk activities, such as swimming in jungle rivers or kayaking in developing countries. Other measures include rodent control, drainage of waters known to be contaminated, and care on the part of those subject to occupational exposure to avoid ingestion or contamination with *L interrogans*. Vaccines are used in cattle and household pets to prevent the disease, and this has reduced its occurrence in humans.

* Penicillin primary treatment

KEY CONCLUSIONS

- Leptospirosis is spread by animal urine contaminating lakes and streams.
- Headache, rash, and meningitis are the primary clinical features.
- The diagnosis is serologic.
- Penicillin, ceftriaxone, and doxycycline are effective therapy.

● *BORRELIA*

Relapsing fever, Lyme disease caused by different species

More than 15 species of *Borrelia* have been associated with human disease, and other species are responsible for similar diseases in animals. *Borrelia burgdorferi* is the cause of Lyme disease. Other members of the genus cause relapsing fever, an illness with intermittent fevers and little else. The relapsing fevers differ in their specific vector and geographic distribution. The human body louse is the vector for *B recurrentis*, but the remainder of the relapsing fevers are linked to several ticks and species of *Borrelia*; these are discussed together here as *B hermsii*, the most common cause of relapsing fever in North America.

Loose spirals take common stains

Many genes in plasmids

Borrelia are long (10-30 μm), slender, spirochetes containing multiple (7-20) axial flagella. In contrast to *Treponema* and *Leptospira*, its spirals form loose, irregular waves. The basic organizational structure of the cell and its motility conform to that of the other Gram-negative spirochetes, but unlike the others, *Borrelia* are readily demonstrated by common staining methods such as the Giemsa or Wright stains. *Borrelia* are microaerophilic and have been successfully grown in specially supplemented (*N*-acetylglucosamine, fatty acids) liquid or semisolid media. A distinct feature of *Borrelia* is the partitioning of the genome between the chromosome and multiple circular and linear plasmids. In some species, a large proportion (>40%) of the genome is in the plasmids, including genes important in animal and human disease.

BORRELIA HERMSII AND BORRELIA RECURRENTIS

OVERVIEW

Multiple species of *Borrelia* spirochetes cause relapsing fever. *Borrelia hermsii* is the most common of the tick borne species and *B recurrentis* the only louse-borne species. Relapsing fever is an illness with fever, headache, muscle pain, and weakness but no signs pointing to any organ system. It lasts about 1 week and returns a few days later. The relapses may continue for as many as four cycles. During each relapse, spirochetes are present in the bloodstream.

 ## BACTERIOLOGY

✳ Proteins undergo antigenic variation

Recombination between linear plasmids

The outer membrane of all *Borrelia* species contains abundant OMPs and lipoproteins. In some species, these surface proteins have been observed to vary antigenically too abundantly to be explained by simple mutation. Experiments with *B hermsii* have demonstrated up to 40 antigenically distinct variants of the same protein arising from a single cell. The genetic mechanism for this antigenic variation involves recombination between genes located in the distinctive linear plasmids. Multiple copies of the genes for these proteins are present. Some genes express the protein, whereas others are "silent" because they lack crucial promoter sequences. When structural sequences from a silent gene are transferred by recombination to an expressing gene on another plasmid, the protein expressed is altered, which may make it antigenically different. This recombination mechanism resembles that described for antigenic variation of gonococcal pili (see Chapter 30, Figures 22–5, 30–7), but the number of possible *B hermsii* variants is more limited than with *N gonorrhoeae*.

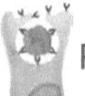 ## RELAPSING FEVER

EPIDEMIOLOGY

Relapsing fever occurs in two forms linked to the mode of transmission and the *Borrelia* species involved. The louse-borne form usually appears in epidemics, because of circumstances connected with body lice, whereas the tick-borne form does not. For this reason, the two forms are sometimes called epidemic (louse-borne) and endemic (tick-borne) relapsing fever. Here they are identified simply by the insect involved.

✳ Body lice or ticks transmit spirochete

The occurrence and distribution of tick-borne relapsing fever are determined by the biology of multiple species of a single tick genus (*Ornithodoros*) and their relation to the primary *Borrelia* reservoir in rodents and other small animals (rabbits, birds, lizards). *Borrelia hermsii* is one of at least 15 *Borrelia* species associated with this cycle. Humans are infected when they accidentally enter this cycle and are bitten by an infected tick. The bite is painless and the feeding period is brief (less than 20 minutes). Because the ticks usually feed at night, cases of relapsing fever are most often associated with overnight recreational forays into wild, wooded areas. A large outbreak in the United States involved National Park employees and tourists who slept in tick- and rodent-infested cabins on the Northern Rim of the Grand Canyon.

* Ticks feed on rodents, small animals

* Painless tick bite transmits bacteria

The epidemiologic conditions associated with louse-borne relapsing fever are much more exacting. The human body louse has no other host, infected lice live no more than 2 months, and there is no transovarial passage to progeny. *B recurrentis* is the only species involved. Lice are infected from human blood, but the spirochetes multiply in their hemolymph, not any of the feeding parts or excrement. This means they can infect another human only if the louse is crushed by scratching and the *Borrelia* reach a superficial wound or mucosal surface. Infected lice must be passed human to human for the disease to persist. These conditions are met by circumstances that combine overcrowding with extremely low levels of general hygiene. War, other kinds of social breakdown, and dire poverty are the prime associates. Currently, this variety of relapsing fever appears to be limited to East and Central Africa and the Peruvian Andes.

* Body lice infected from human blood

* Lice transferred human to human

PATHOGENESIS

The disease manifestations develop at times when thousands of spirochetes are circulating per milliliter of blood. The febrile illness has endotoxin-like features, but the exact mechanisms of disease are unknown. Between episodes, the organisms disappear from the blood and are sequestered in internal organs only to reappear during relapses. The OMPs are antigenically different with each relapse. The relapsing cycles correlate with antibody production to the new protein generated by recombination between plasmids.

* Spirochetes in blood

* OMPs altered by recombination

IMMUNITY

Immunity to relapsing fever is largely humoral and appears to involve lysis of the organism in the presence of complement. The disease is controlled when number of variants from the antigenic repertoire are no longer able to escape the immune response.

Antibody controls disease

 ## RELAPSING FEVER: CLINICAL ASPECTS

MANIFESTATIONS

After a mean incubation period of 7 days, massive spirochetemia develops, with high fever, rigors, severe headache, muscle pains, and weakness. The febrile period lasts about 1 week and terminates abruptly with the development of an adequate immune response. The disease relapses 2 to 4 days later, usually with less severity, but following the same general course. Tick-borne relapsing fever is usually limited to one or two relapses, but up to 30 may occur.

* Fever, headache, muscle pain

Louse-borne relapsing fever is more severe than tick-borne disease, possibly because of predisposing social conditions. Fatalities are rare in tick-borne disease but may be as high as 40% in untreated louse-borne fever. There is usually not more than one or two relapses. Fatal outcomes are due to myocarditis, cerebral hemorrhage, and hepatic failure.

Louse-borne more severe

DIAGNOSIS

Diagnosis of relapsing fever is readily made during the febrile period by Giemsa or Wright staining of blood smears. The appearance of the spirochete among the red cells is characteristic. Culture and serologic tests are available only in reference laboratories.

* Blood smears demonstrate *Borrelia*

TREATMENT

Patients with relapsing fever respond well to doxycycline, tetracycline, or penicillin therapy. If the level of spirochetes is high at the time treatment is initiated, a systemic febrile reaction (Jarisch-Herxheimer) resembling Gram-negative sepsis may ensue. This is felt to be due to rapid lysis of the organisms with release of outer membrane LPS. It is more common in louse-borne than tick-borne relapsing fever.

* Doxycycline primary treatment

PREVENTION

Attention to general hygiene important

Prevention of tick-borne relapsing fever involves attention to deticking, insecticide treatment, and rodent control around habitations such as mountain cabins, which are known to be associated with infection. Control of louse-borne relapsing fever involves delousing, particularly dusting of clothing with appropriate insecticides. Ultimately, improved hygiene stops outbreaks and prevents further occurrences.

KEY CONCLUSIONS

- *Borrelia hermsii* and other species of *Borrelia* cause tick-borne relapsing fever.
- *Borrelia recurrentis* causes louse-borne relapsing fever in lice, which must be passed human to human.
- Relapses are related to antigenic variation of OMPs.
- Spirochetes are seen in routine blood smears.

BORRELIA BURGDORFERI

OVERVIEW

B burgdorferi is transmitted to humans by *Ixodes* ticks following a complex life cycle involving ticks, mice, and deer. The spirochete has multiple classes of OMPs, which undergo antigenic variation in the multiple stages of the life cycle and in human infection. Acute Lyme disease is characterized by fever, a migratory "bull's eye" skin rash, muscle and joint pains, often with evidence of meningeal irritation. In a chronic form evolving over several years, meningoencephalitis, myocarditis, and a disabling recurrent arthritis may develop.

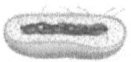 **BACTERIOLOGY**

Osps differ at stages of infection

B burgdorferi consists of at least 20 subspecies which differ in geographic distribution and some clinical manifestations. Three of these are the primary causes of Lyme disease. All these are referred to here as *B burgdorferi*. As with other species of *Borrelia*, there are multiple classes of OMPs, many of which undergo antigenic variation. Recent studies have focused on a class called outer surface proteins (Osps), which have been linked to aspects of pathogenesis and immunity. In response to environmental signals (temperature, pH) two of these proteins, OspA and OspC, are differentially expressed, depending on the stage of tick or mammalian infection.

LYME DISEASE

EPIDEMIOLOGY

❋ Transmitted in tick–mouse–deer cycle

❋ Infect humans in the woods

B burgdorferi exists in a complex cycle involving ticks, mice, and deer (**Figure 37–8**). Lyme disease occurs when the ticks feed on humans who enter their wooded habitat. The disease is endemic in several regions of the United States, Canada, and temperate Europe and Asia. Approximately 90% of the more than 30,000 cases reported each year in the United States occur in areas along the northeastern and mid-Atlantic seaboard, including Old Lyme, Connecticut, where the disease was first recognized.

❋ Adult and nymph stages infect humans

❋ No deer, no disease

The primary reservoir of *B burgdorferi* is rodents, particularly white-footed mice. Infection is transmitted by *Ixodes* ticks (**Figure 37–9**), whose complete life cycle involves rodents for the early stages and deer for adult maturation. In the spring, fertile female ticks, engorged from their blood meals, fall from their deer hosts to the ground and deposit their eggs. During the summer, the tick larvae seek out and obtain a blood meal from mice and the *B burgdorferi* ingested by the larvae are maintained through the subsequent development stages of the tick. The following spring or summer, the small (1-2 mm) nymphs feed again on vertebrate hosts to obtain the blood required for maturation to adulthood. The engorged, satiated nymphs fall off their hosts and mature into adults by parasitizing available deer, thus completing a life cycle that has occupied a full 2 years. Vertebrates other than deer can be infected by both the adult and nymph stages of

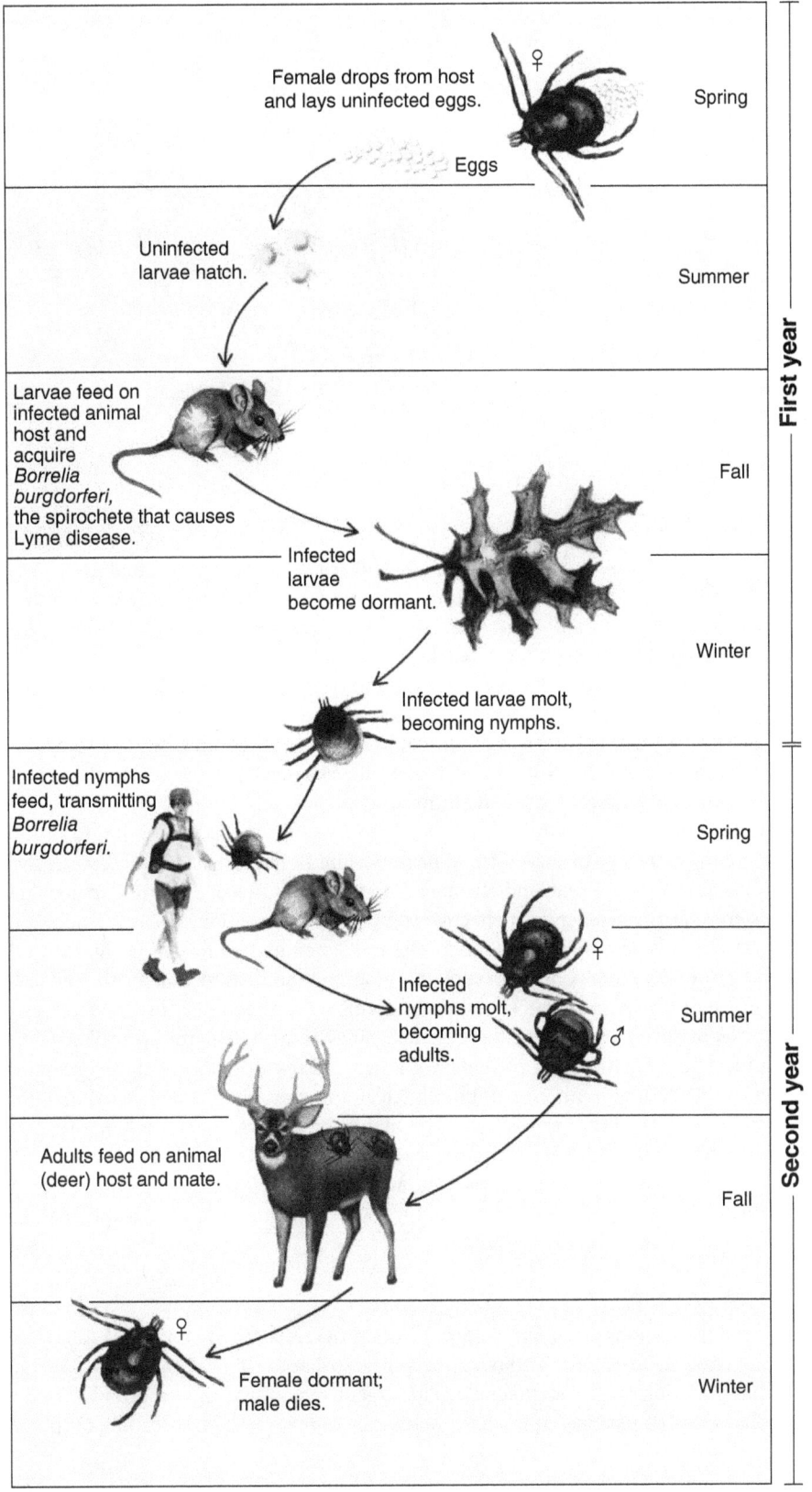

Female drops from host
and lays uninfected eggs. — Spring

Eggs

Uninfected
larvae hatch. — Summer

Larvae feed on
infected animal
host and
acquire
*Borrelia
burgdorferi*,
the spirochete that causes
Lyme disease. — Fall

Infected
larvae
become dormant.

Infected larvae molt,
becoming nymphs. — Winter

Infected nymphs
feed, transmitting
*Borrelia
burgdorferi*.

Infected
nymphs molt,
becoming
adults. — Spring

Adults feed on animal
(deer) host and mate. — Summer

Female dormant;
male dies. — Fall / Winter

First year

Second year

FIGURE 37-8. **Lyme disease life cycle.** The life cycle covers 2 years during which the tick obtains three blood meals. The males die soon after mating; the females die after depositing their eggs in the following spring. Variations depend on climate and food availability for the natural hosts. (Reproduced with permission from Nester EW, Anderson DG, Roberts CE Jr, et al: *Microbiology: A Human Perspective*, 6th ed. New York, NY: McGraw Hill; 2008.)

the tick, but human Lyme disease is acquired primarily from nymphs, because they are active at the time of year when humans are most likely to invade their ecosystem. The infecting dose is very low (<20 organisms), making even a single tick bite a risk for disease. Deer are essential to the mating and survival of the tick, and thus the disease does not occur in areas in which deer are not abundant.

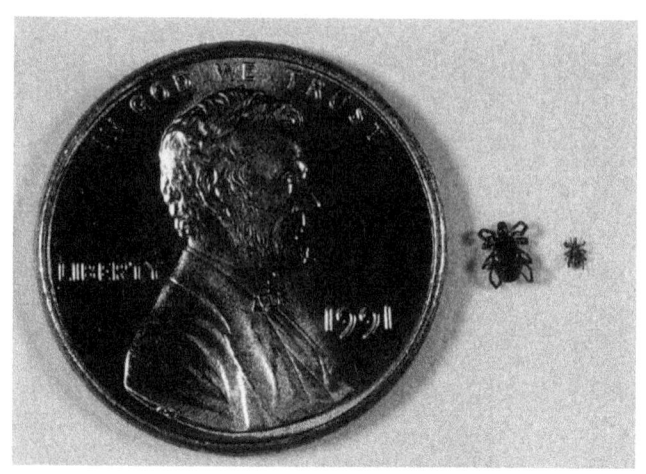

FIGURE 37–9. The deer tick (*Ixodes scapularis*) adult and nymph. (Reproduced with permission from Nester EW, Anderson DG, Roberts CE Jr, et al: *Microbiology: A Human Perspective*, 6th ed. New York, NY: McGraw Hill; 2008.)

2 mm

PATHOGENESIS

Because Lyme disease is a recently discovered disease with a complex biology, it is not surprising that the pathogenic mechanisms in humans remain to be established clearly. Studies in ticks have shown changes in the antigenic makeup of *B burgdorferi* as it migrates from the midgut and salivary glands and again after it reaches mammalian tissue. OspA is the major outer surface protein expressed when *B burgdorferi* resides in ticks, where it mediates binding to midgut cells. OspA expression diminishes during tick feeding and engorgement, whereas OspC increases, so that by the time of transmission to animal hosts, OspC predominates. OspC binds mammalian plasminogen and has been shown to protect the spirochetes from macrophage ingestion. Antibody against OspC is protective in animals.

After infection, the *B burgdorferi* surface proteins that mediate adhesion to fibronectin or elements of the extracellular matrix could be important in the early stages of disease. By analogy with other bacterial proteins that bind serum factor H, similar Osps of *B burgdorferi* are likely to facilitate persistence by interference with effective complement deposition. The spirochete is not known to produce digestive enzymes, but tissue spread and dissemination may be facilitated by the utilization of host proteases. As the organism spreads, inflammation is stimulated by the cell wall peptidoglycan and possibly by elements of the outer membrane, although *B burgdorferi* lacks classic LPS. When deposited in joint tissues, these elements may contribute to the arthritis of Lyme disease.

Clinical investigations in patients with Lyme disease have noted modulation of immune responses, including inhibition of mononuclear and natural killer cell function, lymphocyte proliferation, and cytokine production. The ability of *B burgdorferi* to downregulate deleterious immune responses could serve as a survival strategy or play a role in chronic disease. Chronic disease, particularly Lyme arthritis, has aspects of autoimmunity. A subcategory of arthritis patients refractory to antimicrobial therapy have been shown to have heightened and persistent humoral immune responses to OspA.

IMMUNITY

The immune response to *B burgdorferi* infection develops slowly, with IgM followed by IgG antibody over weeks to months. Although immune-mediated killing by the classical complement pathway has been demonstrated, the molecular target is unknown. Host neutrophils and macrophages can phagocytose opsonized spirochetes and induce a metabolic burst leading to spirochetal death.

LYME DISEASE: CLINICAL ASPECTS

MANIFESTATIONS

Lyme borreliosis is a highly variable disease involving many body systems. It occurs in overlapping patterns that come and go at different times. The skin lesion spreading from the site of the tick bite is its most distinctive feature. Relapsing arthritis is the most persistent finding and

OspA in ticks

✳ OspC in mammals

Proteins bind to fibronectin, factor H

✳ Peptidoglycan stimulates inflammation

Downregulation of immune function

✳ Arthritis may be autoimmune

Target of antibody unclear

✳ Spreading from bite site

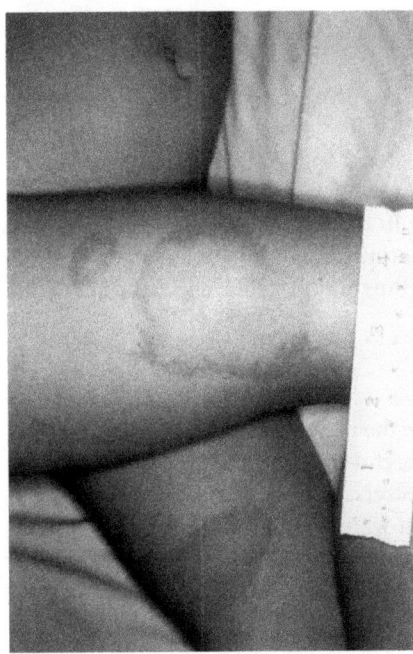

FIGURE 37-10. **Erythema migrans.** The typical rash of Lyme disease is shown evolving in concentric rings around the site of the tick bite. (Reproduced with permission from Willey JM: *Prescott, Harley, & Klein's Microbiology*, 7th ed. New York, NY: McGraw Hill; 2008.)

the one most likely to become chronic. Lyme disease is rarely fatal, but if untreated, it is often a source of chronic ill health.

The primary lesion begins sometime in the first month after a tick bite, which is often unnoticed. A macule or papule appears at the site of the bite and expands to become an annular lesion with a raised, red border and central clearing forming a bull's-eye pattern. As the bull's-eye ring expands and evolves, it forms the complex known as **erythema migrans (Figure 37–10)**. Along with the skin lesions, fever, fatigue, myalgia, headache, joint pains, and mild neck stiffness are often present. Approximately 50% of untreated patients develop secondary skin lesions that closely resemble the primary one, but are not at the site of the tick bite. In untreated patients, the skin lesions usually disappear over a period of weeks, but constitutional symptoms may persist for months.

⁕ Expanding rings called erythema migrans

⁕ Febrile aches mark acute disease

Days to months after the onset of the primary lesion, a second stage may develop in which involvement of the nervous or cardiovascular system is superimposed. Neurologic abnormalities include a fluctuating meningitis, cranial nerve palsies, and peripheral neuropathy. Cardiac disease is usually limited to conduction abnormalities (atrioventricular block), but in some cases acute myocarditis can lead to cardiac enlargement. Both neurologic and cardiac abnormalities fluctuate in intensity, but generally resolve completely in a matter of weeks.

Nerve palsies, cardiac findings

Weeks to years after the onset of infection, arthritis marks the continuing state of the disease. It develops in almost two-thirds of untreated patients. Without therapy, the spirochetes may persist in localized niches for years. Typically, this too follows a fluctuating or intermittent course, generally involving the large joints, particularly the knees. The arthritis may become chronic with erosion of the bone and cartilage, although the spirochetes are rarely demonstrable in the lesions. Less common chronic neurologic dysfunctions include subtle encephalitis affecting memory, mood, or sleep, and peripheral neuropathies.

⁕ Fluctuating arthritis becomes chronic

DIAGNOSIS

Presently, the diagnosis of early Lyme disease is based on exposure and typical clinical findings. Although *B burgdorferi* can be cultured from erythema migrans skin lesions, blood, joint fluid, and CSF, few laboratories have the skill to accomplish this or even stock the special medium required. The spirochetes are seldom detected on any kind of direct microscopic examination. Nucleic acid amplification procedures able to detect *B burgdorferi*-specific DNA sequences in body fluids (joint, CSF) have been developed.

Culture not practical

With culture generally unavailable, the diagnosis in later stages of disease usually rests on the demonstration of circulating antibodies to *B burgdorferi*. The current recommendation is to first perform a sensitive screening test (EIA) followed by a confirmatory immunoblot (Western blot),

*EIA followed by immunoblot

which detects specific antigens of the organism. For persons who lack a typical clinical or epidemiologic history, great caution should be exercised before making a diagnosis of Lyme disease based only on positive serologic tests.

TREATMENT

Doxycycline, amoxacillin primary treatment

Doxycycline is the primary treatment for persons 8 years and above. Amoxicillin is used in children and pregnant women. Cefuroxime is a third choice in the face of allergy. The response to treatment is typically slow, requiring the continuation of antimicrobials for 30 to 60 days. Chronic Lyme disease is most probably an autoimmune state, and thus antimicrobial agents would not be effective.

PREVENTION

Preventing bites, removing ticks

The most useful preventive measures in endemic areas are the use of clothes that reduce the likelihood of the infected nymph reaching the legs or arms, careful search for nymphs after potential exposure, and removal of the tick by its head with tweezers. Duration of tick attachment to humans is also a factor in transmission; the risk is greatest when the tick has been feeding for at least 48 to 72 hours. Some insect repellents may provide added protection. Prophylactic doxycycline may be used following a tick bite, but only in a highly endemic region.

 Why no vaccine? What would you use as an immunogen?

KEY CONCLUSIONS

- *Borrelia burgdorferi* has a complex life cycle involving ticks, mice, and deer in the woods.
- Erythema migrans, the primary Lyme disease manifestation, is a dramatic moving annular rash.
- Chronic Lyme disease involves inflammation of joints, cardiovascular and nervous systems which may be immunopathologic.
- A two-step serologic diagnosis must be interpreted together with clinical and epidemiologic observations.

CASE STUDY

A Rash and Facial Paralysis

This 39-year-old man was in his usual state of good health and had just returned from a summer trip to Rhode Island. One week after returning home, he developed a fever and muscle aches, which resolved and were followed 2 weeks later with a rash on his right forearm, right hip, and left knee. At each site, the rash was initially localized but then over a few days moved outward forming large erythematous rings. Two weeks after the rash started, he felt a numbness on the left side of his face followed by a sagging and inability to move the facial muscles below his eye.

On physical examination, the patient was afebrile and had normal vital signs. A skin examination demonstrated the three skin lesions noted above, which had, according to the patient, faded significantly. A neurologic examination demonstrated left facial nerve weakness. The remainder of the examination was normal.

Laboratory studies included a normal complete blood count. A lumbar puncture was performed. CSF contained 78 nucleated cells/mm³ with 88% lymphocytes and 12% monocytes. CSF glucose level was 60 mg/dL, and protein level was 55 mg/dL.

 Think ▸▸ Apply 37-2: A vaccine using OspC as the antigen was developed and marketed. Its approach was novel as it would have to be effective during the tick bite. It has now been withdrawn. Antigenic variation could be a problem.

QUESTIONS

1. To consider a diagnosis of Lyme disease, what additional history would be most helpful from this patient?
   A. Food consumption
   B. Swimming in lakes or streams
   C. Sexual contact
   D. Hiking locales
   E. Illness of friends

2. What laboratory test would be most likely to confirm this diagnosis?
   A. *Borrelia burgdorferi* immunoassay
   B. *Borrelia burgdorferi* immunoblot
   C. *Borrelia burgdorferi* immunoassay plus immunoblot
   D. Darkfield examination of rash
   E. PCR of CSF

3. What molecular structure of *B burgdorferi* facilitates its life cycle in ticks?
   A. OspA
   B. OspB
   C. OspC
   D. LPS
   E. Peptidoglycan

ANSWERS

1. (D)

2. (C)

3. (A)

APPENDIX 37–1	Nonvenereal Treponemes				
DISEASE	CAUSE	MAJOR GEOGRAPHIC LOCATION	PRIMARY LESION	SECONDARY LESIONS	TERTIARY LESIONS
Bejel	*T pallidum*, subspecies *endemicum*[a]	Middle East; arid, hot areas	Oral cavity[b]	Oral mucosa	Rare; gummatous lessions of skin, periosteum, bone, and joint
Yaws	*T pallidum*, subspecies *pertenue*	Humid, tropical belt	Skin, papillomatous	Systemic; resemble syphilis	Rare; gummatous lesions of skin, periosteum, bone, and joint[c]
Pinta	*T carateum*	Central and South America	Skin, erythematous papule	Skin; merge into primary lesion; altered pigmentation	Areas of altered skin pigmentation and hyperkeratoses

[a]Probably a variant of that causing venereal syphilis.
[b]Often inapparent.
[c]Neurologic manifestations usually absent.

chapter 38

Mycoplasma

mycopla ...n do not have cell walls

Mycoplasma pneumoniae · Mycoplasma genitalium · Mycoplasma hominis

OVERVIEW

Mycoplasma are tiny bacteria that lack a cell wall. Their outer cell membrane contains sterols that they obtain from the tissues in which they grow. *Mycoplasma pneumoniae* is second only to the pneumococcus as a cause of community-acquired pneumonia. However, *M pneumoniae* has a predilection for younger persons and spreads person-to-person in families or closed groups, whereas the elderly are at greatest risk for pneumococcal pneumonia. Mycoplasmal infection presents as tracheobronchitis or pneumonia with headache and a persistent nonproductive cough, often worse at night. Chest radiographs usually show unilateral patchy infiltrates without lobar consolidation, hence the term atypical pneumonia. The course is almost always benign, but improvement is accelerated by treatment with doxycycline or azithromycin. In the past, diagnosis was confirmed if at all by serology or rarely by culture. Multiplex PCR platforms for respiratory pathogens and pneumonia have changed the approach to diagnosis.

There has been a resurgence interest and research in *Mycoplasma genitalium* (MG), which is second only to *Chlamydia trachomatis* as a cause of cervicitis, urethritis, and pelvic inflammatory disease (PID). The recognition of MG as a major cause of sexually transmitted infection (STI) has been transformed by NAA testing, since it does not grow in culture. Gene variations that result in resistance to macrolides and fluoroquinolones are an emerging problem globally.

Mycoplasma hominis is a resident of the genitourinary tract; however, its clinical manifestations are uncommon and extragenital. It can cause transient bacteremia with parturition, localized infection in joints, including prosthetic ones, and sternal wound infections after cardiac surgery. *M hominis* can be grown on chocolate agar from tissue or aspirated fluid obtained sterilely from these sites. Confirmed infections are treated with doxycycline or a fluoroquinolone; they are resistant to macrolides and β-lactams.

The role of *Ureaplasma* in human disease syndromes remains ill-defined.

T his chapter includes two genera of unique microbes that lack a cell wall but otherwise resemble bacteria. They differ from viruses by having both DNA and RNA and by the ability to grow in cell-free media. They are ubiquitous in nature as the smallest of free-living microorganisms. Numerous *Mycoplasma* species have been isolated from animals and humans, but *M pneumoniae* stands out as the clearest and most important human pathogen. The other species associated with human disease are summarized in **Table 38–1**.

GENERAL FEATURES

Mycoplasma and *Ureaplasma* are taxonomically placed in the Mollicutes, a class of prokaryotes that lack a cell wall. Although their DNA does not resemble any other prokaryote, evolutionary studies suggest they are derived from Gram-positive bacteria by reductive evolution. They are very small (diameter 0.2-0.3 μm), highly pleomorphic, and appear as coccoid bodies, filaments, and bottle-shaped forms. The cells are bounded only by a single trilaminar membrane which, unlike bacteria, contains sterols. The sterols are not synthesized by the organism but are acquired as essential components from the tissue in which the organism is growing. Flagella and pili are lacking, but surface organelles mediating attachment have been identified for some species. Lacking a cell wall, *Mycoplasma* and *Ureaplasma* stain poorly or not at all with the usual stains.

✳ No cell wall

✳ Cell membrane contains sterols

[handwritten note top:] B lactams (penicillin/cephalosporin ineffective due to no cell wall).

[handwritten note left margin:] Doxycycline & azithromycin preferred for children.

[handwritten note left margin:] Fluoroquinolone is good.

[handwritten note:] rise during summer months.

TABLE 38–1	Features of Pathogenic *Mycoplasma* and *Ureaplasma*			
	PRIMARY SITE	**MOTILITY**	**ATTACHMENT (PROTEINS)**	**DISEASE**
M pneumoniae	Respiratory	Gliding	Terminal organelle (P1, P30)	Pneumonia
M hominis	Genitourinary			Extra-intestinal infections
M genitalium	Genitourinary	Gliding	Terminal organelle (MgPa)	Urethritis, cervicitis, PID
Ureaplasma sp.	Genitourinary			Role ill-defined as yet

PID, Pelvic inflammatory disease.

Their double-stranded DNA genome is small, in part due to the lack of genes encoding a complex cell wall. *M pneumoniae* is an aerobe, but most other species are facultatively anaerobic. Although possible to isolate with special media, the laborious techniques required have been supplanted by NAATs. The exception is *M hominis*, which grows on chocolate agar. As the center of a colony grows into the agar and looks denser, it takes on the appearance of an inverted "fried egg."

Not stained by common methods

* NAA useful

● *MYCOPLASMA PNEUMONIAE*

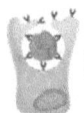 ### MYCOPLASMA PNEUMONIAE — *causes pneumonia*

In addition to the general features of *Mycoplasma*, *M pneumoniae* has a terminal organelle that is a membrane-bound protrusion of the cytoplasm capped by a button. This structure contains a number of proteins (P1, P30) that are involved in attachment to cell surfaces. It also mediates a form of movement called gliding motility in which the organism advances over smooth surfaces in the direction of the protrusion. *M pneumoniae* also produces an ADP-ribosylating toxin.

* Organelle mediates attachment and gliding motility

MYCOPLASMAL PNEUMONIA

EPIDEMIOLOGY

M pneumoniae accounts for approximately 10% of all cases of pneumonia. Infection is acquired by droplet spread. Experimental challenges indicate that the human infectious dose is very low, possibly less than 100 organisms. Infections with *M pneumoniae* occur worldwide, but they are especially prominent in temperate climates. Epidemics at 4- to 6-year intervals have been noted in both civilian and military populations. The most common age range for symptomatic *M pneumoniae* infection is between 5 and 15 years, and the disease accounts for more than one-third of all cases of pneumonia in teenagers (but is also seen in older persons). Infections in children younger than 6 months are uncommon. The disease often appears as a sporadic, endemic illness in families or closed communities because its incubation period is relatively long (2-3 weeks) and because prolonged shedding in nasopharyngeal secretions may cause infections to be spread over time. In families, attack rates in susceptible persons approach 60%. Asymptomatic infections occur, but most studies have suggested that more than two-thirds of infected cases develop some evidence of respiratory tract illness.

* Infecting dose very low

* Worldwide, often in teenagers

Outbreaks in families, closed communities

PATHOGENESIS

M pneumoniae infection involves the trachea, bronchi, bronchioles, and peribronchial tissues and may extend to the alveoli and alveolar walls. The organism appears to thrive on the phospholipids present in lung epithelia. Initially, *M pneumoniae* attaches to the cilia and microvilli of the cells lining the bronchial epithelium. This attachment is mediated by protrusion-associated proteins

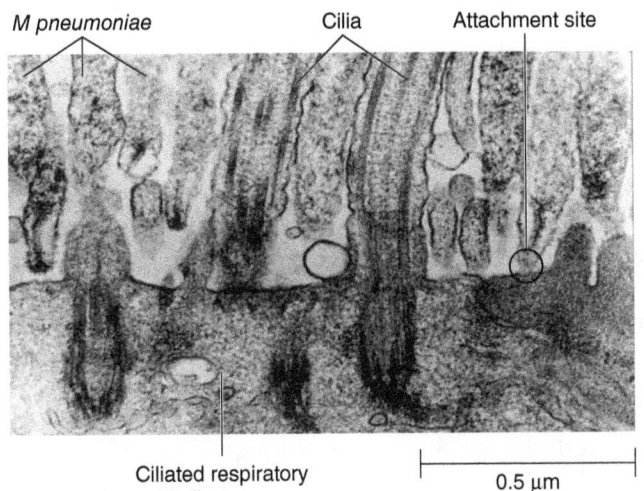

M pneumoniae   Cilia   Attachment site

Ciliated respiratory
epithelium   0.5 μm

FIGURE 38–1. *Mycoplasma pneumoniae* **infecting respiratory epithelium.** Transmission electron micrograph. Note the distinctive appearance of the tips of the mycoplasmas adjacent to the host epithelium. The tips probably represent a site on the microorganism that is specialized for attachment. (Reproduced with permission from Nester EW, Anderson DG, Roberts CE Jr, et al: *Microbiology: A Human Perspective*, 6th ed. New York, NY: McGraw Hill; 2008.)

(P1, P30) which bind to complex oligosaccharides containing sialic acid found in the apical regions of bronchial epithelial cells (**Figure 38–1**). The oligosaccharide receptors are chemically similar to antigens on the surface of erythrocytes and are not found on the nonciliated goblet cells or mucus, to which *M pneumoniae* does not bind. Other proteins bind to elements of the extracellular matrix-like fibronectin. The ADP-ribosylating toxin interferes with ciliary action and causes nuclear vacuolization and fragmentation of tracheal epithelial cells. This leads to inflammation and desquamation of the involved mucosa (**Figure 38–2**). The inflammatory response is most pronounced in the bronchial and peribronchial tissue and is composed of lymphocytes, plasma cells, and macrophages, which may infiltrate and thicken the walls of the bronchioles and alveoli. Organisms are shed in upper respiratory secretions for 2 to 8 days before the onset of symptoms, and shedding continues for as long as 14 weeks after infection.

Adherence mediated by protrusion-associated proteins

✳ ADPR toxin interferes with ciliary action, leads to desquamation

IMMUNITY

Both T- and B-cell–mediated immune responses occur, and generally appear to be effective in preventing reinfection. Complement-fixing serum antibody titers reach a peak 2 to 4 weeks after infection and gradually disappear over 6 to 12 months. Also, nonspecific immune responses to the glycolipids of the outer membrane of the organism often develop, which can be detrimental to the host. For example, cold hemagglutinins are IgM antibodies that react with an altered antigen on human RBCs and are seen in about two-thirds of symptomatic patients infected with *M pneumoniae*.

Immunity is not complete, and reinfection with *M pneumoniae* may occur. Clinical disease appears to be more severe in older than in younger children, which has led to the suggestion that many of the clinical manifestations of disease are the result of immune responses rather than invasion by the organism. High titers of cold agglutinins may be associated with hemolysis and Raynaud phenomenon.

Antibody peaks at 2 to 4 weeks

✳ Cold agglutinins are IgM

Immunity is incomplete

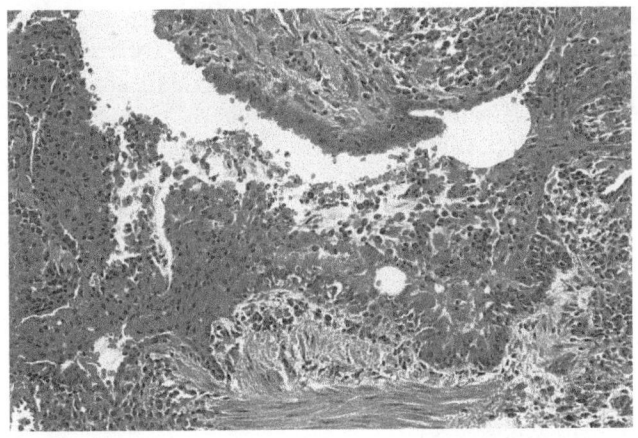

FIGURE 38–2. *Mycoplasma pneumoniae* **bronchiolitis.** This lung section shows destruction of the bronchiolar wall and mucosal ulceration. (Reproduced with permission from Connor DH, Chandler FW, Schwartz DQ, et al: *Pathology of Infectious Diseases*. Stamford CT: Appleton & Lange; 1997.)

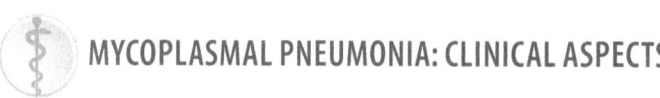

MYCOPLASMAL PNEUMONIA: CLINICAL ASPECTS

MANIFESTATIONS

A mild tracheobronchitis with fever, cough, headache, and malaise is the most common syndrome associated with acute *M pneumoniae* infection. The pneumonia is typically less severe than other bacterial pneumonias. It has been described as walking pneumonia because most cases do not require hospitalization. The disease is of insidious onset, with fever, headache, and malaise for 2 to 4 days before the onset of respiratory symptoms. Pulmonary symptoms are generally limited to a non- or minimally productive cough. Radiographs show a unilateral or patchy pneumonia, usually in a lower lobe, although multiple lobes are sometimes involved. Small pleural effusions are seen in up to 25% of cases. The average duration of untreated illness is 3 weeks. The severity of pulmonary involvement is greater in patients with immune deficiencies.

Pharyngitis with fever and sore throat may also occur. Nonpurulent otitis media or myringitis may occur concomitantly in up to 15% of patients with *M pneumoniae* pneumonitis, but bullous myringitis is rare. A variety of other extrapulmonary complications have been described, involving skin (erythema multiforme), peripheral vasospasm (Raynaud phenomenon), central nervous system (encephalitis, myelitis), joints (arthralgias), and other sites.

* Walking pneumonia has insidious onset

* Nonproductive cough

Pharyngitis, otitis common

DIAGNOSIS

Clinical diagnosis of *M pneumoniae* infection may be difficult because the manifestations overlap with those of other respiratory infections. Gram-stained sputum usually shows some mononuclear cells, but because it lacks a cell wall, *M pneumoniae* is not seen. The absence of bacteria suggests a viral or *Mycoplasma* etiology. The organism can be isolated from throat swabs or sputum of infected patients using special culture media and methods, but growth is slow, and isolation usually requires incubation for a week or longer. Thus, serologic tests rather than culture were used historically for specific diagnosis. A fourfold rise of serum antibody titer or seroconversion in acute and convalescent sera indicated *M pneumoniae* infection. The most widely used serologic method was complement fixation. With the relatively long incubation period and insidious onset of the disease, many patients already had high antibody titers at the time they were first seen. Consequently, a single high titer, such as a complement fixation titer greater than 1:128 or IgM-specific antibody (measured by enzyme immunoassay or immunofluorescence), supported recent infection. These methods have been replaced by multiplex PCR panels in most clinical microbiology laboratories.

* Serologic diagnosis now replaced by PCR

TREATMENT

Doxycycline and azithromycin for children are the preferred agents used for treatment of *M pneumoniae* pneumonia. Fluoroquinolones are effective alternatives. β-Lactams are ineffective because *M pneumoniae* lacks a cell wall. Almost all patients with *M pneumoniae* pneumonia recover, but treatment markedly shortens the course of illness.

Doxycycline, azithromycin, fluoroquinolones

● OTHER *MYCOPLASMA* AND *UREAPLASMA*

Mycoplasma genitalium has emerged as a sexually transmitted infection (STI) second only to *Chlamydia trachomatis* as an established cause of nongonococcal urethritis in men and pelvic inflammatory disease in women (Table 38-1). The increased recognition and diagnosis of *M genitalium* as an important STI is the result of wider use of NAA testing, since it does not grow in culture. The optimal sample for NAA testing is a first-voided urine specimen that is leucocyte esterase-positive. Gene variations that result in resistance to macrolides and fluoroquinolones are a growing problem for treatment globally, since doxycycline-moxifloxacin or doxycycline-azithromycin are recommended for therapy.

M hominis is a resident the genitourinary tract; however, its clinical manifestations are uncommon and extragenital. It can cause amnionitis, transient bacteremia with parturition, localized infection in joints (including prosthetic ones), sternal wound infections after cardiac surgery, and pericardial infections. *M hominis* can be grown on chocolate agar from tissue or aspirated fluid obtained sterilely from these sites. Confirmed infections are treated with doxycycline or a fluoroquinolone; they are resistant to macrolides and β-lactams.

The role of *Ureaplasma* in human disease syndromes remains ill-defined.

KEY CONCLUSIONS

- *Mycoplasma* lack a cell wall and cell membrane contains sterols.
- *Mycoplasma pneumoniae* causes tracheobronchitis and atypical pneumonia in youth.
- Persistent dry cough, fever, and headache with patchy infiltrates on chest radiographs are common features.
- Doxycycline and azithromycin (for children) shorten the course of illness.
- *Mycoplasma genitalium* causes urethritis and pelvic inflammatory disease.
- *Mycoplasma hominis* causes extragenital infections (joints, sternal wounds).

CASE STUDY

A Teenager with Respiratory Complaints

In July, a 14-year-old girl presents with cough and fever to 102°F. She does not appear seriously ill. Chest examination is abnormal and chest radiograph shows bilateral, patchy infiltrates. Her brother, aged 12, had a similar illness 3 weeks earlier.

QUESTIONS

1. Which is the most likely cause of this girl's illness?
   A. *Legionella pneumophila*
   B. *Chlamydiophila pneumoniae*
   C. *Mycoplasma pneumoniae*
   D. Influenza A virus
   E. *Metapneumovirus*

2. Which is the most appropriate diagnostic test?
   A. Culture
   B. Immunofluorescent assay on sputum
   C. Serology

3. Which is the treatment of choice for this patient?
   A. Penicillin
   B. Ribavirin
   C. Oseltamivir
   D. Azithromycin
   E. Ceftriaxone

ANSWERS

1. (C)

2. (C)

3. (D)

chapter 39

Chlamydia

Chlamydia trachomatis · Chlamydophila psittici · Chlamydophila pneumoniae

OVERVIEW

Chlamydiae are obligate intracellular bacteria whose cells lack peptidoglycan and who share a common replicative cycle that involves two forms: elementary and reticulate bodies (**Figure 39–1**). Elementary bodies (EBs) are smaller, have rigid cell walls, can survive outside cells, and are infectious. Once EBs attach to the cell membranes of susceptible cells, they enter the cell by endocytosis and transform into larger, but fragile reticulate bodies (RBs) that multiply by binary fission and form more EBs that are released by exocytosis or cell rupture to infect adjacent cells and begin the cycle anew. Despite their biologic similarities, the *Chlamydia* are diverse in their tropisms and clinical features even within a single species. *Chlamydia trachomatis* primarily produces infections of the conjunctiva or genital tract depending on which biovar is involved. Trachoma is a progressive conjunctivitis with inflammation and scarring resulting in blindness and is caused by *C trachomatis* biovars A, B, and C. Sexually transmitted biovars D-K cause urethritis, cervicitis, salpingitis, and neonatal infections of the eye and respiratory tract after vaginal delivery by infected mothers. L biovars of *C trachomatis* cause lymphogranuloma venereum (LGV), a sexually transmitted disease that manifests as painless genital ulcers followed by painful suppuration of regional inguinal lymph nodes. LGV biovars can also cause ulcerative proctitis, rectal fistulae, and strictures.

Chlamydophila species cause atypical pneumonia. *Chlamydophila psittici* causes psittacosis, a zoonotic pneumonia contracted by inhalation of respiratory secretions or aerosols of cloacal droppings of infected birds of diverse species. *Chlamydophila pneumoniae* causes community-acquired pneumonia that mimics *Mycoplama pneumoniae* in its person-to-person transmission, clinical features, and treatment.

Members of the genus *Chlamydia* are obligate intracellular bacteria that lack peptidoglycan in their cell wall. *Chlamydia trachomatis* is the most important human pathogen and is a major cause of conjunctivitis and genital tract infections. A chronic form of *C trachomatis* conjunctivitis, called trachoma, is the leading preventable cause of blindness in the world. *Chlamydophila pneumoniae* and *Chlamydophila psittaci* are respiratory pathogens. Our knowledge of biology and pathogenesis of these bacteria is based primarily on the study of *C trachomatis*.

CHLAMYDIA TRACHOMATIS

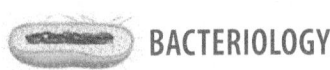

BACTERIOLOGY

C trachomatis are round cells between 0.3 and 1 μm in diameter depending on the stage in the replicative cycle (see below). Their envelope is of the Gram-negative type, including an outer membrane that contains lipopolysaccharide and proteins. A major difference is that chlamydiae lack the thin peptidoglycan layer between the outer membrane and the plasma membrane. Although there is no detectable peptidoglycan in chlamydial cells, genomic studies have demonstrated an almost complete set of genes for peptidoglycan synthesis. The outer membrane includes a major outer membrane protein (MOMP) that is immunogenic. *Chlamydia* are obligate intracellular

✱ No peptidoglycan layer

✱ Requires host cell metabolism

FIGURE 39–1. **Chlamydia life cycle. A.** Fluorescence light micrograph of human cells (red) infected with *Chlamydia trachomatis* (green). **B.** A transmission electron micrograph of human cells that contain reticulate bodies (white arrows), elementary bodies (black arrows), and an intermediate form called "aberrent bodies" (black arrowhead). **C.** A schematic representation of the infectious cycle of Chlamy.

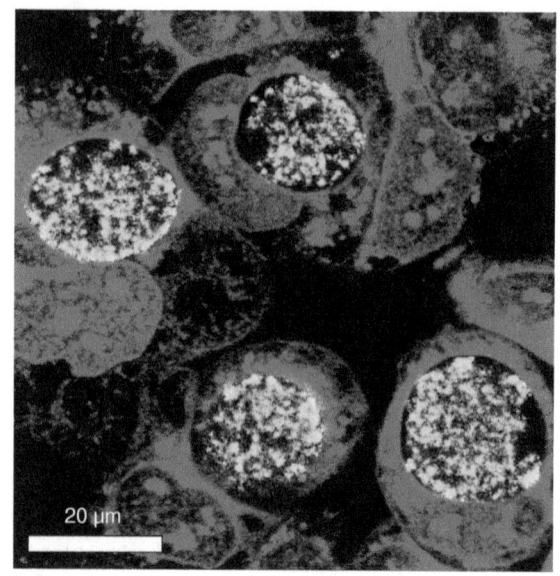

A

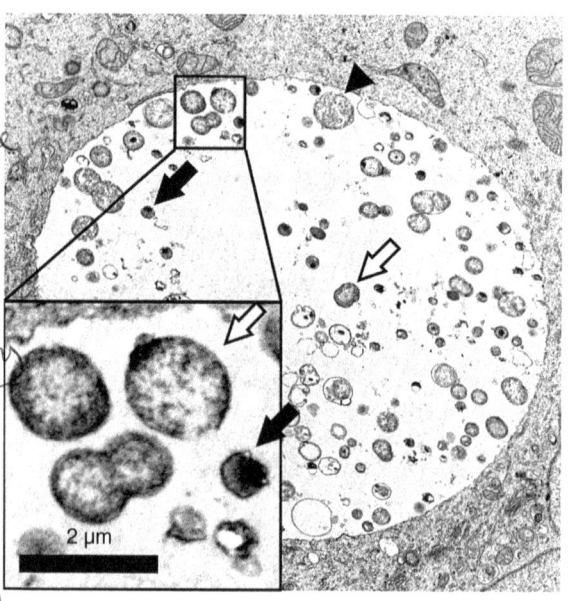

B

- will cause infections
 of the eye.
 (erythromycin drops)

- silent infection in
 over 75% of ppl.

- can cause pelvic
 inflammatory
 disease → scar tissue
 → blocks fallopian
 tubes → infertility.

- Ectopic pregnancy
 (tubal) life threatening
 for woman (massive
 hemmorhaging)

- Chlamydia infectious
 lead to male inferti-
 lity as well, attacking
 the vas deferense.

Elementary body

Size about 0.3 µm
Rigid cell wall
Relatively resistant to sonication
Resistant to trypsin
RNA:DNA content = 1:1
Toxic for mice
Isolated organisms infectious
Adapted for extracellular survival

Reticulate body (initial body)

Size 0.5-1.0 µm
Fragile cell wall
Sensitive to sonication
Lysed by trypsin
RNA:DNA content = 3:1
Nontoxic for mice
Isolated organisms not infectious
Adapted for intracellular growth

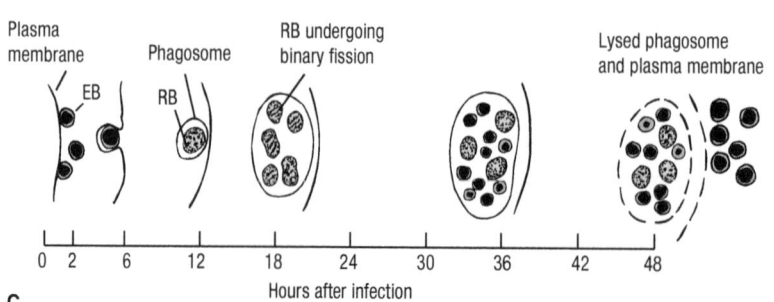

Plasma membrane   RB undergoing   Lysed phagosome
                     Phagosome   binary fission   and plasma membrane

EB   RB

0   2   6   12   18   24   30   36   42   48

Hours after infection

C

TABLE 39–1	Features of Human *Chlamydia* and *Chlamydophila* Infection					
SPECIES	**BIOVARS**	**CELL TROPISM**	**RESERVOIR**	**TRANSMISSION**	**DISEASE**	**COMPLICATIONS**
Chlamydia trachomatis	A-C	Conjunctiva	Humans	Hand-eye, fomites, flies	Conjunctivitis	Blindness
C trachomatis	D-K	Urogenital	Humans	Sexual, perinatal	NGU, cervicitis, proctitis	PID, infertility
C trachomatis	L_1, L_2, L_3	Urogenital, colorectal	Humans	Sexual	LGV, ulcers, lymphadenopathy	
Chlamydophila psittaci	Many	Respiratory, systemic	Birds	Aerosol inhalation	Pneumonia	
Chlamydophila pneumoniae	One	Respiratory	Humans	Respiratory droplets	Pneumonia	

LGV, lymphogranuloma venerum; NGU, nongonococcal urethritis; PID, pelvic inflammatory disease.

parasites because they rely on the host cell for key amino acids and energy-generating metabolites like ATP. Among bacteria only the mycoplasmas have a smaller genome.

DNA homology between *C trachomatis*, *C psittaci*, and *C pneumoniae* is less than 30%, although 16S rRNA sequence analysis suggests they share a common origin. The three species share a common group antigen. Their major differential features are shown in **Table 39–1**. *C trachomatis* has multiple biovars, each with a different tissue tropism. Biovars A-C infect ocular epithelial cells and cause trachoma; biovars D-K target urogenital epithelial cells and cause nongonococcal urethritis (NGU), mucopurulent cervicitis, and inclusion conjunctivitis; and biovars L_1-L_3 infect genital colorectal tissues and cause lymphogranuloma venereum (LGV).

REPLICATIVE CYCLE

The replicative cycle of chlamydiae is illustrated in Figure 39–1. It involves two major forms of the organism: a small, hardy infectious form termed the elementary body (EB), and a larger fragile intracellular replicative form called the reticulate body (RB). The EB is a metabolically inert form that neither expends energy nor synthesizes protein. The cycle begins when the EB attaches to the plasma membrane of susceptible target cells and induces its own endocytosis. This is accomplished in part by the secretion of a preformed translocated actin recruiting protein (Tarp) which induces actin cytoskeletal rearrangements in the target cell. Utilizing stores of ATP the EB then begins the process of converting to the replicative RB. With inhibition of lysosomal fusion in the host cell, the organism forms its own membrane-bound vesicle called the inclusion. After RBs increase in number, the process reverses and the RBs reorganize and condense to yield multiple EBs. They are then released by exocytosis, extrusion of intact inclusions, or cell lysis to infect adjacent cells. The efficiency of this cycle is optimized by a chlamydial protease-like activity factor (CPAF) which regulates cellular apoptosis signals. In the growth phase apoptosis is inhibited, but at the release stage cell death proceeds. Both Tarp and CPAF are injected by secretion systems (type III). Tarp is injected across the plasma membrane, CPAF across the inclusion membrane. A variant in the overall replicative cycle is called the persistent state in which the EBs and RBs become dormant but are still able to resume multiplication. This state can be induced by some cytokines (IFN-γ), nutrient restriction, and interestingly, penicillin. As indicated earlier, *Chlamydia* lacks the peptidoglycan target of penicillin but still has a set of genes for its synthesis.

✳ EB induces endocytosis, cytoskeletal rearrangement

✳ RBs replicate forming inclusion then EBs

Cell apoptosis regulated

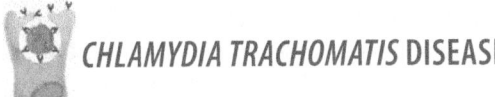

CHLAMYDIA TRACHOMATIS DISEASE

EPIDEMIOLOGY

C trachomatis causes disease in several sites, primarily the conjunctiva and genital tract. In its various forms, this infection is one of the most frequent in the world. Humans are the sole reservoir. Person-to-person spread is through direct contact or via fomites. Inclusion conjunctivitis is of two types: biovars A-C cause trachoma (see below) in children and adults whereas neonatal conjunctivitis is seen among population groups in whom the strains (biovars D-K) causing genital

✳ Finger and fomite eye transmission

infections are common. Newborns acquire *C trachomatis* through direct contact with infective cervical secretions of the mother at delivery. Adults can also develop conjunctivitis by contact with genital secretions.

Trachoma, a chronic follicular conjunctivitis, afflicts an estimated 500 million persons worldwide and blinds 7 to 9 million, particularly in Africa. The disease is usually contracted in infancy or early childhood from the mother or other close contacts. Spread is by contact with infective human secretions, directly via hands to the eye or via fomites..

High rate of sexual transmission

The prevalence of chlamydial urethral infection in U.S. men and women ranges from 5% in the general population to 20% in those attending sexually transmitted disease clinics. Approximately one-third of male sexual contacts of women with *C trachomatis* cervicitis develop urethritis after an incubation period of 2 to 6 weeks. The proportion of men with mild to absent symptoms is higher than in gonorrhea.

PATHOGENESIS

Chlamydiae have a tropism for columnar epithelial cells of the endocervix and upper genital tract of women, and the urethra, rectum, and conjunctiva of both sexes. Depending on the biovar a wide range of other cells may be infected including endothelium, smooth muscle, lymphocytes, and macrophages. Initial attachment is probably mediated by MOMP and possibly other outer membrane proteins followed by cellular invasion by the mechanisms described above. The LGV biovars can also enter through breaks in the skin or mucosa. Once the replication cycle is established, the primary injury is due to inflammation secondary to the release of proinflammatory cytokines such as interleukin-8 by infected epithelial cells. Chlamydial lipopolysaccharides probably also play an important role in initiation of the inflammatory process. This results in early tissue infiltration by polymorphonuclear leukocytes, later followed by lymphocytes, macrophages, plasma cells, and eosinophils. If the infection progresses further (because of lack of treatment and/or failure of immune control), aggregates of lymphocytes and macrophages may form in the submucosa; these can progress to necrosis, followed by fibrosis and scarring. The chronic progressive inflammation with scarring seen in trachoma is due to persistent or recurrent infections over many years beginning in childhood. In the later stages the process may be primarily immunopathologic. Live *Chlamydia* may not be present and inflammation can be triggered by *C trachomatis* antigens to which the patient has been sensitized.

Early release of cytokines

Fibrosis and scarring later

❋ Recurrent infections cause trachoma

IMMUNITY

Immunity to *C trachomatis* infections seems to take a long time to develop and even then is incomplete. Up to 50% of women with genital infections may still be shedding the organism a year later. The intracellular location and the prospect that low levels of cytokines may induce the persistent state are complicating features. T_H1 responses seem to be the most protective. T_H2 responses directed at MOMP may participate as well but antibody is also associated with immunopathologic injury in the chronic forms like trachoma.

Immunity incomplete

❋ T_H1 responses most protective

CHLAMYDIA TRACHOMATIS: CLINICAL ASPECTS

MANIFESTATIONS

■ Eye Infections

Trachoma and inclusion conjunctivitis are distinct diseases of the eye that have some overlap in their clinical manifestations. Trachoma, a chronic conjunctivitis caused by *C trachomatis* biovars A-C, is usually seen in poor countries and often leads to blindness. Neonatal inclusion conjunctivitis, an acute infection commonly caused by biovars D-K, is usually not associated with chronicity or permanent eye damage.

❋ Trachoma and neonatal conjunctivitis due to different serotypes

Trachoma

Chronic inflammation of the eyelids and increased vascularization of the corneal conjunctiva are followed by severe corneal scarring and conjunctival deformities (**Figure 39–2**). Visual loss often occurs 15 to 20 years after the initial infection as a result of repeated scarring of the cornea.

Conjunctival vascularization then scarring

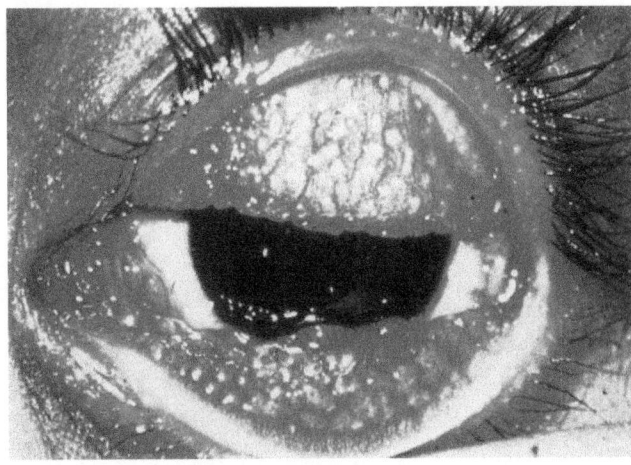

FIGURE 39-2. **Trachoma.** An active infection showing follicular hypertrophy. The inflammatory nodules cover the thickened conjunctiva. (Reproduced with permission from Willey JM: *Prescott, Harley, & Klein's Microbiology*, 7th ed. New York, NY: McGraw Hill; 2008.)

Inclusion Conjunctivitis

Neonatal inclusion conjunctivitis usually presents as an acute, watery then mucopurulent eye discharge 5 to 12 days after birth. Infection occurs in roughly one-third of infants born vaginally to infected mothers. The infection is not prevented by prophylaxis with topical erythromycin or tetracycline. Untreated, it may persist for 3 to 12 months. Inclusion conjunctivitis is clinically similar in adults and is usually associated with concomitant genital tract disease. Diagnosis can be made quickly by demonstrating characteristic cytoplasmic inclusions in smears of conjunctival scrapings (**Figure 39-3**). In both neonates and adults, systemic therapy is preferred because the nasopharynx, rectum, and vagina may also be colonized and other forms of disease may develop, such as aspiration pneumonia in neonates. More than 50% of all infants born to mothers excreting *C trachomatis* during labor show evidence of infection during the first year of life. Most develop inclusion conjunctivitis, but 5% to 10% develop neonatal pneumonia. *C trachomatis* accounts for about one-third to one-half of all cases of interstitial pneumonia in infants. The illness usually develops in a child between 6 weeks and 6 months of age and has a gradual onset. The infant is usually afebrile, but develops difficulty in feeding, a characteristic staccato (pertussis-like) cough, and shortness of breath. The disease is rarely fatal, but may be associated with decreased pulmonary function later in life.

Pneumonia in infants has delayed, gradual onset

 Why does inclusion conjunctivitis not lead to trachoma?

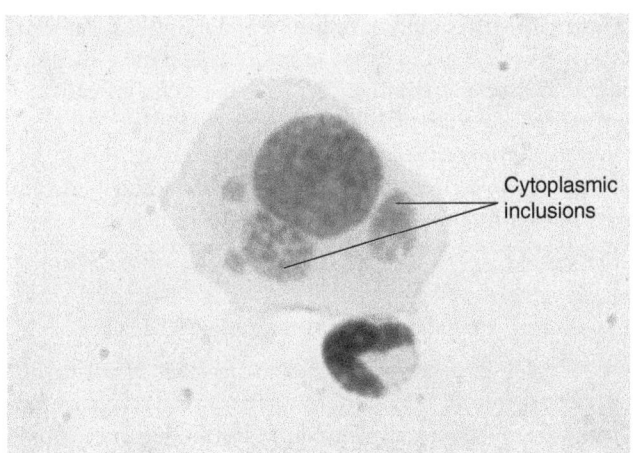

FIGURE 39-3. *Chlamydia trachomatis* cytoplasmic inclusion bodies in a conjunctival epithelial cell. (Reproduced with permission from Willey J, Sherwood L, Woolverton C: *Prescott's Principles of Microbiology*. New York, NY: McGraw Hill; 2008.)

Cytoplasmic inclusions

 Think ▸▸ Apply 39-1: The differences in disease spectrum between the *C trachomatis* biovars is based on epidemiologic evidence. A biologic difference is presumed but not proven. Trachoma follows chronic, repeated eye infection, and immunopathologic events. It is possible that due to the perinatal mode of transmission followed by treatment, subsequent infections fail to occur with inclusion conjunctivitis.

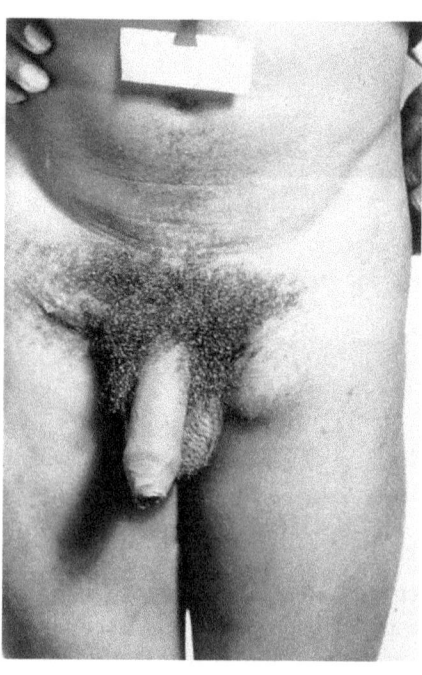

FIGURE 39–4. **Lymphogranuloma venerum.** Ulcerated inguinal lymph node. (Reproduced with permission from Connor DH, Chandler FW, Schwartz DQ, et al: *Pathology of Infectious Diseases.* Stamford CT: Appleton & Lange; 1997.)

■ Genital Infections

The clinical spectrum of sexually transmitted infections with *C trachomatis* is similar to that of *Neisseria gonorrhoeae*. *C trachomatis* can cause urethritis and epididymitis in men and cervicitis and salpingitis in women. In addition, three biovars of *C trachomatis* cause LGV, a distinctly different sexually transmitted disease (Table 39–1).

C trachomatis urethritis is manifested by dysuria and a thin urethral discharge akin to that of *Mycoplasma genitalium*. Infections of the uterine cervix may produce vaginal discharge but are usually asymptomatic. Ascending infection in the form of salpingitis and pelvic inflammatory disease (PID) occurs in an estimated 5% to 30% of infected women. The scarring produced by chronic or repeated infection is an important cause of sterility and ectopic pregnancy.

LGV is a sexually transmitted infection caused by *C trachomatis* strains L$_1$, L$_2$, or L$_3$. It occurs principally in South America, Africa, Southeast Asia, India, and Caribbean countries. The clinical course is characterized by a transient genital lesion followed by multilocular suppurative involvement of the inguinal lymph nodes (**Figure 39–4**). The primary genital lesion is usually a small painless ulcer or papule, which heals in a few days and may go unnoticed. The most common presenting complaint is inguinal adenopathy. Nodes are initially discrete, but as the disease progresses, they become matted and suppurative. The skin over the node may be thinned, and multiple draining fistulas develop. Systemic symptoms such as fever, chills, headaches, arthralgia, and myalgia are common. Late complications include urethral or rectal strictures and perirectal abscesses and fistulas. In homosexual men, LGV strains can cause a hemorrhagic ulcerative proctitis. Lymph nodes may need to be aspirated to prevent rupture.

DIAGNOSIS

Appropriate specimen collection is the first step in making an etiologic diagnosis of chlamydial infections, which are now done by molecular methods. Because *C trachomatis* is an obligate intracellular microorganism, swab specimens from conjunctiva, urethra, and endocervix should include epithelial cells for detection by nucleic acid hybridation with DNA probes for chlamydial 16S rRNA. Nucleic acid amplification (NAA) tests are rapid, sensitive, and specific for genital *Chlamydia* infections. An ideal specimen is the first 20 mL of voided urine; some platforms also are validated for use with vaginal, cervical, urethral, and rectal swabs. NAATs that detect both *C trachomatis* and *N gonorrhoeae* are commonly used.

Chlamydial serology may be useful in the diagnosis of LGV, where a single high complement fixation (CF) antibody titer (1:64 or greater) or a fourfold rise supports a presumptive diagnosis.

✳ Clinical spectrum similar to N gonorrhoeae

✳ Salpingitis and PID cause sequelae

✳ Papule and inguinal adenopathy

✳ Chronic abscesses, strictures, fistulas

Epithelial cells required

✳ NAA sensitive and specific

In 80% to 90% of patients, the LGV CF test is positive shortly after the appearance of inguinal lesions. The most satisfactory method for diagnosis of LGV is isolation of an LGV strain of *C trachomatis* from tissue or lymph node aspirates, but cultures are rarely done now.

✳ Serodiagnosis limited to LGV

TREATMENT

Strains of *C trachomatis* are susceptible to macrolides and doxycycline. Azithromycin is the preferred therapy, because it is given as a single oral dose for non-LGV *C trachomatis* infection. Doxycycline is an alternative for *C trachomatis* and is the drug of choice for treating LGV. For trachoma, a single dose of azithromycin is the treatment of choice.

✳ Azithromycin, doxycycline effective

PREVENTION

Prophylaxis for infants using topical erythromycin or silver nitrate on the conjunctiva has limited effectiveness for *Chlamydia*, because 15% to 25% of exposed infants still develop inclusion conjunctivitis. The primary approach to prevention of all forms of genital and infant *C trachomatis* infection entails detection of this infection in sexually active individuals and appropriate treatment with azithromycin, including infected women late in pregnancy. For trachoma, corrective surgery may prevent blindness and is required for severe corneal and conjunctival scarring. Control of trachoma is directed toward prevention of continued reinfection during early childhood. Improvement in general hygienic practices is the most important factor in decreasing transmission of infection within families, but one of the most difficult to implement on a broad scale.

Treat high-risk individuals

Reinfection prevention essential

● *CHLAMYDOPHILA PSITTACI*

■ Epidemiology

Human psittacosis (ornithosis) is a zoonotic pneumonia contracted through inhalation of respiratory secretions or dust from droppings of infected birds. It was initially described in psittacines, such as parrots and parakeets, but was subsequently shown to occur in over 100 avian species, including turkeys. The disease is usually latent in its natural host, but may become active, particularly with the stress of recent captivity or transport; *C psittaci* is then excreted in large amounts. Until recently classified with the genus *Chlamydia*, the closely related *C psittaci* (and *C pneumoniae*) were splint off based on differences in ribosomal RNA sequence analysis.

✳ Pneumonia contracted from birds

Psittacosis in humans is seen mainly as an occupational hazard of poultry workers and bird fanciers, particularly owners of psittacine birds. Reported cases of human psittacosis in the United States decreased during the 1950s, in association with the use of antimicrobials in poultry feeds and quarantine regulations for imported psittacine birds. Currently, 100 to 200 cases of psittacosis are reported each year. *C psittaci* is highly infectious and its airborne infectious potential is enough for *C psittaci* to be placed on lists of potential bioterrorism weapons. Nonetheless, human-to-human transmission is rare.

Associated with poultry processing and many birds

CLINICAL DISEASE AND TREATMENT

The incubation period for psittacosis is 5 to 15 days. Psittacosis in humans is an acute infection of the lower respiratory tract, usually presenting with acute onset of fever, headache, malaise, muscle aches, dry hacking cough, and bilateral interstitial pneumonia. Occasionally, systemic complications such as myocarditis, encephalitis, endocarditis, and hepatitis may develop. The liver and spleen are often enlarged. The diagnosis of psittacosis should be suspected in any patient with acute onset of febrile lower respiratory illness who gives a history of close exposure to birds. Indeed, a history of bird exposure should be especially sought in patients who appear to have a bilateral pneumonia not proven to be caused by other agents. Spread can occur from both symptomatic and asymptomatic infections of birds. The specific diagnosis is usually made by demonstrating a fourfold rise in the titer of microimmunofluorescence or CF antibodies or a single IgM titer of higher than 1:32 or greater A drawback of CF titers are cross-reactions with *C trachomatis* and *C pneumoniae*. Treatment with doxycycline (preferred) or azithromycin is effective if given early in the course of illness.

Bilateral interstitial pneumonia

✳ Diagnosis serologic

Treatment with doxycycline

● *CHLAMYDOPHILA PNEUMONIAE*

Manifestations similar to *M pneumoniae*

Azithromycin, levofloxacin, or doxycycline preferred treatment

C pneumoniae has been shown to be as common a cause of community-acquired pneumonia that mimics the features of *M pneumoniae* infection. Since this agent has been recognized as a cause of pneumonia for little more than a decade, its clinical features and disease mechanisms are still in development. It is estimated that 10% of pneumonia and 5% of bronchitis cases are due to this agent. Epidemiologic evidence indicates that infection occurs throughout the year and is spread between humans by person-to-person contact. Outbreaks of community-acquired pneumonia caused by *C pneumoniae* have been reported as has apparent nosocomial spread. Reinfections occur, and clinically evident *C pneumoniae* infection may occur more often in the elderly than in younger individuals. Most infections manifest as pharyngitis, lower respiratory tract disease, or both, and the clinical spectrum is similar to that of *M pneumoniae* infection. Pharyngitis or laryngitis may occur 1 to 3 weeks before bronchitis or pneumonia, and cough may persist for weeks. The diagnosis is established by NAATs; both *C pneumoniae* and *M pneumoniae* are included in widely available respiratory and pneumonia multiplex PCR panels, whereas *C. psittaci* is not. Treatment with azithromycin, doxycycline, or levofloxacin is effective in ameliorating the signs and symptoms of *C pneumoniae* infection.

KEY CONCLUSIONS

- The chlamydiae share a common mode of replication but differ in tropisms.
- *Chlamydia trachomatis* biovars A-C cause trachoma, a leading cause of blindness in impoverished populations.
- *C trachomatis* biovars D-K are sexually transmitted, cause urogenital disease, and neonatal infection after vaginal delivery to infected mothers.
- *C trachomatis* biovars L_1-L_3 cause genital and rectal disease by sexual transmission.
- Both *Chlamydophila* species cause pneumonia.
- *Chlamydophila psittaci* is a zoonotic pathogen that causes psittacosis and is acquired from birds.
- *Chlamydophila pneumoniae* resembles *Mycoplama pneumoniae* in its clinical features with nonproductive cough and patchy lung infiltrates.
- Apart from *C psittaci,* all the chlamydiae are exclusively human pathogens.
- Azithromycin or doxycycline are used for therapy of infections with the chlamydiae.

CASE STUDY

An Unanticipated Result

A 29-year-old man presents with a 2-day history of burning on urination and a thin, watery urethral discharge. He had unprotected sex with a new female partner 4 weeks ago. A Gram stain reveals 50% polymorphonuclear (PMN) and 50% mononuclear leukocytes. No microorganisms are visible.

QUESTIONS

1. Which is the most likely cause of this man's urethritis?
   A. *Neisseria gonorrhoeae*
   B. *Ureaplasma urealyticum*
   C. *Chlamydia trachomatis*
   D. *Trichomonas vaginalis*
   E. *Mycoplasma hominis*

2. Which is the most sensitive test to detect the pathogen?
   A. Culture
   B. Serology
   C. Immunofluorescent assay
   D. Nucleic acid amplification assay

3. To which is the causative microbe susceptible?
    A. Not susceptible to antibiotics
    B. Most susceptible to β-lactam antibiotics
    C. Resistant to quinolones
    D. Susceptible to macrolides

ANSWERS

1. **(C)**
2. **(D)**
3. **(D)**

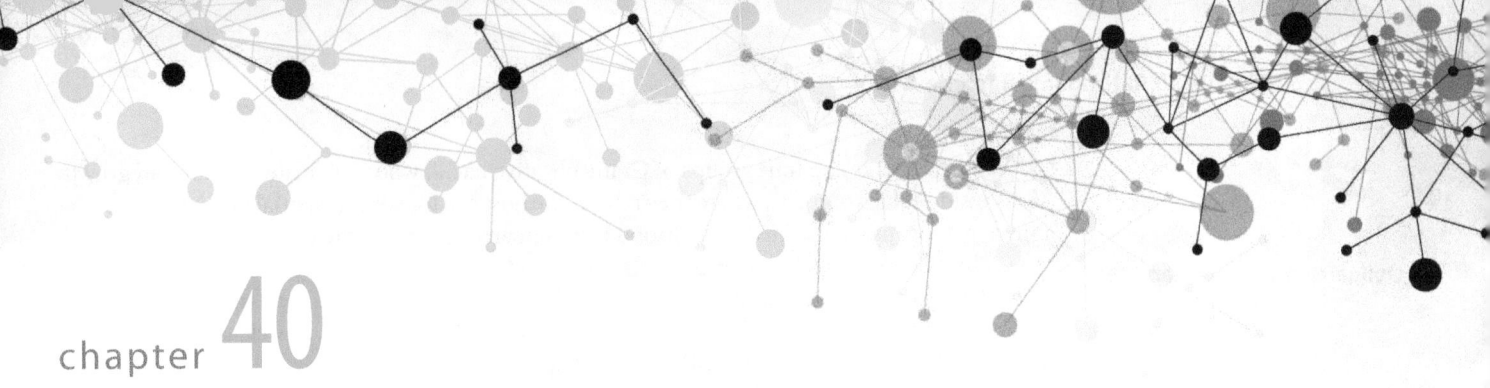

chapter 40

Rickettsia, Orientia, Ehrlichia, Anaplasma, and Bartonella

Rickettsia rickettsii · *Rickettsia akari* · *Rickettsia prowazekii* · *Rickettsia typhi* · *Orientia tsutsugamushi* · *Ehrlichia chaffeensis*

Anaplasma phagocytophilum · *Bartonella quintana* · *Bartonella bacilliformis* · *Bartonella henselae*

His mouth was dry and sticky; a heavy fog weighed down his brain.

—Anton Chekhov (a physician): *Typhus*

OVERVIEW

The agents covered in this chapter are all small, Gram-negative, if they stain at all, intracellular coccobacilli that are arthropod-borne to humans. Their epidemiology, however, is determined largely by the distribution and habits of their arthropod vectors (ticks, fleas, mites, and sandflies). Clinical features also differ by pathogen, but all respond to doxycycline therapy. The rickettsioses fall into two categories: spotted fever group (SFG) and typhus group (TG). With molecular tools, including sequencing, many new rickettsia are being described in both groups, but only the most important currently or historically are presented here.

In the SFG are tick-transmitted *Rickettsia rickettsii* that causes Rocky Mountain spotted fever (RMSF) and mite-borne *Rickettsia akari* that causes rickettsialpox. In the TG is louse-borne *Rickettsia prowazekii* that causes epidemic typhus, flea-transmitted *Rickettsii typhi* that causes murine typhus, and mite-borne *Orientia tsutsugamushi* that causes scrub typhus. By far the most important rickettsiosis in the United States in both incidence and severity is RMSF, whereas epidemic typhus ranks foremost historically in Europe. Both RMSF and typhus are characterized by fever, headache, myalgia, and rash. In RMSF, the rash appears first on the palms and soles, wrists, and ankles and migrates centripetally; whereas in epidemic typhus, the rash moves in the opposite direction beginning on the trunk and spreading to the extremities. Both diseases may be fatal as the result of severe vascular collapse.

Ehrlichia and *Anaplasma* are both transmitted by ticks. *Ehrlichia chaffeensis* primarily infects monocytes and causes human monocytic ehrlichiosis (HME) and *Anaplasma phagocytophilum* infects polymorphonuclear granulocytes and causes human granulocytic anaplasmosis (HGA). Both HME and HGA manifest with fever, headache, malaise, leukopenia, and thrombocytopenia. A rash may be seen, but is neither common nor prominent.

Bartonella species are louse-borne *Bartonella quintana* that causes trench fever, sandfly-borne *Bartonella bacilliformis* that invades red blood cells and causes Oroya fever and verruga peruana, and *Bartonella henselae* (bacillary angiomatosis and cat-scratch disease) that is transmitted by scratches or bites of cats or their fleas.

Obligate intracellular parasites

This chapter takes up four groups of Gram-negative bacilli whose obligate or preferred growth is inside eukaryotic cells where they rely on the host cell for some essential nutrients. They are animal pathogens transmitted by arthropods to humans who are in the wrong place at the wrong time. The diseases vary depending on whether the target is endothelial cells, phagocytes, or erythrocytes. Most have prolonged fevers, often with vasculitis. These include classic ones like Rocky Mountain spotted fever (RMSF), typhus, and cat-scratch disease (CSD), as well as recently recognized infections like human ehrlichiosis and anaplasmosis.

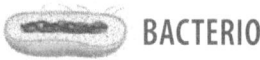 **RICKETTSIA**

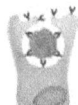 **BACTERIOLOGY**

STRUCTURE

Gram-negative coccobacilli stained best by immunofluorescence

Abundant outer membrane proteins

Rickettsiae are small coccobacilli, which measure no more than 0.3 to 0.5 μm. Although the Gram reaction is negative, rickettsiae take the usual bacterial stains poorly and are better demonstrated by specific immunofluorescence. The ultrastructural morphology, which is similar to that of other Gram-negative bacteria, includes a Gram-negative type of cell envelope, ribosomes, and a nuclear body. Chemically, the cell wall contains lipopolysaccharide and at least two large proteins in the outer membrane, as well as peptidoglycan. The outer membrane proteins extend to the cell surface, where they are the most abundant protein present. They are discussed here as members of either the SFG or TG. Due to differences in protein composition and its lack of lipopolysaccharide, *Orientia tsutsugamushi* (formerly *R tsutsugamushi*) has been placed in a separate genus.

METABOLISM

Rickettsia grows freely in the cytoplasm of eukaryotic cells to which they are highly adapted, in contrast to *Ehrlichia* and *Bartonella* that replicate in cytoplasmic vacuoles. Rickettsiae can be grown only in the living eukaryotic cells found in cell cultures, organ cultures, and embryonated eggs. *Rickettsia* is able to adhere to a wide variety of cell types through the binding of outer membrane proteins. They enter cells by induced phagocytosis and escape to the cytoplasms by elaboration of a phospholipase. In the cytoplasm the SFG *rickettsiae* move about utilizing an actin-based motility similar to that already described for *Listeria* and *Shigella* (see Chapters 26 and 33). Intracytoplasmic growth eventually produces lysis of the cell.

✳ Grow in cytoplasm following induced endocytosis

✳ Exogenous cofactors and ATP required

✳ Lose infectivity outside host cell

The obligate intracellular parasitism of *Rickettsiae* has several interesting features. Failure to survive outside the cell is related to requirements for nucleotide cofactors (coenzyme A, NAD), amino acids, phosphorylated sugars, and ATP. Outside the host cell, *Rickettsiae* not only cease metabolic activity, but leak protein, nucleic acids, and essential small molecules. This instability leads to rapid loss of infectivity because the penetration of another cell requires energy. Over time, *Rickettsiae* have lost some of their core metabolic capabilities by reductive evolution and instead use transport systems which extract these essential elements from their host cells.

RICKETTSIAL DISEASE

EPIDEMIOLOGY

Most rickettsiae have animal reservoirs and are spread by ticks, lice, fleas, or mites, which are prominent components of their life cycles (**Table 40–1**). The global distribution of specific rickettsial infections is determined by climate, reservoir, vector, and human interactions as detailed under the clinical aspects of each entity. These epidemiologic differences of rickettsial infections are important despite their shared features in pathogenesis. Rickettsial infections of humans usually result in clinical illness.

PATHOGENESIS

Following transmission from the salivary gland of infected ticks the bacteria spread locally creating a necrotic eschar. The major rickettsial species have a tropism for vascular endothelium. The primary pathologic lesion is a vasculitis in which they multiply in the endothelial cells lining the

TABLE 40-1   Features of *Rickettsia, Ehrlichia, Anaplasma,* and *Bartonella*

ORGANISM	TARGET	DISEASE	DISTRIBUTION	VECTOR	RESERVOIR
Rickettsia rickettsii	Vascular endothelium	Rocky Mountain spotted fever	North, Central, and South America	Tick	Rodents, dogs
R conorii, R africae, R australis	Vascular endothelium	Other spotted fevers	Worldwide	Tick	Rodents, dogs
R akari	Vascular endothelium	Rickettsialpox	Worldwide	Mite	Mouse
R prowazekii	Vascular endothelium	Typhus	Worldwide	Body louse	Human
R typhi	Vascular endothelium	Murine (endemic) typhus	Worldwide	Flea	Rodents esp. rats
Orientia tsutsugamushi	Mononuclear cells	Scrub typhus	Far East, China, India	Mite larvae (chiggers)	
Ehrlichia chaffeensis	Mononuclear cells	Human monocytic ehrlichiosis	United States	Tick	Deer
Anaplasma phagocytophilum	PMNs	Human granulocytic anaplasmosis	United States, Europe, Asia	Tick	Deer
Bartonella quintana	Vascular endothelium, RBCs	Trench fever, bacillary angiomatosis	Worldwide	Body louse	Humans
B henselae	Vascular endothelium, RBCs	Cat-scratch disease, bacillary angiomatosis	Worldwide	Cat to cat by fleas	Cats
B bacilliformis	Vascular endothelium, RBCs	Oroya fever, verruga peruana	South America[a]	Sandfly	

[a]Only at elevations between 1 and 3 km in the Andes mountains.

small blood vessels (**Figure 40–1**). Pathophysiologically, this leads to increased vascular permeability, hypovolemia, and hypotension. Focal areas of endothelial proliferation and perivascular infiltration leading to thrombosis and leakage of red blood cells into the surrounding tissues account for the rash and petechial lesions. Vascular lesions occur throughout the body and produce the systemic manifestations of the disease. These lesions are most apparent in the skin but are most lethal in the adrenal glands. *Orientia tsutsugamushi* infects mononuclear cells but still produces fever and rash.

✳ Infect vascular endothelium with vasculitis, thrombosis

✳ Increased vascular permeability leads to hypotension

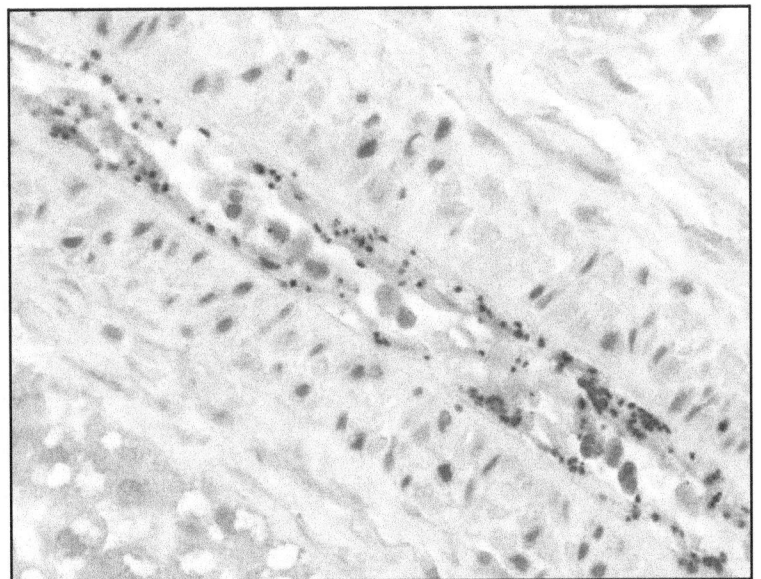

FIGURE 40–1. **Rickettsial vasculitis.** Immunohistochemical stain shows *Rickettsia rickettsia* (red) in endothelial cells that line the blood vessel. (Reproduced with permission from Biggs HM, Behravesh CB, Bradley KK, et al: Diagnosis and Management of Tickborne Rickettsial Diseases: Rocky Mountain Spotted Fever and Other Spotted Fever Group Rickettsioses, Ehrlichioses, and Anaplasmosis - United States, MMWR Recomm Rep 2016 May 13;65(2):1-44.)

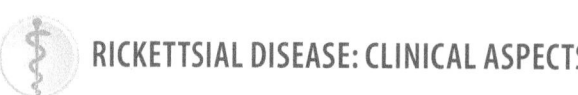

RICKETTSIAL DISEASE: CLINICAL ASPECTS

SPOTTED FEVER GROUP

Tick-borne rickettsioses worldwide

The most important rickettsial disease in North America is RMSF, which is caused by *Rickettsia rickettsii*. A number of other spotted fever rickettsioses are found in other parts of the world (Table 40–1); the name often reveals the locale (eg, Mediterranean spotted fever, Marseilles fever). They are caused by *Rickettsia species*, serologically related to, but distinct from, *R rickettsii* (eg, *R conorii* and *R africae*). Another less severe spotted fever, rickettsialpox, also occurs in North America.

■ Rocky Mountain Spotted Fever

RMSF is an acute febrile illness that occurs in association with residential and recreational exposure to wooded areas where infected ticks exist. The frequency of reported cases of spotted fever group (SFG) rickettsia in the United States has increased 10-fold in the past 2 decades (**Figure 40–2**).

Epidemiology

✳ Transovarial spread perpetuates tick infection

Rickettsia rickettsii is primarily a parasite of ticks. In the western United States, the wood tick (*Dermacentor andersoni*) is the primary vector. *Dermacentor variabilis* is the most common tick vector in the eastern, central, and Pacific coastal U.S. The brown dog tick *Rhipicephalus sanguineus* is found throughout the United States and northern Mexico and is an emerging vector in the Southwest. Various *Amblyomma* ticks are vectors of SFG rickettsiae from Mexico to Argentina. *Rickettsia rickettsii* does not kill its arthropod host, so the parasite is passed through unending generations of ticks by transovarial spread. Adult females require a blood meal to lay eggs and thus may transmit the disease. Infected adult ticks have been shown to survive as long as 4 years without feeding.

Children at greatest risk

Rickettsia rickettsii is found in North, Central, and South America. Cases of RMSF have been reported from every state in the continental U.S., have increased markedly in recent years (**Figure 40–2**), and have extended their geographical range (**Figure 40–3**) in concert with changes in climate and tick habitat. The highest incidence now occurs in persons over the age of 40 years, whereas the highest case-fatality rate is among children less than 10 years old. Men outnumber

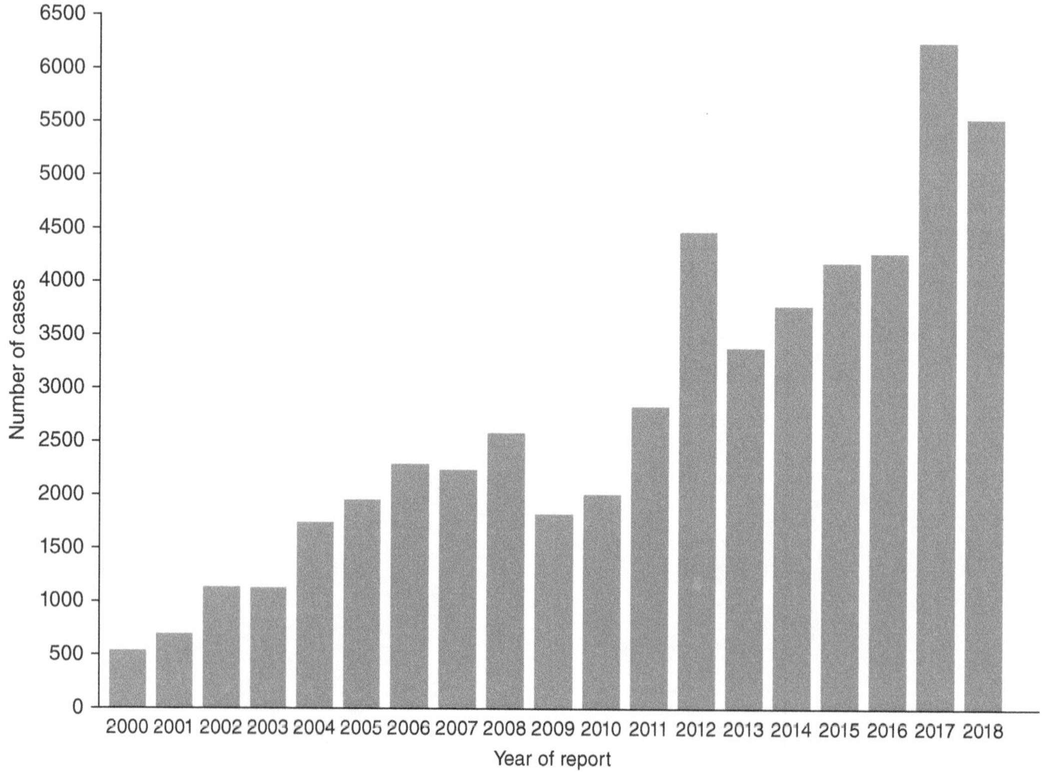

FIGURE 40–2. **Yearly reported cases of spotted fever rickettsioses (SFR) in the United States, 2000-2018** (Reproduced with permission from Centers for Disease Control and Prevention. U.S. Department of Health & Human Services. Rocky Mountain Spotted Fever (RMSF). April, 2020.)

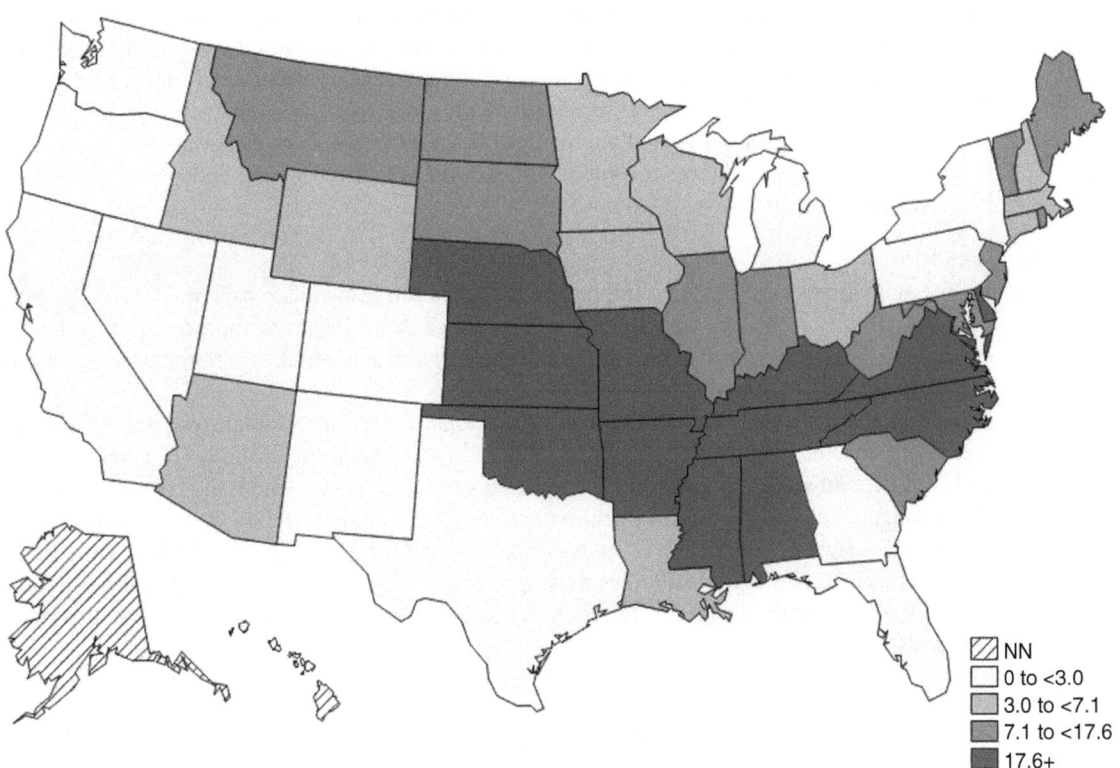

FIGURE 40–3. Geographical distribution and annual incidence of spotted fever rickettsioses (SFR) in the United States, 2018. The geographical range and annual incidence (per million persons) for cases of SFR in the United States for 2018 are shown. Both the range and frequency of RMSF are increasing. (Reproduced with permission from Centers for Disease Control and Prevention. U.S. Department of Health & Human Services. Rocky Mountain Spotted Fever (RMSF). April, 2020.)

women in SFG cases. The illness is generally seen between April and September because of increased exposure to ticks, but RMSF has occurred in all months. A history of tick bite can be elicited in approximately 70% of cases.

Manifestations

The incubation period between the tick bite and the onset of illness is usually 6 to 7 days, but it may be from 2 days to 2 weeks. Fever, headache, rash, toxicity, mental confusion, and myalgia are the major clinical features. The rash is the most characteristic feature of the illness, but may not occur in up to one-third of cases. Rash usually develops on the second or third day of illness as small erythematous macules that rapidly become petechial (**Figure 40–4**). The lesions appear

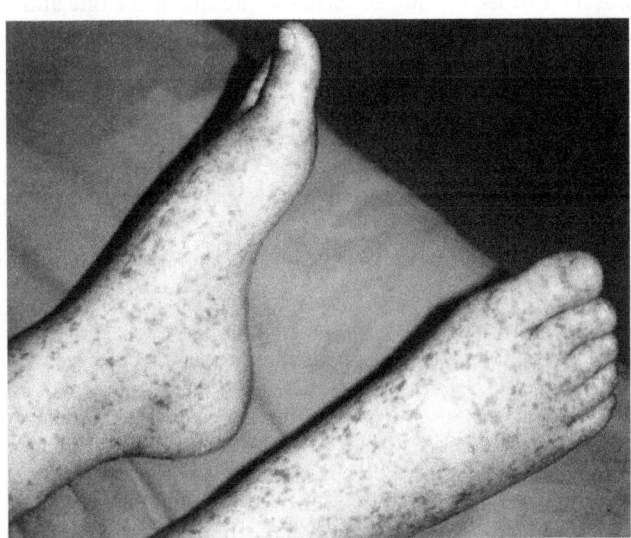

FIGURE 40–4. Rocky Mountain spotted fever. The rash begins on the arms and legs and spreads centrally. (Reproduced with permission from Nester EW, Anderson DG, Roberts CE Jr, et al: *Microbiology: A Human Perspective,* 6th ed. New York, NY: McGraw Hill; 2008.)

initially on the wrists and ankles and then spread up the extremities to the trunk in a few hours. A diagnostic feature of RMSF is the frequent appearance of the rash on the palms and soles, a finding not usually seen in maculopapular eruptions associated with other rickettsial infections, including typhus. Muscle tenderness, especially in the gastrocnemius, is characteristic and may be extreme. If untreated, or occasionally in patients despite therapy, complications such as disseminated intravascular coagulation, thrombocytopenia, encephalitis, vascular collapse, and renal and heart failure may ensue.

Diagnosis

Unlike many infections, the most important consideration in the diagnosis of RMSF is the early initiation of doxycycline therapy solely on the basis of clinical signs, symptoms, and epidemiologic features. Doing so can be life saving. All the diagnostic methods have limitations in speed, sensitivity, specificity, or availability.

Culture of rickettsiae is both difficult and hazardous. Therefore, serologic tests are the primary means of a specific diagnosis of *R rickettsii*. The indirect fluorescent antibody (IFA) test on acute and convalescent serum specimens is the most sensitive and specific and is the reference method. IFA is usually available only in state health or reference laboratories. RT-PCR is relatively insensitive for the diagnosis of RMSF. It is often difficult to establish the diagnosis of RMSF early in the course of illness. However, antibodies may appear by the sixth or seventh day of illness, and a fourfold rise in antibody titer between acute serum and convalescent serum establishes the diagnosis.

Treatment

Appropriate antibiotic therapy is highly effective if given during the first week of illness. If delayed into the second week or when pathologic processes such as disseminated intravascular coagulation are present, therapy may be futile. The antibiotic of choice is doxycycline for both children and adults. Sulfonamides may worsen the disease process and are thus contraindicated. Before specific therapy became available, the mortality rate associated with RMSF was approximately 25%. Treatment has reduced this figure to between 5% and 7%. Death results primarily in patients in whom clinical recognition and therapy are delayed into the second week of illness.

Prevention

The major means of preventing RMSF is avoidance or reduction of tick contact. Frequent tick removal in tick-infested areas is important, because ticks generally must feed for 6 hours or longer before they can transmit the disease. Tick surveys in the Carolinas have shown infection in about 5% of samples.

■ Rickettsialpox

Rickettsialpox was first recognized in 1946 in New York City, where an average of five cases per year continue to occur. It has been reported in other U.S. cities and in Eastern Europe, Korea, and South Africa. It is a benign rickettsial illness caused by *Rickettsia akari* and transmitted by a rodent mite. Distinguishing features of the disease include an eschar at the site of the bite and a vesicular rash. The house mouse and other semi-domestic rodents are the primary reservoirs. Humans acquire infection when the mite seeks an alternative host.

Rickettsialpox is a biphasic illness. The first phase is the local lesion at the bite, which starts as a papulovesicle and develops into a black eschar in 3 to 5 days. Fever and constitutional symptoms appear as the organism disseminates. The second phase of the disease is a diffuse rash distributed randomly in the body, which, like the local lesion, becomes vesicular and develops into eschars. However, the rash does not occur on the palms or soles. Rickettsialpox is self-limiting after 1 week, and no deaths have been reported. Doxycycline therapy shortens the course to 1 to 2 days.

TYPHUS GROUP

■ Epidemic Louse-Borne Typhus Fever

Primary louse-borne typhus fever is caused by *R prowazekii*, which is transmitted to humans by the body louse. Historically, it has appeared during times of misery (war, famine) that create conditions favorable to human body lice (crowding, infrequent bathing). This is the only rickettsial disease that can occur as an epidemic. Foci of typhus persist in parts of Africa, Latin America, and

Asia. After the Civil War in Burundi in 1993, upwards of 100,000 cases of epidemic typhus occurred in refugees with case-fatality rates exceeding 5%. In disrupted countries, the homeless population is a focus. Epidemic typhus has not been seen in the United States for more than half a century. *R prowazekii* has been recovered from flying squirrels and their ectoparasites in the southeastern United States, and a few human cases of sylvatic typhus have occurred in these areas.

The chain of epidemic typhus infection starts with *R prowazekii* circulating in a patient's blood during an acute febrile infection. The human body louse becomes infected during one of its frequent blood meals, and after 5 to 10 days of incubation, large numbers of rickettsiae appear in its feces. Since the louse defecates while it feeds, the organisms can be rubbed into the louse bite wounds when the host scratches the site. Dried louse feces are also infectious through the mucous membranes of the eye or respiratory tract. The louse dies of its infection in 1 to 3 weeks, and the rickettsiae are not transmitted transovarially.

Fever, headache, and rash begin 1 to 2 weeks after the bite. A maculopapular rash occurs in 20% to 80% of patients and appears first on the trunk and then spreads centrifugally to the extremities, a pattern opposite to that of RMSF. Headache, malaise, and myalgia are prominent components of the illness. Complications include myocarditis and central nervous system dysfunction. In untreated disease, the fatality rate increases with age from 10% to as high as 60%. The diagnostic test of choice is serology, but therapy must be initiated immediately on clinical suspicion. Treatment with doxycycline is effective. Louse control is the best means of prevention and is particularly important in controlling epidemics. No effective vaccine is available.

* Epidemic louse-borne due to *R prowazekii*

* Human blood feeding plus louse defecation

No transovarial transmission

* Fever, headache, rash, high mortality

* Rash begins on trunk not extremities

Endemic (Murine) Typhus

Endemic or murine typhus is caused by *Rickettsia typhi* and transmitted to humans by the rat flea (*Xenopsylla cheopis*). Human illness is incidental to the natural transmission of the disease among urban rats, which serve as the reservoir. The disease occurs worldwide but only 50 to 100 cases of murine typhus are reported in the United States each year. These typically occur along the Gulf Coast of Texas and in Southern California.

The pathogenesis is similar to that of louse-borne typhus, but the history includes exposure to rats, rat fleas, or both. The flea defecates when it takes a blood meal, and the infected feces gain access through the bite wound. After an incubation period of 1 to 2 weeks, illness begins with headache, myalgia, and fever. The rash is maculopapular, not petechial; it starts on the trunk and then spreads to the extremities in a manner similar to typhus. Because of antigens shared by *R typhi* and *R prowazekii*, serologic tests may not separate the two diseases. In the untreated patient, fever may last 12 to 14 days. With doxycycline therapy, the course is reduced to 2 to 3 days. Mortality and complications are rare, even if the disease is untreated.

* Transmitted by rat fleas

* Resembles typhus but less severe

Shares antigens with *R prowazekii*

Scrub Typhus

Scrub typhus is found predominantly in South Asia, China, and Indonesia (the scrub typhus triangle). The causative organism is *Orientia tsutsugamushi*, a rickettsial organism. The geographic range of scrub typhus is expanding with many cases now documented in India, Micronesia, and the Maldives. In 2016, it was elegantly documented by IFA, ELISA, and polymerase chain reaction (PCR) in southern Chile. Mites that infest rodents are the reservoir as well as vectors and transmit the rickettsiae to their own progeny via infected ova. Humans pick up the mites as they pass by low trees or brush. The mite larvae (chiggers) deposit rickettsiae as they feed. The typical initial lesion, a necrotic eschar at the site of the bite on the extremities, develops in only 50% to 80% of cases. Fever increases slowly over the first week, sometimes reaching 40.5°C. Headache, rash, and generalized lymphadenopathy follow later.

The maculopapular rash, which appears after about 5 days, is more evanescent than that seen with louse-borne or murine typhus. Hepatosplenomegaly and conjunctivitis may also appear. Specific diagnosis requires demonstration of a serologic response with the IFA test or PCR on blood or biopsy. The prognosis is good with doxycycline therapy, but the mortality rate of untreated patients is as high as 30%.

* Transmitted by rodent mite larvae

* Local eschar, fever, headache, rash, lymphadenopathy

Serologic diagnosis by IFA

Ehrlichia and Anaplasma

Ehrlichia and *Anaplasma* include several species of tick-borne Gram-negative bacteria that cause animal and human disease. The principal diseases are HME, which is due to *E chaffeensis,* and HGA, which is due to *Anaplasma phagocytophilum*. The structure of these species does not include lipopolysaccharide or peptidoglycan, but they can independently carry out basic metabolic tasks such as the Krebs cycle and generation of ATP. All are obligate intracellular pathogens that infect WBCs. The preferred bone marrow derived lineage of WBC varies with the animal species infected. In humans, *E chaffeensis* primarily infects mononuclear cells and *A phagocytophilum* polymorphonuclear cells (PMNs). They enter their preferred cell type by receptor-induced endocytosis and multiply in the endocytotic vacuole. The replicative cycle includes replicative forms and denser infectious forms in inclusions (morulae) similar to those seen in *Chlamydia*. Replication and survival are enhanced by blocking lysosomal fusion with their vacuole and resistance to killing by reactive oxygen species. No toxins or other virulence factors have been described. Injury in human disease is primarily related to inflammatory host responses and can be especially severe in HIV-positive patients.

E chaffeensis infections tend to occur in the southeastern and lower Midwestern United States and are transmitted by *Amblyomma* ticks, whereas HGA tends to cluster in the northern states with a distribution similar to Lyme disease and is also transmitted by *Ixodes* ticks (**Figures 40–5 and 40–6**). It has also been reported from other areas of the world, including Asia and Europe. HGA exceeds the frequency of ehrlichiosis and is second only to Lyme disease (see Chapter 37) as a tick-borne infection in the United States but both are increasing. HME is transmitted by the lone star tick (*Amblyomma americanum*), and the white-tailed deer is the animal reservoir. HGA is transmitted by *Ixodes* ticks, as is Lyme disease, and the animal reservoir is small mammals (eg, mice, rats, voles). The findings are clinically similar to RMSF, but rashes are less commonly seen. Although rash is rare in anaplasmosis, it can be seen in 33% of cases of ehrlichiosis, especially later in the disease course. Mortality can exceed 3% in untreated ehrlichiosis, which is more severe in the elderly and may have neurologic (meningoencephalitis) findings.

A preliminary diagnosis of ehrlichiosis or anaplasmosis may be suggested by observation of characteristic intracytoplasmic inclusions (morulae) in mononuclear cells (HME) or granulocytes (HGA), respectively (**Figure 40–7**). The diagnosis of either is usually made serologically by a fourfold or greater rise in IFA antibody or a titer greater than or equal to 1:64 to the specific antigen. PCR for both ehrlichiosis or anaplasmosis is more sensitive than it is for RMSF. Both IFA and PCR methods are the province of public health or reference laboratories. Clinical laboratory clues to human ehrlichiosis or anaplasmosis include a falling leukocyte count, thrombocytopenia,

* No LPS or peptidoglycan

* Intracellular parasites of monocytes or PMNs

Endocytotic vacuole resists lysosomal fusion

* Tick-borne and WBC associated

Inclusions in monocytes (*Ehrlichia*) or granulocytes (*Anaplasma*)

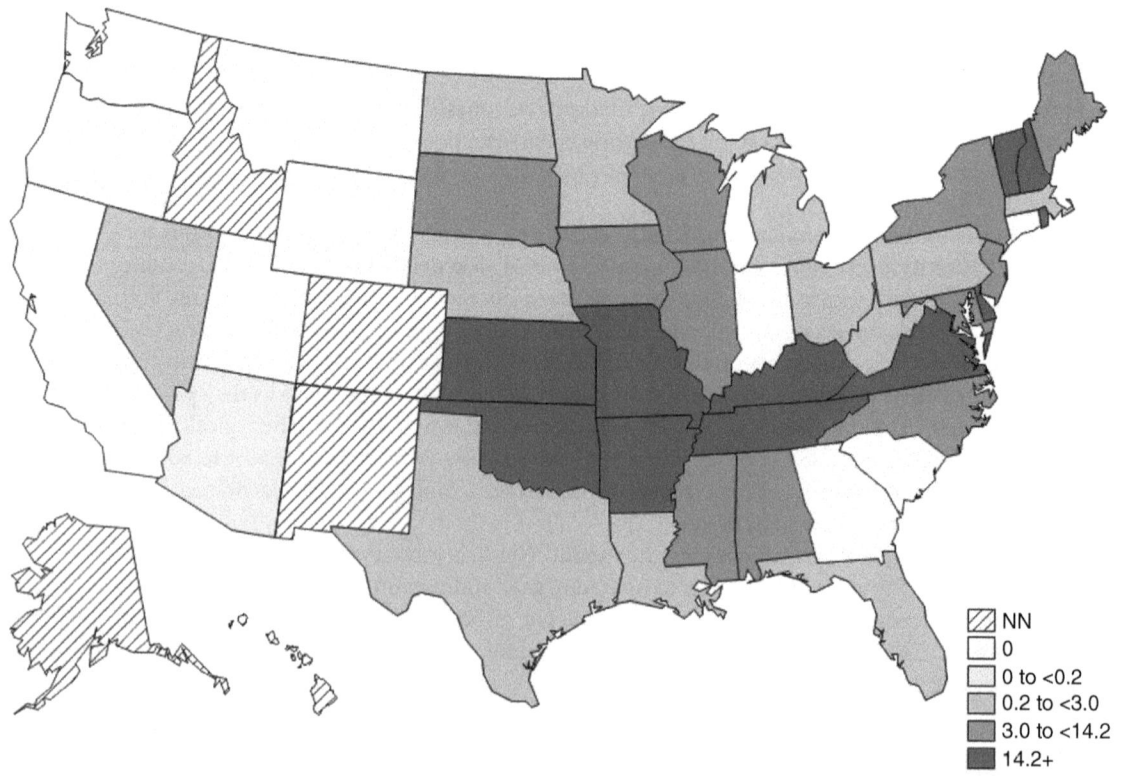

NN
0
0 to <0.2
0.2 to <3.0
3.0 to <14.2
14.2+

FIGURE 40–5. Geographical distribution and annual incidence of ehrlichiosis in the United States, 2018. The geographical range and annual incidence (per million persons) for cases of ehrlichiosis in the United States for 2018 are shown. (Reproduced with permission from Centers for Disease Control and Prevention. U.S. Department of Health & Human Services. Ehrlichiosis. March, 2020.)

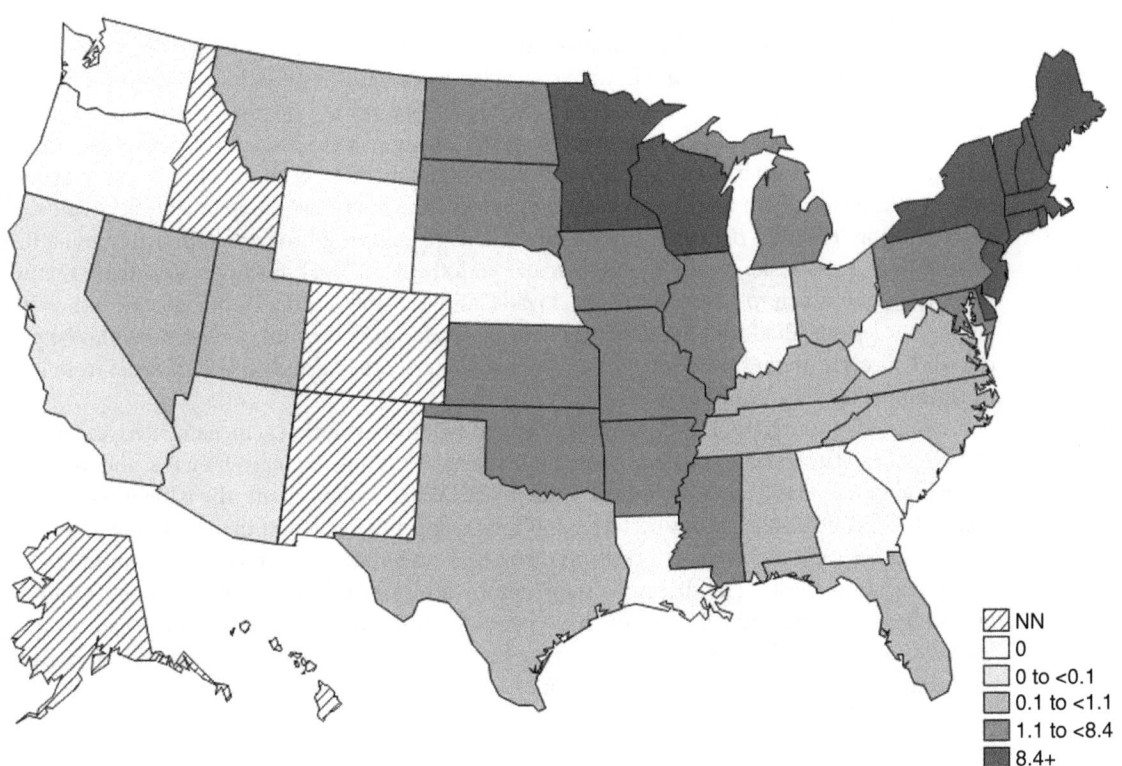

FIGURE 40–6. **Geographical distribution and annual incidence of anaplasmosis in the United States, 2018.** The geographical range and annual incidence (per million persons) for cases of Anaplasmosis in the United States for 2018 are shown. (Reproduced with permission from Centers for Disease Control and Prevention. U.S. Department of Health & Human Services. Anaplasmosis. March, 2020.)

anemia, and impaired liver and renal function. Doxycycline is the drug of choice for both. The risk of infection can be reduced by avoiding wooded areas and tick bites.

Treatment is doxycycline

 Why is PCR useful for the diagnosis of ehrlichiosis and anaplasmosis but not RMSF?

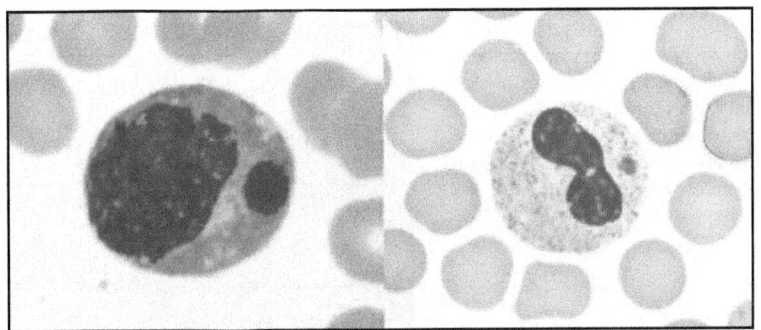

FIGURE 40–7. **Peripheral blood smears of ehrlichiosis and anaplasmosis.** Wright stain of peripheral blood smears showing intramonocytic morula associated with *Ehrlichia chafeensis* infection (left) and an intragranulocytic morula (right) associated with *Anaplasma phagocytophilum* infection. (Reproduced with permission from Biggs HM, Behravesh CB, Bradley KK, et al: Diagnosis and Management of Tickborne Rickettsial Diseases: Rocky Mountain Spotted Fever and Other Spotted Fever Group Rickettsioses, Ehrlichioses, and Anaplasmosis - United States, MMWR Recomm Rep 2016 May 13;65(2):1-44.)

 Think ▸▸ Apply 40-1: The location of *Rickettsia rickettsia* is in endothelial cells (see Figure 40–1), but Ehrlichia and Anaplasma are found circulating in the bloodstream (see Figure 40–7). Similarly, blood-smear microscopy may disclose diagnostic circulating monocytes (ehrlichiosis) or granulocytes (anaplasmosis) with inclusions (morulae), whereas these are not found with RMSF.

Bartonella

Bartonella species cause a variety of diseases, the best known of which are trench fever (*Bartonella quintana*) and CSD (*B henselae*). They are coccobacillary Gram-negative bacilli genomically most closely related to the genus *Brucella* (see Chapter 36). Contrary to other bacteria discussed in this chapter, *Bartonella* species can be cultured on artificial media. Pathogenically they employ a unique strategy that involves persistence in an intraerythrocytic niche in both the bloodsucking arthropods that transmit them and the animals they infect. The mammalian reservoirs vary with each species. Upon infection *Bartonella* species are unable to enter erythrocytes directly but must first mature in a primary site thought to be vascular endothelial cells. Following release from the primary site, they attach to RBCs, form pits, invade, and multiply inside. Pathologically, tumor-like angiogenic lesions filled with immature capillaries, swollen endothelium, and bacteria may be produced. This cycle of multiplication within two vascular cell types also shields *Bartonella* from both innate and adaptive immune responses.

B quintana causes **trench fever,** which has a worldwide distribution. The name derives from its prominence in the trenches of World War I. This disease has a reservoir in humans, and its vector is the body louse. Most cases are mild or subclinical. When symptomatic, the patient has sudden onset of chills, headache, relapsing fever, and a maculopapular rash on the trunk and abdomen. Illness can last for 4 to 5 days, can recur in repeated 4- to 5-day bouts, or can persist uninterruptedly for up to 6 weeks. The disease is suggested by a history of louse contact. More recently, *B quintana* bacteremia and endocarditis have been described in homeless alcoholic men in both France and the United States. The diagnosis can be made by culturing the organism on special agar medium or by demonstrating seroconversion.

Bartonella bacilliformis, the first discovered *Bartonella*, is the cause of Oroya fever, an acute hemolytic anemia and, in its chronic phase, verruga peruana which features nodular, highly vascular skin lesions. The link between the two was not known until a Peruvian medical student inoculated himself with blood from a verruga peruana lesion and tragically died from Oroya fever. Infections with this agent are seen only in South America at intermediate altitudes, in keeping with the distribution of its sandfly vector.

Another species, *B henselae*, has been associated with a number of diseases, the most common of which is CSD. CSD is a febrile lymphadenitis with systemic symptomatology that sometimes persists for weeks to months. Approximately 25,000 cases occur in the United States each year. The disease is transmitted by cat scratches or bites and perhaps by the bites of cat fleas. Manifestations may include skin rashes, conjunctivitis, encephalitis, and prolonged fever. Occasionally endocarditis and granulomatous or suppurative hepatosplenic and osseous lesions occur. In up to 10% of patients with CSD, ocular complications ensue of which the most dramatic is neuroretinitis with acute loss of vision. Its hallmark is the macular star (**Figure 40–8**). Fortunately, the

* Persist in vascular endothelium, RBCs

* Tumor-like vascular lesions filled with bacteria

* *B quintana* causes trench fever

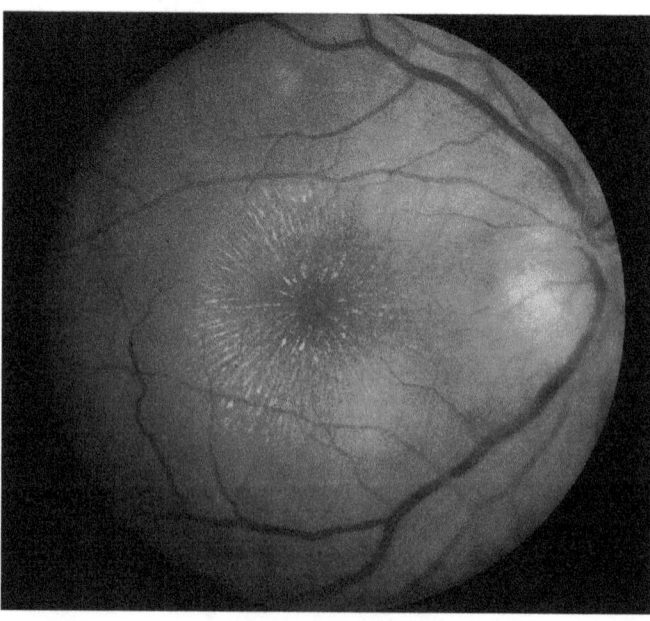

FIGURE 40–8. **Macular star in retina of eye.** Macular star associated with *Bartonella henselae* neuroretinis shows stellar macular exudation. (Used with permission from Steven R. Conlon, Sr. Photographer, Department of Pathology, Duke University, School of Medicine.)

blindness from the optic disk edema and retinal inflammation usually resolves over weeks to months with azithromycin therapy.

Bartonella henselae has been isolated directly from the blood of cats, although the latter do not appear ill. It can also be isolated from human blood, lymph nodes, and other materials using special media. Organisms can sometimes be directly demonstrated in infected tissues by using the Warthin-Starry silver impregnation stain. A serologic response to *B henselae* antigens is the primary method of diagnosis. Azithromycin may reduce the duration of lymph node enlargement and symptoms.

Bacillary angiomatosis, a proliferative disease of small blood vessels of the skin and viscera, seen in patients with AIDS and other immunocompromised hosts, has been linked with *Bartonella* by molecular methods used to amplify ribosomal RNA gene fragments directly from tissue samples. Subsequently, both *B henselae* and *B quintana* have been cultured from patients with bacillary angiomatosis. Other conditions seen primarily in patients with AIDS, such as hepatitis and bacteremia with fever, have also been associated with *B henselae. Bartonella* infections in AIDS and other immunosuppressed patients, as well as the bacteremia observed in alcoholic and homeless men, generally respond to prolonged courses of azithromycin or doxycycline. *Bartonella* endocarditis usually requires valve replacement as well.

* CSD common in children

* Persistent lymphadenitis

Neuroretinitis with transient blindness

Untreated AIDS with severe, protracted infections

KEY CONCLUSIONS

- *Rickettsia, Ehrlichia, Anaplasma,* and *Bartonella* are all small, Gram-negative bacilli that are arthropod-borne and dwell inside target cells on which they depend for survival.
- *Rickettsia* consists of two groups: SFG and TGR.
- SFG includes tick-borne *R rickettsii* (RMSF) and mite-borne *R akari* (rickettsialpox).
- TG includes louse-borne *R prowazekii* (epidemic typhus) and flea-borne *R typhi* (endemic or murine typhus).
- Geographical range of mite-borne *Orientia tsutsugamushi* (scrub typhus) is increasing.
- Both RMSF and typhus are characterized by fever, headache, myalgia, and rash.
- Rash of RMSF begins on extremities and spreads to the trunk, whereas in typhus the rash begins centrally and moves to the periphery.
- *Ehrlichia* targets monocytes (HME) and *Anaplasma* targets granulocytes (HGA); both are tick-borne.
- HME and HGA both present with fever, headache, and malaise and cause diminished WBCs and platelets: rash is infrequent.
- *Bartonella* species are louse-borne *B quintana* (trench fever), sandfly-transmitted *B bacilliformis* (Oroya fever), and *B henselae* (bacillary angiomatosis and cat-scratch disease). They are transmitted by scratches or bites of cats or their fleas.
- Doxycycline or azithromycin is effective for all the infections above and may be life saving.

CASE STUDY

Fever and Rash Following Tick Bite

A 6-year-old girl from North Carolina was in her usual state of good health until 10 days before admission, when she had a tick removed from her scalp. She developed a sore throat, malaise, and a low-grade fever 8 days after tick removal. She was seen by her pediatrician when she began developing a pink, macular rash, which started on her palms and lower extremities and spread to cover her entire body. The pediatrician's diagnosis was viral exanthem. One day before admission, she developed purpura, emesis, diarrhea, myalgias, and increased fever. On the day of admission, she was taken to her local hospital emergency room because of mental status changes. Her physical examination was significant for diffuse purpura; periorbital, hand, and foot edema; cool extremities with weak pulses; and hepatosplenomegaly. Her laboratory studies revealed: Na+ level of 125 mmol/L, platelet count 26,000/mm³, WBC count 14,900/mm³, hemoglobin level of 8.8 g/L, and greatly increased coagulation times. Ampicillin therapy was begun, and she was intubated but died soon after transfer to another institution.

QUESTIONS

1. What feature in this patient's history is most helpful?
   A. Sore throat
   B. Rash
   C. Tick bite
   D. Diarrhea
   E. Leukocytosis

2. To confirm a diagnosis of Rocky Mountain spotted fever, what would be the most useful laboratory test?
   A. Culture
   B. Gram stain
   C. Serology
   D. Darkfield examination

3. The primary cause of the fatal outcome in this patient is the tropism of *Rickettsia* for:
   A. Skin
   B. WBCs
   C. Enterocytes
   D. Muscle
   E. Blood vessels

ANSWERS

1. (C)

2. (C)

3. (E)

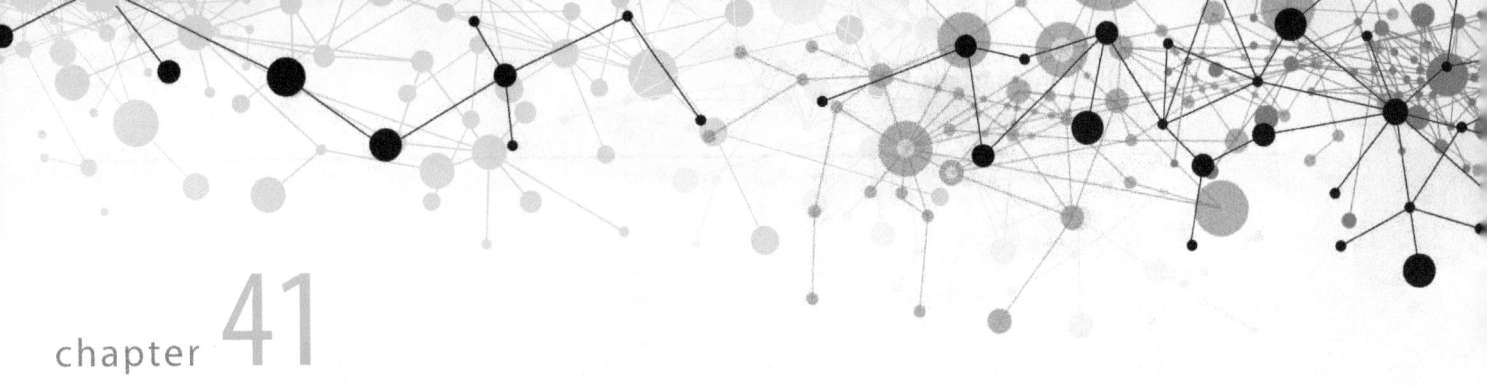

chapter 41

Dental and Periodontal Infections

Dental caries, periodontitis, and the tooth loss and other sequelae that follow are secondary to the microbial build-up on teeth called plaque. The prevention and/or halting of the progression of these diseases relies on the elimination of dental plaque from the tooth surfaces. In addition to causing caries and chronic periodontitis, the bacteria of dental plaque play a role in more aggressive forms of periodontitis and necrotizing periodontal diseases.

DENTAL PLAQUE

Dental plaque is an adherent dental deposit that forms on the tooth surface composed almost entirely of bacteria derived from the resident microbiota of the mouth. From a microbial pathogenesis standpoint, dental plaque is the most prevalent and densest of human biofilms (**Figure 41–1**). The biofilm first forms in relation to the dental pellicle, which is a physiologic thin organic film covering the mineralized tooth surface composed of proteins and glycoproteins derived from saliva and other oral secretions. As the plaque biofilm evolves, it does so in relation to the pellicle, not the mineralized tooth itself. The formation of plaque takes place in stages and layers at two levels. The first is the anatomic location of the plaque in relation to the gingival line. The earliest plaque is supragingival, which may then extend to subgingival plaque. The second level is the layering within the plaque, the bacterial species involved, and the bacteria/pellicle and bacteria/bacteria binding mechanisms required.

> Dental plaque is a bacterial biofilm
>
> Plaque forms in stages

The initial supragingival plaque primarily involves Gram-positive bacteria using specific ionic and hydrophobic interactions as well as lectin-like (carbohydrate binding) surface structures to adhere to the pellicle and to each other. The prototype early colonizer is *Streptococcus sanguis*, but other streptococci (*S mutans*, *S mitis*, *S salivarius*, *S oralis*, *S gordonii*), lactobacilli, and *Actinomyces* species are usually present. If the early colonizers are undisturbed, the late colonizers appear in the biofilm in as little as 2 to 4 days. These are primarily Gram-negative anaerobes including anaerobic spirochetes. These include *Fusobacterium*, *Porphyromonas*, *Prevotella*, *Veillonella*, *Treponema denticola*, and more *Actinomyces* species. These bacteria use similar mechanisms to bind to the early colonizers and to each other. This sets up a highly complex biofilm in which coaggregation involves structures that the bacteria brought with them (lectins), quorum sensing, and new metabolic activity. An example of the latter is the formation of extracellular glucan polymers, which act like a cement binding the plaque biofilm together. The biofilm also fastens nutrient and growth regulatory relationships between its members and provides a shield from the outside. In all, there are thought to be 300 to 400 bacterial species present in mature dental plaque. The structure of the involved bacteria is shown in Figure 41–1 and its gross and microscopic appearance in **Figure 41–2.**

> Attachment of bacteria to dental pellicle begins colonization
>
> Early and late colonizers differ
>
> Adhesion mechanisms create biofilm

Dental plaque would coat the tooth surfaces uniformly but for its physical removal during chewing and other oral activities. Characteristically, plaque remains in the non–self-cleansing areas of the teeth such as pits and fissures, along the margins of the gingiva, and between the teeth. For this reason, plaque-related diseases—caries, gingivitis, and periodontitis—occur most frequently and most severely at these locations. Subgingival plaque extends below the gum line to

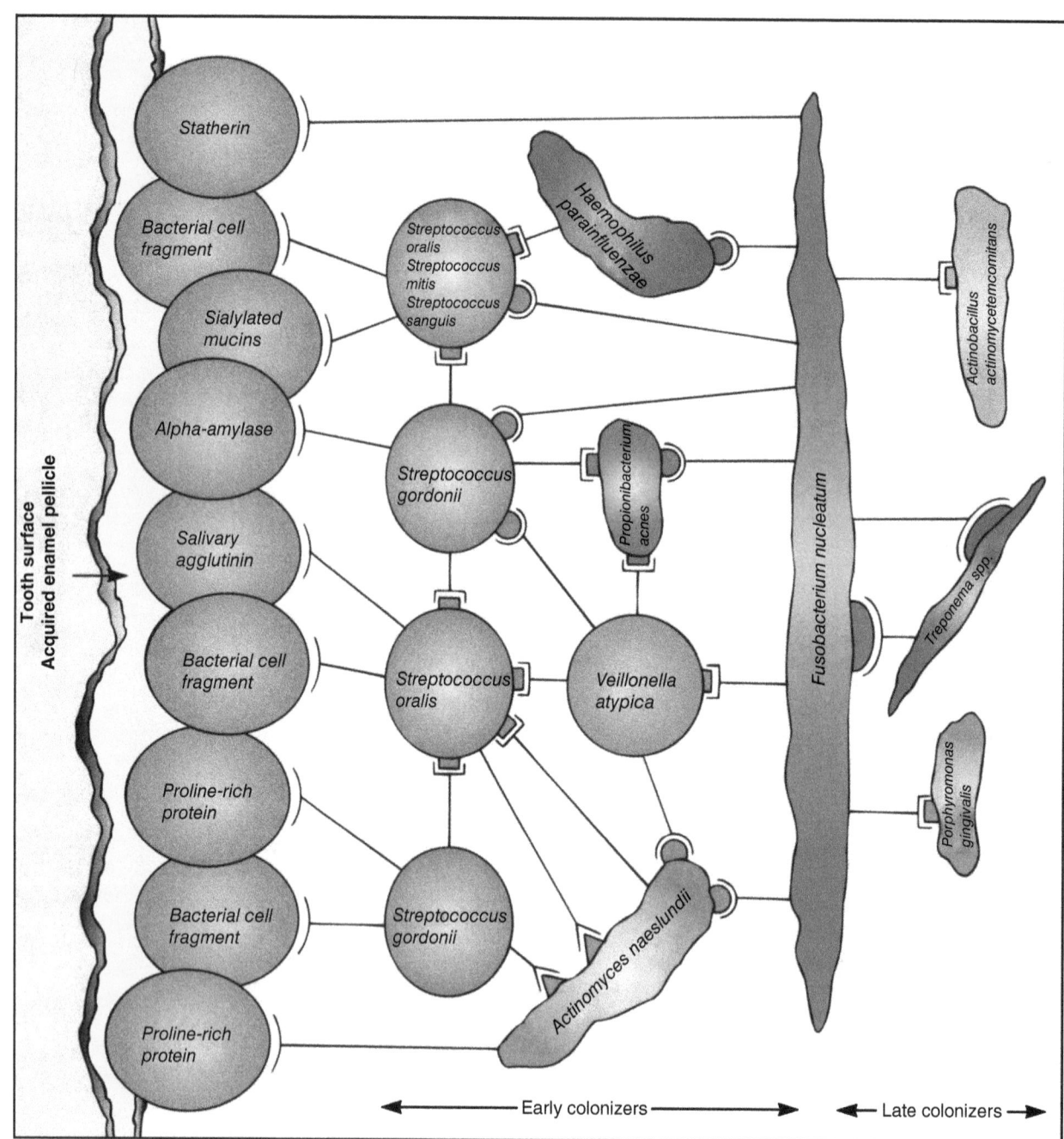

FIGURE 41–1. **Dental plaque biofilm.** The stages of formation of the bacterial biofilm called dental plaque are shown. Early colonizers bind to the enamel pellicle and late colonizers bind to the other bacteria. (Reproduced with permission from Willey J, Sherwood L, Woolverton C: *Prescott's Principles of Microbiology*. New York, NY: McGraw Hill; 2008.)

Plaque accumulates in non–self-cleansing areas

Subgingival plaque differs in bacterial composition

the sulcus around the tooth and periodontal pockets, which are pathologic extensions of the sulcus. This plaque has a thin adherent layer attached to the tooth surface and a nonadherent bacterial zone between that and the epithelial cells lining the sulcus. Supragingival plaque lacks such a distinct nonadherent zone. The bacterial composition of subgingival plaque is shifted toward the Gram-negative anaerobic bacteria and spirochetes. In addition to the late colonizers cited above, it may also include members of the *Campylobacter*, *Capnocytophagia*, and *Eikenella* genera.

Because the causative organisms of both dental caries and chronic periodontitis are believed to be in the dental plaque, a prime method for maintaining oral health is regular home care practices for plaque removal. Dental plaque cannot be effectively removed from the teeth solely by chemical or enzymatic means, and the use of antibiotics for prophylactic inhibition of plaque formation cannot be clinically justified, although patients undergoing long-term antibiotic treatment for other medical reasons demonstrate a lower incidence of caries and periodontal disease.

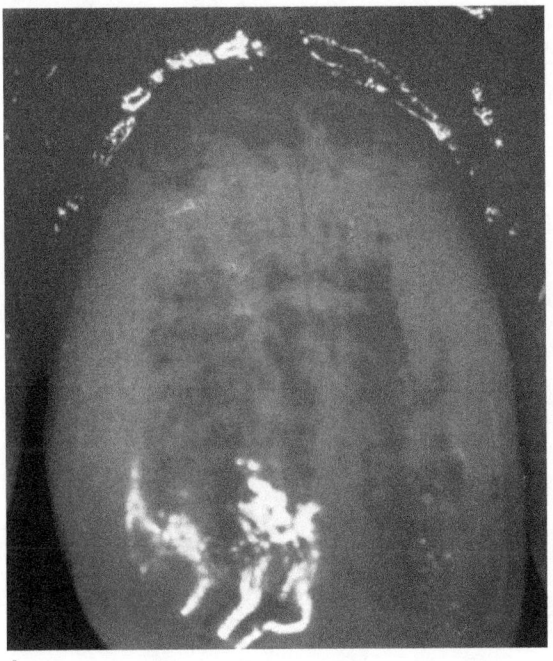
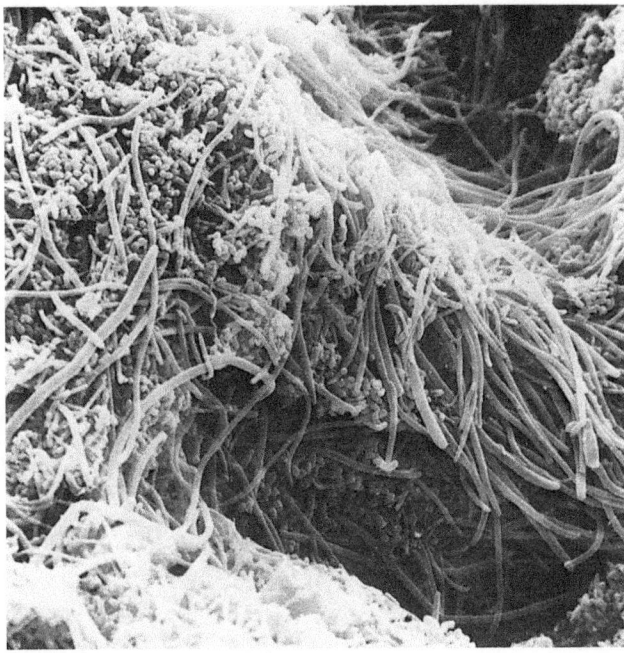

A   B

FIGURE 41-2. **Dental plaque. A.** Disclosing tablets containing vegetable dye stain heavy plaque accumulation at the junction of the tooth and gingiva. (Reproduced with permission from Willey JM: *Prescott, Harley, & Klein's Microbiology*, 7th ed. New York, NY: McGraw Hill; 2008.)

Antiseptic substances that bind to tooth surfaces and inhibit plaque formation, such as the bis-biguanides, chlorhexidine, and alexidine, have been shown to be effective in reducing plaque, caries, and gingival inflammation. A commercial preparation containing 0.12% chlorhexidine can be used in controlling dental plaque and associated disease. Toothpaste and mouth rinse additives such as phenolic compounds, essential oils, triclosan, fluorides, herbal extracts, and quaternary ammonium compounds have been shown to have some plaque-reducing ability as well. The use of these substances must be accompanied by proper tooth brushing, flossing, and periodic professional cleaning to ensure effective disease prevention.

Removal of plaque prime element of oral hygiene

Chemicals may be used along with brushing and flossing

DENTAL CARIES

Dental caries are the result of progressive destruction of the mineralized tissues of the tooth. This is primarily caused by the acid products of glycolytic metabolic activity when the plaque bacteria are fed the right substrate. The basic characteristic of the carious lesion is that it progresses inward from the tooth surface, either the enamel-coated crown or the cementum of the exposed root surface, involving the dentin and finally the pulp of the tooth (**Figures 41-3** and **41-4**). From there, infection can extend into the periodontal tissues at the root apex or apices.

Caries produced by plaque bacteria

The microbial basis of dental caries has been long established based on work first with *Lactobacillus acidophilus* and then *S mutans*. Although *S mutans* is now regarded as the dominant organism for the initiation of caries, multiple members of the plaque biofilm participate in the evolution of the lesions. These include other streptococci (*S salivarius, S sanguis, S sobrinus*), lactobacilli (*L acidophilus, L casei*), and actinomycetes (*A viscosus* and *A naeslundii*). The acid products produced by the interaction of *S mutans* with multiple species in the biofilm are the underlying cause of dental caries.

Members of biofilm produce acid

S mutans is most cariogenic

Dietary monosaccharides and disaccharides such as glucose, fructose, sucrose, lactose, and maltose provide an appropriate substrate for bacterial glycolysis and acid production to cause tooth demineralization. A possible edge for *S mutans* is its ability to metabolize sucrose more efficiently than other oral bacteria. It also has regulatory systems which stimulate the conversion of dietary carbohydrates to acid and intracellular storage polymers. Ingested carbohydrates permeating the dental plaque are absorbed by the bacteria, and are metabolized so rapidly that organic acid products accumulate and cause the pH of the plaque to drop to levels sufficient to react with the hydroxyapatite of the enamel, demineralizing it to soluble calcium and phosphate ions. Production of acid and the decreased pH are maintained until the substrate supply is

Demineralization is by acid production from dietary carbohydrate

FIGURE 41–3. **Cariogenesis.** A microscopic view of pellicle and plaque formation, acidification, and destruction of tooth enamel. (Reproduced with permission from Willey JM: *Prescott, Harley, & Klein's Microbiology*, 7th ed. New York, NY: McGraw Hill; 2008.)

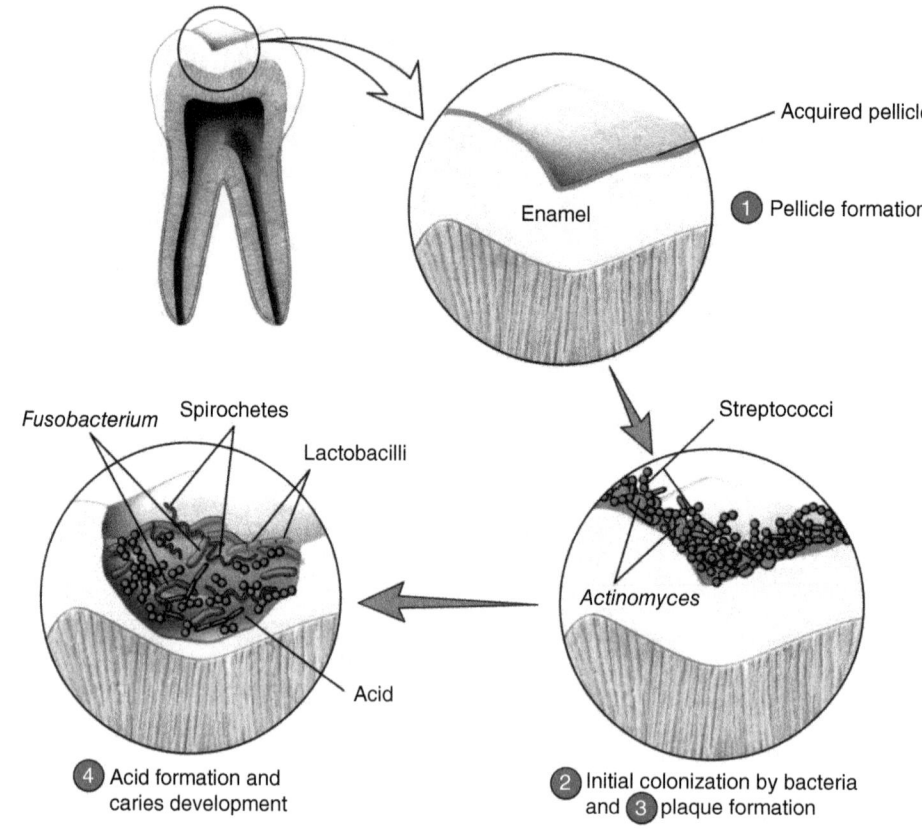

FIGURE 41–4. **Hemisected human tooth showing an advanced carious lesion on the right side of the crown and a much smaller lesion on the left side.** Note the progression of the lesion through the enamel and dentin, pointing toward the pulp chamber in the center of the tooth.

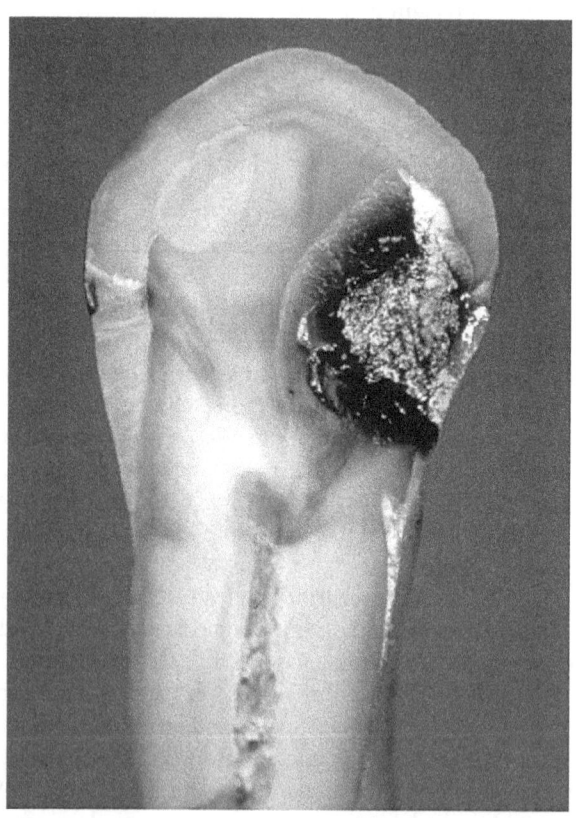

exhausted. Upon exhaustion of the immediate source *S mutans* is able to survive long periods of sugar starvation. Obviously, foods with high sugar content, particularly sucrose, which adhere to the teeth and have long oral clearance times are more cariogenic than less retentive foodstuffs such as sugar-containing liquids. Once the substrate is exhausted, the plaque pH returns slowly to its more neutral pH resting level and some recovery can take place. This sets up a demineralization–remineralization cycle, which depends on carbohydrate refueling from the diet. With repeated snacking between meals, the plaque pH may never return to normal and demineralization dominates.

An additional factor with sucrose is that it is also used in the synthesis of extracellular polyglycans such as dextrans and levans by transferase enzymes on the bacterial cell surfaces. This polyglycan production by *S mutans* contributes to aggregation and accumulation of the organism on the tooth surface. Extracellular polyglycan may also increase cariogenicity by serving as an extracellular storage form of substrate. Certain microorganisms synthesize extracellular polyglycan when sucrose is available but then break it down into monosaccharide units to be used for glycolysis when dietary carbohydrate is exhausted. Some oral bacteria also use dietary monosaccharides and disaccharides internally to form glycogen, which is stored intracellularly and used for glycolysis after the dietary substrate has been exhausted; thus, the period of acidogenesis is again prolonged and the cariogenicity of the microorganism increased. These microorganisms can prolong acidogenesis beyond the oral clearance time of the substrate.

The most common complications of dental caries are extension of the infection into the pulp chamber of the tooth (pulpitis), necrosis of the pulp, and extension of the infection through the root canals into the periapical area of the periodontal ligament. Periapical involvement may take the form of an acute inflammation (periapical abscess), a chronic nonsuppurating inflammation (periapical granuloma), or a chronic suppurating lesion that may drain into the mouth or onto the face via a sinus tract. A cyst may form within the chronic nonsuppurating lesion as a result of inflammatory stimulation of the epithelial rests normally found in the periodontal ligament. If the infectious agent is sufficiently virulent or host resistance is low, the infection may spread into the alveolar bone (osteomyelitis) or the fascial planes of the head and neck (cellulitis). Alternatively, it may ascend along the venous channels to cause septic thrombophlebitis. Because most carious lesions represent a mixed infection by the time cavities have developed, it is not surprising that most oral infections resulting from the extension of carious lesions are mixed and frequently include anaerobic organisms.

Dental caries is the single greatest cause of tooth loss in the child and young adult. Its onset can occur very soon after the eruption of the teeth. The first carious lesions usually develop in pits or fissures on the chewing surfaces of the deciduous molars and result from the metabolic activity of the dental plaque that forms in these sites. Later in childhood, the incidence of carious lesions on smooth surfaces increases; these lesions are usually found between the teeth. The factors involved in the formation of a carious lesion are (1) a susceptible host or tooth, (2) the proper microflora on the tooth, and (3) a substrate from which the plaque bacteria can produce the organic acids that result in tooth demineralization.

The newly erupted tooth is most susceptible to the carious process. It gains protection against this disease during the first year or so by a process of posteruptive maturation believed to be attributable to improvement in the quality of surface mineral on the tooth. Saliva provides protection against caries, and patients with dry mouth (xerostomia) suffer from high caries attack rates unless suitable measures are taken. In addition to the mechanical flushing and diluting action of saliva and its buffering capacity, the salivary glands also secrete several antibacterial products. Thus, saliva is known to contain lysozyme, a thiocyanate-dependent sialoperoxidase, and immunoglobulins, principally those of the secretory IgA class. The individual importance of these antibacterial factors is unknown, but they clearly play some role in determining the ecology of the oral microbiota.

Proper levels of fluoride, either systemically or topically administered, result in dramatic decreases in the incidence of caries (50-60% reduction by water fluoridation, 35-40% reduction by topical application). In the case of systemic fluoridation, the protective effect is thought to result from the incorporation of fluoride ions in place of hydroxyl ions of the hydroxyapatite during tooth formation, producing a more perfect and acid-resistant mineral phase of tooth structure. Topical application of fluoride is believed to achieve the same result on the surface of the tooth by initial dissolution of some of the hydroxyapatite, followed by recrystallization of apatite,

Acid production facilitated by sticky carbohydrates

Demineralization–remineralization related to snacking

Polyglycans from sucrose important in adherence, carbohydrate storage

Acidogenesis prolonged by intracellular glycogen stores

Extension to pulp and periapical locations complicate infections

Severe complications spread to bone or local fascia

Greatest cause of tooth loss in children and young adults

Require microflora and suitable substrates for organic acid production

Saliva protects by mechanical flushing and multiple chemical actions

which incorporates fluoride ions into its lattice structure. Another important mode of action, namely, the inhibition of demineralization, and the promotion of remineralization of incipient carious lesions by fluoride ions in the oral fluid, has more recently been proposed as an important anticaries mechanism of fluoride, perhaps more important than the other proposed mechanisms. In any event, fluoridation represents the most effective means known for rendering the tooth more resistant to the carious process.

CHRONIC PERIODONTITIS

Plaque-induced periodontal disease encompasses two separate disease entities: gingivitis and chronic periodontitis. These diseases are believed to be related, in that gingivitis, although a reversible condition, is thought to be an early stage leading ultimately to chronic periodontitis in the susceptible subject. The term **gingivitis** is used when the inflammatory condition is limited to the marginal gingiva and bone resorption around the necks of teeth has not yet begun. Gingivitis develops within 2 weeks in individuals who fail to practice effective tooth cleansing. **Chronic periodontitis** is used to describe the stage of chronic periodontal disease in which there is progressive loss of tooth support owing to resorption of the alveolar bone and periodontal ligament. Periodontitis can also lead to periodontal abscess when the chronic inflammatory state around the necks of the teeth becomes acute at a specific location.

Both gingivitis and chronic periodontitis are caused by bacteria in the dental plaque that lie in close proximity to the necks of the teeth and marginal gingival tissues. Thus, subgingival plaque found within the gingival crevice or the sulcus around the necks of the teeth is thought to house the etiologic agent(s). The characteristic histopathologic picture of gingivitis is of a marked inflammatory infiltrate of polymorphonuclear leukocytes, lymphocytes, and plasma cells in the connective tissue that lies immediately adjacent to the epithelium lining the gingival crevice and attached to the tooth. Collagen is lost from the inflamed connective tissue. There does not seem to be any direct invasion of the gingival tissues by large numbers of intact bacteria, at least in the early stages of the disease.

All forms of periodontitis are polymicrobial infections primarily involving anaerobic bacteria in much the same way described for other anaerobes in Chapter 29. The agents involved are derived from the predominantly Gram-negative anaerobic flora of the subgingival plaque (see previous text) led by *Aggregatibacter actinomycetemcomitans*, *Porphyromonas gingivalis*, and *Treponema denticola*. Just as bacteria–bacteria interactions determine the plaque, cross-feeding and growth stimulation have been observed between these two organisms when grown together. This kind of synergism between *P gingivalis*, *T denticola*, and other plaque members is felt to foster progression of gingivitis to chronic periodontitis. Some of these organisms have also been shown to produce virulence factors similar to those associated with other invasive bacterial pathogens. *T denticola* is able to bind serum factors that interfere with complement deposition, and *P gingivalis* is a potent producer of extracellular proteases. The former facilitates survival in tissues and the latter injury to those tissues. Recent studies indicate bacterial interactions with Toll-like receptors (TLRs) may trigger these inflammatory responses.

Chronic periodontitis is responsible for most tooth loss in people older than 35 to 40 years. The disease progresses slowly and results in the progressive destruction of the supporting tissues of the tooth (periodontal ligament and alveolar bone) from the margins of the gingiva toward the apices of the roots of the teeth. Progression may occur as a series of acute episodes separated by quiescent periods of indeterminate duration. More aggressive forms of periodontitis result in more rapid loss of tooth support. Aggressive types of disease called localized aggressive periodontitis occur in adolescents, and generalized aggressive periodontitis occurs in young adults. There is some evidence that the causative agents may differ in this form of periodontitis. A small capnophilic (carbon dioxide-requiring) Gram-negative rod (*Actinobacillus actinomycetemcomitans*) has been indicted based on studies of the flora of disease sites. A virulence factor found in those strains of *A actinomycetemcomitans* that are associated with this disease is the production of a leukotoxin by the bacteria.

As the disease progresses, a point may be reached at which the alveolar bone around the necks of the teeth is resorbed; the condition is then no longer termed gingivitis but periodontitis. With resorption of the bone, the attachment of the periodontal ligament is lost and the gingival sulcus deepens into a periodontal pocket. Periodontitis is not considered to be a reversible disease in that the lost alveolar bone and periodontal ligament do not regenerate with cessation of the

Fluoride produces more acid-resistant mineral phase of tooth

Causes destruction of supporting tissues

Subgingival plaque causes collagen loss

Polymicrobial anaerobic infection from subgingival plaque

Synergistic interactions facilitate growth

Virulence factors cause disease

Chronic periodontitis causes tooth loss

Acute juvenile periodontitis associated with *Actinobacillus*

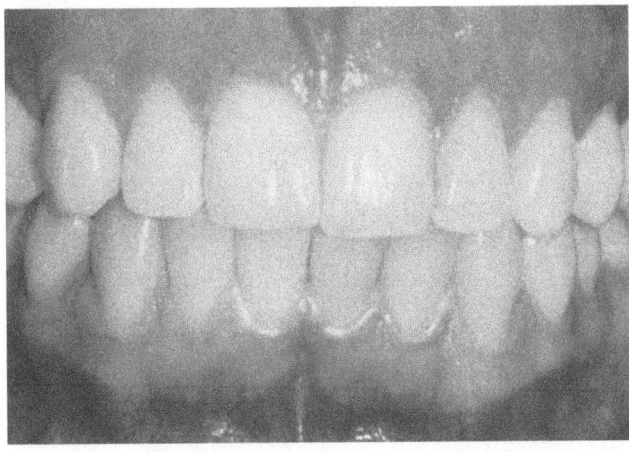
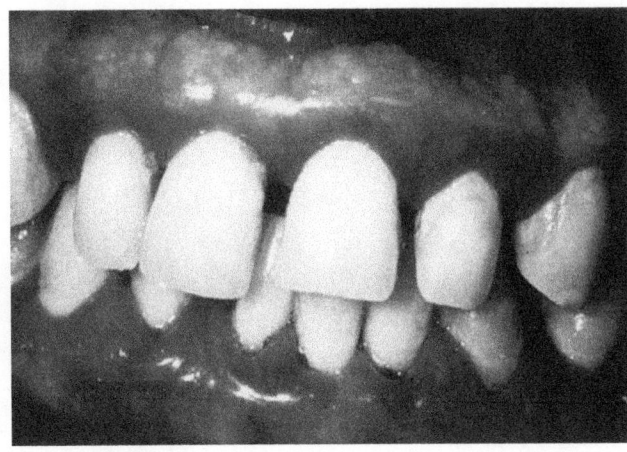

A   B

FIGURE 41–5. **Periodontitis. A.** Normal gingival. **B.** Periodontal disease, with plaque, inflammatory changes, bleeding, and shortening of the gingival between the teeth. (Reproduced with permission from Nester EW, Anderson DG, Roberts CE Jr, et al: *Microbiology: A Human Perspective*, 6th ed. New York, NY: McGraw Hill; 2008.)

inflammation, even though further progression may be halted. If unchecked, bone resorption progresses to loosening of the tooth, which may ultimately be exfoliated. **Figure 41–5** shows a case of advanced chronic periodontitis. Occasionally, the neck of a periodontal pocket becomes constricted, the bacteria proliferate causing an acute inflammatory response in the occluded pocket, and a periodontal abscess results. This acute exacerbation requires drainage in the same way as abscesses elsewhere for the patient to obtain symptomatic relief.

With continued progress, periodontitis and bone resorption develop

Periodontal abscess may result

NECROTIZING PERIODONTAL DISEASES

Necrotizing ulcerative gingivitis (also called acute necrotizing ulcerative gingivitis, Vincent infection, or trench mouth) and necrotizing ulcerative periodontitis represent a spectrum of acute inflammatory disease starting with destruction limited to the soft tissues (gingivitis) and extending to destruction of the alveolar bone and periodontal ligament (periodontitis). This disease spectrum is distinctly different from gingivitis–chronic periodontitis. It has an acute onset, frequently associated with periods of stress and poor oral hygiene. Rapid ulceration of the interdental areas of the gingiva results in destruction of the interdental papillae. The inflammatory condition initially confined to the gingival tissues can quickly extend into pathologic bone resorption. Unlike gingivitis and chronic periodontitis, acute necrotizing periodontal disease is painful. As the oral epithelium is destroyed, the causative bacteria come into direct contact with the underlying tissues and may invade them. Spirochetes and fusiform bacteria have been implicated; thus, the term **fusospirochetal disease** has been used to describe this infection, which can also be manifested as ulceration in other areas of the pharynx or oral cavity. *Prevotella intermedia* has also been found in high numbers in the lesions. Morphologic studies have shown that the spirochetes actually appear to invade the tissues. The disease may be treated with systemic antibiotics and topical antimicrobials for immediate relief of symptoms, but resolution depends on thorough professional cleaning of the teeth and institution of good home care.

Acute onset with painful ulcerative lesions

Fusospirochetal etiology together with other anaerobes

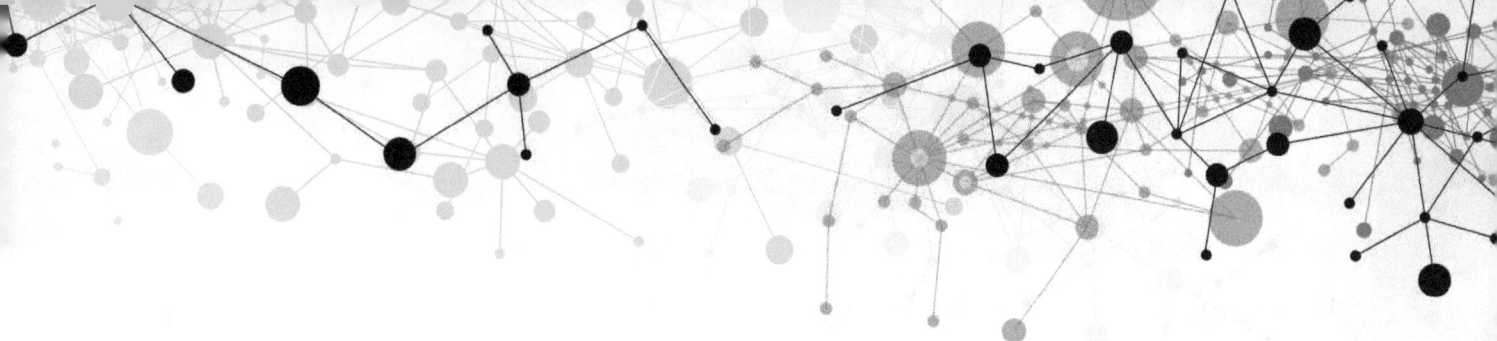

PART IV
Pathogenic Fungi

J. Andrew Alspaugh · Julie M. Steinbrink

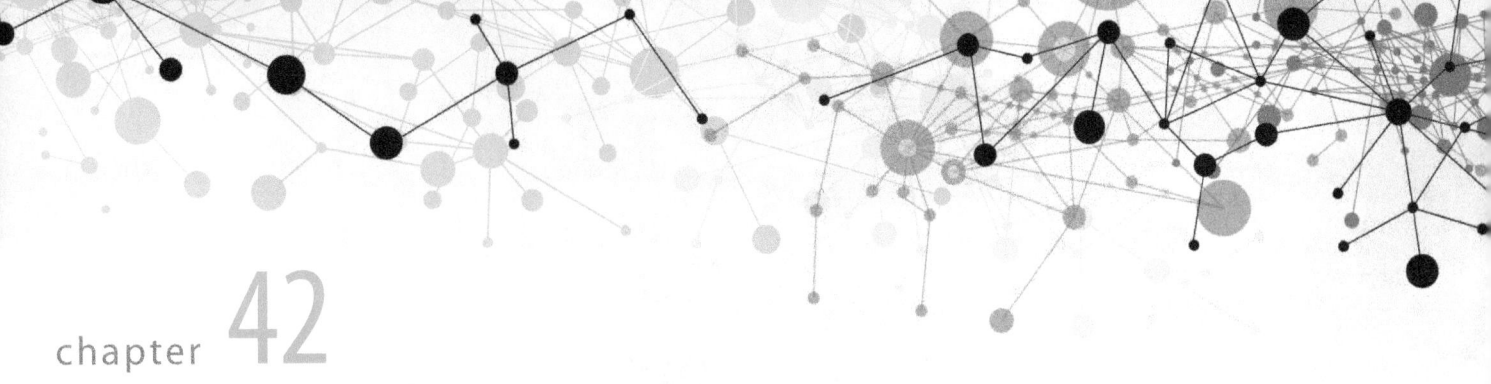

chapter 42

Fungi—Basic Concepts

OVERVIEW

The fungal kingdom encompasses a diverse and rich group of organisms ranging from microscopic yeasts to mushrooms. Most fungi are free-living in nature where they function as decomposers in the energy cycle. Of the more than 90,000 known fungal species, fewer than 200 have been reported to produce disease in humans. Once considered clinical rarities, human fungal infections are becoming increasingly common, especially among immunocompromised patients. Therefore, it is important to understand the unique clinical and microbiological features of these diseases.

CLINICAL CONTEXT

A "yeast" is identified growing from a patient's blood culture.

1. What are fungi, and do they commonly cause important human diseases?
2. How does the lab technologist identify the species of this fungus?
3. How does the clinician know if this microorganism is relevant to the care of the patient?

● MYCOLOGY

Fungi are eukaryotes with a higher level of biologic complexity than bacteria. Fungi may be unicellular or may differentiate and become multicellular by the development of long, branching filaments. They lack the chlorophyll of plants and therefore need to acquire nutrients from the external environment. The diseases caused by fungi are called mycoses. These infections vary greatly in their manifestations but tend to present with subacute or chronic features, often relapsing over time. Acute disease, such as that produced by many viruses and bacteria, is less common with fungal infections.

✳ Fungal cell organization is eukaryotic

STRUCTURE

The fungal cell has many typical eukaryotic features, including a nucleus with a nucleolus, nuclear membrane, and linear chromosomes (**Figure 42–1**). The cytoplasm contains a cytoskeleton with actin microfilaments and tubulin-containing microtubules. Ribosomes and organelles, such as mitochondria, endoplasmic reticulum, and the Golgi apparatus, are also present. Fungal cells have a rigid cell wall external to the cytoplasmic membrane, which differentiates them from mammalian cells. In addition to the cell wall, another important difference from mammalian cells is the sterol composition of the cytoplasmic membrane. In mammalian cells, the dominant membrane sterol is cholesterol; in fungi, it is ergosterol. Fungi are usually haploid in their DNA content, although diploid nuclei are formed through nuclear fusion in the process of sexual reproduction. Interestingly, the generation of polyploid/aneuploid nuclei is a strategy used by some fungi to generate genetic diversity as a response to cell stress, such as antifungal therapy.

Presence of a nucleus, mitochondria, and endoplasmic reticulum

✳ Fungal cell wall distinguishes from mammalian cells

✳ Ergosterol, not cholesterol, makes up cell membrane

The chemical structure of the cell wall in fungi is markedly different from that of bacterial cells in that it does not contain peptidoglycan, glycerol, teichoic acids, or lipopolysaccharide. In their place are complex polysaccharides such as **mannans, glucans,** and **chitins** in close association with each other and with structural proteins (**Figure 42–2**). Mannoproteins are composed of mannose-based polymers (mannan) linked to various proteins embedded in the external structural matrix of the cell wall. Mannoproteins are very important since antibodies are readily

FIGURE 42-1. **A yeast cell showing the cell wall and internal structures of the fungal eukaryotic cell plan.** (Reproduced with permission from Willey JM: *Prescott, Harley, & Klein's Microbiology,* 7th ed. New York, NY: McGraw Hill; 2008.)

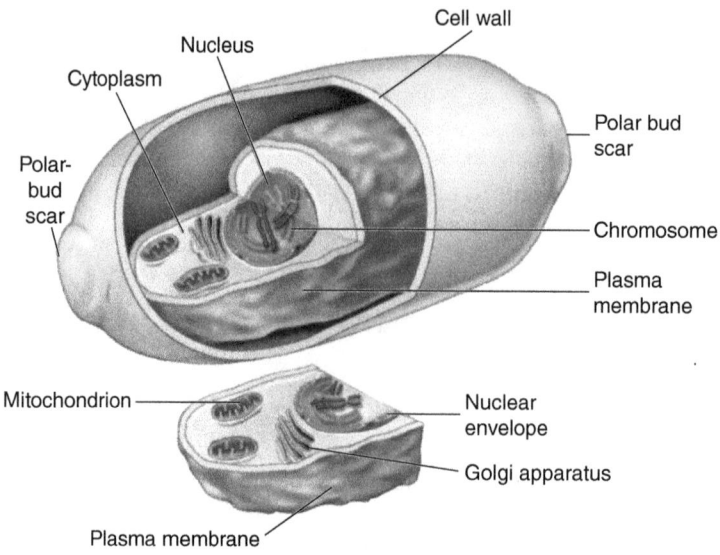

Cell wall mannan linked to surface proteins

Chitin and glucans give rigidity to cell wall

developed against these molecules on the cell surface. The potential variations in the composition and linkages of the mannan side chains allow fungi to generate a complex and adaptable cell surface to avoid easy immune detection by an infected host. The identification of different antibodies directed against specific mannoproteins also allows laboratories to "serologically" distinguish between individual strains within a fungal species. The alpha- and beta-glucans are polymers of glucose found abundantly throughout the cell wall. Additionally, chitin, composed of long chains of *N*-acetylglucosamine, provides rigid structural support to the fungal cell in a manner analogous to the chitin in crab shells or cellulose in plants. In addition to their structural roles, these cell wall carbohydrates serve complex cell functions, often simultaneously activating and inhibiting various arms of the host immune response.

FIGURE 42-2. **The fungal cell wall.** The overlapping mannan, glucan, chitin, and protein elements are shown. Proteins complexed with the mannan (mannoproteins) extend beyond the cell wall.

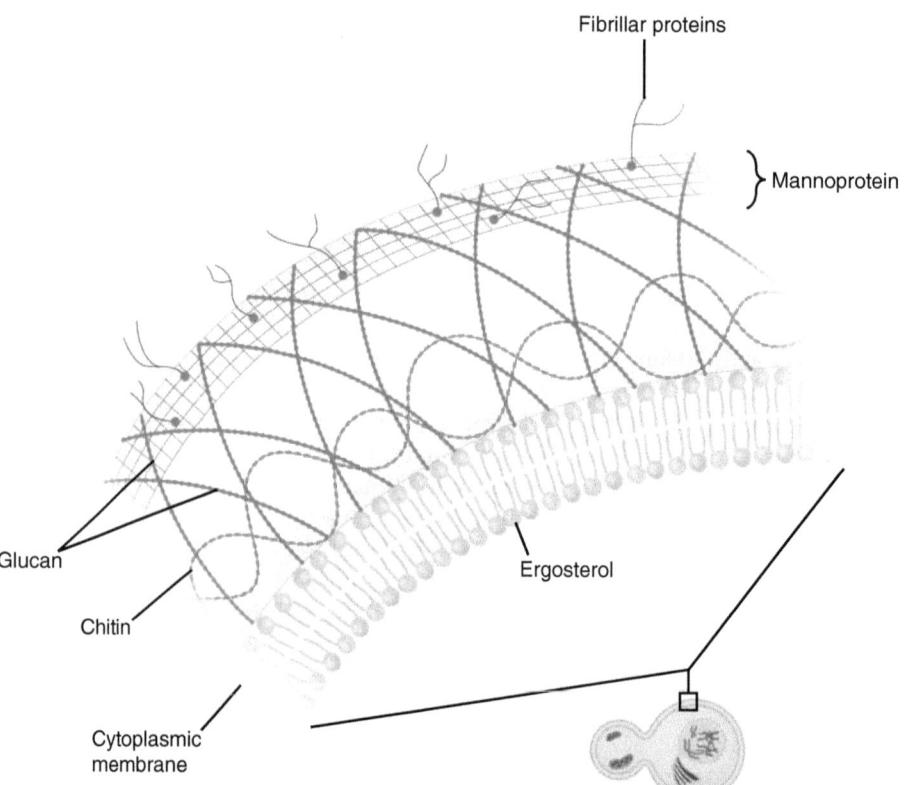

METABOLISM

In contrast to plants, fungi lack chloroplasts and photosynthetic energy-producing mechanisms. Therefore, fungi must acquire nutrients from exogenous sources. Metabolic diversity among fungi is great, but most are able to grow with very simple carbon and nitrogen sources. In nature, nutrients for free-living fungi are derived from decaying organic matter. Most fungi are strict aerobes, although some can grow under anaerobic conditions.

Heterotrophic metabolism uses available organic matter

● FUNGAL MORPHOLOGY AND GROWTH

The size of fungi varies immensely. A single cell without transverse septa may range from bacterial size (2-4 μm) to a macroscopically visible structure. The morphologic forms of growth vary from colonies superficially resembling those of bacteria to some of the most complex, multicellular, colorful, and beautiful structures seen in nature. Mushrooms are an example of the potential higher structural differentiation among fungi.

Vary in size from single cells to multicellular mushrooms

Mycology, the science devoted to the study of fungi, has various terms to describe the morphologic components that comprise these structures. The terms and concepts that must be mastered can be limited by considering only the fungi of medical importance and accepting some simplification.

YEASTS AND MOLDS

Fungi that cause human infections can be broadly divided based on their morphological forms. **Yeasts** are fungi that primarily grow in a round cellular form. **Molds** are fungi that primarily grow as filamentous, tube-like structures called hyphae (**Figure 42–3A and B**). Although it is useful to consider this basic distinction based on cell shape, it is important to remember that some fungi can transition between yeast-like and hyphal morphologies. Often, this plasticity of shape is directly related to pathogenesis since different forms may be better suited for different microenvironments. The yeasts tend to have the simplest cellular forms, reproducing by a process of asexual budding, constriction, and cell separation similar to many bacteria.

Fungal forms include *yeasts* (single cells) and *molds* (elongated, filamentous hyphae)

Fungi may also grow through the development of **hyphae** (singular, hypha), which are tube-like extensions of the cell with thick, parallel walls. As the hyphae extend, they form an intertwined mass called a **mycelium**. Most molds form hyphal **septa** (singular, septum), which are cross-walls perpendicular to the cell walls, dividing the hypha into subunit cells (**Figure 42–4**). The structure of these septa varies among species and may contain pores and incomplete walls that allow movement of nutrients, organelles, and nuclei between adjacent cells. Some species,

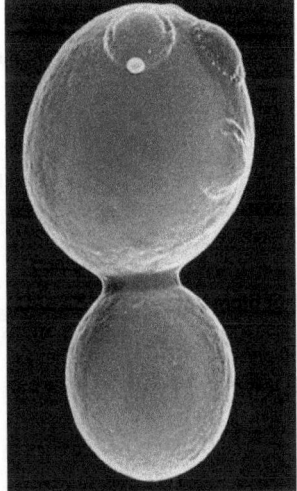

A *Saccharomyces cerevisiae:* budding division

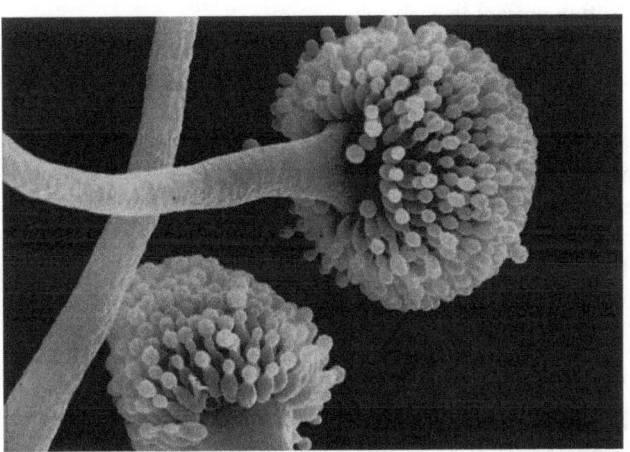

B

FIGURE 42–3. Yeast and mold forms of fungal growth. A. This oval yeast cell is budding to form a daughter cell. Scars from prior cell separations can be seen on other parts of the cell. **B.** The mold form is highly variable. Here tubular stalks called conidiophores arising from hyphae (not seen) bear a "Medusa head" crop of reproductive conidia. (Reproduced with permission from Willey JM: *Prescott, Harley, & Klein's Microbiology*, 7th ed. New York, NY: McGraw Hill; 2008.)

FIGURE 42–4. **Hyphae. A.** Nonseptate hyphae with multiple nuclei. **B.** Septate hyphae divide nuclei into separate cells. **C.** Electron micrograph of septum with a single pore. **D.** Multipore septum structure within fungal hyphae. (Reproduced with permission from Willey JM: *Prescott, Harley, & Klein's Microbiology*, 7th ed. New York, NY: McGraw Hill; 2008.)

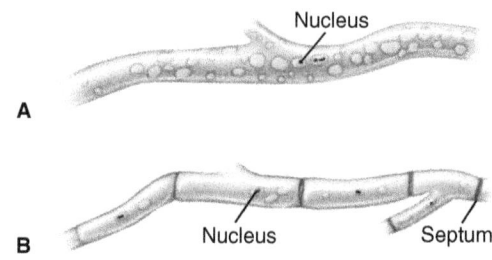

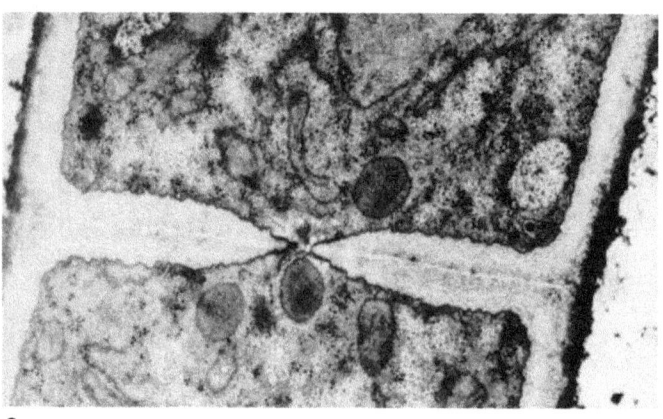

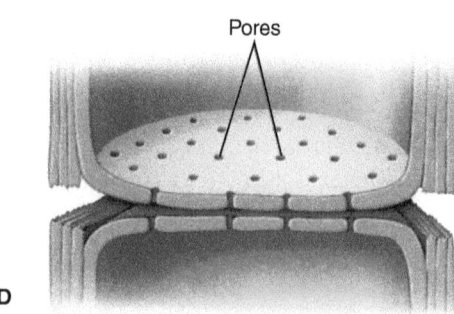

including some human pathogens, form septae that are very distant from each other. Because their microscopic appearance, therefore, suggests a single, continuous hyphal cell, these particular species are often called "aseptate" molds. In both septate and aseptate hyphae, multiple nuclei are often present in each cell.

A portion of the mycelium (vegetative mycelium) usually grows into the medium or organic substrate (eg, soil) and functions like the roots of plants as a collector of nutrients and moisture. The more visible surface growth may assume a fluffy character as the mycelium becomes aerial. The hyphal walls are rigid in order to support this extensive, intertwining network. Different molds often have unique sexual and asexual structures associated with their hyphae (**Figure 42–5A-D**). These sexual structures are often unique to each species, allowing microbiology laboratories to distinguish among molds based on their morphological features. Some fungi also form **pseudohyphae,** which are actually elongated yeast cells growing end-to-end. Therefore, pseudohyphae are distinguished from true hyphae by having recurring bud-like constrictions and less rigid cell walls.

✳ Molds produce septate or aseptate hyphae

Aerial mycelium bears reproductive conidia or spores—the basis for species identification

✳ Pseudohyphae are elongated yeast-like cells

DIMORPHISM

Although many fungi tend to grow as either yeasts or molds, some species can transition between morphological forms depending on environmental conditions. These species are known as **dimorphic fungi.** Many fungi, including the most common human fungal pathogen *Candida albicans*, display a striking ability to modify their cellular shape and structure in order to adapt to new environments. These morphological transitions are often very important for the pathogenesis of human infections.

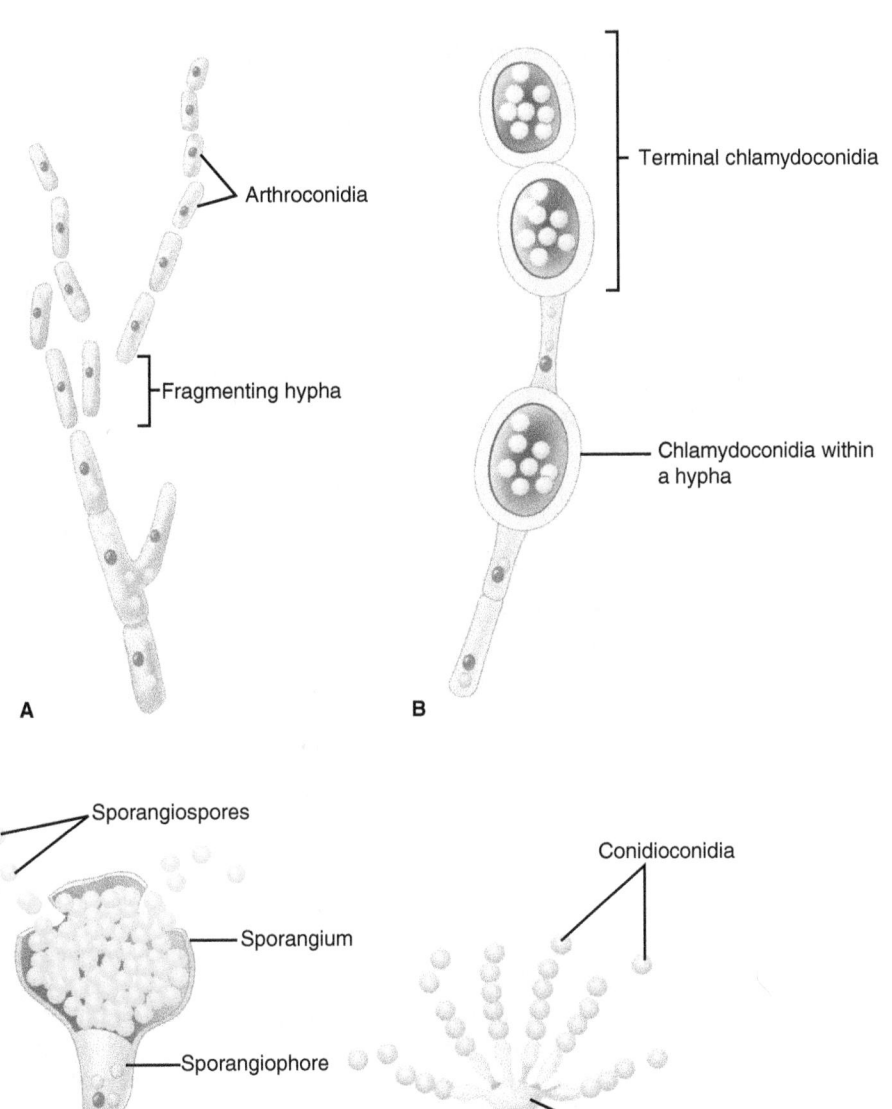

FIGURE 42-5. **Asexual mold forms. A.** Arthroconidia develop within the hyphae and eventually break off. **B.** Chlamydoconidia are larger than the hyphae and develop with the cell or terminally. **C.** Sporangioconidia are borne terminally in a sporangium sac. **D.** Simple conidia arise directly from a conidiophore. (Reproduced with permission from Willey JM: *Prescott, Harley, & Klein's Microbiology*, 7th ed. New York, NY: McGraw Hill; 2008.)

A distinct group of human pathogens are the **thermally dimorphic fungi**, shifting from yeast-like to hyphal growth based on temperature. These fungal species tend to grow in the mold form in their environmental reservoir as well as when incubated in culture at ambient temperatures. However, they convert to a yeast-like growth form in the mammalian host or when incubated in culture at 37°C. Importantly, the conidia produced in the mold phase may be infectious and serve to disseminate the fungus during growth in the environment.

Fungal dimorphism in fungi is reversible, a feature that distinguishes it from developmental processes such as embryogenesis seen in higher eukaryotes. The importance of the dimorphism in fungal virulence has been demonstrated in several fungi, including *C albicans* and *Histoplasma capsulatum*. Strains that are locked in one growth phase are often markedly reduced in their ability to produce disease and persist in the host.

Dimorphism: growth of a fungus in either a yeast or mold form

In thermally dimorphic fungi, temperature triggers a shift between phases

Dimorphism reversible, linked to virulence

CLASSIFICATION

Fungal classification has historically relied upon observable cellular characteristics such as the septation of hyphae and the appearance of the sexual structures. However, nucleic acid sequence-based and protein-based classification methods are becoming more common, allowing fungi to be grouped by genetic and biochemical relatedness. Molecular classification techniques have also

TABLE 42–1	Classification of medically important fungi		
GENUS	**TYPICAL GROWTH**	**SEPTATION**[a]	**PHYLUM**
Superficial Fungi			
Epidermophyton	Mold	+	Ascomycota
Microsporum	Mold	+	Ascomycota
Trichophyton	Mold	+	Ascomycota
Subcutaneous Fungi			
Sporothrix	Dimorphic	+	Ascomycota
Opportunistic Fungi			
Aspergillus	Mold	+	Ascomycota
Candida	Dimorphic	+	Ascomycota
Mucor	Mold	–	Zygomycota
Rhizopus	Mold	–	Zygomycota
Pneumocystis	Cysts[b]		Ascomycota
Systemic Fungi			
Blastomyces	Dimorphic	+	Ascomycota
Coccidioides	Dimorphic	+	Ascomycota
Histoplasma	Dimorphic	+	Ascomycota
Cryptococcus	Yeast		Basidiomycota

[a]For those that form hyphae.
[b]Tissue forms but does not grow in culture.

Taxonomy based on visual identification of fungal features, genome sequencing, protein identification

Medical grouping organized by biologic behavior in humans

Systemic fungi infect previously healthy persons

demonstrated that several microbial species are actually fungi despite having few fungal growth characteristics (eg, *Pneumocystis* species and Microsporidia).

Fungi have historically been organized into five phyla: Ascomycota, Basidiomycota, Zygomycota, Chytridiomycota, and Glomeromycota. The medically important genera fall mostly within the Ascomycota, with a few in Basidiomycota, and Zygomycota, as shown in **Table 42–1**.

The grouping of medically important fungi used in the following chapters is based on the types of tissues they parasitize and the diseases they produce, rather than on the principles of basic mycologic taxonomy. The **superficial** fungi, such as the dermatophytes, cause indolent lesions of the skin and its appendages, commonly known as ringworm and athlete's foot, without typically spreading to deeper tissues. The **subcutaneous** pathogens characteristically cause infection through the skin, followed by subcutaneous or lymphatic spread. The **opportunistic** fungi are those found in the environment or in the resident flora that produce disease primarily in immunocompromised hosts. The **systemic** pathogens are the most virulent fungi and may cause serious and progressive systemic disease in previously healthy persons. These fungal species are not found in the human microbiota. Although their major potential is to produce deep-seated visceral infections and systemic spread (systemic mycoses), they may also produce superficial infections as part of their disease spectrum or as the initiating event. As with all clinical classifications, overlaps and exceptions occur. In the end, the interplay between host and microorganism defines the disease.

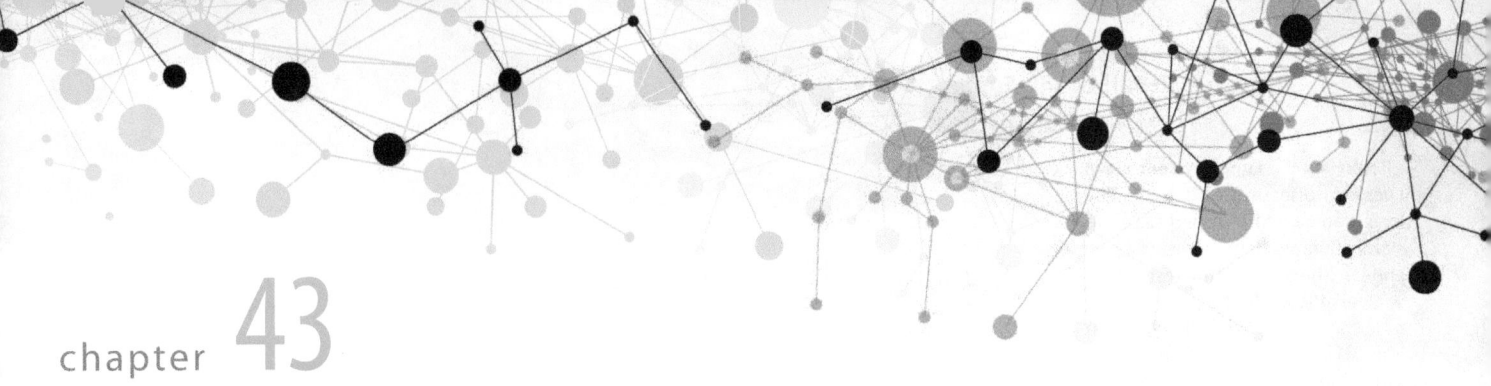

chapter 43

Pathogenesis and Diagnosis of Fungal Infections

We all have regular contact with fungi. They are so widely distributed in our environment that thousands of fungal spores are inhaled or ingested every day. Some species are so well adapted to humans that they are common members of the microbiota. Despite this ubiquity, clinically apparent systemic fungal infections are uncommon. However, systemic fungal infections pose some of the most difficult diagnostic and therapeutic problems in infectious disease, particularly among immunocompromised patients. The purpose of this chapter is to provide an overview of the pathogenesis and immunology of fungal infections. Details relating to specific fungi are provided in Chapters 45 to 47.

● GENERAL ASPECTS OF FUNGAL DISEASE EPIDEMIOLOGY

Fungal infections are most often acquired from the external environment. One common mechanism of infection is by the inhalation of conidia generated from environmental molds. Some of these fungi are ubiquitous, whereas others are restricted to specific **endemic** areas, geographic regions whose climate favors their growth. Many fungi produce disease only after they are accidentally injected past the skin/mucosal barrier, especially in immunocompromised patients. Other pathogenic fungi have more sophisticated means of tissue penetration and invasion. Infection can result from systemic invasion by a fungal species that is typically an endogenous member of the resident flora, such as that seen with systemic candidiasis (**Figure 43–1**).

Environmental conidia inhaled

* Some endemic to geographic regions

PATHOGENESIS

Compared with bacterial, viral, and parasitic disease, less is known about the pathogenic mechanisms and virulence factors involved in fungal infections. Analogies to bacterial diseases come closest because of similarities in microbial adherence to mucosal surfaces, invasion into deeper tissue layers, production of extracellular compounds, and interaction with phagocytes (**Figure 43–2**). In general, the principles discussed in Chapter 22 also apply to fungal infections. Most fungi are opportunists, causing serious disease only in individuals with impaired host defense systems. Only a few fungi are able to cause disease in previously healthy persons.

Fungi have mechanisms for adherence and invasion

Most fungi are opportunists

■ Adherence

Several fungal species, particularly the yeasts, are able to colonize the mucosal surfaces of the gastrointestinal and female genital tracts. It has been shown experimentally that the ability to adhere to buccal or vaginal epithelial cells is associated with both colonization and virulence. Within the genus *Candida*, the species that best adhere to epithelial cells are those most frequently

FIGURE 43–1. **Fungi system view.** Localized disease (*left*) is caused by local trauma or the superficial invasion of flora resident on the oropharyngeal (thrush), gastrointestinal, or vaginal mucosa. Systemic fungal disease (*right*) most often begins with inhalation of conidia followed by dissemination to other sites.

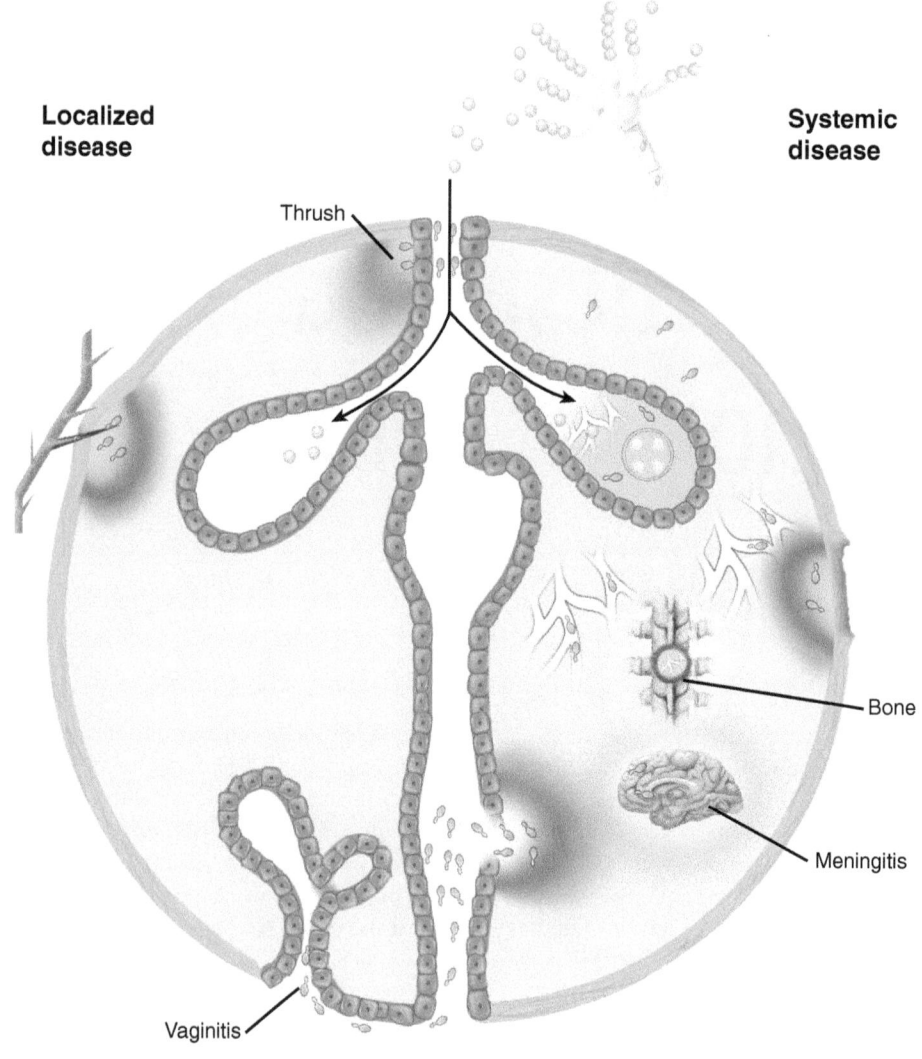

isolated from clinical infections. Adherence usually requires surface adhesins on the fungus and a receptor on the epithelial cell. In the case of *Candida albicans*, mannoprotein components extending from the cell wall have been implicated as specific adhesins, interacting with host fibronectin and other components of the extracellular matrix. Other fungal/host binding mediators have been identified, and this process can help to explain why certain tissue are targeted by specific fungal pathogens. For example, the neuropathogen *Cryptococcus neoformans* displays a unique interaction with proteins on the endothelium of the brain microvasculature, perhaps explaining how this species specifically invades the central nervous system.

Adherence is mediated by fungal adhesins to host cell receptors

FIGURE 43–2. **Immunity to fungal infections. A.** Pathogenic fungi are able to survive and multiply slowly in nonactivated macrophages. **B.** When macrophages are activated by cytokines from T cells, the growth is restricted and the fungi digested.

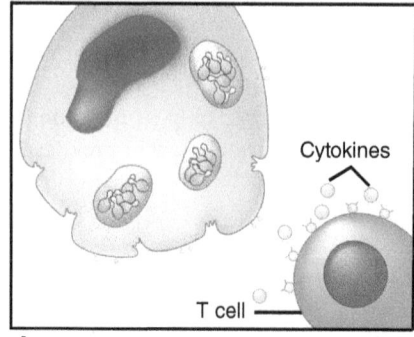

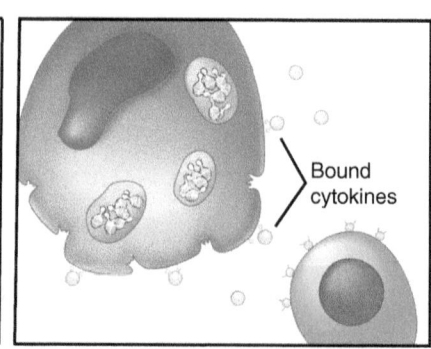

■ Invasion

Passing an initial surface barrier—skin, mucous membrane, or respiratory epithelium—is an important step for most successful pathogens. Some fungi are introduced through mechanical breaks. For example, *Sporothrix schenckii* infection typically follows a traumatic injury to the skin. Fungi that initially infect the lung must produce conidia small enough to be inhaled past the upper airway defenses. For example, arthroconidia of *Coccidioides immitis* (2-6 μm) can remain suspended in air for a considerable period of time, their size allowing efficiency delivery to the terminal bronchioles to initiate pulmonary coccidioidomycosis.

Triggered by temperature and possibly other cues, dimorphic fungi from the environment undergo a metabolic shift similar to the heat shock response, completely changing their morphology to a more invasive form. Invasion directly across mucosal barriers by the endogenous yeast *C albicans* is similarly associated with a morphologic change, the formation of hyphae. For this species, the ability to transition between yeast-like and hyphal forms allows it to effectively penetrate tissue, form adherent biofilms, and disseminate to distant sites. Extracellular enzymes (eg, proteases, elastases) are also associated with the advancing edge of the hyphal form of *Candida* species, as well as with the invasive forms of many of the dimorphic and other pathogenic fungi.

> Introduced through breaks in skin
>
> Conidia may bypass airway defenses
>
> Invasion may involve enzymes
>
> Dimorphic fungi change to more invasive form

■ Injury

There are many mechanisms of tissue injury during fungal infection. Although many fungi produce secondary metabolites and **mycotoxins** in the environment, most of these extracellular toxins do not appear to be directly related to pathogenesis in human infections. Cell surface components contributing to host damage, analogous to the endotoxin of Gram-negative bacteria, are lacking in most fungi. Moreover, only the most immunocompromised patients, such as those with neutropenia, appear to have extensive injury due to direct fungal destruction of the surrounding tissue. In contrast, the injury experienced by the host during most fungal infections seems to be due primarily to the immune response against the infecting microorganism. As the immune system attempts to clear the fungal pathogens, there is often collateral damage to the host.

> No classic exotoxins
>
> Injury due to inflammatory responses of host

IMMUNITY

■ Innate Immunity

Healthy persons have effective innate immunity to most fungal infections, especially the opportunistic molds. This resistance is mediated by the professional phagocytes (neutrophils, macrophages, and dendritic cells), the complement system, and pattern recognition receptors. Important receptors recognizing fungal elements include lectin-like structures on phagocytes (eg, dectin-1) that bind glucans on fungal cells, as well as Toll-like receptors (TLR2, TLR4). In most instances, neutrophils and alveolar macrophages are able to kill the conidia of fungi if they reach the tissues.

Fungal species that cause human infections have developed strategies to avoid immune recognition and to thwart various aspects of immune-mediated clearance. The polysaccharide capsule of *C neoformans* shields immunogenic epitopes on the cell surface from being sensed by pattern recognition receptors and complement proteins. Moreover, capsule material secreted by the cryptococcal cell specifically inhibits the function of many immune cells. Similarly, *C albicans* is able to bind complement components in a way that interferes with phagocytosis. As the thermally dimorphic fungi convert to the pathogenic yeast-like state, they too become more resistant to killing by phagocytes because of changes in surface structures subject to pattern recognition.

In addition to preventing immune recognition, many fungal pathogens are also able to survive once sensed and engulfed by immune cells. The yeast-to-hyphal transition by *C albicans* favors its escape from phagocytic immune cells. As the hyphae of the thermally dimorphic fungus *C immitis* convert to the spherule (tissue) phase, they also become resistant to phagocytic killing because of their size and surface characteristics. Some fungi produce substances such as melanin, which interfere with oxidative killing by phagocytes. The yeast forms of *Histoplasma capsulatum* and *C neoformans* are adapted to live and multiply within macrophages by interfering with lysosomal killing mechanisms.

> Most fungi are readily killed by neutrophils
>
> Pathogenic fungi resist phagocytic killing

■ Adaptive Immune Response

A recurrent theme with fungal infections is the importance of an intact immune response in preventing infection and progression of disease. The small number of species that are able to cause clinically apparent infection are usually cleared from the host, most often through a combination of the innate activity of neutrophils and through the development of an adaptive, T_H1-mediated

> T-cell–mediated responses of primary importance
>
> Progressive disease in immunocompromised

immune response. Progressive, debilitating, or life-threatening fungal infections are commonly associated with depressed or absent cellular immune responses.

■ Humoral Immunity

Antibodies may not correlate with resistance

Opsonizing antibody effective for some yeast

Antifungal antibodies can be detected at some time during the course of almost all fungal infections, but the appearance of antibodies does not necessarily correlate with antifungal resistance. In coccidioidomycosis, for example, high titers of *C immitis*-specific antibodies are associated with dissemination and a worsening clinical course; antibody titers decrease as the infection is cured. In contrast, antibodies directed against the *C neoformans* capsule may actually contribute to the cell-mediated clearance of this encapsulated yeast from the site of infection. Antibody may also play a role in control of *C albicans* infections by enhancing fungus–phagocyte interactions.

■ Cellular Immunity

Systemic disease with deficiencies in neutrophils and T$_H$1 immunity

Considerable clinical and experimental evidence points toward the importance of cellular immunity in the resolution of fungal infections. Most patients with invasive mycoses have neutropenia, defects in neutrophil function, or depressed T$_H$1 immune responses. These can result from factors such as steroid treatment, hematologic malignancies, transplantation, and AIDS.

Fungi escaping neutrophils grow in macrophages

A basic schema for fungal-host interactions is illustrated in Figure 43–2. When hyphae or yeast cells of the fungus reach deep tissue sites, they are either killed by neutrophils or resist destruction by one of the antiphagocytic mechanisms described earlier. Surviving cells continue to grow slowly within the host in their tissue-adapted fungal forms (spherules for *C immitis*, hyphae for *Aspergillus fumigatus*, intracellular yeasts for *C neoformans* and *H capsulatum*). The growth of these invasive forms may be slowed or killed by phagocytes such as neutrophils and macrophages. In healthy persons, the extent of infection is minimal, and any symptoms are instead caused by the host inflammatory response.

Immune defects lead to progressive disease

Everything awaits the specific adaptive immune response to the invader. In fungal infections, antigen-presenting cells such as dendritic cells and macrophages help to activate adaptive immune response, including antifungal antibody production and T$_H$1-mediated cellular immunity. Defects that disturb this cycle lead to progressive disease. To the extent that they are known, the specifics of these reactions are discussed in the following chapters.

LABORATORY DIAGNOSIS

■ Direct Examination

KOH digests tissue, but not fungal wall

Calcofluor white enhances detection by staining fungal chitin

Fungi can often be identified by directly observing their distinctive morphologic features on direct microscopic examination of infected pus, fluids, or tissues. The simplest method is to mix a clinical specimen, such as skin scrapings, with a 10% solution of potassium hydroxide (KOH) on a microscope slide under a coverslip. The strong alkali digests the tissue elements (epithelial cells, leukocytes, debris) but not the rigid cell walls of either yeasts or molds. After digestion of the material, the fungi can be observed under the light microscope with or without staining (**Figure 43–3**). Direct examinations can be aided by the use of calcofluor white, a dye that binds to

FIGURE 43–3. KOH (potassium hydroxide) preparation. Scalp scrapings from a suspected ringworm lesion have been mixed with 10% KOH and viewed under low power. The skin has been dissolved, revealing tubular branching hyphae.

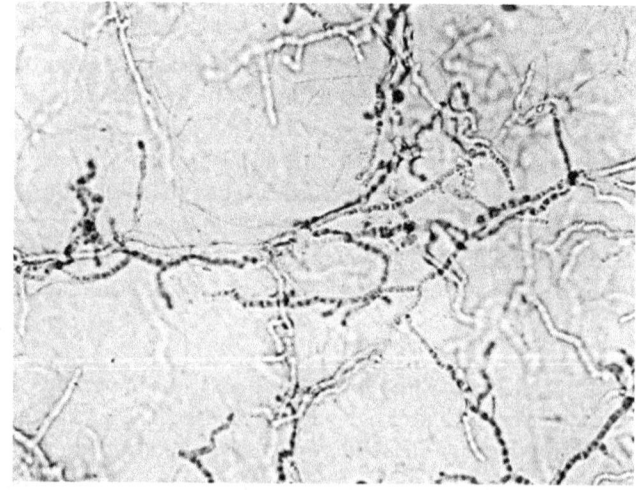

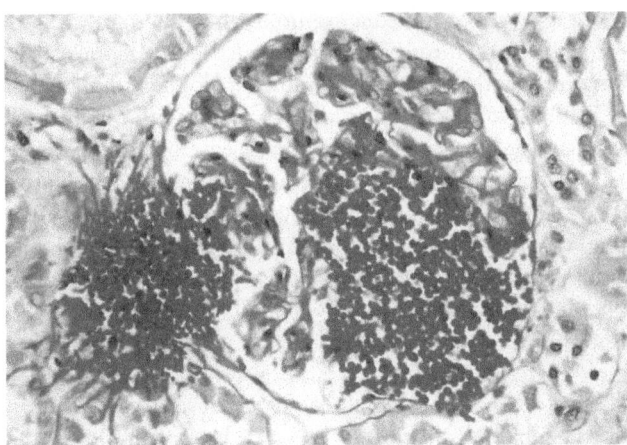

FIGURE 43–4. **Disseminated candidiasis.** *Candida albicans* (stained red by H and E stain) has invaded a kidney glomerulus. Most cells are in the yeast form, but some hyphae are seen at the lower left. (Reproduced with permission from Connor DH, Chandler FW, Schwartz DQ, et al: *Pathology of Infectious Diseases.* Stamford CT: Appleton & Lange; 1997.)

polysaccharides in cellulose and chitin. Under ultraviolet light, calcofluor white fluoresces, enhancing detection of fungi in fluids or tissue sections. A few yeasts including *C albicans* can be visualized using the Gram stain (Gram positive).

Histopathologic examination of tissue biopsy specimens is widely used to diagnose fungal infections and shows the relation of the organism to tissue elements and host responses (blood vessels, phagocytes, granulomatous reactions). Most fungi can be seen in sections stained with the basic hematoxylin and eosin (H&E) method used in histology laboratories (**Figure 43–4**). Specialized staining procedures such as silver impregnation methods are frequently used because they stain almost all fungi strongly, but only a few tissue components (**Figure 43–5**). The pathologist should be alerted to the possibility of fungal infection when tissues are submitted because fungal-specific stains are not used routinely.

Often visible in H&E preparations

Silver stains enhance detection

■ Culture

Fungi can be grown by methods similar to those used to isolate bacteria. The growth of many fungal species occurs readily on enriched bacteriologic media commonly used in clinical laboratories (eg, blood agar and chocolate agar). Many fungal cultures, however, require days to weeks of incubation for initial growth; bacteria present in the specimen grow more rapidly and may interfere with isolation of a slow-growing fungus. Therefore, the culture procedures of diagnostic mycology are designed to favor the growth of fungi over bacteria and to allow incubation to continue for a sufficient time to isolate slower growing strains.

Culture simple but slow

Selective media enhance isolation

The most commonly used medium for cultivating fungi is Sabouraud's agar, which contains only glucose and peptones as nutrients. Its pH is 5.6, which is optimal for growth of dermatophytes and satisfactory for growth of many other fungi. Most bacteria fail to grow, or grow poorly, on Sabouraud's agar. A wide variety of media are used for isolating specific fungi, many of which use either Sabouraud's medium or brain-heart infusion as their base.

Sabouraud's agar optimal for many fungi

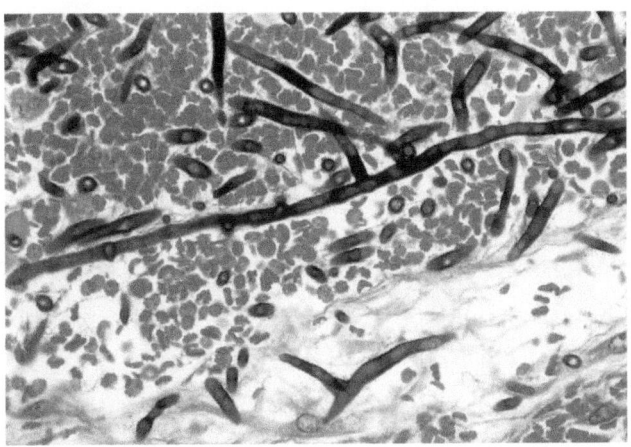

FIGURE 43–5. **Fusarium invasion.** The branching septate hyphae are stained black by this silver stain. (Reproduced with permission from Connor DH, Chandler FW, Schwartz DQ, et al: *Pathology of Infectious Diseases.* Stamford CT: Appleton & Lange; 1997.)

Blood agar or other types of enriched bacteriologic media are used when pure cultures are expected, such as sub-culturing yeasts from blood cultures. These media can be made more fungal-selective by the addition of antibacterial antibiotics such as chloramphenicol and gentamicin. Cycloheximide, an antimicrobial that inhibits some saprophytic fungi, is sometimes added to Sabouraud's agar to prevent overgrowth of contaminating molds from the environment, particularly for skin cultures. However, media containing these selective agents cannot be relied on exclusively because they can interfere with growth of some pathogenic fungi or because the "contaminant" may be producing an opportunistic infection. For example, cycloheximide inhibits *C neoformans*, and chloramphenicol may inhibit the yeast forms of some dimorphic fungi. In contrast to most pathogenic bacteria, many fungi grow best at 25°C to 30°C, and temperatures in this range are used for primary isolation. Paired cultures incubated at 30°C and 35°C may be used to demonstrate dimorphism.

Once a fungus is isolated from a clinical sample, identification procedures often depend on whether the growing fungus is a yeast or a mold. Historically, yeasts have been identified to the species level by biochemical tests analogous to those tests used for bacteria. The observation of specific fungal structures such as pseudohyphae is also diagnostically useful among the yeasts. More recently, biochemical assessments using mass spectroscopy have been increasingly used for microbial identification.

Molds are most often identified by the morphology of their conidia and conidiophores. Other features such as the size, texture, and color of the colonies help characterize molds, but without demonstrating conidiation they are not sufficient for identification. Conidium production may not occur for days or weeks after the initial growth of the mold. It is similar to waiting for flowers to bloom, and it can be frustrating when the result has immediate clinical application. Similar to yeasts, mass spectroscopy-based identification of mold species is likely to complement morphological assessments.

It is desirable, but not always possible, to demonstrate the yeast and mold phases with dimorphic fungi. In some cases, this result can be achieved with parallel cultures at 30°C and 35°C. The tissue form of *C immitis* is not readily produced *in vitro*. Demonstration of dimorphism has become less important with the development of specific DNA probes for the major systemic pathogens. These probes are rapid and can be applied directly to the mycelial growth of the readily grown mold phases of these fungi.

■ Antigen and Antibody Detection

Serum antibodies directed against a variety of fungal antigens can be detected in patients infected with those agents. These tests are most helpful for determining prior exposure to various fungi, and they are rarely useful for diagnosing acute infections, except for *C immitis* in which antibody levels often correlate with extent of infection. Immunoassays to detect fungal antigens attempt to identify fungal-specific components including mannans, mannoproteins, glucans, chitin. Two of these tests are extremely sensitive and specific for systemic infection: (1) the *C neoformans* capsular polysaccharide antigen test (cryptococcal antigen) and (2) the *H capsulatum* surface antigen test (*Histoplasma* antigen). Serum antigen tests for *Aspergillus* species (galactomannan) and other fungal pathogens (β-D-glucan) are less sensitive and specific for diagnosing infection but can be useful in some cases. PCR-based assays also offer promise for nonculture-based identification of fungal nucleic acid in clinical samples.

Selective media make use of antimicrobials

Cultures are incubated at 30°C

Yeasts identified biochemically

Molds identified by morphology, culture features

Temperature variation induces dimorphism

DNA probes more rapid

Serologic tests useful for some fungi

Antigen detection shows promise

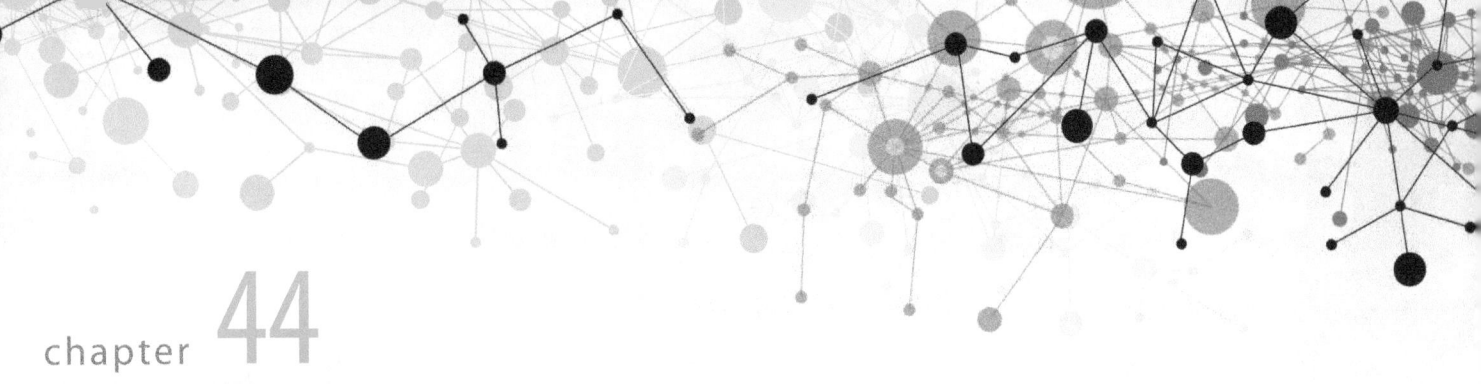

chapter 44

Antifungal Agents and Resistance

Compared with antibacterial agents, relatively few antimicrobials are available for treatment of fungal infections. Many substances with antifungal activity have proven to be unstable, to be toxic to humans, or to have undesirable pharmacologic characteristics, such as poor diffusion into tissues. Newer antifungal agents target fungal-specific cellular features and demonstrate lower toxicity than older drug classes.

Many antifungals are too toxic for use

Many fungal infections are self-limiting and require no therapy. However, there are also circumstances in which either topical or systemic antifungal agents are used. Superficial mycoses are often treated with topical therapy, limiting toxicity to the host. Invasive or systemic fungal infections that are not controlled by the host's immune system often require the prolonged use of systemic antifungals. Given that most of the patients with these infections also have underlying immunosuppression, invasive mycosis can be among the most difficult of all infectious diseases to treat successfully. The characteristics of currently used antifungal agents are summarized in **Table 44–1**. They are also discussed in the text that follows in relation to their target of action, as illustrated in **Figure 44–1**.

Treatment is needed for invasive fungal infections in immunocompromised persons

● ANTIFUNGAL AGENTS

CYTOPLASMIC MEMBRANE

■ Polyenes

The polyenes **nystatin** and **amphotericin B** are lipophilic and bind to ergosterol, the dominant sterol in the cytoplasmic membrane of fungal cells. Sterol-binding by the polyenes has many adverse effects on the fungal cell, including the formation of annular channels that penetrate the membrane and lead to leakage of essential small molecules from the cytoplasm and cell death. Their binding affinity for the ergosterol in fungal membranes is not completely specific, cross-reacting with mammalian sterols such as cholesterol. This cross-binding is the basis for the considerable toxicity that limits their use. Almost all fungi are susceptible to amphotericin B, and the development of resistance is rare.

＊Amphotericin B binds ergosterol, forms membrane channels

Cross-reactivity with mammalian sterols basis for toxicity

At physiologic pH, amphotericin B is insoluble in water and must be administered intravenously as a colloidal suspension. It is not absorbed from the gastrointestinal tract. Infusion is commonly followed by chills, fever, headache, and dyspnea. The major limitation to amphotericin B therapy is the toxicity created by its affinity for mammalian as well as fungal membranes. The most serious toxic effect is renal dysfunction, observed in virtually every patient receiving a prolonged therapeutic course. Experienced clinicians learn to titrate the dosage for each patient to minimize the nephrotoxic effects. For obvious reasons, use of amphotericin B is limited to progressive, life-threatening fungal infections. In such cases, despite its toxicity, it retains a prime initial position in treatment and is often followed by the use of a less toxic agent. Preparations that complex amphotericin B with lipids have been used as a means to limit toxicity. The even greater toxicity of nystatin limits its use in topical preparations.

Amphotericin B must be infused in suspension

Therapy titrated against toxicity

TABLE 44–1	Features of Antifungal Agents			
AGENT	**ACTION**	**RESISTANCE**	**ROUTE**	**CLINICAL USE**
Polyenes				
Nystatin	Cell membrane pores	Sterol modification	Topical	Most fungi
Amphotericin B	Cell membrane pores	Sterol modification	Intravenous	*Aspergillus, Candida, Cryptococcus, Histoplasma, Sporothrix, Coccidioides, Zygomycetes*
Azoles				
Fluconazole	Ergosterol synthesis (demethylase)	Efflux, demethylase alteration, overproduction of target[a]	Oral, intravenous	*Candida, Cryptococcus, Histoplasma,[c] Coccidioides[c]*
Itraconazole	Ergosterol synthesis (demethylase)	Efflux, demethylase alteration, overproduction of target[a]	Oral, intravenous	*Aspergillus, Sporothrix, Candida, Blastomyces, Histoplasma, Coccidioides*
Voriconazole	Ergosterol synthesis (demethylase)		Oral, intravenous	*Candida, Aspergillus,* some saprophytic molds
Posaconazole	Ergosterol synthesis (demethylase)		Oral, intravenous	*Candida, Aspergillus* (prophylaxis), *Zygomycetes*
Isavuconazole	Ergosterol synthesis (demethylase)		Oral, intravenous	*Candida, Aspergillus* (prophylaxis), *Zygomycetes*
Clotrimazole	Ergosterol synthesis (demethylase)		Topical	*Candida*, dermatophytes
Ketoconazole	Ergosterol synthesis (demethylase)		Topical	*Candida*, dermatophytes
Miconazole	Ergosterol synthesis (demethylase)		Topical	*Candida*, dermatophytes
Allylamines				
Terbinafine	Ergosterol synthesis (squalene epoxidase)	?Efflux	Oral, topical	Dermatophytes
Flucytosine (5-FC)				
	DNA synthesis, RNA transcription	Permease or modifying enzymes[b] mutation	Oral	*Candida* and *Cryptococcus[d]*
Echinocandins				
Caspofungin	Glucan synthesis (β-glucan synthase)	Altered synthase	Intravenous	*Candida, Aspergillus*
Micafungin	Glucan synthesis (β-glucan synthase)	Altered synthase	Intravenous	*Candida, Aspergillus*
Anidulafungin	Glucan synthesis (β-glucan synthase)	Altered synthase	Intravenous	*Candida, Aspergillus*
Griseofulvin	Microtubule disruption	Unknown	Oral	Dermatophytes
Potassium iodide	Unknown	Unknown	Oral	*Sporothrix schenckii*

5-FC, 5-Flucytosine.
[a]Most work is with fluconazole and *Candida*; other azoles are to be assumed to be similar.
[b]Cytosine deaminase and uracil phosphoribosyltransferase (the enzymes that modify 5-FC to active forms).
[c]Itraconazole generally preferred.
[d]Only in combination with amphotericin B owing to developing resistance.

■ Azoles

The azoles are a large family of synthetic organic compounds, which include members with antibacterial, antifungal, and antiparasitic properties. Their activity is based on inhibition of the enzyme (14 α-demethylase) responsible for conversion of lanosterol to ergosterol, the major sterol of the fungal cell membrane. This enzyme inhibition results in ergosterol depletion and lanosterol accumulation, thereby leading to defective fungal membranes. All antifungal azoles have the same basic mechanism of action. The differences among them are in avidity of enzyme binding,

Inhibit enzyme crucial for synthesis of membrane ergosterol

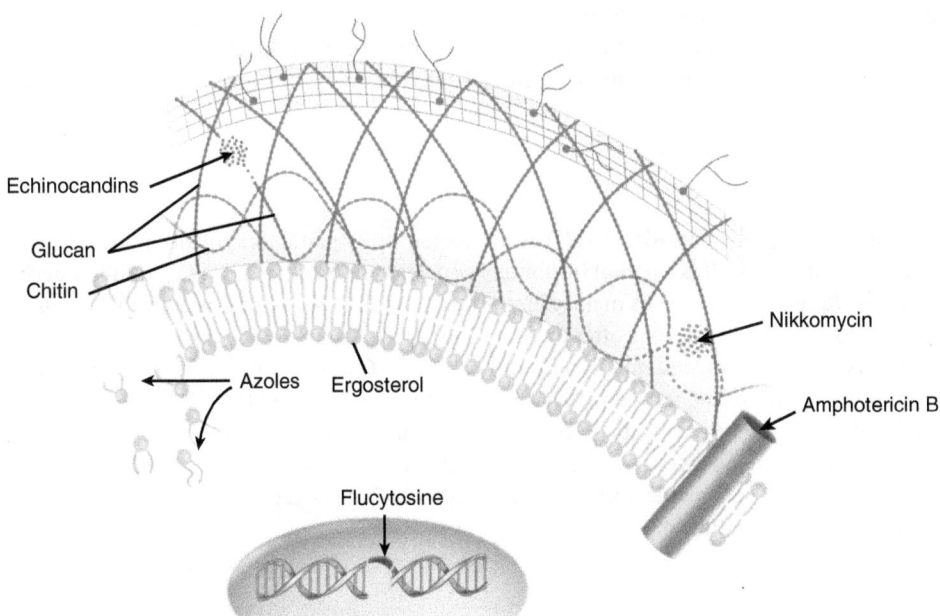

FIGURE 44-1. Sites of action of antifungal agents. This figure demonstrates the cellular targets of the major antifungal agents: (1) cell wall (echinocandins and nikkomycin—an experimental chitin synthase inhibitor), (2) cell membrane (azoles, amphotericin B), and (3) nucleic acid synthesis (flucytosine).

pharmacology, and side effects. Azoles can also affect the precursors of some hormones and may therefore cause endocrinological side effects, restricting their use in pregnancy.

The systemic azoles are generally grouped based on antifungal spectrum. **Fluconazole** is primarily active against yeasts, including many *Cryptococcus* and *Candida* species. In contrast, newer azole compounds have extended activity against molds such as *Aspergillus* species, as well as the thermally dimorphic fungi (eg, *Coccidioides*, *Blastomyces*, *Histoplasma*). These mold-active azoles include **itraconazole, voriconazole, posaconazole,** and **isavuconazole**. Most of these agents can be given orally or parenterally. Although generally well tolerated, the antifungal azoles can cause varying degrees of liver toxicity. Additionally, all systemic azoles can adversely affect cardiac myocyte repolarization and therefore prolong the QTc interval on an EKG, placing patients at increased risk for cardiac arrhythmias. Among the systemic azoles, isavuconazole has the least potential for QTc prolongation. **Ketoconazole**, **clotrimazole,** and **miconazole** are available in over-the-counter topical preparations for superficial mycoses.

Azoles less nephrotoxic than amphotericin B

Divided between yeast-active and mold-active agents

Allylamines

The allylamines are a group of synthetic compounds that act by inhibition of an enzyme (squalene epoxidase) in the early stages of ergosterol synthesis. The allylamine group includes **terbinafine**, available in oral and topical forms for the treatment of dermatophyte (ringworm) infections.

Terbinafine inhibits ergosterol synthesis

CELL WALL SYNTHESIS

The unique chemical nature of the fungal cell wall, with its interwoven layers of mannans, glucans, and chitin (Figure 44–1), makes it an ideal target for chemotherapeutic attack. The echinocandins, which block glucan synthesis, are now in widespread clinical use due to their potent antifungal effect and comparatively low adverse effect profile. Other cell wall-active antifungals are in preclinical development.

Echinocandins

Echinocandins inhibit a glucan biosynthetic enzyme (β-1,3-D-glucan synthase) required for the synthesis of a structural cell wall carbohydrate of many fungi. Echinocandin administration, therefore, causes morphologic distortions and osmotic instability in yeasts and molds, similar to the effect of β-lactams on bacteria. The first such agent to be licensed was **caspofungin,** which has activity against *Candida* and *Aspergillus*. Although highly active against many *Candida* species, the echinocandins tend to be used as second-line agents for invasive aspergillosis. *Cryptococcus neoformans* and the thermally dimorphic fungi, whose cell wall glucans have a slightly different structure, are more tolerant of echinocandins. Therefore, echinocandins should not be used as

Inhibit enzyme crucial for glucan synthesis

Indications for *Candida*, *Aspergillus*

primary therapy for these infections. Since there are no similar glucans in humans, echinocandin toxicity is minimal. Newer echinocandins, **micafungin** and **anidulafungin,** have the same mode of action and a similar spectrum of antifungal activity.

NUCLEIC ACID SYNTHESIS

■ Flucytosine

5-Fluorocytosine (flucytosine/5-FC) is an analog of cytosine, one of the pyrimidine bases in both DNA and RNA. It is a potent inhibitor of nucleic acid synthesis. 5-FC requires a permease to enter the fungal cell, where its metabolites interfere with DNA synthesis and RNA transcription.

5-FC inhibits RNA and DNA synthesis

Active against yeasts but not molds

Resistance develops if used alone

Flucytosine is well absorbed after oral administration. It is active against most clinically important yeasts, including *Candida albicans* and *C neoformans*, but it has little activity against molds or dimorphic fungi. The frequent development of mutational resistance during therapy limits its application to mild yeast infections or its use in combination with amphotericin B for cryptococcal meningitis. The primary toxic effect of flucytosine is a reversible bone marrow suppression that can lead to neutropenia and thrombocytopenia. This effect is dose related and can be controlled by drug monitoring.

OTHER ANTIFUNGAL AGENTS

Griseofulvin is a product of one of the *Penicillium* species of molds. Griseofulvin is actively taken up by susceptible fungi and acts on the microtubules and associated proteins that make up the mitotic spindle. It interferes with cell division and possibly other cell functions associated with microtubules. Griseofulvin is absorbed from the gastrointestinal tract after oral administration and concentrates in the keratinized layers of the skin. It is active only against the agents of superficial mycoses. Clinical effectiveness has been demonstrated for many causes of dermatophyte infection, but the response is slow. Prolonged therapy may be required.

Microtubule disruption interferes with cell division

Active against dermatophytes

Potassium iodide is the oldest known oral chemotherapeutic agent for a fungal infection. It is effective only for cutaneous sporotrichosis. Its activity is somewhat paradoxical because the mold form of the etiologic agent, *Sporothrix schenckii*, can grow on medium containing 10% potassium iodide. The pathogenic yeast form of this dimorphic fungus appears to be susceptible to molecular iodine.

Iodide inhibits *Sporothrix*

● RESISTANCE TO ANTIFUNGAL AGENTS

DEFINITION OF RESISTANCE

The concepts, definitions, and laboratory methods described in Chapter 23 for bacterial resistance are generally applicable to fungi. Quantitative susceptibility is determined by measuring the minimal inhibitory concentration (MIC) of a drug under conditions that favor the growth of fungi. The wide range of growth rates and diversity of growth forms (yeast, hyphae, conidia) in the various fungi have added technical variables to testing, but standardized methods are now available. Comparison of MICs with drug pharmacology allows classification of fungi as susceptible or resistant, but these results do not yet predict clinical outcome with the same certainty they do with bacteria. Because of its specialized nature, the availability of antifungal susceptibility testing is restricted to major centers and reference laboratories.

Fungal resistance similar to bacteria

Fungal MICs labor intensive

MECHANISMS OF RESISTANCE

Many of the same resistance mechanisms observed in bacteria are also found in fungi. Fungi tend to primarily inactivate drug activity using efflux pumps and by altering their biosynthetic pathways. In contrast to bacteria, fungi do not make hydrolytic enzymes to inactivate antibiotics to the same extent as bacteria. In part this may be due to the reduced ability for horizontal gene transfer between species.

■ Polyene Resistance

Amphotericin B resistance rare

Because amphotericin B binds directly to the ergosterol in the fungal cell membrane, the only means to resist this action is to change the membrane sterol composition. Therefore, only a few rare fungal species are intrinsically resistant to amphotericin B.

■ Flucytosine Resistance

5-FC requires a permease for entry into the cell and then multiple enzymes to modify it to the active metabolites that inhibit nucleic acid synthesis. Mutation in any one of these enzymes renders the drug ineffective. It is one of the few antimicrobials in which emergence of resistance is predictable *during* therapy of an acute infection. This is the reason that its use is mostly limited to combination therapy with other antifungals.

Multiple enzyme mutations cause flucytosine resistance

■ Azole Resistance

There are several mechanisms by which fungi can become resistant to the azoles. The most well-characterized mechanism is through the induction of efflux pumps that transport the drug out of the cell. Some pumps act on all azoles, and others act on only one. Fungal species can also alter the subunits of the demethylase enzyme by mutation, effectively decreasing the affinity of the azole for its enzyme target. Multiple mutations can have an additive effect.

Azole pumped out by efflux pumps

Enzyme target altered

Additionally, some fungi are able to decrease the effect of the azoles by increasing the production of the drug target. Some azole-resistant strains of *Candida* and *Cryptococcus* species actually duplicate regions of their genome to increase the number of copies of the demethylase-encoding genes. This results in the requirement of higher concentrations of the azole drug to inhibit fungal growth. Some azole-resistant strains have also been shown to accomplish ergosterol synthesis by an alternate pathway, thus bypassing the azole target enzyme. Of particular concern is the widespread agricultural use of azole fungicides in many countries. This practice may result in the transfer of azole resistance mechanisms to medically important fungi as azole resistance increases among environmental isolates.

Demethylase enzyme upregulated or bypassed

■ Echinocandin Resistance

Resistance to echinocandins has significantly increased in recent years. One resistance mechanism is an altered target. Mutations in subunits of the glucan synthetase have been correlated with increases in MIC more than a thousand-fold.

Mutant glucan synthetase

SELECTION OF ANTIFUNGALS

As with all chemotherapy, the selection of antifungal agents for treatment of superficial, subcutaneous, and systemic mycoses involves balancing expected efficacy against toxicity. The factors to be considered are the following: (1) the threat of morbidity or mortality posed by the specific infection, (2) the immune status of the patient, (3) the toxicity of the antifungal, and (4) the probable activity of the antifungal agent against the fungus. In the case of superficial mycoses, the risks of appropriate therapy are small, and various topical agents may be safely used. At the other extreme, an immunocompromised patient will most likely be treated aggressively with systemic agents for proven or even suspected systemic fungal infection. Since cultures and susceptibility tests may not be available at the time of presumptive diagnosis, the decisions regarding which agents to use are often made and sustained on an empiric basis. Even when guided by *in vitro* testing, treatment failures are common, particularly in highly immunocompromised patients, emphasizing the importance of the immune system in preventing and clearing systemic fungal infections.

KEY CONCLUSIONS

- Topical antifungal therapy can often be used for superficial infections, but invasive infections require systemic therapy.
- Antifungal agents act on several fungal cell targets, including the cell membrane (polyenes and azoles), the cell wall (echinocandins), and nucleic acid synthesis (flucytosine).
- Amphotericin B resistance is rare among fungi, but its use is limited by toxicity, especially nephrotoxicity.
- Azoles are frequently divided into those with activity primarily against yeasts (fluconazole) and those with expanded activity against molds (itraconazole, voriconazole, posaconazole, isavuconazole).
- Echinocandins are well-tolerated systemic antifungals that are most frequently used for infections due to *Candida* species, and as secondary agents for aspergillosis.
- Flucytosine is active against many yeasts, but resistance can develop during therapy if used as a single agent.

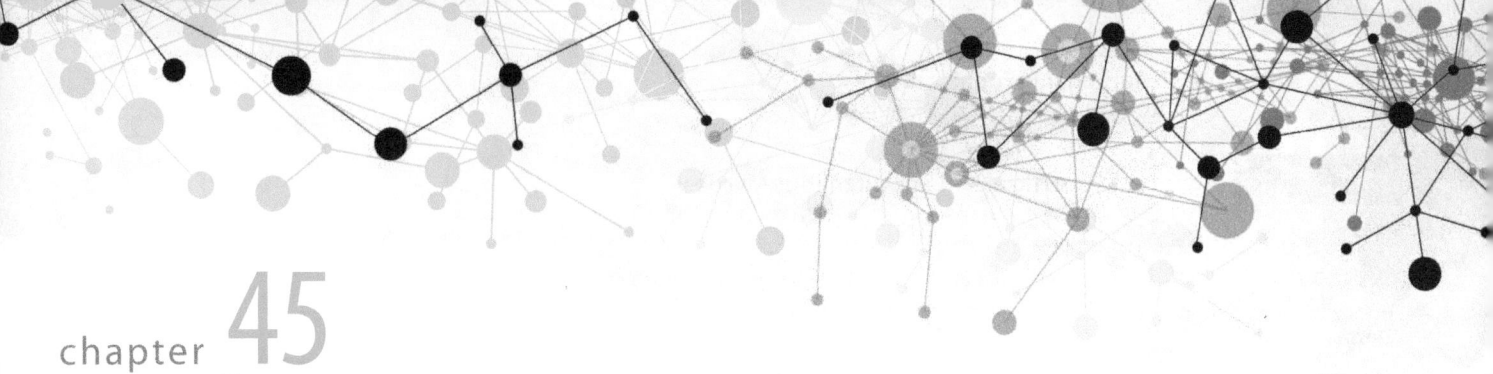

chapter 45

The Superficial and Subcutaneous Fungi: Dermatophytes, *Malassezia*, *Sporothrix*, and Pigmented Molds

Epidermophyton species · *Microsporum* species · *Trichophyton* species · *Malassezia furfur* · *Hortaea werneckii* ·

Sporothrix schenckii · *Fonsecaea* species · *Phialophora* species · *Cladophialophora* (*Cladosporium*) species

The least invasive of the pathogenic fungi are the dermatophytes and other superficial fungi that are adapted to the keratinized outer layers of the skin. Subcutaneous fungi go a step farther by extending infection to the tissue beneath the skin but rarely invading deeper structures (**Table 45–1**).

● SUPERFICIAL FUNGI

DERMATOPHYTES

OVERVIEW

Dermatophytoses are superficial infections of the skin and its appendages. Common names for these infections include ringworm (**Figure 45–1**), athlete's foot, and jock itch. They are caused by species of three genera collectively known as dermatophytes. These fungi are highly adapted to the nonliving, keratinized tissues of nails, hair, and the stratum corneum of the skin. The source of infection may be humans, animals, or the soil.

TABLE 45–1	Agents of Superficial and Subcutaneous Mycoses				
		FUNGAL GROWTH			
FUNGUS	**IN LESION**	**IN CULTURE (25°C)**	**INFECTION SITE**	**DISEASE**	
Dermatophytes					
Microsporum canis	Septate hyphae	Mold	Hair,[a] skin	Ringworm	
Microsporum audouini	Septate hyphae	Mold	Hair[a]	Ringworm	
Microsporum gypseum	Septate hyphae	Mold	Hair, skin	Ringworm	
Trichophyton tonsurans	Septate hyphae	Mold	Hair, skin, nails	Ringworm	
Trichophyton rubrum	Septate hyphae	Mold	Hair, skin, nails	Ringworm	
Trichophyton mentagrophytes	Septate hyphae	Mold	Hair, skin	Ringworm	
Trichophyton violaceum	Septate hyphae	Mold	Hair, skin, nails	Ringworm	
Epidermophyton floccosum	Septate hyphae	Mold	Skin	Ringworm	
Other superficial fungi					
Malassezia furfur[b]	Yeast (mycelia)[c]	Yeast	Skin (pink to brown)[d]	Pityriasis (tinea) versicolor	
Hortaea werneckii[e]	Septate hyphae, ellipsoidal cells	Yeast (mold)	Skin (brown–black)[d]	Tinea nigra	
Trichosporon cutaneum	Septate hyphae	Mold	Hair (white)[b]	White piedra	
Piedraia hortae	Septate hyphae	Mold, ascospores	Hair (black)[b]	Black piedra	
Subcutaneous fungi					
Sporothrix schenckii	Cigar-shaped yeast (rare)	Mold	Subcutaneous, lymphatic spread	Sporotrichosis	
Fonsecaea pedrosoi	Muriform body[f]	Mold	Wart-like foot lesions	Chromoblastomycosis	
Phialophora verrucosa	Muriform body[f]	Mold	Wart-like foot lesions	Chromoblastomycosis	
Cladophialophora (Cladosporium) carrionii	Muriform body[f]	Mold	Wart-like foot lesions	Chromoblastomycosis	

[a]Specimens fluoresce under ultraviolet light.
[b]Previously known as *Pityrosporum orbiculare*.
[c]Denotes less frequent findings.
[d]Color of clinical lesions.
[e]Previously known as *Cladosporium werneckii*.
[f]Multicompartment yeast-like structure.

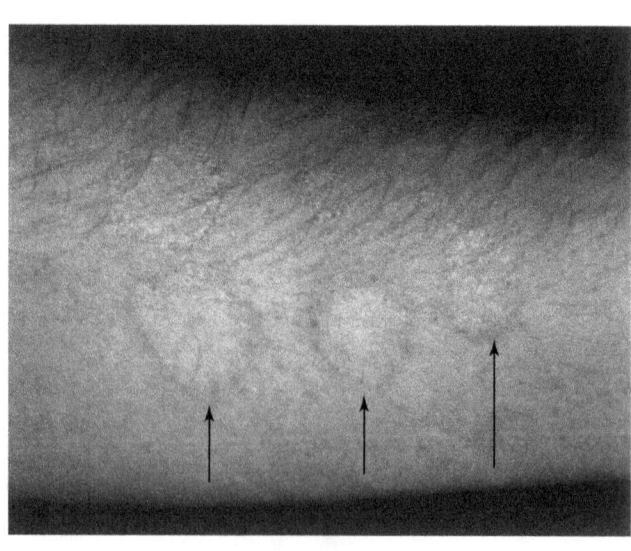

FIGURE 45–1. **Ringworm.** The ring-like lesions on this forearm are due to advancing growth of *Trichophyton mentagrophytes*. (Reproduced with permission from Willey JM: *Prescott, Harley, & Klein's Microbiology*, 7th ed. New York, NY: McGraw Hill; 2008.)

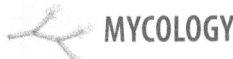 MYCOLOGY

The three genera of medically important dermatophytes (literally, skin-plants) are *Epidermophyton*, *Microsporum*, and *Trichophyton* (Table 45–1). Most dermatophyte infections are diagnosed and treated as a clinical syndrome since determining the causative species will not usually affect therapeutic choices.

✳ *Epidermophyton*, *Microsporum*, and *Trichophyton* major genera

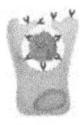 DERMATOPHYTE DISEASE

CLINICAL CAPSULE

Dermatophytoses are slowly progressive eruptions of the skin and its appendages. Although often unsightly, they are not typically painful or life-threatening. The manifestations vary depending on the site of infection and vigor of the host response, but they often involve erythema, induration, itching, and scaling. The most familiar name is "ringworm," describing the annular shape of the advancing edge of this cutaneous infection.

Transmission can occur after close contact with an infected person or animal. However, exposure to detached skin scales or hair containing the fungal elements (fomites) may also result in new infections. Dermatophyte transmission has been described in many shared spaces, including locker room floors, barbershops, hotel carpets, and movie theater/airplane seats. However, health care workers do not need to take special precautions beyond handwashing after contact with an infected patient.

✳ Transmission requires contact with intact or detached skin or hair

PATHOGENESIS

Dermatophytoses begin when the infecting fungus comes in contact with skin, especially if there are minor breaks in the skin integrity. Detached hair and skin scales containing dermatophytes can remain infectious for months in the environment. Once the stratum corneum is penetrated, the organism can proliferate in the keratinized layers of the skin, with a variety of proteinases helping to establish infection. The course of the infection depends on many factors: the anatomic location, the degree of skin moisture, the dynamics of skin growth and desquamation, the speed and extent of the inflammatory response, and the infecting species. For example, if the organism grows very slowly in the stratum corneum and if skin turnover by desquamation is rapid, the infection will probably be short-lived and cause minimal signs and symptoms. Inflammation tends to increase desquamation rates and helps to limit infection, whereas immunosuppressive agents such as topical corticosteroids decrease shedding of the keratinized layers and tend to prolong infection. Invasion of any deeper structures is extremely rare.

Most dermatophyte infections are self-limited. However, those infections in which fungal growth rates and skin desquamation are balanced, and in which the inflammatory response is poor, tend to become chronic. The lateral spread of infection and its associated inflammation produce the characteristic sharp advancing margins that were once believed to be the burrows of worms. This characteristic is the origin of the common English name **ringworm**, as well as the Latin term *tinea* (worm), which is often applied to the clinical forms of the disease (Figure 45–1).

Infection may spread from skin to other keratinized structures, such as hair and nails, or may invade them primarily. The hair shaft is penetrated by hyphae (**Figure 45–2**), which extend either exclusively within the shaft (endothrix) or both within and outside the shaft (ectothrix). The end result is damage to the hair shaft structure, which often breaks off. Loss of hair at the root and plugging of the hair follicle with fungal elements may result. Invasion of the nail plate causes a hyperkeratotic reaction, which dislodges or distorts the nail (**onychomycosis**).

Occasionally, dermatophyte infections become chronic and widespread. This progression has been related to both host and organism factors. Approximately half of these patients have underlying diseases affecting their immune responses or are receiving treatments that compromise T-lymphocyte function. These chronic infections are particularly associated with *Trichophyton rubrum*, to which both normal and immunocompromised persons appear to be hyporesponsive. Interestingly, the clinical manifestations of these infections are largely due to delayed-type hypersensitivity responses rather than from direct effects of the fungus on the host.

Initial infection through skin breaks

Fungal growth, skin desquamation determine outcome

Poor inflammatory response leads to chronic infection

Hair shaft penetrated and broken

Infected nails thickened, dislodged

Widespread infection with T-lymphocyte defects and *T rubrum*

FIGURE 45-2. **Black piedra.** Note invasion by *Piedraia hortae* both within (endothrix) and outside (ectothrix) the hair shaft. Dermatophyte invasion would be similar. (Reproduced with permission from Willey JM: *Prescott, Harley, & Klein's Microbiology*, 7th ed. New York, NY: McGraw Hill; 2008.)

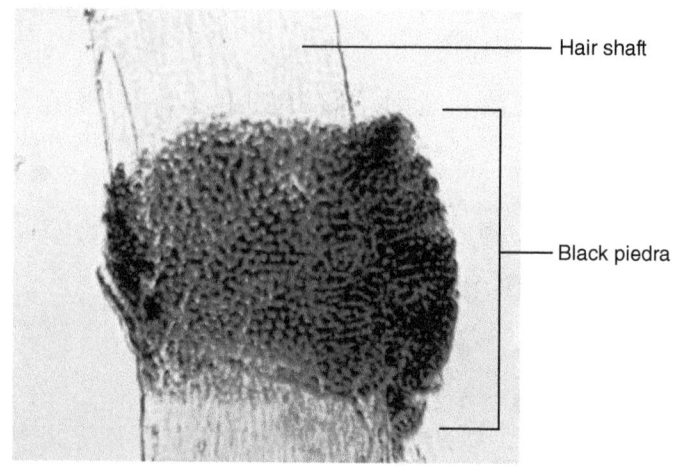

Hair shaft

Black piedra

DERMATOPHYTOSES: CLINICAL ASPECTS

MANIFESTATIONS

Dermatophyte infections range from inapparent colonization to chronic progressive eruptions that last months or years, causing considerable discomfort and disfiguration. Dermatologists often give each infection its own "disease" name based on the Latin name for the anatomic site at which the infection is found. For example, these names include *tinea capitis* (scalp; **Figure 45–3A**), *tinea pedis* (feet, athlete's foot), tinea manuum (hands), *tinea cruris* (groin), *tinea barbae* (beard, hair), and *tinea unguium* (nail beds). Skin infections otherwise not included in this anatomic list are called *tinea corporis* (body). There are certain clinical, etiologic, and epidemiologic differences among these syndromes, but they are basically the same disease in different locations. The primary differences among etiologic agents that infect different sites are shown in Table 45–1.

Tinea capitis. Infection of hair and the scalp begins with an erythematous papule around the hair shaft, which progresses to scaling of the scalp, and discoloration/fracture of the shaft. Spread to adjacent hair follicles progresses in a ring-like fashion, leaving behind broken, discolored hairs, and sometimes black dots where the hair is absent but the infection has invaded the follicle. In most cases, symptoms beyond itching are minimal, but the degree of inflammatory response markedly affects the clinical appearance and, in rare cases, can cause constitutional symptoms.

 *Involved skin site defines type of "tinea"

Scalp infection leads to itching, hair loss

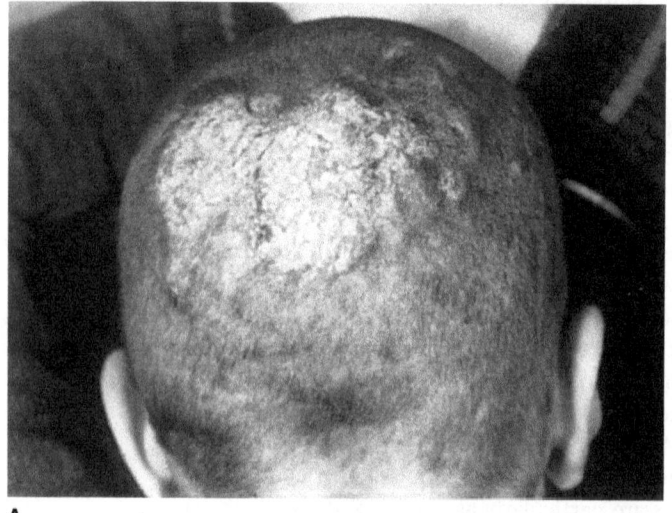

A

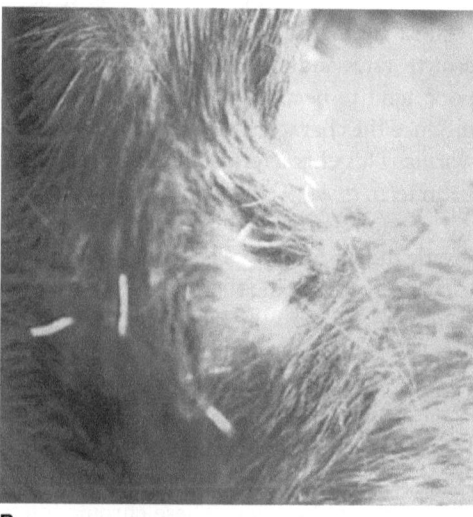

B

FIGURE 45-3. **Tinea capitis. A.** Ringworm of the scalp with superficial lesions and loss of hair. **B.** Close-up using an ultraviolet lamp (Wood's light) reveals fluorescing hair fragments. The culture grew *Microsporum audouinii*. (Reproduced with permission from Willey JM: *Prescott, Harley, & Klein's Microbiology*, 7th ed. New York, NY: McGraw Hill; 2008.)

Other sites. Skin lesions on other parts of the body begin in a similar manner and enlarge to form sharply delineated erythematous patches with central clearing (nearly normal skin appearance in the center). Multiple lesions can fuse to form unusual geometric patterns on the skin. Lesions may appear in any location, but they are particularly common in moist, sweaty skin folds. Obesity and the wearing of tight apparel increase susceptibility to infection in the groin and beneath the breasts. Another form of infection, which involves scaling and splitting of the skin between the toes, is commonly known as **athlete's foot**. Again, excessive moisture and maceration of the skin provide the mode of entry.

＊ Skin infection favors moist areas, skin folds

Nail bed infections first cause discoloration of the subungual tissue, followed by hyperkeratosis and discoloration of the nail plate. Progression of infection causes disfigurement of the nail but few symptoms until the nail plate is so dislodged or distorted that it exposes or compresses adjacent soft tissue. All dermatophyte infections provide a potential site of entry for skin bacteria, predisposing to more acute and painful lesions around the nail, or to more extensive bacterial cellulitis.

＊ Hyperkeratosis can dislodge the nail plate

 Why is it especially important to aggressively treat tinea pedis in patients with diabetes mellitus?

DIAGNOSIS

The goal of diagnostic procedures is to distinguish dermatophytoses from other causes of skin inflammation. Infections caused by bacteria, other fungi, as well as noninfectious disorders (eg, psoriasis and contact dermatitis) may have similar features. The most important step of fungal detection is microscopic examination of material taken from the lesions. Potassium hydroxide (KOH) or calcofluor white preparations of skin scrapings from the advancing edge of a dermatophyte lesion often demonstrate septate hyphae. Examination of infected hairs reveals hyphae and arthroconidia penetrating the hair shaft. Some species of dermatophyte fluoresce when exposed to ultraviolet (UV) light, and selection of hairs for examination can be aided by the use of a UV (Wood's) lamp (Figure 45–3B).

KOH mounts demonstrate hyphae

Some species fluoresce under UV light

Mild infections with typical clinical findings and positive KOH preparations are often not cultured because clinical management is not influenced significantly by the identity of the etiologic species. Suspected dermatophyte infections with negative KOH preparations, especially those that fail to respond to empiric antifungal therapy, often require culture. The same material used for direct examination can be cultured for isolation of the offending dermatophyte (**Figure 45–4**).

Culture is used when KOH preparations are negative

TREATMENT AND PREVENTION

Dermatophyte infections can usually be prevented simply by observing general hygiene measures. When they occur, many local skin infections resolve without specific antifungal therapy. Those that do not resolve may be treated with topical terbinafine or azoles (miconazole, ketoconazole). More extensive skin infections, especially those involving the scalp, often require systemic therapy with griseofulvin, itraconazole, or oral terbinafine, often combined with topical therapy. Nail infections are especially difficult to cure, likely due to the slow turnover of the infected nail and poor penetration of antifungal agents. Therapy for nail infections must be continued over weeks to months, and relapses may occur. Keratolytic agents (Whitfield's ointment) may be useful for reducing the size of hyperkeratotic lesions.

Topical terbinafine or azoles usually sufficient

Systemic antifungal agents used in refractory cases

 Think▶▶Apply 45-1: Many chronic changes occur in the skin of the feet of patients with diabetes mellitus. Due to diabetes-associated microvascular changes, the skin can become thin and dystrophic. Also, diabetes-associated peripheral neuropathy can prevent diabetic patients from noticing microtrauma to the skin that occurs during daily activity. Together, these changes predispose many diabetic patients to develop bacterial cellulitis of the lower extremities. This condition is more likely if the skin barrier is compromised by tinea pedis, allowing bacteria ready access to deeper skin layers.

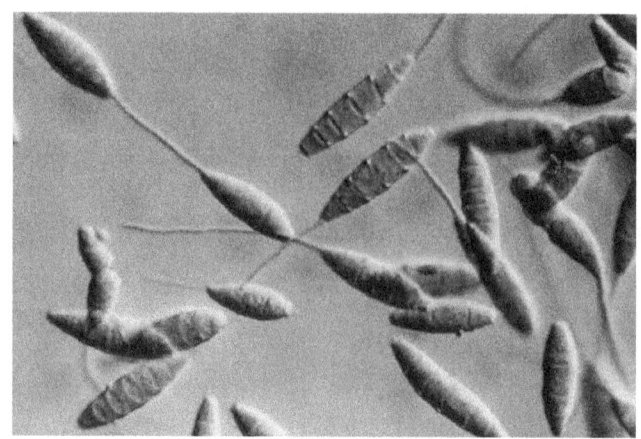

FIGURE 45–4. Large boat-shaped macroconidia of *Microsporum gypseum*. (Reproduced with permission from Nester EW, Anderson DG, Roberts CE Jr, et al: *Microbiology: A Human Perspective*, 6th ed. New York, NY: McGraw Hill; 2008.)

20 m

■ Other Superficial Mycoses

Pityriasis (tinea) versicolor is a very common superficial fungal infection of the skin. It is characterized by discrete patches of either hypopigmentation or hyperpigmentation, especially on the skin of the torso and upper arms. These lesions are associated with some scaling but minimal induration. Pityriasis versicolor is most commonly caused by fungi of the genus *Malassezia*, especially *Malassezia furfur*. These fungal species are common components of the skin microbiome, but they are present more abundantly in the setting of clinical infection. In scrapings of infected skin, they appear as clusters of budding yeast cells mixed with hyphae. *Malassezia* species grow in the yeast form in culture media enriched with lipids.

M furfur requires lipids for growth

Tinea nigra, another superficial skin infection, is characterized by brown to black macular lesions, usually on the palms or soles. There is little associated inflammation or scaling, and skin architecture is well preserved since the infection is confined to the stratum corneum. This feature distinguishes tinea nigra from other pigmented lesions such as melanomas, which tend to change the lines and markings of the skin. This infection is caused by melanized, black-pigmented fungi ("dematiaceous" fungi) such as *Hortaea werneckii*, commonly found in soil and other environmental sites. Scrapings of the lesion show brown- to black-pigmented septate hyphae.

H werneckii causes superficial pigmented lesions of hands and feet

Piedra is an infection of the hair characterized by black or white nodules attached to the hair shaft. White piedra (caused by *Trichosporon cutaneum*) infects the shaft in a hyphal form that can fragment into component buds. Black piedra (caused by *Piedraia hortae*) grows as branched hyphae in the hair shaft (Figure 45–2).

Black or white piedra infections of the hair shaft

SUBCUTANEOUS FUNGI

Many fungal pathogens can produce subcutaneous lesions as part of their disease spectrum. However, those considered here are introduced traumatically through the skin, with infection typically limited to subcutaneous tissues, lymphatic vessels, and contiguous tissues. These fungi rarely spread to distant organs. The diseases they cause include *sporotrichosis*, *chromoblastomycosis*, and *mycetoma*. Only sporotrichosis has a single specific etiologic agent, *Sporothrix schenckii*. Chromoblastomycosis and mycetoma are clinical syndromes with multiple fungal etiologies.

SPOROTHRIX

SPOROTHRIX SCHENCKII

Mold forms convert to cigar-shaped yeasts during infection

Sporothrix schenckii is a dimorphic fungus that grows as a cigar shaped, 3- to 5-mm yeast in tissues and in culture at 37°C. The mold, which grows in cultures incubated at 25°C, is presumably the infectious form in nature.

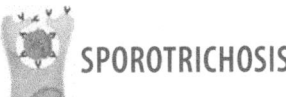 SPOROTRICHOSIS

Sporothrix schenckii is widely present in soil and other organic matter. Sporotrichosis begins with injection of the organism's conidia into the subcutaneous tissue, typically by a thorn prick or splinter in the hand. *Sporothrix schenckii* induces a slowly progressive infection that follows the lymphatic drainage from the original site (lymphangitis). Superficial ulcers may occur, but the infection rarely involves deeper structures.

EPIDEMIOLOGY

Sporothrix schenckii is a ubiquitous saprophyte particularly found in hay, moss, soil (including potting soil), and decaying vegetation, as well as the surfaces of various plants. Infection is acquired by traumatic inoculation of the fungus through the skin, often affecting gardeners, farmers, and rural laborers.

❋ Inoculated by gardener, farmer trauma

 SPOROTRICHOSIS: CLINICAL ASPECTS

MANIFESTATIONS

Skin lesions due to *S schenckii* begin as painless papules developing a few weeks to a few months after inoculation. Its location can usually be explained by occupational exposure, most often involving the hand. The initial papule enlarges slowly and eventually ulcerates, leaving an open sore. Pustular or firm nodular lesions may appear around the primary site of infection or at other sites along the lymphatic drainage route (**Figure 45–5**). The spread of infection along lymphatic channels is so characteristic for this infection that lymphangitic progression of any infection is often referred to as having a "sporotrichoid" appearance. Ulcerated lesions can become chronic, and multiple ulcers develop if the disease is untreated. Symptoms are directly related to the local areas of infection. Constitutional signs and symptoms in sporotrichosis are rare.

Skin papule ulcerates

❋ Lymphatic involvement creates multiple lesions

DIAGNOSIS

Direct microscopic examination for *S schenckii* is usually unrewarding because there are too few organisms to detect readily with KOH preparations. Even specially stained biopsy samples and serial sections are usually negative, although the presence of a histopathologic structure, the asteroid body, is suggestive. This structure is composed of *S schenckii* yeast cells surrounded by

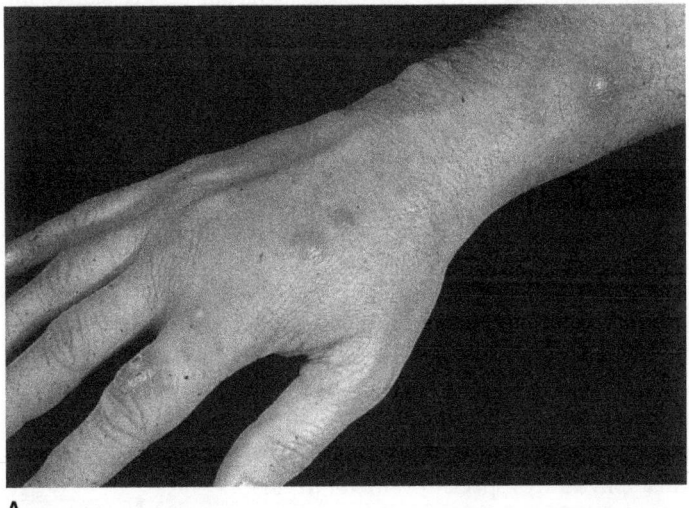 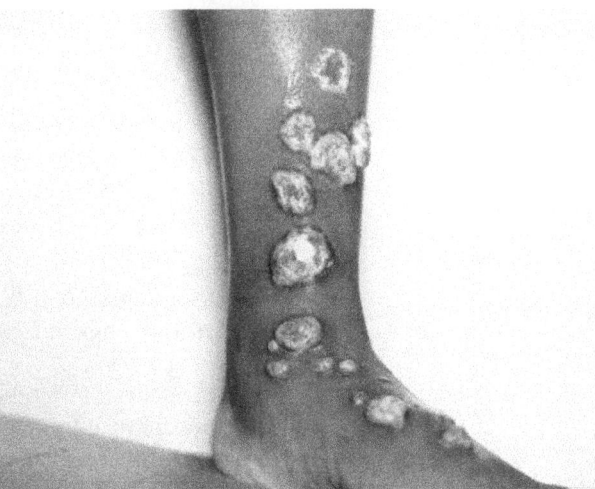

A   B

FIGURE 45–5. Sporotrichosis. A. This infection began on the finger and has started to spread up the lymphatic channels of the arm, leaving satellite lesions behind. If untreated, these lesions will evolve into ulcers. **B.** A more advanced case beginning with inoculation in the foot. (Reproduced with permission from Connor DH, Chandler FW, Schwartz DQ, et al: *Pathology of Infectious Diseases*. Stamford CT: Appleton & Lange; 1997.)

amorphous eosinophilic "rays." Definitive diagnosis depends on culture of infected pus or tissue. The organism grows within 2 to 5 days on all commonly used mycology media. Identification requires demonstration of both the typical conidia and of dimorphism.

TREATMENT AND PREVENTION

Potassium iodide replaced by itraconazole

Historically, cutaneous sporotrichosis was treated with a saturated solution of potassium iodide (SSKI) administered orally. Itraconazole is now preferred for all forms of disease, with oral terbinafine and SSKI as alternatives. Pulmonary and systemic infections may require the additional use of amphotericin B. Eradication of the environmental reservoir of *S schenckii* is not usually practical.

● CHROMOBLASTOMYCOSIS

Multiple species produce wart-like pigmented lesions in tropics

Chromoblastomycosis is a chronic form of skin infection caused by multiple species of pigmented saprophytic fungi, also known as melanized or "dematiaceous" fungi. Disease caused by *Fonsecaea*, *Phialophora*, and *Cladophialophora* (*Cladosporium*) species typically occurs on the foot or leg, the sites of skin inoculation by the fungus. Primary lesions appear as papules that develop into scaly, wart-like structures, usually under the feet. Fully developed lesions have been likened to the tips of a cauliflower. Extension occurs through painless, slowly progressive satellite lesions. The organisms are found in the soil of endemic areas, and most infections occur in individuals who work barefoot. Disseminated infections due to the dematiaceous molds are uncommon, observed almost exclusively in highly immunocompromised patients. In these patients, certain pigmented molds have a predilection for infecting the central nervous system. Therefore, in highly immunocompromised patients, the isolation of a pigmented mold from a clinical specimen cannot necessarily be ignored as a contaminant.

Brown pigmented bodies seen in chromoblastomycosis

The outstanding mycologic feature in chromoblastomycosis is the presence in histological sections of brown-pigmented, thick-walled, multiseptate, 5 to 12 mm globose structures called muriform bodies. Branching septate hyphae may also be demonstrated in KOH preparations of tissue scrapings. In culture these fungi grow as darkly pigmented molds. Surgery and antifungal therapy have been used in treatment, but cure rates of advanced disease are disappointing. Itraconazole and other mold-active azoles are the systemic antifungal agents most frequently used for this infection.

● MYCETOMA

Mycetoma is the clinical term for a chronic, disfiguring infection associated with prior trauma to the foot. This infection is caused by varied microorganisms, with more than a dozen fungi described as potential etiologies. Bacterial species such as actinomycetes and *Nocardia* species (Chapter 28) may produce a similar disease. The typical clinical appearance of mycetoma is that of massive induration with draining sinuses. Some of the fungi that cause mycetoma are geographically widespread. Most cases, however, occur in the tropics, probably because the chronically damp, macerated skin of the feet among those who go barefoot. An illustrative case of mycetoma occurred in a college rower in Seattle; he was the only member of his shell who insisted on rowing barefoot.

❋ Massive inflammatory lesions of feet with draining sinuses

Multiple species involved

Trauma to bare feet injects fungi

Once infection is established, treatment of mycetoma is difficult, often requiring combined surgical and antimicrobial therapy depending on the causative microbe. Mycetomas cause by environmental molds may demonstrate hyphae in biopsied tissue. However, these fungal elements may be difficult to demonstrate because of a tendency to form microcolony granules. The definitive diagnosis of the etiological agent often requires culture of infected tissue.

SUMMARY

- Superficial fungal infections are frequently self-limited and can often be treated with topical antifungal therapy.
- Dermatophytes infect the superficial, keratinized layers of the skin.
- Dermatophyte infections are generally diagnosed as a clinical syndrome, named for the infected body site (eg, tinea capitis, tinea pedis).
- Nail infections caused by dermatophytes are especially difficult to cure.
- Pityriasis (tinea) versicolor, caused by *M furfur*, manifests as patches of hypo- or hyper-pigmented lesions of the skin of the torso and proximal extremities.
- Sporotrichosis begins by inoculation of the skin with soil or plant material, and often spreads along regional lymphatics as nodules and ulcers.

CLINICAL CASE
Head Bump

A 4-year-old boy was taken by his mother to the family doctor for evaluation of a 2-month history of a slowly growing "bump" on the back of his head. The boy had no other siblings or any pets at home. He attended a day care center each weekday. Examination revealed a happy, alert child in no distress. A raised, scaling lesion 3.5 cm in diameter with a few pinpoint pustules was present on the posterior scalp. A KOH preparation of material from the lesion was negative. A fungal culture of material from the lesion was later positive for a fungus with numerous microconidia and macroconidia typical of *Microsporum* species.

QUESTIONS

1. What is the most likely source of this child's infection?
   A. Parents
   B. Child at day care center
   C. Animal
   D. Insect
   E. Food

2. What is the human niche where this organism proliferates best?
   A. Fibronectin
   B. Macrophages
   C. M cells
   D. Keratin

3. What additional examination might have revealed this infection while the child was in the doctor's office?
   A. X-ray
   B. Serologic test
   C. Ultraviolet light
   D. Biopsy
   E. DNA probe

ANSWERS

1. (B)
2. (D)
3. (C)

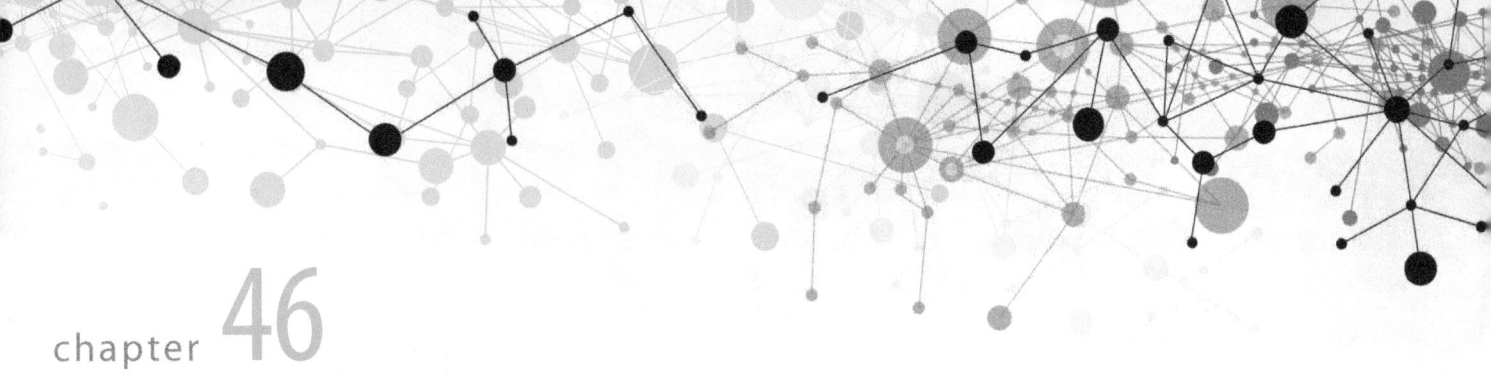

chapter 46

The Opportunistic Fungi: *Candida, Aspergillus,* the Zygomycetes, and *Pneumocystis*

Candida albicans • Candida glabrata • Candida krusei • Candida tropicalis • Candida parapsilosis • Candida auris •

Aspergillus fumigatus • Absidia species • Rhizopus species • Mucor species • Pneumocystis jirovecii

The "opportunistic fungi" are usually found as members of the resident human microbiota or on decaying matter in the environment. With the breakdown of host defenses, they can cause infections ranging from skin/mucous membrane involvement to life-threatening, systemic disease. The most common opportunistic infections are caused by two species: the yeast *Candida albicans,* a common inhabitant of the gastrointestinal and genital microbiota; and the mold *Aspergillus fumigatus* which is widespread in the environment. *Pneumocystis,* a frequent cause of pneumonia in AIDS patients, is an unusual fungus that used to be considered a parasite on morphologic grounds. However, it too is a frequent colonizer of the human respiratory tract. The diseases caused by these opportunistic fungi are summarized in **Table 46–1**.

● CANDIDA

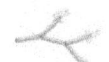 **MYCOLOGY**

Candida species grow in multiple morphologic forms, most often as a budding yeast. *C albicans* is also able to form hypha-like structures triggered by changes in conditions such as temperature, pH, and available nutrients. When observed in their initial stages of germination from the yeast cell, these nascent hyphae resemble sprouts and are called "germ tubes" (**Figure 46–2A**). Most *C albicans* strains produce germ tubes when incubated in the presence of serum, allowing a rapid means of distinguishing this species from other *Candida* species. Other elongated forms with restrictions at regular intervals are called **pseudohyphae** because they lack the parallel walls and septation of true hyphae. Germ tube–negative strains may be further identified biochemically or reported as "yeast not *C albicans*," depending on their apparent clinical significance.

✳ *C albicans* morphologies: yeast, hyphae, and pseudohyphae

TABLE 46–1				
ORGANISM	TISSUE	CULTURE AT 37°C	SOURCE	INFECTION
Candida	Yeast (hyphae)*ᵃ*	Yeast	Endogenous	Skin, mucous membranes, urinary tract, disseminated
Aspergillus	Hyphae (septate)	Mold	Environment	Lung, disseminated
*Zygomycetes*ᵇ	Hyphae (nonseptate)	Mold	Environment	Rhinocerebral, lung, disseminated
Pneumocystis	Elliptical spores	Noneᶜ	Unknown	Pneumonia

ᵃLess common feature; pseudohyphae are produced as well.
ᵇCommon genera include Absidia, Mucor, Rhizopus.
ᶜHas not been grown in culture.

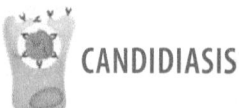

CANDIDIASIS

OVERVIEW

Candidiasis occurs in localized and disseminated forms. Localized disease often presents as erythema and white plaques in moist skinfolds (diaper rash/intertrigo) or on mucosal surfaces (oral thrush). It may also cause the itching and thick white discharge of vulvovaginitis. *Candida* bloodstream and urinary tract infections (UTIs) are especially common among hospitalized patients with intravenous and urinary catheters. Deep tissue and disseminated infections are limited almost exclusively to the immunocompromised.

EPIDEMIOLOGY

C albicans is present in the microbiota of 30% to 50% of healthy persons, especially common in the oropharyngeal, gastrointestinal, and female genital tracts. Most infections, even those occurring in hospitalized patients, are thought to arise from one's own resident species. However, transmission and new acquisition of *Candida* colonization can occur by direct mucosal contact with others (eg, through sexual intercourse). Other factors that increase the risk of *Candida* infections include invasive procedures, indwelling intravascular devices, and the prolonged use of antibacterial agents.

✳ Infections from endogenous flora entering deep tissues via intravascular devices

PATHOGENESIS

The ability of *Candida* species to change between the yeast and hyphal forms is strongly associated with its pathogenic potential, and these different morphological forms are likely required for different phases of candidiasis (**Figure 46–1**). In histologic preparations, hyphal structures are seen during *Candida* invasion, either superficially into the mucosa or within deep tissues (Figure 46–3). However, systemic dissemination in the bloodstream most likely occurs by smaller

Transitions between yeast and hyphae important for invasion, dissemination

FIGURE 46–1. *Candida albicans.* This scanning electron micrograph demonstrates dimorphism with both yeast-like cells and hyphae. (Reproduced with permission from Willey JM: *Prescott, Harley, & Klein's Microbiology*, 7th ed. New York, NY: McGraw Hill; 2008.)

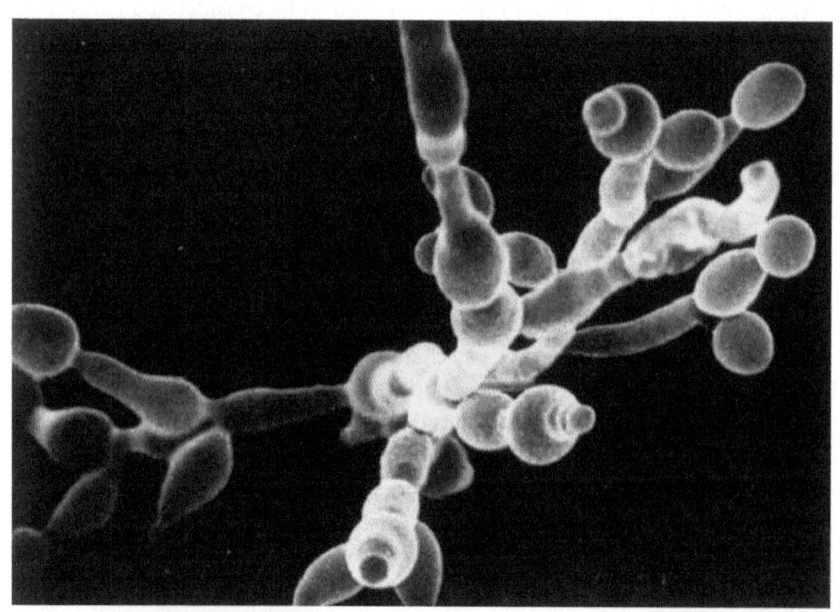

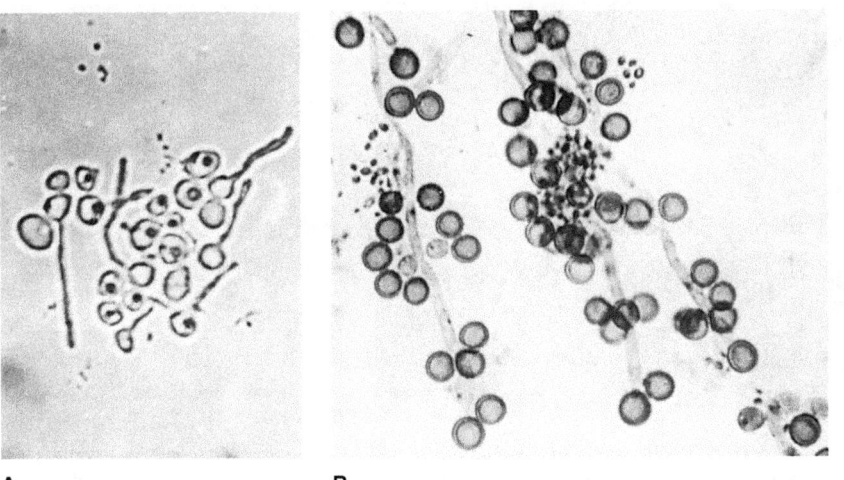

A   B

FIGURE 46–2. *Candida albicans.* **A.** When incubated at 37°C and in the presence of serum, *C albicans* rapidly forms elongated hyphae called germ tubes. **B.** On specialized media, *C albicans* forms thick-walled chlamydoconidia, which differentiate it from other *Candida* species.

yeast-like forms. Therefore, it is the plasticity between yeast and hyphal forms, rather than one morphology or the other, that results in the ability of *C albicans* to so effectively colonize and infect the host (**Figure 46–4**). The yeast-hyphal switch can be controlled *in vitro* by the manipulation of a wide variety of environmental conditions (serum, pH, temperature, amino acids). Various sensors and signaling pathways for morphogenesis have been described, including those in which *C albicans* induces its own morphological change by directly altering the local pH.

Switch triggered by environment

One of the most important pathogenic features of *C albicans* is its ability to form biofilms. These complex structures include yeast and hyphal forms of the fungus along with host-derived proteins. Once formed, the biofilm strongly adheres to components of the extracellular matrix (ECM) as well as to plastics. Neither host immune cells nor antifungal agents are able to penetrate *Candida* biofilms well, making this structure an important source of microbial persistence during infection. In a very practical sense, fungal biofilms that develop on prosthetic surfaces (eg, intravenous catheters, prosthetic joints, prosthetic heart valves) are almost impossible to sterilize without device removal.

Fungal biofilms adhere to surfaces and inhibit immune cell function and antifungal penetration

Many factors predispose to both local and invasive *Candida* infections. Antibacterial therapy reduces microbial competition on mucosal surfaces and increases the relative abundance of *C albicans* within the microbiota. Alterations in innate immunity (eg, leukopenia or corticosteroid therapy) or adaptive immunity (eg, AIDS) are important contributing factors to systemic and mucosal candidiasis. Additionally, anatomic disruptions of the skin and mucosa may enhance the invasion process by exposing *Candida* binding sites in the ECM, and by allowing direct access to deeper tissues. Biofilm formation on medical devices also contributes to fungal persistence in this host. Diabetes mellitus predisposes to *C albicans* infection, possibly due to greater production of surface mannoproteins in the presence of high glucose concentrations.

Antimicrobials, immunosuppression increase risk

Disruptions provide access to ECM

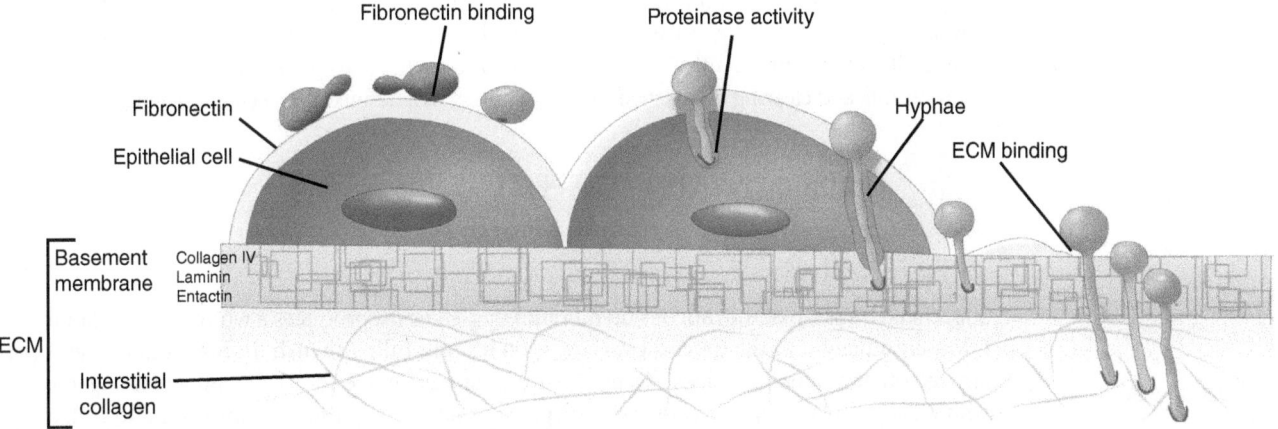

FIGURE 46–3. **Pathogenesis of *Candida albicans* infections.** Proposed mechanisms of *C albicans* attachment and invasion are shown. Surface glycoproteins on the yeast may bind to fibronectin covering the host epithelial cell, or to elements of the extracellular matrix (ECM) when the epithelial surface is disrupted. Invasion is associated with formation of hyphae and production of proteinases, which may digest tissue elements.

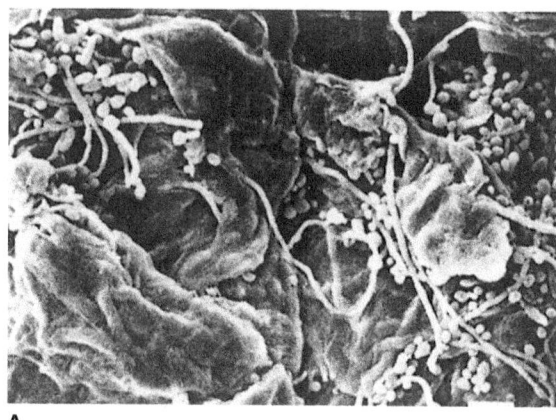 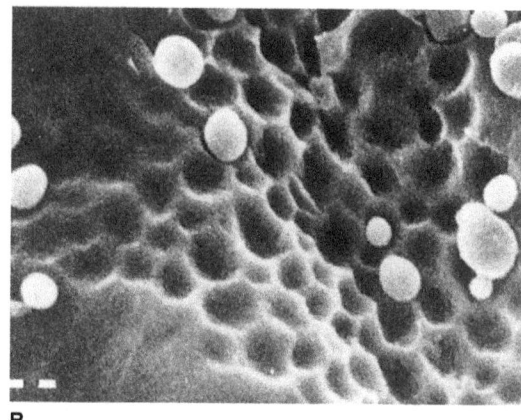

A   **B**

FIGURE 46–4. Invasiveness of *Candida albicans*. Two features of *C albicans* invasiveness are seen in these scanning electron micrographs taken from experiments with murine corneocytes. **A.** Both yeast-like and hyphal elements are present. The filamentous elements spread over the surface and invade the cell cuticle. **B.** A *C albicans* strain that produces a protease is seen producing cavity-like depressions in the cell surface. This activity could play a role in invasion of host tissue. (Reproduced with permission of Ray TL, Payne CD: Scanning electron microscopy of epidermal adherence and cavitation in murine candidiasis: a role for Candida acid proteinase, *Infect Immunol* 1988;Aug;56(8):1942–1949.)

IMMUNITY

As a mucosal colonizer, *C albicans* is in continuous contact with epithelial cells and innate immune effectors. At this interface, the epithelial cells secrete potent antifungal peptides, such as candidalysin, that nonspecifically inhibit fungal growth. These mucosal lining cells are also the initiators of more specific antifungal immunity mediated by the binding of host receptors (EphA2, EGFR/Her2, E-cadherin) to fungal surface features such as β-glucans and Als adhesin proteins. These receptor-ligand interactions result in NF-kB and MAP kinase-mediated activation of proinflammatory cytokines and chemokines leading to the recruitment of macrophages, polymorphonuclear neutrophils (PMNs), and Th17 cells. These latter cells also induce further antimicrobial peptides such as β-defensins.

Many immunodeficiency syndromes involving T-lymphocyte dysfunction result in severe mucocutaneous candidiasis, emphasizing the importance of this arm of the immune system in defense against mucosal *Candida* infections. For example, patients with AIDS develop frequent episodes of oral and esophageal candidiasis, suggesting that protection against mucosal infections involves CD4-mediated immune responses.

Systemic candidiasis is most frequently a disease involving device biofilms and the disruption of protective anatomic barriers. Once introduced into distant sites through the bloodstream, *C albicans* cells are readily recognized by innate immune cells such as neutrophils and resident macrophages. This occurs through the recognition of fungal surface components such as β-glucans by host pattern recognition receptors, including dectin-1. Innate humoral elements, including complement proteins, play an important role in enhancing fungal cell phagocytosis and recruiting additional immune cells to local sites of infection. Anti-*Candida* antibodies are readily detected in most people, but their role in preventing and clearing established infections is less well defined than cellular defenses.

Epithelial cells secrete antifungal peptides

Th17 immunity mediator of protection

Host pattern recognition receptors identify fungal surface features, activate immunity

 ## CANDIDIASIS: CLINICAL ASPECTS

MANIFESTATIONS

Superficial invasion of the mucous membranes by *C albicans* produces a white, cheesy plaque that is loosely adherent to the mucosal surface. Oral lesions, called **thrush,** occur on the tongue, palate, and other mucosal surfaces as ragged white patches (**Figure 46–5**). Scraping the fungal plaque with a tongue blade will reveal varying degrees of underlying mucosal invasion and inflammation, helping to differentiate this infectious process from other causes of superficial oral films. Similarly, **vulvovaginal candidiasis** presents with a thick, curd-like vaginal discharge and itching. Although many women have at least one episode of vulvovaginal candidiasis in a lifetime, a small proportion suffers chronic, recurrent infections.

✳ White mucosal plaque called thrush

✳ Vaginitis may be recurrent

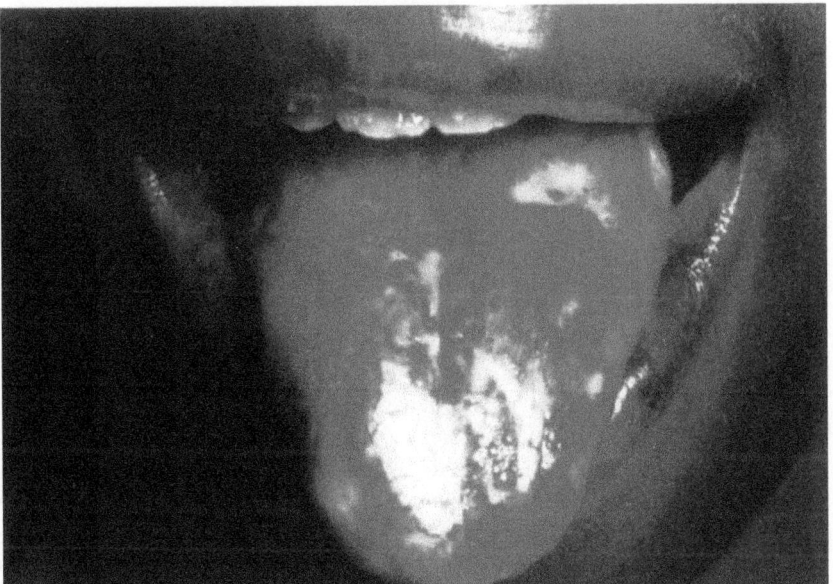

FIGURE 46–5. **Thrush.** The white plaques on this AIDS patient's tongue are caused by *Candida albicans*. (Reproduced with permission from Willey JM: *Prescott, Harley, & Klein's Microbiology,* 7th ed. New York, NY: McGraw Hill; 2008.)

Superficial *C albicans* infections also occur in skin folds and other areas in which wet, macerated skin surfaces are opposed. For example, one type of diaper rash is caused by *C albicans* (**Figure 46–6A**). Other infections of the skinfolds and appendages occur in association with recurrent immersion in water (eg, dishwashers). The initial lesions are erythematous papules or confluent areas of erythema, tenderness, and skin fissures. Infection usually remains confined to the chronically irritated area with adjacent "satellite" lesions.

✴ Macerated skin a common site of infection

Rarely, chronic and relapsing *Candida* infections occur in patients with a specific defect in T_H1 immune defenses. This condition, known as **chronic mucocutaneous candidiasis (CMC)**, manifests with recurrent severe skin and mucosal lesions. With time, patients with CMC experience considerable skin disfigurement. Although lesions may become extensive, they usually do not result in fungal dissemination.

In contrast, most people live their entire lives in constant contact with *C albicans* but without developing symptomatic infections. This observation largely reflects the ability of normal hosts to effectively control the growth of this fungus. However, *Candida* colonization without associated symptomatic inflammation may also represent a clinical example of immunologic tolerance—to be able to be exposed to a microorganism without developing an excessive immune response. Therefore, it is possible that a subset of patients with frequent episodes of symptomatic candidiasis (eg, recurrent vulvovaginal candidiasis) actually fails to appropriately suppress an over-exuberant immune reaction to resident fungi, as opposed to defects controlling microbial growth.

Chronic mucocutaneous candidiasis is associated with specific T-cell defects

Inflammatory patches similar to those in thrush may also develop in the esophagus and upper GI tract. These lesions occur most frequently in immunocompromised patients and are characterized

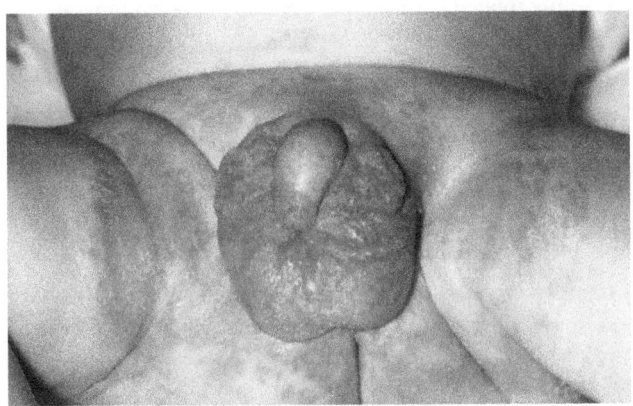

A

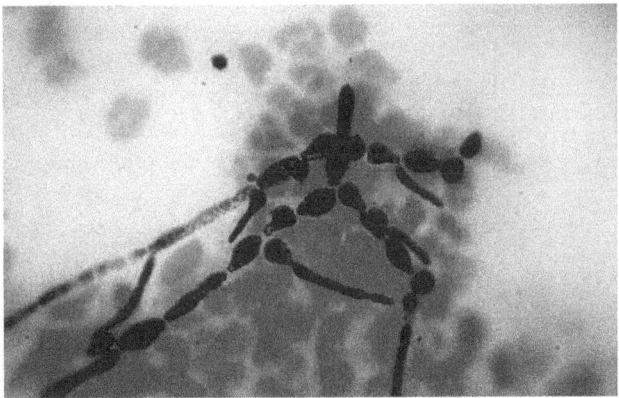

B

FIGURE 46–6. *Candida albicans* **skin infection. A.** This rash is preceded by chronically damp skin in the diaper area. **B.** This Gram stain demonstrates yeast cells and pseudohyphae. (Reproduced with permission from Nester EW, Anderson DG, Roberts CE Jr, et al: *Microbiology: A Human Perspective,* 6th ed. New York, NY: McGraw Hill; 2008.)

* Esophagitis, intestinal candidiasis similar to thrush

by painful swallowing or substernal chest pain. Extensive ulcerations, scarring, and occasionally perforation of the esophagus may ensue.

In addition to infection of mucosal surfaces, Candida infection often involve the urinary tract. Ascending infections may produce cystitis, pyelonephritis, renal abscesses, or expanding fungus ball lesions in the renal pelvis. Patients with urinary catheters, kidney transplants, or other types of chronic urinary devices are at risk for these infections.

UTIs ascending or hematogenous

Disseminated candidiasis associated with high mortality

Endophthalmitis appears as white cotton-like retinal lesions

Disseminated infections are the most serious forms of candidiasis, associated with a very high attributable mortality. These infections occur most frequently in hospitalized patients, and the fungus often gains access to the bloodstream through disruptions of the skin (eg, burns, intravascular catheters), alterations of the GI tract (eg, intestinal perforations, abdominal surgery), or prosthetic devices colonized with *Candida* biofilms. Once in the bloodstream, *Candida* species can infect many organs, including the kidneys, brain, and heart valves. Patients with candidemia typically have fever and a sepsis-like syndrome. However, these symptoms are generally not sufficiently characteristic to suggest *C albicans* over bacterial pathogens. Importantly, disseminated candidiasis frequently involves the eye. *Candida* **endophthalmitis** has the characteristic funduscopic appearance of a white cotton ball expanding on the retina or floating free in the vitreous humor. Endophthalmitis and infections of other eye structures can lead to blindness, and ocular complications must be considered in cases of disseminated candidiasis.

- **What specific interventions might limit the incidence of mucosal candidiasis (oral thrush and vaginal candidiasis) in immunologically normal hosts?**
- **What specific interventions might limit the incidence of candidemia in hospitalized patients?**

DIAGNOSIS

KOH and Gram smears show yeast and hyphae

Readily grown in routine culture

Exudate or epithelial scrapings examined by KOH preparations (Figure 46–6B) demonstrate abundant budding yeast cells; if associated hyphae/pseudohyphae are present, the infection is almost certainly caused by *C albicans*. *C albicans* is readily isolated in culture from clinical specimens including blood. Cultures from respiratory specimens, such as sputum, run the risk of contamination from yeasts present in the normal oropharyngeal flora.

Deep organ involvement is difficult to prove without a direct aspirate or biopsy. However, *Candida* species often grow in routine blood cultures, and every episode of candidemia must be carefully evaluated for evidence of dissemination, endophthalmitis, and involvement of prosthetic devices.

TREATMENT

* Topical nystatin or azoles for superficial lesions

* Amphotericin B, fluconazole, and echinocandins for invasive disease

C albicans is usually susceptible to amphotericin B, nystatin, flucytosine, the echinocandins, and the azoles. Superficial infections are generally treated with topical nystatin or azole preparations. Measures to decrease moisture and chronic trauma are important adjuncts in treating *Candida* skin infections. All *C albicans* infections may also require addressing predisposing conditions. For example, removal of an infected catheter, control of diabetes, or optimizing underlying medical conditions can be important aspects of the complete treatment of infection. Systemic therapy with amphotericin B, echinocandins, or azoles is required for disseminated or deep tissue infections.

Think ▸▸ Apply 46-1: **Many cases of oral thrush could be prevented by limiting unnecessary antibacterial use, avoiding the associated disruption of the mucosal microbiota that predisposes to yeast overgrowth. Candidemia can be limited by minimizing unnecessary intravenous and urinary catheter use in hospitalized patients. In healthcare settings, adherence to good hand-hygiene limits spread from person to person.**

The choice of treatment is often guided by speciation and antifungal susceptibility testing. Fluconazole has been effective treatment for CMC and recurrent mucosal infections, although antifungal resistance can develop with the prolonged use of this agent.

OTHER CANDIDA SPECIES

Candida species other than *C albicans* can produce very similar infections to those described above, especially disseminated and UTI. However, these non-albicans *Candida* species are isolated almost exclusively from patients with nosocomial infections. Antibiotic use, wounds, and prosthetic devices predispose hospitalized patients to infections with diverse *Candida* species. Some species, such as *C glabrata, C krusei,* and *C auris* display increased levels of resistance to the azole antifungals. Therefore, these species may selectively colonize patients previously treated with azoles. Other *Candida* species, including *C tropicalis* and *C parapsilosis,* are often more susceptible to standard antifungals, but they are also isolated mostly from hospitalized patients, perhaps arising from the altered microbiota resulting from the hospital environment. Nosocomial transmission of *Candida* species may occur with poor adherence to proper handwashing and other infection control practices.

* Hospitalization increases risk for non-*albicans Candida*

* *C glabrata, C krusei, C auris* often resistant to azoles

● *ASPERGILLUS*

 **MYCOLOGY**

Aspergillus species are rapidly growing molds that are frequently isolated from the environment and thus are common causes of infections in patients with severe immune compromising conditions. Both in culture and during infection, *Aspergillus* species grow as branching **septate hyphae**. With prolonged culture in the laboratory, fruiting bodies develop as sites of spore (conidia) formation. Individual species are identified based on differences in the structure of the **conidiophore** and the arrangement of the **conidia**. (**Figure 46-7A–C**). The most common cause of infections in humans is *A fumigatus,* but others species, such as *A flavus, A niger,* and *A terreus* may less frequently cause human disease. For all of these species, fluffy colonies appear in 1 to 2 days; by 5 days, hyphal growth may cover an entire culture plate.

Species are distinguished based on arrangement of conidia on the conidiophore

● ASPERGILLOSIS

OVERVIEW

Invasive aspergillosis occurs in highly immunocompromised persons, often rapidly resulting in death. Patients at highest risk for this infection typically have prolonged neutropenia due to treatments for hematological malignancies, or perhaps those undergoing hematopoietic stem cell transplantation. Most infections are acquired by inhaling infectious spores from the environment. Fever and a dry cough may be the only clinical signs of early aspergillosis, even before lung consolidation is demonstrated radiologically. Finding definitive evidence for *Aspergillus* infections is challenging. Therefore, many patients are treated empirically for this condition when suspicious lung infiltrates are observed in the setting of profound immunosuppression.

EPIDEMIOLOGY

Aspergillus species are widely distributed in nature and throughout the world. They seem to adapt to a wide range of environmental conditions, and the heat-resistant conidia provide a good mechanism for dispersal. Like bacterial spores, the fungal conidia survive well in the environment, and human infection is most commonly caused by inhalation. Outbreaks of pulmonary aspergillosis in hospitals have been traced to fungal spores transmitted through air ducts, emphasizing the potential for environmental acquisition of infection. Similarly, building construction and remodeling have also been associated with increased frequency of *Aspergillus* infections. Hospital wards with highly immunocompromised patients often use specialized air filtration devices to limit patient exposure to these environmental fungi.

Conidia may be spread through air ducts in hospital units

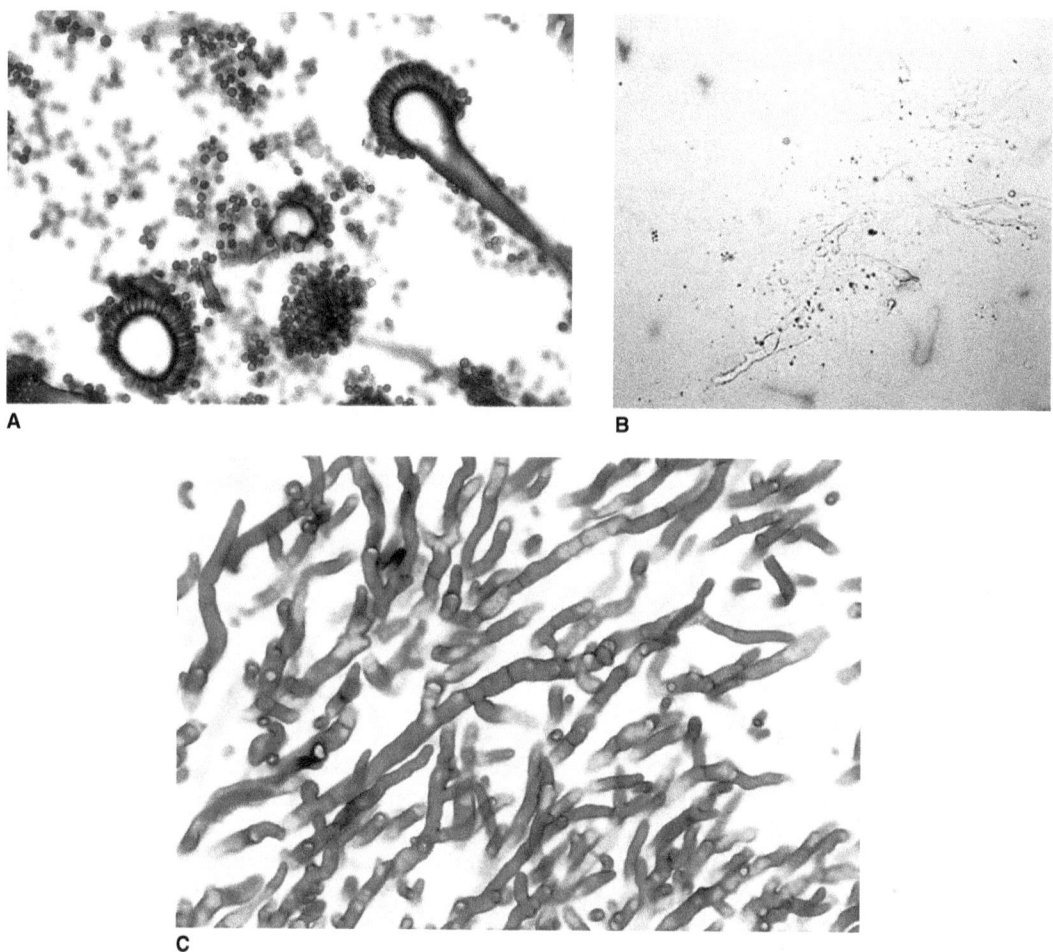

FIGURE 46–7. ***Aspergillus.* A.** This asexual conidium-forming structure is characteristic of *Aspergillus* species. The conidia are borne at the end of the finger-like extensions at the end of the conidiophore. These structures are rarely produced *in vivo.* **B.** This tissue aspirate mixed with KOH shows branching, septate hyphae. **C.** Histologic sections also show branching, septate hyphae, but because the conidia shown in A are not seen, the findings are not diagnostic of *Aspergillus.* (A and C, Reproduced with permission from Connor DH, Chandler FW, Schwartz DQ, et al: *Pathology of Infectious Diseases.* Stamford CT: Appleton & Lange; 1997.)

PATHOGENESIS

Once inhaled, *Aspergillus* conidia are small enough to readily reach the terminal airways and alveoli. However, the resident innate immune cells are able to suppress the germination of these cells into growing hyphae. Therefore, lung infections due to *Aspergillus* species are exceeding rare in people with normal immune systems. Host factors favoring *Aspergillus* growth include anatomic abnormalities of the lungs (eg, bronchiectasis, severe emphysema) and immunosuppression (neutropenia, lung transplantation).

Inhaled conidia reach terminal airways

IMMUNITY

Macrophages, particularly pulmonary alveolar macrophages, are the first line of defense against inhaled *Aspergillus* conidia, phagocytosing and killing them prior to germination. For the conidia that survive and germinate, PMNs become the primary defense. They are able to attach to the growing hyphae, generate an oxidative burst, and secrete reactive oxygen intermediates. Patients with AIDS rarely develop pulmonary or disseminated aspergillosis, suggesting that adaptive, T-cell mediated immunity is less important than innate immune mechanisms in controlling and preventing this infection. Antibodies to *Aspergillus* fungal elements are formed during infection, but their protective value is incompletely defined.

✴ Alveolar macrophages kill conidia

✴ PMNs attack hyphae

ASPERGILLOSIS: CLINICAL ASPECTS

MANIFESTATIONS

Aspergillus infections typically present in one of four major ways, with the clinical findings completely dependent on the immune status of the host. These clinical presentations include: (1) *Aspergillus* pneumonia, (2) disseminated aspergillosis, (3) allergic respiratory disease, and (4) aspergilloma (fungus ball).

***Aspergillus* pneumonia.** As the main site of fungal cell entry into the body, the lung is the primary organ involved in most cases of aspergillosis. Although innate immune responses in the lung are usually able to clear *Aspergillus* spores as they are inhaled, anatomic and immune defects can allow this fungus to grow and establish infection. Patients with severe forms of emphysema and bronchiectasis, including those with cystic fibrosis, have regions of anatomic abnormalities within their lungs that offer protected sites for fungal germination and growth. Resident lung macrophages and neutrophils are less effective at controlling fungal growth in these regions of scarring and tissue destruction within the airways and lung parenchyma. In the presence of an intact immune system, the infection is unable to deeply penetrate into the surrounding lung tissue or to disseminate. However, this smoldering infection can result in symptoms of chronic bronchopneumonia, with flares of cough and worsening respiratory function.

In contrast, patients with severe defects of immunity, such as solid-organ transplantation or neutropenia, can develop a progressive and immediately life-threatening pneumonia due to *Aspergillus* species. This rapidly progressive infection does not require prior lung anatomic abnormalities, and it emphasizes the importance of the innate immune system in preventing fungal colonization and growth. During invasive pulmonary aspergillosis, the fungal hyphae penetrate intact lung tissue and blood vessels, leading to local necrosis (Figure 46–7C). Symptoms include fever, cough, hemoptysis, and respiratory failure. Rapidly progressive lung infiltrates are often observed radiographically. Untreated, this infection quickly leads to death. Even in the presence of antifungal therapy, cure of this infection often requires restoration of immune function (eg, recovery from neutropenia, reduction of transplant immunosuppression). When feasible, surgical debridement of infected tissue combined with antifungals may favor patient survival.

* Pulmonary aspergillosis in immunocompromised patient highly invasive

Disseminated aspergillosis. Once a primary *Aspergillus* infection is established in an immunocompromised patient, the fungus can disseminate through the bloodstream to affect any organ system in the body. The most dreaded site of spread is the central nervous system. The symptoms of disseminated infection will depend on the organs affected. However, changes in mental status, or other specific organ dysfunction, should always prompt a thorough clinical investigation in immunosuppressed patients. isseminated aspergillosis carries a high mortality rate. Therefore, much effort has gone into developing rapid diagnostic and preventive strategies in neutropenic patients, since delays in the treatment of invasive aspergillosis (IA) are associated with worse survival.

Allergic respiratory disease. As ubiquitous components of the air, fungal spores are typically captured by mucus present in our respiratory tract. In patients with allergic tendencies, the accumulation of excessive mucus in the airways may provide a growth substrate for inhaled fungi. After germinating, these fungal elements are not able to invade the underlying respiratory tissue, nor are they able to disseminate from this initial growth site. However, as potent allergens, the fungi may induce a cycle of progressive inflammation, creating enhanced mucinous substrate for fungal growth. The growth of environmental *Aspergillus* species in the sinuses and larger airways can cause chronic allergic symptoms in susceptible patients. Allergic sinus disease due to fungi is thought to be an especially common cause of chronic sinusitis.

Of note, children with severe forms of asthma are especially prone to develop a condition known as allergic bronchopulmonary aspergillosis (ABPA), characterized by eosinophilia, symptomatic asthma flares, cough, and respiratory distress. Anti-*Aspergillus* antibodies can often be detected in the bloodstream. During flares of ABPA, fleeting infiltrates may be seen on chest radiographs. These infiltrates do not reflect invasive fungal disease, but rather extensive inflammation due to the allergic reaction to fungal antigens. This condition is treated with antiallergy therapy (eg, inhaled/systemic corticosteroids, antihistamines, immunotherapy) rather than antifungals.

Allergic disease marked by eosinophilia and specific anti-*Aspergillus* IgG

Treated with antiallergy therapy and not antifungals

Aspergilloma (fungus ball). Patients with prior lung infections can develop pulmonary scarring and cavities. Historically, this was especially common in patients with old, healed pulmonary tuberculosis. Fungal spores that found their way into these cavities were often able to grow into macroscopic fungal colonies. These "balls" of fungal hyphae appear radiographically as round regions of consolidation inside of old lung cavities. Unable to penetrate into the surrounding tissues, these fungus balls nonetheless are often able to induce mechanical trauma to the wall of the lung cavity. Patients with aspergillomas therefore often experience recurrent episodes of hemoptysis. If large blood vessels are present near these cavities, life-threatening bleeding can occur. Antifungal therapy may help some patients with this condition. However, cavity removal or catheter-guided embolization of involved lung vessels may be required for recurrent hemorrhages due to aspergillomas.

Fungus ball in lung cavities can injure surrounding blood vessels, cause hemoptysis

DIAGNOSIS

Aspergillus can often be isolated and identified in cultures of infected tissue. The diagnostic problem is distinguishing *Aspergillus* contamination and colonization from invasive disease. However, the isolation of a pathogenic *Aspergillus* species from a susceptible host with a consistent clinical setting is highly suggestive of IA. The diagnosis often requires invasive techniques such as lung biopsy or bronchoalveolar lavage (BAL). Fungal growth from infected material is demonstrated by the presence of branching, septate hyphae (Figure 46–7B and C). Infrequently, the complete fruiting bodies are produced *in vivo*, creating a striking and diagnostic histologic picture (Figure 46–7A). Serological demonstration of anti-*Aspergillus* antibodies may be helpful in suggesting allergic aspergillosis, but they have little value in defining invasive disease. Immunoassays detecting circulating *Aspergillus* antigens (galactomannan, glucans) are also helpful, especially when used serially in neutropenic patients to detect preclinical infections.

Direct aspirate or biopsy often required

Serodiagnosis useful for allergic disease

Antigen testing helpful in neutropenic patients

 Why would rapid and noninvasive diagnostic tests be important advances for invasive aspergillosis?

TREATMENT AND PREVENTION

The mold-active azoles are the preferred treatments for IA. Echinocandins and amphotericin B are alternatives. No regimen is considered highly effective because the mortality rate of invasive disease is high; therefore, azoles are often used as prophylactic agents in susceptible patients. Surgical removal of infected tissue is sometimes helpful, even in the brain. Construction of rooms with filtered air has been effective in reducing exposure to environmental conidia.

✳ **Mold-active azoles, amphotericin B, echinocandins, and surgery**

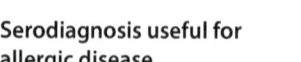 **ZYGOMYCETES AND ZYGOMYCOSIS/MUCORMYCOSIS**

Zygomycosis (mucormycosis) refers to infection with the zygomycete fungi, including *Absidia*, *Rhizopus*, and *Mucor* species. These fungi are ubiquitous decomposers in soil and are commonly found growing on bread and many other foods. Infections are most common in patients with neutropenia. Zygomycetes occasionally cause disease in persons with diabetes mellitus (especially those with frequent episodes of diabetic ketoacidosis) and in immunosuppressed patients receiving corticosteroid therapy.

Similar to aspergillosis, pulmonary or rhinocerebral mucormycosis is acquired by inhalation of conidia from the environment. The pulmonary form has clinical findings similar to those of other

Absidia, Rhizopus, and *Mucor* soil saprophytes

✳ **Immunocompromised hosts infected**

 Think▶▶Apply 46-2: **Due to the devastated immune system of most patients with IA, this infection can progress rapidly, leading to patient death. Culture-based diagnostic tests are rarely positive in this infection, perhaps due to poor access to adequate specimens. Patients with neutropenia (low neutrophils) are also frequently thrombocytopenic (low platelets), making clinicians hesitant to biopsy infected tissue due to concerns for hemorrhage. Delays in diagnosis and treatment of IA are associated with poor survival.**

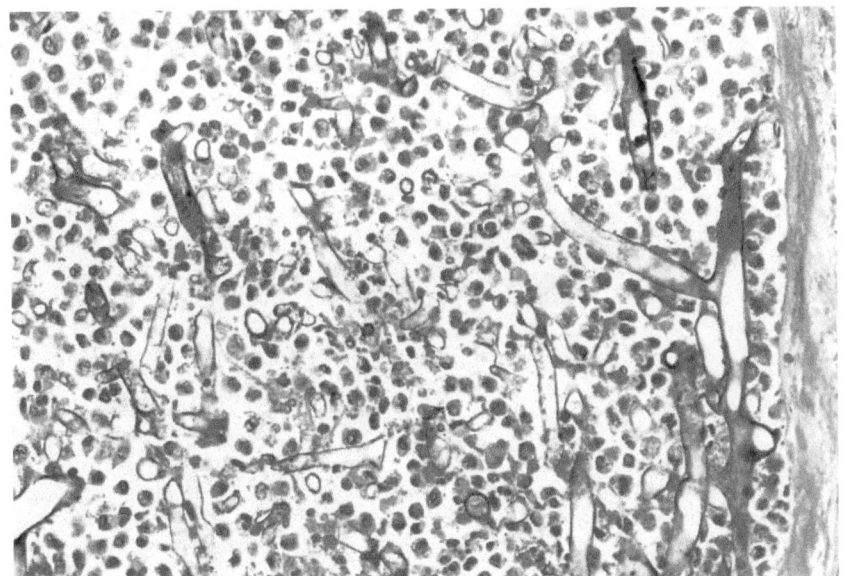

FIGURE 46–8. Zygomycosis. This zygomycete has invaded a blood vessel. Note the ribbon-like hyphae without septation. (Reproduced with permission from Connor DH, Chandler FW, Schwartz DQ, et al: *Pathology of Infectious Diseases.* Stamford CT: Appleton & Lange; 1997.)

fungal pneumonias, with dense pulmonary consolidation. In rhinocerebral mucormycosis, the infecting fungi penetrate the mucosa of the nose, paranasal sinuses, or palate, often resulting in ulcerative lesions. Once beyond the mucosa, they progress through tissue, nerves, blood vessels, and fascial planes, potentially reaching the base of the brain. This clinical syndrome typically begins with sinus symptoms and headache, rapidly progressing to orbital cellulitis, cranial nerve palsy, vascular thrombosis, coma, and death.

Pulmonary disease similar to other fungi

Sinus infections can erode to the brain

The pathologic findings in mucormycosis are distinctive: zygomycetes all show ribbon-like, **nonseptate (aseptate) hyphae** in tissue which are so large that their branch points can be difficult to visualize (**Figure 46–8**). As with *Aspergillus* infections, tissue biopsies are usually necessary to demonstrate the invasive hyphae, unless they can be seen on scrapings from palatal or nasal ulcers. For reasons that are unclear, cultures are sometimes negative, even those from tissue containing characteristic hyphae. Therapy involves control of underlying disease (eg, recovery from neutropenia, treatment of hyperglycemia) and high-dose antifungal therapy (lipid-associated amphotericin B, selected azoles). Surgical debridement is the most important intervention favoring survival and cure of infection.

❋ **Large ribbon-like, aseptate hyphae seen in tissues**

● *PNEUMOCYSTIS*

Pneumocystis jirovecii is a ubiquitous colonizer of the human airway. It does not cause infections in most people, but it can cause a lethal pneumonia in immunocompromised persons, particularly those with AIDS. The more familiar name to many clinicians, *P carinii*, is now used for a *Pneumocystis* species found in rats. *P jirovecii* has not been grown in culture and was long considered a parasite rather than a fungus based on the morphology of forms seen in infected tissue.

⅄ MYCOLOGY

Because it has not been possible to cultivate *Pneumocystis*, our knowledge about its basic biology is limited. Observations rest on the study of organisms purified from infected lungs and genomic analysis of *Pneumocystis* DNA. The *Pneumocystis* "life cycle" is deduced from static images seen in infected tissues. The observed stages include delicate 5 to 8 μm cystic structures (**Figure 46–9**). The trophic form is bounded by a cell wall and cytoplasmic membrane that enclose a nucleus and several mitochondria. As the precyst matures, the nuclei divide to form eight "spores" within the original structure to form the cyst. The spores have an eccentric nucleus, a nucleolus, and a single mitochondrion in the cytoplasm. No filamentous form has been observed.

Life cycle is deduced from static images

FIGURE 46–9. *Pneumocystis* pneumonia. A methenamine silver stain of material from an infected lung reveals folded cysts, some of which contain comma-shaped spores. (Reproduced with permission from Connor DH, Chandler FW, Schwartz DQ, et al: *Pathology of Infectious Diseases*. Stamford CT: Appleton & Lange; 1997.)

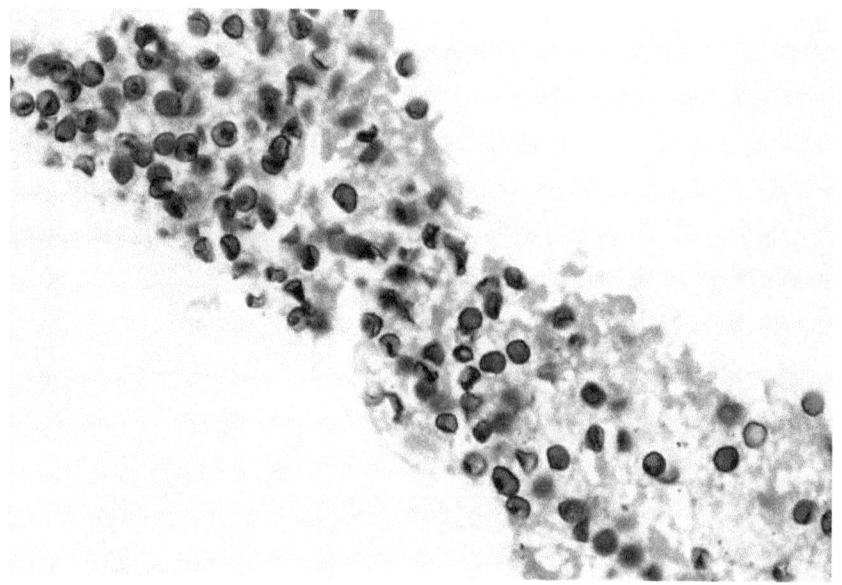

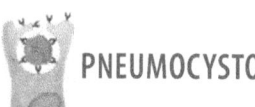 PNEUMOCYSTOSIS

OVERVIEW

Pneumocystis pneumonia is an opportunistic infection with nonspecific initial symptoms, including fever or malaise. Respiratory symptoms come later with nonproductive cough and shortness of breath. Radiographs reveal symmetric alveolar pulmonary infiltrates, which spread outward from the hilar regions. Untreated progressive hypoxia can lead to death in a 3- to 4-week period. The observation of an increased incidence of *Pneumocystis* pneumonia in the early 1980s was one of the first clinical clues to the identification of HIV/AIDS.

EPIDEMIOLOGY

Worldwide distribution in humans and animals

Airborne transmission probable

Lung colonization with *Pneumocystis* species occurs worldwide in humans and in a broad spectrum of animal life. Exposure is nearly ubiquitous; specific antibodies are present in most children by the age of 4. The reservoir and mode of transmission remain unknown, but laboratory rodents acquire *Pneumocystis* colonization with the first breaths of life. Perhaps due to low organism burden, *Pneumocystis* is not typically observed in the respiratory tract of asymptomatic persons. However, its frequent presence in the human lung was suggested by nucleic acid amplification techniques in over half of asymptomatic victims of automobile accidents. Among HIV-infected individuals, the strains involved in second and third episodes of *Pneumocystis* infection are frequently antigenically different, suggesting frequent reacquisition of new strains.

✳ PCP is a complication of immunodeficient states

✳ AIDS patients are at high risk

Before the AIDS pandemic, *Pneumocystis* pneumonia (PCP) occurred sporadically among infants with congenital immunodeficiencies and in older children and adults as a complication of immunosuppressive therapy. Now AIDS has become the most common predisposing condition, and PCP is often a presenting manifestation of late-stage HIV infection. In fact, before the development of effective chemoprophylactic regimens (see Treatment and Prevention), PCP occurred in approximately 50% of all AIDS patients at the time of initial diagnosis.

PATHOGENESIS

Low CD4 counts increase the risk in AIDS

Pneumocystis is an organism of low virulence, which seldom produces disease in a host with normal T-lymphocyte function. In experimental animals, progressive infection can be initiated with starvation or corticosteroid administration. In AIDS patients, the risk of developing pneumocystosis increases dramatically once the CD4+ T-lymphocyte count has fallen below 200 cells/mm^3. Concurrent viral, bacterial, fungal, and protozoan infections are found frequently in humans with PCP, suggesting that *Pneumocystis* may require the presence of another microbial agent for its multiplication.

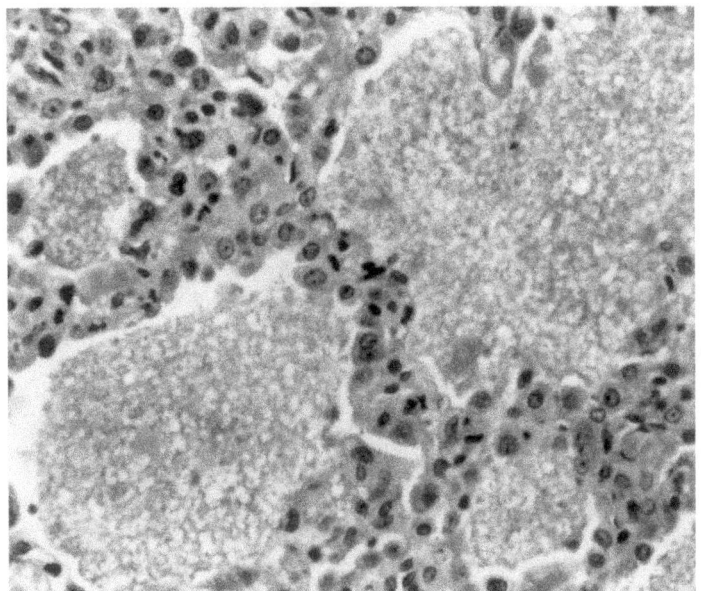

FIGURE 46–10. **Lung biopsy specimen from** *Pneumocystis* **pneumonia, showing "foamy" contents of alveoli.** (Reproduced with permission from Connor DH, Chandler FW, Schwartz DQ, et al: *Pathology of Infectious Diseases*. Stamford CT: Appleton & Lange; 1997.)

Histologically, PCP is characterized by alveoli filled with desquamated alveolar cells, monocytes, organisms, and fluid, producing a distinctive foamy, honeycombed appearance (**Figure 46–10**). Hyaline membranes suggestive of ARDS may be present. *Pneumocystis* is not easily visualized by routine histological strains, but its presence is more apparent by methenamine silver or similar silver-containing stains.

Alveoli filled with foamy exudate

IMMUNITY

The nature of the immunodeficiencies in patients with pneumocystosis points to the primacy of T_H1 immune responses in resolution of infection with *Pneumocystis*. Alveolar macrophages are the first line of defense, with activated macrophages and CD4+ lymphocytes playing essential roles in the resolution of the infection.

Activated macrophages and cytokines mediate CMI

PNEUMOCYSTOSIS: CLINICAL ASPECTS

MANIFESTATIONS

In the immunocompromised host, the disease presents as a progressive, diffuse pneumonitis. Illness may begin after discontinuation or a decrease in the dose of corticosteroids or, in the case of acute lymphocytic leukemia, during a period of remission. These observations suggest that the immune response to the organism results in many of the symptoms accompanying the infection. In infants and patients with AIDS, symptom onset is typically insidious, and the clinical course is often 3 to 4 weeks in duration. Fever is mild or absent. In older persons and patients who have previously been on high doses of corticosteroids, the onset can more abrupt. In both populations, the cardinal manifestations are progressive dyspnea and tachypnea; cyanosis and hypoxia eventually supervene. A nonproductive cough is present in 50% of all patients. Lung infiltrates on chest radiographs typically spread out symmetrically from the hilar regions of the lungs, eventually affecting most of the lung. Occasionally, unilateral infiltrates, coin lesions, lobar infiltrates, cavitary lesions, or spontaneous pneumothoraces are observed. Pleural effusions are uncommon. Clinical and radiographic abnormalities are generally accompanied by a decrease in arterial oxygen saturation, diffusion capacity of the lung, and vital capacity. Death occurs by progressive hypoxia.

✳ **Diffuse pneumonitis with insidious onset**

Nonproductive cough, dyspnea, and cyanosis develop later

Alveolar infiltrates spread out from the hila

Lesions outside the lung were rarely seen before the AIDS epidemic, but they now appear with some regularity in this patient population. The sites most often involved are lymph nodes, bone marrow, spleen, liver, eyes, thyroid, adrenal glands, gastrointestinal tract, and kidneys. The extrapulmonary clinical manifestations range from incidental autopsy findings to progressive multisystem disease.

Extrapulmonary lesions seen in AIDS

DIAGNOSIS

Diagnostic yield from sputum low

BAL best of invasive procedures

Definite diagnosis of pneumocystosis depends on finding organisms of typical morphology in appropriate specimens. Because the pathologic process is alveolar rather than bronchial, the organisms are not readily seen in expectorated specimens such as sputum. The diagnostic yield is much better from specimens obtained by more invasive procedures. Of these, BAL gives the best results with the least morbidity. Percutaneous needle aspiration of the lung, transbronchial biopsy, and open lung biopsy, though somewhat more sensitive techniques, are accompanied by more complications, including pneumothorax and hemothorax.

 Silver and other stains readily demonstrate *Pneumocystis*

DNA amplification from BAL, a means of diagnosis

Pneumocystis can be demonstrated by a variety of staining procedures. The standard stain is methenamine silver (Figure 46–9), but direct fluorescent antibody (DFA) method, if available, is slightly more sensitive. Laboratories often perform a rapid stain (Wright, Giemsa, Papanicolaou) first and confirm by methenamine silver or DFA later. Detection of *Pneumocystis* DNA in BAL fluid by polymerase chain reaction is also routinely used in many clinical laboratories. The detection of fungal antigens in the blood, such as beta-D glucan, supports the diagnosis.

> **To prevent missed diagnoses, should tests for PCP be routinely added to standard clinical microbiological panels used to evaluate respiratory samples from all patients with pneumonia?**

TREATMENT AND PREVENTION

The fixed combination of trimethoprim and sulfamethoxazole (TMP-SMX) is the treatment of choice for all forms of pneumocystosis. It is administered orally or intravenously for 14 to 21 days. Patients with AIDS often receive the longer course because they start with a higher organism burden, respond more slowly, and suffer relapse more often. Unfortunately, patients with AIDS have a high incidence of adverse effects to TMP-SMX, particularly the sulfonamide component. This requires the use of other antimicrobials (eg, clindamycin, primaquine, dapsone) alone or in combination with trimethoprim. The use of adjunctive corticosteroids in hypoxic patients with PCP results in improved survival, likely due to prevention of an excessive immune reaction to dying microbes.

TMP-SMX is treatment of choice

Chemoprophylaxis prevents PCP in AIDS

Prophylaxis. Low-dose administration of TMP-SMX has been shown to significantly decrease the incidence of PCP in high-risk patients and prevents relapse in patients with AIDS. This chemoprophylaxis is indicated for patients who have CD4+ lymphocyte counts lower than 200/mm³, unexplained fever, or a previous episode of PCP. Chemoprophylaxis for PCP is also used in solid-organ transplant patients immediately after transplantation and during treatment for allograft rejection.

KEY CONCLUSIONS

Candida

- *Candida albicans* is a commensal yeast-like fungus in the normal, human mucosal microbiota.
- Growing in both yeast and hyphal forms, *C albicans* can form nearly impenetrable biofilms on prosthetic material, as well as causing mucosal and disseminated infections.
- Certain *Candida* species are resistant to specific antifungals. Therefore, the particular *Candida* isolate causing systemic infections should be identified to the species level.
- Bloodstream infections due to *Candida* species are very common in hospitalized patients. When present, consider potential sources (eg, IV catheters, intestinal lesions) as well as potential distant sites of spread (eg, retina).

 Think ▶▶ Apply 46-3: Clinicians should maintain a high index of suspicion for PCP in patients with known or suspected defects in cell-mediated immunity (AIDS, transplant patients). This infection is exceedingly uncommon in immunocompetent patients, limiting the effectiveness of general screening for PCP in most cases of pneumonia.

Aspergillus

- Invasive aspergillosis (IA) occurs most commonly in patients with defective neutrophils.
- Immediate antifungal therapy and surgical debridement are important interventions when IA is considered or recognized in immunocompromised patients.
- Environmental controls and prophylactic antifungal therapy may decrease the incidence of IA for selected patient populations (eg, hematopoietic stem cell transplant patients).

Mucormycosis/zygomycosis

- Environmental molds such as the zygomycetes can cause destructive sinus infections in patients with poorly controlled diabetes mellitus.
- Pulmonary infections occur in highly immunocompromised patients and have a high mortality, often requiring combination of antifungal therapy and surgical debridement.

Pneumocystis

- PCP occurs in patients with profound defects in CD4+ lymphocyte function.
- Specific prophylactic therapy will often help to prevent PCP in susceptible patients.
- In addition to antimicrobial therapy, adjunctive corticosteroids may decrease mortality in severe cases of PCP by limiting immune-mediated damage during antimicrobial treatment.

CLINICAL CASE

A Budding Blood Culture

A 71-year-old woman was admitted with a recurrence of poorly differentiated squamous cell carcinoma of the cervix. She underwent extensive gynecologic surgery (excision of the organs of the anterior pelvis) and was maintained postoperatively on broad-spectrum intravenous antibiotics. The woman had a central venous catheter placed on the day of the surgery.

Beginning 3 days postoperatively, the patient had temperatures of 38.0°C to 38.5°C, which persisted without a clear source. Multiple blood cultures grew a yeast-like fungus. When incubated in serum, these round fungal cells sprouted long tubes with parallel sides.

QUESTIONS

1. Which organism is most likely to be identified in this patient's blood culture?
   - A. *Candida albicans*
   - B. *Candida glabrata*
   - C. *Aspergillus*
   - D. *Mucor*
   - E. *Pneumocystis*

2. What feature of the organism might have facilitated its infection in these circumstances?
   - A. Mannoprotein
   - B. Glucan
   - C. Germ tube formation
   - D. Biofilm formation
   - E. Sporocytes

3. Which is the probable origin of the infecting agent?
   - A. Animals
   - B. Hospital air
   - C. Medical devices
   - D. Patient's flora
   - E. Healthcare workers

ANSWERS

1. (A)
2. (D)
3. (D)

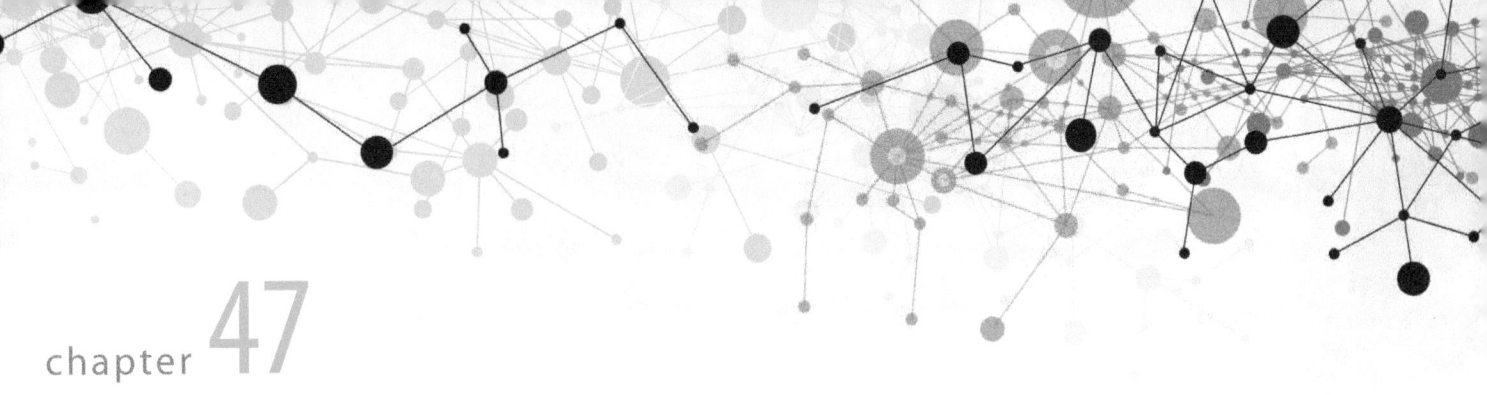

chapter 47

The Systemic Fungal Pathogens: *Cryptococcus, Histoplasma, Blastomyces, Coccidioides, Paracoccidioides*

Cryptococcus neoformans/Cryptococcus gattii · Histoplasma capsulatum · Blastomyces dermatitidis · Coccidioides immitis/Coccidioides posadasii · Paracoccidioides brasiliensis

The fungi discussed in this chapter cause a variety of infections, each ranging in severity from subclinical to progressive, debilitating disease. Some of these species are dimorphic, growing in the infectious mold form in the environment but switching to a round, yeast-like form in infected tissues. They differ from the opportunistic fungi in their ability to cause disease in previously healthy persons. However, the most serious infections still occur in patients with compromised immune systems. With the exception of *Cryptococcus neoformans*, each of these fungi is predominantly restricted to geographic niches corresponding to the environmental habitats of the mold form of the species. None of these infections is transmitted from human to human. The major features of the systemic pathogens are summarized in **Table 47-1**.

● *CRYPTOCOCCUS*

CRYPTOCOCCUS NEOFORMANS AND *CRYPTOCOCCUS GATTII*

Cryptococcus species were first isolated from environmental sources more than a century ago, and they are now recognized as important human pathogens, especially in the setting of HIV infection. The most important clinical manifestation of cryptococcal disease is a life-threatening meningitis in immunocompromised patients.

Found throughout the world, *Cryptococcus* species grow as a budding yeast 4 to 6 μm in diameter. The most characteristic feature of these cells is a large polysaccharide **capsule** (**Figure 47–1**), often extending the overall diameter of these cells to 25 μm or more. Cryptococcal species are basidiomycetes, a group of fungi that includes the mushrooms as well as many agricultural pathogens. The *Cryptococcus* genus contains two pathogenic species complexes, *C neoformans* and the more recently recognized *Cryptococcus gattii*.

The cryptococcal capsule is a unique feature among pathogenic fungi, composed of a complex polysaccharide polymer. The major components of the capsule are glucuronoxylomannan and

Two pathogenic *Cryptococcus* species and multiple varieties

TABLE 47–1	Features of Systemic Fungal Pathogens					
	GROWTH					
ORGANISM	**CULTURE AT 25°C**	**CULTURE AT 37°C**	**TISSUE**	**SOURCE**	**PRIMARY DISEASE**	**DISSEMINATED DISEASE**
Cryptococcus neoformans, C gattii	Encapsulated yeast	Encapsulated yeast	Encapsulated yeast	Environment, worldwide	Pneumonia	Chronic meningitis
Histoplasma capsulatum	Mold, tuberculate macroconidia[a]	Small yeast	Small intracellular yeast[b]	Environment, U.S. Midwest[d]	Pneumonia, hilar adenopathy	RES enlargement
Blastomyces dermatitidis	Mold[a]	Yeast		Environment, U.S. Midwest[c]	Pneumonia	Skin and bone lesions
Coccidioides immitis, C posadasii	Mold, arthroconidia	(Spherules)[e]	Spherules	Environment, Sonoran desert[c,f]	Valley fever	Pneumonia, meningitis, skin, bone
Paracoccidioides brasiliensis	Mold	Yeast, multiple blastoconidia		Environment, Latin America	Pneumonia	Mucocutaneous, RES

RES, reticuloendothelial system (lymph nodes, liver, spleen, bone marrow).
[a]Micoconidia are formed but are not distinctive.
[b]Typically multiple yeast within macrophages.
[c]Ecologic "islands" are found throughout the Americas.
[d]Ecologic islands are found worldwide.
[e]It is difficult to grow the spherule phase in culture.
[f]In the United States and includes parts of Arizona, California, Nevada, and western Texas.

An encapsulated yeast cell is diagnostic for *Cryptococcus* species

glucuronoxylomannogalactan, together referred to as **GXM.** Capsule production is repressed under environmental growth conditions, and it is stimulated by human physiologic conditions and in culture on some laboratory media. Capsular material is also secreted into the surrounding environment, serving to suppress the activity of nearby immune cells. GXM is so potently immunosuppressive that it has been used to treat autoimmune conditions such as rheumatoid arthritis in experimental trials.

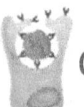 CRYPTOCOCCOSIS

CLINICAL CAPSULE

Cryptococcus species are yeasts distinguished by a surrounding capsule. The primary disease caused by cryptococci is a chronic meningitis. The clinical onset is slow, even insidious, with low-grade fever and headache progressing to altered mental state and seizures. In the cerebrospinal fluid (CSF) and in tissues, the inflammatory response is often remarkably muted. Most patients who develop this infection have some obvious form of immune compromise, although some show no demonstrable immune defect.

FIGURE 47–1. *Cryptococcus neoformans.* This India ink preparation was made by mixing cerebrospinal fluid containing cryptococci with India ink. The yeast cells can be seen within the clear space caused by the large polysaccharide capsule excluding the ink particles. Note that the one on the right is budding. (Reproduced with permission from Nester EW, Anderson DG, Roberts CE Jr, et al: *Microbiology: A Human Perspective,* 6th ed. New York, NY: McGraw Hill; 2008.)

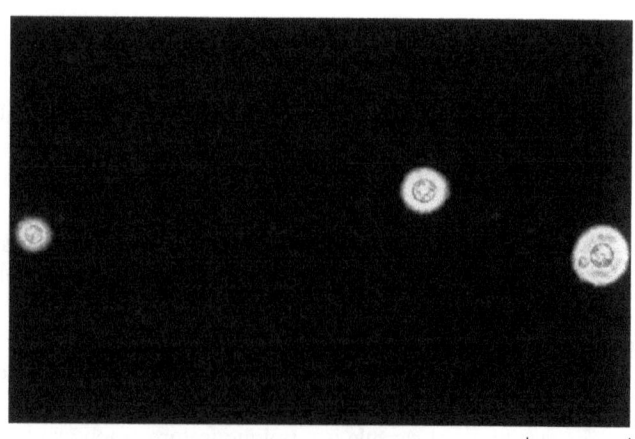

20 m

EPIDEMIOLOGY

Cryptococcus neoformans can be isolated from environmental samples throughout the world, particularly in soil contaminated with bird droppings and decaying vegetable matter. The infectious form is felt to be either desiccated yeast cells or sexual basidiospores stirred up from these sites and subsequently inhaled. The less common species *C gattii* was once felt to be restricted to tropical and subtropical areas, but it has recently been isolated from patients and the environment near the US Pacific Northwest (British Columbia, Washington, Oregon). Person-to-person transmission has not been documented, with most cases likely resulting from reactivation of dormant foci of remote infections, similar to tuberculosis (TB).

Cases of symptomatic cryptococcal infections in immunologically normal people are very rare, although it is well known that most people are exposed to this fungus early in childhood. This suggests that cryptococcal species are well controlled by the immune system after initial infection. Cryptococcosis in immunocompromised patients occurs primarily in those with defects in CD4+ T-lymphocyte function, particularly in patients with AIDS in whom it is the most common systemic fungal infection. Recent data estimated that more than 200,000 deaths occur each year in AIDS patients due to this infection. In countries with well-developed antiretroviral therapy programs, the incidence of cryptococcal disease has markedly declined in recent years. However, this infection remains an important clinical issue in other immunocompromised populations. Life-threatening disease can occur in patients with no known immune defects, although many clinicians believe that poorly characterized immune disorders may explain the majority of these infections.

✳ Associated with soil and bird droppings

Inhaled yeasts, basidiospores initiate infection

PATHOGENESIS

After being inhaled, *Cryptococcus* cells reach the alveoli, where production of the polysaccharide capsule is the prime determinant of virulence. The capsule is antiphagocytic and has various other immunomodulating effects, such as downregulation of cytokines, interference with antigen presentation, inhibition of leukocyte migration, misdirection of specific antibody responses, and delaying the development of T_H1 immune responses. *C neoformans* produces sufficient capsule that the GXM is readily detected in the blood and other body fluids. Therefore, the immune regulatory effects of the released capsule polysaccharide may act both locally and systemically.

✳ "Crypto" is immunologically "hidden" behind its capsule

✳ Circulating GXM interferes with immune function

The affinity of *C neoformans* for the central nervous system (CNS) is striking. Proposed explanations include crossing the blood–brain barrier inside macrophages (Trojan horse model) and the ability of laccase to convert the abundant catecholamines in the CNS to melanin. Similar to other neuropathogens, *C. neoformans* has components on its cell surface may help to target this microbe to the CNS by specific interactions with proteins on the endothelial cells of the brain microvasculature.

Melanin provides oxidative protection in macrophages

CRYPTOCOCCOSIS: CLINICAL ASPECTS

MANIFESTATIONS

Meningitis is the most commonly recognized form of cryptococcal disease. Unlike bacterial infections of the CNS, cryptococcal meningitis usually has a slow, insidious onset with relatively nonspecific findings until late in its course. Common presenting symptoms include intermittent headache, irritability, dizziness, and difficulty with complex cerebral functions, appearing over weeks or months. Behavioral changes have sometimes been mistaken for psychoses. Fever is usually, but not invariably, present. Seizures, cranial nerve defects, and papilledema may appear later in the clinical course, as may dementia and decreased levels of consciousness. A more rapid course may be seen in AIDS patients. Historically, as many as 5% to 15% of untreated patients with AIDS developed symptomatic cryptococcal infections. Although the onset of illness may be subacute, cryptococcal infection of the CNS is usually fatal if not recognized and treated.

✳ Meningitis insidious and chronic

✳ Course more rapid with AIDS

✳ Untreated CNS infection fatal

Like many other pathogenic fungi that enter the host through the lung, most initial pulmonary infections are minimally symptomatic. Infections can be truly clinically inapparent, or they may manifest as a self-limited respiratory illness. However, cryptococcal pneumonia can be progressive and severe in immunocompromised patients. In either case, no clinical findings are sufficiently specific to suggest the etiology.

Dissemination of infection occurs almost exclusively in immunocompromised patients, sometimes targeting the skin and bones. Classically, cryptococcal skin lesions are papular or nodular, often with a central umbilication, and remarkable for their lack of inflammation. The diagnosis is sometimes made when lesions are biopsied as suspected neoplasms.

There are differences in the disease spectrums of the two *Cryptococcus* species. *C gattii* is more likely to produce symptomatic pulmonary infections and less likely to invade the CNS. *C gattii* infection has also been described more frequently in patients with no definable immunological defect. In the CNS, *C gattii* may cause more localized lesions (cryptococcomas) as opposed to the diffuse meningoencephalitis typical of *C neoformans*.

Pneumonia often asymptomatic

CNS involvement varies with species

DIAGNOSIS

Increased intracranial pressure common

Cells, glucose depression in CSF may be minimal

India ink preparation shows encapsulated yeasts

Typical CSF findings in cryptococcal meningitis are increased intracranial pressure, pleocytosis (usually >100 white blood cells/mm^3) with predominance of lymphocytes, and depression of glucose levels. In some cases, one or all of these findings may be absent, yet cryptococci are still isolated on culture. Encapsulated yeast cells (diagnostic of *C neoformans* infection) are demonstrable in CSF in approximately 50% of cases by mixing centrifuged CSF sediment with **India ink** and examining the mixture under the microscope (Figure 47–1). Experience is necessary to avoid confusion of lymphocytes with cryptococci. *C neoformans* stains poorly with routine histologic stains; thus, it is easily missed unless special fungal stains are used (**Figure 47–2**).

For the isolation of *C neoformans* by culture, the volume of CSF sampled is important. The number of organisms present may be small enough to require a substantial volume of fluid (>30 mL) to yield a positive culture. The detection of cryptococcal capsular antigen in the CSF is the most sensitive and specific way to make the diagnosis of cryptococcal meningitis. This test can also be performed on serum where it is especially useful in diagnosing infection in immunocompromised patients due to higher levels of circulating organisms. The cryptococcal antigen test is performed by latex agglutination or enzyme immunoassay (EIA), and its quantitation has prognostic significance. A rising antigen level can indicate progression, and a declining titer is a favorable sign.

Cryptococci may be few

✳ **GXM detectable in CSF and serum**

TREATMENT

Amphotericin B and flucytosine used in combination

Fluconazole for non-CNS infections

Lumbar puncture assesses intracranial pressure

The primary treatment for serious cryptococcal infections includes induction therapy with amphotericin B plus flucytosine, followed by an extended consolidation course with fluconazole. Although 75% of persons with meningitis respond to this treatment, many patients suffer relapses after antifungal therapy is stopped, requiring repeated courses of therapy. In patients with AIDS-associated cryptococcosis, reconstitution of the immune system with antiretroviral therapy is very important to prevent recurrent infection. One-half of patients with a microbiological cure have some kind of residual neurologic damage. The management of CNS cryptococcosis also involves addressing elevated intracranial pressure when present, often with serial lumbar punctures or CSF shunting procedures. Azoles alone can often be used in non-CNS disease; therefore, it is very important to perform lumbar punctures and CSF analysis in all patients with cryptococcal infections to determine if the CNS is involved.

FIGURE 47–2. **Cryptococcal meningitis.** The *C neoformans* cells are stained red by this PAS (periodic acid-Schiff) stain. The capsule is not stained but is creating the halo around the organisms. Note the lack of inflammatory cells. (Reproduced with permission from Connor DH, Chandler FW, Schwartz DQ, et al: *Pathology of Infectious Diseases.* Stamford CT: Appleton & Lange; 1997.)

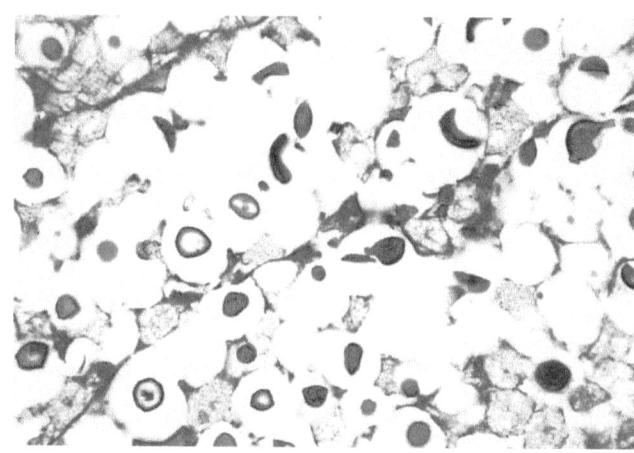

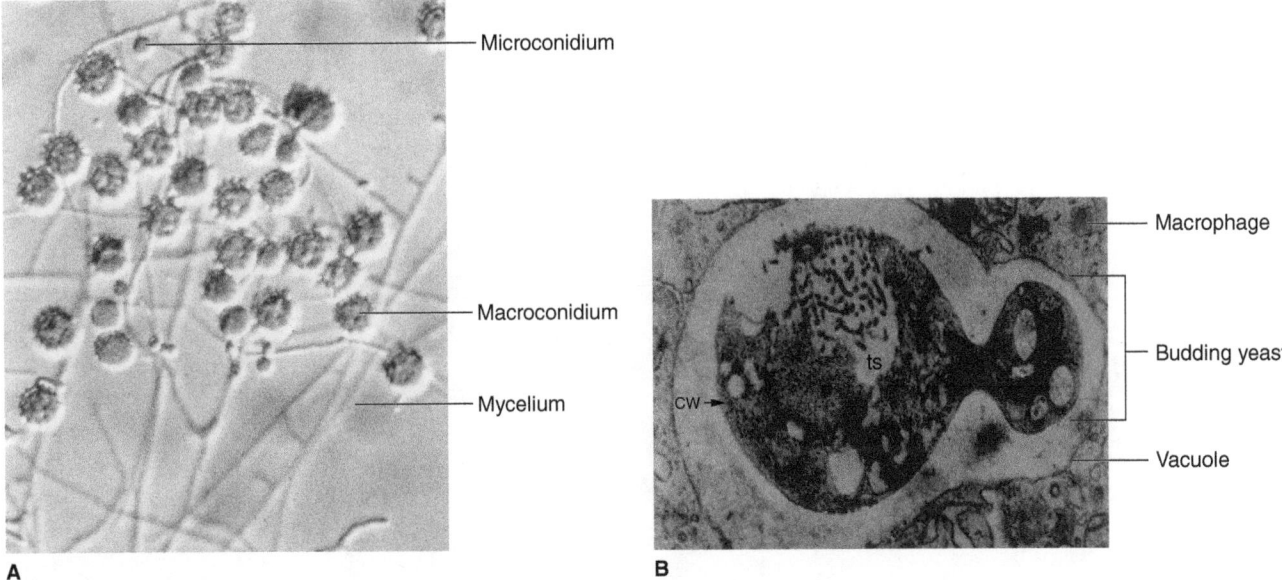

FIGURE 47-3. Histoplasma capsulatum. A. Mold phase with hyphae, microconidia, and tuberculate macroconidia. **B.** A yeast cell is multiplying (note budding) within a macrophage phagocytic vacuole. (Reproduced with permission from Willey JM: *Prescott, Harley, & Klein's Microbiology*, 7th ed. New York, NY: McGraw Hill; 2008.)

● HISTOPLASMA

 ## HISTOPLASMA CAPSULATUM

Histoplasma capsulatum is one example of a thermally dimorphic fungus (**Figure 47-3B**), microorganisms that change growth form depending on the ambient temperature. Common features of this group of fungi include the fact that most are restricted to particular geographic locations (**regions of endemicity**). Additionally, these fungi establish initial infection by the inhalation of environmental spores. Immune competent patients typically spontaneously resolve infections due to these fungi, but they can become chronic or disseminated.

H capsulatum grows in a round, yeast-like phase in tissue and in cultures incubated at 37°C. However, when incubated at lower temperatures, such as those most commonly encountered in the environment, *Histoplasma* species grow as a filamentous mold where it is a saprophyte in soil.

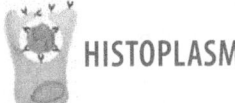 ## HISTOPLASMOSIS

OVERVIEW

Histoplasma capsulatum is a thermally dimorphic fungus that can be isolated from the soil in specific endemic areas. After infection, patients are usually asymptomatic or experience a self-limited illness characterized by fever and cough. During this initial infection, a pulmonary infiltrate and hilar adenopathy may or may not be evident on a radiograph, complicating the initial diagnosis. Progressive infections show extension in the lung or enlargement of lymph nodes, liver, and spleen.

EPIDEMIOLOGY

H capsulatum is particularly prevalent in certain temperate, subtropical, and tropical zones, and endemic areas are present in all continents of the world except Antarctica. The largest and best-defined area of endemicity is the U.S. region drained by the Ohio and Mississippi rivers (**Figure 47-4**). More than 50% of the residents of states in this area have radiologic evidence of previous infection. In some locales, up to 90% demonstrate delayed-type hypersensitivity to *Histoplasma* antigens, suggesting that they have been infected at some point in the past. Point source outbreaks of histoplasmosis have occurred after the inhalational of large amounts of fungi

Microconidia infectious

Mold grows in soil with bird droppings

FIGURE 47–4. Geographic distribution of systemic fungal infections in the United States.

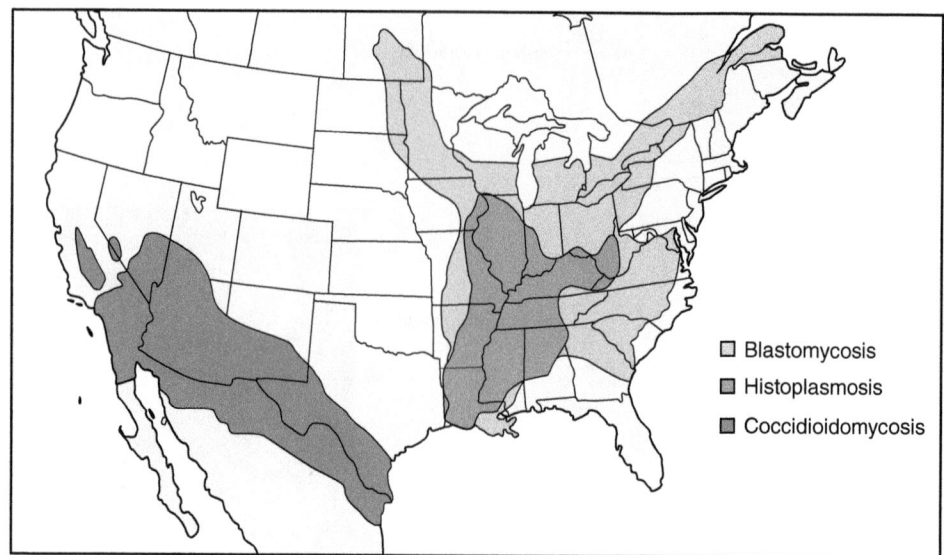

Blastomycosis
Histoplasmosis
Coccidioidomycosis

✳ High prevalence in central United States

following disturbances of bird roosts, bat caves, and soil at construction sites. Persons in endemic areas whose employment (agriculture, construction) or avocation (spelunkers) brings them in contact with aerosolized microconidia are at increased risk. Disease is more common in men, but there are no other known genetic differences in susceptibility.

PATHOGENESIS

✳ Reticuloendothelial system focus of infection

Once infection is established, *H capsulatum* cells live primarily in the lymph nodes, spleen, bone marrow, and other elements of the reticuloendothelial system. This is an example of a microorganism that has adapted to intracellular growth within phagocytic macrophages. Other examples include *M tuberculosis* and *C neoformans*. Like TB and cryptococcosis, the initial infection with *H capsulatum* occurs in the lungs after inhalation of infectious conidia. These fungal spores convert to the yeast form after germinating in the host.

✳ Lymphatic spread and reactivation similar to TB

The initial pulmonary infection of histoplasmosis generally spreads to regional lymph nodes, resulting in a primary focus of paired lung/lymphatic lesions similar to the Ghon complex of TB. Also like TB, most cases never advance beyond the primary stage, leaving only a calcified node and pulmonary calcifications as evidence of prior infection. As in TB, viable fungal cells may remain in these old lesions and reactivate later, particularly if the person becomes immunocompromised.

✳ Granulomas in liver, spleen, bone marrow

Pathologically, histoplasmosis is characterized by granulomatous inflammation with associated necrosis. Even with special fungal stains, *H capsulatum* may be difficult to detect within these infected foci, making a precise pathological diagnosis challenging. Extrapulmonary spread of histoplasmosis occurs primarily in immunocompromised patients, primarily involving the reticuloendothelial system with resulting enlargement of the liver and spleen. In patients with compromised immunity, numerous organisms within macrophages may be found in these organs, in lymph nodes, bone marrow, or even peripheral blood (**Figure 47–5**).

⚕ HISTOPLASMOSIS: CLINICAL ASPECTS

MANIFESTATIONS

Most cases asymptomatic or only fever, cough

Most cases of *H capsulatum* infection in normal hosts are minimally symptomatic, often causing mild fever and cough for a few days or weeks. Mediastinal lymphadenopathy and subtle pulmonary infiltrates may be seen on X-rays. More severe cases are most often characterized by chills, malaise, chest pain, and more extensive lung infiltrates, all of which usually resolve without specific therapy. Most people who resolve the primary infection have scattered calcified pulmonary granulomas as radiographic evidence of healed histoplasmosis. Rarely, residual pulmonary nodules may continue to enlarge over a period of years, causing a differential diagnostic problem with

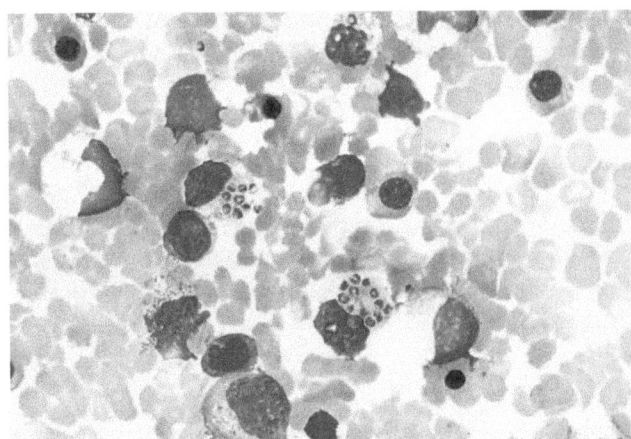

FIGURE 47-5. *Histoplasma capsulatum.* This peripheral blood smear shows two monocytes with multiple organisms filling their cytoplasm. Note the size of the yeast cells, which is very small for fungi. (Reproduced with permission from Connor DH, Chandler FW, Schwartz DQ, et al: *Pathology of Infectious Diseases.* Stamford CT: Appleton & Lange; 1997.)

pulmonary neoplasms. Progressive pulmonary disease can mimic pulmonary TB, with sputum production, night sweats, weight loss, and even the development of lung cavities. The clinical course of pulmonary histoplasmosis may infrequently be chronic and relapsing, with symptoms lasting for several months to years.

⁎ Pulmonary disease shows cavities, weight loss

Disseminated histoplasmosis generally appears as a nonspecific febrile illness in an immunocompromised patient, with enlargement of reticuloendothelial organs. Populations at particular risk for developing disseminated histoplasmosis include patients with advanced AIDS as well as those being treated with tumor necrosis factor-alpha inhibitors. The CNS, skin, gastrointestinal tract, and adrenal glands may also be involved. Painless ulcers on mucous membranes are a common clinical finding; however, given their painless nature, these lesions must be actively sought by clinicians in order to help make the diagnosis. The course of disseminated histoplasmosis is typically chronic, with manifestations that depend on the organs involved. For example, chronic bilateral adrenal failure (Addison disease) may develop when the adrenal glands are affected.

⁎ Dissemination involves RES, mucous membranes, adrenal glands

DIAGNOSIS

In most forms of pulmonary histoplasmosis, the diagnostic yield of direct examinations or culture of sputum is low. In disseminated disease, blood culture or biopsy samples of a reticuloendothelial organ are the most likely to contain *Histoplasma*. Of these cultures, bone marrow culture has the highest yield. Because of their small size, the yeast cells are difficult to see in potassium hydroxide (KOH) preparations, and their morphology is not sufficiently distinctive to be diagnostic. Specimens must therefore be examined carefully under high magnification. Selective fungal stains such as methenamine silver demonstrate the organism but may not differentiate it from other yeasts. Hematoxylin and eosin (H&E)-stained tissue or Wright-stained bone marrow often demonstrates the organisms in their intracellular location in macrophages (Figure 47–5). Identification of culture isolates requires demonstration of the typical conidia and dimorphism. Nucleic acid probes have been developed for culture confirmation.

Blood and bone marrow examination require special stains

Antibodies can be detected during and after infection, but their diagnostic usefulness in endemic areas is limited by false-negative results and cross-reactions with blastomycosis. Rising antibody titers are suggestive of dissemination or relapse. The histoplasmin skin test has been useful in the past to document prior exposure, but the reagents are no longer commercially available. Isolation of the fungus in culture or clear histologic demonstration is often necessary to establish a firm diagnosis of histoplasmosis. The diagnosis of disseminated infection has been greatly aided by the development of a commonly used EIA detecting a *Histoplasma* polysaccharide antigen. This test can be performed on blood or urine samples, and it detects more than 90% of cases of disseminated disease.

⁎ ID of polysaccharide in blood and urine by EIA aids in diagnosing disseminated infection

TREATMENT

Primary infections and localized lung lesions usually resolve without treatment. For mild disease localized to the lung, a systemic azole such as itraconazole is commonly used. For more severe or disseminated disease, initial therapy with amphotericin B is often followed by longer-term therapy with itraconazole. Azoles can be effective in an endemic area for prophylaxis of persons with

✳ Amphotericin B and itraconazole treatments of choice, particularly for disseminated infection

a high risk of disease, including AIDS patients with low CD4 counts and other immunocompromised patients. The echinocandin class of antifungals is decidedly less effective, and these agents should not routinely be used for histoplasmosis.

 Patients with immunocompromising disorders (eg, patients with progressive AIDS, patients receiving anti-tumor necrosis alpha therapy) are at high risk for developing life-threatening complications from invasive infections due to pathogenic fungi. Can you suggest minimally invasive testing strategies that might identify patients with subclinical infections due to these fungi and who are therefore at risk for serious complications with progressive immunosuppression?

● *BLASTOMYCES*

 ### *BLASTOMYCES DERMATITIDIS*

✳ Yeast cells have broad-based buds (rule of "B's")

Mold similar to *Histoplasma*

Blastomyces dermatitidis is a dimorphic fungus with some characteristics similar to those of *Histoplasma*. This fungus grows in yeast-like phase in tissues and in cultures incubated at 37°C. The yeast cells are typically larger (8-15 mm) than those of *H capsulatum*, with broad-based buds (blastoconidia) and a thick wall (**Figure 47–6**). The mold phase appears in culture at 25°C.

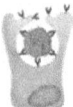 ## BLASTOMYCOSIS

CLINICAL CAPSULE

Blastomyces dermatitidis is a thermally dimorphic fungus similar to *Histoplasma*. Many clinical features of blastomycosis are similar to histoplasmosis. During initial infection, most patients are asymptomatic or have self-limited mild fever and cough. Chronic infections of the lung infrequently occur. Skin lesions are the most common manifestation of disseminated disease. Unlike histoplasmosis, the reticuloendothelial system is not involved.

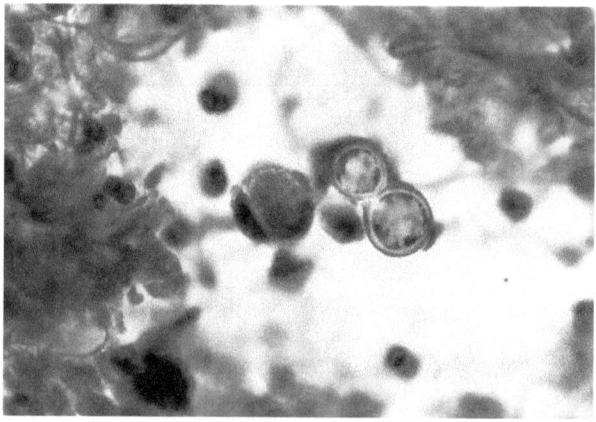

FIGURE 47–6. ***Blastomyces dermatitidis.*** Large thick-walled yeast cells are shown in this sputum. Note how the blastoconidia retain a broad attachment to the mother cell before separating. (Reproduced with permission from Connor DH, Chandler FW, Schwartz DQ, et al: *Pathology of Infectious Diseases.* Stamford CT: Appleton & Lange; 1997.)

 Think►►Apply 47-1: Patients with late-stage AIDS or other forms of immunosuppression can have subclinical infections due to pathogenic fungi that become clinically evident with time. Minimally invasive tests for fungal antigens, such as urine or blood tests for *Cryptococcus* or *Histoplasma* antigens, have been used to identify these infected but asymptomatic patients in order to effectively direct antifungal therapy before serious complications develop.

EPIDEMIOLOGY

Blastomycosis is most commonly observed in geographic regions that overlap with those for histoplasmosis. In North America, this includes the upper Midwestern states and regions around the Great Lakes (Figure 47–4), but infections have been reported in Africa, the Middle East, and Europe as well. A specific skin test for blastomycosis is not routinely available, thus limiting epidemiological mapping of the endemic areas. Unlike histoplasmosis, the causative agent of blastomycosis, *Blastomyces dermatitidis*, is not strongly associated with bird or bat habitats. It is assumed that inhalation of environmental microconidia is the means of infection, as is the case for most endemic fungal pathogens.

❊ Geographic distribution similar to *Histoplasma*

BLASTOMYCOSIS: CLINICAL ASPECTS

MANIFESTATIONS

Because mild cases of blastomycosis are difficult to diagnose, most infections are only recognized if they progress to more advanced or disseminated stages of the disease. Pulmonary infection is evidenced by cough, sputum production, chest pain, and fever. Hilar lymphadenopathy may be present, as may nodular pulmonary infiltrates with alveolar consolidation. This nonspecific clinical picture may mimic a pulmonary tumor, TB, or some other form of chronic pneumonitis. In contrast to histoplasmosis, mucous membrane lesions are rarely observed in blastomycosis. Instead, lesions develop more commonly on exposed skin, often as "grouped microabscesses." Given the chronicity of many untreated cases of cutaneous blastomycosis, the associated extensive necrosis and fibrosis may produce considerable disfigurement. Bone infection has features similar to those of other causes of chronic osteomyelitis. The urinary and genital tracts are the most commonly affected visceral sites; the prostate is especially prone to infection.

❊ Pulmonary blastomycosis similar to other mycoses

❊ Skin lesions on exposed surfaces, often grouped microabscesses

❊ GU tract/prostate frequently involved

DIAGNOSIS

Direct demonstration of typical large yeasts with broad-based buds (blastoconidia) in KOH preparations of infected tissue is the most rapid means of diagnosis (Figure 47–6). Biopsy specimens also have a high yield, and the organisms are visible in histopathology samples stained with either H&E or special fungal stains. *Blastomyces dermatitidis* grows in the clinical microbiology laboratory on routine fungal media, but cultures may take as long as 4 weeks. Conidia are not particularly distinctive, and demonstration of thermal dimorphism and typical yeast morphology is essential to avoid confusion with other fungi. A DNA probe is particularly useful in differentiating cultures from *Histoplasma*. Serological tests are available but are less sensitive than those for other fungal pathogens.

KOH and biopsy show budding yeast

Culture takes weeks, conidia not distinctive

TREATMENT

As with histoplasmosis, itraconazole and other mold-active azoles may be used for mild to moderate disease. Amphotericin B is indicated for more serious or disseminated infections. Fluconazole or voriconazole may be used in meningitis. As with other systemic mycoses, response to treatment is slow, and relapse is common.

Amphotericin B and azoles effective

● COCCIDIOIDES

 COCCIDIOIDES IMMITIS AND COCCIDIOIDES POSADASII

Coccidioides species are dimorphic fungi commonly encountered within North America in the desert regions of the southwestern United States and northern Mexico. In contrast to *Blastomyces* and *Histoplasma* species that grow in the body as budding yeast-like cells, the tissue form of *Coccidioides* species is a large (12-100 μm), round-walled **spherule** (**Figure 47–7A**). This structure is quite distinctive and unique among the pathogenic fungi. Its formation takes place in a process illustrated in **Figure 47–8.** The spherule eventually ruptures, releasing 200 to 300 endospores (**Figure 47–9**), each of which can differentiate into another spherule.

Dimorphism with unique spherule

❊ Spherules form and release endospores

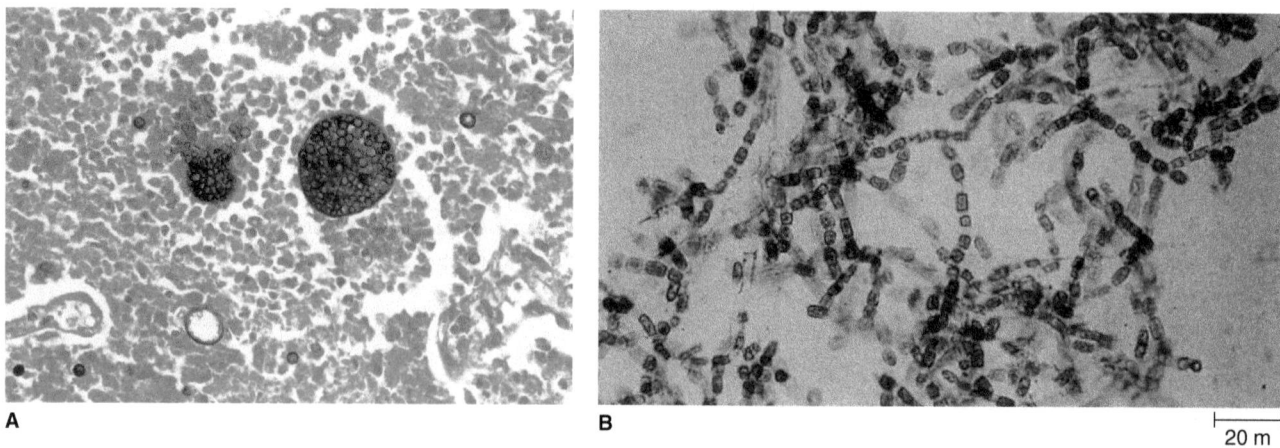

20 m

FIGURE 47–7. *Coccidioides immitis.* **A.** Lung tissue with a large thick-walled spherule containing multiple endospores. The smaller spherule to its left has ruptured releasing endospores. **B.** Mold phase in which alternate cells have differentiated to form barrel-shaped arthroconidia. (A, Reproduced with permission from Connor DH, Chandler FW, Schwartz DQ, et al: *Pathology of Infectious Diseases*. Stamford CT: Appleton & Lange; 1997. B, Reproduced with permission from Nester EW, Anderson DG, Roberts CE Jr, et al: *Microbiology: A Human Perspective*, 6th ed. New York, NY: McGraw Hill; 2008.)

FIGURE 47–8. Life cycle of *Coccidioides immitis*. The nature cycle takes place in desert climates with modest rainfall. Hyphae differentiate into arthroconidia, which break loose and may be suspended in the air. Soil disruptions and wind facilitate spread and the probability of inhalation into human lungs. In the human host environment, *in vivo* differentiation produces cleavage planes and eventually huge spherules. The spherules rupture, releasing endospores, which can then repeat the *in vivo* cycle.

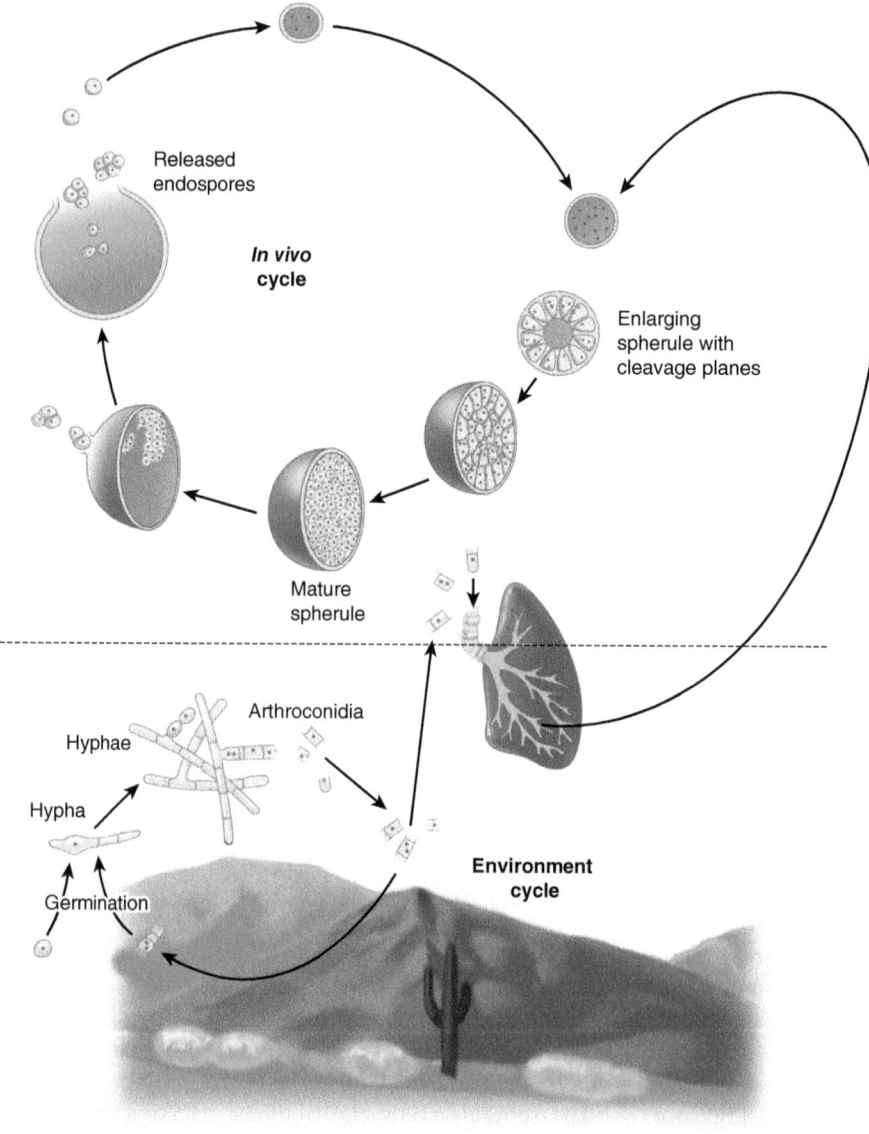

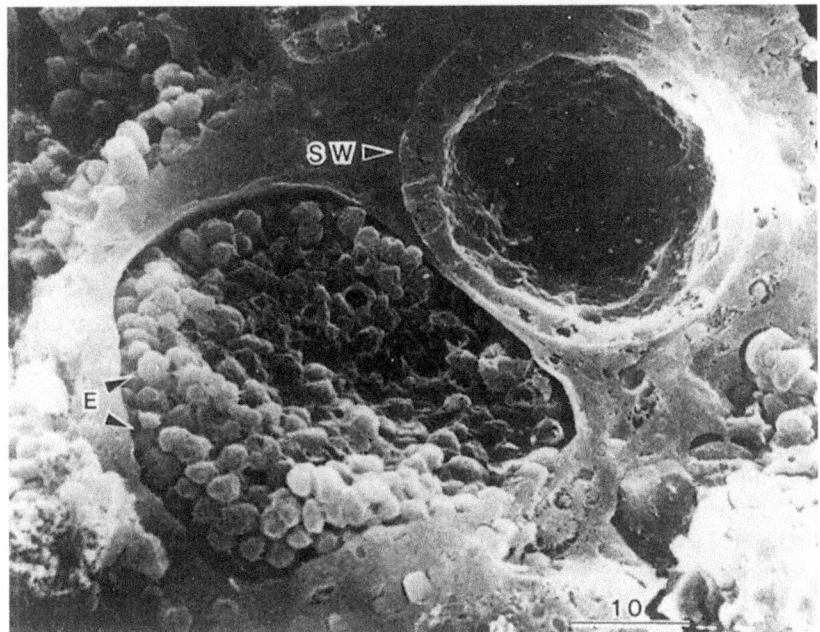

FIGURE 47–9. *Coccidioides immitis.* This electron micrograph of infected mouse lung shows a spherule filled with endospores (E) and one that has discharged its endospores into the surrounding tissue. Note the thickness of the spherule wall (SW). (Reproduced with permission from Drutz DJ, Huppert M: Coccidioidomycosis: factors affecting the host-parasite interaction, *J Infect Dis* 1983; Mar;147(3):372-390.)

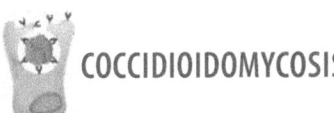 COCCIDIOIDOMYCOSIS

OVERVIEW

Coccidioides species are thermally dimorphic fungi endemic in parts of the American West. Acute primary infection with *C immitis* is most often asymptomatic, but it can manifest as a complex of symptoms called "Valley Fever" by residents of the endemic areas. Valley Fever includes fever, malaise, dry cough, joint pains, and sometimes a rash. Red, inflamed nodules on the extremities (erythema nodosum) are suggestive of Valley Fever. Disseminated forms of the disease can involve the bones, joints, skin, and a progressive chronic meningitis.

EPIDEMIOLOGY

Coccidioidomycosis is the most geographically restricted of the systemic mycoses because *C immitis* grows only in the alkaline soil of semiarid climates known as the Lower Sonoran life zone (Figure 47–4). These areas are characterized by hot, dry summers, mild winters with few freezes, and annual rainfall of about 10 inches during brief rainy seasons. Ecologic "islands" with these conditions are found scattered throughout Central and South America. The primary endemic zones in the United States are in Arizona, Nevada, New Mexico, western Texas, and the arid parts of central and southern California. Three unrelated cases in the eastern half of Washington State could give this zone its most northern extension. The area between the Cascade and Rocky Mountains is also dry and arid, but prolonged winter freezes make it less hospitable for *Coccidioides* species. Persons living in the endemic areas are at high risk of infection, and positive skin test rates of 50% to 90% occur in long-time residents of highly endemic areas. Coccidioidomycosis is not transmissible from person to person.

Infection cannot typically be acquired without at least visiting an endemic area, although some interesting examples have been recorded in which the endemic zone itself "paid a visit" and resulted in infections. In 1978, a storm originating in Bakersfield, California (endemic zone), carried a thick cloud of dust all the way to San Francisco. This weather event was followed by cases of coccidioidomycosis in persons who had never left the Bay Area. Similarly, infection in a patient who had never left the southeastern United States was epidemiologically associated with exposure to preprocessed cotton grown in Arizona.

Coccidioides immitis is also a notorious cause of infection in laboratory workers. The high infectivity of cultured arthroconidia has caused it to be classified as a significant biohazard and potential bioweapon.

* Restricted to Sonoran Desert

High proportion of locals infected

* Considered potential bioweapon

IMMUNITY

Lifelong immunity to coccidioidomycosis clearly develops in most of those who become infected. This immunity is associated with strong polymorphonuclear leukocyte and T_H1-mediated responses to coccidioidal antigens. In most cases, a mixed inflammatory response is associated with early resolution of the infection and development of a positive delayed-type hypersensitivity skin test. Progressive disease is associated with weak or absent cellular immunity and loss of delayed-type hypersensitivity to coccidioidal antigens. The disease progresses when cell-mediated immunity and consequent macrophage activation do not develop. Such immune deficits may be a result of disease (AIDS) or immunosuppressive therapy, but progressive coccidioidomycosis may infrequently occur in persons with no known immune defects.

Humoral mechanisms are not known to play a major role in immunity to coccidioidomycosis. In fact, *C immitis* is resistant to complement-mediated killing, and levels of complement-fixing antibody are inversely related to the process of disease resolution. Persons with minimal objective indications of tissue involvement (eg, lesions, radiographs) have strong T-lymphocyte responses to *C immitis* antigens and little if any detectable anti-*Coccidioides* antibody. Those with disseminated disease and absent cellular immunity have high titers of antibody. Thus, the levels of antibody seem to indicate the degree of antigenic stimulation rather than any known contribution to resolution of the infection (**Figure 47–10**).

 ## COCCIDIOIDOMYCOSIS: CLINICAL ASPECTS

MANIFESTATIONS

More than 50% of those infected with *C immitis* experience no symptoms, or the disease is so mild that it cannot be recalled when evidence of infection (serology, skin test) is discovered. Others develop malaise, cough, chest pain, fever, and arthralgia 1 to 3 weeks after infection. This illness, dubbed **Valley Fever** by the local San Joaquin Valley residents, lasts 2 to 6 weeks with few distinctive findings. The chest X-ray is usually clear or shows only hilar adenopathy. Red, inflamed skin nodules, known as erythema nodosum, may occur during the course of initial infection, particularly on the extremities, and most frequently in women. In most cases, all clinical symptoms of Valley Fever resolve spontaneously, but often only after considerable discomfort and loss of productivity. In more than 90% of cases, there are no pulmonary residua. A small number of cases progress to a chronic pulmonary infection characterized by cavity formation and a slowly relapsing course that extends over years. Less than 1% of all primary infections and 5% of symptomatic cases disseminate to foci outside the lung.

There is a well-recognized but poorly understood predisposition to chronic infections among distinct patient populations. Disseminated disease is more common in men, as well as people from areas of the world in which malaria is hyperendemic. The genetic determinants of this association have not yet been elucidated. Given the importance of CD_4-mediated immunity in controlling coccidioidomycosis, patients with AIDS or transplants are also at particular risk for disseminated infection. Evidence of extrapulmonary infection almost always appears in the first year after infection. The most commonly involved sites are bones, joints, skin, and the CNS. Coccidioidal meningitis develops slowly with gradually increasing headache, fever, neck stiffness, and other signs of meningeal irritation. The CSF findings are similar to those in TB and other fungal causes of meningitis, such as *C neoformans*. Mononuclear cells predominate in the cell count, but substantial numbers of neutrophils and eosinophils are often present. If untreated, the disease is slowly progressive and fatal.

DIAGNOSIS

With enough persistence, direct examination of infected tissue can reveal diagnostic forms of *C immitis*. The thick-walled spherules are so large and characteristic (Figure 47–7A) that they are difficult to miss in wet mounts (KOH, calcofluor) or biopsy sections. Skin and visceral lesions are most likely to demonstrate spherules; however, these fungal forms are rarely seen in the CSF. Spherules released into expectorated sputum are often small (10-15 mm) and immature without well-developed endospores, thus difficult to visualize. In contrast, spherules stain well in histologic sections of infected tissue using either H&E or special fungal stains.

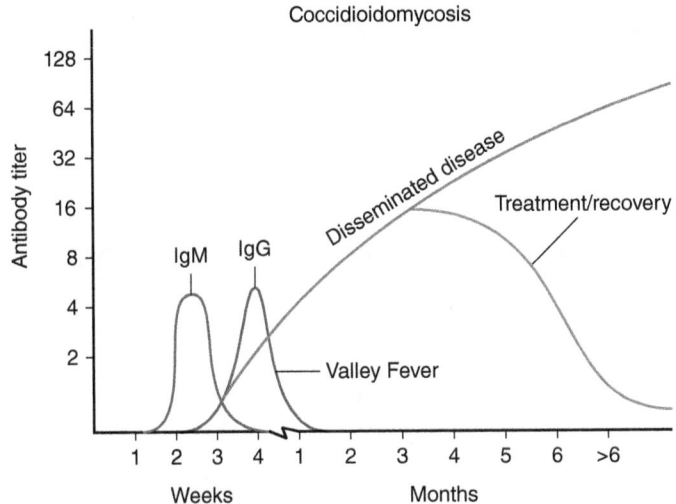

FIGURE 47–10. Serologic tests in coccidioidomycosis.

Culture of *C immitis* from sputum, visceral lesions, or skin lesions is not difficult, but must be undertaken only by those with experience and proper biohazard protection. Cultures of CSF are positive in less than half the cases of meningitis. Laboratories must be warned of the possibility of coccidioidomycosis to ensure diagnosis and prevent inadvertent laboratory infection.

CSF culture difficult

Laboratory infection risk

TREATMENT

Primary coccidioidomycosis is self-limited, and no antifungal therapy is indicated except to reduce the risk of dissemination in patients with risk factors, such as immunocompromise and pregnancy. Itraconazole is preferred for acute or progressive pulmonary disease, with fluconazole as an alternative agent. Disseminated, extrapulmonary infection may require amphotericin B. Fluconazole is often favored as treatment for meningitis because of its enhanced CSF penetration. In cases of refractory meningitis, amphotericin B may be infused directly into the CSF. Unlike other forms of the disease that can be treated for cure, coccidioidomycosis involving the CNS often requires lifelong therapy.

Primary disease treated only with risk factors

Amphotericin B, azoles with progression

● *PARACOCCIDIOIDES BRASILIENSIS*

Paracoccidioides brasiliensis is the cause of paracoccidioidomycosis (South American blastomycosis), a disease limited to tropical and subtropical areas of Central and South America. The organism is a dimorphic fungus, the most noteworthy feature of which is the production of multiple blastoconidia from the same cell. Characteristic 5 to 40 μm cells covered with budding blastoconidia may be seen in tissue or in yeast-phase growth at 37°C. This structure has a morphology reminiscent of a ship's steering wheel, often referred to as a "Captain's wheel" when seen in tissue. The disease manifests primarily as chronic mucocutaneous or cutaneous ulcers. The disfiguring ulcers spread slowly and develop a granulomatous mulberry-like base. Regional lymph nodes, reticuloendothelial organs, and the lungs may also be involved.

Yeast with multiple blastoconidia in ulcerative lesions

Paracoccidioidomycosis has a striking predilection for men, despite skin test evidence that subclinical cases occur at the same rate in both sexes. This may be related to the experimental observation that estrogens but not androgens inhibit conversion of mold-phase conidia to the yeast phase. Treatment is with sulfonamides, amphotericin B, and, more recently, the azole compounds.

Strong predilection for men

KEY CONCLUSIONS

- Remember the "C's" of *Cryptococcus neoformans*
  - Capsule
  - CD4 cell dysfunction predisposes to symptomatic infection
  - CNS infections are most common
  - Cryptococcal antigen is the most sensitive diagnostic test

- The thermally dimorphic fungi each have distinctive tissue forms
  - *Histoplasma*—small, budding yeasts
  - *Blastomyces*—broad-based budding yeasts
  - *Coccidioides*—spherule with endospores
- Infections due to the thermally dimorphic fungi:
  - begin after inhalation of infectious particles
  - cause a minimally symptomatic initial lung infection in most people
  - can disseminate, especially in immunocompromised patients
- Histoplasmosis can mimic tuberculosis with a primary lung infection, granulomatous inflammation, and dissemination in macrophages
- Blastomycosis disseminated disease often manifests as chronic skin lesions
- Coccidioidomycosis can cause a chronic and fatal meningitis
- Paracoccidioidomycosis causes disfiguring skin and mucosal lesions, especially in men

CASE STUDY
A Forgetful Farmer

A 64-year-old farmer was hospitalized because of "progressive dementia." He had been in excellent health and working full time, never having left the state of Montana. Two months before admission, he became uncharacteristically careless and forgetful, and he was increasingly unable to perform his work on the farm. Neither he nor his family noticed other symptoms, except for a chronic frontal headache of 1 month duration.

Physical examination revealed a well-developed man who did not appear ill. His blood pressure, pulse, and respiratory rate were normal, and his temperature was 99.2°F. The rest of the examination was normal except for mild nuchal rigidity, disorientation to time and place, and marked confusion. A complete blood count was normal, and an HIV serological test was negative.

Lumbar puncture revealed clear CSF with an opening pressure of 250 mm; 100 white blood cells (92% lymphocytes); protein of 85 mg% and glucose of 45 mg% (concomitant blood sugar was 90 mg%). Gram stain of the CSF was negative.

QUESTIONS

1. If this is a case of fungal meningitis, the most likely etiologic agent is:
   A. *Candida albicans*
   B. *Cryptococcus neoformans*
   C. *Histoplasma capsulatum*
   D. *Coccidioides immitis*
   E. *Paracoccidioides brasiliensis*

2. If blood and CSF cultures for bacteria, mycobacteria, and fungi are negative, what test is most likely to reveal the diagnosis?
   A. GMX antigen detection
   B. GMX antibody detection
   C. Germ tube test
   D. Silver stain
   E. *Coccidioides immitis* IgG

3. What is the most common route of primary infection for this pathogenic microorganism?
   A. Inoculation
   B. Ingestion
   C. Insect vector
   D. Inhalation
   E. Animal bite

ANSWERS

1. **(B)**

2. **(A)**

3. **(D)**

    Most cases of cryptococcal meningitis/meningoencephalitis occur in patients with defined defects of immunity, such as late-stage HIV infection. However, this infection has been described in otherwise immunocompetent patients, presenting with chronic and progressive CNS symptoms. *C neoformans* is the most common cause of fungal meningitis. *C immitis* can infrequently cause meningitis, but travel to endemic areas is required for infection. *P brasiliensis* is endemic to regions in Central and South America. Detection of the GXM component of the cryptococcal capsule is the most sensitive test for this infection. Like many fungal pathogens, *C neoformans* typically enters the body through the lungs by inhalation.

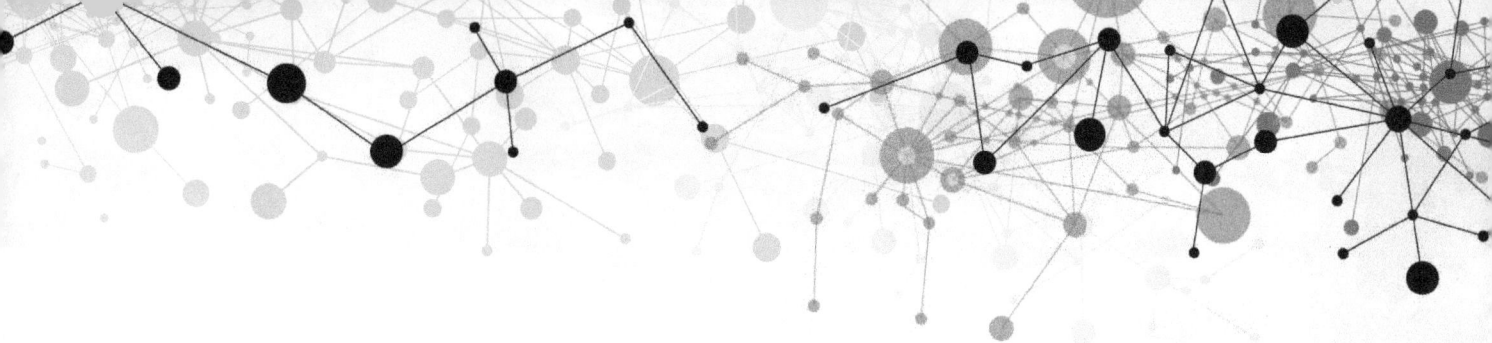

PART V
Pathogenic Parasites

Paul Pottinger · Charles R. Sterling

chapter 48

Parasites—Basic Concepts

The discipline of Medical Parasitology encompasses a broad spectrum of organisms belonging to the kingdoms Protista and Animalia that include diverse phylogenetic groupings such as the subkingdoms Protozoa and Metazoa, respectively. The latter include the trematodes, cestodes (Platyhelminthes), and nematodes (Nemathelminthes). Although often quite dissimilar, many parasites do share some important traits. They are opportunists by nature and exploit environmental niches and lifestyles within their hosts that suit their individual needs. Many have high prevalence rates, given the right set of circumstances, and may cause significant morbidity and mortality. All have exceedingly complex life cycles. The purpose of this chapter, and Chapters 49 and 50 that follow, is to lay a foundation of basic definitions and concepts that hopefully will aid the student in better understanding the specific diseases that will be described in succeeding chapters.

DEFINITION

Within the context of this section of the book, the term **parasite** refers to organisms that are physiologically dependent upon their host for survival and belong to the major taxonomic groupings mentioned earlier: Protozoa, Platyhelminthes, and Nemathelminthes. **Parasitism,** however, denotes a relationship in which one organism, the parasite, usually benefits at the expense of the other, the host. Protozoa are microscopic, single-celled eukaryotes with a membrane-bound nucleus and organelles. Helminths, comprising both Platyhelminthes and Nemathelminthes, in contrast, are macroscopic, multicellular worms possessing differentiated tissues and complex organ systems; they vary in length from more than 1 m to less than 1 mm. The majority of both Protozoa and helminths are free living, play a significant role in the ecology of the planet, and seldom inconvenience the human race. The less common disease-producing species are typically **obligate** parasites, dependent on vertebrate hosts, arthropod hosts, or both for their survival. Most parasites are perfectly happy living in a **commensalistic** relationship with their host, producing little or no injury. Of importance to us are those that disturb this relationship, leading to pathogenesis and, occasionally, to death of both the host and parasite.

※ Eukaryotic, single-celled Protozoa and multicellular, macroscopic helminths

Majority are commensalistic

※ Disease-producing species usually obligate parasites

SIGNIFICANCE OF HUMAN PARASITIC INFECTIONS

The relative infrequency of parasitic infections in the temperate societies of the industrialized world with strict sanitation has sometimes led to the parochial view that knowledge of parasitology has little relevance for physicians practicing in these areas. In spite of this view, parasites such as *Toxoplasma gondii, Cryptosporidium* spp., *Giardia, Trichomonas vaginalis,* and *Enterobius vermicularis* thrive in our midst. Many others pose risks as imported agents and our medical communities are continuously challenged to both identify and treat them. In addition, the continuing presence of parasitic disease among the impoverished, immunocompromised, sexually active, and peripatetic segments of industrialized populations means that most physicians throughout the world regularly encounter those pathogens. Parasitic diseases remain among the major causes of human misery and death in the world today and, as such, are important obstacles to the development of economically less favored nation (**Table 48–1**). Moreover, political, socioeconomic, and medical instabilities in several parts of the world have combined to produce a dramatic recrudescence of several parasitic diseases with important consequences to both the United States and the developing world.

Currently, about half of the world's population lives in areas where malaria transmission could or does occur; of these, approximately 200 to 300 million experience new cases annually, with many individuals being infected more than once during any given year. About 400,000 people, predominantly children living in Sub-Saharan Africa, die of malaria each year. *Plasmodium falciparum*, the deadliest of the malarial organisms and responsible for cerebral malaria, has developed resistance to several categories of antimalarial agents, and resistant strains are now found throughout Southeast Asia, parts of the Indian subcontinent, Southeast China, large areas of tropical America, and tropical Africa. Disturbingly, this parasite is developing increased resistance to artemisinin, the current frontline drug in the treatment of malaria. Although several

TABLE 48–1	Estimated Prevalence of Parasitic Infections
DISEASE	**ESTIMATED POPULATION AFFECTED**
Amebiasis	10% of world population
Annual deaths	120,000
Giardiasis	>200 million
Trichomoniasis	>200 million
Malaria	300 million
Population at risk	3 billion
Annual deaths	<1 million
Leishmaniasis	12 million
African trypanosomiasis	
Population at risk	50 million
New cases per year	100,000
Annual deaths	5000
American trypanosomiasis	15 million
Population at risk	65 million
New cases per year	60,000
Schistosomiasis	207 million
Population at risk	600 million
Annual deaths	0.5–1.0 million
Clonorchiasis and opisthorchiasis	13.5 million
Paragonimiasis	2.1 million
Fasciolopsiasis	10 million
Filiariasis	128 million
Onchocerciasis	18 million
Dracunculiasis	<25,000
Ascariasis	1.3 billion
Hookworm	1.3 billion
Trichuriasis	0.9 billion
Strongyloidiasis	35 million
Enterobius vermicularis	400 million
Cestodiasis	65 million

new drugs are in development, it could take years before they reach the public that needs them the most. Growing resistance of the anopheline mosquito vectors of malaria to the less toxic and less expensive insecticides has resulted in a cutback of many malaria control programs. On top of that, many mosquito vectors of malaria are changing their habits, perhaps in response to our efforts to control them. In countries such as India, Pakistan, and Sri Lanka, where eradication efforts had previously interrupted parasite transmission, the disease incidence has increased 100-fold in recent years. In tropical Africa, the intensity of transmission has been greatly reduced largely due to the compliant use of insecticide-impregnated bed nets. Presently, approximately 2000 cases of imported malaria are reported to the Centers for Disease Control and Prevention. Most of these are the result of individuals traveling to malarious areas and not being compliant in taking prophylactic medicines.

Entamoeba spp., many of which are strictly commensalistic, are intestinal Protozoa that infect about 50% of the world's population, with rates varying substantially depending on sanitary conditions. The pathogenic *Entamoeba* has historically been thought of as *Entamoeba histolytica* and it is estimated that up to 10% of the world's population harbor this parasite. A noninvasive species, *Entamoeba dispar*, which is morphologically similar to *E histolytica* has been recognized and probably accounts for 90% of all reported *E histolytica*-like infections. The invasive *E histolytica*, which is morphologically identical to *E dispar*, produces amebiasis, a disease characterized by intestinal ulcers and liver abscesses. Rates up to 4% are seen in the United States. It is more commonly seen in areas of the world with poor sanitation, but occurs in the United States as well, particularly in institutions for the mentally retarded and among migrant workers and some male homosexuals.

In the poor, rural areas of Latin America, *Trypanosoma cruzi* infects an estimated 8 million individuals, leaving many with the characteristic heart and gastrointestinal lesions of Chagas disease that characterize the chronic phase of this disease. An estimated 300,000 people who have immigrated from endemic areas live with this parasite in the United States. This parasite has a large reservoir host population, including many animals that live in peridomestic situations. This disease is transmitted by triatomine bugs that have also been found to be infected with *T cruzi* in the United States. In Africa, from the Sahara Desert in the north to the Kalahari in the south, related organisms, belonging to subspecies of the ancestral *Trypanosoma brucei*, cause one of the most lethal of human infections, sleeping sickness. Animal strains of this same organism limit food supplies by making the raising of cattle economically unfeasible over vast areas of the African continent. A large part of this latter problem is influenced by the activity of the vectors, members of the tsetse fly genus *Glossina*.

Leishmaniasis, a disease produced by an intracellular protozoan and transmitted by sandflies of the genus *Phlebotomus*, is found in parts of Europe, Asia, Africa, and Latin America. Clinical manifestations range from a self-limiting skin ulcer, known as oriental sore, through the mutilating mucocutaneous infection of espundia, to a highly lethal infection of the reticuloendothelial system (kala-azar).

In 1947, in an article entitled "This Wormy World," Stoll estimated that between the Tropic of Cancer and the Tropic of Capricorn, there were many more intestinal worm infections than people. The prevalence was judged to be far lower in temperate climates. The most serious of the helminthic diseases, schistosomiasis, affects an estimated 140 million individuals in Africa, Asia, and the Americas. These infections tend to be very chronic and persons with heavy worm burdens develop bladder, intestinal, and liver disease, which may ultimately result in death. The pathology accompanying schistosomiasis is largely the result of immune responses directed against eggs that get trapped in various tissues. Unfortunately, the disease is frequently spread because of rural development schemes involving irrigation projects. Egypt, Sudan, Ghana, and Nigeria have seen significant increases in the incidence of the disease in these areas due to extension of the snail vectors into new areas, often mitigating the economic gains of the development program itself.

The parasitic nematodes *Ascaris lumbricoides*, hookworms, and *Trichuris* infect more than 1.5 billion people. Collectively they account for tremendous morbidity that is manifest as reduced growth rates among children, iron deficiency, and anemia. *Ascaris* females can produce up to 250,000 extremely environmentally resistant eggs per day!

Larval tapeworm infections are a far more serious threat to human health than infections with adult tapeworms. This is exemplified by infection with the cysticercus of *Taenia solium*,

---

* Resistance of malaria to chemotherapeutics

* Resistance of insect vectors to insecticides

* Increases in imported malaria

Amebic infections in 10% of world

* Trypanosomiasis produces disease, limits food supplies

Leishmaniasis cutaneous or disseminated

* Worm infections spread by irrigation projects

Intestinal nematodes infect one-fourth of the world's population

which frequently results in neurocysticercosis. Another larval tapeworm infection caused by *Echinococcus granulosus* results in hydatid cyst disease in humans. An endemic pocket of this disease exists in the four corners area of the United States.

Larval and adult nematode infections cause serious illness. Two closely related filarial worms, *Wuchereria bancrofti* and *Brugia malayi*, which are endemic in Asia and Africa and transmitted by many species of mosquitoes, interfere with the flow of lymph and can produce grotesque swellings of the legs, arms, and genitals. Another filarid, transmitted by black flies, produces onchocerciasis (river blindness) in millions of Africans and Americans, leaving thousands blind.

Toxoplasmosis, giardiasis, trichomoniasis, cryptosporidiosis, and pinworm (enterobiasis) infections are five cosmopolitan parasitic infections well known to American physicians. Toxoplasmosis, a protozoan infection of cats, infects possibly one-half of the world's human population. Although it is usually asymptomatic, infection acquired in utero may result in abortion, stillbirth, prematurity, or severe neurologic defects in the newborn. Asymptomatic infection acquired either before or after birth may subsequently produce visual impairment. Immune suppression, such as caused by HIV infection and immunosuppressive therapy may reactivate latent infections, producing severe encephalitis.

Multiple parasitic diseases in United States

CLASSIFICATION, FORM, AND FUNCTION

■ Protozoa

Classification

The classification schemes for the Protozoa seem to be evolving even quicker than the organisms themselves. Within the context of this book a classification scheme used by classical parasitologists in textbooks has been adopted. It is based largely on light and electron microscopy and modes of locomotion, but considers current evolutionary thinking based on comparative genetics. Within the context of this scheme, the Protozoa are considered a subkingdom within the kingdom Protista.

The subkingdom Protozoa includes the following phyla: Sarcomastigophora, including the flagellates and amebas; Apicomplexa, including malaria parasites, *Cryptosporidium* and *Toxoplasma*; Microsporidia, including the microsporidia; and Ciliophora, including the ciliates (**Table 48-2**).

The Sarcomastigophora are an extremely diverse group including true flagellates of the subphylum Mastigophora and parasites such as those belonging to the genera *Leishmania*, *Trypanosoma*, *Giardia*, *Trichomonas*, and *Dientamoeba*. Mastigophorans include those that are obligate intracellular parasites (*Leishmania*), parasites of the blood vascular system (*Trypanosoma*), intestinal track (*Giardia*), or genital–urinary track (*Trichomonas*). The subphylum Sarcodina can also be found within this phylum and include the important genera *Entamoeba*, *Acanthamoeba*, and the ameba–flagellate *Naegleria*.

TABLE 48-2   Classification of Protozoan Parasites

Kingdom—Protista
  Subkingdom—Protozoa
    Phylum—Sarcomastigophora
      Subphylum—Mastigophora
        Genera—*Leishmania, Trypanosoma, Giardia, Trichomonas* and *Dientamoeba*
      Subphylum—Sarcodina
        Genera—*Entamoeba, Acanthamoeba,* and *Naegleria*
    Phylum—Apicomplexa
      Genera—*Plasmodium, Toxoplasma, Cryptosporidium,*
      Cyclospora, Isospora, Sarcocystis, and *Babesia.*
    Phylum—Microsporidia
      Genera—*Enterocytozoon* and *Encephalitozoon*
    Phylum—Ciliophora
      Genus—*Balantidium*

The Apicomplexa also represent a diverse group of organisms that have been placed together phylogenetically because of the presence of complex apical organelles in life cycle stages responsible for cellular invasion. All are obligate intracellular parasites for most of their life cycles. Parasites in this taxonomic grouping include members of the genera *Plasmodium, Toxoplasma, Cryptosporidium, Cyclospora, Isospora, Sarcocystis,* and *Babesia.*

The Microsporidia include an opportunistically important group of parasites called the microsporidia. Many infections in this group are seen in immunocompromised patients with the more important genera being *Enterocytozoon* and *Encephalitozoon.* The Ciliophora include a single genus, *Balantidium,* which is only occasionally encountered in humans.

Form and Function

Protozoa range in size from slightly more than 1 to more than 100 μm. They are single-celled organism and have a true membrane-bound nucleus. The nucleus contains clumped or dispersed chromatin and a central nucleolus or **karyosome.** The shape, size, and distribution of the nucleus can be useful in distinguishing protozoan species from one another.

The cytoplasm is frequently divided into an inner endoplasm and a thin outer ectoplasm. The granular **endoplasm** is concerned with nutrition and often contains food reserves, contractile vacuoles, and undigested particulate matter. The **ectoplasm** may be organized into specialized organelles of locomotion. In some species, these organelles appear as blunt, dynamic extrusions known as pseudopods. In others, highly structured thread-like cilia or flagella arise from intracytoplasmic basal bodies. Flagella are longer and less numerous than cilia and possess a structure and a mode of action distinct from those seen in prokaryotic organisms.

Endoplasm contains nutrients

Ectoplasm has organelles of locomotion

Most parasitic Protozoa are heterotrophic and must assimilate organic nutrients. This assimilation is accomplished by engulfing soluble or particulate matter in digestive vacuoles, processes termed **pinocytosis** and **phagocytosis,** respectively. In some species, food is ingested at a definite site, the peristome or cytostome. Food may be retained in special intracellular reserves, or vacuoles. Undigested particles and wastes are extruded at the cell surface by mechanisms that are the reverse of those used in ingestion. The intracellular location of many of these parasites means that host cells may have to be modified to accommodate for transport and assimilation of nutrients. This is especially true among the apicomplexans and parasites like *Leishmania.* Many parasitic protozoans are facultative anaerobes in their definitive host (*E histolytica* and *Giardia* are excellent examples). The African trypanosomes must switch from an inefficient anaerobic to a more efficient mode of aerobic respiration when they take up residence in their vector. This is accomplished by profound changes that take place within the kinetoplast–mitochondrial complex of these organisms. The malaria parasite *P falciparum* has been found to complete its development within the microaerophilic environment of postcapillary venules. This discovery now allows investigators to extensively cultivate this parasite *in vitro.* Some parasitic Protozoa are amitochondriate and utilize specialized organelles such as mitosomes (*Giardia*) or hydrogenosomes (*T vaginalis*) where terminal events of electron transfer in anaerobic respiration occur.

Many Protozoa are facultative anaerobes

＊ **Nutrients engulfed by phagocytosis or pinocytosis**

Survival is ensured by fastidious reproductive and protective techniques. Reproduction in many parasitic protozoans is accomplished primarily by simple binary fission. In one phylum of Protozoa, the Apicomplexa, a cycle of multiple fission (schizogony) alternates with a period of sexual reproduction (sporogony). A similar mode of reproduction is seen in the microsporidia although somewhat modified. Many Protozoa, when exposed to an unfavorable milieu, become less active metabolically and secrete a cyst wall capable of protecting the organism from physical and chemical conditions that would otherwise be lethal. In this form, the parasite is better equipped to survive passage from host to host in the external environment. *Giardia, Entamoeba, Naegleria, Cryptosporidium, Cyclospora,* and others are all capable of forming environmentally protective cysts or oocysts. The microsporidia produce spores. Immunoevasive mechanisms described in later chapters also contribute to survival of these parasites within the host.

Reproduction usually by binary fission

Protozoa form cysts as survival form

■ Helminths

Classification

As for the Protozoa, the classification of helminth parasites is ever changing. The scheme used in this book is a more classical one and readily accepted and understood by most parasitologists. Accordingly, the various helminth groups discussed are placed into distinct phyla within the subkingdom Metazoa of the kingdom Animalia, which includes all multicellular organisms. These phyla include the Platyhelminthes with the important classes Trematoda (flatworms)

TABLE 48–3	Classification of Helminth parasites

Kingdom—Animalia
  Subkingdom—Metazoa
    Phylum—Platyhelminthes
      Class—Trematoda
        Genera—*Schistosoma, Fasciola, Fasciolopsis, Clonorchis, and Paragonimus*
      Class—Cestoidea
        Genera—*Diphyllobothrium, Taenia, Echinococcus,* and *Hymenolepis*
    Phylum—Nemathelminthes
      Genera—*Trichuris, Trichinella, Capillaria, Strongyloides,*
      Necator, Ancylostoma, Ascaris, Toxocara, Wuchereria, Brugia, and Onchocerca
    Phylum—Acanthocephala
      Genus—*Macrocanthorhynchus*

and Cestoidea (tapeworm), the Nemathelminthes, or roundworms, and the Acanthocephala, or thorny-headed worms (**Table 48–3**).

The class Trematoda includes important parasites belonging to the genera *Schistosoma, Fasciola, Fasciolopsis, Clonorchis,* and *Paragonimus.* Cestoidea includes the tapeworm parasitic genera *Diphyllobothrium, Taenia, Echinococcus,* and *Hymenolepis.*

The Nemathelminthes include important parasites belonging to the genera *Trichuris, Trichinella, Capillaria, Strongyloides, Necator, Ancylostoma, Ascaris, Toxocara, Wuchereria, Brugia,* and *Onchocerca.*

The Acanthocephala contains only one genus, *Macracanthorhynchus,* considered to be of occasional importance to humans.

Form and Function

All helminths are multicellular organisms. The Trematoda vary in size from a few millimeters to several inches and are usually flat in shape. They all are invested in a tegument that is organized as a multicellular syncytium. Absorption of nutrients and excretion of wastes occur across the tegument. They are acoelomate with a body filled with parenchymal tissue. Embedded within this tissue are an incomplete digestive tract composed of ceca and the reproductive organs of both sexes. The schistosomes are an exception to this, have separate sexes, and are tubular in shape. Trematodes usually possess two suckers which help them to locomote and anchor to host tissue. Most trematodes have complex life cycles involving snails as a required first intermediate host in which asexual multiplication of larval stages takes place. Larval stages called cercaria emerge from snail and may either directly penetrate the final definitive host (the schistosomes), or encyst openly in the environment or within a second intermediate host (all other parasitic trematodes).

The Cestoidea, or tapeworms, have a flattened, ribbon-like body, or strobila, composed of segments called proglottids. Like the trematodes, they are invested in a tegument and are acoelomate with proglottids filled with parenchymal tissue. Each proglottid serves as an individual reproductive unit harboring both sets of male and female reproductive organs and are classified as being immature, mature, or gravid (egg filled). At the anterior end of the worm is a scolex (head region) that may or may not be armed with hooks. This body region is anchored to host tissue. Tapeworms continuously produce proglottids, which may be shed individually (apolysis) or as a chain once the eggs are released (anapolysis). They also possess a primitive nervous system that links the scolex to the proglottids. Tapeworms have complex life cycles that vary tremendously and will be discussed in chapters that follow. Infections by larval tapeworms usually result in greater pathogenesis to the host than infection by adult tapeworms. This is true of infections caused by *Diphyllobothrium latum, T solium, E granulosus,* and *Echinococcus multilocularis.*

The Nemathelminthes, or nematodes, have a cylindrical fusiform body and a tubular alimentary tract that extends from the mouth at the anterior end to the anus at the posterior end. They are invested in a tough cuticle that must be shed as they go through molts to become adults. They are considered as pseudocoelomate organisms with a body cavity filled with fluid. These worms possess only longitudinal muscles that allow them to flex and put pressure on internal organs so they can function. The sexes are separate, and the male worm is typically smaller than the female.

An unusual feature in males is that sperms are ameboid and not flagellated. A variety of reproductive modes are used by these worms including oviparity (egg laying), ovoviviparity (egg followed by larval birth in utero), and parthenogenesis. First larval stages are considered as L$_1$ upon hatching and molt four times to become adults. Life cycles vary tremendously within this group from being direct (*Trichuris*), indirect, and complex (*Strongyloides*), to those requiring an intermediate host (all filarial parasites). These life cycles will be discussed in chapters to follow. Helminth parasites are nourished by ingestion (nematodes) or absorption (trematodes and cestodes) of the body fluids, lysed tissue, or intestinal contents of their hosts. Carbohydrates are rapidly metabolized, and the glycogen concentration of the worms is high. Respiration is primarily anaerobic, although larval offspring frequently require oxygen. A large part of the energy requirement is devoted to reproductive needs. The daily output of offspring can be as high as 200,000 for some worms.

Protection from the host's digestive and body fluids is afforded by the tegument or cuticle and the secretion of enzymes. Some worms, such as the schistosomes, can protect themselves from immunologic attack by the incorporation of host antigens into their tegument. The life span of the adult helminth is often measured in weeks or months, but some, such as the hookworms, filariae, and flukes, can survive within their hosts for decades, producing chronic infections with attendant morbidity or mortality.

HOST TYPES AND TRANSMISSION PATTERNS

Parasites usually encounter one or more hosts during their life cycles, but the one host they must visit is the **definitive host.** This is the host in which the parasite reaches sexual maturity. Many protozoa do not have a sexual stage of the life cycle, in which case, if there is more than one host type in the life cycle, the more evolved host is usually considered the definitive host. Purists would argue that the mosquito is the definitive host for malaria because the sexual union of gametes occurs in that host, yet for this book, the definitive host is considered to be man. If some development of a parasite occurs in another host, then that host is considered an **intermediate host.** Snails are intermediate hosts for schistosome parasites and tsetse flies for most African trypanosomes. For one parasite, *Trichinella*, the same host is both a definitive and intermediate host because sexually active adult worms reside in the intestinal tract and the first-stage larvae are nurtured within muscle cells of the same host. Snail and tsetse fly intermediate hosts may also be considered **vectors.** However, there can be vectors in which no development takes place. Such a vector is then considered a **mechanical vector.** Such a host can also be referred to as a **paratenic** or **transport host.** Flies are considered transport hosts for *Giardia, Cryptosporidium,* and *E histolytica.* For many parasites there are also **reservoir hosts.** Such a host is a reservoir of infection from which other hosts can be infected. The East African trypanosomes have many ungulate species as reservoir hosts. These animals are considered as definitive hosts as well.

Some parasites, such as *Cryptosporidium hominis* and *Cyclospora cayetanensis* are highly **host specific.** In these cases, humans are the only hosts. *Cryptosporidium parvum*, on the other hand, is a zoonotic species with many animals serving as reservoirs from which man can become infected. *Trichinella*, mentioned earlier, is an example of a parasite that has loose host specificity. Any carnivorous animal can serve as a host for this parasite.

Parasitic infections that are transmissible from animals to humans are considered **zoonotic.** Many parasitic infections considered in the following chapters fall into this category. Those transmissible from humans to humans or back to animals are considered **anthroponotic.** *Cryptosporidium hominis* is readily transmissible from humans to humans, and some of the primate malarias encountered in South America are thought to have arisen from human malarias brought to the new world after colonization. Transmission patterns that only involve animals are considered **enzootic.** If a transmission pattern occurs in association with man, it is considered **synanthropic.** Many parasitic infections fall into this pattern of transmission. Transmission patterns may also involve life cycles occurring away from man and these usually involve animal hosts and are considered **sylvatic.** *Echinococcus granulosus* has a synanthropic cycle involving dogs, sheep, and man, and a sylvatic cycle involving deer and coyotes or moose and wolves.

■ Single-Host Parasite Life Cycle Examples

As is evident from the previous discussion, many parasites require but a single host species for the completion of their life cycles. The method by which the parasite is transmitted from individual to individual within that species is determined in large part by its viability in the external

TABLE 48–4	Transmission and Distribution of Four Representative Parasites		
ORGANISM	**INFECTIVE FORM**	**MECHANISM OF SPREAD**	**DISTRIBUTION**
Trichomonas vaginalis	Trophozoite	Direct (venereal)	Worldwide
Entamoeba histolytica	Cyst/trophozoite	Direct (venereal)	Worldwide
	Cyst	Indirect (fecal–oral)	Areas of poor sanitation
Ascaris lumbricoides	Egg	Indirect (fecal–oral)	Areas of poor sanitation
Plasmodium falciparum	Sporozoite	*Anopheles* mosquito	Tropical and subtropical areas

environment and, in the case of helminths, by the conditions required for the maturation of eggs or offspring. The mode of transmission, in turn, determines the social, economic, and geographic distribution of the parasite. A few examples are described in **Table 48–4.**

The protozoan *T vaginalis* does not produce a protective cyst form. Although its active or trophozoite form is relatively hardy, it can survive only a few hours outside of its normal habitat, the human genital tract. Thus, for all practical purposes, transmission requires the direct genital contact of sexual intercourse. Thus, trichomoniasis is cosmopolitan, occurring wherever human hosts engage in sexual activity with multiple partners.

Another protozoan, *E histolytica*, inhabits the human gut and produces hardy **cysts** that are passed in the stool. Transmission occurs when another individual ingests these cysts. Like *T vaginalis*, the organism can be passed by direct physical contact, in this case by oral–anal sexual activity. This mode of transmission, in fact, accounts for the high incidence of amebic infections in male homosexuals. Unlike *T vaginalis*, however, the cysts can survive for prolonged periods in the external environment, where they may eventually contaminate food or drinking water. Thus, in environments such as mental institutions, where the level of personal hygiene is low, or in populations in which methods for the sanitary disposal of human wastes are not available, amebiasis is common.

The intestinal helminth *A lumbricoides* illustrates still another transmission pattern. In this infection, highly resistant eggs are passed in the human stool. Unlike the situation with *E histolytica* described previously, the eggs are not immediately infective but must incubate in soil under certain conditions of temperature and humidity before they are fully embryonated and infectious. Thus, this parasite cannot be transmitted directly from host to host. The organism spreads only when indiscriminate human defecation results in deposition of eggs on soil and subsequent exposure of that soil to the climatic conditions required for embryonation of the eggs. For this reason, *Ascaris* infections are most prevalent in areas of the tropics and subtropics and are associated with poor sanitation.

■ Multiple-Host Parasite Life Cycle Examples

A few Protozoa and many helminths require two or more host species in their life cycle. As stated previously, to avoid confusion, it is customary to refer to the species in which the parasite reproduces sexually as the definitive host and that in which asexual reproduction or larval development takes place as the intermediate host. When there is more than one intermediate host, they are known simply as the first and second intermediate hosts. In some cases, such as that of *Taenia saginata*, the beef tapeworm, both host species are vertebrates; humans serve as the definitive host and cattle as the intermediate host. Among parasites that inhabit the blood and tissues of humans, it is more common for a blood-feeding arthropod to serve as a second host and as the transmitting vector. An example is malaria, in which the causative *Plasmodium* is transmitted from person to person by the bite of an infected female mosquito of the genus *Anopheles*. As mentioned previously, people argue whether mosquito or man is the definitive host as the sexual union of gametes occurs in the mosquito.

✳ Transmission by direct sexual contact

✳ Fecal–oral transmission common for intestinal parasites

Infectivity develops in soil

Multiple hosts may be involved

Definitive and intermediate hosts

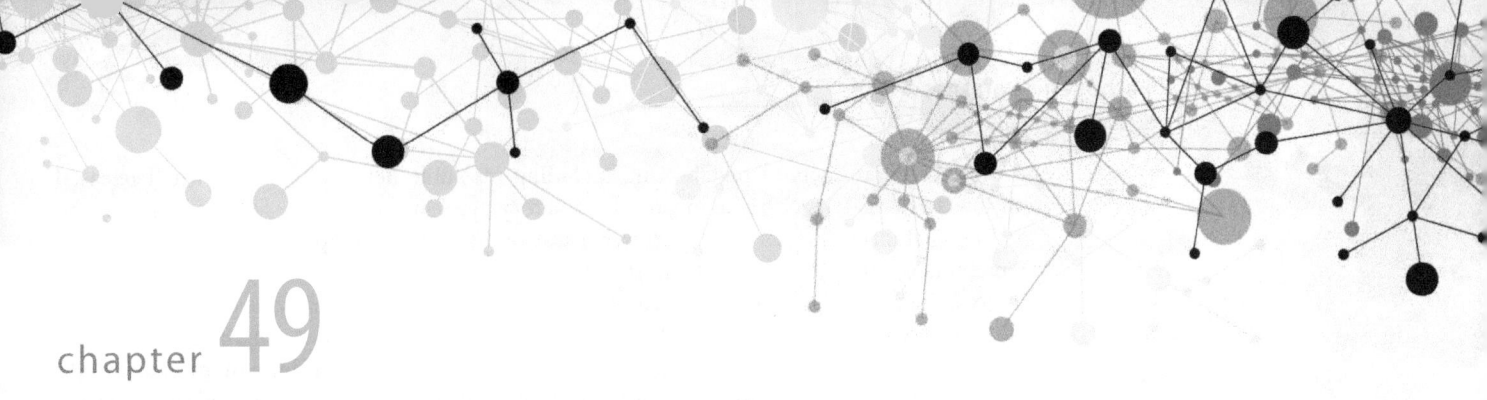

chapter 49

Pathogenesis and Diagnosis of Parasitic Infection

PATHOGENESIS

The pathogenesis of both protozoan and helminthic disease is highly variable. Many factors contribute to this variability and included among them may be parasite size, induced injury, reproductive potential, nutritional requirements (including metabolites or toxins produced), niche selection (often influenced by individual life cycles and migration patterns through the host), and last, but not the least, immunologic consequences of infection.

Parasite size may or may not be a predictor of pathogenesis. Many of the parasitic Protozoa, including those that cause malaria (*Plasmodium*), African sleeping sickness (*Trypanosoma brucei* subspecies), Chagas disease (*Trypanosoma cruzi*), and leishmaniasis (*Leishmania*), are among the smallest and most pathogenic. The giant cestode, *Diphyllobothrium latum*, can reach sizes exceeding 10 m, yet produces a pernicious anemia due to vitamin B12 competition with the host in less than 1% of the infected individuals. *Ascaris lumbricoides*, which can grow up to a foot in length can cause severe intestinal blockage if enough worms are present. The larval hydatid cyst of the tapeworm *Echinococcus granulosus* can achieve considerable size if given long enough to grow and can put tremendous pressure on organs it may be found within.

Parasite-induced injury frequently results from parasite invasion of host tissues. Hookworms, *Strongyloides* and *Trichuris*, repeatedly probe the intestinal or colon lining, promoting and inducing extensive, immunologically mediated inflammatory responses. In these cases, worm burden determines the extent of the pathogenesis. The egg laying of schistosome parasites determines the pathology of this infection as many eggs get trapped in tissues in their attempt to leave the host. The result is extensive inflammation and eventual fibrosis of affected tissues.

The reproductive potential of parasites varies considerably. Protozoa generally have short generational times. In large part, this is due to the asexual nature of their reproduction for much of their life cycles. Rates vary from several hours (African trypanosomes) to several days (malaria). This can place tremendous pressure on host resources with attendant consequences. Helminthes, however, are usually incapable of reproducing within their definitive hosts, so overall worm burden becomes a greater determinant of pathogenesis. This, in turn, will depend on how many eggs, or larvae, initiated the infection. An exception is encountered in *Trichinella*, in which fertile females residing within the intestinal lining give birth to larvae that migrate to the musculature.

Nutritional requirements among parasites vary tremendously, although most tend to be facultative anaerobes. All *Trypanosoma* spp. metabolize carbohydrates from their host, but the metabolites are fermentation-like end products of pyruvate that can affect endothelial linings within the host. Malaria parasites of the genus *Plasmodium* ultimately have rather synchronous infections and produce byproducts of metabolism, including insoluble hemozoin, which when released from infected cells trigger a rise in proinflammatory cytokines that cause fever and impair the functioning of macrophages. Hookworms, because of their voracious appetite and wasteful digestive methods, deplete the iron in the host, resulting in severe anemia if the worm burden is great enough. Hookworms, and many of their allies, also produce powerful enzymes to help predigest what they take in. These enzymes help produce inflammatory responses. *Entamoeba histolytica* and *Trichomonas vaginalis* produce enzymes that help mediate **contact-dependent cytotoxicity** reactions. In the case of *E histolytica*, this helps the parasite establish extraintestinal sites of infection. In one interesting case, the death of filarial parasites or their larvae in a definitive host also releases mutualistic endosymbionts. These are felt to contribute to inflammatory responses seen in such infections as those caused by *Onchocerca volvulus* and resulting in river blindness.

Where the parasite resides, or migrates during establishment in the host, can also be a strong determinant of pathogenesis. Many helminth parasites undergo an obligatory migration through the bloodstream that brings them in contact with lung tissue. This required migration often results in Loeffler syndrome that manifests as an intense eosinophilic inflammatory response. Larval stages of *Taenia solium* are frequently encountered in brain tissue, resulting in neurocysticercosis. Parasites such as *Toxocara canis* may be unable to complete full development in humans, but larvae try to migrate through tissues, causing visceral larval migrans. Many more examples will be expanded upon in chapters that follow.

Finally, there can be numerous immunologic consequences of infection that help promote pathogenesis. Antigen, antibody, and complement complexes combine to cause excessive anemia and glomerulonephritis in African trypanosomiasis. Allergic reactions play a major role in the cutaneous reactions to invading hookworm, *Strongyloides*, and schistosome larvae (ground itch, swimmers' itch). Transient pneumonias induced by the pulmonary migration of *Ascaris* and other nematode larvae (Loeffler syndrome), nocturnal paroxysms of asthma in some patients with filariasis (tropical pulmonary eosinophilia), and the shock, asthma, and urticaria that follow rupture of a hydatid cyst are all immunologically mediated. The latter frequently results in anaphylaxis. Cardiac damage in Chagas disease is thought, at least in part, to reflect immune-induced inflammatory responses, or perhaps autoimmune-related phenomena. Immune complex diseases are seen in schistosomiasis (Katayama syndrome) and malaria (nephrosis). The granulomatous reaction to schistosomal eggs is the result and antibody-dependent, cell-mediated cytotoxic (ADCC) responses. The entire clinicopathologic spectrum of manifestations arising from leishmanial infections appears to be caused by differences in the ability of cell-mediated immune responses to function properly.

✱ Immunopathologic mechanisms contribute to parasitic diseases

IMMUNITY AND IMMUNE EVASION

The large size, complex structure, varied metabolic activity, and synthetic prowess of most parasites provide their human host with an intense antigenic challenge. Generally, the resulting immunologic response is vigorous, but its role in modulating the parasitic invasion differs significantly from that in viral and bacterial infections. It is apparent from the chronic course and frequent recurrences typical of many parasitic diseases that complete acquired resistance resulting in sterile immunity is often absent. Immunity does, however, frequently serve to moderate the intensity of the infection and its associated clinical manifestations. In fact, clinical recovery and resistance to reinfection in some instances require the persistence of viable organisms at low concentration within the body of the host (**premunition = infection immunity**). An excellent example of this is seen in patients infected with *Toxoplasma gondii*.

Immune response vigorous but often ineffective

All those immune responses generally exercised against the more primitive viral and bacterial microorganisms, including **innate responses,** driven by the complement system, dendritic cells and natural killer cells, and **adaptive (acquired) responses,** driven by antibodies, cytokines (lymphokines), cytotoxic T lymphocytes, activated macrophages, memory cells, and ADCC mechanisms, have been shown to play a part in modulating parasitic infection.

Innate immune responses are usually immediate, less specific, and evolutionarily considered older than adaptive responses. Innate responses often depend on pattern recognition molecules leading to the destruction of bound organisms by complement activation and phagocytosis. Receptor engagement and activation are often critical to further involvement by adaptive responses. One example of innate responses manifests against parasite infections including those seen against malaria. The innate immune response to malaria involves multiple mechanisms, but rarely results in clearance of the parasite. Like other protozoan parasites, *Plasmodium falciparum* induces the production of IFN-γ by NK cells and subsequent phagocytosis of free parasites by macrophages. NK cells themselves can also lyse parasite-infected erythrocytes. Complicating the picture, improper activation of innate immune mechanisms during malaria may contribute to the disease. For instance, activation of the complement system is a common finding in human malaria, but excessive complement activation appears to be associated with an increased risk of cerebral malaria and severe malarial anemia in children. Likewise, iron sequestration mediated by hepcidin, another innate immune response against malaria, may also worsen anemia by decreasing erythropoiesis.

Overall, parasites are very capable of resisting host innate defenses. Adaptive responses, therefore, are critical in attempts by the host to control such infections and include both humoral and cell-mediated responses. As already noted, they are usually not perfect.

Antibodies are one line of defense against parasites. They play roles in opsonization, neutralization, complement activation, and ADCC adaptive responses. Antibodies are largely responsible for eliminating populations of trypanosomes from infected individuals. Interestingly, these antibodies are not formed as a result of classical immune stimulation, instead, the antigenic signal coming from the trypanosomes consists of T-independent antigens that can directly stimulate B cells to form antibody. In this case, the antibody is not the classical IgG but IgM. Although this is useful in eliminating the dominant population of trypanosomes present, another wave of parasites arises because of antigenic variation. Antibodies, if present in high enough concentration, can neutralize sporozoites and merozoites of malaria, thereby preventing them from invading their target host cells, hepatocytes, and red blood cells. Antibody generation against malarial sporozoites using attenuated and recombinant vaccines is currently undergoing multiple pilot clinical trials in developing countries where malaria is endemic. Complement activation does not usually result in direct parasite killing. In fact, many protozoan parasites have evolved mechanisms to avoid complement-mediated killing. Instead, complement appears to play a role in cell-mediated and especially ADCC responses against parasites.

All elements of immune response mobilized

On invasion of tissue, many helminths, and the schistosomes in particular, stimulate the production of IgE, the Fc portion of which binds to mast cells and basophils. Interaction of the antibody with parasitic antigen triggers the release of histamine and other mediators from the attached cells. These may injure the worm directly or, by increasing vascular permeability and stimulating the release of chemotactic factors, may lead to the accumulation of other cells and IgE antibodies capable of initiating antibody-dependent, cell-mediated destruction of the parasite. This is augmented by complement. The specific killer cell involved is often the eosinophil. These cells attach by their Fc receptor site to IgE antibody-coated parasites and degranulate, releasing a major basic protein that is directly toxic to the worm.

✳ IgE response to worms attracts eosinophils

Eosinophils release toxic protein

Cellular immunity is likewise important as an adaptive response. It is a hallmark of cutaneous *Leishmania tropica* infections. Skin lesion biopsies show the presence of lymphocytes and macrophages working in synergy to contain parasites. Activated macrophages are quite capable of destroying engulfed leishmanial parasites. However, defects in this type of cooperation can be seen in leishmanial infections that result in mucocutaneal leishmaniasis. Lesions containing these parasites contain plenty of macrophages, but few or no lymphocytes.

Cytotoxic T cells, or CD8+ T cells, play an important part in response to many protozoan infections. These cells not only produce INF-γ but can also produce TNF-α, and recently have been shown to produce IL-17. Collectively, all the cytokines have been shown to have varying roles for protective responses in toxoplasmosis, malaria, Chagas disease, and leishmaniasis.

Many cellular responses also work in consort with antibody responses to assist in modulating parasitic infections. An excellent example of this is seen in the case of many nematode infections such as *Trichinella*, *Ancylostoma*, *Necator*, and *Strongyloides*, where intimate association with intestinal tissue is an integral part of the life cycle. Such interactions lead to inflammatory responses that are the result of antigen signaling through the Peyer patches, movement of cells to mesenteric lymph nodes, and clonal expansion of both T and B cells that migrate back to the intestinal epithelium to promote inflammatory responses that depend on both antibody and cell-mediated constituents. The whole idea of inflammation in this instance is to produce an environment inhospitable for the worms or to induce worm expulsion as in the case of *Trichinella*.

Many parasites are capable of evading host immune responses. The strategies used vary considerably and allow the parasite to successfully propagate and spread to other hosts. If immune responses were completely successful in eliminating parasites, parasites would no longer be a problem. However, if all parasites killed their hosts, transmission would be interrupted. What good is a dead host to a parasite? The techniques by which parasites have been shown to evade the consequences of the host's specific adaptive responses are numerous. Included among them are seclusion within immunologically protected areas of the body, continual alteration of surface antigens (antigenic variation), molecular mimicry, and active evasion or suppression of the host's effector mechanisms. Several protozoa are shielded from the host defenses by virtue of their intracellular location. Some have even found ways to avoid or survive the normally lethal environment of the macrophage, a first-line defense cell normally intent on destroying pathogens it encounters. *T cruzi*, for example, escapes from phagosomes into the cytoplasm early during host infection. *T gondii* inhibits the fusion of phagosomes with lysosomes, thus preventing phagolysosome formation. *Leishmania* species, capable of neither of these feats, are resistant to the action of lysosomal enzymes and survive in macrophage phagolysosomes. Once macrophages have been activated to sufficient levels; however, the tables are somewhat turned on these parasites.

Protozoa escape phagosome, prevent phagosome/lysosome fusion, avoid destruction

In the examples given above, *T cruzi* and *T gondii* have alternate mechanisms for escaping host responses. They do so by becoming intracellular in cell types not normally involved in immune responsiveness. The gut lumen is perhaps the largest immunologic sanctuary within the body, because, unless the integrity of the intestinal mucosa is breached by injury or inflammation, this barrier protects lumen-dwelling parasites, many of which are surrounded by a protective tegument, or cuticle, from most of the effective humoral and cellular immune mechanisms of the host, allowing survival and the opportunity to reproduce.

✳ **Outer covering of parasite may provide protection from host defenses**

Most immune effector mechanisms are directed against the surface antigens of the parasite, and alteration of these antigens may blunt the immunologic attack. Many parasites undergo developmental changes within their hosts that are generally accompanied by alterations in surface antigens. Immune responses directed at an early developmental stage may be totally ineffective against a later stage of the same parasite. Such stage-specific immunity is very evident in malaria because different life cycle stages express different antigens and even give rise to different types of responses. The issue of stage-specific immunity in malaria is further compounded by species-specific immunity. No wonder we still do not have a totally effective vaccine against this disease. Even more intriguing is the ability of some parasites to vary the antigenic characteristics of a single developmental stage. The trypanosomes that cause African sleeping sickness circulate in the bloodstream coated with a thick glycoprotein surface coat. The development of humoral antibody to this coating results in the elimination of parasites from the blood expressing the dominant surface coat. However, within this dominant population of parasites are a few that have undergone antigenic variation and produced a new variant surface glycoprotein coat. This less dominant population gives rise to the next dominant population and this process repeats itself over and over. Over 1000 variant types can arise via this process. The process is genetically and not immunologically driven. The expression of individual genes from this large genetic repertoire is controlled by the sequential transfer of a duplicate copy of each gene to an area of the parasite genome responsible for gene expression. Continued antigenic variation, unfortunately, causes host immunosuppression with attendant consequences.

✳ **Antigenic shifts occur in parasites**

✳ **Trypanosomal variation outpaces immunologic response**

Variants of trypanosomes selected from preexisting repertoire

Several protozoan and helminthic pathogens are thought to be capable of neutralizing antibody-mediated attack by shedding and, later, regenerating specific surface antigens. Adult schistosomes, in addition, may immunologically hide from the host by masking themselves with host blood group antigens and immunoglobulins and through a process known as molecular mimicry by which they produce substances that are transported to their tegument that mimic substances naturally found within the host.

Antigenic shedding, masking with host antigens

Several parasites can destroy or inactivate immunologic mediators. Tapeworm larvae produce anticomplementary chemicals, and *T cruzi* splits the Fc component of attached antibodies, rendering it incapable of activating complement. Several protozoa, most notably *T brucei* species that are responsible for African sleeping sickness, induce polyclonal B-cell activation leading to the production of nonspecific immunoglobulins and eventual exhaustion of the antibody-producing capacity of the host. This and other protozoa can produce nonspecific suppression of both cellular and humoral effector mechanisms, also enhancing the host's susceptibility to a variety of unrelated secondary infections. Patients with disseminated leishmaniasis display a specific inability to mount a cellular immune response to parasitic antigens in the absence of evidence of generalized immunosuppression. Finally, the thick, tough cuticle of many adult helminths renders them impervious to immune effector mechanisms designed to deal with the less robust microbes.

✳ **Destroy immunologic mediators**

✳ **Cause immune suppression**

Cuticle resists immune effectors

DIAGNOSIS

Diagnosing parasitic infections can test the limits of the best physicians and diagnostic laboratories. Many of these infections are not frequently encountered in most of the industrialized world, as they are elsewhere, and many laboratories do not routinely handle requests to diagnose such infections. In addition, personnel may be poorly trained to adequately diagnose these infections.

The continuous arrival of travelers and immigrants from endemic areas, and the fact that parasitic infections may at times be life-threatening, necessitates consideration of these diseases in differential diagnoses. Unfortunately, the clinical manifestations of parasitic infections are highly varied, often mimic other disease conditions, and are seldom sufficiently characteristic to raise this possibility in the clinician's mind. It is incumbent upon the physician to ask questions related to travel history, food and liquid intake, activities, exposure to biting insects, etc, to raise the possibility that the individual might have acquired a parasitic disease.

Consider indigenous, imported infections

Once considered, an appropriate diagnostic test must be ordered. Typically, diagnosis rests on the demonstration and morphologic identification of the parasite or its progeny in the stool, urine, sputum, blood, or tissues of the human host.

✱ *Morphologic demonstration primary diagnostic*

A routine blood differential may raise the specter of such an infection. Eosinophilia has been recognized as an important clue to the diagnosis of parasitic disease. However, this phenomenon is characteristic only of helminthic infection, and even in these cases it is frequently variable. Eosinophilia, which presumably reflects an immunologic response to the complex foreign proteins possessed by worms, is most marked during tissue migration. Once migration ceases, the eosinophilia may decrease or disappear entirely.

In intestinal infections, an O&P or ova and parasite examination may suffice. This may involve concentration procedures such as floatation or sedimentation, followed by a wet mount or stained smear, or both, of the stool sample. Some parasites, such as *Giardia*, however, may be passed in the feces intermittently or in fluctuating numbers and repeated specimens are needed to confirm infection. Occasionally, specimens other than stool must be examined. In the case of small bowel infections, such as giardiasis and strongyloidiasis, aspirates of the duodenum or a small bowel biopsy may be required to establish the diagnosis. Similarly, the recovery of large bowel parasites such as *E histolytica* and *Schistosoma mansoni* may require proctoscopy or sigmoidoscopy, with aspiration or biopsy of suspect lesions. Eggs of pinworms (*Enterobius*) may be found on the perianal skin and require recovery using a specialized scotch tape application technique.

✱ *Stool concentration for intestinal parasites*

Parasites dwelling within the tissue and blood of the host are more difficult to identify. Direct examination of the blood is useful for the detection of malarial parasites, *Leishmania*, trypanosomes, and filarial progeny (microfilariae). The concentration of organisms in the bloodstream may fluctuate, however, and require the collection of multiple specimens over several days. Both wet mount and stained preparations of thin and thick blood smears (see Chapter 51) are used. Timing of blood collection is important in diagnosing filarial infections because they may display marked periodicity. Lung flukes and occasionally other helminths discharge their offspring in the sputum and may be found there with appropriate concentration techniques. In others, larvae can be recovered with skin (onchocerciasis) or muscle (trichinosis) biopsy.

Blood and tissue parasites require timing

In some infections, parasite recovery is uncommon. Immunodiagnostic and nucleic acid hybridization techniques provide diagnostic alternatives for these situations. Although tests for circulating antibodies have long been available for many parasitic diseases, they have often lacked sensitivity and specificity. The replacement of crude, antigenically complex parasitic extracts with purified homologous antigens, together with the adaptation of highly reactive test systems, has significantly increased the sensitivity and specificity of such tests. Currently, reliable serologic procedures are available for amebiasis, cysticercosis, echinococciasis, paragonimiasis, schistosomiasis, strongyloidiasis, toxocariasis, toxoplasmosis, and trichinosis. More will undoubtedly follow in the near future.

Serologic tests available for some parasites

Techniques for the detection of parasitic antigens in blood, body fluids, tissues, and excreta also have been developed. Commercial immunofluorescent and immunosorbent kits for *T vaginalis* (genitourinary fluids), *E histolytica*, *Giardia*, and *Cryptosporidium* (feces) are now commonly found in clinical laboratories. Less generally available are systems for the detection of malaria antigens in blood and *T gondii* in tissue.

Antigen detection becoming available

Even with many recent advances, the acknowledged limitations of both microscopic and serologic techniques in diagnosing parasitic infections have stimulated a widespread interest in resorting to gene amplification techniques to affect a more sensitive and specific diagnosis of

✳ Molecular methods used increasingly

these infections. The advent of the polymerase chain reaction (PCR) in its various formats has had a tremendous impact on detecting many parasite infections. Highly specific probes are available for the detection of malaria, Chagas disease, the African trypanosomes, leishmaniasis, toxoplasmosis, cryptosporidiosis, schistosomiasis, cysticercosis, and the etiologic agents of lymphatic filariasis. In some instances, PCR can be multiplexed and conducted in real time (RT-PCR). This permits the simultaneous detection of several parasites from one sample. The probes for many of these parasites have demonstrated sensitivities that match or exceed those of traditional techniques. The major limitations of PCR probes as diagnostic tools largely relate to the technical aspects of the hybridization procedure and, with time, will undoubtedly be overcome.

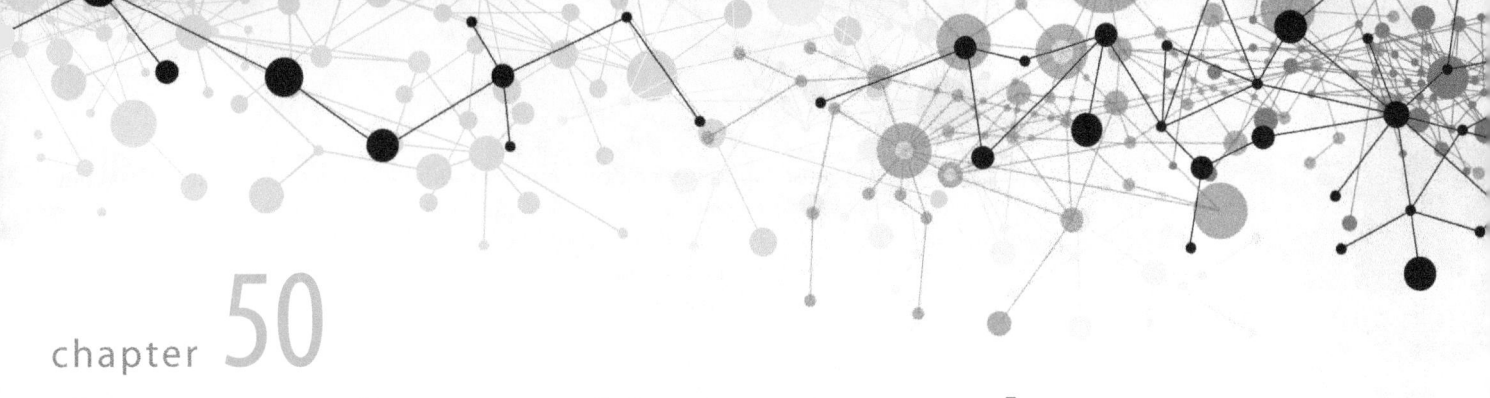

chapter 50

Antiparasitic Agents and Resistance

OVERVIEW

Most parasitic infections can be treated. Generally, drugs are effective against either protozoa or helminths, but not both. Some are well tolerated, while others are toxic or unpleasant for the patient. Antiparasitic resistance is a much more important issue in protozoan infections than helminth infections due to the worms' more complex and slow life cycles. All providers should be familiar with the medications covered here.

Parasites have been with us throughout human history, and the use of natural remedies to treat these infections date to antiquity. Quinine-containing extracts of cinchona tree bark were used to treat malaria hundreds of years ago. In China, a recipe for malaria treatment using Qinghaosu tea was recorded by Ge Hong centuries earlier. Based on what we now know about the chemistry of these natural products, both remedies had a firm biochemical basis for their effectiveness. By 1930, chemically synthesized drugs had been marketed for the treatment of malaria, trypanosomiasis, and schistosomiasis.

Antiparasitic agents among first antimicrobials

In spite of the introduction and explosive increase in the number and variety of antibacterials, antiparasitic medications have lagged far behind. Most antibacterials are ineffective against parasites, which share eukaryotic characteristics of their hosts. Most antiparasitics were only partially effective, toxic, and required prolonged or parenteral administration. In time, newer antiparasitics were developed that overcame many of these problems. Their numbers are still limited, and only recently have their safety and efficacy begun to match those of their antibacterial equivalents.

Newer antiparasitics broader spectrum, less toxic

Antiparasitic drug use and development have been shaped to a significant degree by the concentration of parasitic diseases in impoverished areas of the world. Community-based public health measures aimed at interrupting pathogen transmission—such as provision of sanitary facilities, clean water supplies, and insecticide-treated bed nets—are often beyond the means of tightly constrained local budgets. Consequently, the major burden of mitigating the impact of parasitic illnesses in endemic areas often falls on clinical officers or community health workers who, operating in remote and under-resourced conditions, must examine, diagnose, and treat sick patients with whom they may have only fleeting contact. Given these realities, optimal therapy for parasitic infections requires drugs that are effective in a single oral dose, easily administered, safe enough to be dispensed with limited medical supervision, sufficiently inexpensive to be widely used, and at low risk of accelerating drug resistance. Few such agents exist. Pharmaceutical companies, faced with the enormous costs of drug development and approval, have been reluctant to expend capital they are unlikely to recover. Public–private partnerships, cofinanced and operated by philanthropic organizations, industry, and academia, provide an exciting model that may yield the next wave of effective treatment for parasitic infections.

Treatment programs difficult in emerging economies

STRUCTURE AND ACTION

With few exceptions, antiparasitic agents have been synthesized de novo rather than developed from naturally occurring substances. Most are relatively simple and often contain benzene or other ring structures.

Most antiparasitics are synthetic

It is believed that most antiprotozoan drugs interfere with nucleic acid synthesis or, less commonly, with carbohydrate metabolism. Antihelminthics, on the other hand, apparently act by compromising the worm's glycolytic pathways or neuromuscular function. In most cases, the parasite and host cells have functionally equivalent target sites. Differential toxicity is achieved by preferential uptake, metabolic alteration of the drug by the parasite, or differences in the susceptibility of functionally equivalent sites in parasite and host.

As has been the case for antibacterial agents, the impact of many antiprotozoan agents has been compromised by the development of resistance in the parasite. This seems to have resulted from mutation and selection in the face of intensive drug use. The mechanisms responsible have been studied for only a few parasites, but appear to be related to reduced uptake or increased efflux of the drug.

DRUGS FOR PROTOZOAN INFECTIONS

As with bacteria, most protozoa are usually harmless. However, certain protozoa may cause disease, and for them the goal of treatment is to achieve a full microbiological cure.

■ Antimalarial Quinolines

Cinchona bark was used in Europe for the treatment of malaria beginning in the 1600s. Its active ingredient is a quinoline alkaloid called **quinine.** Synthesis of new quinolines was stimulated by the interruption of quinine supplies during the World War I and World War II and, after 1961, by the growing impact of drug-resistant falciparum malaria in several areas of the world. Among the most effective agents are those that share the double-ring structure of quinine.

Current analogs fall into three major groups: 4-aminoquinolines (including **chloroquine**), 8-aminoquinolines (including **primaquine**), and 4-quinolinemethanols (including **mefloquine**). All of them selectively destroy intracellular parasites by accumulating in parasitized host cells. Most of these agents appear to inhibit heme polymerase, leading to the buildup of toxic hemoglobin metabolites within the malarial parasite.

Quinine, chloroquine, and mefloquine concentrate in parasitized erythrocytes and rapidly destroy the erythrocytic stage of the parasite that is responsible for the clinical manifestations of malaria. Thus, these agents can be used either prophylactically to prevent clinical symptoms or therapeutically to terminate an acute attack. They do not concentrate in tissue cells, and thus organisms sequestered in sites outside the erythrocytes, particularly the liver, survive and may later reestablish erythrocytic infection and produce a clinical relapse. In contrast, primaquine and tafenoquine accumulate in tissue cells, destroy hepatic parasites, and effect a full "radical" cure.

Chloroquine phosphate was the most widely used antimalarial drug for decades. In the doses used for long-term malaria prophylaxis it was remarkably free of untoward effects. Unfortunately, its heavy use led to widespread resistance in *Plasmodium falciparum*, and thus it is no longer recommended for prevention or treatment of falciparum malaria in most parts of the world (see Resistance below). Primaquine phosphate, the 8-aminoquinoline used to eradicate persistent hepatic parasites, has toxic effects related to its oxidant activity. Methemoglobinemia and hemolytic anemia are particularly frequent in patients with glucose-6-phosphate dehydrogenase deficiency because they are unable to generate sufficient quantities of the reduced form of nicotinamide adenine dinucleotide to respond to this oxidant stress. Typically, the anemia is severe in patients of Mediterranean and Far Eastern ancestry and mild in patients of African ancestry. The newer drug tafenoquine carries the same potential risk but is taken more conveniently with a single dose rather than daily for 2 weeks with primaquine.

Quinine is the oldest and most toxic of the quinolines. It is currently used for severe or complicated malaria only when artemisinin combination therapy is not available (see later). Quinidine, a less cardiotoxic optical isomer of quinine, is better tolerated but not readily available in the United States. Mefloquine, an oral 4-quinolinemethanol analog, originally displayed a high level of activity against most chloroquine-resistant parasites; however, mefloquine-resistant strains of *P falciparum* are now widespread in Southeast Asia and are present to a lesser degree in South America and Africa. Concerns regarding psychiatric side effects of mefloquine have been generally overblown, but serve as another reason for the waning use of this medication.

Phenanthrene methanols are not in the strict sense quinine analogs. Nevertheless, they are structurally similar to this group of agents and, together with them, were discovered to have

✳ Differential toxicity based on uptake, metabolic factors

✳ Acquired resistance involves reduced uptake

✳ Quinine and analogs active against malaria

Accumulate, block heme metabolism

✳ Suppress malarial infection in RBCs

✳ 8-aminoquinolones cure by treating liver

✳ Chloroquine less effective

✳ Primaquine, tafenoquine may have hematologic toxicity

Quinine active against chloroquine-resistant malarial strains

antimalarial activity during the World War II. **Halofantrine,**[*] the most effective of the group, is a blood schizonticide effective against both sensitive and multidrug-resistant strains of *P falciparum*. However, because of rare cases of fatal heart arrhythmias, it is not available in the United States. A related drug, **Lumefantrine,** is much safer, but is unreliable when dosed alone. It is always administered as a coformulation with artemisinins (see later).

Phenanthrenes active against multidrug-resistant malaria

▪ Artemisinin

This natural extract of the plant *Artemisia annua* (qing hao, sweet wormwood) is a sesquiterpene lactone peroxide that is structurally distinct from all other known antiparasitic compounds. Extracts of qing hao were recommended for the treatment of fevers in China as early as AD 341; their specific antimalarial activity was defined by Chinese investigators in 1971. Although it has also been shown to be active against the free-living amoeba *Naegleria fowleri* and several trematodes, including *Schistosoma japonicum*, *Schistosoma mansoni*, and *Clonorchis sinensis*, its greatest impact to date has been in the treatment of malaria. Extensive investigations showed it to be schizonticidal for both chloroquine-sensitive and chloroquine-resistant strains of *P falciparum*. Several derivatives, among them **artemether** and **artesunate,** are significantly more active than the parent compound. All are concentrated in parasitized erythrocytes, where they decompose and release free radicals, which are thought to damage parasitic membranes. Artemisinin compounds act more rapidly than other antimalarial agents, stopping parasite development and preventing cytoadherence in falciparum malaria. Because of their relatively short half-life, they should be administered in coformulations with longer-acting agents such as lumefantrine. This "artemisinin combination therapy (ACT)" is so safe and effective that it has become the standard of care for treatment of acute malaria worldwide. Unfortunately, resistance has been detected, especially among *P falciparum* isolates from the Thai–Myanmar border. Although depression of reticulocyte counts has been reported, these agents appear significantly less toxic than quinoline antimalarials. Because there is some evidence that they may possess teratogenic properties, they should be avoided in the first trimester of pregnancy if possible. They may be given orally, rectally (by suppository), or parenterally.

Active against malaria, amoebas, *Schistosoma*

Concentrated in erythrocytes

＊ ACT treatment of choice for falciparum malaria

▪ Quinones

Atovaquone is a novel hydroxynaphthoquinone that shows promise in the treatment of malaria and toxoplasmosis. Its antiparasitic activity appears to result from the specific blockade of pyrimidine biosynthesis secondary to the inhibition of the parasite's mitochondrial electron transport chain.

Efficacy trials established its capacity to affect rapid clearance of parasitemia in patients with chloroquine-resistant falciparum malaria. Frequent parasitic recrudescences were eliminated when atovaquone was administered in combination with the folate antagonist **proguanil** (see later). This coformulation (**Malarone**) is popular in malaria prophylaxis because it is effective, well tolerated, and protects against liver infection, thus can be dosed for just a week following exposure. Atovaquone has also demonstrated activity against toxoplasmosis in patients with acquired immunodeficiency syndrome (AIDS). Unlike other antitoxoplasma agents, atovaquone is active against *Toxoplasma gondii* cysts as well as tachyzoites, suggesting that this agent may produce radical cure. Supporting this is the infrequency with which cessation of atovaquone treatment of toxoplasmic cerebritis in AIDS patients has resulted in relapse. Relapse after atovaquone treatment of the fungus *Pneumocystis jirovecii* in this same patient population appears similarly uncommon.

＊ Atovaquone stable and active against malaria and toxoplasmosis

▪ Folate Antagonists

Folic acid is a critical coenzyme for the synthesis of purines and ultimately DNA. In protozoa, as in bacteria, the active form of folic acid is produced *in vivo* by a simple two-step process. The first step, the conversion of *para*-aminobenzoic acid to dihydrofolic acid, is blocked by sulfonamides. The second step, the transformation of dihydro- to tetrahydrofolic acid, is blocked by folic acid antagonists, which competitively inhibit dihydrofolate reductase. Used together with sulfonamides, folate antagonists may inhibit the growth of some protozoa.

Trimethoprim, an inhibitor of dihydrofolate reductase, is used in combination with sulfamethoxazole to treat toxoplasmosis. Another folate antagonist, **pyrimethamine,** has a high affinity for sporozoan dihydrofolate reductase and has been particularly effective, when used with

Sulfonamide and folate antagonists inhibit protozoa

---

[*]Not available in the United States.

a sulfonamide, in the management of clinical malaria and toxoplasmosis. A third folate antagonist, **proguanil,** is commonly taken in combination with atovaquone for malaria prophylaxis. Acquired protozoal resistance to sulfonamides coformulated with folate antagonists has greatly diminished their effectiveness for malaria prevention and treatment.

Folate antagonists may result in folate deficiency in individuals with limited folate reserves, such as newborns, pregnant women, and the malnourished. This is of greatest concern when large doses are used for prolonged periods, as in the treatment of acute toxoplasmosis. When folate antagonists are used with sulfonamides, the entire range of sulfonamide toxic effects may be seen. Patients with advanced AIDS may suffer an unusually high incidence of toxic side effects to trimethoprim–sulfamethoxazole.

■ Nitroimidazoles

Metronidazole, a nitroimidazole, was introduced in 1959 for the treatment of trichomoniasis. Subsequently, it was found to be effective in the management of giardiasis, amebiasis, and a variety of infections produced by obligate anaerobic bacteria. Energy metabolism in all of them depends on the presence of low-redox–potential compounds, such as ferredoxin, to serve as electron carriers. These compounds reduce the 5-nitro group of the imidazoles to produce intermediate products responsible for the death of the protozoal and bacterial cells, possibly by alkylation of DNA. Resistance, though uncommon, has been noted in strains of *Trichomonas vaginalis* lacking nitroreductase activity. Nausea, dysgeusia (taste perversion), and peripheral neuropathy are notable potential side effects.

Tinidazole, a newer nitroimidazole, appears to be both a more effective and better-tolerated antiprotozoal agent. Its greater lipid solubility improves cerebrospinal fluid levels and *in vitro* activity. Either drug can be used for trichomoniasis, invasive amebiasis, and giardiasis.

Benznidazole, another member of this drug family, is used for the treatment of Chagas disease. A related medication in the nitrofuran class, **nifurtimox,** is also used for this condition. Both may be toxic to the gastrointestinal and neurological systems and these treatments have limited efficacy in chronic Chagas. This disease is an important cause of morbidity and mortality in Latin America, and newer treatments are urgently needed.

■ Nitazoxanide

A member of the thiazolide class, nitazoxanide provides an unusually broad spectrum of activity. It is effective not only against gastrointestinal protozoa such as giardia and amoeba, but in trials has also killed helminths such as human hookworm. In fact, it has demonstrated *in vitro* activity against certain anaerobic bacteria and even some viruses, although it is not used clinically for those purposes. In diarrhea due to giardia or cryptosporidium, for which it is approved in the United States, its mechanism seems to be interfering with the cell's electron transfer enzymes. Unfortunately, its clinical usefulness in cryptosporidiosis among immunocompromised patients is limited, and new medications for this condition are urgently needed.

■ Eflornithine (Difluoromethylornithine)

Eflornithine is an enzyme-activated, irreversible inhibitor of ornithine decarboxylase (ODC). In mammalian cells, decarboxylation of ornithine by ODC is a mandatory step in the synthesis of polyamines, compounds thought to play critical roles in cell division and differentiation. Originally developed as an antineoplastic agent, eflornithine proved ineffective in cancer chemotherapy trials. It was also marketed as a topical depilatory agent (anti hair growth). With the discovery that polyamines of *Trypanosoma* species were also synthesized from ornithine, eflornithine was successfully tested in the treatment of animal trypanosomiasis. It has been used to treat advanced cases of human West African sleeping sickness due to *T brucei gambiense*. However, it is not effective against the more virulent *T brucei rhodesiense*, it is dosed intravenously, and it remains expensive. Eflornithine appears to be cytostatic and requires an intact host immune system for maximum effect.

■ Heavy Metals

Arsenic and antimonial compounds have been used for generations. They form stable complexes with sulfur compounds and probably exert their biologic effects by binding to sulfhydryl (–SH) groups. They are toxic to the host as well as to the parasite, and have their greatest impact on cells

---

✷ Sulfonamides effective in *Toxoplasma* infections

Folate deficiency, sulfonamide toxicities occur during treatment

Active against protozoa at low-redox–potential

Alternative option for giardiasis

Originally an anticancer drug

Active against West African sleeping sickness

that are metabolically active such as neuronal, renal tubular, intestinal epithelial, and bone marrow stem cells. Their differential toxicity and therapeutic value are due to enhanced uptake by the parasite and its intense metabolic activity. However, significant host toxicity remains. Only one trivalent arsenical, **melarsoprol** (Mel B), is now used for African trypanosomiasis of the central nervous system, because of its penetration of the blood–brain barrier. Due to its toxicity, including a roughly 10% chance of fatal arsenic poisoning, it is used only when less toxic agents have failed or when the central nervous system is involved. Safer agents are urgently needed for this deadly disease.

Antimonial agents are now restricted to the management of leishmanial infections. Two pentavalent compounds, **sodium stibogluconate** (Pentostam) and **meglumine antimoniate**† (Glucantime), may be used for all forms of leishmaniasis. In disseminated visceral disease, prolonged therapy is usually required, and relapses often occur. In localized cutaneous leishmaniasis, cure is usually achieved with a relatively brief course. Toxic side effects are similar to those of the arsenicals, although less severe. However, visceral leishmaniasis is usually treated using intravenous **amphotericin-lipid** formulations, which are typically used as antifungal medications. In fact, these drugs are being used more frequently for cutaneous leishmaniasis as well, where they are often effective and better tolerated than the antimonials.

■ Miltefosine

A recent advance in antiprotozoal treatment is the introduction of **miltefosine.** This alkylphosphocholine compound belongs to the phospholipid family. It appears to target protein kinase B, a molecule involved in cellular apoptosis regulation. Blockade of protein kinase B seems to trigger programmed death of infected cells, including many strains of leishmania and free-living amoebas. And, it is dosed orally. As clinical experience grows with this medication, it seems to hold great promise for the treatment of these neglected infections.

KEY CONCLUSIONS

- Antiprotozoan medications act through a variety of mechanisms.
- Some are highly organism specific, while others have a broader spectrum.
- Older medications may be profoundly toxic; newer compounds are better tolerated.
- Resistance is of particular concern for the antimalarial drugs (see later).

DRUGS FOR HELMINTH INFECTIONS

The approach to treatment of most worm infections differs significantly from those applied to prokaryotic or protozoan infections. Helminths, with few exceptions, do not multiply within the human host, and severe infections usually require the repeated acquisition of infectious worms.

For gastrointestinal helminth infections, full eradication is not usually necessary. Interestingly, the intensity of gastrointestinal worm burden does not follow a normal distribution in human populations. Most infected persons harbor fewer than a dozen adult worms in the GI tract; a small minority of "wormy persons" harbor very large worm numbers. Because there is a direct correlation between worm burden and clinical disease, only this minority suffers significant morbidity. Concentrating treatment on those few clinically ill patients could moderate the medical impact of a helminthic disease on the community at a cost dramatically lower than that required for mass treatment. Moreover, it is usually unnecessary to eradicate all gastrointestinal worms from treated patients; a significant decrease in the worm burden may be adequate to alleviate clinical symptoms. This can often be accomplished with entire affected populations by providing short, subcurative doses that further reduce cost and minimize the likelihood of drug toxicity. Because this approach can dramatically decrease the total community worm burden, the number of worm progeny shed into the environment is similarly reduced, and the transmission of the disease slowed or—rarely—eliminated entirely.

For tissue-invasive helminths, full cure is often the goal, although ironically medical treatment may be less effective than in GI infection. In some cases, adult tissue-invasive worms are more susceptible to therapy than immature forms, and in other cases the opposite is true. Even

Arsenic, antimonial compounds inactivate –SH groups

Toxicity based on enhanced uptake

＊ Melarsoprol active against trypanosomiasis, but toxic

＊ Antimonials used only for leishmania infections

Useful in visceral and cutaneous leishmaniasis, amebic encephalitis

Worms treatment efforts concentrate on the most heavily parasitized

†Not available in the United States.

worse, dying tissue invaders may release antigens that lead to an undesired inflammatory state that endangers the patient.

Neither GI-dwelling nor tissue-invasive helminths have demonstrated considerable drug resistance, presumably because their reproduction happens over a longer period of time and because most of them complete their reproductive cycle outside the human host.

Goal is reduced worm burden

■ Benzimidazoles

As their name implies, the basic structure of benzimidazoles consists of linked imidazole and benzene rings. Unlike their antiprotozoal cousins discussed previously, the benzimidazoles are broad-spectrum anthelmintic agents. The prototype drug, **thiabendazole,** acts against both adult and larval nematodes. Soon after its introduction in the early 1960s, it was shown to be useful in the management of cutaneous larva migrans, trichinosis, and most intestinal nematode infections. The mechanism by which it exerts its anthelmintic action is uncertain. It is known to inhibit fumarate reductase, an important mitochondrial enzyme of helminths. The primary mode of action, however, may derive from the known capacity of all benzimidazoles to inhibit the polymerization of tubulin, the eukaryotic cytoskeletal protein. Side effects are related to the gastrointestinal tract or liver, and rapidly resolve with the discontinuation of the drug. Hypersensitivity reactions, induced either by the drug or by antigens released from the damaged parasite, may occur. For this reason, thiabendazole has been replaced by newer, better-tolerated agents of the same class.

Broad-spectrum anthelmintics

Mebendazole, a carbamate benzimidazole introduced in 1972, has a spectrum similar to that of thiabendazole, but also has been found to be effective against a number of cestodes, including *Taenia, Hymenolepsis,* and *Echinococcus.* It irreversibly binds to worm tubulin, thus interfering with the assembly of cytoplasmic microtubules, structures essential for glucose uptake. This results in glycogen depletion, cessation of ATP formation, and worm paralysis or death. Unlike thiabendazole, mebendazole is not well absorbed from the gastrointestinal tract and may owe part of its effectiveness against intestine-dwelling adult worms to its high concentrations in the human gut. It does not appear to affect glucose metabolism in humans, and toxicity is uncommon. Teratogenic effects have been observed in experimental animals; its use in infants and pregnant women is relatively contraindicated.

Blocks glucose uptake by adult and larval worms

Interferes with tubulin, microtubules

Albendazole is a benzimidazole carbamate that is more highly absorbed and thus has a somewhat broader spectrum than that of its close relative, mebendazole. It demonstrates more activity against *Strongyloides stercoralis* and several tissue nematodes. In addition to the vermicidal (adult killing) and larvicidal (immature-form killing) properties that it shares with other benzimidazoles, it is ovicidal (egg killing), enhancing its effectiveness in tissue cestode infections such as echinococcosis and cysticercosis. Its activity against *Giardia,* one of the most common intestinal protozoa, makes it an appealing candidate for the treatment of polyparasitism. Although it shares the teratogenic potential of other benzimidazoles, it is otherwise extremely well tolerated. Single-dose therapy is effective in the management of many intestinal nematode infections.

✳ **Albendazole better absorbed, broader spectrum**

Triclabendazole is another benzimidazole with enhanced activity against hermaphroditic trematodes, especially Fasciola hepatica, the cause of sheep liver rot and human hepatic fascioliasis.

■ Ivermectin

Ivermectin is a member of the avermectin group: macrocyclic lactones produced as fermentation products of *Streptomyces avermitilis.* Structurally similar to the macrolide antibiotics, ivermectin is effective at extremely low concentration against a wide variety of nematodes and arthropods. It appears to induce neuromuscular paralysis by acting on a receptor of the parasite peripheral neurotransmitter, gamma-aminobutyric acid (GABA). In mammals, GABA is confined to the central nervous system, and because ivermectin does not cross the blood–brain barrier in significant concentration, it does not appear to produce significant untoward effects in the mammalian host. A derivative of avermectin B1, ivermectin was originally developed and marketed as a horse dewormer. However, its effect on human health has been tremendous. It is currently the drug of choice for the treatment and suppression of onchocerciasis and is dosed on a massive scale for that purpose in West Africa. It is also effective in the treatment of strongyloidiasis, filariasis, and certain GI helminth infections. It also has activity against ectoparasites, making it useful in the treatment of common syndromes such as head lice and scabies.

Influences nematode neurotransmitters

✳ *Activity against filariae*

✳ *Drug of choice for onchocerciasis*

TABLE 50-1   Miscellaneous Antiparasitic Agents

COMPOUND	DRUG CLASS	ROUTE	MECHANISM OF ACTION	CLINICAL USE	COMMENT
Amphotericin	Polyene	IV	Membrane disruptor	Leishmaniasis	Antifungal agent also harms *Leishmania* spp.
Benznidazole	Nitroimidazole	Oral	DNA binder	Acute Chagas disease	Bone marrow depression peripheral neuropathy, rash, itching
Bithionol	Phenol	Oral	Uncouples phosphorylation	Paragonimiasis	Not commercially available in the United States
Diethylcarbamazine	Piperazine	Oral	Neuromuscular paralysis	Filarial infections	Allergic reactions to filarial antigens
Diloxanide furoate	Acetanilide	Oral	Unknown	Intestinal amebiasis	Used only for asymptomatic carriers
Iodoquinol	Halogenated quinoline	Oral	Unknown	Intestinal amebiasis *Dientamoeba* infections	Related drug has caused optic atrophy
Miltefosine	Phospholipid	Oral	Protein kinase B inhibitor	Viseral and cutaneous leishmaniasis, amebic encephalitis	Only oral option for viseral leishmaniasis
Nifurtimox	Nitrofuran	Oral	Oxidative stress by production of free radicals	Acute Chagas disease	Toxicity, prolonged therapy, marginal effectiveness
Nitazoxanide	Nitrothiazolyl-salicylamide	Oral	Inhibits anaerobic metabolism	*Cryptosporidium*, *Giardia*	Occasional vomiting, abdominal pain, diarrhea
Paromomycin	Aminoglycoside	Oral	Similar to other aminoglycosides	Intestinal cryptosporidiosis	Not absorbed, marginal effectiveness
Pentamidine	Diamidine	IV	Binds DNA	Leishmaniasis trypanosomiasis	Toxic
Pyrantel pamoate	Tetrahydropyrimidine	Oral	Neuromuscular blockade; inhibits fumarate reductase	Pinworm infection, hookworm infection, ascariasis	Single-dose therapy
Spiramycin	Macrolide	Oral	Blocks protein synthesis	Toxoplasmosis	Used to treat pregnant women
Suramin	Sulfated naphthylamine	IV	Inhibits glycerophosphate oxidase and dehydrogenase	African trypanosomiasis onchocerciasis	Not effective in central nervous system disease Renal toxicity

IV, intravenous.

■ Praziquantel

Praziquantel, a heterocyclic pyrazinoisoquinoline, is an important anthelmintic, effective against a broad range of cestodes and trematodes, many of which are poorly responsive to previously available agents. It is given in one to three doses. The drug is rapidly taken up by susceptible helminths, in which it appears to induce the loss of intracellular calcium, tetanic muscular contraction, and destruction of the tegument. The differential toxicity of this agent may be related to the inability of susceptible worms to metabolize the drug. Aside from transient, mild gastrointestinal symptoms, praziquantel appears remarkably free of side effects in humans. It is currently the drug of choice for the treatment of most trematode infections, including schistosomiasis, clonorchiasis, and opisthorchiasis. Its side effects are minor, and its overall high level of safety suggests that it may play a significant role in future worldwide mass therapy campaigns.

Loss of intracellular calcium in cestodes, trematodes

Used in mass therapy

■ Diethylcarbamazine

Diethylcarbamazine (DEC) is a derivative of piperazine, used to kill tissue-invasive helminths of the microfilarial family. It is believed to work via inhibition of arachidonic acid metabolism. DEC is usually well tolerated, and has even been added to cooking salt in areas endemic to lymphatic

Use for microfilarial infections with caution

filariasis, in order to assist in disease control. On the other hand, it is so deadly to another micro-filarial infection, onchocerciasis, that it is *avoided* in endemic areas to prevent severe allergic reactions triggered by overwhelming microfilaricidal action.

■ Other Antiparasitic Agents

A number of antiparasitic agents, their properties, and their clinical uses are listed in **Table 50–1.**

KEY CONCLUSIONS

- Anthelminthic drugs usually have a broad spectrum of activity.
- Most are very well tolerated.
- The goals of treatment may differ between GI-dwelling worms (where a few adult survivors are often well tolerated) and tissue-invasive worms (where full cure is more desirable).

ANTIPARASITIC RESISTANCE

✴ *Plasmodium falciparum* resistance a major problem

The major problem with antiparasitic resistance relates to *Plasmodium* species, specifically *P falciparum.* This organism divides asexually within the human host, under the selective pressure of drug treatment, thus fostering an environment in which drug-resistant mutants may be selected. The crisis of drug-resistant malaria is widespread throughout sub-Saharan Africa, Asia, and Latin America, but resistance has also appeared in other areas. The most common is chloroquine resistance, wherein the parasite reduces the amount of drug that accumulates in its digestive vacuoles. This involves mutations in a transport molecule of the digestive membrane called *P falciparum* chloroquine resistance transporter (PfCRT). This mutation is now the rule, rather than the exception, and chloroquine is only effective with acceptable reliability against *P falciparum* in areas of northern Latin America. Other parasite point mutations can similarly result in resistance to sulfadoxine–pyrimethamine and atovaquone–proguanil (the latter by mutations in the cytochrome b gene) and reduced susceptibility to mefloquine, quinine, and quinidine. Resistance to artemisinin combination therapy has emerged in Southeast Asia, and is of great concern globally; if this highly effective treatment class falls, we currently have no reliable, nontoxic drug to take its place.

Helminth resistance to antiparasitic agents has been less of a concern, although this may be due to the relatively lower use of this class of drugs, as well as the helminths' longer and more complex reproductive cycles. As antihelminthics are used more widely and intensively, in the long run, resistant populations may be selected.

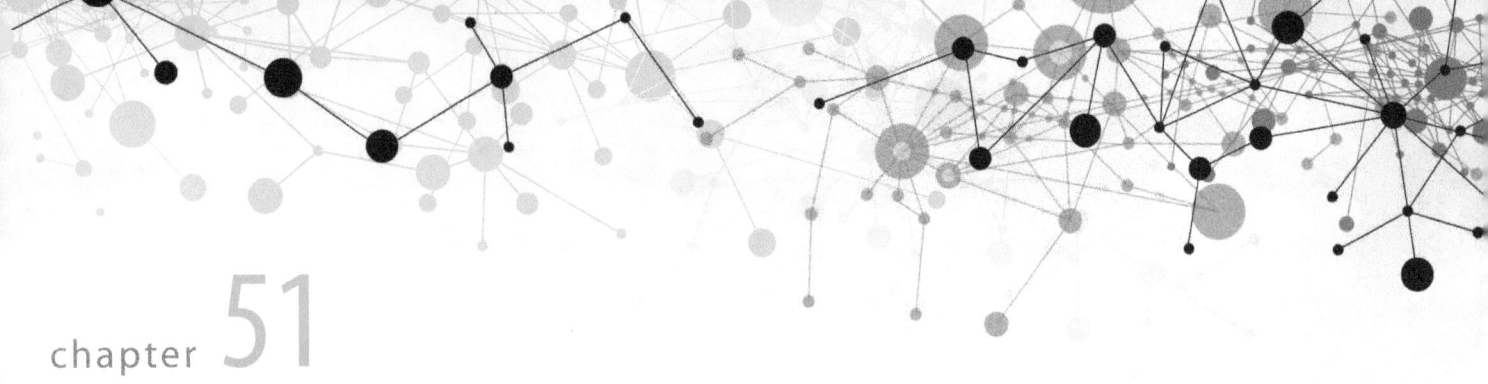

chapter 51

Apicomplexa and Microsporidia

Plasmodium falciparum • Plasmodium vivax • Plasmodium ovale • Plasmodium malariae • Plasmodium knowlesi
• Babesia spp. • Toxoplasma gondii • Cryptosporidium spp. • Cyclospora cayetanensis • Isospora belli

A man can be riddled with malaria for years on end, with its chills and its fevers and its nightmares, but if one day he sees that the water from his kidneys is black, he knows he will not leave that place again, wherever he is, or wherever he hoped to be.

—Beryl Markham: *West with the Night* (1942)

● APICOMPLEXA

When the paroxysms fall on even days, the crises will be on even days; and when the paroxysms fall on odd days, the crises will be on odd days. Furthermore, it is necessary that one know that if crises fall on days other than those mentioned above, there will be a relapse, and this may be deadly. But it is essential to pay attention and know at which times the crises will lead to death and in which to recovery, or during which is there tendency to fair better or worse.

—Hippocrates (Translated from the ancient Greek in his work—Epidemics)

GROUP CHARACTERISTICS

The Apicomplexa are obligate intracellular protozoan parasites. The name of this group of parasites derives from the complex of organelles located at the apical end of parasite life cycle stages that are involved in penetrating cells. These organelles include the rhoptries, micronemes, and associated microtubular complexes located in this region of the parasite. The Apicomplexa have alternating cycles of sexual and asexual reproduction. Asexual multiplication within the host occurs by a process of multiple fission termed schizogony. The nucleus of a trophozoite divides into several parts, forming a multinucleated schizont. The cytoplasm then condenses around each nuclear portion to form new daughter cells, or merozoites, which burst from their intracellular location to invade new host cells. After the completion of one or more of these asexual cycles, some merozoites differentiate into male and female gametocytes, initiating the sexual phase of the life cycle. In the case of malaria, the gametocytes reach maturity in the mosquito host and effect fertilization, forming a zygote, or motile ookinete. In other Apicomplexa, this process may occur in intestinal cells. The zygote then becomes an oocyst for these parasites. Sporozoites are formed within the oocyst by an asexual process of sporogony and when released, penetrate host tissue cells, and begin another asexual cycle as trophozoites. The only phase of this life cycle that is diploid is when the zygote is formed. All other stages in the life cycle are haploid. The general apicomplexan cell plan is illustrated in **Figure 51–1.**

Intracellular protozoa alternate sexual, asexual cycles

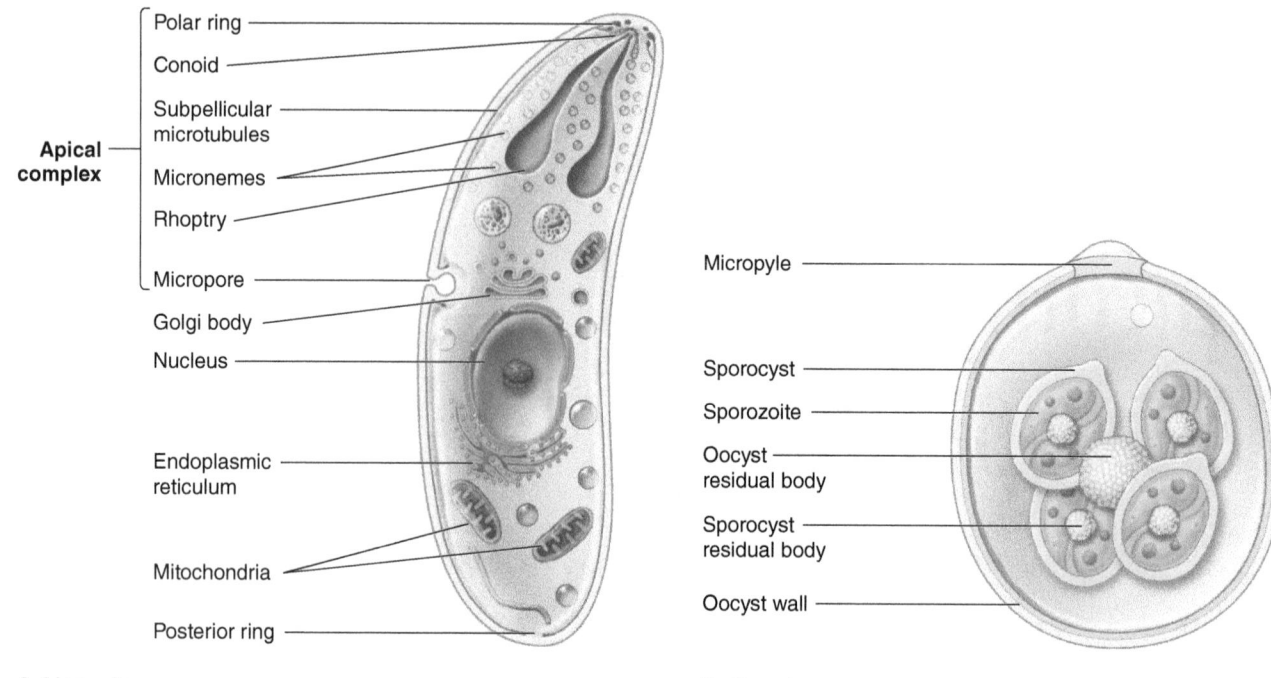

A. Merozoite

B. Oocyst

FIGURE 51–1. The apicomplexan cell. (Reproduced with permission from Willey JM: *Prescott, Harley, & Klein's Microbiology*, 7th ed. New York, NY: McGraw Hill; 2008.)

Cause malaria, toxoplasmosis, cryptosporidiosis, cyclosporiasis, isosporiasis, and babesiosis

Two Apicomlexan infections, malaria and toxoplasmosis, are common diseases in humans; together, they affect more than one-third of the world's population and kill or deform perhaps one-half million neonates and children each year. *Cryptosporidium, Cyclospora*, and *Isospora* are Apicomplexa that can cause diarrhea, particularly in the immunocompromised. *Babesia*, a relative of malaria, and transmitted by ticks, is also a member of this group.

● *PLASMODIUM* SPP.

Of all infectious diseases there is no doubt that malaria has caused the greatest harm to the greatest number.

—*Laderman, 1975*

OVERVIEW

Plasmodium is a parasite species with a sexual cycle in mosquitoes and an asexual cycle in humans. Malaria is a febrile illness caused by a *Plasmodium* spp. infection of human erythrocytes. Malaria is transmitted by female mosquitoes of the genus *Anopheles*. Malaria infection is followed by a period of patency while the parasite develops in the liver and is species dependent. Patency begins with fevers that are accompanied by headache, chills, sweats, and malaise, and typically appear in paroxysmal episodes lasting hours and recurring for weeks. Fever episodes usually become synchronous and can be used to help in identifying the malarial species. Anemia may also be present. Cerebral malaria, caused by *Plasmodium falciparum*, is due to capillary blockage in the brain and can be fatal. Children suffer the greatest from this complication.

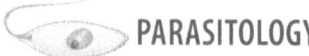 PARASITOLOGY

✳ Sexual phase in mosquito, asexual in humans

Five species infect humans

The plasmodia are Apicomplexa in which the sexual and asexual cycles of reproduction are completed in different host species. The sexual phase occurs within the gut of mosquitoes and results in the formation of a motile zygote, the ookinete. These arthropods subsequently transmit the parasite as sporozoites while feeding on a vertebrate host. Within the vertebrate, the plasmodia reproduce asexually, first in the liver and then in erythrocytes; they eventually burst from the erythrocyte and invade other uninvolved RBCs. This event produces periodic fever and anemia in the host, a disease process known as malaria. Of the many species of plasmodia, five are known to infect humans and are considered here: *Plasmodium vivax, Plasmodium ovale, Plasmodium malariae, Plasmodium knowlesi,* and *Plasmodium falciparum.*

LIFE CYCLE OF MALARIAL PARASITES

> This day relenting God
> Hath placed within my hand
> A wondrous thing; and God
> Be praised. At his command,
>
> Seeking his secret deeds
> With tears and toiling breath,
> I find thy cunning seeds,
> O million-murdering Death.
>
> I know this little thing
> A myriad men will save,
> O Death, where is thy sting?
> Thy victory, O Grave?

—Sir Ronald Ross, August 22, 1897, in a poem to Sir Patrick Manson on the discovery of sporozoites in mosquito salivary glands.

The life cycle in the female *Anopheles* mosquito begins with the ingestion of male and female gametocytes from the circulation of a malaria-infected individual. In the gut of the mosquito, the gametocytes reach full maturation, are released from infected erythrocytes, and effect fertilization. The resulting zygote, an ookinete, is the only stage in the life cycle that is diploid, is motile, and penetrates the mosquito's gut wall, lodges beneath the basement membrane facing the mosquito's hemocoel, undergoes a postzygotic reduction division, and vacuolates to form an oocyst. Within this structure, thousands of sporozoites are formed by asexual division. The enlarging cyst eventually ruptures, releasing the sporozoites into the body cavity of the mosquito. Some penetrate the salivary glands, rendering the mosquito infectious for humans. The time required for the completion of the cycle in mosquitoes varies from 1 to 3 weeks, depending on the species of insect and parasite as well as on the ambient temperature and humidity.

* Mosquito ingests gametocytes from human blood

* Sporozoites reach mosquito salivary glands

Sporozoites from the mosquito's salivary glands are injected into the human's subcutaneous capillaries when the female mosquito feeds. Within minutes and up to 1 hour, they attach to and invade liver cells (hepatocytes), a process mediated by a ligand present in the outer protein coat of the sporozoites (circumsporozoite protein). In *P vivax* and *P ovale* infections, some of the sporozoites enter a dormant state immediately after cell invasion to become hypnozoites. These stages are responsible for the **relapse** phenomenon seen in malarial infections caused by these species. In all malarial infections, the remaining sporozoites initiate exoerythrocytic schizogony, each producing about 2000 to 40,000 daughter cells, or merozoites, depending on the infecting species. After 1 to 2 weeks, the infected hepatocytes rupture, releasing merozoites into the general circulation.

* Humans infected by mosquito bite

* Infection of hepatocytes starts asexual cycle

The erythrocytic phase of malaria starts with the attachment of a released hepatic merozoite to a specific receptor on the RBC surface. After attachment, the merozoite releases substances from its apical organelles, the rhoptries, which affect red cell membrane fluidity resulting in invagination of the cell membrane and entry of the parasite into a parasitophorous vacuole. The intracellular parasite initially appears as a small ring-shaped trophozoite, which enlarges and becomes more active and irregular in outline. Within a few hours, nuclear division occurs, producing the multinucleated schizont. The cytoplasm eventually condenses around each nucleus of the schizont to form an intraerythrocytic cluster of 6 to 24 merozoite daughter cells. About 24 (*P knowlesi*), 48 (*P vivax, P ovale,* and *P falciparum*) to 72 (*P malariae*) hours after initial invasion, infected erythrocytes rupture, releasing the merozoites and producing the first clinical manifestations of disease. The newly released merozoites invade other RBCs, where most repeat the asexual cycle. Other merozoites are transformed into sexual forms or gametocytes. These latter forms do not produce RBC lysis and continue to circulate in the peripheral vasculature until ingested by an appropriate mosquito. The recurring asexual cycles continue, involving an ever-increasing

* Erythrocytic cycle begins with merozoite attachment to RBC

* Trophozoites multiply in RBCs, form new merozoites

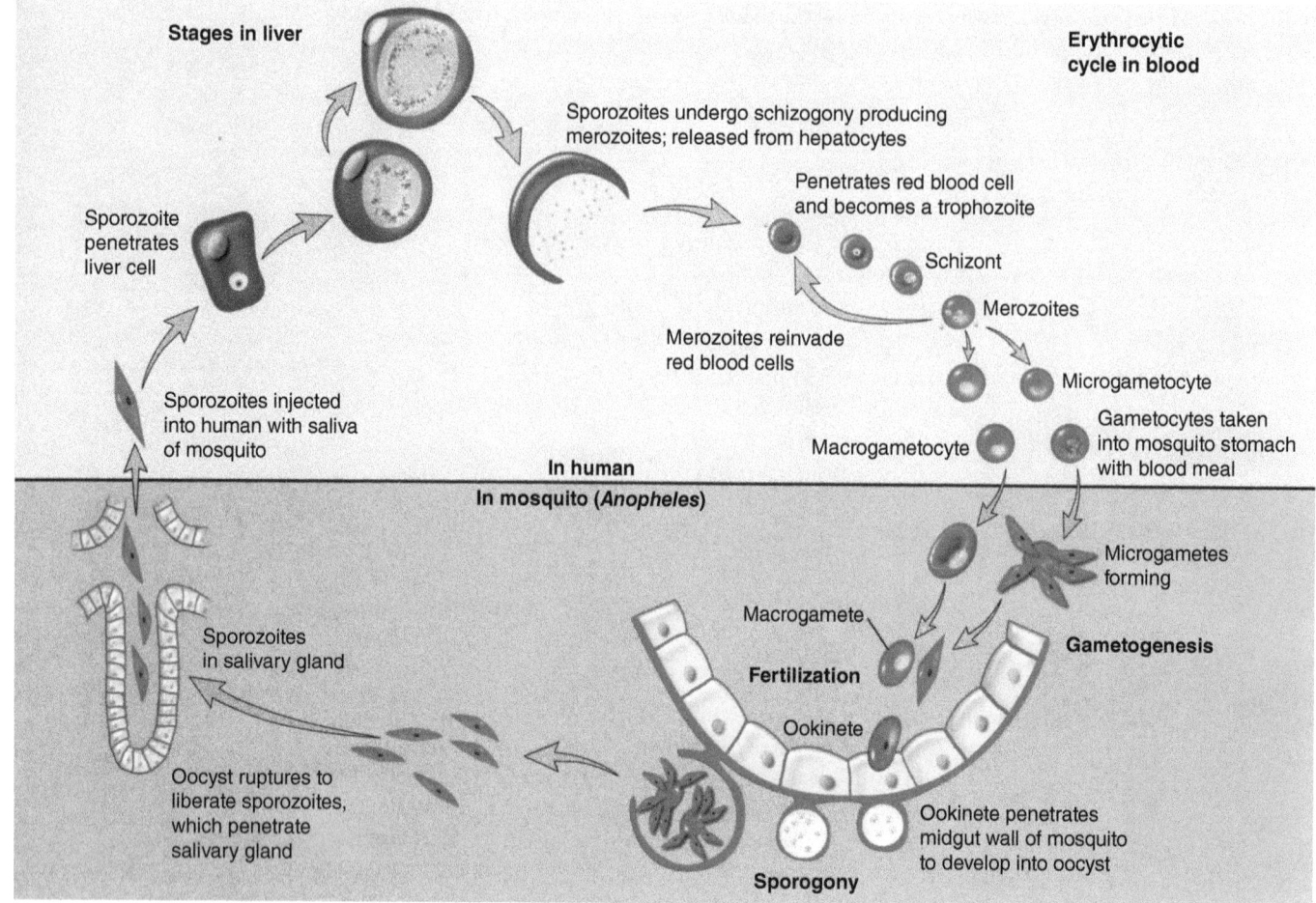

FIGURE 51–2. Malaria. Life cycle of *Plasmodium vivax*. (Reproduced with permission from Willey JM: *Prescott, Harley, & Klein's Microbiology*, 7th ed. New York, NY: McGraw Hill; 2008.)

RBCs rupture, releasing merozoites to infect new RBCs

✳ Dormancy causes relapses with *P vivax* and *P ovale*

number of erythrocytes until the development of host immunity helps contain the erythrocytic cycle. The dormant hepatic sporozoites of *P vivax* and *P ovale* survive the host's immunologic attack and may, after a latent period of months to years, resume intrahepatic multiplication. This leads to a second release of hepatic merozoites and the initiation of another erythrocytic cycle, a phenomenon known as relapse. The life cycle of malarial parasites is summarized in **Figure 51–2** and variations in the differential characteristics of the parasites infecting humans are summarized in **Table 51–1**.

TABLE 51–1	Differential Characteristics of *Plasmodium* Species				
CHARACTERISTICS	*P VIVAX*	*P OVALE*	*P MALARIAE*	*P FALCIPARUM*	*P KNOWLESI*
Erythrocyte					
Enlarged, pale	+	+	–	–	–
Oval, fimbriated	–	+	–	–	–
Schüffner dots	+	+	–	–	–
Maurer dots	–	–	–	+	–
Parasite					
All asexual stages seen	+	+	+	–	+
Band forms	–	–	+	–	+
Double infections	–	–	–	+	–
Double chromatin dots	–	–	–	+	–
Banana-shaped gametocytes	–	–	–	+	–

MORPHOLOGY OF ERYTHROCYTIC PARASITES

The morphology of the stained intraerythrocytic *Plasmodium* parasites is shown in **Figure 51–3.** In stained smears, three characteristic features aid in the identification of plasmodia: Red nuclear chromatin; blue cytoplasm; and brownish-black malarial pigment, or hemozoin, consisting largely of a hemoglobin degradation product, ferriprotoporphyrin IX. The change in the shape of the cytoplasm and the division of the chromatin at different stages of parasite development are obvious. Gametocytes can be differentiated from the asexual forms by their large size and lack of nuclear division. Some of the infected erythrocytes develop membrane invaginations or caveolae-vesicle complexes, which are thought to be responsible for the appearance of the dark Schüffner dots or granules (see following text).

The appearance of each of the five species of plasmodia that infect humans is sufficiently different to allow their differentiation in stained smears, although some similarities in some stages exist between the different species. The parasitized erythrocyte in *P vivax* and *P ovale* infections is pale and enlarged and contains numerous Schüffner dots. All asexual stages (trophozoite, schizont, merozoite) may be seen simultaneously. Cells infected by *P ovale* are elongated and frequently irregular or fimbriated in appearance. In *P malariae* infections, the RBCs are not enlarged and contain no granules. The trophozoites often present as "band" forms, and the merozoites are arranged in rosettes around a clump of central pigment. In *P falciparum* infections, the rings are very small and may contain two chromatin dots rather than one. There is often more than one parasite per cell, and parasites are frequently seen lying against the margin of the cell. Intracytoplasmic granules known as Maurer dots may be present, but are often cleft shaped and fewer in number than Schüffner dots. Schizonts and merozoites of *P falciparum* are not present in the peripheral blood as they are sequestered in postcapillary venules. Gametocytes are large and banana shaped. *P knowlesi* shares many of

Morphology of the parasite and the infected RBCs vary by stage and species

Morphologic differences, primary means of diagnosis

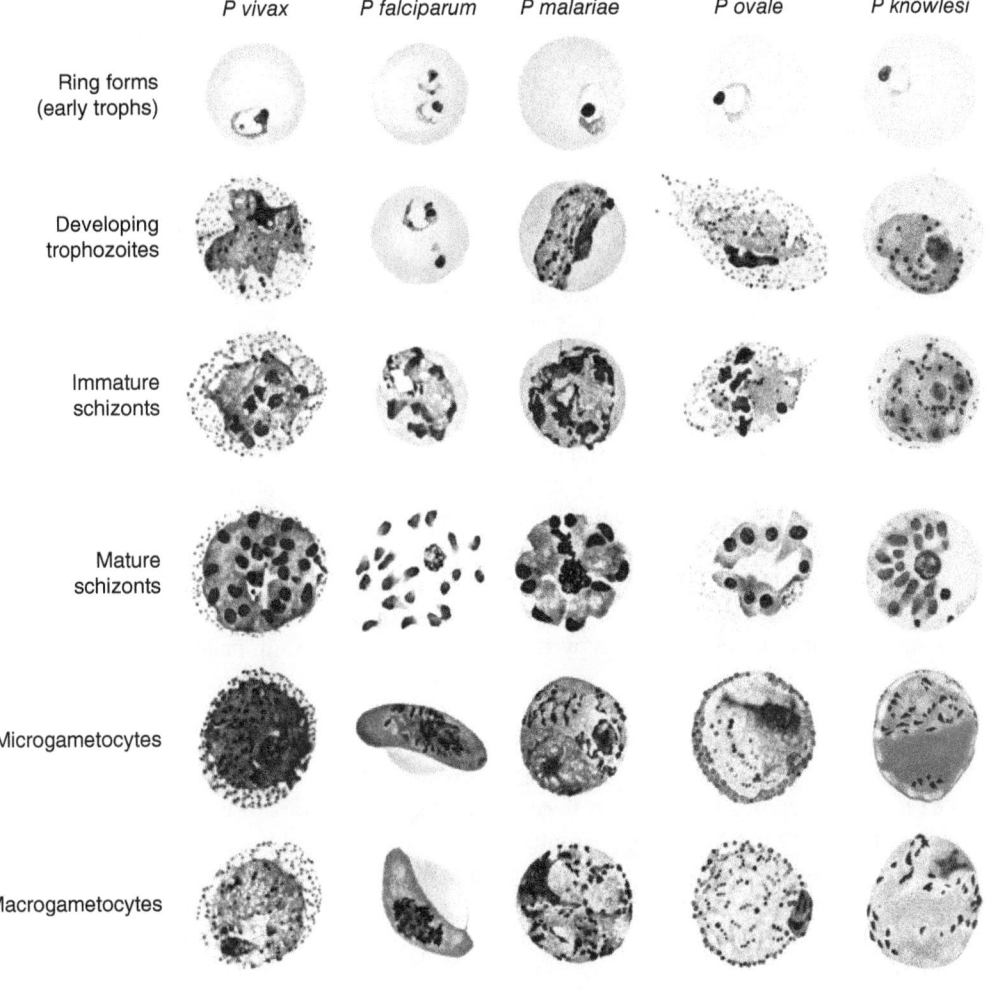

	P vivax	P falciparum	P malariae	P ovale	P knowlesi
Ring forms (early trophs)					
Developing trophozoites					
Immature schizonts					
Mature schizonts					
Microgametocytes					
Macrogametocytes					

FIGURE 51–3. Drawings of erythrocytic stages of malarial parasites. Note that trophozoite and schizont forms of *Plasmodium falciparum* occur in visceral capillaries rather than in blood. Female gametophytes have morphologic differences from the male forms shown. (Reproduced with permission from Centers for Disease Control, Coatney GR, Collins WE, et al: *The Primate Malarias*. National Institutes of Health; 1971.)

the morphologic characteristics of *P malariae*, but can be distinguished from the latter by its fever cycle and diagnostically by using polymerase chain reaction (PCR). These characteristics are summarized in Table 51-1.

PHYSIOLOGY

Vary in ability to attack erythrocytes

Duffy antigen, glycoprotein A RBC receptors

Species of plasmodia differ significantly in their ability to invade subpopulations of erythrocytes; *P vivax* and *P ovale* attack only immature cells (reticulocytes), whereas *P malariae* attacks only senescent cells. During infection with these species, therefore, no more than 1% to 2% of the cell population is involved. *P falciparum*, in contrast, invades RBCs, regardless of age, and may produce very high levels of parasitemia and particularly serious disease. In part, these differences may be related to the known differences in the RBC receptor sites available to the individual *Plasmodium* species. In the case of *P vivax*, the site is closely related to the Duffy blood group antigens (Fy^a and Fy^b). Duffy-negative individuals, who constitute most people of West African ancestry, are therefore resistant to vivax malaria. RBC sialoglycoproteins, particularly glycoprotein A, have been implicated as the *P falciparum* receptor site.

✱ Sickle cell trait limits *P falciparum*

Hemoglobinopathies exert protection

Certain RBC genetic polymorphisms may also affect parasitism. The altered hemoglobin (hemoglobin S) associated with the sickle cell trait limits the intensity of the parasitemia caused by *P falciparum*, and thereby provides a selective advantage to individuals who are heterozygous for the sickle cell gene. Thus, the sickle cell gene, which would otherwise be disadvantageous, is common in populations living in malarious areas. Parasite growth appears to be retarded in RBCs heterozygous for hemoglobin S (SA) when they are exposed to conditions of reduced oxygen tension such as those which might be present in the visceral capillaries. These conditions cause the hemoglobin in infected cells to polymerize, rendering it unusable by the parasite. In essence, the parasite starves to death. Sickling may also render the erythrocyte more susceptible to phagocytosis or directly damage the parasite. A similar protective effect may be exerted by hemoglobins C, D, and E; thalassemias; and glucose-6-phosphate dehydrogenase (G6PD) or pyridoxal kinase deficiencies, because these abnormalities have also been found more frequently in malarious areas. The protection in these conditions may be related to the increased susceptibility of such RBCs to oxidant stress. In thalassemia, the protection may also be related in part to the production of fetal hemoglobin, which retards maturation of *P falciparum*, as well as an increased binding of antibodies to modified parasitic antigens (neoantigens) presenting on the surface of the erythrocytes.

Changes induced in erythrocyte

Endothelium binding causes microinfarcts

Once invasion has occurred, malaria parasites may induce several changes in the erythrocytic membrane. These include alteration of its lipid concentration, modification of its osmotic properties, and incorporation of parasitic neoantigens, rendering the RBCs susceptible to immunologic attack. *P vivax* and *P ovale* stimulate the production of caveolae–vesicle complexes, which are visualized as Schüffner dots in stained smears. In *P falciparum* infections, electron-dense elevated knobs or excrescences form on the RBC surface. These produce a strain-specific, high–molecular-weight adhesive protein (PfEMP1), which mediates binding to receptors on the endothelium of capillaries and postcapillary venules of the brain, placenta, and other organs, where they can produce obstruction and microinfarcts.

Metabolize anaerobically, synthesize own folate

Malarial parasites generate energy by the anaerobic metabolism of glucose. They appear to satisfy their protein requirements by the degradation of hemoglobin within their acidic food vacuoles, resulting in the formation of the malarial pigment (hemozoin) mentioned previously. It has been estimated that the average plasmodium destroys between 25% and 75% of the hemoglobin of its host erythrocyte. Unlike their vertebrate hosts, malarial parasites synthesize folates de novo. Thus, antifolate antimicrobials such as pyrimethamine are effective antimalarial agents.

GROWTH IN THE LABORATORY

Continuous *in vitro* cultivation of plasmodia in human erythrocytes was first achieved in 1976. More recently, the sporogonic cycle has been propagated in laboratory-reared mosquitoes. These twin developments provide new opportunities for studying the biology, immunology, and chemotherapy of human malaria. The most immediate impact of these advances has been on the introduction of methods for testing the sensitivity of *P falciparum* to chemotherapeutic agents. Ultimately, these developments will play critical roles in the generation of effective antimalarial vaccines.

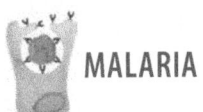

MALARIA

EPIDEMIOLOGY

Malaria has a worldwide distribution between 45°N and 40°S latitude, generally at altitudes below 1800 m. *P vivax* is the most widely distributed of the four species, and together with the uncommon *P malariae*, is found primarily in temperate and subtropical areas. *P falciparum* is the dominant organism of the tropics. *P ovale* is rare and found principally in Africa. *P knowlesi*, first recognized in humans in 1965, accounts for up to 70% of the infections recorded in some areas of Southeast Asia. It is also a zoonotic species, with long-tailed macaques being the dominant reservoir.

Distribution in tropical areas worldwide

The intensity of malarial transmission in an endemic area depends on the density and feeding habits of suitable mosquito vectors and the prevalence of infected humans, who serve as parasite reservoirs. In hyperendemic areas (areas where more than half of the population is parasitemic), transmission is usually constant, and disease manifestations are moderated by the development of immunity. Mortality is largely restricted to infants and to nonimmune adults who migrate into the region and is primarily caused by *P falciparum*. When the prevalence of disease is lower, transmission is typically intermittent. In this situation, solid immunity does not develop, and the population suffers repeated, often seasonal, epidemics, the impact of which is shared by people of all ages.

Manifestations muted with hyperendemicity

Presently, an estimated 2 billion people live in malaria-endemic areas in 103 of the poorest countries of Africa, Asia, Latin America, and Oceania. Within these areas, malaria transmission has been reduced significantly over the last 15 years, largely as the result of the compliant use of insecticide impregnated bed nets (**Figure 51–4**). Still, many within these areas are thought to be carrying the malaria parasite at any given time. Approximately 400,000 individuals, primarily African children, die of malaria annually. Although endemic malaria disappeared from the United States decades ago, imported cases continue to be reported. An increase in international travel has resulted in an increase in the number of U.S. cases to approximately 1500 to 2000 annually as reported by the Centers for Disease Control and Prevention (CDC). Forty-five percent of the patients with imported malaria have acquired the disease in Africa, 30% in Asia, and 10% in the Caribbean or Latin America. Fifty percent of recent infections have involved American travelers: Nearly 60%

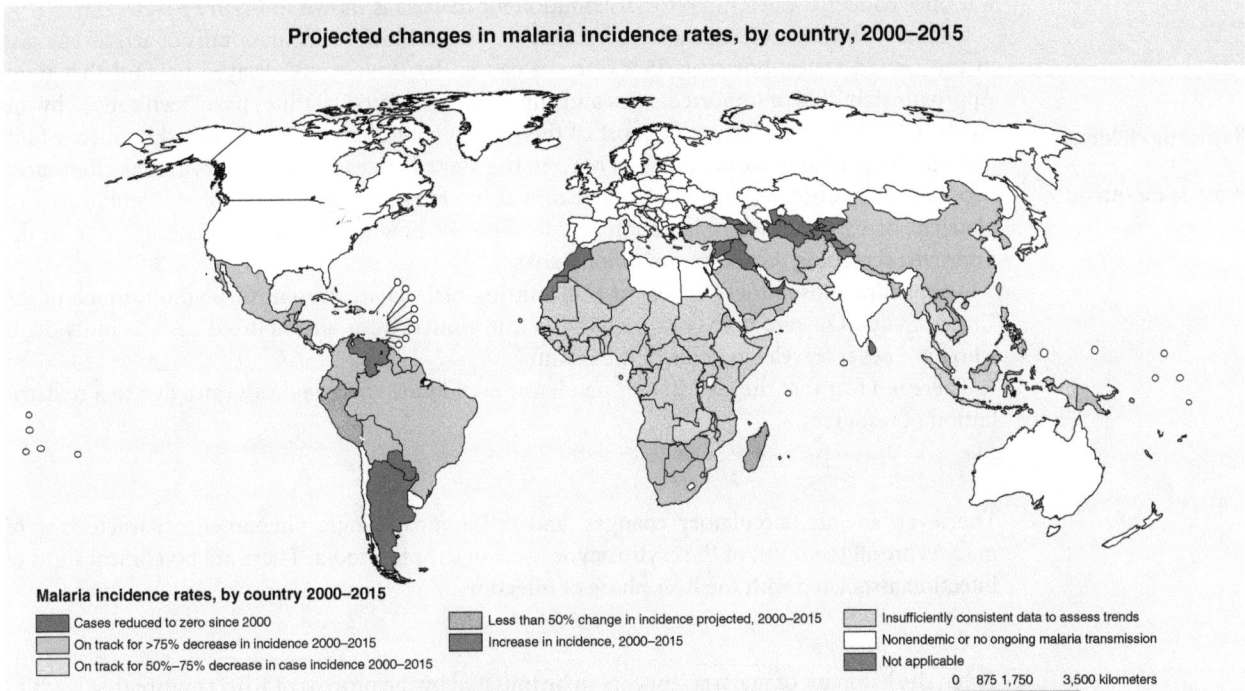

FIGURE 51–4. Worldwide changes in malaria incidence 2000-2015: http://www.who.int/gho/malaria/en/ Geographic distribution of malaria. (Data from Thacker SB, Parrish RG, Trowbridge FL. A method for evaluating systems of epidemiological surveillance, *World Health Stat Q* 1988;41(1):11–18.)

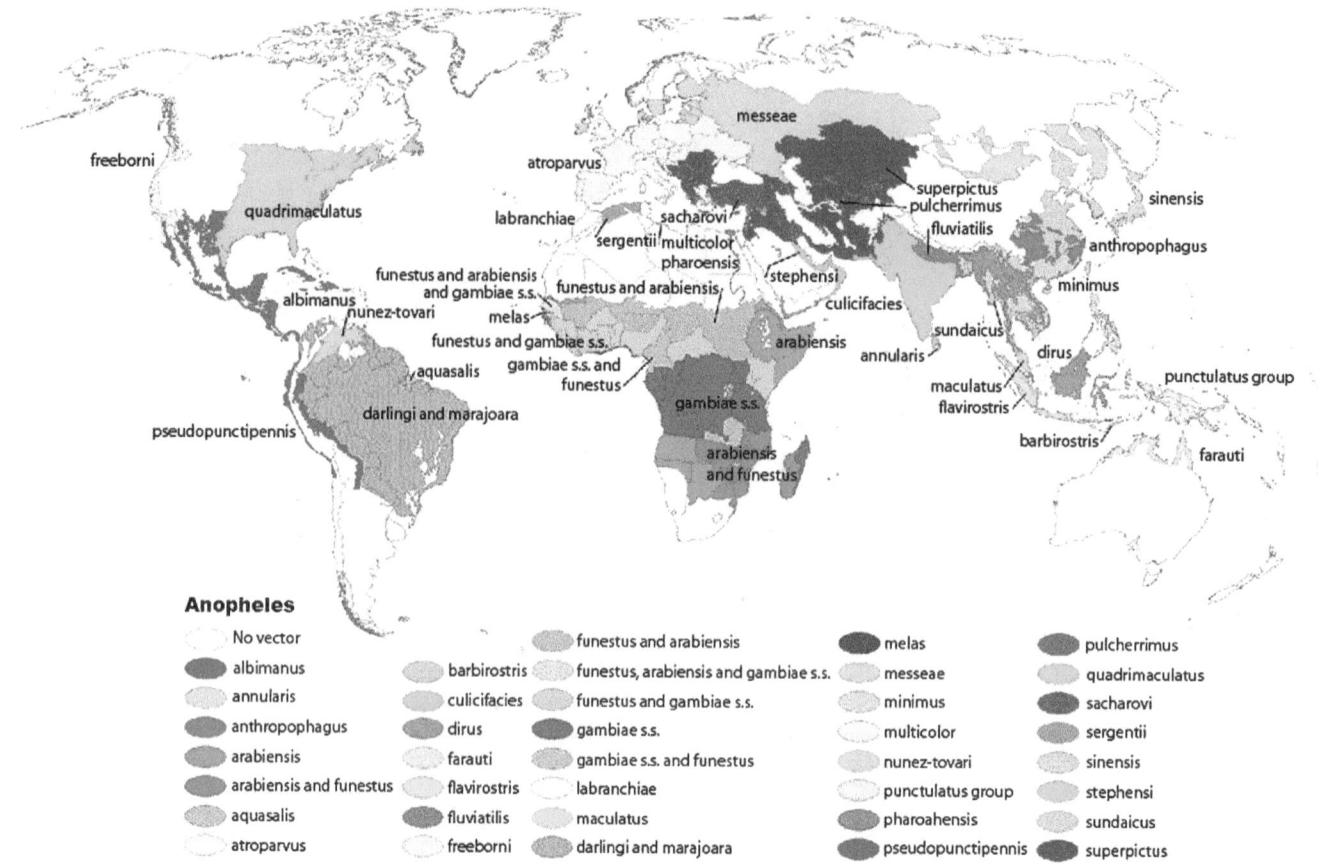

FIGURE 51–5. Current distribution of malaria vectors. (Reproduced with permission from Kiszewski A, Mellinger A, Spielman A, et al: A global index representing the stability of malaria transmission, *Am J Trop Med Hyg* 2004 May;70(5):486–498.)

of these acquired their infection in Africa. Climatologists and epidemiologists warn that global warming could enhance mosquito and therefore malaria transmission into areas where malaria was once endemic. Current vector distribution for malaria is shown in **Figure 51–5**.

Clinical manifestations of malaria typically develop within weeks to months of arrival of cases in the United States; however, 25% of cases caused by *P vivax* are delayed beyond that time. Approximately 40% of imported cases and almost all associated fatalities have been caused by the virulent *P falciparum*. Tragically, most of these cases could have been prevented or successfully treated. Congenital malaria in infants born in the United States of mothers from malarious areas is occasionally observed. Infections transmitted by transfusions of whole blood, leukocytes, or platelets, or by organ transplantation are, fortunately, now unusual in this country due to the improved screening procedures of blood banks.

Anopheline mosquitoes capable of transmitting malaria are present throughout much of the United States. On rare occasions, malaria is transmitted from an imported case to individuals who have never traveled outside of the country.

There is a fear that the COVID-19 pandemic could raise malaria death rates due to a redistribution of resources.

Malaria kills mostly children

Imported malaria months after travel

PATHOGENESIS

The fever, anemia, circulatory changes, and immunopathologic phenomena characteristic of malaria are all the result of the erythrocytic cycle of the plasmodia. There are no clinical signs of infection associated with the liver phase of infection.

■ Fever

Fever, the hallmark of malaria, appears to be initiated by the process of RBC rupture that leads to the liberation of a new generation of merozoites. It is possible that parasite-derived pyrogens are released at the time of red cell rupture; alternatively, the fever might result from the release of proinflammatory cytokines such as interleukin-1 (IL-1) and/or tumor necrosis factor (TNF) from macrophages involved in the ingestion of parasitic or erythrocytic debris. Early in malaria, RBCs appear to be infected with malarial parasites at several different stages of development, each inducing erythrocyte destruction at a different time. The resulting fever is irregular and hectic. Because temperatures higher than 40°C destroy mature parasites, a single population eventually emerges, parasite replication is synchronized, and fever occurs in distinct paroxysms at 24-hour (*P knowlesi*), 48-hour (*P falciparum, P vivax, P ovale*) or, in the case of *P malariae,* 72-hour intervals. Periodicity is seldom seen in patients who are rapidly diagnosed and treated. Periodicity is also not always a hallmark of *P falciparum* infections. Fever-induced modifications to membrane architecture and infected-cell sequestration events are thought to play a role in disrupting periodicity in these infections. Sometimes, the fever in *P falciparum* infections can more or less be continuous.

✴ Fever with RBC rupture

✴ Synchronization of replication causes cyclic fever

Anemia

Parasitized erythrocytes are phagocytosed by a stimulated reticuloendothelial system or are destroyed at the time of parasite-induced cell rupture, releasing toxic products. This not only results in destruction of infected cells but noninfected ones as well, resulting in an anemia that may be disproportionate to the degree of parasitism. Depression of marrow function, sequestration of erythrocytes within the enlarging spleen, and accelerated clearance of nonparasitized cells all appear to contribute to the anemia. So too might cytokine imbalances brought about by overstimulation of innate immune responses. Such imbalances can influence erythropoiesis. Intravascular hemolysis, though uncommon, may occur, particularly in *P falciparum* malaria. When hemolysis is massive, hemoglobinuria develops, resulting in the production of dark urine. This process in conjunction with malaria is known as **blackwater fever.**

Destruction of RBCs causes anemia

Massive intravascular hemolysis

Circulatory Changes

The high fever results in significant vasodilatation. In falciparum malaria, vasodilatation leads to a decrease in the effective circulating blood volume and hypotension, which may be aggravated by other changes in the small vessels and capillaries. The intense parasitemias of *P falciparum* is capable of producing comas and the adhesion of infected RBCs to the endothelium of visceral capillaries can impair the microcirculation and precipitate tissue hypoxia, lactic acidosis, and hypoglycemia. Although all deep tissues are involved, the brain is the most intensely affected resulting in what has been described as **cerebral malaria (Figure 51–6)**.

Blood flow decreased to vital organs

Cytokines

Elevated levels of IL-1 and TNF are consistently found in patients with malaria. Probably released at the time of parasite rupture from erythrocytes, these proteins are certainly an essential part of

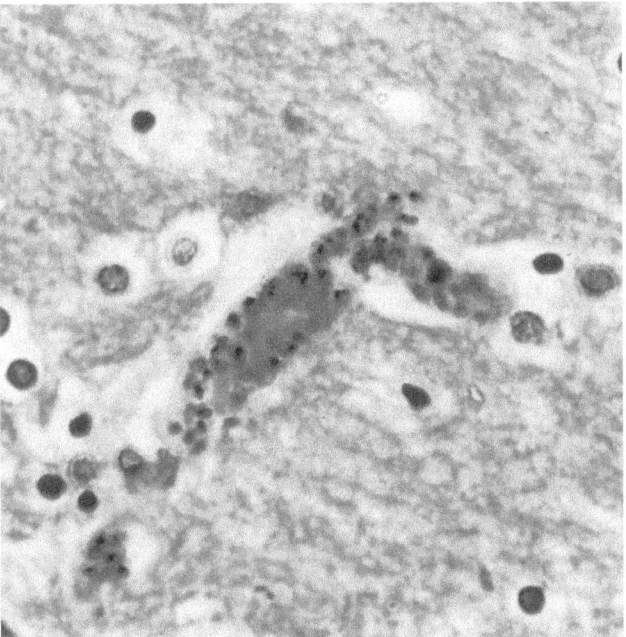

FIGURE 51–6. **Central nervous system malaria.** This small cerebral blood vessel is blocked with many parasitized erythrocytes adherent to the endothelium. (Reproduced with permission from Connor DH, Chandler FW, Schwartz DQ, et al: *Pathology of Infectious Diseases.* Stamford CT: Appleton & Lange; 1997.)

the host's immune response to malaria. By modulating the effects of endothelial cells, macrophages, monocytes, and neutrophils, they may play an important role in the destruction of the invading parasite. However, TNF levels increase with parasite density, and high concentrations appear harmful. TNF has been shown to cause upregulation of endothelial adhesion molecules; high concentrations might precipitate cerebral malaria by increasing the sequestration of *P falciparum*-parasitized erythrocytes in the cerebral vascular endothelium. Alternatively, excessive TNF levels might precipitate cerebral malaria by directly inducing hypoglycemia and lactic acidosis.

Elevated cytokines contribute to injury

■ Other Pathogenic Phenomena

Thrombocytopenia is common in malaria and appears to be related to both splenic pooling and a shortened platelet lifespan. Both direct parasitic invasion and immune mechanisms may be responsible. There may be an acute transient glomerulonephritis in falciparum malaria and progressive renal disease in chronic *P malariae* malaria. These phenomena probably result from the host immune response, with deposition of immune complexes in the glomeruli.

Thrombocytopenia and nephritis

IMMUNITY

Once infected, the host quickly mounts a stage-, species-, and strain-specific immunologic response that typically limits parasite multiplication and moderates the clinical manifestations of disease, without eliminating the infection. A prolonged recovery period marked by recurrent exacerbations in both symptoms and number of erythrocytic parasites follows. Recrudescences are marked by periods in which the parasitemia drops below the threshold of detection, only to surge again. Fluctuations in immunity probably account for this phenomenon. With time, these recrudescences become less severe and less frequent, and eventually may stop altogether.

＊Immune response limits, does not eliminate infection

The exact mechanisms involved in this recovery are uncertain. In simian and probably in human malaria, recovery is known to require the presence of both T and B lymphocytes. It is probable that the T lymphocytes act partially through their helper effect on antibody production. Some authorities have suggested that they also play a direct role through cytokine production by stimulating effector cells to release nonspecific factors capable of inhibiting intraerythrocytic multiplication. The B lymphocytes begin production of stage- and strain-specific antiplasmodial antibodies within the first 2 weeks of parasitemia. With the achievement of high levels of antibodies, the number of circulating parasites decreases. The infrequency with which malaria occurs in young infants has been attributed to the transplacental passage of such antibodies. It is uncertain whether they are directly lethal, act as opsonizing agents, or block merozoite invasion of RBCs. Antibody responses are also detectable against sporozoites and, because of this, much attention has been given to develop a vaccine against this parasite stage. Because sporozoites clear so quickly from the peripheral circulation, however, they may escape immune detection and all it would take is one to initiate hepatic schizogony resulting in blood stage infection. Antibodies against sporozoites have no effect on erythrocytic stages of infection.

Antibody-mediated immunity important

In simian malaria, the parasite can undergo antigenic variation and thereby escape the suppressive effect of the antibodies. This antigenic variation leads to cycles of recrudescent parasitemia, but ultimately to production of specific antibodies to the variants, and cure. In *P falciparum* malaria, chronic infection is maintained through the insertion of highly polymorphic variant antigens that are inserted into the infected erythrocyte membrane. With *P falciparum*, the disease typically does not exceed 1 year, but with *P malariae* the erythrocytic infection can be extremely persistent, lasting in one case up to 53 years. How erythrocytic parasites circulating in numbers too small to be detected on routine blood films escape immunologic destruction remains a puzzle. In a closely related simian malaria, splenectomy results in rapid cure, suggesting that suppressor T lymphocytes in the spleen may play a protective role. In infection with *P vivax* and *P ovale*, latent hepatic infection may result in the discharge of fresh merozoites into the bloodstream after the disappearance of erythrocytic forms. This phenomenon, known as **relapse**, can maintain infection for 3 to 5 years or longer.

Antigenic variation could play a role in persistence

In almost all cases, immunity to malaria is usually short lived and does not result in a sterile immunity. Many individuals, living in areas where transmission is sporadic, can be infected multiple times by the same species of parasite. A question often asked: if natural infection with malaria does not result in a lasting or sterile immunity, can a vaccine be developed that will?

MALARIA: CLINICAL ASPECTS

MANIFESTATIONS

The incubation period between the bite of the mosquito and the onset of disease is approximately 2 weeks. With *P malariae* and with strains of *P vivax* in temperate climates, however, this period is often more prolonged. Individuals who contract malaria while taking antimalarial suppressants may not experience illness for many months. In the United States, the interval between entry into the country and onset of disease exceeds 1 month in 25% of *P falciparum* infections and 6 months in a similar proportion of *P vivax* cases.

The clinical manifestations of malaria vary with the species of plasmodia but typically include chills, fever, splenomegaly, and anemia. The hallmark of disease is the malarial paroxysm. This manifestation begins with a cold stage, which persists for 20 to 60 minutes. During this time, the patient experiences continuous rigors and feels cold. With the consequent increase in body temperature, the rigors cease and vasodilatation commences, ushering in a hot stage. The temperature continues to rise for 3 to 8 hours, reaching a maximum of 40°C to 41.7°C before it begins to fall. The wet stage consists of a decrease in fever and profuse sweating. It leaves the patient exhausted but otherwise well until the onset of the next paroxysm.

Typical paroxysms first appear in the second or third week of fever, when parasite replication within erythrocytes becomes synchronized. In falciparum malaria, synchronization may never take place, and the fever may remain hectic and unpredictable. The first attack is often severe and may persist for weeks in the untreated patient. Eventually the paroxysms become less regular, less frequent, and less severe. Symptoms finally cease with the disappearance of the parasites from the blood.

In falciparum malaria, capillary blockage can lead to several serious complications. When the central nervous system is involved (cerebral malaria), the patient may develop delirium, convulsions, paralysis, coma, and rapid death. Acute pulmonary insufficiency frequently accompanies cerebral malaria, killing about 80% of those involved. When splanchnic capillaries are involved, the patient may experience vomiting, abdominal pain, and diarrhea with or without bloody stools. Jaundice and acute renal failure are also common in severe illness. These pernicious syndromes generally appear when the intensity of parasitemia exceeds 100,000 organisms per cubic millimeter of blood. Most deaths occur within 3 days.

DIAGNOSIS

Malarial parasites can be demonstrated in stained smears of the peripheral blood in virtually all symptomatic patients. Typically, capillary or venous blood is used to prepare both thin and thick smears, which are stained with Wright or Giemsa stain and examined for the presence of erythrocytic parasites. Thick smears, in which erythrocytes are lysed with water before staining, concentrate the parasites and allow detection of very mild parasitemia. Nonetheless, it may be necessary to obtain several specimens before parasites are seen. Artifacts are numerous in thick smears, and correct interpretation requires experience. The morphologic differences among the five species of plasmodia may allow their speciation on the stained thin smear by the skilled observer.

Several attempts have been made to improve the standard thin and thick smear method. One such procedure involves acridine orange staining of centrifuged parasites in quantitative buffy coat (QBC) tubes. Although it is expensive, this requires a fluorescence microscope and permits less reliable parasite speciation; its rapidity and ease of use make it attractive to laboratories that are only occasionally called on to identify patients with malaria. Simple, specific card antigen detection procedures are now available. The most widely used test, ParaSight F, detects a protein (HRP2) excreted by *P falciparum* within minutes. The test can be performed under field conditions and has a sensitivity of more than 95%. A second rapid test, OptiMAL, detects parasite lactate dehydrogenase, and, unlike ParaSight F, can distinguish between *P falciparum* and *P vivax*. Numerous PCR assays have also been developed for the laboratory diagnosis of malaria.

Serologic tests for malaria are offered at a few large reference laboratories but are used primarily for epidemiologic purposes. They are occasionally helpful in speciation and detection of otherwise occult infections. The recently completed sequencing of the malaria genome will lead to newer diagnostic methods.

Incubation prolonged by suppressants

Malarial paroxysm: cold, hot, wet stages

✷ *Paroxysms when parasite replication synchronized*

✷ *Cerebral falciparum malaria often lethal*

✷ *Thick and thin blood smears detect parasites*

Acridine orange stains, other methods available

TREATMENT

The indications for treatment rest on several factors. These include the severity of disease, the infecting species of *Plasmodium*, and the part of the world in which the infection was acquired. The immune status of the afflicted patient may also factor into this equation. The species and area of infection acquisition are likely to help determine if the parasite is resistant to any antimalarials or not. Falciparum malaria is potentially lethal in nonimmune individuals, such as new immigrants or travelers to a malarious area, and immunosuppressed indigenous individuals, such as pregnant women. These individuals must receive urgent treatment.

The complete treatment of malaria requires the destruction of erythrocytic schizonts, hepatic schizonts, and erythrocytic gametocytes. The first terminates the clinical attack, the second prevents relapse, and the third renders the patient noninfectious to *Anopheles* and thus breaks the cycle of transmission. Unfortunately, no single drug accomplishes all three goals. The present strategy for the diagnosis and treatment of malaria is shown in **Figure 51–7**.

Need to destroy all forms of the parasite

■ Termination of Acute Attack

Several agents can destroy asexual erythrocytic parasites. Chloroquine, a 4-aminoquinoline, has been the most commonly used. It acts by inhibiting the degradation of hemoglobin, thereby limiting the availability of amino acids necessary for growth. It has been suggested that the weak basic nature of chloroquine also acts to raise the pH of the food vacuoles of the parasite, inhibiting their acid proteases and effectiveness. When originally introduced, it was rapidly effective against all four species of plasmodia and, in the dosage used, free of serious side effects. However, chloroquine-resistant strains of *P falciparum* are now widespread in Africa and Southeast Asia; they are also found, though less frequently, in other areas of Asia and in Central America and South America. Chloroquine-resistant strains of *P vivax* have been reported from Papua New Guinea, India, and Pakistan, but overall remains poorly defined worldwide.

✳ **Chloroquine inhibits hemoglobin degradation**

✳ **Artemisinins prevent gametocyte development**

Other schizonticidal agents include quinine/quinidine, antifolate–sulfonamide combinations, mefloquine, halofantrine, and the artemisinins. Unfortunately, resistance to these agents is increasing, particularly in Southeast Asia. The artemisinins work by binding to proteins in many of the organism's key biochemical pathways. The artemisinins are also unique in their capacity to reduce transmission by preventing gametocyte development. Resistance to this latter first-line drug is increasing in areas of Southeast Asia.

✳ **Chloroquine, other resistance common with *P falciparum***

Strains of *P malariae*, *P ovale*, and *P vivax* (except for some acquired in the South Pacific and South America) remain sensitive to chloroquine and may be treated with this agent. *P vivax* infections acquired in New Guinea and Sumatra, however, should be assumed to be chloroquine-resistant and managed with mefloquine alone or in combination with other agents. *P falciparum* has now become variably resistant to all drug groups, including the artemisinin compounds.

Combination therapy necessary

There is a growing consensus that the most effective way to slow the further development of drug-resistant strains of *P falciparum* is to use one of the artemisinins in combination with quinine/quinidine, antifolate–sulfonamide compounds, mefloquine, or halofantrine.

■ Radical Cure

In *P vivax* and *P ovale* infections, hepatic schizonts persist and must be destroyed to prevent reseeding of circulating erythrocytes with consequent relapse. Primaquine, an 8-aminoquinoline, is used for this purpose. Some *P vivax* infections acquired in Southeast Asia and New Guinea fail initial therapy owing to relative resistance to this 8-aminoquinoline. Retreatment with a larger dose of primaquine is usually successful. Unfortunately, primaquine may induce hemolysis in patients with G6PD deficiency. Persons of Asian, African, and Mediterranean ancestry should thus be screened for this abnormality before treatment. Chloroquine destroys the gametocytes of *P vivax*, *P ovale*, and *P malariae* but not those of *P falciparum*. Primaquine and artemisinins, however, are effective for this latter species.

✳ **Primaquine destroys hepatic schizonts of *P vivax* and *P ovale***

PREVENTION

■ Personal Protection

In endemic areas, mosquito contact can be minimized with the use of house screens, insecticide bombs within rooms, and/or insecticide-impregnated mosquito netting around beds. Those who must be outside from dusk to dawn, the period of mosquito feeding, should apply insect repellent and wear clothing with long sleeves and pants. In addition, it is possible to suppress clinical manifestations of infection, if they occur, with a weekly dose of chloroquine. In areas where

Algorithm for Diagnosis and Treatment of Malaria in the United States*

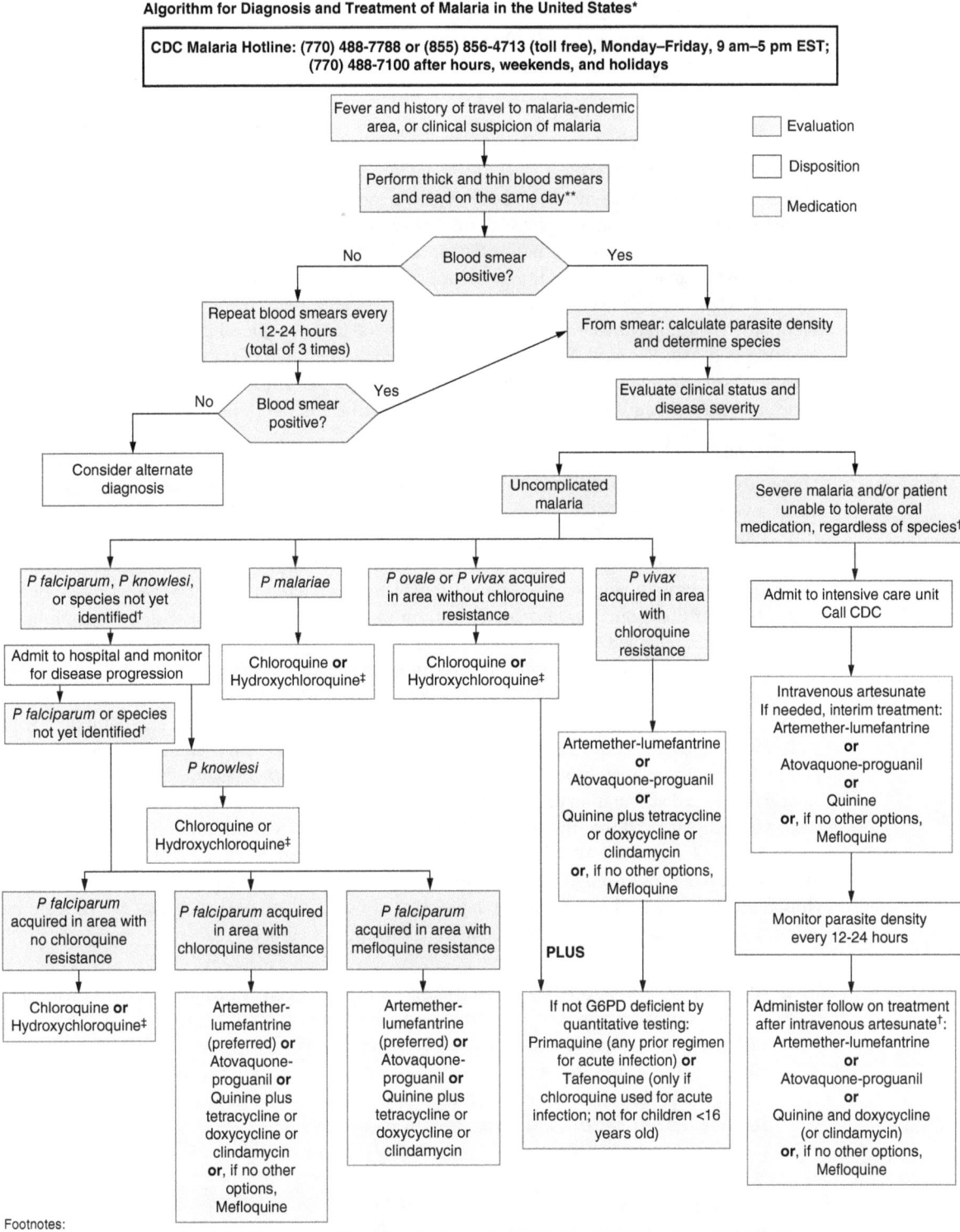

FIGURE 51-7. Algorithm for diagnosis and treatment of malaria in the United States. (Reproduced with permission from Centers for Disease Control and Prevention. U.S. Department of Health & Human Services. Algorithm for Diagnosis and Treatment of Malaria in the United States. May, 2020. https://www.cdc.gov/malaria/resources/pdf/Malaria_Treatment_Guidelines.pdf.)

chloroquine-resistant strains are common, an alternative schizonticidal agent should be used. Mefloquine, Malarone, or doxycycline are usually preferred. The antifolate pyrimethamine plus a sulfonamide can be taken as well. However, use of this combination is occasionally accompanied by serious side effects, so it is recommended only when mefloquine- and doxycycline-resistant

✳ Mosquito protection with screens and repellents

✳ Chemoprophylaxis considers resistance in area

strains are present in the area, and then only for individuals residing in areas of intense transmission for prolonged periods of time. On leaving an endemic area, it is necessary to eradicate residual hepatic parasites with primaquine before discontinuing suppressive therapy.

■ General

Reduce contact with and eradicate mosquitoes

Complete eradication has failed

Malaria control measures have been directed toward reducing the infected human and mosquito populations to below the critical level necessary for sustained transmission of disease. The techniques used include those mentioned previously, treatment of febrile patients with effective antimalarial agents, chemical or physical disruption of mosquito breeding areas, and residual insecticide sprays. An active international cooperative program aimed at the eradication of malaria resulted in a dramatic decline in the incidence of the disease between 1956 and 1968. Eradication was not achieved, however, because mosquitoes became resistant to many of the chemical agents used, and today malaria annually still infects 200 to 300 million inhabitants of Africa, Latin America, and Asia. Tropical Africa alone accounts for 100 million of the afflicted and for most of the 400,000 deaths that occur annually because of this disease. The long-term hope for progress in these areas now depends on the compliant use of existing and development of new technologies.

■ Vaccines

Subunit vaccines fused with a hepatitis B protein have shown promise

Three advances in the last decade have produced the hope for the first time that an effective malaria vaccine might be within reach of medical science. The establishment of a continuous *in vitro* culture system and the successful propagation of malaria in laboratory-raised mosquitoes have provided the large quantities of parasite needed for antigenic analysis. Development of the hybridoma technique allowed the preparation of monoclonal antibodies with which antigens responsible for the induction of protective immunity could be identified. Finally, recombinant DNA procedures enabled scientists to clone and sequence the genes encoding such antigens, permitting the amino acid structure to be determined and peptide sequences suitable for vaccine development to be identified. In 2012, a phase III clinical trial consisting of a protein fragment from the outer surface of *P falciparum*, fused with a hepatitis B virus protein, and combined with an immune adjuvant reduced episodes of both clinical and severe malaria in children aged 5 to 17 months by approximately 30%. This vaccine, named Mosquirix, has now been approved for a closely monitored vaccination program in Malawi, Ghana, and Kenya, targets the preerythrocytic stage of the disease and requires four injections. Overall efficacy is low and offers protection for no more than 4 years. The WHO does not recommend vaccinating young children under 1 year of age. Studies are continuing, with development of new adjuvants that may be even more potent. Hopefully, this may lead to vaccine strategies that are sorely needed throughout the developing world. Other attenuated sporozoite vaccines are currently in clinical trial.

 As a physician, you have been asked to make recommendations to a student who comes from the western highland area of Kenya to do undergraduate work at Harvard, has experienced multiple episodes of malaria all through his childhood and teenage years, has not been home in 2 years, and wants to return to his home in Kenya for a 1-month visit before coming back to the United States to resume his education. What would you recommend?

KEY CONCLUSIONS

- Human malaria is transmitted only by female *Anopheles* mosquitoes.
- Malaria symptoms are preceded for a prepatent period involving multiplication of parasites in the liver.
- *Plasmodium vivax* and *ovale* can relapse due to dormant hypnozoites in the liver.
- *Plasmodium knowlesi* is a zoonotic malarial species.
- Malaria parasites eventually replicate in synchronous fashion, producing fevers at regular intervals. An exception to this is *Plasmodium falciparum* whose replication may be asynchronous.
- Cerebral malaria, due to *P falciparum*, can result in coma and death if not treated.
- Immunity to malaria is short lived and stage- and species-specific.
- Malaria is increasingly becoming resistant to drugs.
- Mosquitoes are increasingly becoming resistant to insecticides.

BABESIA SPP.

The genus *Babesia* is represented by species that are close relatives of malaria belonging to the order Piroplasmida. They are small parasites of the mammalian host RBCs and are transmitted by ticks. These parasites were the first shown to be transmitted by an arthropod intermediate host. The organism involved in this instance was *B bigemina*, the causative agent of redwater fever in cattle.

Babesia microti is one of the parasites of interest to human health. It was first reported from a patient on Nantucket Island, Massachusetts. Since then there have been hundreds of cases reported from New England and in the states of Wisconsin, Washington, and California. Hard ticks of the genus *Ixodes* are the principal vectors. These ticks are also capable of transmitting Lyme disease. Within the tick vector, the disease can also be transmitted between stages of development (transstadial transmission) or across generations through the ova (transovarial transmission). *Babesia divergens* is the primary species infecting humans in Europe. It is also transmitted by *Ixodes* ticks. Unlike malaria, *Babesia* only infects the RBCs of its human host. Resulting symptoms can be flu like with attendant symptoms of fevers, chills, sweats, etc; not too unlike malaria. Diagnosis is affected by finding the small piroplasms in blood smears **(Figure 51–8)**. Because they resemble malaria it is often necessary to send smears to a reference laboratory or to have serologic or PCR testing performed.

Patients usually respond well to treatment with a combination of quinine and clindamycin. Because these may be poorly tolerated, atovaquone plus azithromycin can also be used. Preventive measures include avoidance of areas known to be tick infected, using appropriate insecticides, wearing appropriate clothing, and performing daily tick inspections if one ventures into wooded areas where ticks live.

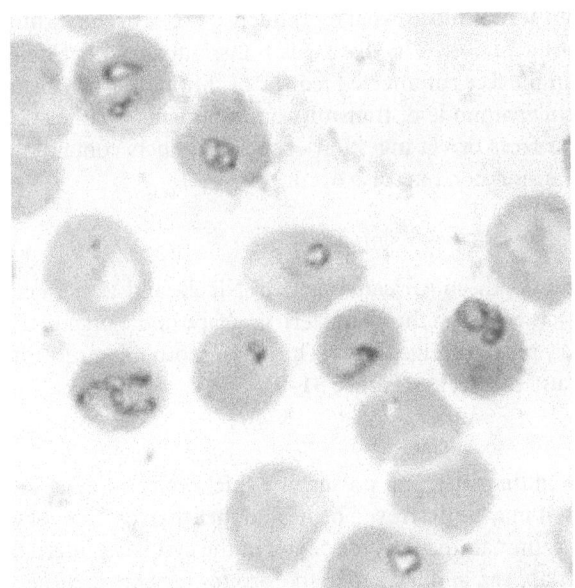

FIGURE 51–8. *Babesia* spp. in human blood. (Reproduced with permission from Centers for Disease Control and Prevention. U.S. Department of Health & Human Services. DPDx - Laboratory Identification of Parasites of Public Health Concern, Babesiosis. October, 2017.)

 Think▸▸ Apply 51-1: The western highland area of Kenya is endemic for *P falciparum* which causes almost all cases of malaria in the region. Because the student has not been home in 2 years, he most likely has lost all immunity to the disease. Because of this he will need to be on chemoprophylaxis for his visit to home. Recommended drugs include Mefloquine (helps arrest tissue phase development), Malarone (works against erythrocytic stages of infection), or doxycycline (usually used in combination with another schizonticide, but shows action against both liver and blood stages). Each is useful, but some show more side effects than others. Patients should be informed of plus and minus uses for each.

- *Babesia* spp. are transmitted to humans by hard ticks that also transmit Lyme disease.
- Symptoms of babesiosis closely resemble those of malaria without the cerebral involvement.
- Babesiosis is usually found in temperate zones where malaria is not endemic.

TOXOPLASMA GONDII

Overview

Toxoplasma gondii is an obligate intracellular parasite transmitted to humans from felines, but more commonly via infected meat products. *Toxoplasma* can infect most warm-blooded animals, both domestic and wild; it is thus the most cosmopolitan of parasites. Cats, however, are the only definitive hosts. Approximately 50% of the world population has been infected as defined serologically. In the United States, this rate is approximately 23%. In the overwhelming majority of persons, infection is chronic, asymptomatic, and self-limiting. Clinical disease manifests in three major forms: (1) self-limiting febrile lymphadenopathy; (2) highly lethal infection of immunocompromised patients, usually manifest as meningoencephalitis; and (3) congenital infection of infants, which may have fatal consequences.

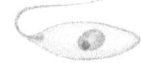 PARASITOLOGY

Asexual and sexual cycles in felines

Like the plasmodia, *T gondii*, the cause of toxoplasmosis, is an obligate intracellular apicomplexan. It differs from *Plasmodium* in that both sexual and asexual reproductive cycles occur within the gastrointestinal tract of felines, the definitive host. The disease is transmitted to other host species by the ingestion of oocysts passed in the feces of infected felines, or through carnivorism from one infected host to another. The principal mode of transmission to humans is either via ingestion of oocysts from contaminated cat feces or via ingestion of meat products containing tissue cysts (bradyzoites). Transplacental transmission may also occur.

＊Human spread via fecal–oral route, ingestion of meat

MORPHOLOGY

T gondii was first demonstrated in 1908 in the gondi, an African rodent, by Nicolle and Manceaux. Its name, derived from the Greek *toxo* (arc), is based on the characteristic shape of the organism. All strains of this parasite appear to be closely related antigenically. The major morphologic forms of the parasite are the oocyst, trophozoite, and tissue cyst (**Figure 51–9**).

■ Oocyst

The oocyst is ovoid, measures 10 to 12 μm in diameter, and possesses a thick wall that makes it resistant to most environmental challenges. It may be destroyed by heat higher than 66°C and by chemicals such as iodine and formalin. In its immature form, the center of the cyst lacks internal structure. With maturation, two sporocysts appear, and later four sporozoites may be discerned within each sporocyst. Sporulation does not occur at temperatures lower than 4°C or higher than 37°C. Complete sporulation may occur within 24 to 48 hours outside the host. This form is responsible for the fecal–oral route of transmission of the parasites from felines to other warm-blooded animals.

＊Tissue cysts killed by cooking

■ Tachyzoite (Trophozoite)

The term "trophozoite" is used in its broadest sense to refer to the asexual proliferative forms responsible for cell invasion and clinical disease. In different stages of the asexual cycle, it is referred to by several other terms, including merozoite and **tachyzoite**. It is crescent or arc shaped, measures 3 by 7 μm, and can invade all nucleated cell types. Although tachyzoites are obligate intracellular organisms, they may survive extracellularly in a variety of body fluids for periods of hours to days. They cannot, however, survive the digestive activity of the stomach and, therefore, are not infective on ingestion.

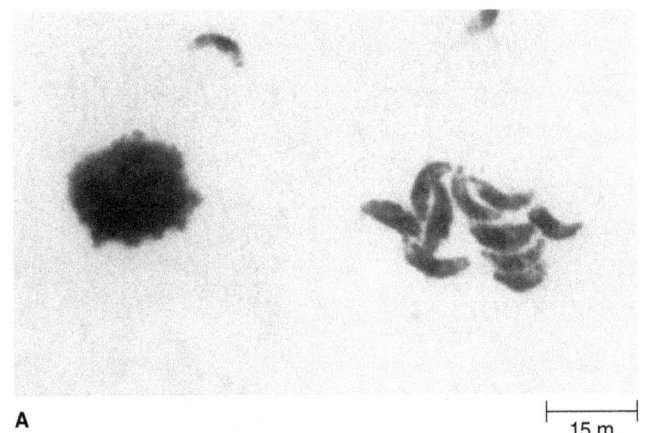

FIGURE 51–9. ***Toxoplasma gondii.*** **A.** Invasive trophozoite forms. **B.** Cyst in tissue. (Reproduced with permission from Nester EW, Anderson DG, Roberts CE Jr, et al: *Microbiology: A Human Perspective*, 6th ed. New York, NY: McGraw Hill; 2008.)

A

15 m

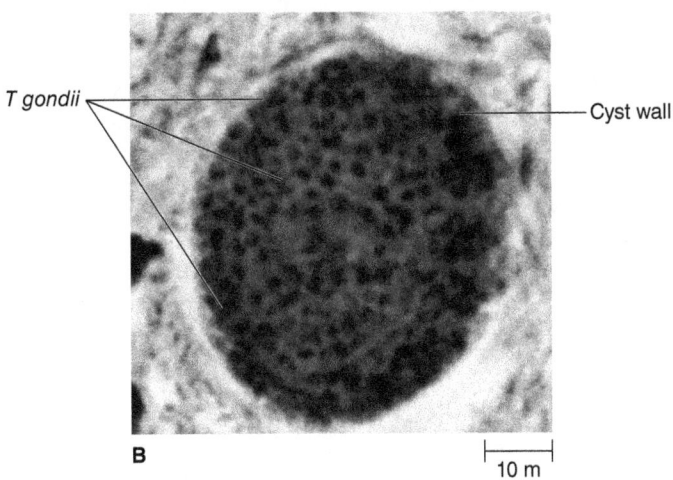

T gondii

Cyst wall

B

10 m

Tissue Cysts

Cysts measure 10 to 200 μm in diameter. The contained organisms, referred to as **bradyzoites,** are like tachyzoites, but are smaller and divide more slowly. Tissue cysts are resistant to digestive enzymes and, like oocysts, are infectious to the animal that ingests them. They survive normal refrigerator temperatures but are killed by freezing and thawing and by normal cooking temperatures.

LIFE CYCLE (FIGURE 51–10)

Definitive Host

Sexual reproduction of *T gondii* occurs only in the intestinal tract of felines, most commonly in the domestic cat. Ingested parasites enter the epithelial cells of the ileum by mechanisms like that of other apicomplexan parasites. Intracellularly, the trophozoites reside within a membrane-bound vacuole and undergo schizogony. With cell rupture, merozoites are released. The merozoites infect adjacent epithelial cells; they then repeat another asexual cycle or eventually differentiate into gametocytes, initiating sexual reproduction. Fusion of the mature male and female gametes leads to the formation of an oval, thick-walled oocyst that is then shed in the feces. In the typical infection, millions of these structures are released daily for 1 to 3 weeks. The oocysts are immature at the time of shedding and must complete sporulation in the external environment. In this process, two sporocysts, each containing four sporozoites, develop within each oocyst. The time required for sporulation typically takes 2 to 3 days, but may vary depending on the ambient temperature and moisture. Once mature, the resistant oocysts may remain viable and infectious for many months in soil.

* Infection in cat ileal cells

* Fusion of gametes leads to oocysts; shed in feces

* Sporulate in environment

Intermediate Hosts

Many animal species, including humans, are considered intermediate hosts for this infection. Infection may be acquired via ingestion of oocysts or via carnivorism of tissue-containing bradyzoites. After ingestion by a susceptible warm-blooded animal, sporozoites or bradyzoites are

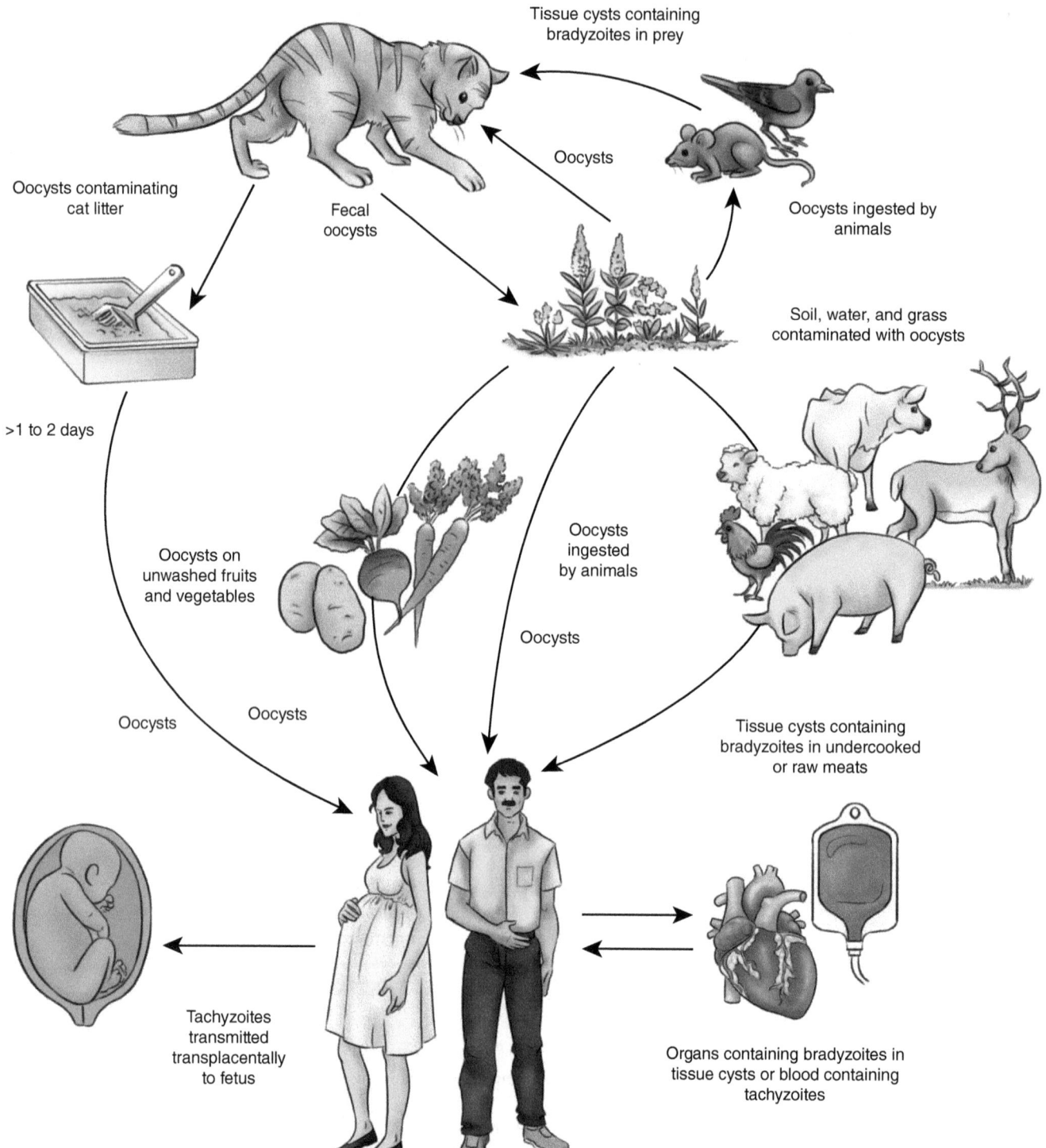

FIGURE 51-10. **Toxoplasmosis.** Pathways for *Toxoplasma gondii* infection: http://www.aafp.org/afp/2003/0515/
p2131.html Fig. 1. *Toxoplasma gondii* life cycle shows oocysts from cat feces or cysts from inadequately cooked meat
as infectious to humans and other animals. (Reproduced with permission from Nester EW, Anderson DG, Roberts CE
Jr, et al: *Microbiology: A Human Perspective*, 6th ed. New York, NY: McGraw Hill; 2008.)

released from the disrupted oocyst or tissue and enter macrophages. Within these cells they are
transported through the lymphohematogenous system to all organ systems. Survival within macrophages early in infections is because lysosomes are prevented from fusing with phagosomes
containing the parasite. Continued intracellular division, termed endodyogeny results in the
formation of 8 to 32 tachyzoites, which rupture from the macrophage and may invade any adjacent nucleated host cell to continue the asexual cycle. With the development of host immunity,
many of the parasites are destroyed as macrophages become competent killers of the parasite.

Within the cells of certain organs, particularly the brain, heart, and skeletal muscle, the trophozoites produce a membrane that surrounds and protects them: Within this tissue cyst, multiplication continues at a slower pace. Eventually, cysts that measure up to 200 μm in diameter are produced and contain more than 1000 bradyzoites. These cysts persist intact for the life of the host or rupture, producing parasitologic relapse. If they are ingested by a carnivore, they survive the digestive enzymes and initiate infection in the new host. The persistence of cysts confers protection against superinfection. This is referred to as **premunition**.

Oocysts, bradyzoites infect host orally

✳ Sporozoites invade macrophages

✳ Cysts can persist for life

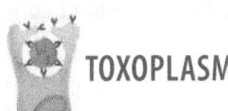

TOXOPLASMOSIS

EPIDEMIOLOGY

■ Prevalence and Distribution

Toxoplasmosis occurs in almost all mammals and many birds. Human infections are found in every region of the globe; in general, the incidence is higher in the tropics and lower in cold and/or arid regions. In the United States, the prevalence of positive serologic evidence for the disease increases with age. By adulthood, approximately 50% of individuals worldwide can be shown to have circulating antibodies against *T gondii*. Seroprevalence in cats may range from about 20% in countries like Japan, where cats are more likely to be kept indoors, to over 70% in some countries where cats are likely to live in rural areas or be feral.

Worldwide distribution among mammals and birds

■ Transmission

Although it is known that humans may acquire toxoplasmosis in a variety of ways, data on their relative frequency are both meager and conflicting. It is likely that the route of transmission varies from population to population, and perhaps from age to age, within any given area. The most important transmission mechanisms of toxoplasmosis are discussed below.

Ingestion of Oocysts

Persons with felinophobia are inclined to believe that the deposition of oocysts in the feces of cats and their subsequent ingestion by the unsuspecting owner is the most common way in which humans acquire this important infection. Disease epidemics of toxoplasmosis associated with exposure to infected cats have been reported. Unfortunately, data from studies relating the frequency of feline exposure to the prevalence of positive serologic tests are conflicting. Acutely infected cats shed oocysts for only a few weeks. It has been shown, however, that chronically infected felines can occasionally reshed oocysts, and prevalence studies have demonstrated that 1% of domestic cats excrete oocysts at any given time. The large number of these structures passed during active shedding and their prolonged survival in the external environment greatly enhance their chance of transmission. Particularly at risk are children at play, who may come in close contact with areas likely to be contaminated with cat feces, and adults responsible for changing a cat's litter box. It is also possible that insects can mechanically transfer oocysts to human food.

✳ Hazard to children by contact with contaminated areas

Ingestion of Tissue Cysts

Tissue cysts have been frequently demonstrated in meat produced for human consumption. They are most common in pork (25%) and mutton (10%) and less so in beef and chicken (<1%). Although such cysts are killed at normal (well-done) cooking temperatures, an impressive array of epidemiologic information links the handling and/or ingestion of raw or undercooked meat with serologic and, occasionally, clinical evidence of disease. Confounding these data is an Indian study that demonstrated no difference between meat eaters and vegetarians in the incidence of positive serologic tests.

✳ Cysts present in meat

Congenital

Approximately 1 of every 500 pregnant women acquires acute toxoplasmosis, and approximately 10% to 20% of the involved women become symptomatic. Regardless of the clinical status of the infected mother, the parasite involves the fetus in 33% to 50% of all acute maternal infections. The risk of transplacental transmission is independent of the clinical severity of the disease in the mother but does correlate with the stage of gestation at which she is exposed. Fetal involvement

❋ Transplacental transmission highest in third trimester

occurs in 17% of first-trimester and 65% of third-trimester infections. Conversely, the earlier a fetal infection is acquired, the more severe it is likely to be. Overall, 20% of fetuses experienced severe consequences; a similar proportion develops mild disease. The remainder are asymptomatic.

Miscellaneous

❋ Transmitted by transfusions, organ transplants

In addition to causing congenital infection, tachyzoites have been responsible for disease transmission in several other situations, including laboratory accidents, transfusions of whole blood and leukocytes, and organ transplantation. Because tachyzoites may survive for several hours in body fluids or exudates of acutely infected humans, it is possible for infection to occur after contact with such materials.

PATHOGENESIS AND IMMUNITY

Dissemination in immunosuppressed subjects

In primary infection, the proliferation of tachyzoites results in the death of involved host cells, stimulation of a mononuclear inflammatory reaction, and parasite-specific antibody and cellular responses. In immunodeficient hosts, such as those with human immunodeficiency virus (HIV)/ acquired immunodeficiency syndrome (AIDS), latent infections reactivate and rapid organism proliferation ensues, producing numerous widespread foci of tissue necrosis. The consequences are most serious in organs such as the brain, where the potential for cell regeneration is limited.

Immunity primarily cell-mediated

In normal hosts, acute infection is rapidly controlled with the development of humoral and cellular immunity. Extracellular parasites are destroyed, intracellular multiplication is hindered, and tissue cysts are formed. Except for lysis of extracellular parasites by antibody and complement, cell-mediated immunity appears to play the principal role in this process, mediated in part by IL-2, interferon-α, and cytotoxic T cells. Immunity appears to be lifelong, most likely due to the persistence of the parasite in the tissue cysts. The cysts, which are found most frequently in the brain, retina, heart, and skeletal muscle, normally produce little or no tissue reaction. The suppression of cell-mediated immunity that accompanies serious illness, or the administration of immunosuppressive agents, may lead to the rupture of a cyst and the release of trophozoites. Their subsequent proliferation and the intense antibody reaction to their presence result in an acute exacerbation of the disease.

 ## TOXOPLASMOSIS: CLINICAL ASPECTS

MANIFESTATIONS

In most patients, infection with *T gondii* is completely asymptomatic. Clinical manifestations, when they do appear, vary with the type of host involved. In general, they may be grouped into one of the three syndromes listed below.

■ Congenital Toxoplasmosis

Immune mechanisms are poorly developed in utero. Thus, a large proportion of fetal infections results in clinical illness. If the infection spreads to the central nervous system, the outcome is often catastrophic. Abortion and stillbirth are the most serious consequences. Liveborn children may demonstrate microcephaly, hydrocephaly, cerebral calcifications, convulsions, and psychomotor retardation. Disease of this severity is usually accompanied by evidence of visceral involvement, including fever, hepatitis, pneumonia, and skin rash. Infants infected with toxoplasmosis later in prenatal development demonstrate milder disease. Many appear healthy at birth but develop epilepsy, retardation, or strabismus months or years later. Probably the most common delayed manifestation of congenital toxoplasmosis is chorioretinitis. This condition, which is thought to result from the reactivation of latent tissue cysts, typically presents during the second or third decade of life as recurrent bouts of eye pain and loss of visual acuity. The lesions are usually bilateral but focal. If the retinal macula is not involved, vision improves as the inflammation subsides. *Toxoplasma gondii* accounts for 25% of all cases of granulomatous uveitis seen in the United States.

❋ Infection in utero produces malformations, chorioretinitis, stillbirth

■ Normal Host

The most common clinical manifestation of toxoplasmosis acquired after birth is asymptomatic localized lymphadenopathy. The cervical nodes are most frequently involved, but nontender enlargement of other regional groups, including the retroperitoneal nodes, also occurs. At times, adenopathy is accompanied by fever, sore throat, rash, hepatosplenomegaly, and atypical lympho-cytosis, thus mimicking the clinical and laboratory manifestations of infectious mononucleosis. Occasionally, the normal host develops severe visceral involvement, which may be manifested as meningoencephalitis, pneumonitis, myocarditis, or hepatitis. Chorioretinitis after postnatally acquired infection, though documented, is uncommon. Unlike congenitally acquired ocular dis-ease, it occurs during midlife and is generally unilateral.

■ Immunocompromised Host

In the immunocompromised host, toxoplasmosis is a serious, often fatal disease. If primary infec-tion is acquired while a patient is undergoing immunosuppressive therapy for malignancy or organ transplantation, widespread dissemination of the infection with necrotizing pneumonitis, myocarditis, and encephalitis may occur. More commonly, acute disease in this population results from the activation of chronic, latent infection by immunosuppressive therapy, or from the acqui-sition of a concurrent immunosuppressive infection, particularly AIDS. Encephalitis occurs in 50% of such cases and in more than 90% of fatal cases. Toxoplasmic encephalitis is particularly common in AIDS patients; it is seen in approximately 10% of those with circulating toxoplasma antibodies. As such, it is a major cause of morbidity and mortality in this patient population. Clin-ically, encephalitis may present as a meningoencephalitis, diffuse encephalopathy, or mass lesion. Acute toxoplasmosis has been seen as a result of organ transplantation in which immunosuppres-sive drugs were given to prevent organ rejection but resulted in a reactivation of latent cyst forms.

Primary infection or reactivation can produce widespread disease

AIDS patients develop encephalitis

DIAGNOSIS

The diagnosis of toxoplasmosis may be established by a variety of methods. In acute toxoplasmic lymphadenitis, the histologic appearance of the involved nodes is often pathognomonic. The tro-phozoite may be demonstrated in tissue with Wright or Giemsa stain. Electron microscopy and indirect fluorescent antibody techniques have also been used successfully on heart transplant or brain tissue obtained by biopsy. Although tissue cysts are selectively stained by periodic acid–Schiff, their presence is not indicative of acute disease. Isolation of the organism can be accom-plished by inoculating blood or other body fluids into mice or tissue cultures. Inoculation of other tissues is not usually helpful because a positive result may only reflect the presence of latent tissue cysts.

Demonstration in histopathologic specimens

Serologic procedures are the primary method of diagnosis. To establish the presence of acute infection, it is usual to demonstrate a fourfold rise in the IgG antibody titer between acute and convalescent serum specimens. Peak titers are often reached within 4 to 8 weeks, so the acute serum must be collected early during illness. Of the many tests developed for the detection of IgG antibodies, indirect hemagglutination, indirect fluorescent antibody, or enzyme immunoassay (EIA) tests are the tests most frequently used. Titers may remain high for many years.

✳ Serodiagnosis the primary approach

The detection of IgM antibodies provides a more rapid confirmation of acute infection. These antibodies appear within the first week of infection, peak in 2 to 4 weeks, and may slowly revert to negative. It also appears that immunoglobulin-M (IgM) antibodies are produced after reactiva-tion of latent disease. EIA for IgM antibody is now commonly used. Examination of tissues, urine, and other body fluids for the presence of toxoplasma antigen, or DNA by the PCR, have been shown to be useful adjunctive tests in immunocompromised individuals and in the diagnosis of congenital infections.

Rising titers of IgG or detection of IgM suggest acute infection or reactivation

TREATMENT AND PREVENTION

Usually, patients infected with toxoplasmosis do not require therapy unless symptoms are partic-ularly severe and persistent or unless vital organs, such as the eye, are involved. Immunocompro-mised and pregnant women, however, should be treated if acute infection (or reactivation) is documented (**Table 51–2**). Routine serial serologic testing of such individuals would allow early detection of infected persons and enhance the prospects of a successful outcome. It is now clear that early treatment of acutely infected pregnant women significantly reduces the incidence of severe congenital infections and reduces the ratio of benign to subclinical forms in infants. At present, the most commonly used therapeutic regimen in the United States for toxoplasmosis is the combination of pyrimethamine and sulfadiazine plus folinic acid. Unfortunately, the former drug is teratogenic and should not be used in the first trimester of pregnancy; spiramycin, a cytostatic macrolide, is often substituted in this setting.

✳ Spiramycin to prevent congenital infection

TABLE 51-2	Indications for Treatment of Toxoplasmosis[a]
SEROLOGIC CRITERIA	**CLINICAL CRITERIA**
Elevated IgM titers	Recently acquired infection
Fourfold rise in IgG titers	Pregnant woman
Very high IgG titers (>1:1000)	Neonate
	Immunocompromised patient (including AIDS)
	Severe constitutional symptoms
	Vital organ involvement (including active chorioretinitis)

Ig, immunoglobulin.
[a]Must satisfy one serologic plus one clinical criterion.

✳ **Atovaquone active against tachyzoites and cysts**

Although the pyrimethamine–sulfonamide combination is very effective against trophozoites, it is inactive against the cyst forms. Because both parasitic forms are present in patients with toxoplasmic encephalitis, recrudescence of illness generally follows completion of standard therapy in patients with AIDS. This may be prevented by initiating chronic, low-dose suppressive therapy after completion of the standard regimen. Atovaquone, a recently introduced hydroxynaphthoquinone, possesses activity against both trophozoites and cysts. Its use, therefore, may result in radical cure of toxoplasma encephalitis, eliminating the need for chronic suppression.

Prevention of toxoplasmosis should be directed primarily at pregnant women and immunologically compromised hosts. Hands should be carefully washed after handling uncooked meat. Cysts in meat can be destroyed by proper cooking (56°C for 15 minutes) or by freezing to –20°C. Cat feces should be avoided, particularly the changing of litter boxes.

A transplant recipient develops signs of acute meningitis within 2 weeks of receiving a donor heart. Acute toxoplasmosis is suspected. (1) How would you diagnose this possibility? (2) How might the recipient have acquired this infection and how might you prove your point? (3) What course of action would you take to treat this patient?

KEY CONCLUSIONS

- Cats are the only definitive host for *Toxoplasma*. All other infected animals are intermediate hosts.
- Transmission to humans is via cat feces, meat products, and congenitally.
- Approximately 50% of the world's population is serologically positive for this infection.
- Cell-mediated immunity appears to be most important in controlling this infection.
- Infection immunity or premonition is due to persistence of bradyzoites and prevents reinfection of the same person as long as that person does not become immunocompromised.
- Congenital transmission is most common during the third trimester, but the most severe symptoms are associated with transmission during the first trimester.
- Most individuals are asymptomatic, but severe disease is often seen in the immunocompromised.

CRYPTOSPORIDIUM SPP.

Overview

Cryptosporidia are small parasites that infect the intestinal cells of mammals. Cryptosporidiosis is an intestinal illness acquired from domestic and wild animals and from other humans. The course includes profuse watery diarrhea, vomiting, and weight loss. Spontaneous complete recovery is the usual outcome, except in immunocompromised persons, in whom debilitating illnesses can occur.

Cryptosporidia ("hidden-spore") are small parasites that can infect the intestinal tract of a wide range of mammals, including humans. Like many other apicomplexan parasites, they are obligate intracellular organisms that exhibit alternating cycles of sexual and asexual reproduction within the gastrointestinal tract of the same host. Long recognized as an important cause of diarrhea in animals, cryptosporidia were not identified as causes of human enteritis until 1976, when first observed in a patient with a congenital IgA immunodeficiency. The advent of the AIDS epidemic sparked an intense interest in this parasite as a problem in humans. There are at least 26 different species of *Cryptosporidium* currently recognized. Of 20 species and genotypes that infect humans, the most common are zoonotic species, *Cryptosporidium parvum*, and a species, *Cryptosporidium hominis*, that only infects humans. The former is more likely to be encountered in rural populations, whereas the latter dominates in urban settings.

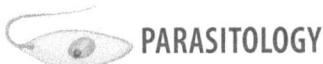 **PARASITOLOGY**

MORPHOLOGY

Regardless of animal host, all species of this tiny (2-6 μm) parasite appear morphologically identical. The organisms appear as small spherical structures arranged in rows along the microvilli of the epithelial cells. They are readily stained with Giemsa and hematoxylin–eosin. Although they remain external to the cytoplasm of the intestinal epithelial cell, they are clearly enveloped by a membrane of host cell origin. They are thus said to be intracellular but extracytoplasmic. The parasite replicates at this site giving rise to oocysts. Oocysts shed into the intestinal lumen contain four sporozoites that are not contained within sporocyst structures like their relative, *Toxoplasma*. Their cell wall provides the unusual property of acid-fastness, allowing them to be visualized with stains generally employed for mycobacteria. Oocysts are typically 5 to 6 μm in diameter.

Small spherical particles associated with microvilli

❋ Oocysts acid-fast

LIFE CYCLE

Infective oocysts are excreted in the stool of the parasitized animal. Unlike those of *Toxoplasma*, cryptosporidia oocysts are fully mature and immediately infective to the next host on passage in the feces. After ingestion by another animal, sporozoites are released from the oocyst and attach to the microvilli of the small intestinal epithelial cells, where they are transformed into trophozoites. These divide asexually by multiple fission (schizogony) to form schizonts containing eight daughter cells known as type 1 merozoites. On release from the schizont, each daughter cell attaches itself to another epithelial cell, where it repeats the schizogony cycle, producing another generation of type 1 merozoites. In the absence of effective immunity, this phase may constitute an autoinfective portion of the life cycle allowing perpetuation of the infection.

❋ Mature, infective oocysts excreted in stools

A second generation of schizonts follows with the formation of four merozoites. These merozoites are destined to invade intestinal cells and give rise to male (microgametocyte) and female (macrogametocyte) sexual forms. Gamete development ensues and after fertilization, the

 Think ▸▸ Apply 51-2: **(1) Since toxoplasmosis was suspected, a serologic test could be performed to see if IgM antibodies are present. This usually signals acquisition of a recent infection. In addition, PCR testing of cerebrospinal fluid and neuroradiology might be performed. (2) Two likely possibilities: (a) The patient could have received the organisms from the donor's heart. Serology should be performed in both patients and obtained from blood specimen of donor before transplant. If recipient is seronegative and donor is seropositive then you know the parasite was present in the donor's heart. (b) Patient had reactivation of a latent infection due to immunosuppressive therapy to prevent heart rejection. In this case, pre- and postpatient serum is likely IgG-positive with titer rising. (3) Patient should be put on pyrimethamine and sulfadiazine or another suitable drug if patient allergic to sulfa drugs. In addition, immunosuppressive therapy should probably be dampened. This latter therapy is meant to prevent tissue rejection, but may help exacerbate toxoplasmosis.**

Cell wall ensures survival of oocysts

resulting zygote develops into an oocyst that is shed into the lumen of the bowel. The majority, approximately 80%, possesses a thick protective cell wall that ensures their intact passage in the feces and survival in the external environment.

Approximately 20% fail to develop the thick protective wall. The cell membrane ruptures, releasing infective sporozoites directly into the intestinal lumen and initiating a new "autoinfective" cycle within the original host. In the normal host, the presence of innate or acquired immunity dampens both the cyclic production of type 1 merozoites and the formation of thin-walled oocysts, halting further parasite multiplication and terminating the acute infection. In the immunocompromised, both presumably continue, explaining why such individuals develop severe, persistent infections in the absence of external reinfection.

Thin-walled oocysts can autoinfect

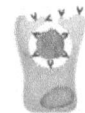 # CRYPTOSPORIDIOSIS

EPIDEMIOLOGY

Cryptosporidiosis appears to involve most vertebrate groups. In all species, infection rates are highest among the young and immature. Experimental and epidemiologic data suggest that domestic animals constitute an important reservoir of disease in humans. Transmission from young animals at petting zoos to children has been documented. Outbreaks of human disease in day care centers, swimming pools, hospitals, and urban family groups indicate that most human infections result from person-to-person transmission. In Western countries, between 1% and 4% of small children presenting to medical centers with gastroenteritis have been shown to harbor cryptosporidia oocysts. In Third World countries, the rates have varied from 4% to 11%. In some outbreaks of diarrhea in day care centers, most attendees were found to have oocysts in their stool.

✳ Animal reservoirs, person-to-person transmission important

Infection rates of cryptosporidiosis in adults suffering from gastroenteritis is approximately one-third of that reported in children; it has been highest in family members of infected children, medical personnel caring for patients with cryptosporidiosis, male homosexuals, and travelers to foreign countries. In the United States, the parasite was identified in 15% of patients with AIDS and diarrhea at the onset of the epidemic. Because of the advent of antiretroviral therapies, this has been reduced to 1% to 2%; in Haiti and Africa, high percentages of such individuals who do not have access to antiretroviral therapies may be involved. Asymptomatic carriage is uncommon in these populations. In many developing countries, most children may acquire multiple infections with *Cryptosporidium* before the age of 5 years. After that infections can still be detected, but symptoms may be absent suggesting that constant exposure may help maintain a measure of immunity.

Infection rates highest in young children

Because oocysts are found almost exclusively in stool, the principal transmission route of cryptosporidiosis is undoubtedly by direct fecal–oral spread. Transmission via contaminated water has been documented. Most noteworthy was the outbreak involving municipal water in the city of Milwaukee in 1993. An estimated 403,000 people were infected via primary and then secondary spread of the organism. The hardy nature of the oocysts, which do not respond to conventional chlorine treatment of water and many other commonly used disinfectants, makes it likely that there is also indirect transmission via contaminated food and fomites. Flies and shellfish have been incriminated as transport hosts for this parasite.

Transmitted via contaminated water

PATHOGENESIS AND IMMUNITY

Although the jejunum is most heavily involved, cryptosporidia have been found throughout the gastrointestinal, and even in the respiratory, tract, particularly in immunocompromised patients. Cryptosporidial cholecystitis is seen with some frequency in AIDS patients with enteritis. By light microscopy, bowel changes appear minimal, consisting of mild-to-moderate villous atrophy, crypt enlargement, and a mononuclear infiltrate of the lamina propria. The pathophysiology of the diarrhea is unknown. The vital role played by the host's immune status in the pathogenesis of the disease is indicated by both the enhanced susceptibility of the young to infection and the prolonged severe clinical disease seen in immunocompromised patients. Indirect evidence suggests that antibodies in the intestinal lumen exert a protective effect against initial *C parvum* infection. Experimental animal studies indicate that CD4+ T lymphocytes and interferon play independent roles in the immunologic clearance of the parasite.

Minimal intestinal pathology

Prolonged disease in AIDS

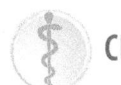

CRYPTOSPORIDIOSIS: CLINICAL ASPECTS

MANIFESTATIONS

Immunocompetent patients usually note the onset of explosive, profuse, watery diarrhea 1 to 2 weeks after exposure. Typically, cryptosporidiosis persists for 5 to 11 days and then rapidly abates. Occasionally, purging, accompanied by a mild malabsorption and weight loss, continues for up to 1 month. A few patients complain of nausea, anorexia, vomiting, and low-grade fever. Except for its shorter duration, more prominent abdominal pain, and relative lack of flatulence, the clinical manifestations of cryptosporidiosis closely resemble those produced by *Giardia lamblia*. Radiographic and endoscopic examinations of the gut are either normal or demonstrate mild, nonspecific abnormalities. Recovery is complete.

Self-limiting diarrhea in normal hosts

Cryptosporidiosis has been described in patients with a broad range of immunodeficiencies, including childhood malnutrition in the Third World countries, AIDS, congenital hypogammaglobulinemia, and in those resulting from cancer chemotherapy and immunosuppressive management of organ transplantations. In such patients, cryptosporidiosis is usually indolent at onset, and manifestations are like those seen in normal hosts, but the diarrhea is more severe. Fluid losses of up to 17 L/day have been described. Patients with biliary cryptosporidiosis present with typical manifestations of cholecystitis and cholangitis. Unless the immunologic defect is reversed, the disease usually persists for the duration of the patient's life. Weight loss is often prominent. The prognosis depends on the nature of the underlying immunologic abnormality; 50% of the patients with AIDS die within 6 months. Although other intercurrent infections are usually the direct cause of death, malnutrition and complications of parenteral nutrition contribute.

✳ Diarrhea more severe in immunocompromised

DIAGNOSIS

The diagnosis of cryptosporidiosis is established by the recovery and identification of *Cryptosporidium* oocysts in a recently passed or preserved diarrheal stool. Oocyst excretion is most intense during the first week of illness, tapers during the second week, and generally stops with the cessation of diarrhea. Because cryptosporidia oocysts are acid-fast, a presumptive identification can be established with any one of the acid-fast staining procedures developed for mycobacteria (**Figure 51–11**). This is best used in the hands of a competent diagnostician with experience. A direct immunofluorescence antibody stain using a monoclonal antibody to oocyst wall has been introduced, and is superior to acid-fast stains, but more time consuming and expensive. When direct examinations are negative, concentration procedures are used and the concentrate restained. Immunofluorescence and EIAs for the detection of anticryptosporidial antibodies are available as are EIAs and PCR methods for application to stool samples.

✳ Oocysts detected by acid-fast, immunofluorescent stains

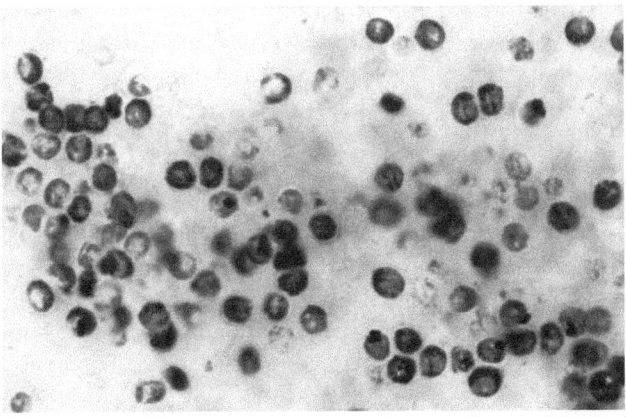

FIGURE 51–11. *Cryptosporidium parvum.* This acid-fast stain demonstrates oocysts in the feces of a diarrheal patient. (Reproduced with permission from Nester EW, Anderson DG, Roberts CE Jr, et al: *Microbiology: A Human Perspective*, 6th ed. New York, NY: McGraw Hill; 2008.)

10 m

TREATMENT AND PREVENTION

Specific treatment remains problematic

In the immunocompetent patient, the disease is self-limited and attempts at specific antiparasitic therapy are not warranted; rehydration may be required in small children. In the immunocompromised host, the severity and chronicity of the diarrhea warrant therapeutic intervention. Unfortunately, there is no uniformly effective anticryptosporidial agent available now. Paromomycin, a luminal antimicrobial, has been shown to reduce the intensity of diarrhea in some patients, and parenteral octreotide acetate, a somatostatin analog, has been useful in decreasing stool volumes. Macrolide antimicrobials have also been suggested in difficult cases. Nitrazoxanide, a synthetic drug, has been approved for use in all patients over 1 year of age in the United States and is reported to have a cure rate of 72% to 88% by the CDC. Parasitologic cure with this drug approaches 80%. The only uniformly successful approach has been the reversal of underlying immunologic abnormalities. When appropriate, withdrawal of cancer chemotherapy agents or immunosuppressive drugs may result in a cure.

Strict stool precautions for symptomatic patients

The stools of patients with cryptosporidiosis are infectious. Stool precautions should be instituted at the time the diagnosis is first suspected; for the immunosuppressed patient, this should be whenever diarrhea, regardless of the presumed cause, is first noted. This is particularly important in cancer chemotherapy and transplantation units, where spread of the disease from a symptomatic patient to other immunosuppressed patients can have life-threatening consequences. Oocysts can survive for many months in the external environment and have been found in most water sources across the United States. The infectious dose for this parasite is acknowledged to be very low.

KEY CONCLUSIONS

- Humans are infected by many zoonotic spp. of *Cryptosporidium* and *Cryptosporidium hominis*, which only infect humans.
- Infection is predominately fecal–oral, either directly or indirectly.
- Oocysts are immediately infective when released in feces and very few oocysts are required to initiate infection of another host.
- Oocysts are highly resistant to most commonly used disinfectants, accounting for numerous waterborne outbreaks.
- Infections are usually resolved in the immunocompetent, but can be life-threatening to the immunocompromised.

● OTHER INTESTINAL PROTOZOA

CYCLOSPORA AND ISOSPORA

Cyclospora was first recognized in the 1980s, but it was not until 1993 that it was shown to be closely related to both *Cryptosporidium* and *Toxoplasma*. The species that infects humans is *Cyclospora cayetanensis*. The species name was derived from the University in Lima, Peru, where much initial work was done on this parasite. This parasite gained notoriety because of foodborne outbreaks of illness that were ultimately linked to raspberries imported into the United States. Similar outbreaks have now been documented in many countries. Humans appear to be the only host for this parasite and its normal endemicity is usually linked to underdeveloped countries.

The parasite has an oocyst that measures 8 to 10 µm in diameter and stains acid-fast variable. It is remarkably like *Cryptosporidium* in its appearance but is larger (**Figure 51–12**). A big difference between the two is that it takes a week or longer for the oocyst to complete sporulation outside the host. Because of this, direct person-to-person transmission is unlikely. Complete sporulation results in an oocyst with two sporocysts each containing two sporozoites. Where both parasites are present in populations, *Cryptosporidium* has both a greater incidence and prevalence.

Symptoms of cyclosporiasis mimic those of *Cryptosporidium*. *Cyclospora* is treatable with trimethoprim–sulfamethoxazole and for this reason it is important to correctly identify this parasite in stool sample since *Cryptosporidium* does not respond to this drug.

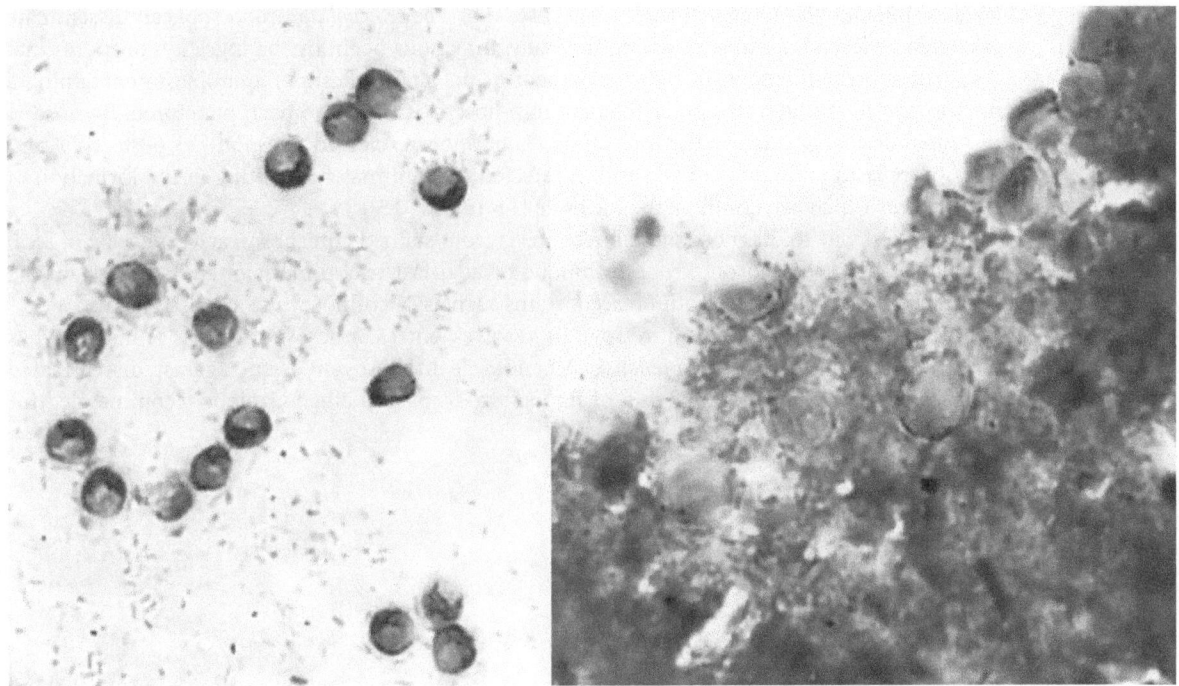

FIGURE 51–12. Side-by-side comparison of staining and size differences between *Cryptosporidium* and *Cyclospora*. *Cyclospora* is on the right.

Isospora belli, now named *Cystoisospora belli*, is another protozoan closely related to *Toxoplasma*. Like *Toxoplasma*, oocysts contain two sporocysts, each with four sporozoites. Oocysts, however, are much larger in size (25-30 µm) and almost football shaped (Figure 51–14). They can be stained with modified acid-fast and trichrome procedures. Clinical disease resembles that of cryptosporidiosis and this parasite responds to treatment with trimethoprim–sulfamethoxazole. This parasite has a worldwide distribution in subtropical areas, but is not that prevalent. It is recognized as a problem in the immunocompromised.

KEY CONCLUSIONS

- Cyclospora cayetanensis occurs only in humans and has been linked to foodborne consumption in outbreak situations.
- Symptoms are like those for cryptosporidiosis.
- This parasite should be carefully distinguished from *Cryptosporidium* because it is easily treatable whereas *Cryptosporidium* is not.
- *Isopora* infection is mostly recognized as a problem in the immunocompetent where it can produce profuse diarrheal disease.

MICROSPORIDIA

The inclusion of this parasite group in this chapter is because at one time they were placed in the same taxonomic grouping (Sporozoa) as were the other organisms discussed in this chapter. Once classified among the Protozoa they are now known to be fungi and are placed in their own phylum, the Microspora. As the name implies, this group of organisms is characterized by producing small spores. There are over 1200 known species parasitizing a very wide variety of eukaryotic hosts.

These parasites came to our attention because of the advent of the HIV/AIDS pandemic and they are still recognized largely as parasites of the immunocompromised. There have, however, been reports of infections caused by these organisms in children of certain African countries.

At least 14 different species have been recorded from humans. The principal ones of concern are *Enterocytozoon bieneusi* and three different species of *Encephalitozoon*. *Enterocytozoon bieneusi* inhabits the intestinal tract and causes diarrhea. *Encephalitozoon* spp. can disseminate to a wide variety of organ sites within the body. Infections begin by the ingestion of spores that discharge a polar filament in the environment of the small intestine. Sporoplasm containing a nucleus travels through this polar filament into host cells that have been punctured. Because of this rapid discharge process, the microsporidia have been referred to as nature's perfect syringe. The sporoplasm and nuclei divide within infected cells ultimately resulting in the formation of more spores which can continue the life cycle (**Figure 51–13**).

The easiest way to diagnose these infections is from stained clinical smears, especially of fecal samples. A quick hot chromotrope technique or acid-fast trichrome is often used to stain the spores (**Figure 51–14**). Chemofluorescent stains such as calcofluor white are also useful.

Immune resolution using antiretrovirals resolves enteric microsporidiosis. Fumagillin has proven efficacious against *E bieneusi*. Albendazole has proven useful against disseminated microsporidiosis and a combination of fumagillin drops and albendazole is recommended for ocular infections.

FIGURE 51–13. Life-cycle diagram of a representative Microsporidian.

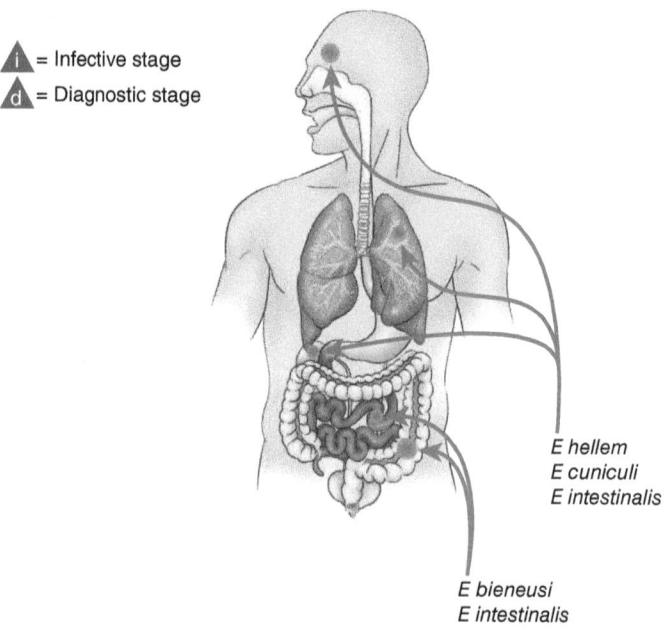

🔺 = Infective stage
🔺 = Diagnostic stage

E hellem
E cuniculi
E intestinalis

E bieneusi
E intestinalis

Intracellular development of *E bieneusi* and *E intestinalis* spores.

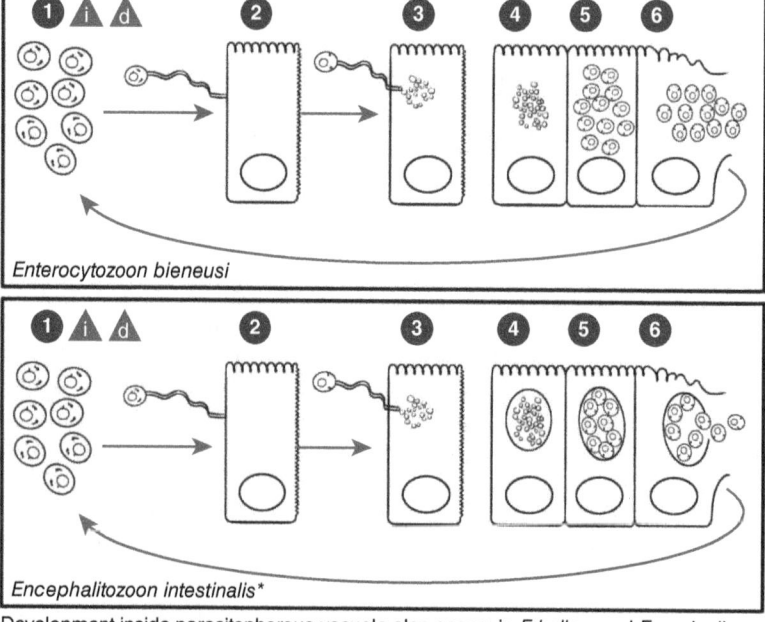

Enterocytozoon bieneusi

*Encephalitozoon intestinalis**

*Development inside parasitophorous vacuole also occurs in *E hellem* and *E cuniculi*.

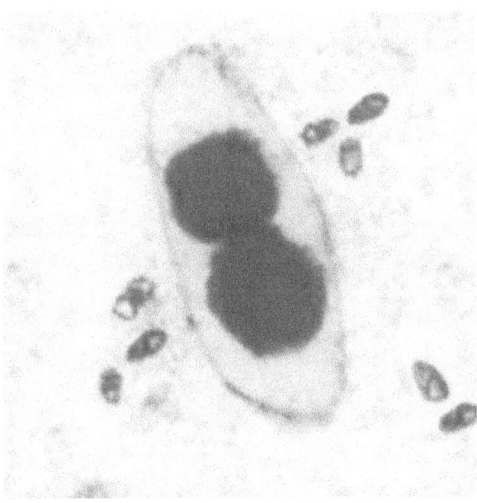

FIGURE 51–14. Fecal smear stained both with modified acid-fast and trichrome stains and showing and Isospora oocyst (large) and microsporidian spores (small). (Reproduced with permission from Garcia LS. Laboratory identification of the microsporidia, *J Clin Microbiol* 2002 Jun;40(6):1892–1901.)

KEY CONCLUSIONS

- Microsporidian infections in humans primarily occur in the immunocompromised.

- *Enterocytozoon bieneusi* infects the gastrointestinal tract while many other microsporidian infections have the ability to disseminate to other organs.

CASE STUDY

Fever After an Excursion

A 30-year-old man returned to the United States 3 weeks ago from a guided tour of Thailand. On advice of his physician, he took oral chloroquine prophylaxis beginning 1 week before departure and ending 1 week after his return. Over the last 4 days, he has developed repeated episodes of fever to 40°C, preceded by chills and associated with a severe headache. The duration of these symptoms has been about 8 hours, ending with profuse sweating, only to recur again within 48 hours.

Physical examination is unremarkable, except for fever.

Laboratory studies reveal only a mild anemia, with a platelet count of 100,000/mm³ (normal 200,000-400,000).

QUESTIONS

1. Which is the most likely diagnosis for this patient?
   A. Vivax malaria
   B. Falciparum malaria
   C. Toxoplasmosis
   D. Ovale malaria
   E. Malariae malaria

2. The diagnostic test of choice is:
   A. Peripheral blood smears
   B. PCR of red blood cells
   C. IgM ELISA serology
   D. Paired sera for IgG antibody quantitation

3. In some malarial infections, treatment to prevent relapse (by destroying persistent hepatic schizonts) is necessary in which two of the following?
   A. *Plasmodium malariae*
   B. *Plasmodium ovale*
   C. *Plasmodium falciparum*
   D. *Plasmodium knowlesi*

4. After primary infection, *T gondii* may persist as cyst forms in all of the following tissues *except* which of the following:
    A. Brain
    B. Heart
    C. Skin
    D. Skeletal muscle
    E. Retina

ANSWERS

1. **(B)**

2. **(A)**

3. **(B) and (D)**

4. **(C)**

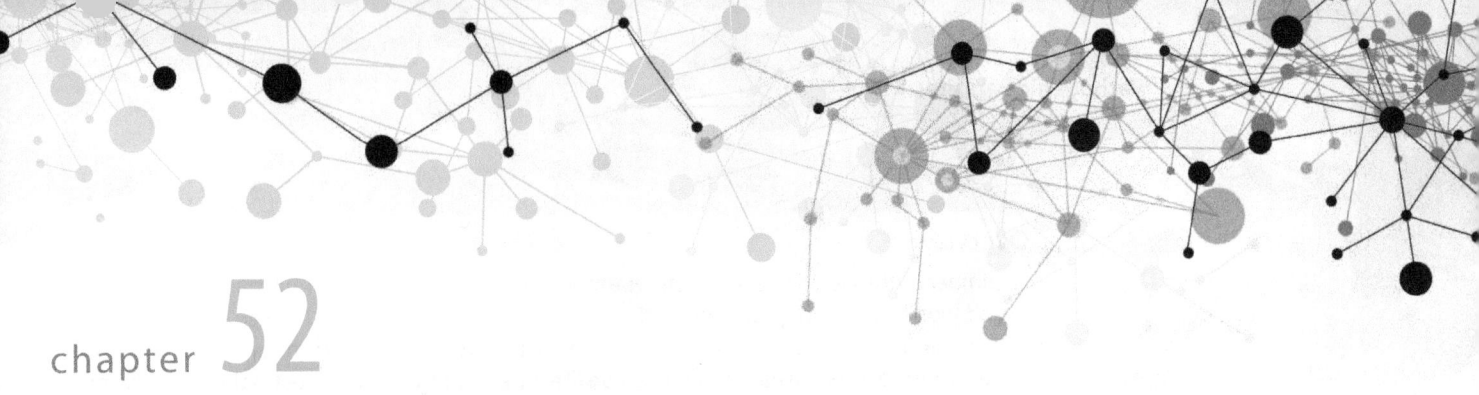

chapter 52

Sarcomastigophora— The Amebas

Entamoeba histolytica · *Entamoeba dispar* · *Naegleria fowleri* · *Acanthamoeba* spp. · *Balamuthia* spp.

> *Amoebas at the start*
> *Were not complex;*
> *They tore themselves apart*
> *And started sex.*
> —Arthur Guiterman: *The Light Guitar*

SARCOMASTIGOPHORA—THE AMEBAS—GROUP CHARACTERISTICS

The Sarcomastigophora include both the amebas and flagellate groups. Because of their divergent organization and medical importance, they are considered in separate chapters. The amebas are characterized by movement involving cytoplasmic streaming dependent upon **pseudopodia** formation. These projections of the relatively solid ectoplasm are formed by streaming of the inner, more liquid endoplasm. They move the ameba forward and, incidentally, engulf and internalize food sources found in its path. Amebas multiply by simple binary fission. Most amebas, when faced with a hostile environment, can produce an external cyst wall that surrounds and protects them. These cysts may survive for prolonged periods under conditions that would rapidly destroy the motile trophozoite. Most amebas belong to free-living genera. They are widely distributed in nature, being found in literally all bodies of standing fresh water. Few free-living amebas produce human disease, although two genera, *Naegleria* and *Acanthamoeba*, have been implicated occasionally as causes of meningoencephalitis and keratitis.

Several genera of amebas, including *Entamoeba*, *Endolimax*, and *Iodamoeba*, are obligate commensalistic parasites of the human alimentary tract and are passed as cysts from host to host by the fecal–oral route. Most amebas are amitochondriate, presumably because of the anaerobic conditions under which they exist in the colon. Only one, *Entamoeba histolytica*, regularly produces disease; it has been recently subdivided into two morphologically identical but genetically distinct species, an invasive pathogen that retains the species appellation "histolytica" and a commensal organism, now designated *Entamoeba dispar*. The two species can be differentiated by isoenzyme analysis, antibodies to surface antigens, and DNA markers.

ENTAMOEBA HISTOLYTICA

Overview

Entamoeba histolytica is an intestinal ameba transmitted between humans. Amebiasis is found worldwide and is caused by the potentially pathogenic *E histolytica*. Approximately 10% of patients with this parasite will have gastrointestinal symptoms and 1% will experience extraintestinal disease which can be life-threatening. Gastrointestinal symptoms may include intermittent diarrhea with abdominal pain. Occasionally, severe dysentery with abdominal cramping and a high fever can occur. Extraintestinal extension depends on the presence of a galactose-specific lectin (Gal/GalNAc) capable of mediating attachment of the organism to colonic mucosa followed by contact dependent cytotoxicity and blood passage of trophozoites to various organs. *Entamoeba dispar*, which is morphologically identical to *E histolytica*, accounts for the vast majority of *E histolytica*-like infections. Treatment is not required for *E dispar*.

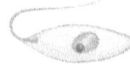 PARASITOLOGY

E histolytica is found throughout the world and is the causative agent of diarrhea and amebic dysentery. Infections may spread to extraintestinal sites and become life-threatening. Close to 500 million people are thought to be infected at any one time, but most of these are likely due to the morphologically identical *E dispar*. Because methods are now available to distinguish *E histolytica* from *E dispar*, the figure of 500 million infected with *E histolytica* may actually be closer to 50 million. Transmission is fecal–oral, either directly or indirectly through contaminated water.

LIFE CYCLE, MORPHOLOGY, AND PHYSIOLOGY

Humans are the principal hosts and reservoirs of *E histolytica*. Transmission from person to person occurs when a cyst passed in the stool of one host is ingested directly or indirectly, such as through food or water, by another. Human hosts may pass up to 45 million cysts daily. Although the average infective dose exceeds 1000 organisms, ingestion of a single cyst has been known to produce infection. After passage through the stomach, the cyst eventually reaches the distal small bowel. Here, the cyst wall disintegrates, releasing the quadrinucleate parasite, which divides to form eight small trophozoites that are carried to the colon. Colonization is most intense in areas of fecal stasis such as the cecum and rectosigmoid, but may be found throughout the large bowel.

E histolytica possesses both trophozoite and cyst forms (**Figure 52–1**). The trophozoites are microaerophilic, dwell in the lumen or wall of the colon, feed on bacteria and tissue cells, and multiply rapidly in the anaerobic environment of the gut. Even though they are called amitochondriate, they do possess nuclear-encoded mitochondrial genes and a remnant organelle. They do have unusual features including polyploid chromosomes, repetitive DNA, multiple origins of DNA replication, genes lacking introns, and unique endocytic pathways. Trophozoites are passed unchanged in the liquid diarrheic stool. Here they can be recognized by their size (12-20 μm in diameter); directional motility; granular, vacuolated endoplasm; and sharply demarcated, clear ectoplasm with finger-like pseudopods. Invasive strains tend to be larger and may contain ingested erythrocytes within their cytoplasm (**Figure 52–2**). Appropriate stains reveal a 3 to 5 μm nucleus with a small central karyosome or nucleolus and fine regular granules evenly distributed around the nuclear membrane (peripheral chromatin). Electron microscopic studies demonstrate microfilaments, an external glycocalyx, and cytoplasmic projections thought to be important for attachment.

Trophozoites are facultative anaerobes that require complex media for growth. Sterile culture techniques (axenic) have been developed and are essential for the preparation of the purified antigens required for serologic testing, zymodeme typing, and characterization of virulence factors. Such techniques are generally available only in research laboratories.

With normal stool transit time, trophozoites usually encyst before leaving the gut. Initially, a cyst contains a single nucleus, a glycogen vacuole, and one or more large, cigar-shaped ribosomal

* Humans hosts and reservoir; fecal–oral transmission

Trophozoites multiply rapidly in the gut

Facultative anaerobes

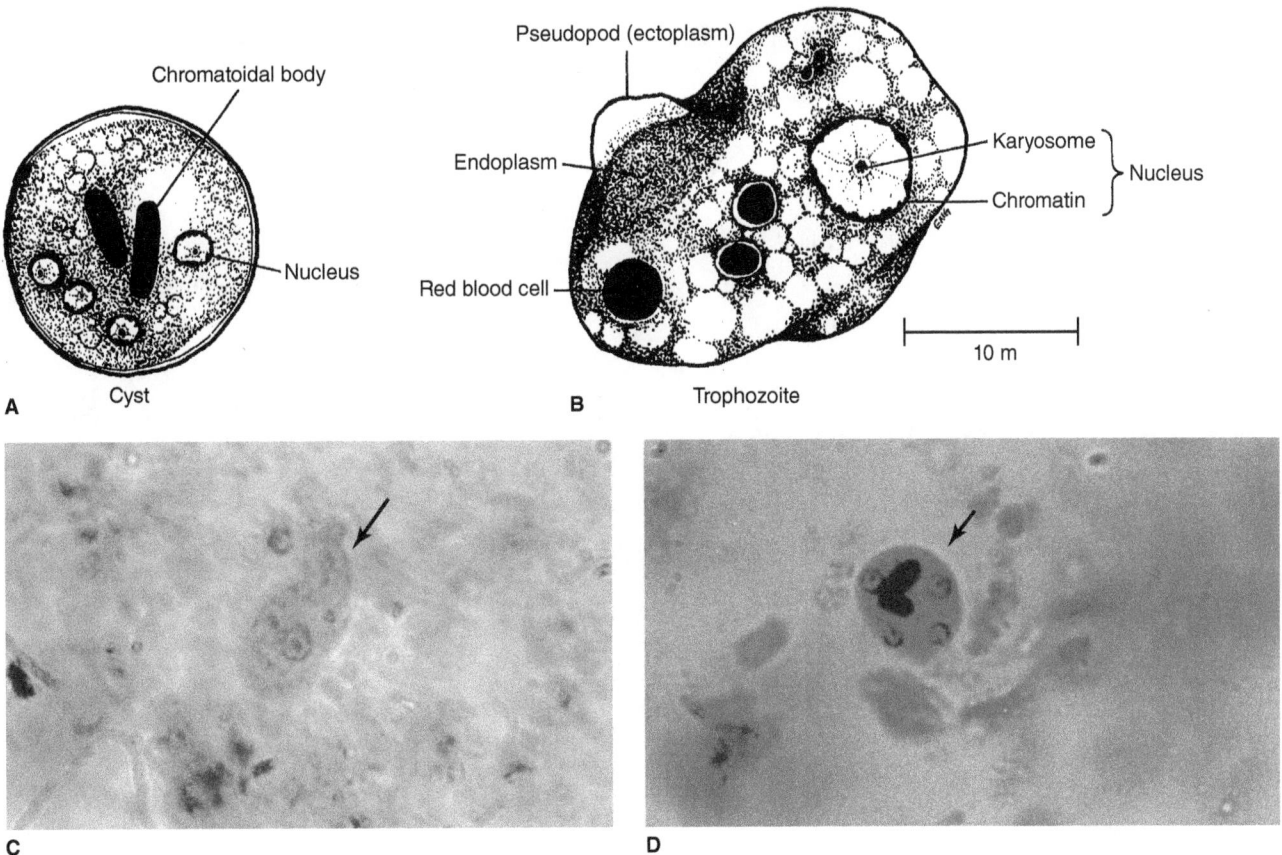

FIGURE 52–1. *Entamoeba histolytica.* **A.** Cyst structures. **B.** Trophozoite structures. **C.** Trophozoite in stool (*arrow*). **D.** Cyst (*arrow*) in stool iodine preparation and cysts in stool iodine preparation.

clusters known as chromatoid bodies. With maturation, the cyst becomes quadrinucleate, and the cytoplasmic inclusions are absorbed. In contrast to the fragile trophozoite, mature cysts can survive environmental temperatures up to 55°C, chlorine concentrations normally found in municipal water supplies, and normal levels of gastric acid. *E histolytica* can be differentiated from the other amebas of the gut by its size, nuclear detail, and cytoplasmic inclusions (**Table 52–1**).

✳ Hardy cysts survive in chlorinated water

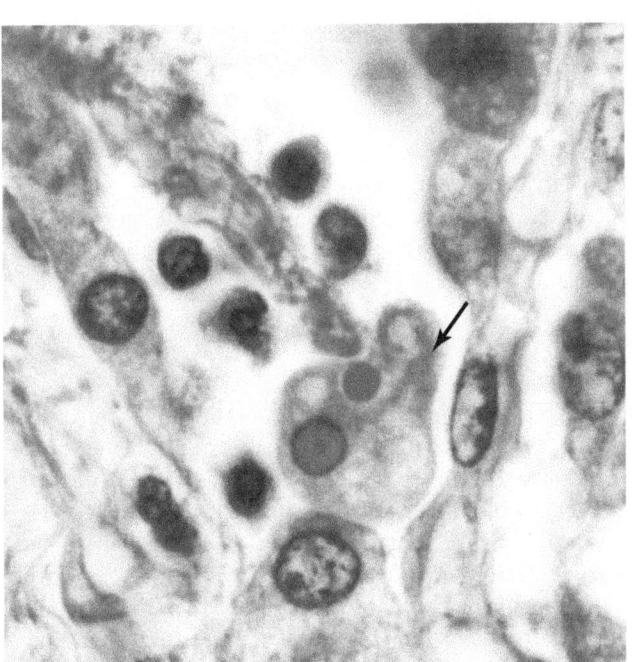

FIGURE 52–2. **Amebiasis.** An *E histolytica* trophozoite (*arrow*) is invading tissue. Note the extending pseudopod and engulfed erythrocyte. (Reproduced with permission from Connor DH, Chandler FW, Schwartz DQ, et al: *Pathology of Infectious Diseases.* Stamford CT: Appleton & Lange; 1997.)

TABLE 52–1	Some Differential Characteristics of *Entamoeba* Species		
CHARACTERISTICS	*E HISTOLYTICA*	*E HARTMANNI*	*E COLI*
TROPHOZOITES			
Cytoplasm	Differentiated[a]	Differentiated	Undifferentiated
Nucleus			
Peripheral chromatin	Fine	Fine	Coarse, irregular
Karyosome	Small, central	Small, central	Large, eccentric
Ingested particles			
Bacteria	No	—	Yes
Red blood cells	Yes	No	No
Size (µm)	>12	<12	>12
CYSTS			
Nuclei[b]	1-4	1-4	1-8
Chromatoid bodies	Rods	Rods	Splinters
Size (µm)	>10	<10	>10

[a]Sharp differentiation between ectoplasm and endoplasm.

[b]Fine structure similar to that of trophozoites.

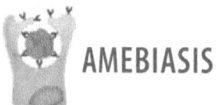 AMEBIASIS

EPIDEMIOLOGY

E histolytica infection rates are higher in warm climates, particularly in areas where the level of sanitation is low. Worldwide, this organism is thought to produce more deaths than any other parasite, except those that cause malaria and schistosomiasis. Reports of amebic liver abscess, for instance, emanate primarily from Mexico, western South America, South Asia, and West and South Africa. For reasons apparently unrelated to exposure, symptomatic illness is much less common in women and children than in men.

Although stool surveys in the United States indicate that 1% to 5% of the population harbors *Entamoeba*, most of these are now known to be colonized with the nonpathogenic *E dispar*. The incidence of invasive amebiasis in the United States decreased sharply over several decades, reaching a nadir in 1974. Since then, the numbers have increased, but remain relatively low. It is now seen particularly in institutionalized individuals, Indian reservations, migrant labor camps, victims of acquired immunodeficiency syndrome (AIDS), and travelers to endemic areas.

Symptomatic amebiasis is usually sporadic, the result of direct person-to-person fecal–oral spread under conditions of poor personal hygiene. Venereal transmission is seen in male homosexuals, presumably the result of oral–anal sexual contact. Food- and waterborne spread occurs, occasionally in epidemic form. Such outbreaks, however, are seldom as explosive as those produced by pathogenic intestinal bacteria. One outbreak of intestinal amebiasis was due to colonic irrigation at a chiropractic clinic.

PATHOGENESIS

Several virulence factors have been identified in *E histolytica*. In an experimental setting, invasiveness correlates well with endocytic capacity, the production of extracellular proteinases capable of activating complement and degrading collagen, the presence of a galactose-specific lectin (Gal/GalNAc) capable of mediating attachment of the organism to colonic mucosa, and—perhaps most important—the capacity to lyse host cells on contact. This has been termed parasite-mediated or **contact-dependent cytotoxicity**. The latter phenomenon is initiated by the galactose-specific, lectin-mediated adherence of the trophozoite to a target cell. After adherence, the ameba releases a pore-forming protein that polymerizes in the target cell membrane, forming large

Worldwide infection; highest rates in warmer climates

Invasive disease rare in the United States

✳ Fecal–oral spread via poor hygiene

Food and water transmission

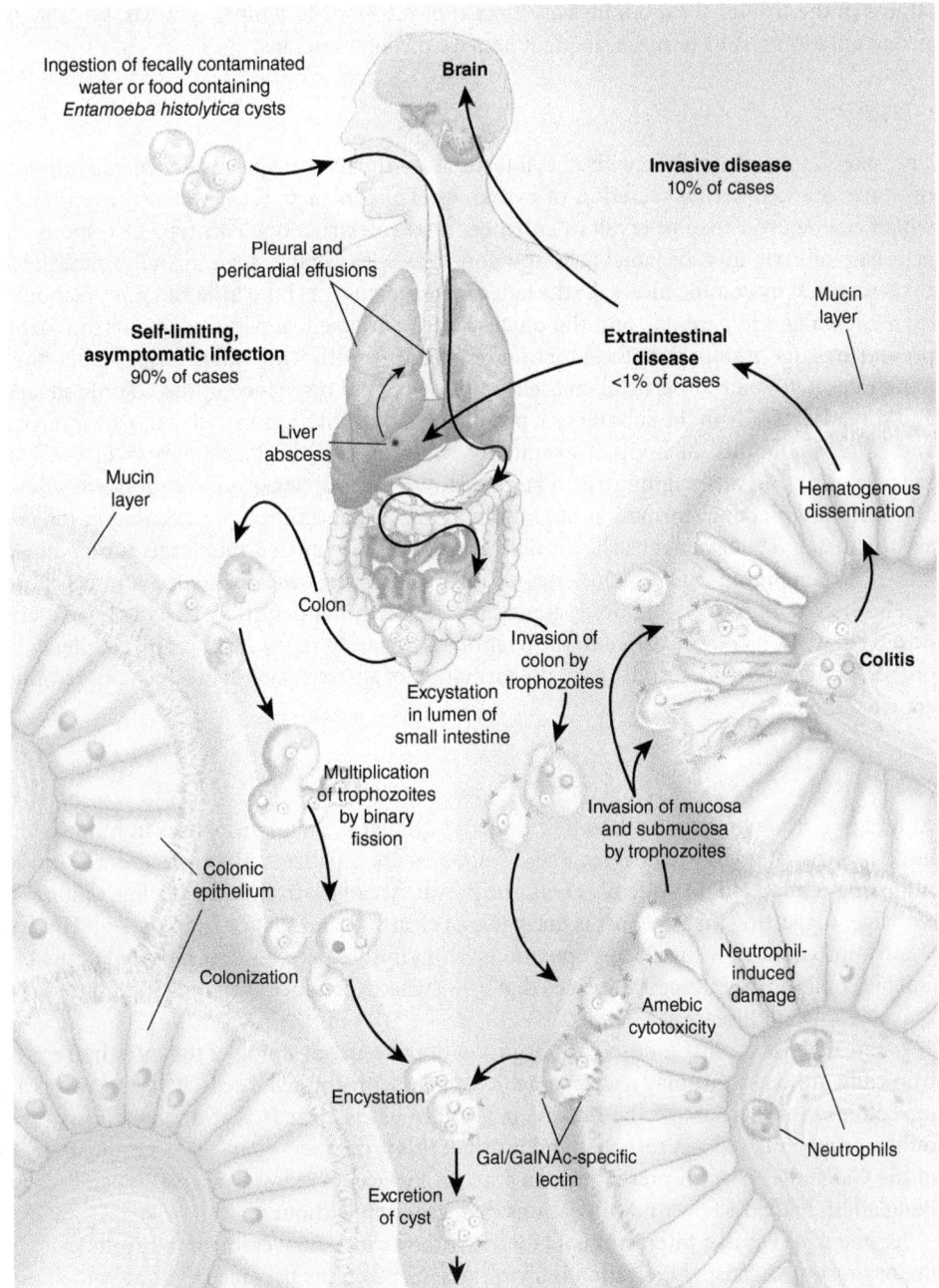

FIGURE 52–3. **Pathways of *E histolytica* colonization within the gastrointestinal tract.** (Reproduced with permission from Connor DH, Chandler FW, Schwartz DQ, et al: *Pathology of Infectious Diseases.* Stamford CT: Appleton & Lange; 1997.)

tubular lesions. Cytolysis rapidly follows. Cysteine proteinases, secreted by the amebas, have also been identified as a major virulence factor. They can degrade portions of the extracellular matrix, including fibronectin, laminin, and type I collagen, and they can interfere with the complement pathway and humoral IgA and IgG responses. Ultimately, this may lead to extraintestinal spread of the trophozoites which may occur in approximately 1% of established infections (**Figure 52–3**). Cyst formation does not take place at extraintestinal sites.

In most cases of *E histolytica* infections, however, tissue damage is minimal, and the host remains symptom-free, suggesting that host factors may modulate the invasiveness of virulent strains. These factors are still poorly understood, but changes in host resistance, the colonic milieu, or the parasite itself may amplify tissue damage and clinical manifestations. Protein malnutrition, high-carbohydrate diets, corticosteroid administration, childhood, and pregnancy all appear to render the host more susceptible to invasion. Certain colonic bacteria appear to enhance invasiveness, possibly by providing a more favorable redox potential for survival and multiplication or by facilitating the adherence of the parasite to colonic mucosa. Finally, it is known that the pathogenic

✳ Lectin-mediated adherence to mucosa and capacity to lyse host cells

Most symptom free

Colonic flora influences invasiveness

strains in the tropics are more invasive than those isolated in temperate areas, possibly because poor sanitation results in more frequent passage through humans.

PATHOLOGY

The interaction of amebas with the intestinal epithelial barrier results in an inflammatory response marked by the secretion of cytokines. This, in turn, results in neutrophil activation which can be protective or result in enhanced tissue destruction. This type of response is characteristic of early invasive amebiasis and contrasts with what is seen in well-established infections manifest by colonic ulcers. In the latter instance, there is little inflammatory response other than edema and hyperemia, and the mucosa between ulcers appears normal. Trophozoites are present in large numbers at the junction between necrotic and viable tissue. Once the lesion penetrates below the superficial epithelium, it meets the resistance of the colonic musculature and spreads laterally in the submucosa, producing a flask-like lesion with a narrow mucosal neck and a large submucosal body. It eventually compromises the blood supply of the overlying mucosa, resulting in sloughing and a large necrotic ulcer. Extensive ulceration leads to secondary bacterial infection, formation of granulation tissue, and fibrotic thickening of the colon. In approximately 1% of patients, the granulation tissue is organized into large, tumor-like masses known as **amebomas.** The major sites of involvement, in order of frequency, are the cecum, ascending colon, rectum, sigmoid, appendix, and terminal ileum. Amebas may also enter the portal circulation and be carried to the liver or, more rarely, to the lung, brain, or spleen. In these organs, liquefaction necrosis leads to the formation of abscess cavities in which only trophozoites are encountered.

IMMUNITY

Although *E histolytica* elicits both humoral and cellular immune responses in humans, it is still not clear which and to what degree, these responses are capable of modulating initial infection or thwarting reinfection. In endemic areas, the prevalence of gastrointestinal colonization increases with age, suggesting that the host is incapable of clearing *E histolytica* from the gut. However, the relative infrequency with which populations living in these areas suffer repeated bouts of severe amebic colitis or liver abscess indicates that those who experience such infections have protection against recurrent disease.

Innate defense against *E histolytica* begins with the mucous lining of the intestinal epithelium. Ironically, although this may restrict amebic contact with epithelial cells, it also provides a milieu for colonization because of the mucins present. What is clear is that infected hosts produce a rather strong mucosal IgA response and much of this is directed against the carbohydrate domain of the Gal/GalNAc lectin present on the ameba's surface. Children with this type of response in Bangladesh had 86% fewer new infections than children without it.

As stated previously, interaction of amebas with the intestinal epithelium results in an inflammatory response causing activation of cytokines. Neutrophils become involved, which may help promote further damage because of their destruction by cysteine proteases released by the amebas and resulting in release of superoxide radicals, or they may help mediate protection following activation via TNF-α.

Patients with invasive disease are known to produce high levels of circulating antibodies. Nevertheless, no correlation exists between the presence or concentration of such antibodies and protective immunity, possibly because pathogenic *E histolytica* trophozoites have the capacity to aggregate and shed attached antibodies and are resistant to the lytic action of complement. Cell-mediated responses have been described in patients with amebic liver abscess and are associated with lymphocyte proliferation and cytokine secretion. Activated macrophages also have the capacity to kill amebas, presumably through nitric oxide or peroxidase production. The susceptibility to invasive amebiasis of malnourished populations, pregnant women, and steroid-treated individuals or patients indicates that cell-mediated immune mechanisms may be directly involved in the control of tissue invasion. The picture is less clear in patients with AIDS and requires further study.

Pathogenic *E histolytica* strains produce a lectin-like substance that is mitogenic for lymphocytes. It has been suggested that this substance could stimulate viral replication of human immunodeficiency virus-infected lymphocytes as does another mitogen, phytohemagglutinin.

Mucosal ulceration, little inflammation

✳ Flask-like ulcers in submucosa

Amebomas, amebic abscesses in a few

Immunity incomplete, not correlated with antibody

Trophozoites shed antibody, resist complement lysis

AMEBIASIS: CLINICAL ASPECTS

MANIFESTATIONS

Individuals who harbor *E histolytica* are usually clinically well. In most cases, particularly in the temperate zones, the organism is avirulent, living in the bowel as a normal commensal inhabitant. Spontaneous disappearance of amebas, over a period of weeks to months, among such patients is common. Serologic data, however, suggest that some asymptomatic carriers possess virulent strains and incur minimal tissue invasion. In this population, the infection may eventually progress to produce overt disease.

Diarrhea, flatulence, and cramping abdominal pain are the most common complaints of symptomatic patients. The diarrhea is intermittent, alternating with episodes of normality or constipation over a period of months to years. Typically, the stool consists of one to four loose to watery, foul-smelling passages that contain mucus and blood. Physical findings are limited to abdominal tenderness localized to the hepatic, ascending colonic, and cecal areas. Sigmoidoscopy reveals the typical ulcerations with normal intertwining mucosa.

Fulminating amebic dysentery is less common. It may occur spontaneously in debilitated or pregnant individuals or may be precipitated by corticosteroid therapy. Its onset is often abrupt, with high fever, severe abdominal cramps, and profuse diarrhea. Most commonly, abscesses occur singly and are localized to the upper outer quadrant of the right lobe of the liver. This localization results in the development of point tenderness overlying the cavity and elevation of the right diaphragm. Liver function is usually well preserved. Isotopic or ultrasound scanning confirms the presence of the lesion. Needle aspiration results in the withdrawal of reddish-brown, odorless fluid free of bacteria and polymorphonuclear leukocytes; trophozoites may be demonstrated in the terminal portion of the aspirate since they are likely colonizing the intact tissue at the periphery of the abscess.

Approximately 5% of all patients with symptomatic amebiasis present with a liver abscess. Ironically, fewer than one-half can recall significant diarrheal illness. Although *E histolytica* can be demonstrated in the stools of 72% of patients with amebic liver abscess when a combination of serial microscopic examinations and culture is used, routine microscopic examination of the stool detects less than half of these. Complications relate to the extension of the abscess into surrounding tissue, producing pneumonia, empyema, or peritonitis. Extension of an abscess from the left lobe of the liver to the pericardium is the single most dangerous complication. It may produce rapid cardiac compression (tamponade) and death or, more commonly, a chronic pericardial disease that may be confused with congestive cardiomyopathy or tuberculous pericarditis.

DIAGNOSIS

The microscopic diagnosis of intestinal amebiasis depends on the identification of the organism in stool or sigmoidoscopic aspirates. Because trophozoites appear predominantly in liquid stools or aspirates, a portion of such specimens should be fixed immediately to ensure preservation of these fragile organisms for stained preparations. The specimen may then be examined in wet mount for typical motility, concentrated to detect cysts, and stained for definitive identification. If trophozoites or cysts are seen, they must be carefully differentiated from those of the commensal parasites, particularly *E hartmanni* and *Escherichia coli* (Table 52–1). *E histolytica* trophozoites can be differentiated from those of *E dispar* only by the presence of ingested erythrocytes in the former and by molecular methods; the cysts appear identical.

Recently, sensitive and specific stool antigen tests for *E histolytica* have become commercially available; their value in the clinical diagnosis of amebiasis, when compared with microscopic examination, is not clear. Although cultural and polymerase chain reaction techniques are somewhat more sensitive and are used by reference laboratories, they are not widely available in many clinical laboratories in developing countries where amebiasis is endemic.

The diagnosis of extraintestinal amebiasis is more difficult because the parasite usually cannot be recovered from stool or tissue. Serologic tests are therefore of paramount importance. Typically, results are negative in asymptomatic patients, suggesting that tissue invasion is required for antibody production. Most patients with symptomatic intestinal disease and more than 90% with hepatic abscess have high levels of antiamebic antibodies. Unfortunately, these titers may persist for months to years after an acute infection, making the interpretation of a positive test difficult

Relationship usually commensal

＊ Diarrhea, flatulence, abdominal pain, ulcerations

＊ Hepatic abscess acute or insidious

Hepatic abscess may extend

＊ Stools trophozoites, cysts in stained or wet preparations

＊ *E histolytica* ingests erythrocytes

Antigen detected in stool

* Extraintestinal amebiasis demonstrates high antibody levels

in endemic areas. At present, the indirect hemagglutination test and enzyme immunoassays using antigens derived from axenically grown organisms appear to be the most sensitive. Several rapid tests, including latex agglutination, agar diffusion, and counterimmunoelectrophoresis, are available to smaller laboratories.

TREATMENT

* Metronidazole combined with other agents

Treatment for noninvasive infection differs from treatment for invasive infection. Paromomycin is useful for noninvasive infection and should probably be used if it is certain that it is truly *E histolytica* and not *E dispar*. Treatment is directed toward relief of symptoms, blood and fluid replacement, and eradication of the organism. The drug of choice for eradication in the case of invasive amebiasis is metronidazole or tinidazole followed by treatment with iodoquinol or paromomycin. Metronidazole and its derivatives are effective against many forms of amebiasis, but should be combined with a second agent, such as iodoquinol or paromomycin, to improve cure rates in intestinal disease and diminish the chance of recrudescent disease in hepatic amebiasis. It may be prudent to also administer a broad-spectrum antibiotic in severe cases of intestinal amebiasis to treat intestinal bacteria that have the potential to spill into the peritoneum. In severe extraintestinal infections, parenteral dehydroemetine treatment may be considered.

 Should all patients diagnosed with an *E histolytica*-like infection be treated?

PREVENTION

Because the disease is transmitted by the fecal–oral route, efforts should be directed toward sanitary disposal of human feces, improvement in personal hygienic practices, and the provision of safe drinking water. In the United States, this applies particularly to institutionalized patients and to camps for migrant farm workers. Male homosexuals should be made aware that certain sexual practices substantially increase their risk of amebiasis and other infections.

KEY CONCLUSIONS

- Transmission of *E histolytica* is fecal–oral, both direct and indirect.
- The majority of *E histolytica* infections are asymptomatic.
- Intestinal symptoms develop in about 10% of infected individuals and extension in 1% of infected individuals.
- Extraintestinal extension depends on the presence of a Gal/GalNAc lectin present on the ameba's surface. Contact-dependent cytotoxicity mediated by many factors allows tissue invasion.
- Immunity involves both antibody and cell-mediated responses, but is poorly understood. IgA antibody, various cytokines, and neutrophils are involved.
- Cysts and trophozoites may be passed in infected individuals, but only trophozoites are found in extraintestinal lesions.
- *Entamoeba dispar* is morphologically identical to *E histolytica* and accounts for approximately 90% of all *E histolytica*-like infections.

 Think ►► Apply 52-1: Keep in mind that the majority of infections caused by *E histolytica*-like infections are caused by the nonpathogenic *E dispar*. With this in mind, and if a reference laboratory can perform PCR on stool specimens, confirmed *E histolytica* should be treated, but not *E dispar*. The question to treat or not in endemic areas where reference laboratories are not as common becomes more difficult. Does the patient exhibit symptoms of intestinal or extraintestinal amebiasis?—then definitely treat. Is the patient from an area where amebiasis is common?—likely treat. Seek differentiation of pathogenic versus nonpathogenic spp. when possible.

PATHOGENIC AND OPPORTUNISTIC FREE-LIVING AMEBAS

Overview

Pathogenic and opportunistic free-living amebas belong to the genera *Acanthamoeba*, *Balamuthia*, *Naegleria*, and *Sappinia*. These organisms are widespread in nature and have been found in soil, drinking water, swimming pools, sewage, draining ditches, thermal pools, eyewash solutions, and even dialysis units. *Naegleria fowleri* is the causative agent of primary amebic meningoencephalitis which results in death within 5 to 6 days following full-body contact with contaminated water sources. *Acanthamoeba* and *Balamuthia* are considered opportunistic because they occur primarily in immunocompromised patients and are the causative agents of chronic granulomatous encephalitis, keratitis, and skin lesions. *Naegleria* and *Sappinia* infections, on the other hand, have been described from healthy patients, and are therefore considered nonopportunistic.

PRIMARY AMEBIC MENINGOENCEPHALITIS

Primary amebic meningoencephalitis is caused by the free-living ameba *Naegleria fowleri*. This parasite largely affects children and young adults through full-body contact with warm fresh water, and is almost always fatal. *Naegleria* species are found in large numbers in shallow fresh water, particularly during warm weather. The organism exists in trophozoite, flagellate, and cyst forms. The trophozoite is an active feeding form that feeds on bacteria and organic matter. It transforms into a bi-flagellate form when deprived of nutrients, but may revert to a trophozoite if conditions become favorable. Under adverse environmental conditions it will encyst **(Figure 52–4)**.

> ❋ Meningoencephalitis due to free-living amebas
>
> ❋ Warm weather, brackish water favor *Naegleria*

More than 300 cases of *Naegleria* meningoencephalitis have been reported, mostly in the United States, Australia, and Europe. Serologic studies suggest that inapparent infections are much more common. Most cases in the United States have occurred in the southern states. Characteristically, patients have fallen ill during the summer after swimming or in small, shallow, warm freshwater lakes. A Czechoslovakian case followed swimming in a chlorinated indoor pool, and several cases worldwide have occurred after bathing in hot mineral water.

> **Naegleria associated with freshwater swimming**

Infection results from full-body contact with water containing the bi-flagellate parasite form. The parasite enters the body through the nasal passages and traverses the nasal mucosa and the cribriform plate as an ameboid form to the olfactory nerves of the central nervous system (CNS). Here, the amebas, which are the only form found in tissue, produce a severe purulent, hemorrhagic inflammatory reaction, which extends perivascularly from the olfactory bulbs to other regions of the brain. The infection is characterized by the rapid onset of severe bifrontal headache, seizures, and at times abnormalities in taste or smell. The disease runs an inexorably downhill course to coma, ending fatally within a few days.

> ❋ Passage to CNS across cribriform plate

A striking feature of this infection is the rapid onset of symptoms following exposure. Because there are no distinctive clinical features to differentiate this infection from acute pyogenic bacterial meningoencephalitis or viral meningoencephalitis, it is imperative for the physician to obtain information regarding the patient's contact with water within the past few days. A careful examination of the cerebrospinal fluid (CSF) may often provide a presumptive diagnosis of *Naegleria* infection. The fluid is usually bloody and demonstrates an intense neutrophilic response. The protein level is elevated, and the glucose level decreased. No bacteria can be demonstrated on stain or culture. Early examination of a wet mount preparation of unspun spinal fluid reveals typical trophozoites. Staining with specific fluorescent antibody confirms the identification. The organism can usually be isolated on agar plates seeded with a Gram-negative bacillus (to feed the amebas) or grown axenically in tissue culture. Unfortunately, most diagnosis of amebic meningoencephalitis is made postmortem **(Figure 52–5)**. To date, there are reports of only six patients who have survived a *Naegleria* infection. All were diagnosed early and treated with high-dose amphotericin B along with rifampin. An investigational drug, miltefosine, is now available for emergency treatment of naegleria infection.

> ❋ Purulent bloody CSF contains *Naegleria* trophozoites

What is one of the most important questions for a physician to ask when presented with symptoms of meningoencephalitis?

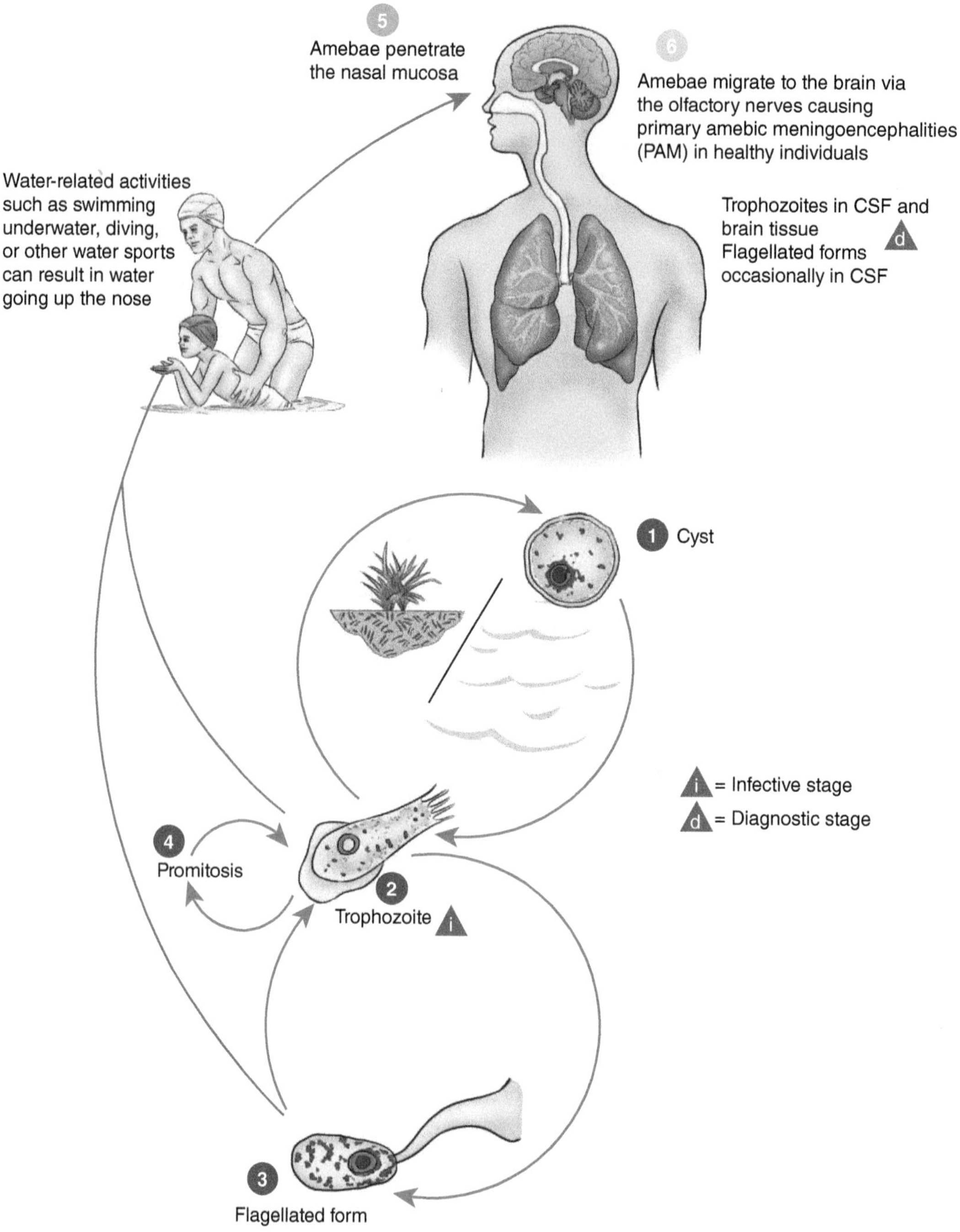

⑤
Amebae penetrate
the nasal mucosa

⑥
Amebae migrate to the brain via
the olfactory nerves causing
primary amebic meningoencephalities
(PAM) in healthy individuals

Water-related activities
such as swimming
underwater, diving,
or other water sports
can result in water
going up the nose

Trophozoites in CSF and
brain tissue
Flagellated forms △d
occasionally in CSF

① Cyst

▲i = Infective stage
△d = Diagnostic stage

④
Promitosis

② Trophozoite ▲i

③
Flagellated form

FIGURE 52–4. **Life cycle** *of Naegleria fowleri.*

Think ▸▸ Apply 52-2: **Where have you been and who or what have you been in contact with. With respect to the contact the issue of contact with warm water should be considered. Full body contact is required because the flagellated stage must make contact via the nasal mucosa. Also, symptoms develop very rapidly. *Naegleria* is usually not transmitted via hot tubes because of the high chlorine content. One case was linked to consumption of water from a municipal water source, but this is highly unusual or unlikely.**

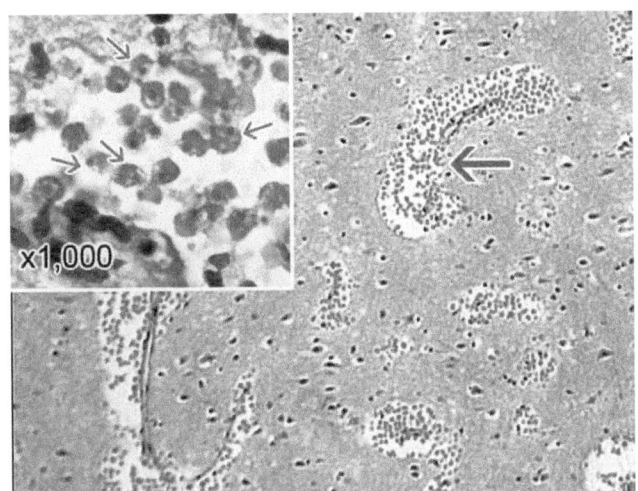

FIGURE 52-5. **Primary amebic meningoencephalitis—*Naegleria fowleri*.** Large clusters of *Naegleria fowleri* trophozoites and the destruction of the normal brain tissue architecture. Cysts are not seen. (Reproduced with permission from Centers for Disease Control and Prevention. Naegleria fowleri—Primary Amebic Meningoencephalitis (PAM)—Amebic Encephalitis. November, 2013.)

KEY CONCLUSIONS

- *Naegleria fowleri* infections are acquired by full-body contact with warm (greater than 40°C) water sources.
- Infections are caused by flagellated trophozoites contacting the nasal mucosa and migrating to the brain.
- Death due to meningoencephalitis usually follows in 5 to 6 days.
- Presumptive diagnosis is usually bacterial or viral meningoencephalitis.

GRANULOMATOUS AMEBIC ENCEPHALITIS

Granulomatous amebic encephalitis (GAE) is caused by one of seven species of free-living amebas belonging to the genus *Acanthamoeba*. These amebas are ubiquitous worldwide and have been described from soil, fresh and brackish waters, cooling towers of electric and nuclear power plants, heating, ventilating and air conditioning units, humidifiers, Jacuzzis, hydrotherapy pools, dental irrigation units, dialysis machines, dust, cell cultures, and various clinical samples. They have also received attention because they may serve as hosts for a wide variety of bacterial pathogens.

Acanthamoeba spp. exist in two forms, trophozoite and cyst. The trophozoite feeds on bacteria and detritus in the environment and divides by binary fission. If environmental conditions become unfavorable, the trophozoite encysts. Cysts have been known to survive for up to 20 years *in vitro*.

The epidemiology of *Acanthamoeba* encephalitis has not been clearly defined. Infections usually involve older, immunocompromised persons, and a history of freshwater swimming is generally absent. The ameba probably reaches the brain by hematogenous dissemination from an unknown primary site, possibly the respiratory tract, skin, or eye. Metastatic lesions have been reported. Histologically, *Acanthamoeba* infections produce a diffuse, necrotizing, granulomatous encephalitis (**Figure 52-6**), with frequent involvement of the mid-brain. Both cysts and

Acanthamoeba affects older immunocompromised

✳ Granulomatous encephalitis with cysts and trophozoites

FIGURE 52-6. **Acanthamoebic granulomatous encephalitis.** A trophozoite (*arrow*) entering an epithelioid cell is seen at the right. The empty ovals in other cells are collapsed cysts. (Reproduced with permission from Connor DH, Chandler FW, Schwartz DQ, et al: *Pathology of Infectious Diseases*. Stamford CT: Appleton & Lange; 1997.)

trophozoites can be found in the lesions. Cutaneous ulcers and hard nodules containing amebas have been detected in patients with AIDS.

The clinical course of *Acanthamoeba* disease is more prolonged than that of *Naegleria* infection and occasionally ends in spontaneous recovery; the disease in immunocompromised hosts is invariably fatal. The spinal fluid usually demonstrates a mononuclear response. Amebas can occasionally be visualized in or cultured from the CSF or biopsy specimens. Fluorescein-labeled antiserum is available from the Centers for Disease Control and Prevention. Definitive diagnosis is usually made histologically after death. Treatment of GAE using a wide variety of therapeutic agents has been attempted, but only rarely has that led to a successful prognosis. Recently, miltefosine has been shown to have amebicidal activity and was used successfully to treat a patient with disseminated acanthamoebiasis.

Prolonged disease, occasional spontaneous recovery

OTHER *ACANTHAMOEBA* INFECTIONS

Skin lesions, uveitis, and corneal ulcerations have also been reported with *Acanthamoeba* disease. The latter are serious, producing a chronic progressive ulcerative lesion that may result in blindness. In recent years, there has been a rise in such infections correlated with the increased number of contact lens wearers. Infection commonly follows mild corneal trauma; most recently reported cases have been in users of soft contact lenses. Clinically, severe ocular pain, a paracentral ring infiltrate of the cornea, and recurrent epithelial breakdown are helpful in distinguishing this entity from the more common herpes simplex keratitis. Trophozoites must be present to bind to the corneal epithelium. The diagnosis can be confirmed by microscopic examination of corneal scraping or corneal biopsy and/or fluorescent antibody techniques. Culture of corneal tissue and contact lenses is frequently successful when the laboratory is given time to prepare satisfactory media. Nucleic acid amplification methods have recently been found more sensitive than culture. Chemotherapy has generally been ineffective unless given very early in the course of infection. Although a combination of corneal transplantation and chemotherapy may be successful later in the course of the disease, enucleation of the eye may be necessary to cure advanced infections. The drugs of choice are propamidine and neomycin eye drops administered alternately for a period of several months. Successful use of clotrimazole has been recently reported. Topical application of steroid is common to relieve pain and lessen inflammation.

Corneal ulcerations associated with use of contact lens

KEY CONCLUSIONS

- The primary routes of exposure to *Acantamoeba* and *Balamuthia* infections are not well defined by may be oral or through the skin and rarely involve water contact.
- Infections with these parasites are more prolonged than those involving *Naegleria*.
- Granulomatous encephalitis, keratitis, and skin lesions are most commonly reported.
- The investigational drug, miltefosine, has been used successfully to treat patients.

CASE STUDY

Weight Loss, Abdominal Discomfort, and a Tender Liver

A 21-year-old college student volunteered for a 2-year assignment as a missionary in a rural area of Central Mexico. Within 4 months of arrival, he developed a mild diarrheal illness with flatulence and abdominal discomfort that subsided spontaneously within a few weeks. Six months later, he noted progressive weight loss over several weeks, a low-grade fever, and right upper abdominal tenderness.

He returned to the United States for medical consultation. The primary physical finding was an enlarged right lobe of the liver, which was tender on palpation. An ultrasound study confirmed the presence of an abscess at that site.

The diagnosis of an amebic hepatic abscess was seriously considered.

QUESTIONS

1. Which of the following laboratory findings would be most likely to be helpful in supporting this patient's diagnosis?
   A. Demonstration of cyst forms in the stool
   B. Demonstration of trophozoites containing erythrocytes in the stool
   C. Isolation of the organism from the abscess
   D. Demonstration of high-serum antibody titers to *E histolytica*

2. Your choice of treatment would usually be:
   A. Tetracycline
   B. Amphotericin B
   C. Clotrimazole
   D. Metronidazole

3. A diagnosis of amebic meningoencephalitis is suggested by a recent history of the following, *except*:
   A. Exposure to a household contact with a similar illness
   B. Swimming in a freshwater lake
   C. Bathing in hot springs
   D. Swimming in a chlorinated pool

ANSWERS

1. (D)

2. (D)

3. (A)

chapter 53

Sarcomastigophora— The Flagellates

Trichomonas vaginalis · *Giardia duodenalis (syn. lamblia)* · *Leishmania* spp. ·
Trypanosoma brucei gambiense and *rhodesiense* · *Trypanosoma cruzi*

SARCOMASTIGOPHORA—THE FLAGELLATES—GROUP CHARACTERISTICS

The flagellated protozoa are widespread in nature, multiply by binary fission, and move about by means of a primary organelle of locomotion, the flagellum. This organelle arises from an intracellular focus known as a kinetosome (basal body), extends to the cell wall as a filamentous axoneme composed of microtubules arranged in the typical 9 pairs + 2 central microtubular pattern, and continues extracellularly as the free flagellum. A pair of dynein arms extends from each outer microtubule of a pair to an adjacent microtubular pair and is responsible for flagellar beating through ATP hydrolysis. The long, whip-like free flagella may be single or multiple. The number is distinctive for individual species. When more than one flagellum is present, each has its own associated basal body and axoneme. The entire flagellar unit and any associated organelles are referred to as a mastigont system.

In some flagellates, such as the trypanosomes, the flagellum becomes part of the cell surface and creates a structure called an undulating membrane. Movement occurs in helical waves and seems to be suited for organisms living within a viscous fluid environment such as that found in the bloodstream.

In other flagellates, the mastigont system includes a rod-like costa, which may serve as a supporting structure for the undulating membrane, or a tube-like axostyle, which arises from the base of a flagella and probably functions in rotational motility and support. Trichomonads possess both these structures.

Although several flagellate genera parasitize humans, only four, *Trichomonas*, *Giardia*, *Leishmania*, and *Trypanosoma*, commonly induce disease. *Trichomonas* and *Giardia* are noninvasive organisms that inhabit the lumina of the genitourinary or gastrointestinal tract and spread without the benefit of an intermediate host. Disease is of low morbidity and cosmopolitan distribution. *Leishmania* and *Trypanosoma*, on the other hand, are invasive tissue and blood parasites that produce highly morbid, frequently lethal diseases. These hemoflagellates require an intermediate insect host for their transmission. Thus, their associated disease states are limited to the semitropical and tropical niches of these intermediate hosts.

● NONINVASIVE LUMINAL FLAGELLATES

Luminal flagellates can be found in the mouth, vagina, or intestine of almost all vertebrates, and it is common for an animal host to harbor more than one species. Humans may serve as host and reservoir to eight species (**Table 53–1**), but only two cause disease. Of these, *Giardia duodenalis* (=*lamblia*) inhabits the intestinal tract, and *Trichomonas vaginalis* inhabits the vagina and genital tract.

＊ Found in flora of vertebrates

TABLE 53–1	Luminal Flagellates Infecting Humans	
FLAGELLATE	**PATHOGENICITY TO HUMANS**	**SITE**
Giardia lamblia	+	Intestine
Dientamoeba fragilis	?	Intestine
Chilomastix mesnili	–	Intestine
Enteromonas hominis	–	Intestine
Retortamonas intestinalis	–	Intestine
Trichomonas hominis	–	Intestine
Trichomonas tenax	–	Mouth
Trichomonas vaginalis	+	Vagina

These organisms are elongated or oval and typically measure 10 to 20 μm in length. They often possess a rudimentary cytostome (mouth aperture) and organelles, such as ventral discs or axostyles, which help maintain their intraluminal position. They are readily recognized in body fluid or excreta by their rapid motility and some can be specifically identified in unstained preparations. All can be cultivated on artificial media.

Some luminal flagellates, most notably *T vaginalis*, possess only a trophozoite stage and are sexually transmitted. Most, including *G duodenalis*, possess both trophozoite and cyst forms. The latter, which is the infective form, is transmitted via the direct or indirect fecal–oral route. Human-to-human infection is thus found in populations where inadequate sanitation or poor personal hygiene favors spread.

* Morphology and rapid motility are distinctive

* May or may not have the cyst stage

TRICHOMONAS VAGINALIS

Overview

Trichomonas vaginalis is an oval flagellate which exists only in the trophozoite stage. Trichomoniasis, caused by *T vaginalis*, is a sexually transmitted disease that has a worldwide distribution. Infection may be asymptomatic, particularly in men, but often produces vaginitis with pain, discharge, and dysuria in women. The infection fluctuates over weeks to months. Men may have urethritis or prostatitis. It is recommended that both sexual partners in a relationship be treated.

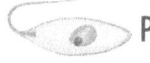 PARASITOLOGY

Three members of the genus *Trichomonas* parasitize humans (Table 53–1), but only *T vaginalis* is an established pathogen. The three species closely resemble one another morphologically, but confusion in identification is rare because of the specificity of their habitats.

The *T vaginalis* trophozoite (**Figure 53–1**) is oval and typically measures 7 by 15 μm. Organisms up to twice this size are occasionally recovered from asymptomatic patients and from cultures. In stained preparations, a single, elongated nucleus and a small cytostome are observed anteriorly. Five flagella arise nearby. Four immediately exit the cell. The fifth bends back and runs posteriorly along the outer edge of an abbreviated undulating membrane. Lying along the base of this membrane is a cross-striated structure known as the costa. A conspicuous microtubule containing a supporting rod or axostyle bisects the trophozoite longitudinally and protrudes through its posterior end. It is thought that the pointed tip of this structure is useful for attachment. In unstained wet mounts, *T vaginalis* is identified by its axostyle and jerky, nondirectional movements.

The organism can be grown on artificial media under anaerobic conditions at pH 5.5 to 6.0. Soluble nutrients are absorbed across the cell membrane. A variety of carbohydrates are degraded to short-chained organic acids. Pyruvate is produced via glycolysis and reduced to lactate, part of which enters structures called hydrogenosomes. Molecular hydrogen and ATP are produced in the hydrogenosomes. These structures are analogous to mitochondria, which *T vaginalis* lacks.

Three *Trichomonas* species have similar morphology

* Protruding axostyle may mediate attachment

Cultivable *in vitro*

* Lacks cyst form, may survive hours outside host

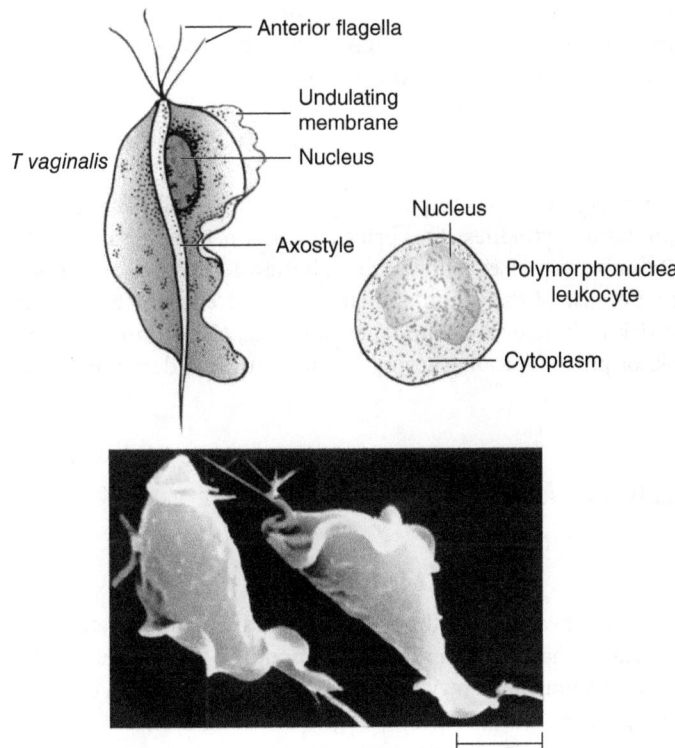

FIGURE   53–1. *Trichomonas vaginalis.* The parasite and its structures are shown in relation to the size of a polymorphonuclear leukocyte (*top*). The micrograph below illustrates their use for motility. (Reproduced with permission from Nester EW, Anderson DG, Roberts CE Jr, et al: *Microbiology: A Human Perspective*, 6th ed. New York, NY: McGraw Hill; 2008.)

Although *T vaginalis* lacks a cyst form, the trophozoite can survive outside of the human host for 1 to 2 hours on moist surfaces. In urine, semen, and water, it may be viable for up to 24 hours, making it one of the most resistant of protozoan trophozoites. Attempts to infect laboratory animals have met with limited success.

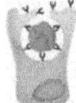 ## TRICHOMONIASIS

EPIDEMIOLOGY

Trichomoniasis is a cosmopolitan disease usually transmitted by sexual intercourse. An estimated 8 million infections occur in the United States annually. Worldwide this figure reaches >200 million cases. Twenty-five percent of sexually active women become infected at some time during their lives and 30% to 70% of their male sexual partners are also parasitized, at least transiently. As would be expected, the likelihood of acquiring the disease correlates directly with the number of sexual contacts. Infection is rare in adult virgins, whereas rates as high as 70% are seen among prostitutes, sexual partners of infected patients, and individuals with other venereal diseases. In women, the peak incidence of trichomoniasis is between 16 and 35 years of age, but there is still a relatively high prevalence in the 30- to 50-year age group.

* Transmission usually sexual

Prevalence linked to sexual activity

Nonvenereal transmission is uncommon. Transfer of organisms on shared washcloths may explain, in part, the high frequency of infection seen among institutionalized women. Female neonates are occasionally noted to harbor *T vaginalis*, presumably acquiring it during passage through the birth canal. High levels of maternal estrogen produce a transient decrease in the vaginal pH of the child, rendering it more susceptible to colonization. Within a few weeks, estrogen levels drop, the vagina assumes its premenarcheal state, and the parasite is eliminated.

Nonvenereal transmission uncommon

PATHOGENESIS AND IMMUNITY

Direct contact of *T vaginalis* with the squamous epithelium of the genitourinary tract results in destruction of the involved epithelial cells and the development of a neutrophilic inflammatory reaction and petechial hemorrhages. Attachment appears to be mediated by adhesins, laminin-binding proteins, and lectin-binding carbohydrates. Trophozoites can secret a variety of proteinases that undoubtedly help initiate contact-dependent cytolytic events. These proteinases are also capable of degrading immunoglobulin-G (IgG) and IgA. A contact-independent mechanism of cell damage has also been shown to correlate with the presence of a 200 kDa glycoprotein that is heat and acid labile. Changes in the microbial, hormonal, and pH environment of the vagina as well as factors inherent to the infecting parasite are thought to modulate the severity of the pathologic changes.

Infection of the vaginal epithelium triggers innate responses by stimulating Toll-like receptors that trigger secretion of proinflammatory cytokines. This brings about a neutrophil and CD4+ response. Humoral and cellular immune responses follow, although they do not appear to result in clinically significant immunity. Because of the proinflammatory response produced, women with this infection are at greater risk of human immunodeficiency virus (HIV) infection. *Trichomonas vaginalis* is also capable of phenotypically varying surface antigenic determinants to help it escape immune detection.

Damages epithelial cells on contact

TRICHOMONIASIS: CLINICAL ASPECTS

MANIFESTATIONS

In women, *T vaginalis* produces a persistent vaginitis. Although up to 50% are asymptomatic at the time of diagnosis, most develop clinical manifestations within 6 months. Approximately 75% develop a discharge, which is typically accompanied by vulvar itching or burning (50%), dyspareunia (50%), dysuria (50%), and a disagreeable odor (10%). Although fluctuating in intensity, symptoms usually persist for weeks or months. Commonly, manifestations worsen during menses and pregnancy. Eventually, the discharge subsides, even though the patient may continue to harbor the parasite. In symptomatic patients, physical examination reveals reddened vaginal and endocervical mucosa. In severe cases, petechial hemorrhages and extensive erosions are present. A red, granular, friable endocervix (strawberry cervix) is a characteristic but uncommon finding. An abundant discharge is generally seen pooled in the posterior vaginal fornix. Although classically described as thin, yellow, and frothy in character, the discharge more frequently lacks these characteristics. Trichomoniasis may increase the risk of preterm birth and enhance susceptibility to HIV infections.

The urethra and prostate are the usual sites of trichomoniasis in men; the seminal vesicles and epididymis may be involved on occasion. Infections are usually asymptomatic, possibly because of the efficiency with which the organisms are removed from the urogenital tract by voided urine. Symptomatic men complain of recurrent dysuria and scant, nonpurulent discharge. Acute purulent urethritis has been reported rarely. Trichomoniasis should be suspected in men presenting with nongonococcal urethritis, or a history of either prior trichomonal infection or recent exposure to trichomoniasis.

* Chronic vaginitis lasting weeks to months

* Urethral, prostatic infection in men asymptomatic

DIAGNOSIS

The diagnosis of trichomoniasis rests on the detection and morphologic identification of the organism in the genital tract. Identification is accomplished most easily by examining a wet mount preparation for the presence of motile organisms. In women, a drop of vaginal discharge is the most appropriate specimen; in men, urethral exudate or urine sediment after prostate massage may be used. Although highly specific when positive, wet mounts have a sensitivity of only 50% to 60%. They are most likely to be negative in asymptomatic or mildly symptomatic patients and in women who have douched in the previous 24 hours. Giemsa- and Papanicolaou-stained smears provide little additional help. The recent introduction of a commercial system that allows direct, rapid microscopic examination without the need for daily sampling may ameliorate this situation. Direct immunofluorescent antibody staining has a sensitivity of 70% to 90%. Parasitic culture, though more sensitive, requires several days to complete and is frequently unavailable. Nucleic acid amplification (NAA) methods have been shown to be the most sensitive for diagnosis.

* Wet mount trophozoite examination sufficient in most

TREATMENT

Oral metronidazole or tinidazole is extremely effective in recommended dosage, curing more than 95% of all *Trichomonas* infections. It may be given as a single dose or over 7 days. Simultaneous treatment of sexual partners may minimize recurrent infections, particularly when single-dose therapy is used for the index case. Because of the disulfiram-like activity of the nitroimidazoles, alcohol consumption should be suspended during treatment. The drug should never be used during the first trimester of pregnancy because of its potential teratogenic activity. Use in the last two trimesters is unlikely to be hazardous but should be reserved for patients whose symptoms cannot be adequately controlled with local therapies. High-dose, long-term metronidazole treatment has been shown to be carcinogenic in rodents. No association with human malignancy has been described to date. NAA-based studies have shown that this infection is underdiagnosed, and therefore infections are undertreated contributing to the continued high incidence of this parasite.

✳ Metronidazole cures 95%

KEY CONCLUSIONS

- *Trichomonas vaginalis* is a common sexually transmitted disease.
- Infected women may experience vaginitis, discharge, and dysuria.
- In females, parasites induce contact-dependent cytotoxicity that leads to inflammation.
- Infection with *T vaginalis* may predispose to HIV infection.
- Infected men are mostly asymptomatic.
- All sexual partners should be treated.

GIARDIA DUODENALIS, SYN. LAMBLIA

Overview

Giardia duodenalis is a sting-ray shaped flagellate which also has a cyst stage. Giardiasis, caused by *G duodenalis*, is an intestinal infection that is fecally-oral transmitted, either directly or indirectly via untreated water sources. It is a common infection worldwide and is most frequent in children. Infection is most often symptomatic, especially in adults. When disease occurs, it is in the form of a diarrhea lasting up to 4 weeks with foul-smelling, greasy stools. Abdominal pain, nausea, and vomiting are also present.

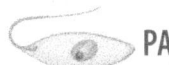 PARASITOLOGY

G duodenalis was first described by Anton von Leeuwenhoek 300 years ago when he examined his own diarrheal stool with one of the first primitive microscopes. It was not until the last several decades, however, that this cosmopolitan flagellate became widely regarded in the United States as a pathogen. Of the six other flagellated protozoans known to parasitize the alimentary tract of humans, only one, *Dientamoeba fragilis*, has been credibly associated with disease. Definitive confirmation or refutation of its pathogenicity will, it is hoped, not require the passage of another three centuries.

Unlike *T vaginalis*, *Giardia* possesses both a trophozoite and a cyst form (**Figure 53–2**). It is a stingray-shaped trophozoite 9 to 21 μm in length, 5 to 15 μm in width, and 2 to 4 μm in thickness. When viewed from the top, the organism's two nuclei and central parabasal bodies give it the appearance of a face with two bespectacled eyes and a crooked mouth. It is uncertain why this organism has two nuclei, but both are transcriptionally active. Four pairs of flagella—anterior, lateral, ventral, and posterior—reinforce this image by suggesting the presence of hair and chin whiskers. These distinctive parasites reside in the duodenum and jejunum, where they thrive in the alkaline environment and absorb nutrients from the intestinal tract. They move about the unstirred mucous layer at the base of the microvilli (**Figure 53–3**) with a peculiar tumbling or "falling leaf" motility or, with the aid of a large ventral disk, attach themselves to the brush border of the intestinal epithelium. The exact molecular mechanism by which the ventral disk mediates attachment has not been resolved but is thought, in part, to involve flagellar motility. Unattached organisms may be carried by the fecal stream to the large intestine.

✳ Trophozoite and cyst stages

✳ Moves about duodenum, jejunum with tumbling motility

In the descending colon, if transit time allows, the flagella are retracted into cytoplasmic sheaths and a smooth, clear cyst wall is secreted. These forms are oval and somewhat smaller than the trophozoites. With maturation, the internal structures divide, producing a quadrinucleate organism harboring two ventral discs, four kinetosomes, and eight axonemes. When fixed and stained,

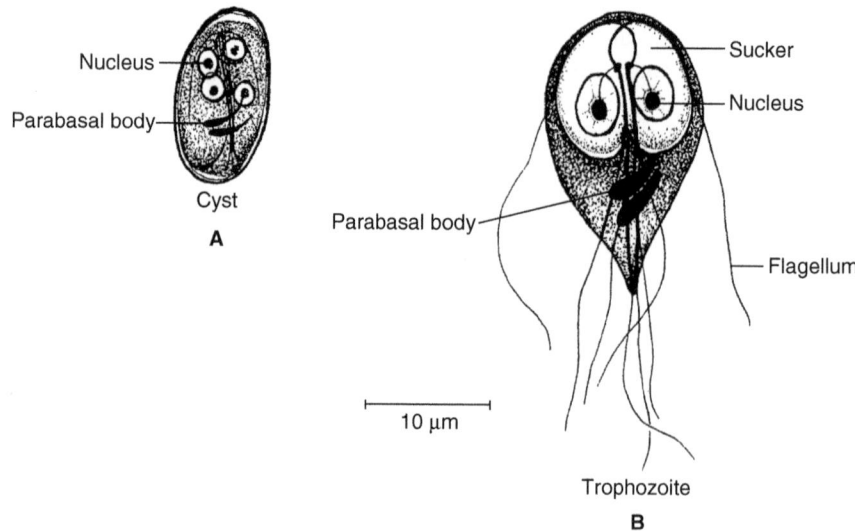

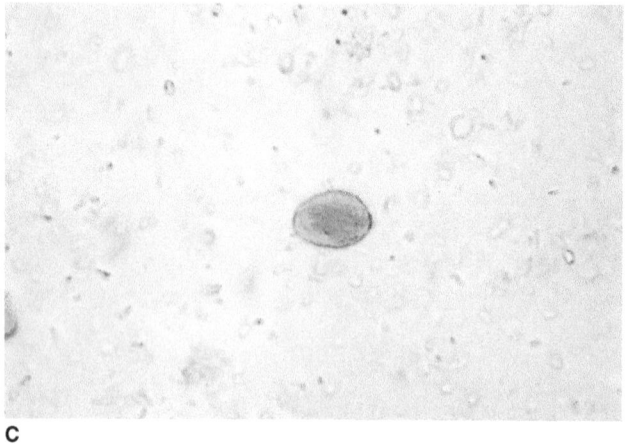

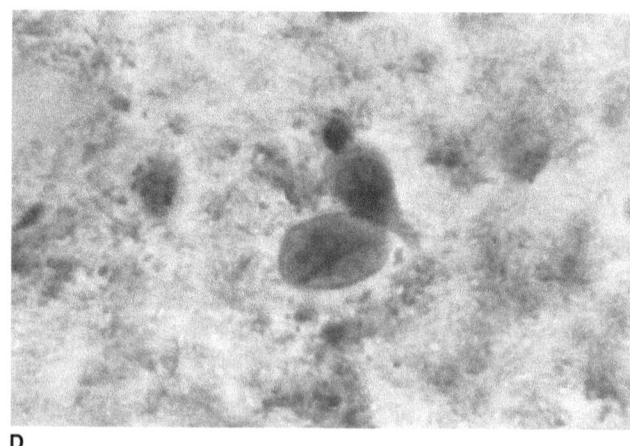

FIGURE 53–2. *Giardia lamblia.* **A.** Cyst structures. **B.** Trophozoite structures. **C.** Cyst in stool iodine preparation. **D.** Trophozoite in stool. (**C and D,** Reproduced with permission from Connor DH, Chandler FW, Schwartz DQ, et al: *Pathology of Infectious Diseases.* Stamford CT: Appleton & Lange; 1997.)

✳ Cystic forms in colon

✳ Resistant cysts transmitted host to host

the cytoplasm pulls away from the cyst wall in a characteristic fashion. The mature cysts, which are the infective form of the parasite, may survive in cold water for more than 2 months and are resistant to concentrations of chlorine generally used in municipal water systems. They are transmitted from host to host by direct and indirect fecal–oral routes. In the duodenum of a new host, the cytoplasm divides to produce two binucleate trophozoites.

Giardia is amitocondriate like *Trichomonas.* Instead, *Giardia* possesses mitosomes, which like the hydrogenosomes of *Trichomonas* are thought to represent mitochondrial adaptations in these aerotolerant anaerobe parasites. *Giardia* can respire aerobically or anaerobically with glucose as the main substrate for respiration. Axenic cultivation of this organism has been achieved *in vitro.* Bile salts enhance the parasite's growth. Although *Giardia* has largely been thought to be an asexual parasite, evidence for genetic recombination, hinting at a form of sexual recombination, has recently been reported.

Organisms of the genus *Giardia* are among the most widely distributed of intestinal Protozoa; they are found in fish, amphibians, reptiles, birds, and mammals. At first, it was assumed that *Giardia* strains found in different animals were host-specific; on this basis, some 40 different species were described. Since it is now recognized that some strains can infect multiple animal hosts, the practice of assigning species status by the host from which the parasite was recovered is considered invalid. At present, only five species are considered valid and of these, only *G duodenalis* infects humans. This parasite is also commonly referred to as *G lamblia* or *G intestinalis* in much of the current literature.

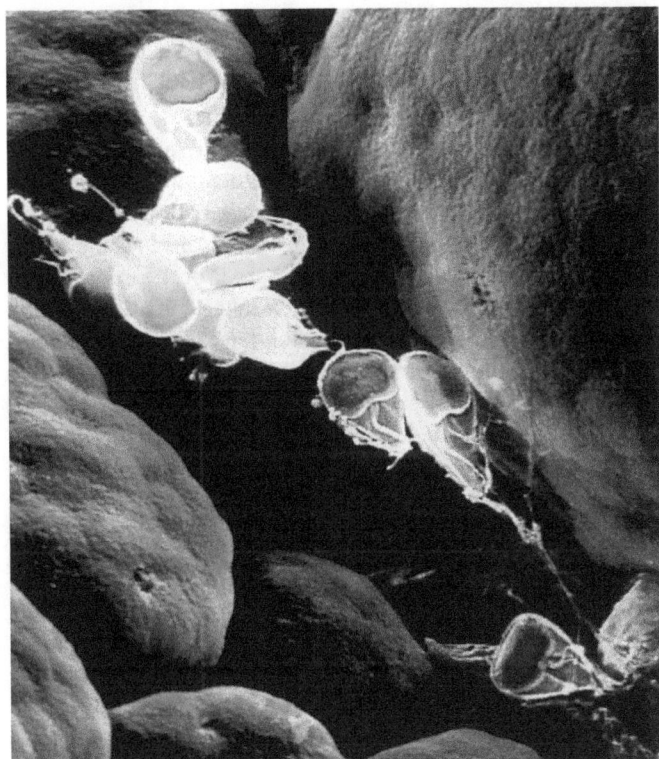

FIGURE 53–3. **Giardiasis.** Scanning electron micrograph of *G lamblia* trophozoites in human intestine. (Reproduced with permission from Nester EW, Anderson DG, Roberts CE Jr, et al: *Microbiology: A Human Perspective*, 6th ed. New York, NY: McGraw Hill; 2008.)

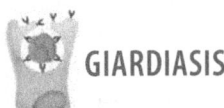 GIARDIASIS

EPIDEMIOLOGY

Giardiasis has a cosmopolitan distribution; its prevalence is highest in areas with poor sanitation and among populations unable to maintain adequate personal hygiene. In developing countries, infection rates may reach 25% to 30%; in the United States, *G duodenalis* is found in 4% of stools submitted for parasitologic examination, making it, along with *Cryptosporidium*, this country's most frequently identified intestinal parasite. All ages and economic groups are represented, but young children and young adults are preferentially involved. Children with immunoglobulin deficiencies are more likely to acquire the flagellate, possibly because of a deficiency in intestinal IgA. Giardiasis is also common among attendees of day care centers. Attack rates of over 90% have been seen in the ambulatory non–toilet-trained population (age 1-2 years) of these institutions, suggesting direct person-to-person transmission of the parasite. The frequency with which secondary cases are seen among family contacts reinforces this probability. Undoubtedly, direct fecal spread is also responsible for the high infection rate among male homosexuals. In several recent studies, the prevalence of giardiasis and/or amebiasis in that population has ranged from 11% to 40% and is correlated closely with the number of oral–anal sexual contacts.

※ Transmission facilitated by poor hygiene, IgA deficiency

High rates in day care centers

Common among male homosexuals

Waterborne and, less frequently, foodborne transmission of *G duodenalis* has also been documented, and probably accounts for the frequency with which American travelers to Third World nations acquire infection. Unlike the typical bacterial diarrhea syndrome seen in travelers, the diarrhea begins late during travel and may persist for several weeks. More than 20 waterborne outbreaks of giardiasis have also been reported in the United States. The sources have included swimming pools, untreated pond or stream water, sewage-contaminated municipal water supplies, and chlorinated but inadequately filtered water. In a few of these outbreaks, epidemiologic data have suggested that wild mammals, particularly beavers, served as the reservoir hosts. Despite the evidence for zoonotic transmission, this remains a controversial topic. In some areas of the world, where different animals, including man's closest friend, the dog, and many have been shown to be infected with *Giardia*, the infecting genotypes differed. In others, the same genotypes were demonstrated in man and animals. In most cases, humans sampled were shown

※ Water- or foodborne traveler's diarrhea lasts for weeks

※ Beavers, other mammals possible sources

to predominantly harbor human genotypes. Extensive infectivity studies using human genotypes have not been conducted.

PATHOGENESIS

Disease manifestations appear related to intestinal malabsorption, particularly of fat and carbohydrates. Disaccharidase deficiency with lactose intolerance, altered levels of intestinal peptidases, and decreased vitamin B12 absorption have been demonstrated. The precise pathogenetic mechanisms responsible for these changes remain poorly understood. Mechanical blockade of the intestinal mucosa by large numbers of *Giardia*, damage to the brush border of the microvilli by the parasite's ventral disc, organism-induced deconjugation of bile salts, altered intestinal motility, accelerated turnover of mucosal epithelium, and mucosal invasion have all been suggested. None of these correlates well with clinical manifestations. Patients with severe malabsorption have jejunal colonization with enteric bacteria or yeasts, suggesting that these organisms may act synergistically with *Giardia*. Eradication of the associated microorganism, however, has not uniformly resulted in clinical improvement. Jejunal biopsies sometimes reveal a flattening of the microvilli and an inflammatory infiltrate, the severity of which correlates roughly with that of the clinical disease. Generally, both malabsorption and the jejunal lesions have been reversed with specific treatment. The demonstration of occasional trophozoites in the submucosa raises the possibility that these changes reflect T-lymphocyte–mediated damage.

Malabsorption, jejunal pathology mechanisms uncertain

IMMUNITY

Susceptibility to giardiasis has been related to several factors, including strain virulence, inoculum size, achlorhydria or hypochlorhydria, and immunologic abnormalities. In one experimental study, humans were challenged with varying doses from as few as 10 cysts. They were uniformly parasitized when 100 or more were ingested. Several workers have noted the frequency with which giardiasis occurs in achlorhydric and hypochlorhydric individuals. *Giardia* infection produces little or no host inflammation suggesting that local responses may help control the infection. Both innate responses involving nitric oxide, defensins, phagocytic, mast and dendritic cells, and adaptive responses involving IgA and T cells have been identified in mouse models of infections and are thought to operate in human infections as well. Animal studies have demonstrated that *Giardia*-specific, secretory IgA (sIgA) antibodies inhibit attachment of trophozoites to intestinal epithelium, perhaps by blocking parasite surface lectins. Moreover, antitrophozoite IgM or IgG antibodies, plus complement, are known to be capable of killing *Giardia* trophozoites. Another indication that antibodies play a role in controlling infections is that humans with immunodeficiencies involving antibody production are more likely to suffer from chronic giardiasis. *Giardia* trophozoites are also capable of changing their surface coat variant surface proteins (VSPs). VSP switching appears to be transcriptionally controlled. Over 200 VSP genes have been identified for this organism. This process occurs once every 6 to 16 generations. The process of VSP switching undoubtedly helps the organism evade host responses.

Predisposing factors include hypochlorhydria, immunocompromise

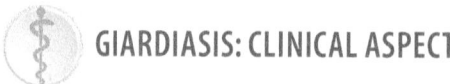 **GIARDIASIS: CLINICAL ASPECTS**

MANIFESTATIONS

In endemic situations, over two-thirds of persons infected with giardiasis are asymptomatic. In acute outbreaks, this ratio of asymptomatic to symptomatic patients is usually reversed. When they do occur, symptoms begin 1 to 3 weeks after exposure and typically include diarrhea, which is sudden in onset and explosive in character. The stool is foul-smelling, greasy in appearance, and floats. It is devoid of blood or mucus. Upper abdominal cramping is common. Large quantities of intestinal gas produce abdominal distention, sulfuric eructations, and abundant flatus. Nausea, vomiting, and low-grade fever may be present. The acute illness generally resolves in 1 to 4 weeks; in children, however, it may persist for months, leading to significant malabsorption, weight loss, and malnutrition.

Subclinical infections common

⁎ Diarrhea, cramping, flatus, greasy stools

In many adults, the acute phase of giardiasis is often followed by a subacute or chronic phase characterized by intermittent bouts of mushy stools, flatulence, "heartburn," and weight loss that persist for weeks or months. At times, patients presenting in this fashion deny having experienced

Subacute and chronic with weight loss

the acute syndrome described previously. In the majority, symptoms and organisms eventually disappear spontaneously. It is not uncommon for lactose intolerance to persist after eradication of the organisms. This condition may be confused with an ongoing infection, and the patient may be subjected to unnecessary treatment.

Lactose intolerance

DIAGNOSIS

The diagnosis of giardiasis is made by finding the cyst in formed stool or the trophozoite in diarrheal stools, duodenal secretions, or jejunal biopsy specimens. In acutely symptomatic patients, the parasite can usually be demonstrated by examining one to three stool specimens after appropriate concentration and staining. In chronic cases, excretion of the organism is often intermittent, making parasitologic confirmation more difficult. Many of these patients can be diagnosed by examining specimens taken at weekly intervals over 4 to 5 weeks. Another approach is to perform an enterotest, in which a bead encapsulated in a gelatinous capsule and attached to a thread is swallowed and then retrieved. The recovered bead is washed onto a slide and examined for active trophozoites. Alternatively, duodenal secretions can be collected and examined for trophozoites in trichrome or Giemsa-stained preparations. There are now several reliable, commercially available, enzyme immunoassays (EIAs) for the direct detection of parasite antigen in stool. They appear to be as sensitive and specific as microscopic examinations. Immunofluorescent assays for the detection of cysts are also available. The organism can be grown in culture, but the methods are not currently adaptable to routine diagnostic work. NAA assays are highly sensitive and can distinguish infecting genotypes.

* Trophozoites and cysts in stool, duodenal aspirates

* EIAs detect *Giardia* antigen in stool

TREATMENT

Five drugs are currently available for the treatment of giardiasis in the United States: quinacrine hydrochloride, metronidazole, tinidazole, furazolidone, and paromomycin. Quinacrine and metronidazole are effective (70-95%) and are preferred for patients capable of ingesting tablets. Furazolidone is used by pediatricians because of its availability as a liquid suspension, but it has the lowest cure rate. These three agents require 5 to 7 days of therapy. Tinidazole, an oral agent that has been widely used in many countries for more than 25 years outside the United States, is safe and effective as a single-dose treatment. This drug has been shown to be the most effective. It has been available in the United States since 2004. Because of the potential for person-to-person spread, it is important to examine and, if necessary, treat close physical contacts of the infected patient, including playmates at nursery school, household members, and sexual contacts. None of the aforementioned agents should be used in pregnant women because of their potential teratogenicity. Paromomycin, a nonabsorbed but somewhat less effective agent, may be used in this circumstance.

Several drugs available

Close contacts should be examined

 Should all patients diagnosed with *G duodenalis* be treated?

PREVENTION

Hikers should avoid ingestion of untreated surface water, even in remote areas, because of the possibility of contamination by feces of other people and potentially by feces of infected animals. Adequate disinfection can be accomplished with halogen tablets yielding concentrations higher than that generally achieved in municipal water systems. The safety of the latter results from additional flocculation and filtration procedures. Use of portable filtration units having a nominal pore size of 1 μm is even more effective. Boiling of water, if possible, is even better.

Avoid drinking untreated surface water

 Think ▸▸ Apply 53-1: Since this infection is easily spread, especially in children, many schools mandate that children with a diagnosis of giardiasis stay at home and not return until symptoms have abated. Hopefully they receive treatment as well. Family members of sick children should monitor themselves for signs of disease and receive treatment if they come down with giardiasis. Since this is such a common disease in developing countries, it may not be possible to treat all who are infected. However, drugs are usually available over the counter and relatively cheap.

- *Giardia* infections occur worldwide but are most common in underdeveloped countries lacking good sanitation practices.

- Infection is fecal–oral, either directly or indirectly, and can be caused by ingesting as few as 10 cysts.

- Children are more likely to be symptomatic compared to adults.

- Malabsorption is often linked to symptoms which may include persistent diarrhea, foul-smelling stools, abdominal pain, nausea, and vomiting.

- Cyst shedding may be intermittent, making microscopic detection difficult based on a single stool sample.

■ Blood and Tissue Flagellates

Two of the many genera of hemoflagellates, *Leishmania* and *Trypanosoma*, are pathogenic to humans. They reside and reproduce within the gut of specific insect hosts. When these vectors feed on a susceptible mammal, the parasite penetrates the feeding site, invades the blood and/or tissue of the new host, and multiplies to produce disease. American trypanosomes differ somewhat in that the infective parasite is passed in the feces of the specific vector during the act of feeding on its host and later rubbed into the feeding site wound. The life cycle is completed when a second insect ingests the infected mammalian blood or tissue fluid. During their passage through insect and vertebrate hosts, flagellates undergo developmental change. Within the gut of the insect (and in culture media), the organism assumes the promastigote (*Leishmania*) or epimastigote (*Trypanosoma*) form (**Figure 53–4**). These protozoa are motile and fusiform and have a blunt posterior end and a pointed anterior end from which a single flagellum projects. They measure 15 to 30 μm in length and 1.5 to 4.0 μm in width. In the promastigote form, the kinetoplast complex is located in the anterior extremity, and the flagellum exits from the cell immediately. The kinetoplast complex of the epimastigote form, in contrast, is located centrally, just in front of the vesicular nucleus. The flagellum runs anteriorly in the free edge of an undulating membrane before passing out of the cell. In the mammalian host, hemoflagellates appear as trypomastigotes (*Trypanosoma*) or amastigotes (*Leishmania, T cruzi*). The former circulate in the bloodstream and closely resemble the epimastigote form, except that the kinetoplast complex is in the posterior end of the parasite. The amastigote stage is found intracellularly.

✳ Life cycle includes insect host

✳ Promastigote, epimastigote in insects

✳ Trypomastigote, amastigote in humans

FIGURE 53–4. Stages in the life cycle of the hemoflagellates (Trypanosomidae).

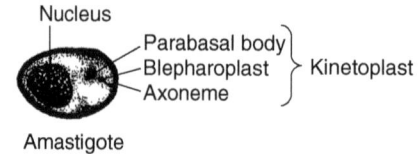

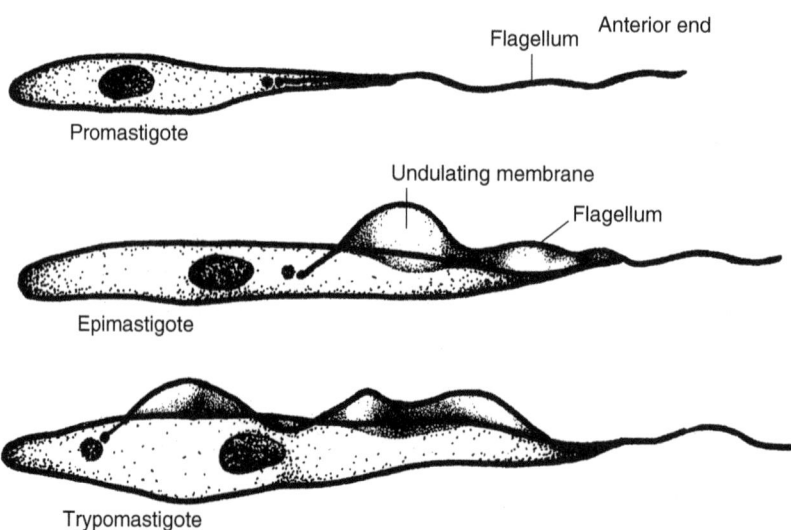

It is round or oval, measures 1.5 to 5.0 µm in diameter, and contains a clear nucleus with a central karyosome. Although it has a kinetoplast complex and an axoneme, there is no free flagellum.

The flagellated forms move in a spiral fashion, and all reproduce by longitudinal binary fission. The flagellum itself does not divide; rather, a second one is generated by one of the two daughter cells. The organisms use carbohydrate obtained from the body fluids of the host in aerobic respiration. Glycolysis is carried out in structures called glycosomes. In addition, these organisms possess a kinetoplast/mitochondrion complex. Up to 15% of total cellular DNA is found within the kinetoplast. Profound changes occur in this complex as the parasite transits from its vertebrate to invertebrate host since the parasite needs to respire more efficiently under conditions encountered in the latter host.

LEISHMANIA SPP.

Overview

Leishmania are obligate intracellular parasites distinguished by a slender body and polar flagellum. Leishmaniasis is caused by different species of *Leishmania* and results in a variety of clinical presentations dependent upon the infecting species. The most common forms of the disease are classified as cutaneal or visceral with accompanying disease manifestations. Cutaneal lesions may or may not heal depending on the infecting species and immune status of the host. Visceral leishmaniasis is often acute and highly lethal.

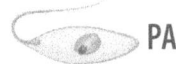 **PARASITOLOGY**

Leishmania species are obligate intracellular parasites of mammals. Several strains can infect humans; they are all morphologically similar, resulting in some confusion over their proper speciation. Definitive identification of these strains requires isoenzyme analysis, monoclonal antibodies, kinetoplast DNA buoyant densities, DNA hybridization, and DNA restriction endonuclease fragment analysis or chromosomal karyotyping using pulse-field electrophoresis. The many strains can be more simply placed in four major groups based on their serologic, biochemical, cultural, nosologic, and behavioral characteristics. For the sake of clarity, these groups are discussed as individual species. Each, however, contains a variety of strains that have been accorded separate species or subspecies status by some authorities. The organisms can be propagated in hamsters and in a variety of commercially available liquid media.

Species morphologically similar; differ in molecular features

DISEASE TRANSMISSION

It is estimated that over 20 million people worldwide suffer from leishmaniasis, and 1 to 2 million additional individuals acquire the infection annually. *Leishmania tropica* in the Old World and *Leishmania mexicana* in the New World produce a localized cutaneous lesion or ulcer, known popularly as oriental sore or chiclero ulcer; *Leishmania braziliensis* is the cause of American mucocutaneous leishmaniasis (espundia); and *Leishmania donovani* and *Leishmania infantum* are the etiologic agents of kala azar, a disseminated visceral disease.

Cutaneous ulcer or visceral infection (kala azar)

All five groups are transmitted by phlebotomine sandflies. These small, delicate, short-lived insects are found in animal burrows and crevices throughout the tropics and subtropics. At night, they feed on a wide range of mammalian hosts. Amastigotes ingested during a meal assume the flagellated promastigote form, multiply within the gut, and eventually migrate to the proboscis. When the fly next feeds on a human or animal host, the promastigotes are injected into the skin of the new host together with salivary peptides capable of inactivating host macrophages. Here, they activate complement by the classic (*L donovani*) or alternative pathway and are opsonized with C3, which mediates attachment to the CR1 and CR3 complement receptors of macrophages. After phagocytosis, the promastigotes lose their flagella and multiply as the rounded amastigote form within the phagolysosome. In stained smears, the parasites take on a distinctive appearance and have been termed Leishman–Donovan bodies. Intracellular survival is mediated by a surface lipophosphoglycan and an abundance of membrane-bound acid phosphatase, which inhibits the macrophage's oxidative burst and/or inactivates lysosomal enzymes. Continued multiplication leads to the rupture of the phagocyte and release of the daughter cells. Some may be taken up by a feeding sandfly; most invade neighboring mononuclear cells.

✴ Transmitted by nocturnally feeding sandflies

✴ Complement mediates macrophages attachment

✴ Inhibit macrophage killing

Amastigotes infect sandfly

		LEISHMANIN	NUMBER OF	NUMBER OF		HUMORAL
HUMAN DISEASE	**PARASITE**	**SKIN TEST**	**LYMPHOCYTES**	**PARASITES**	**PROGNOSIS**	**ANTIBODY TITER**
Localized skin ulcer (oriental sore, chiclero ulcer, uta)	*L tropica* *L mexicana*	Positive	Many	Few	Good	Low
Mucocutaneous lesions (espundia)	*L braziliensis*	Positive	Many	Few	Poor	Low
Disseminated cutaneous						
Ethiopian	*L tropica*[a]	Negative	Few	Many	Poor	High
American	*L mexicana*[a]					
Disseminated visceral (kala azar)	*L donovani*	Negative	Few	Many	Poor	High

TABLE 53–2   Immune Response to Leishmaniasis

[a]Different subspecies from those causing localized skin ulcers.

Cellular immune responses produce cure

Mucocutaneous metastases in *L braziliensis*

Continuation of this cycle results in extensive histiocytic proliferation. The course of the disease at this point is determined by the species of parasite and the response of the host's T cells. CD4+ T cells of the T$_H$1 type secrete interferon (IFN)-γ in response to leishmanial antigens. This, in turn, activates macrophages to kill intracellular amastigotes by the production of toxic nitric oxide. In the localized cutaneous forms of leishmaniasis, this immune response results in the development of a positive delayed skin (leishmanin) reaction, lymphocytic infiltration, reduction in the number of parasites, and, eventually, spontaneous disappearance of the primary skin lesion. In infections with *L braziliensis*, this sequence may be followed weeks to months later by mucocutaneous metastases. These secondary lesions are highly destructive, presumably because of the host's hypersensitivity to parasitic antigens. Scrapings from these lesions show a noticeable absence of lymphocytes indicating that the cell-mediated immune response has been impaired.

Some strains of *L tropica* and *L mexicana* fail to elicit an effective intracellular immune response in certain hosts. Such patients appear to have a selective suppressor T-lymphocyte–mediated anergy to leishmanial antigens. Consequently, there is no infiltration of lymphocytes or decrease in the number of parasites. The skin test remains negative, and the skin lesions disseminate and become chronic (diffuse cutaneous leishmaniasis). In infections with *L donovani*, there is a more dramatic inhibition of the T$_H$1 response. The leishmanial organisms can disseminate through the bloodstream to the visceral organs, possibly because of a relative resistance of *L donovani* to the natural microbicidal properties of normal serum, and/or their ability to better survive at 37°C than strains of *Leishmania*, causing cutaneous lesions. Although dissemination is associated with the development of circulating antibodies, they do not appear to serve a protective function and may, via the production of immune complexes, be responsible for the development of glomerulonephritis. A simplified outline of the immune responses in different forms of leishmaniasis is presented in **Table 53–2**.

✳ **Lack of cellular immune response in disseminated, chronic infections**

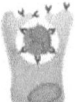 # LOCALIZED CUTANEOUS LEISHMANIASIS

EPIDEMIOLOGY

Cutaneous leishmaniasis is a zoonotic infection of tropical and subtropical rodents. It is particularly common in areas of Central Asia, the Indian subcontinent, Middle East, Africa, the Mediterranean littoral, and Central and South America. In the latter area, *L mexicana* infects several species of arboreal rodents. Humans become involved when they enter forested areas to harvest chicle for chewing gum and are bitten by infected sandflies. In the Eastern Hemisphere, the desert gerbil and other burrowing rodents serve as the reservoir hosts of *L tropica*. Human infection occurs when rural inhabitants come in close contact with the burrows of these animals. In the

Mediterranean area, southern Russia, and India, human disease involves urban dwellers, primarily children. In this setting, the domestic dog serves as the reservoir, although sandflies may also transmit *L tropica* directly from human to human.

Distribution related to human, rodent reservoirs

Urban reservoir is canine

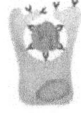 LOCALIZED CUTANEOUS LEISHMANIASIS

MANIFESTATIONS

Lesions usually appear on the extremities or face (the ear in cases of chiclero ulcer) weeks to months after the bite of the sandfly (**Figure 53–5**). They first appear as pruritic papules, often accompanied by regional lymphadenopathy. In a few months, the papules ulcerate, producing painless craters with raised erythematous edges, sharp walls, and a granulating base. Satellite lesions may form around the edge of the primary sore and fuse with it. Multiple primary lesions are seen in some patients. Spontaneous healing occurs in 3 to 12 months, leaving a flat, depigmented scar. Occasionally, the lesions fail to heal, particularly on the ears, leading to progressive destruction of the pinna. A permanent strain-specific immunity usually follows healing. Multiple, disseminated nonhealing lesions may be seen in patients with acquired immunodeficiency syndrome (AIDS).

✳ Chronic, self-limiting skin ulceration

Strain-specific immunity

DIAGNOSIS AND TREATMENT

In endemic areas, the diagnosis of localized cutaneous leishmaniasis is made on clinical grounds and confirmed by the demonstration of the organism in the advancing edge of the ulcer. Material collected by biopsy, curettage, or aspiration is smeared and/or sectioned, stained, and examined microscopically for the pathognomonic Leishman–Donovan bodies. Material should also be cultured in liquid media. The leishmanin skin test becomes positive early during the disease and remains so for life. Recently, it has been demonstrated that small numbers of *Leishmania* may be detected in tissue by NAA methods, and strains distinguished with probes to kinetoplast DNA. These techniques, though not widely available, permit direct, rapid, and specific diagnosis of all leishmanial infections.

✳ Demonstrate Leishman–Donovan bodies or culture from tissue

Patients with small, cosmetically minor lesions that do not involve the mucous membrane may be carefully followed without treatment. Pentavalent antimonial agents and liposomal amphotericin B have proved to be effective chemotherapeutic agents for individuals with more consequential lesions. Recently, ketoconazole and itraconazole, alone or in combination with the previously mentioned agents, have been found to be effective in some forms of cutaneous leishmaniasis. Paromomycin has also proved to be useful. What has become clear is that what works for one form of cutaneal leishmaniasis may not work for another. Combinations of thermotherapy and drugs have also been tried. Bacterial superinfections are treated with appropriate antibiotics. Prophylactic measures include the control of the sandfly vector by use of insect repellents and fine mesh screening on dwellings.

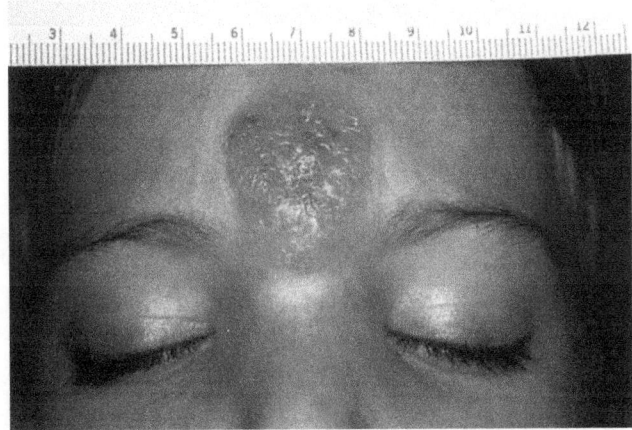

FIGURE 53–5. Cutaneous leishmaniasis. A well-developed lesion on the forehead of a 7-year-old girl. This more closely resembles a lesion that is progressing toward healing. See comments associated with this figure in the text. (Reproduced with permission from Connor DH, Chandler FW, Schwartz DQ, et al: *Pathology of Infectious Diseases.* Stamford CT: Appleton & Lange; 1997.)

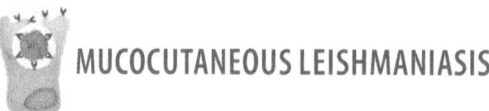

MUCOCUTANEOUS LEISHMANIASIS

❋ Rodent reservoir of
   L braziliensis

Leishmania braziliensis causes a natural infection in the large forest rodents of tropical Latin America. Sandflies transmit the infection to humans engaged in military activities, road builders, opening jungle areas for new settlements, and others.

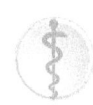

MUCOCUTANEOUS LEISHMANIASIS

MANIFESTATIONS

❋ Primary metastasizes to oral,
   nasal areas

A primary skin lesion similar to oriental sore develops 1 to 4 weeks after sandfly exposure. Occasionally, it undergoes spontaneous healing. More commonly, it progressively enlarges, often producing large vegetating lesions. After a period of weeks to years, painful, destructive, metastatic mucosal lesions of the mouth, nose, and occasionally the perineum, appear in 2% to 50% of the patients. Sometimes, decades pass and the primary lesion totally resolves before the metastases manifest themselves. Destruction of the nasal septum produces the characteristic tapir nose. Erosion of the hard palate and larynx may render the patient aphonic. In blacks, the lesions are often large, hypertrophic, polypoid masses that deform the lips and cheeks. Fever, anemia, weight loss, and secondary bacterial infections are common. Mucosal lesions caused by other *Leishmania* species may be seen after visceral dissemination in AIDS patients.

Detection of organisms as with
cutaneous leishmaniasis

The diagnosis of mucocutaneous leishmaniasis is made by finding the organisms in the lesions as described for localized cutaneous leishmaniasis. Because the propensity to metastasize to mucocutaneous sites is specific to certain species and subspecies, precise identification of the responsible organism as described in the introduction is of clinical importance. The leishmanin skin test yields positive results, and most patients have detectable antibodies. As described for cutaneous leishmaniasis, it is now possible to provide a rapid, direct, species-specific diagnosis using NAA methods and probes to kinetoplast DNA.

TREATMENT

Treatment is accomplished with the agents described later in the chapter for kala azar. Advanced lesions are often refractory and relapse is common. Cured patients are immune to reinfection. Control measures, other than insect repellents and screening of dwellings, are impractical because of the sylvatic nature of the disease.

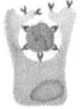

DISSEMINATED VISCERAL LEISHMANIASIS (KALA AZAR)

Kala azar is caused by *L donovani* and *L infantum*. *L donovani* is found in East Africa and the Indian subcontinent, whereas *L infantum* is found in Europe, North Africa, and Latin America. Its epidemiologic and clinical patterns vary from area to area. In Africa, rodents serve as the primary reservoir. Human cases occur sporadically, and the disease is often acute and highly lethal. In Eurasia and Latin America, the domestic dog is the most common reservoir. Human disease is endemic, primarily involves children, and runs a subacute to chronic course. In India, the human is the only known reservoir, and transmission is carried out by anthropophilic species of sandflies. The disease recurs in epidemic form at 20-year intervals, when a new cadre of nonimmune children and young adults appears in the community. There appears to be a high incidence of visceral leishmaniasis in patients with HIV infection. Presumably, HIV-induced immunosuppression either facilitates acquisition of the disease and/or allows reactivation of latent infection.

Geographic differences in reservoirs and disease severity

PATHOGENESIS

After the host is bitten by an infected sandfly, the parasites disseminate in the bloodstream and are taken up by the macrophages of the spleen, liver, bone marrow, lymph nodes, skin, and small intestine. Histiocytic proliferation in these organs produces enlargement with atrophy or replacement of the normal tissue.

✳ Invade macrophages of reticuloendothelial system

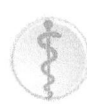 ## KALA AZAR: CLINICAL ASPECTS

MANIFESTATIONS

Most kala azar infections are asymptomatic; these become symptomatic years later during periods of host immunocompromise. Symptomatic disease most commonly manifests itself 3 to 12 months after acquisition of the parasite. It is often mild and self-limited. A minority of infected individuals develop the classic manifestations of kala azar. Fever, which is usually present, may be abrupt or gradual at the onset. It persists for 2 to 8 weeks and then disappears, only to reappear at irregular intervals during the disease. A double-quotidian pattern (two fever spikes in a single day) is a characteristic but uncommon finding. Diarrhea and malabsorption are common in Indian cases, resulting in progressive weight loss and weakness. Physical findings include enlarged lymph nodes and liver, massively enlarged spleen, and edema. In light-skinned persons, a grayish pigmentation of the face and hands is commonly seen, which gives the disease its name (kala azar, black disease). Anemia with resulting pallor and tachycardia are typical in advanced cases. Thrombocytopenia induces petechial formation and mucosal bleeding. The peripheral leukocyte count is usually less than 4000/mm³; agranulocytosis with secondary bacterial infections contributes to lethality. Serum IgG levels are enormously elevated but play no protective role. Circulating antigen–antibody complexes are present and are probably responsible for the glomerulonephritis seen so often in this disease.

✳ Delayed onset, recurrent fever, chronic disease, diarrhea

Immune complex glomerulonephritis

DIAGNOSIS AND TREATMENT

The diagnosis of kala azar is made by demonstrating the presence of the organism in aspirates taken from the bone marrow, liver, spleen, or lymph nodes. In the Indian form of kala azar, *L donovani* is also found in circulating monocytes. The specimens may be smeared, stained, and examined for the typical Leishman–Donovan bodies (amastigotes in mononuclear phagocytes) or cultured in artificial media and/or experimental animals. As described for cutaneous leishmaniasis, a limited number of reference laboratories can provide a rapid, direct, species-specific diagnosis using NAA and probes to kinetoplast DNA. Results of the leishmanin skin test are negative during active disease but become positive after successful therapy.

✳ Demonstrate Leishman–Donovan bodies or culture

The mortality rate in untreated cases of kala azar is 75% to 90%. Treatment with pentavalent antimonial drugs lowers this rate dramatically. Initial therapy, however, fails in up to 30% of African cases, and 15% of those that do respond eventually relapse. Resistant cases are treated with the more toxic pentamidine, amphotericin B, or liposomal amphotericin B. Allopurinol and IFN-γ have proved to be useful adjunctive therapies in resistant cases. A new oral drug, miltefosine, has been shown to be very efficient and safe for both cutaneal and visceral leishmaniasis. Post-Kala azar dermal leishmaniasis, a condition marked by hypopigmented macules, papules, nodules, or facial erythema may appear many years after partial or even successful treatment of visceral leishmaniasis, particularly caused by *L donovani*. The lesions can be confused with those caused by leprosy. The lesions coincide with IFN-γ–producing cells causing skin inflammation as a reaction to persisting parasites in the skin. Patients need to be treated as those for visceral leishmaniasis. Control measures are directed at the *Phlebotomus* vector, with the use of residual insecticides, and at the elimination of mammalian reservoirs by treating human cases and destroying infective dogs.

Up to 90% mortality without treatment

AFRICAN *TRYPANOSOMA*

Overview

Three species of *Trypanosoma* are morphologically the same. African trypanosomiasis is a highly lethal meningoencephalitis transmitted to humans by bloodsucking flies of the genus *Glossina*. It occurs in two distinct clinical and epidemiologic forms: West African or Gambian (chronic) sleeping sickness caused by *Trypanosoma brucei gambiense*, and East African or Rhodesian (acute) sleeping sickness caused by *T brucei rhodesiense*. Both of these organisms use antigenic variation to escape immune elimination. This, in turn, causes overall immune depression, leading to disease exacerbation. Nagana, a disease of cattle caused by a closely related trypanosome, renders over 10 million square kilometers of Central Africa unsuitable for animal husbandry.

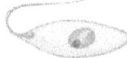 PARASITOLOGY

The trypanosomes that comprise this group are all related to an ancestral *T brucei*. They are morphologically identical, but vary in their disease-producing capabilities in animals and humans. The three subspecies, known as *T brucei brucei*, *T brucei gambiense*, and *T brucei rhodesiense*, can be distinguished by their biologic characteristics, host preferences, zymodeme types, and DNA hybridization patterns. *Trypanosoma brucei* only infects animals due to the presence of a lytic factor in human serum, while *T brucei gambiense* and *T brucei rhodesiense* give rise to West African and East African Sleeping Sickness in humans, respectively. All of them undergo similar developmental changes during their passage between their insect (tsetse fly) and mammalian host. On ingestion by the tsetse fly (*Glossina* spp.) and after a period of multiplication in the midgut, the parasites migrate to the insect's salivary glands and assume the epimastigote form. After a period of time they are transformed into metacyclic trypomastigotes, rendering them infectious to mammals. When the fly again takes a meal, the parasites are inoculated with the fly's saliva. Newly emerged and young flies are more efficient transmitters of the disease than older flies. A highly variable surface glycoprotein (VSG) coat, which is acquired in the tsetse fly, accounts for this organism's ability to undergo a process of antigenic variation in its mammalian host. The parasite enters the bloodstream and trypomastigote stage parasites referred to as slender forms divide by longitudinal fission every 5 to 10 hours. For reasons independent of the host's immune response, multiplication eventually slows and some parasites of a dominant population of organisms assume a short, stumpy appearance. These forms have a more developed kinetoplast–mitochondrial complex and constitute the parasites that are infective to the tsetse fly. Near the end of the episode of parasitemia, both slender and stumpy types may be seen in a single blood specimen. Metacyclic trypomastigotes inoculated by a tsetse fly usually contain a population of organisms dominated by a distinctive antigenic type. After a period of time in the vertebrate host, usually a week or so, the antigenic variant type changes. This change is under the control of up to 1000 genes that have been identified in some strains of these organisms that can account for a change in the variant surface glycoprotein antigenic type. Each dominant population usually contains a few organisms that have already undergone antigenic change so that when the host responds immunologically to the dominant population there will be survivors that give rise to the next dominant population. Expression of individual genes largely appears to be controlled by the sequential duplication and subsequent transfer of each gene (expression-linked copy) to one or more areas of the genome responsible for gene expression. Genes located near expression loading sites and referred to as nonduplication activated genes also can give rise to new, and sometimes repeat, antigenic types.

✳ Epimastigote and trypomastigote forms in tsetse fly

✳ Trypomastigote form injected into blood from fly's saliva

✳ Antigenic variation of glycoprotein coat due to shifting expression of preexisting genes

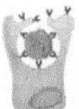

AFRICAN TRYPANOSOMIASIS (SLEEPING SICKNESS)

EPIDEMIOLOGY

The tsetse fly, and consequently sleeping sickness, is confined to the central area of Africa between the continent's two great deserts, the Sahara in the north and the Kalahari in the south. The disease is also separated into West and East African forms and is loosely divided by the Rift Valley. Approximately 50 million people live in this area, and presently about 1000 acquire sleeping sickness annually. At the height of its resurgence, this number was near 40,000 in 1998. Because of the activity of many species of tsetse flies that transmit sleeping sickness and other trypanosome infections of animals, it has been estimated that an additional 100,000,000 cattle cannot be raised in this tsetse-infested area. Major outbreaks of human infection have been reported in several locations within the endemic area over the past two decades, partly because of the internecine wars in this area that have interrupted control programs. Although an estimated 20,000 Americans travel to endemic areas each year, less than two dozen cases of African trypanosomiasis have been diagnosed in Americans since 1967.

Riverine tsetse flies found in the forest galleries that border the streams of West and Central Africa serve as the vectors of the Gambian disease. Although these flies are not exclusively anthropophilic, humans are thought to be the major reservoirs of the parasite. The infection rate in humans is affected by proximity to water but seldom exceeds 2% to 3% in nonepidemic situations. Nevertheless, the extreme chronicity of the human disease ensures its continued transmission.

Rhodesian sleeping sickness, in contrast, is transmitted by flies indigenous to the great savannas of East Africa that feed on the blood of the small antelope and other ruminants inhabiting these areas. The antelope serves as a principal parasite reservoir, although human-to-human and cattle-to-human spread has been documented. Humans typically become infected when they enter the savanna to hunt or to graze their domestic animals. The Sudan is one country where both the Gambian and Rhodesian forms of sleeping sickness are still found. Continued civil strife and deforestation in other countries could change that picture. At present, there is little evidence of coinfections with African trypanosomes and HIV, possibly because the former is primarily rural in distribution and the latter is concentrated in cities and because major immune responses to trypanosomes are largely antibody-mediated and bypass T cells.

PATHOGENESIS AND IMMUNE RESPONSIVENESS

Multiplication of the trypomastigotes at the inoculation site produces a localized inflammatory lesion. After the development of this chancre, organisms spread through lymphatic channels to the bloodstream, inducing a proliferative enlargement of the lymph nodes. The subsequent parasitemia is typically low grade and recurrent. Replicating organisms of the dominant antigenic type continuously produce surface glycoproteins. Much of this is shed from the parasite's surface and serves as a T-cell–independent antigen to directly stimulate B cells to produce antibody. The antibody produced in this fashion is IgM which can bind to the organism, leading to its destruction by lysis and opsonization. The trypomastigotes disappear from the blood, reappearing 3 to 8 days later as a new dominant antigenic variant arises. The recurrences gradually become less regular and frequent, but may persist for weeks to years before finally disappearing. During parasitemia, trypanosomes localize in the small blood vessels of the heart and central nervous system (CNS). This localization results in endothelial proliferation and a perivascular infiltration of plasma cells and lymphocytes. In the brain, hemorrhage and a demyelinating panencephalitis may follow.

The mechanism by which the trypanosomes elicit vasculitis is uncertain. The infection stimulates a massive, nonspecific polyclonal activation of B cells, the production of large quantities of IgM (typically 8-16 times the normal limit), and the suppression of other immune responses. Most of this reaction represents specific protective antibodies that are ultimately responsible for the control of the parasitemia. Some, however, consist of nonspecific heterophile antibodies, antibodies to DNA, and rheumatoid factor. Antibody-induced destruction of trypanosomes releases invariant nuclear and cytoplasmic antigens with the production of circulating immune complexes. Many authorities believe that these complexes are largely responsible for anemia and vasculitis seen in this disease.

Tsetse fly confined to Central Africa

Humans reservoir of West African sleeping sickness

Antelopes reservoir of East African trypanosomiasis; humans infected incidentally

❋ Local chancre, lymphadenitis at inoculation site

❋ Intermittent parasitemia with antigenic shifts

❋ Localize in blood vessels of heart and CNS with vasculitis

IgM levels specific and nonspecific

❋ Immune complexes cause anemia, vasculitis

Is vaccine development likely to provide a rationale approach to controlling African trypanosomiasis?

 ## AFRICAN TRYPANOSOMIASIS (SLEEPING SICKNESS): CLINICAL ASPECTS

MANIFESTATIONS

The trypanosomal chancre appears 2 to 3 days after the bite of the tsetse fly as a raised, reddened nodule on one of the exposed surfaces of the body. With the onset of parasitemia 2 to 3 weeks later, the patient develops recurrent bouts of fever, tender lymphadenopathy, skin rash, headache, and impaired mentation. In the Rhodesian form of disease, myocarditis and CNS involvement begin within 3 to 6 weeks. Heart failure, convulsions, coma, and death follow in 6 to 9 months. Gambian sleeping sickness usually progresses more slowly, but in some areas of Africa clinical manifestations of disease may overlap with the Rhodesian form of the disease. Bouts of fever often persist for years before CNS manifestations gradually appear. Spontaneous activity progressively diminishes, attention wavers, and the patient must be prodded to eat or talk. Speech grows indistinct, tremors develop, sphincter control is lost, and seizures with transient bouts of paralysis occur. In the terminal stage, the patient develops a lethal intercurrent infection or lapses into a final coma. Recent studies have shown great variability in the progression of both the Rhodesian and Gambian forms of the disease.

❋ Raised red papule on exposed surface

❋ Parasitemic manifestations 2 to 3 weeks later

❋ Late CNS involvement

DIAGNOSIS

A definitive diagnosis is made by microscopically examining lymph node aspirates, blood, or cerebrospinal fluid for the presence of trypomastigotes (**Figure 53–6**). Early in the disease, actively motile organisms can often be seen in a simple wet mount preparation smear; identification requires examination of an appropriately stained smear. If these tests prove negative, the

FIGURE 53–6. **African sickness.** *Trypanosoma brucei* in a routine blood smear. (Reproduced with permission from Nester EW, Anderson DG, Roberts CE Jr, et al: *Microbiology: A Human Perspective*, 6th ed. New York, NY: McGraw Hill; 2008.)

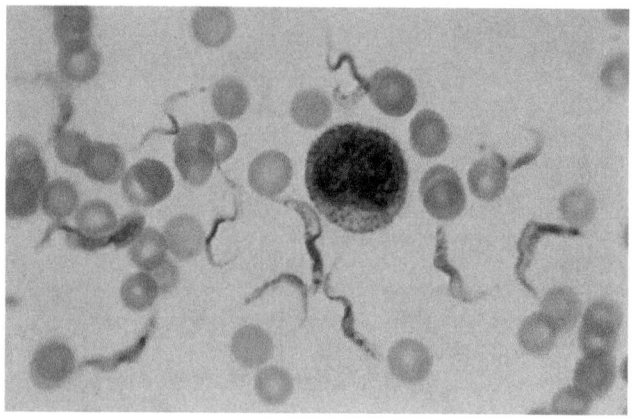

 Think ▸▸ Apply 53-2: Presently, the answer is no. Antibodies can destroy dominant populations of trypanosomes in the bloodstream, but antigenic variation helps the parasite escape total destruction and gives rise to new dominant populations. It would be impossible to raise a vaccine against the complete genetic variant types possible—more than 1000. In addition, such an approach will result in stimulation of IgM antibodies, which are short lived. Experimental vaccination studies in animal models have also shown that the host's capacity to mount an efficient immune response and to maintain its immunological memory may be undermined. Despite all of this, the fact that some animal species become trypanotolerant suggests that a vaccine strategy can eventually be developed.

blood can be centrifuged and the stained buffy coat examined. Inoculation of rats or mice can also prove helpful in diagnosing the Rhodesian disease. The patient may also be screened for elevated levels of IgM in the blood and spinal fluid or specific trypanosomal antibodies by a variety of techniques. A card agglutination test for trypanosomiasis (CATT), which can be performed on fingerstick blood, can provide serologic confirmation within minutes. Subspecies-specific DNA probes may eventually prove useful for the identification of organisms in clinical specimens.

✳ **Trypomastigotes in lymph nodes, blood, and CSF**

Animal inoculation in Rhodesian disease

TREATMENT

Lumbar puncture must always be performed before initiation of therapy for sleeping sickness. If the specimen reveals evidence of CNS involvement, agents that penetrate the blood–brain barrier must be included. Unfortunately, the most effective agent of this type is a highly toxic arsenical, melarsoprol (Mel B). Although this agent occasionally produces a lethal hemorrhagic encephalopathy, the invariably fatal outcome of untreated CNS disease warrants its use. The ornithine decarboxylase inhibitor, eflornithine (DFMO) appears capable, when used alone, or in combination with suramin, of curing CNS disease caused by *T brucei gambiense* without the serious side effects associated with melarsoprol. Unfortunately, it is very expensive and is only variably effective in *T brucei rhodesiense* infections. If the CNS is not yet involved, less toxic agents, such as suramin, pentamidine, or eflornithine, can be used. In such cases, the cure rate is high and recovery complete.

Drugs depend on CNS involvement

Without CNS recovery often complete

PREVENTION

Although a variety of tsetse fly control measures, including the use of insecticides, deforestation, and the introduction of sterile males into the fly population, have been attempted, none has proved totally practicable. The tsetse fly is larviparous and carries a larva within its body until mature and ready to pupate. This means flies have a better chance of survival. In addition, adults are strong fliers. Similarly, eradication of disease reservoirs by the early detection and treatment of human cases and the destruction of wild game has had limited success. Attempts to develop effective vaccines are currently underway but are complicated by the antigenic variability of the trypanosomes. A degree of personal protection can be achieved with insect repellents and protective clothing. Although prophylactic use of pentamidine was once advocated, enthusiasm for this treatment has waned.

Neither vector or reservoir control has been successful

KEY CONCLUSIONS

- The tsetse flies of several species are the vectors of all species of African trypanosomes.
- The unique life cycle of this fly makes fly control very difficult.
- Humans are the predominant reservoirs of *T brucei gambiense*, while wild ungulates are the predominant reservoirs of *T brucei rhodesiense*.
- Antigenic variation in trypanosome is a genetically controlled process.
- Immune responses are largely driven by T-independent antigens resulting in IgM antibody production which eliminates dominant homotype populations, but not the heterotypes which give rise to the next dominant homotype population.
- Immune depression often accompanies disease because of B-cell depletion.
- Invasion of the central nervous system by parasites gives rise to the "sleeping sickness" phase of the disease.

AMERICAN TRYPANOSOMA

Overview

Trypanosoma cruzi is a small curved trypanosome. American trypanosomiasis is a disease produced by *T cruzi* and transmitted by true bugs of the family Reduviidae, also known as kissing bugs. About 7 to 10 million people, predominantly in Central and South America are infected. Clinically, the infection may present as an acute phase with febrile illness such as seen in children, an indeterminant phase in which symptoms may largely be absent, and a chronic phase in which heart or gastrointestinal maladies are manifest, largely in adults.

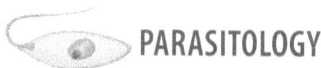 **PARASITOLOGY**

The trypomastigotes of *T cruzi* are smaller than those of *T brucei* and typically assume a C shape when seen in the peripheral circulation. Their developmental cycle differs in several respects from that of *T brucei*. Most significant, *T cruzi* does not multiply in the bloodstream. The circulating trypomastigotes must invade tissue cells, lose their flagella, and assume the amastigote form before binary fission can occur. Continued multiplication as amastigotes and epimastigotes in intracellular nests leads to distention and eventual rupture of the tissue cell. Released trypomastigotes regain the bloodstream. This new generation of trypomastigotes may invade other host cells, thus continuing the mammalian cycle. Alternatively, they may be ingested by a feeding reduviid and develop into epimastigotes within its midgut. On completion of the invertebrate cycle, the parasites migrate to the hindgut and are discharged as infectious metacyclic trypomastigotes when the reduviid defecates in the process of taking another blood meal. This process can recur at each feeding for as long as 2 years. Infection in the new host is initiated when the trypomastigotes contaminate either the feeding site or the mucous membranes.

Trypanosoma cruzi comprises several strains, each with its own distinct geographic distribution, tissue preference, and virulence. These strains may be distinguished from one another with specific antisera and by differences in their isoenzyme and DNA restriction patterns. All are somewhat morphologically similar. In blood specimens, the trypomastigotes can be distinguished from those of *T brucei* by their characteristic C or U shape, narrow undulating membrane, and large posterior kinetoplast. *T cruzi* does not undergo antigenic variation.

* Mammalian cycle with nondividing extracellular trypomastigotes, dividing intracellular amastigotes and epimastigotes

Invertebrate cycle produces trypomastigotes in bug

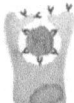 **AMERICAN TRYPANOSOMIASIS (CHAGAS DISEASE)**

EPIDEMIOLOGY

Chagas disease affects 7 to 10 million people in a geographic area extending from Mexico to southern Argentina, producing death in 50,000 annually. Within these areas, it is the leading cause of chronic heart disease, accounting for 25% of all deaths in the 25- to 44-year age group. Transmission occurs primarily in rural settings, where the reduviid can find harborage in animal burrows and in the cracked walls and thatch of poorly constructed buildings. This large (3 cm) insect leaves its hiding place at night to feed on its sleeping hosts. Its predilection to bite near the eyes or lips has earned this pest the nicknames of "kissing bug" and "assassin bug." Most new infections in these areas occur in children. Infections can also be acquired transplacentally and through blood transfusions or organ transplantations. As many as 300,000 individuals who have immigrated from Central and South America to the United States are infected with *T cruzi* and likely do not know it!

In addition to humans, several wild and domestic animals, including rats, cats, dogs, opossums, racoons, and armadillos, serve as reservoirs for Chagas disease. The close association of many of these hosts with human dwellings tends to amplify the incidence of disease in humans and the difficulty involved in its control.

Organ transplantation and transfusion-related infections are rapidly increasing problems in urban settings within endemic areas. Recrudescence of the latent infection is increasingly seen in immunosuppressed individuals, including patients with HIV infections. More effective blood bank screening provides hope that transmission of this disease will be substantially curtailed in the near future.

Recently, oral/foodborne transmission of Chagas disease has gained attention. For this to occur, the parasite must survive in the feces of its natural vector on foods that are consumed. Outbreaks in Brazil have been linked to the consumption of açai juice prepared from a reddish/purple fruit from the açai palm tree. In total, more than 1000 cases of infection with *T cruzi* has been linked with oral infection in different regions of Brazil, Columbia, Bolivia, Guyana Francesa, Argentina, and Ecuador.

An estimated 300,000 infected Latin American immigrants are currently living in the United States. Because *T cruzi* has been found in both vertebrate and invertebrate hosts in the southern United States, there is a possibility of sustained transmission of this organism within this country. Although serologic evidence suggests that the acquisition of human infection in this area

* Chagas disease in South and Central America

* "Kissing bug" feeds at night

* Infected Immigrants from Central and South America

Wild and domestic animal reservoirs amplify transmission

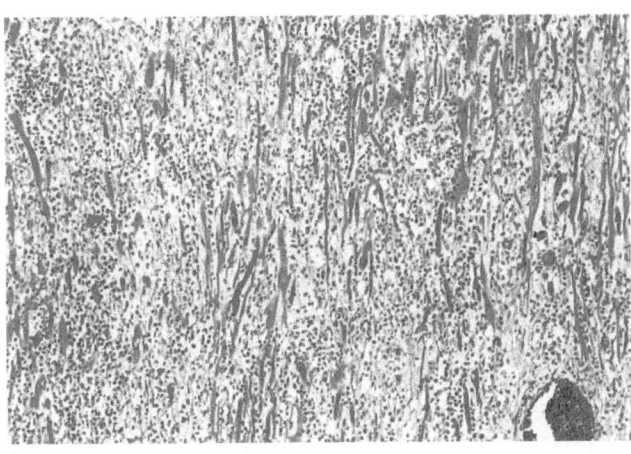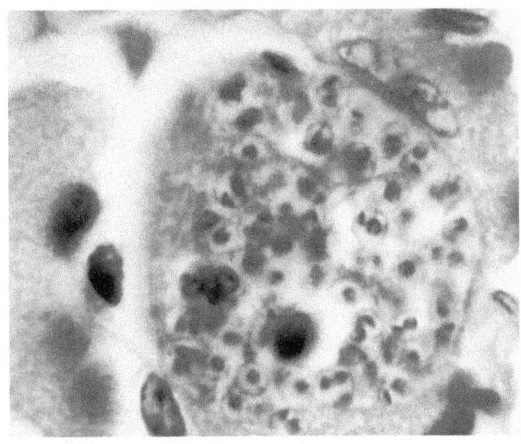

A   B

FIGURE 53-7. **Chagas disease. A.** Acute myocarditis with atrophic myofibers separated by inflammatory cells. **B.** *Trypanosoma cruzi* amastigotes clustered in myofiber from the same case. (Reproduced with permission from Connor DH, Chandler FW, Schwartz DQ, et al: *Pathology of Infectious Diseases.* Stamford CT: Appleton & Lange; 1997.)

is not uncommon, clinically apparent autochthonous cases have been rare. Most of these acquired the infection through blood–blood transfusions.

PATHOGENESIS

Multiplication of the parasite at the portal of entry stimulates the accumulation of neutrophils, lymphocytes, and tissue fluid, resulting in the formation of a local chancre or chagoma. The subsequent dissemination of the organism with invasion of tissue cells produces a febrile illness that may persist for 1 to 3 months and result in widespread organ damage. Any nucleated host cell may be involved, but those of mesenchymal origin, especially the heart, skeletal muscle, smooth muscle, and ganglion neural cells, are particularly susceptible. Cell entry is facilitated by binding to host cell fibronectin; a 60-kDa *T cruzi* surface protein (penetrin) appears to promote adhesion. After penetration, the trypomastigote escapes the phagosome via the production of a pore-forming protein, transforms to the amastigote form, and multiplies freely within the cytoplasm to produce a pseudocyst, a greatly enlarged and distorted host cell containing masses of organisms (**Figure 53–7**). With the rupture of the pseudocyst, many of the released parasites disintegrate, eliciting an intense inflammatory reaction with destruction of surrounding tissue. The development of an antibody-dependent, cell-mediated immune response leads to the eventual destruction of the *T cruzi* parasites and the termination of the acute phase of illness.

❋ Local chancre at inoculation site

❋ Entry to mesenchymal cells facilitated by fibronectin-binding protein

❋ Pore-forming protein aids escape from phagosome

Pseudocysts from cytoplasmic multiplication

Parasitic antigens released during this acute phase may bind to the surface of tissue cells, rendering them susceptible to destruction by the host's immune response. It has been suggested by some that this results in the production of antibodies that cross-react with host tissue, initiating a sustained autoimmune inflammatory reaction in the absence of systemic manifestation of illness. In the heart, this reaction leads to changes in coronary microvasculature, loss of muscle tissue, interstitial fibrosis, degenerative changes in the myocardial conduction system, and loss of intracardiac ganglia. In the digestive tract, loss of both ganglionic nerve cells and smooth muscle results in dilatation and loss of peristaltic movement, particularly of the esophagus and colon.

Heart damage may be autoimmune

Ganglionic, smooth muscle loss in GI tract

 ## AMERICAN TRYPANOSOMIASIS (CHAGAS DISEASE): CLINICAL ASPECTS

MANIFESTATIONS

Serologic studies suggest that only one-third of the persons newly infected with Chagas disease develop clinical illness. Acute manifestations, when they occur, are seen primarily in children. They begin with the appearance of the nodular, erythematous chagoma 1 to 3 weeks after the bite of the reduviid. If the eye served as a portal of entry, the patient presents with Romaña sign: reddened eye, swollen lid, and enlarged preauricular lymph node. The onset of parasitemia is signaled by the development of a sustained fever; enlargement of the liver, spleen, and lymph nodes;

Most asymptomatic; acute disease in children

Myocardial injury indicated by tachycardia and ECG

signs of meningeal irritation; and the appearance of peripheral edema or a transient skin rash. In a small percentage of symptomatic patients, heart involvement results in tachycardia, electrocardiographic (ECG) changes, and occasionally arrhythmia, enlargement, and congestive heart failure. Newborns may experience acute meningoencephalitis. Clinical manifestations persist for weeks to months. In 5% to 10% of untreated patients, severe myocardial involvement or meningoencephalitis leads to death.

✳ Chronic cardiomyopathy leads to heart block, failure

Dilatation of esophagus and colon seen in southern latitudes

Chronic disease, the result of end-stage organ damage, is usually seen only in adulthood. Ironically, most patients with late manifestations have no history of acute illness. The most serious of the late manifestations is heart disease. Studies of asymptomatic, seropositive patients in endemic areas have shown that a significant proportion have cardiac abnormalities demonstrated by electrocardiographic, echocardiographic, or cineangiographic techniques, suggesting that Chagas cardiomyopathy is a progressive, focal disease of the myocardium and conduction system, leading eventually to clinical disease. This may present as arrhythmia, thromboembolic events, heart block, enlargement with congestive heart failure, and cardiac arrest. In some areas of rural Latin America, up to 10% of the adult population may show cardiac manifestations. In the United States, chagasic heart disease in immigrants is usually initially misdiagnosed as coronary artery disease or idiopathic dilated cardiomyopathy. Megaesophagus and megacolon, which are less devastating than the heart disease, are typically seen in more southern latitudes. This geographic variation in clinical manifestations is thought to be attributable to a difference in tissue tropism between individual strains of *T cruzi*. Megaesophagus leads to difficulty in swallowing and regurgitation, particularly at night. Megacolon produces severe constipation with irregular passage of voluminous stools. *T cruzi* brain abscess has been described in a small number of AIDS patients.

DIAGNOSIS

✳ Trypomastigotes in peripheral blood

Xenodiagnosis involves allowing bugs to feed

Organisms difficult to recover in chronic disease

The diagnosis of acute Chagas disease rests on finding the trypomastigotes in the peripheral blood or buffy coat, and their morphologic identification as *T cruzi*. The methods are like those described for diagnosis of African trypanosomiasis. If the results are negative, a laboratory-raised reduviid can be fed on the patient, then dissected and examined for the presence of parasites, a procedure known as **xenodiagnosis**. Alternatively, the blood may be cultured in a variety of artificial media or experimental animals. In the diagnosis of chronic disease, recovery of the organisms is the exception rather than the rule, and diagnosis depends on the clinical, epidemiologic, and immunodiagnostic findings. A variety of serologic tests are available; small numbers of false-positive results limit their usefulness, particularly when used as screening procedures in nonendemic areas. The recent production of specific recombinant proteins and synthetic peptides for use as antibody targets may improve the reliability of these procedures. Polymerase chain reaction techniques for the amplification of trypomastigote DNA are available.

TREATMENT

Treatment may reduce acute disease

The role of treatment in Chagas disease remains unsettled. Two agents, nifurtimox and benznidazole, effectively reduce the severity of acute disease but appear to be ineffective in chronic infections. Both drugs must be taken for prolonged periods of time, may cause serious side effects, and do not always result in parasitologic cure. Allopurinol, a hypoxanthine oxidase inhibitor devoid of serious side effects, has recently been shown to be capable of suppressing parasitemia and reversing the serostatus of patients with acute disease. Additional studies to confirm these encouraging results are necessary.

PREVENTION

The reduviid vector can be controlled by applying residual insecticides to rural buildings at 2- or 3-month intervals. The addition of latex to the insecticide creates a colorless paint that prolongs activity. This approach has proven effective because larval instar stages of the kissing bug lack wings and, therefore, stay close to their source of blood. A strong initiative using this approach has been undertaken in the southern portion of South America. Fumigants can be used to prevent reinfection. Patching wall cracks, cementing floors, and moving debris and woodpiles away from human dwellings reduces the number of reduviids within the home. Transfusion-induced disease, a major problem in endemic areas, has been partially controlled by the addition of gentian violet to all blood packs before use or by screening potential donors serologically for Chagas disease.

The large number of infected immigrants now entering nonendemic countries presents an increasing risk of transfusion-mediated parasite transmission in these areas as well. Cases of acute Chagas disease have been reported in the United States in immunosuppressed patients who received blood from donors unaware of their infection status; the resulting diseases were particularly fulminant. Immunodiagnostic tests for Chagas disease are neither readily available nor sufficiently specific for use in nonendemic areas; prevention will probably require deferral of blood donations from persons who have recently emigrated from endemic areas. Immunoprophylaxis is not available at present.

✱ Control of reduviid bugs in homes most important

KEY CONCLUSIONS

- *Trypanosoma cruzi* infections are transmitted primarily through the feces of infected kissing bugs.
- Infection is manifest by acute, indeterminant, and chronic phases.
- Chronic disease is manifest as cardiomyopathies and/or gastrointestinal maladies in about 25% of infected individuals.
- Chagas disease can be transmitted congenitally and via blood transfusion and organ transplantation.
- At present, therapies are only available during acute phase infection.

CASE STUDY

A Child With Recurrent Fever and Diarrhea

This 3-year-old girl who resides in Central Africa has had recurrent fevers for the last 6 weeks, accompanied by persistent diarrhea and weight loss. A physical examination reveals her to be alert but with significant generalized weakness, widespread lymphadenopathy, hepatomegaly, and massive splenomegaly.

Laboratory findings include anemia, leukopenia, thrombocytopenia, and hematuria.

QUESTIONS

1. Which is the most likely cause of this child's illness?
   A. *Leishmania donovani*
   B. *Leishmania tropica*
   C. *Trypanosoma cruzi*
   D. *Trypanosoma brucei*

2. Which is the insect vector involved?
   A. Mosquito
   B. Tsetse fly
   C. Sandfly
   D. Reduviid bug

3. *Trypanosoma cruzi* can significantly affect all of the following tissues, *except*:
   A. Heart
   B. Smooth muscle
   C. Skin
   D. Skeletal muscle
   E. Neural tissue

ANSWERS

1. **(A)**

2. **(C)**

3. **(C)**

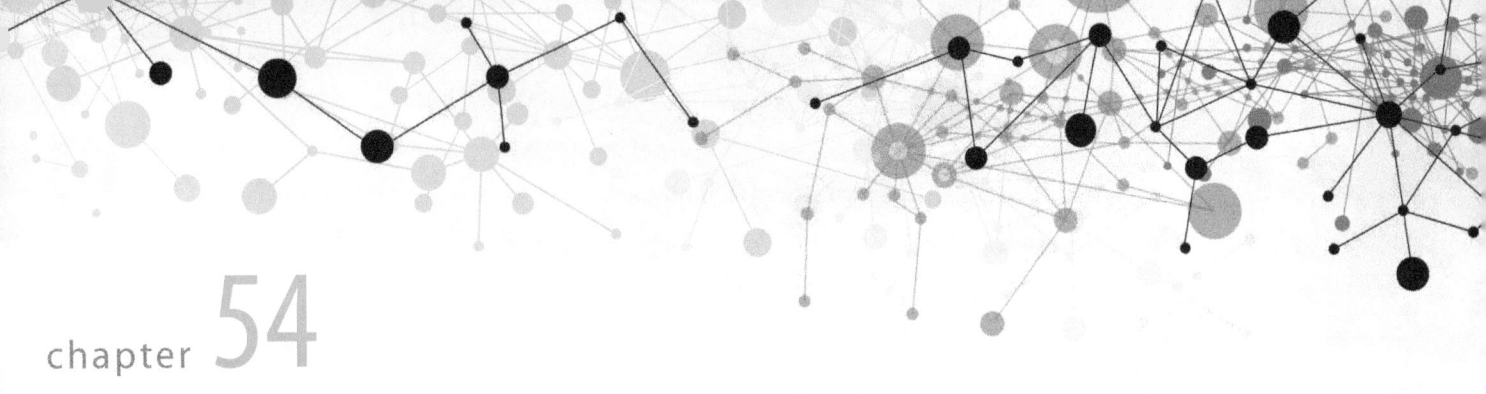

chapter 54

Intestinal Nematodes

Enterobius vermicularis • *Trichuris trichiura* • *Ascaris lumbricoides* • *Necator americanus* •

Ancylostoma duodenale • *Strongyloides stercoralis*

> *Life is dear to every living thing; the worm that crawls upon the ground will struggle for it.*
>
> — Solomon Northup

OVERVIEW

Nematodes are worms with bodies that are round in cross-section. They come in two broad categories: Intestinal nematodes (covered here) and tissue nematodes (covered in Chapter 55). The distinction between these groups may seem arbitrary because some intestinal nematodes migrate through tissue on their way to the gut, and some tissue nematodes spend part of their lives in the intestines! However, the difference between the groups will be clear if you focus on whether the *adult* form spends its time chiefly in the intestines or in other body tissues.

■ Impact

Six intestinal nematodes commonly infect humans: *Enterobius vermicularis* (pinworm), *Trichuris trichiura* (whipworm), *Ascaris lumbricoides* (large roundworm), *Necator americanus* and *Ancylostoma duodenale* (human hookworms), and *Strongyloides stercoralis*. Together, they infect more than 25% of all humans. Most people who carry a small number of any of these intestinal roundworms have no symptoms whatsoever. However, people with large numbers of adult worms may suffer from abdominal discomfort, malnutrition, anemia, and occasionally death. Other closely related nematodes of animals that occasionally infect humans are also listed in **Table 54–1**, but are not discussed here.

■ Morphology

All intestinal nematodes have cylindrical, tapered bodies covered with a tough, acellular cuticle. Sandwiched between this tegument and the body cavity are layers of muscle, longitudinal nerve trunks, and an excretory system. A tubular alimentary tract consisting of a mouth, esophagus, midgut, and anus runs from the anterior to the posterior extremity. Highly developed reproductive organs fill the remainder of the body cavity. The sexes are separate; the male worm is generally smaller than its mate, and may be distinguished by a more curled posterior end than the tapered end in females.

■ Life Cycles

Helminth life cycles have confused and frustrated generations of students. They may seem arcane, but they reveal how the pathogen will be transmitted to a new host. Therefore, physicians and public health experts who aim to develop strategies for prevention and control must understand life cycle fundamentals. The life cycles of the six main human intestinal nematodes are summarized in **Table 54–2**.

   Life is difficult for worm offspring, most of which will die before reaching adulthood. Thus, female worms are extremely prolific, and may produce thousands of offspring every day, generally

TABLE 54–1	Intestinal Nematodes		
HUMAN PARASITE		**ANIMAL PARASITE**	**HUMAN DISEASE**
Enterobius vermicularis (pinworm)			Enterobiasis
Trichuris trichiura (whipworm)			Trichuriasis
		Capillaria philippinensis	Intestinal capillariasis
Ascaris lumbricoides (large roundworm)			Ascariasis
		Ascaris suum	Ascariasis
		Anisakis spp.	Anisakiasis
Necator americanus (hookworm)			Hookworm disease
Ancylostoma duodenale (hookworm)			
		Ancylostoma braziliense	Cutaneous larva migrans
Strongyloides stercoralis			Strongyloidiasis

in the form of eggs. In most cases, eggs are fertilized and then carried from the adult to the environment in human feces. Typically, the eggs must incubate or "embryonate" outside of the human host before they become infectious to another person; during this time, the embryo repeatedly segments, eventually developing into an adolescent form known as a **larva**. The egg may then be ingested with contaminated food. In some species, the egg hatches outside of the host, releasing a larva capable of penetrating the skin of a person who comes in direct physical contact with it. Obviously, intestinal nematodes are principally found in areas where human feces are deposited indiscriminately or used for fertilizer.

■ Pathogenesis

The adults of each of the six nematodes listed previously can survive for months or years within the lumen of the human gut. The severity of illness produced by each depends on the level of adaptation to the host it has achieved. Some species have a simple life cycle that can be completed without serious consequences to the host. Less well-adapted parasites, on the other hand, have more complex cycles, often requiring tissue invasion and/or production of enormous numbers of offspring to ensure their continued survival and dissemination. Within a given species, disease severity is related directly to the number of adult worms harbored by the host. The greater the worm load or worm burden, the more serious the consequences. Because most nematodes do not multiply within the human, small worm loads may remain asymptomatic and undetected throughout the lifespan of the parasite. Repeated infections, however, progressively increase the worm burden and at some point may cause symptomatic disease. Although humans can mount an immune response that may eventually contribute to the expulsion of worms, it is slow to develop and incomplete. It is therefore the frequency and intensity of reinfection more than the

Long survival in gut lumen

✱ Worm load, repeated infection important to severity

TABLE 54–2	Life Cycles of Intestinal Nematodes					
PARASITE	**ROUTE OF INFECTION**	**MIGRATION IN BODY**	**DIAGNOSTIC FORM**	**SITE OF EMBRYONATION**	**INFECTIVE FORM**	**FREE-LIVING CYCLE**
Enterobius vermicularis (pinworm)	Mouth	Intestinal	Egg	Perineum	Egg	No
Trichuris trichiura (whipworm)	Mouth	Intestinal	Egg	Soil	Egg	No
Ascaris lumbricoides (giantworm)	Mouth	Pulmonary	Egg	Soil	Egg	No
Necator americanus[a] (hookworm)	Skin	Pulmonary	Egg	Soil	Filariform larvae	No
Strongyloides stercoralis	Skin	Pulmonary	Rhabditiform larvae	Soil; intestine[b]	Filariform larvae	Yes

[a]Same for *A duodenale*, the other human hookworm.
[b]Intestine in cases of autoinfection.
Reproduced with permission from Harrison TR, Isselbacher KJ: *Harrison's Principles of Internal Medicine,* 9th ed. New York, NY: McGraw Hill; 1980.

host's immune response that determine the worm burden. This burden is seldom uniform within affected populations, but rather "aggregated" within subgroups of "wormy persons," presumably related to their exposure or perhaps undefined immunologic factors.

● PARASITES AND DISEASES

ENTEROBIUS

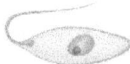 ### ENTEROBIUS VERMICULARIS (PINWORM): PARASITOLOGY

The adult female pinworm is 10 mm long, cream colored, with a sharply pointed tail; such characteristics have given rise to the common name pinworm, or threadworm. Running longitudinally down both sides of the body are small ridges that widen anteriorly to fin-like alae. The seldom-seen male is smaller (3 mm) and possesses a ventrally curved tail and copulatory spicule. The clear, thin-shelled, ovoid eggs are flattened on one side and measure 25 by 50 μm (**Figure 54–1**).

❋ Common name pinworm or threadworm

LIFE CYCLE (FIGURE 54–2)

Enterobius has the simplest life cycle of the intestinal nematodes. The adult worms lie attached to the mucosa of the cecum, where the male inseminates the female. As her period of gravidity draws to a close, the female migrates down the colon, slips unobserved through the anal canal in the dark of the night, and deposits as many as 20,000 sticky eggs on the host's perianal skin, bedclothes, and linens. The eggs are near maturity at the time of deposition and become infectious shortly thereafter. Handling of bedclothes or scratching of the perianal area results in adhesion of the eggs to the fingers and fingernails; subsequently the eggs are ingested during eating or thumb sucking. Alternatively, the eggs may be shaken into the air (eg, during making of the bed), inhaled, and swallowed. The eggs subsequently hatch in the upper intestine, and the larvae migrate to the cecum, where they mature to adults and mate. The entire adult-to-adult cycle is completed in 2 weeks.

Adults inhabit cecum

❋ Female transits anus at night to deposit eggs on perineum

Eggs infectious shortly after deposition

Larvae mature in intestine

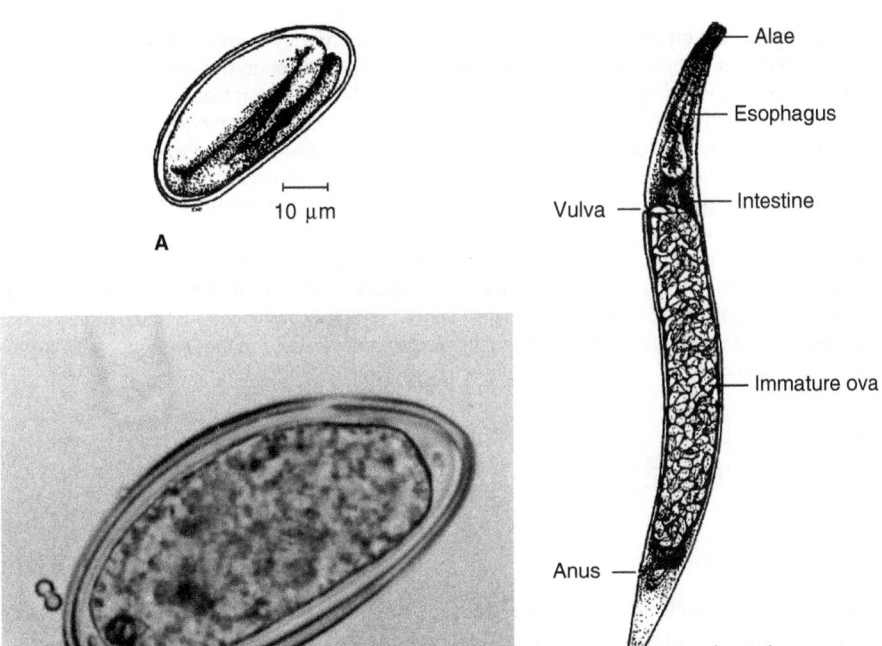

FIGURE 54–1. *Enterobius vermicularis.* **A.** Egg structure. **B.** Structure of adult female pinworm. **C.** Embryonated egg recovered from stool. (C, Reproduced with permission from Connor DH, Chandler FW, Schwartz DQ, et al: *Pathology of Infectious Diseases.* Stamford CT: Appleton & Lange; 1997.)

FIGURE 54–2. *Enterobius vermicularis* life cycle.

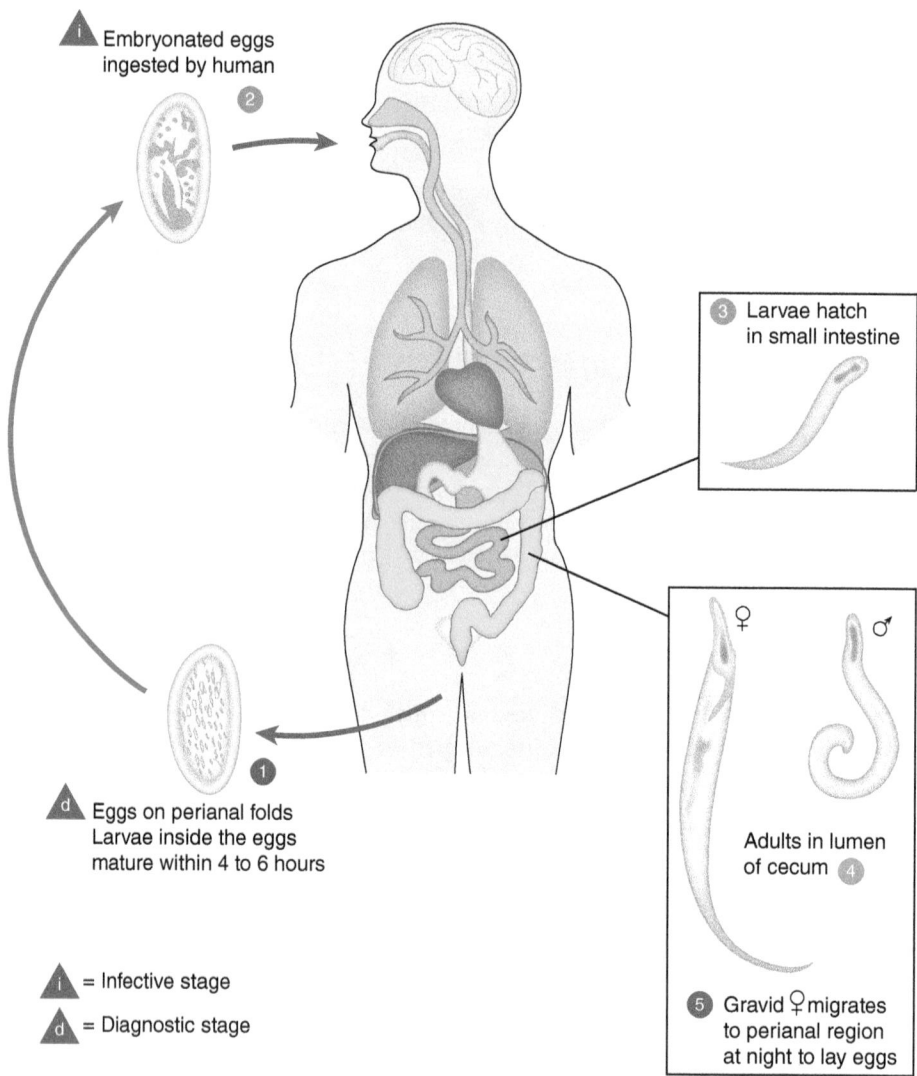

Eggs are deposited on perianal folds ①. Self-infection occurs by transferring infective eggs to the mouth with hands that have scratched the perianal area ②. Person-to-person transmission can also occur through handling of contaminated clothes or bed linens. Enterobiasis may also be acquired through surfaces in the environment that are contaminated with pinworm eggs (eg, curtains, carpeting). Some small number of eggs may become airborne and inhaled. These would be swallowed and follow the same development as ingested eggs. Following ingestion of infective eggs, the larvae hatch in the small intestine ③ and the adults establish themselves in the colon ④. The time interval from ingestion of infective eggs to oviposition by the adult females is about 1 month. The life span of the adults is about 2 months. Gravid females migrate nocturnally outside the anus and oviposit while crawling on the skin of the perianal area ⑤. The larvae contained inside the eggs develop (the eggs become infective) in 4 to 6 hours under optimal conditions ①. Retroinfection, or the migration of newly hatched larvae from the anal skin back into the rectum, may occur but the frequency with which this happens is unknown.

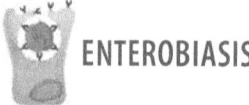 ENTEROBIASIS

EPIDEMIOLOGY

The pinworm is well adapted to the human host. Eggs have been found in a 10,-000-year-old coprolith, making this nematode the oldest demonstrated infectious agent of humans. It has been estimated to infect at least 200 million people worldwide, particularly children, including millions in the United States alone. Despite evidence that its prevalence is now decreasing in the United States, it remains the single most common cause of human helminthiasis in industrialized nations. Infection is more common among children.

The eggs are relatively resistant to desiccation and may remain viable in linens, bedclothes, or house dust for several days. Once infection is introduced into a household, other family members are often rapidly infected.

PATHOGENESIS AND IMMUNITY

The adult worms produce no significant intestinal pathology and do not appear to induce protective immunity.

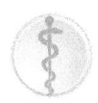 ## ENTEROBIASIS: CLINICAL ASPECTS

MANIFESTATIONS

E vermicularis seldom produces serious disease. Many carriers have no complaints at all, but when symptoms do develop, the most common presentation is pruritus ani (anal itching). This symptom is most severe at night and has been attributed to the migration of the gravid female. It may lead to irritability in children. In severe infections, the intense itching may lead to excoriation and secondary bacterial infection. In female patients, the worm may enter the genital tract, producing vaginitis, granulomatous endometritis, or even salpingitis. Adult worms may be found in the appendix of patients with acute appendicitis, although it is unclear whether they have triggered the attack or are merely bystanders. It has also been suggested that errant worms might carry enteric bacteria into the urinary bladder in young women, triggering acute bacterial cystitis.

✳ Nocturnal pruritus ani

Occasional infection of female GU tract

DIAGNOSIS

Eosinophilia is usually absent. The diagnosis is suggested by the clinical manifestations and confirmed by the recovery of the characteristic eggs from the perianal skin. This is accomplished by applying the sticky side of cellophane tape to the mucocutaneous junction, then transferring the tape to a glass slide and examining the slide for eggs (Figure 54–1C) under the low-power lens of a microscope. Occasionally, adult females are seen by the parent of an infected child or recovered with the cellophane tape procedure.

✳ Perianal cellophane tape test detects ova

TREATMENT AND PREVENTION

Several highly satisfactory agents, including pyrantel pamoate, mebendazole, and albendazole are available for treatment of enterobiasis. Many experts believe that all members of a family or other cohabiting group should be treated simultaneously. Although cure rates are high, reinfection is extremely common. In severe infections, retreatment after 2 weeks is recommended. Enhanced hygiene, including scrubbing under children's fingernails, may help to break the chain of transmission.

Family members may need treatment

✳ Reinfection common

TRICHURIS

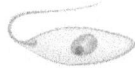 ## *TRICHURIS TRICHIURA* (WHIPWORM): PARASITOLOGY

The adult whipworm is 30 to 50 mm in length. The anterior two-thirds is thin and thread-like, whereas the posterior end is bulbous, giving the worm the appearance of a tiny whip. The tail of the male is coiled; that of the female is straight. The female produces 3000 to 10,000 oval eggs each day. They are of the same size as pinworm eggs, but have a distinctive thick brown shell with translucent knobs on both ends (**Figure 54–3**).

Produces up to 10,000 eggs a day

LIFE CYCLE (FIGURE 54–4)

Trichuris trichiura has a life cycle slightly more complex than that of the pinworm. The adults live attached to the colonic mucosa by their thin anterior end, using the larger ends for copulation. While retaining its position in the cecum, the gravid female releases its eggs into the lumen of the gut. These pass out of the body with the feces and, in poorly sanitized areas of the world, are deposited on soil. The eggs are immature at the time of passage and must incubate for at least 10 days (longer if soil conditions, temperature, and moisture are suboptimal) before they become

FIGURE 54-3. *Trichuris trichiura.* **A.** Egg structure. **B.** Structure of female adult whipworm. **C.** Embryonated egg with bipolar plugs from stool. (**C**, Reproduced with permission from Connor DH, Chandler FW, Schwartz DQ, et al: *Pathology of Infectious Diseases.* Stamford CT: Appleton & Lange; 1997.)

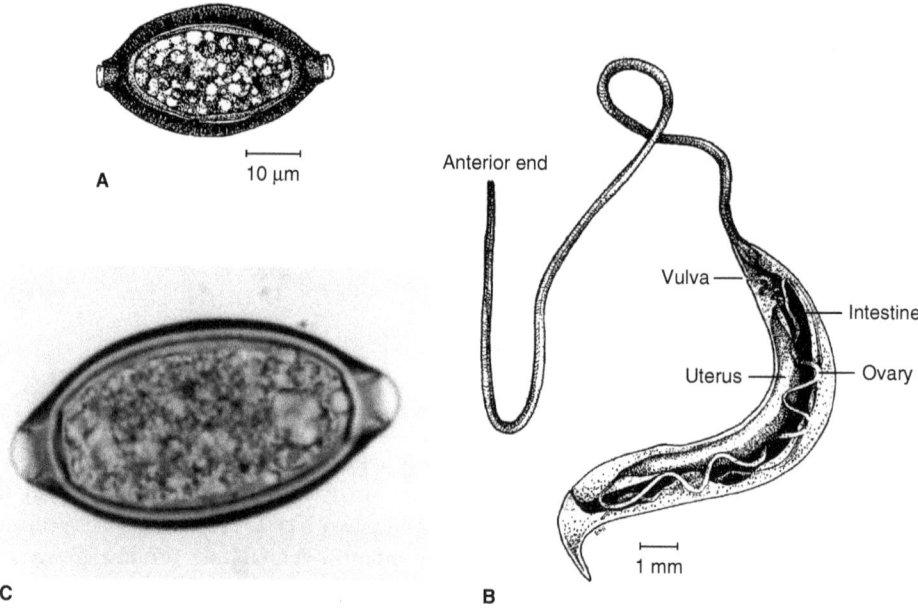

Adults inhabit cecum, release eggs to lumen

✳ **Complexity: eggs must mature in soil 10 days**

fully embryonated and infectious. Once in this state, they are ingested unknowingly by the next human host—picked up on the hands of children at play, or by agricultural workers, or diners in areas where human feces are used as fertilizer. After ingestion, the eggs hatch in the duodenum, and the released larvae mature for approximately 1 month in the small bowel before migrating to their adult habitat in the cecum.

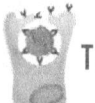

TRICHURIASIS

EPIDEMIOLOGY

Soil defecation in warm, humid climate

Adult worms live for years

Although it is less widespread than the pinworm, the whipworm is a cosmopolitan parasite, infecting approximately 800 million people globally. It is concentrated in areas where indiscriminate defecation and a warm, humid environment produce extensive seeding of soil with infectious eggs. In some communities in tropical climates, infection rates may be as high as 80%. Although the incidence is much lower in temperate climates, trichuriasis affects individuals throughout the rural areas of the southeastern United States. Although the intensity of infection is generally low, adult worms may live 4 to 8 years.

PATHOGENESIS AND IMMUNITY

Colonic ulceration provides bacterial bloodstream entry

Attachment of adult worms to the colonic mucosa and their subsequent feeding activities produce localized ulceration and hemorrhage (0.005 mL blood per worm per day). The ulcers provide enteric bacteria with a portal of entry to the bloodstream, and occasionally a sustained bacteremia results. Decreased prevalence of trichuriasis in the postadolescent period and the demonstration of acquired immunity in experimental animal infections suggest that immunity may develop in human infections. An IgE-mediated immune mucosal response is demonstrable in humans, but is insufficient to cause appreciable parasite expulsion.

TRICHURIASIS: CLINICAL ASPECTS

MANIFESTATIONS

Colonic damage, abdominal pain, diarrhea

Light infections of trichuriasis are asymptomatic. With moderate worm loads, damage to the intestinal mucosa may induce nausea, abdominal pain, diarrhea, and stunting of growth. Occasionally, a child may harbor 800 adult worms or more. In these situations, the entire colonic lumen is parasitized, with significant mucosal damage, blood loss, and anemia (**Figure 54–5**). This may cause a "dysentery syndrome" with bloody diarrhea that mimics infection with bacterial

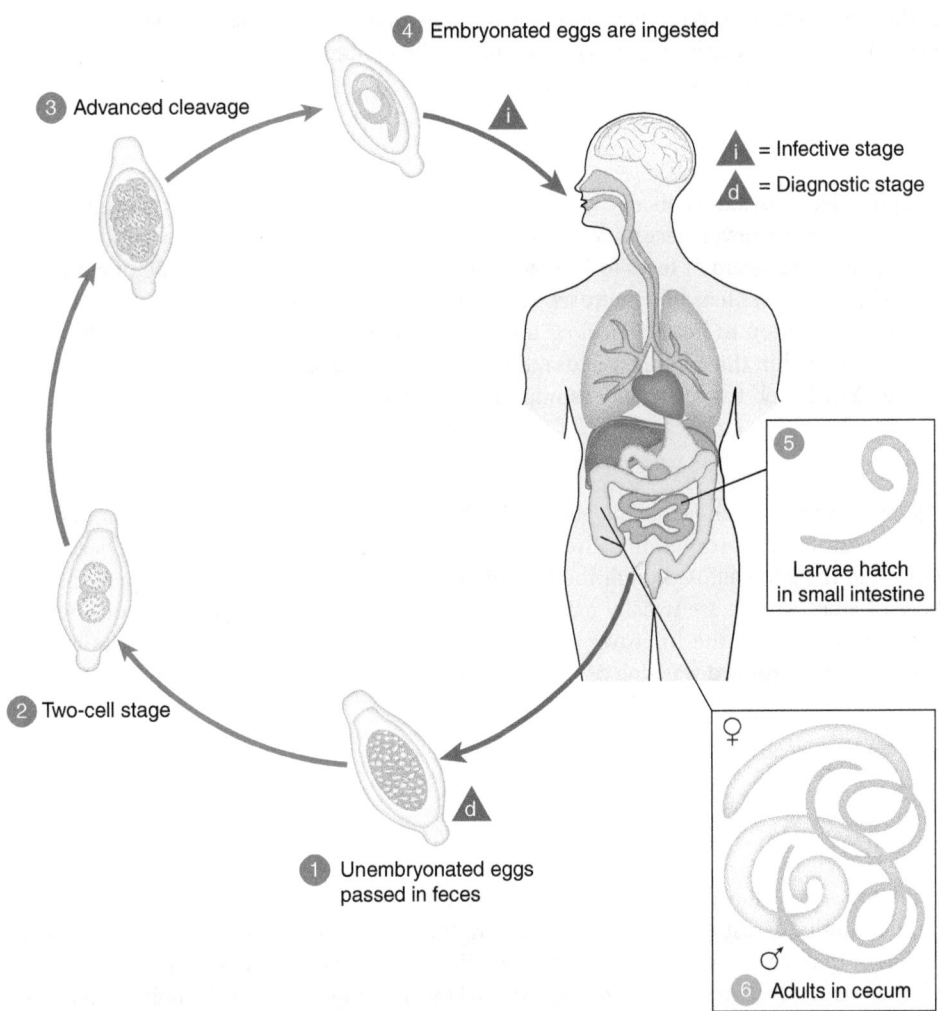

④ Embryonated eggs are ingested

③ Advanced cleavage

FIGURE 54–4. *Trichuris trichiura* **life cycle.**

▲i = Infective stage

▲d = Diagnostic stage

⑤ Larvae hatch in small intestine

② Two-cell stage

♀

① Unembryonated eggs passed in feces

♂

⑥ Adults in cecum

The unembryonated eggs are passed with the stool ①. In the soil, the eggs develop into a two-cell stage ②, an advanced cleavage stage ③, and then they embryonate ④; eggs become infective in 15 to 30 days. After ingestion (soil-contaminated hands or food), the eggs hatch in the small intestine, and release larvae ⑤ that mature and establish themselves as adults in the colon ⑥. The adult worms (approximately 4 cm in length) live in the cecum and ascending colon. The adult worms are fixed in that location, with the anterior portions threaded into the mucosa. The females begin to oviposit 60 to 70 days after infection. Female worms in the cecum shed between 3000 and 20,000 eggs per day. The lifespan of the adults is about 1 year.

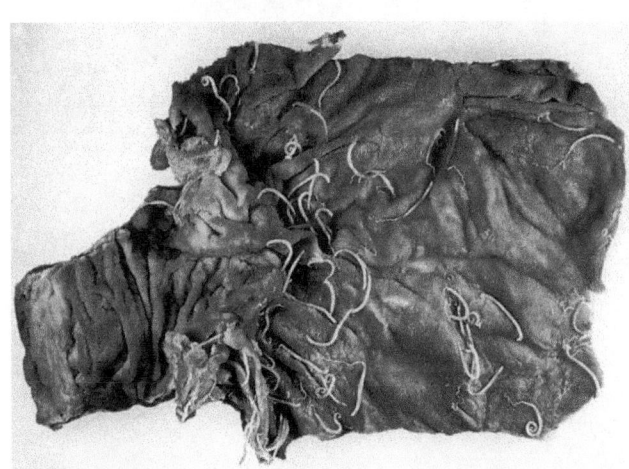

FIGURE 54–5. Whipworm infestation. Terminal ileum covered with adult *Trichuris trichiura.* (Reproduced with permission from Connor DH, Chandler FW, Schwartz DQ, et al: *Pathology of Infectious Diseases.* Stamford CT: Appleton & Lange; 1997.)

* Worm load causes dysentery, rectal prolapse

pathogens such as *Shigella*. Heavy worm burdens may cause tenesmus, the sensation that one needs to defecate, which may trigger prolapse of the rectum through the anus, particularly when the host strains during a bowel movement.

DIAGNOSIS

Stools examined for characteristic eggs

In light infections, stool concentration methods may be required to recover the eggs. Such procedures are almost never necessary in symptomatic infections, because they produce more than enough eggs per gram of feces to be readily detected by examining 1 to 2 mg of emulsified stool with the low-power lens of a microscope (Figure 54–3C). Unlike enterobiasis, a moderate eosinophilia is common in heavy *Trichuris* infections, presumably because the adults have anchored themselves within the colonic mucosa, thus presenting antigens to the gut-associated lymphatic tissue (GALT) and triggering an eosinophilic response.

TREATMENT AND PREVENTION

* Treatment effective

* Prevention via sanitation

Albendazole or mebendazole may be used; albendazole may have slightly superior efficacy, perhaps because it is absorbed into the bloodstream and thus reaches the worm's head where it is buried in the gut wall. Although the full microbiologic cure rate is less than perfect, more than 90% of adult worms are usually expelled with treatment, rendering the patient asymptomatic. Prevention requires the improvement of sanitary facilities, both for waste disposal and hand hygiene, and improved washing or cooking of contaminated fruits and vegetables.

ASCARIS

ASCARIS LUMBRICOIDES: PARASITOLOGY

Earthworm-sized roundworm produces elliptical eggs

Viable in soil 6 years

A lumbricoides, a short-lived worm (6-18 months), is the largest and most common of the intestinal helminths. Measuring 15 to 30 cm in length, it dwarfs its fellow gut roundworms. Its firm, creamy cuticle and more pointed extremities differentiate it from the common earthworm, which it otherwise resembles in both size and external morphology. The male is slightly smaller than the female and possesses a curved tail with copulatory spicules. The female passes 200,000 eggs daily, whether or not she is fertilized. Eggs are elliptical, measure 35 by 55 µm, and have a rough, mammillated, albuminous coat over their chitinous shells (**Figure 54–6**). These eggs are highly resistant to environmental conditions and may remain viable for up to 6 years in mild climates.

FIGURE 54–6. *Ascaris lumbricoides.* **A.** Structure of fertile and infertile egg. **B.** Fertilized egg in stool. **C.** Adult female worm. (B, Reproduced with permission from Connor DH, Chandler FW, Schwartz DQ, et al: *Pathology of Infectious Diseases.* Stamford CT: Appleton & Lange; 1997.)

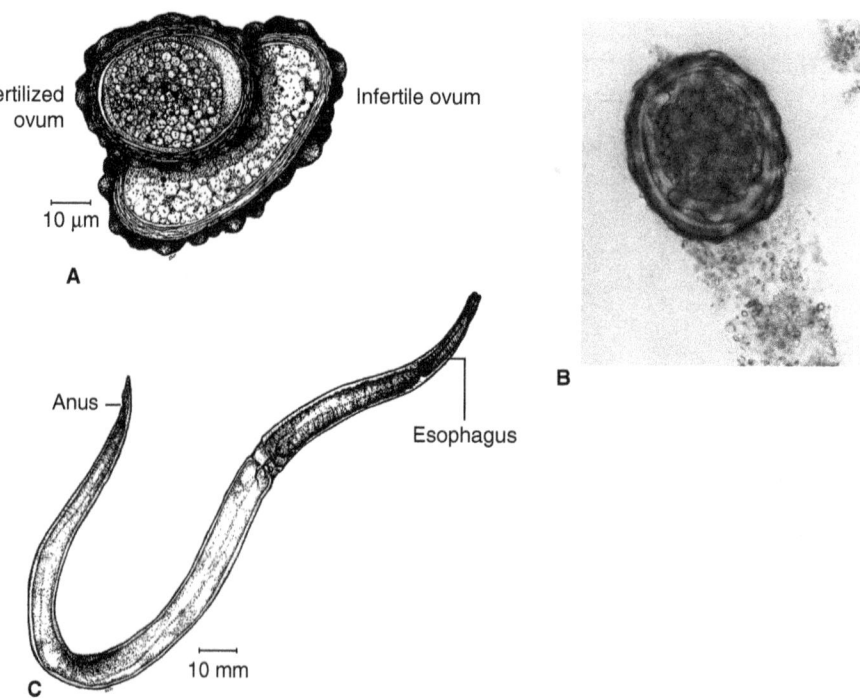

LIFE CYCLE (FIGURE 54–7)

The adult ascarids live high in the small intestine, where they actively maintain their position not by burrowing into the mucosa, but rather by sheer strength of muscular activity, swimming against the stream of stool to avoid being expelled. The eggs are deposited into the intestinal lumen and passed in the feces. Like those of *Trichuris*, the eggs must embryonate in soil, usually for a minimum of 3 weeks, before becoming infectious. And, like *Trichuris*, the eggs of *Ascaris* must be ingested, but the similarity to *Trichuris* ends after ingestion. Once they hatch in the intestines, *Ascaris* larvae penetrate the intestinal mucosa and invade the portal venules. They are carried to the liver, where they are still small enough to squeeze through that organ's capillaries and exit in the hepatic vein. They are then carried to the right side of the heart and pumped out to the lung. By the time they reach the pulmonary capillaries, they are too large to pass through to the left side of the heart. Finding their route blocked, they rupture into the alveolar spaces, are coughed up, and subsequently swallowed. After regaining access to the upper intestine, they complete their maturation and mate. Their reasons for making this circuitous journey are unknown, although the high oxygen tension in the alveoli may provide a growth advantage.

Adults inhabit small intestine

Eggs mature 3 weeks in soil

✳ Complexity: larvae enter blood, pass through alveoli, respiratory tract, esophagus to intestines

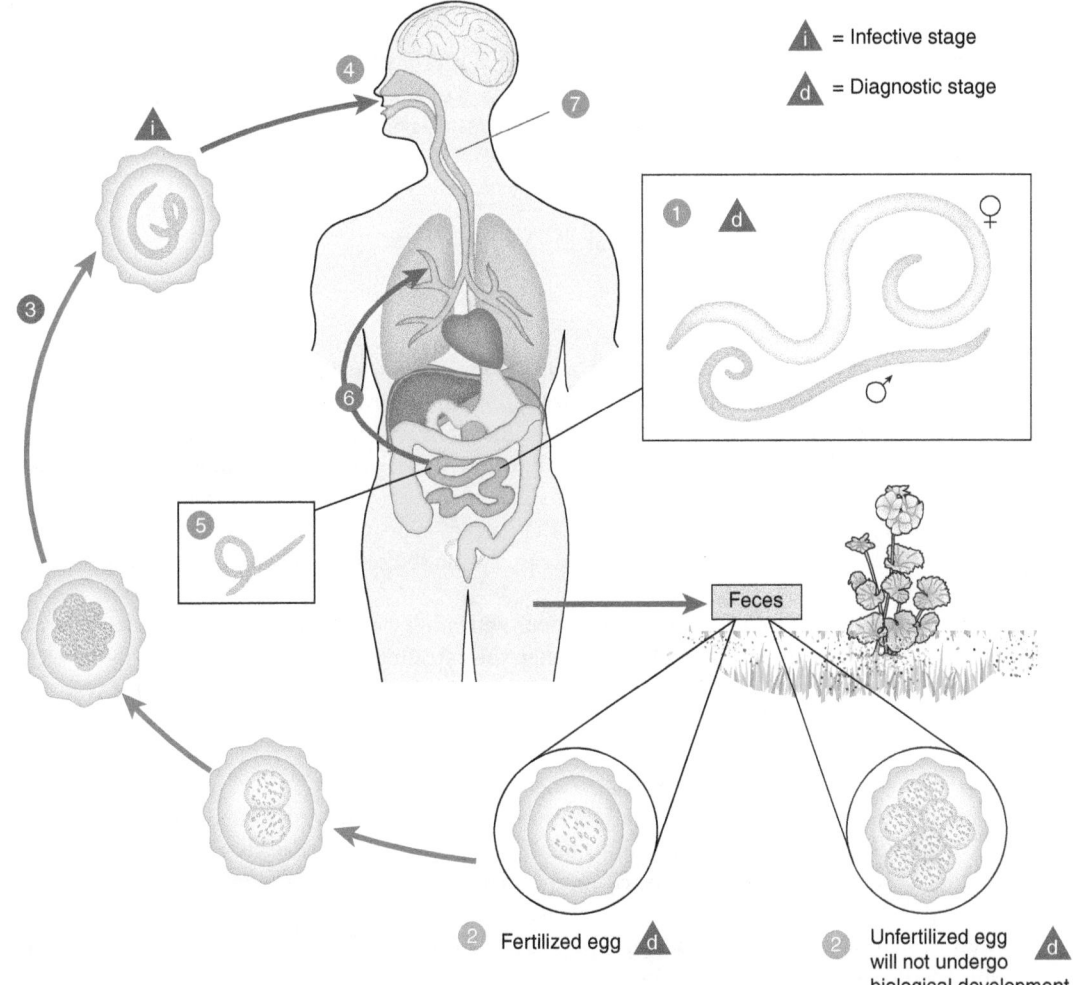

Adult worms ① live in the lumen of the small intestine. A female may produce approximately 200,000 eggs per day, which are passed with the feces ②. Unfertilized eggs may be ingested but are not infective. Fertile eggs embryonate and become infective after 18 days to several weeks ③, depending on the environmental conditions (optimum: moist, warm, shaded soil). After infective eggs are swallowed ④, the larvae hatch ⑤, invade the intestinal mucosa, and are carried via the portal, then systemic circulation to the lungs ⑥. The larvae mature further in the lungs (10-14 days), penetrate the alveolar walls, ascend the bronchial tree to the throat, and are swallowed ⑦. Upon reaching the small intestine, they develop into adult worms ①. Between 2 and 3 months are required from ingestion of the infective eggs to oviposition by the adult female. Adult worms can live for 1 to 2 years.

FIGURE 54–7. *Ascaris lumbricoides* **life cycle.**

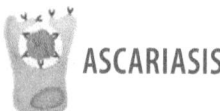

ASCARIASIS

EPIDEMIOLOGY

Epidemiology similar to *Trichuris*

More than 1 billion of the world's population, including millions of Americans, are infected with *A lumbricoides*. Together they have been estimated to pass tons of *Ascaris* eggs into the environment annually. Like trichuriasis, with which it often coexists, ascariasis is a disease of warm climates and poor sanitation. It may be maintained by small children who defecate in the immediate vicinity of the home and pick up infectious eggs on their hands during play, and by adults who consume contaminated uncooked vegetables. In dry, windy climates, eggs may become airborne and then inhaled and swallowed. In tropical areas, the entire population may be involved; most worms, however, appear to be aggregated in a minority of the population, suggesting that some "wormy persons" are predisposed to heavy infections for reasons unknown. Isolated infected family clusters are more common in temperate climates.

PATHOGENESIS AND IMMUNITY

✱ **Hypersensitivity to larval migration**

There is evidence that ascariasis induces a partially protective immune response in the host. Moreover, the severity of pulmonary damage induced by the migration of larvae through the lung appears to be related in part to an immediate hypersensitivity reaction to larval antigens.

ASCARIASIS: CLINICAL ASPECTS

MANIFESTATIONS

Clinical manifestations of ascariasis may result from larvae when they migrate through the lung or from adults in the intestinal lumen. During migration through the lungs, larvae may induce fever, cough, wheezing, and shortness of breath. Laboratory studies may reveal eosinophilia, oxygen desaturation, and migratory pulmonary infiltrates. This syndrome is sometimes called Loeffler's syndrome. The severity of these symptoms related to the degree of hypersensitivity induced by previous infections and the intensity of the current exposure. Death from respiratory failure has been noted occasionally, but this is a rare exception to the rule of spontaneous improvement in most patients.

Asymptomatic with small worm loads

✱ **Larval migration through lungs mimics pneumonia**

✱ **Malabsorption, occasional obstruction with heavy adult worm loads**

If the worm load is small, intestinal infections with adult worms may be completely asymptomatic. They often come to clinical attention when the parasite is vomited up or passed in the stool. This situation is most likely during episodes of fever due to other causes, which appear to stimulate the worms to increase motility. Many physicians who have worked in highly endemic regions have had the disconcerting experience of observing an ascarid crawl out of a patient's mouth or nose during an otherwise uneventful evaluation of fever. Occasionally, an adult worm may migrate to the appendix, bile duct, or pancreatic duct, causing obstruction and inflammation of the organ. After intestinal surgery, adults may migrate through the surgical anastomosis and into the peritoneum, causing peritonitis. Heavy worm loads may produce abdominal pain and malabsorption of fat, protein, carbohydrate, and vitamins. The overall growth of marginally nourished children may be restricted. Occasionally, a bolus of worms may form and cause intestinal obstruction, particularly in young children (**Figure 54–8**). Worm loads of 50 are not uncommon, although 2000 worms have been recovered from a single child. WHO estimates 60,000 may die from ascariasis annually worldwide.

DIAGNOSIS

Stool reveals characteristic eggs

When it happens, the passage of an adult worm makes the diagnosis easy. Otherwise, ascariasis is generally confirmed by finding its characteristic eggs (Figure 54–7B) in feces. The extreme productivity of the female ascarid generally makes this easy, except when atypical-appearing unfertilized eggs predominate. The pulmonary phase of ascariasis is diagnosed by the finding of larvae and eosinophils in the sputum.

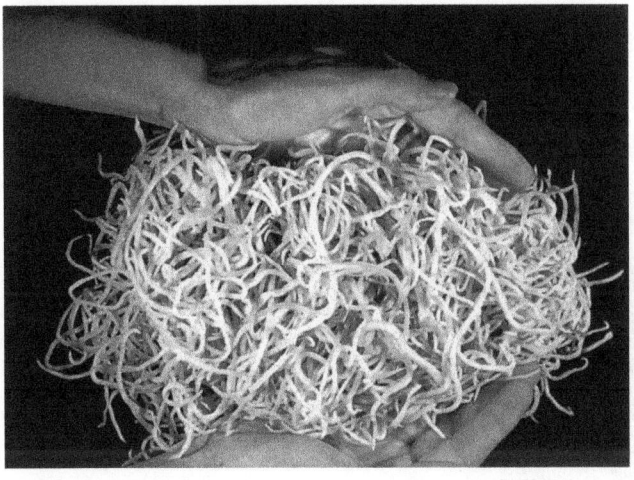

FIGURE 54-8. Ascariasis intestinal obstruction. Mass of adult worms recovered from infant at autopsy. (Reproduced with permission from Connor DH, Chandler FW, Schwartz DQ, et al: *Pathology of Infectious Diseases.* Stamford CT: Appleton & Lange; 1997.)

TREATMENT AND PREVENTION

Albendazole, mebendazole, and pyrantel pamoate are highly effective; albendazole is preferred when *T trichiura* is also present, which happens commonly. Community-wide control of ascariasis can be achieved with mass drug administration every 6 months. Ultimately, durable control requires adequate sanitation facilities.

✳ Prevention via sanitation

 Why do we not expect eosinophilia in patients with longstanding infection with adult ascaris worms?

HOOKWORMS

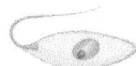 ## *ANCYLOSTOMA* AND *NECATOR*: PARASITOLOGY

Two species, *Necator americanus* and *A duodenale*, infect humans. Adults of both species are pinkish-white and measure about 10 mm in length (**Figure 54–9**). The head is often curved in a direction opposite to that of the body, giving these worms the hooked appearance from which their common name is derived. The males have a unique fan-shaped copulatory bursa, rather than the curved, pointed tail common to the other intestinal nematodes. The two species can be readily differentiated by the morphology of their oral cavity. *A duodenale* possesses four sharp tooth-like structures, whereas *N americanus* has dorsal and ventral cutting plates. With the aid of these structures, the hookworms attach to the mucosa of the small bowel and suck minute quantities of blood. The fertilized female releases 10,000 to 20,000 eggs daily. They measure 40 by 60 μm, possess a thin shell, and are usually in the two- to eight-cell stage when passed in the feces (Figure 54–9A).

N americanus, A duodenale infect humans

Oral cavity morphology distinctive

LIFE CYCLE (FIGURE 54–10)

The life cycles of the two hookworms, *N americanus* and *A duodenale*, are identical. Adults live attached to the small bowel mucosa, where they suck blood, mate, and shed eggs. The eggs are passed in the feces at the four- to eight-cell stage of development. On reaching soil, the eggs hatch within 48 hours, releasing microscopic **rhabditiform larvae**. These move actively through the surface layers of soil, feeding on bacteria and debris. After doubling in size, they molt to become infective **filariform larvae**, which may survive in moist conditions without feeding, for

 Think ▸▸ Apply 54-1: Although the larvae may trigger short-term eosinophilia when they transit the lungs, adult worms live in the patient's gut lumen, where they are relatively shielded from the immune system.

FIGURE 54–9. **Necator americanus. A.** Structure of hookworm egg in stool. **B.** Structure of female adult hookworm.

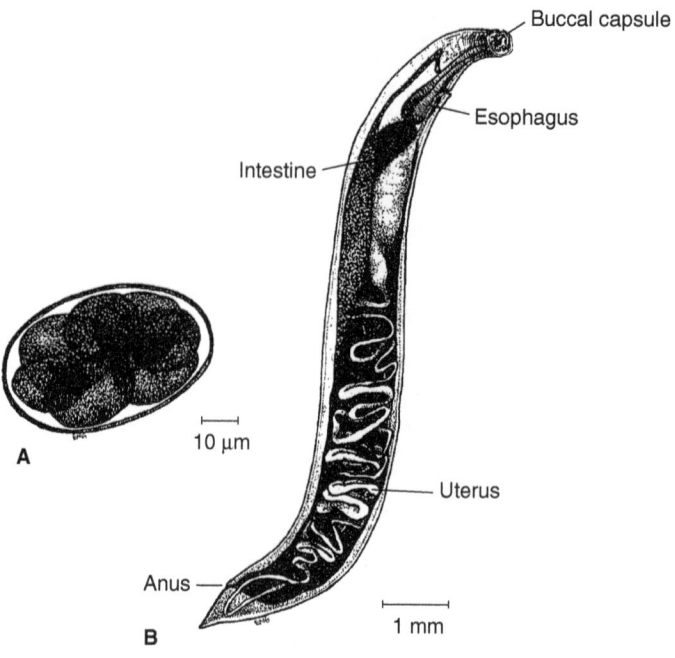

FIGURE 54–10. **Hookworm life cycle.**

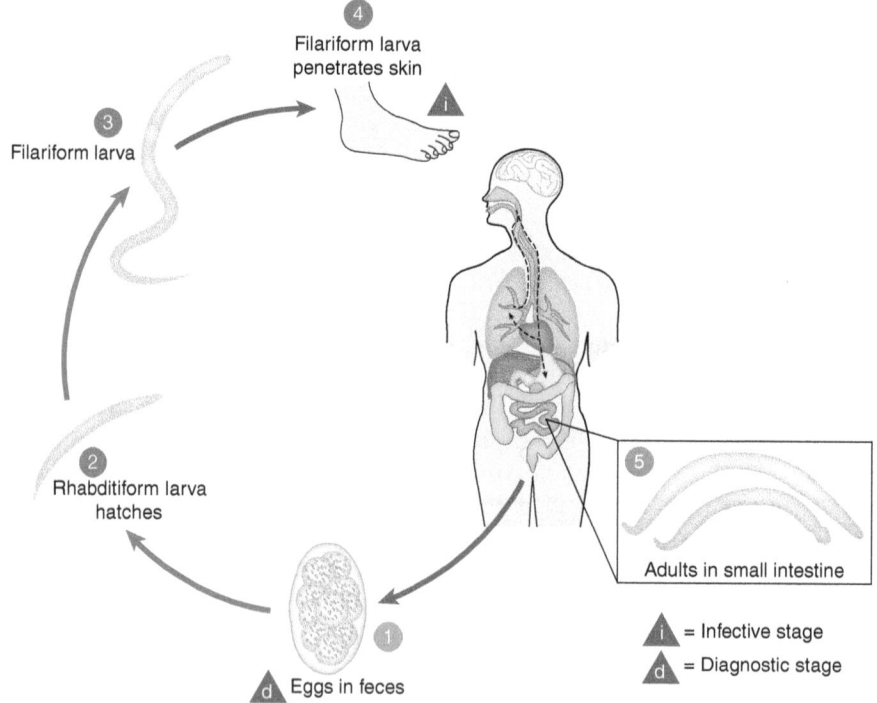

Eggs are passed in the stool ①, and under favorable conditions (moisture, warmth, shade), larvae hatch in 1 to 2 days. The released rhabditiform larvae grow in the feces and/or the soil ②, and after 5 to 10 days (and two molts) they become filariform (third-stage) larvae that are infective ③. These infective larvae can survive 3 to 4 weeks in favorable environmental conditions. On contact with the human host, the larvae penetrate the skin and are carried through the blood vessels to the heart and then to the lungs. They penetrate into the pulmonary alveoli, ascend the bronchial tree to the pharynx, and are swallowed ④. The larvae reach the small Intestine, where they reside and mature into adults. Adult worms live in the lumen of the small intestine, where they attach to the intestinal wall with resultant blood loss by the host ⑤. Most adult worms are eliminated in 1 to 2 years, but the longevity may reach several years. Some *A duodenale* larvae, following penetration of the host skin, can become dormant (in the intestine or muscle). In addition, infection by *A duodenale* may probably also occur by the oral and transmammary route. *Necator americanus*, however, requires a transpulmonary migration phase.

up to 6 weeks. On contact with human skin, these hookworms penetrate the epidermis, reach the lymphohematogenous system, and are passively transported to the right side of the heart and onward to the lungs. Here, like juvenile ascarids, they develop and ultimately rupture into alveolar spaces, are coughed up, swallowed, and pass into the small intestine, where they mature into adults.

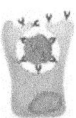

HOOKWORM DISEASE

EPIDEMIOLOGY

Hookworm transmission requires deposition of egg-containing feces on shady, well-drained soil; development of larvae under conditions of abundant rainfall and high temperatures (23-33°C); and direct contact of unprotected human skin with filariform larvae. Infections become particularly intense in closed, densely populated communities, such as tea and coffee plantations. *Necator americanus* is found in the tropical areas of South Asia, Africa, and America, as well as the southern United States. *A duodenale* is seen in the Mediterranean basin, the Middle East, northern India, China, and Japan. It has been estimated that together these two worms may cause 50,000 to 60,000 deaths annually, and extract over 1 million liters of blood each day from 700 million people scattered around the globe, including hundreds of thousands in the United States.

PATHOGENESIS AND IMMUNITY

Each adult *A duodenale* extracts 0.2 mL of blood daily, *N americanus* 0.03 mL of blood. Additional blood loss may be related to the worms' tendency to migrate within the intestine, leaving bleeding points at old sites of attachment. Because the adults may survive 2 to 14 years, the accumulated blood loss in heavy infections may be substantial, especially in patients with other reasons for iron deficiency. Infection elicits both a humoral antibody response and immediate hypersensitivity reaction in the host, but evidence that these influence the infection is lacking. Eosinophils in the blood and gut may play a role in the destruction of worms and/or modulation of the immediate hypersensitivity reaction.

HOOKWORM DISEASE: CLINICAL ASPECTS

MANIFESTATIONS

In most patients infected with hookworms, the adult worm burden is small and the infection asymptomatic. Clinical manifestations, when they do occur, may be related to the penetration of the skin by the filariform larvae, the migration of the larvae through the lung, and/or the presence of adult worms in the gut. Skin penetration may produce a pruritic erythematous rash and swelling, known as "ground itch." This manifestation is more common in infection with *N americanus*, and happens on any skin that has come into contact with the ground, generally occurs between the toes or on the ankle, and may persist for days before resolving spontaneously.

Pulmonary manifestations of hookworm disease may mimic those seen in ascariasis, but are generally less frequent and less severe. In the gut, the adult worm may produce epigastric pain and abnormal peristalsis. The major manifestations, however, are the result of chronic blood loss: anemia and hypoalbuminemia. The severity of the anemia depends on the worm burden, other concurrent causes of blood loss such as menses, and the intake of dietary iron. If iron intake exceeds iron loss resulting from hookworm infection, a normal hemoglobin will be maintained. Commonly, however, dietary iron is ingested in a form that is poorly absorbed. As a result, severe anemia may develop over a period of months or years. In children, this condition may precipitate heart failure or kwashiorkor. Neurocognitive and physical development may be impacted.

DIAGNOSIS

The diagnosis of hookworm disease is made by examining direct or concentrated stool specimens for the distinctive eggs (Figure 54–9A). Because these eggs are nearly identical in the two species and because treatment of both species is the same, precise identification of the causative worm is not important. Quantitative egg counts permit estimation of worm load, information of epidemiological rather than clinical use. If the stool is allowed to stand too long before it is examined, the

---

Margin notes:

✳ Complexity: Filariform larvae penetrate skin and then follow same path as *Ascaris* larvae to gut

Larvae require hot, moist conditions, human skin

Limited to tropical areas, southern United States.

Adults live in gut for years

✳ Blood loss in heavy infections

Peripheral and gut eosinophilia

✳ Asymptomatic depending on worm load

✳ Pruritus, rash at skin penetration site

Iron-deficiency anemia caused by blood loss from intestinal worms

✳ Diagnose by eggs in human stool

Eggs of both look the same

eggs may hatch, releasing rhabditiform larvae. These larvae closely resemble those of *S stercoralis* and must be differentiated from them (see below).

TREATMENT AND PREVENTION

✳ **Treatment highly effective**

✳ **Prevention via improved sanitation**

The anemia must be corrected. When it is mild or moderate, iron replacement is adequate. More severe anemia may require blood transfusions. The three most widely used anthelmintic agents, albendazole, mebendazole, and pyrantel pamoate are all highly effective. As with *Trichuris* and *Ascaris*, prevention of hookworm infection requires improved sanitation. However, an additional prevention benefit may be afforded by wearing shoes, because this provides defense against skin invasion by filariform larvae. Attempts to develop effective vaccines against human hookworm infection have not yet borne fruit.

STRONGYLOIDES

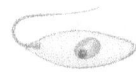 ## *STRONGYLOIDES STERCORALIS*: PARASITOLOGY

S stercoralis has the most complex life cycle of all the intestinal nematodes—and the greatest risk of life-threatening, overwhelming infection. The adults measure only 2 mm in length, making them the smallest of the intestinal nematodes. The male is seldom seen within the human host, suggesting that the female can conceive parthenogenetically in this environment. Strongyloides eggs are not diagnostically important because they usually hatch within the intestinal wall, releasing microscopic rhabditiform larvae. These larvae then develop into larger infectious filariform larvae. These larvae, which measure about 16 by 200 μm, can be distinguished from the similar larval stage of the hookworms by their short buccal cavity and large genital primordium (**Figure 54–11**).

LIFE CYCLE (FIGURE 54–12)

Three different life cycles have been described for the *Strongyloides* nematode. The first, or **direct cycle**, is similar to that observed with the hookworms. Adult females live in the small intestinal mucosa, where they lay eggs. These eggs often hatch within the intestinal tissue, releasing

FIGURE   54–11. *Strongyloides stercoralis*. A–C. Structure of rhabditiform larvae, filariform larvae, and adult worm. **D.** Filariform larvae (arrow) in lung surrounded by fibrin and inflammatory cells. (D, Reproduced with permission from Connor DH, Chandler FW, Schwartz DQ, et al: *Pathology of Infectious Diseases*. Stamford CT: Appleton & Lange; 1997.)

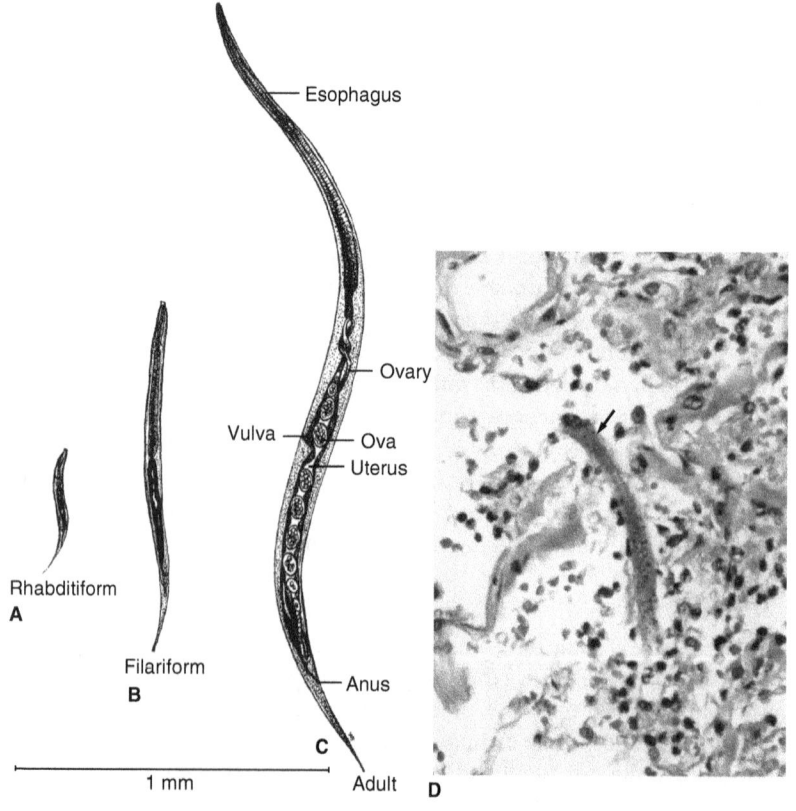

Esophagus

Rhabditiform
A

Filariform
B

Vulva

Ovary

Ova
Uterus

Anus

C

1 mm

Adult   **D**

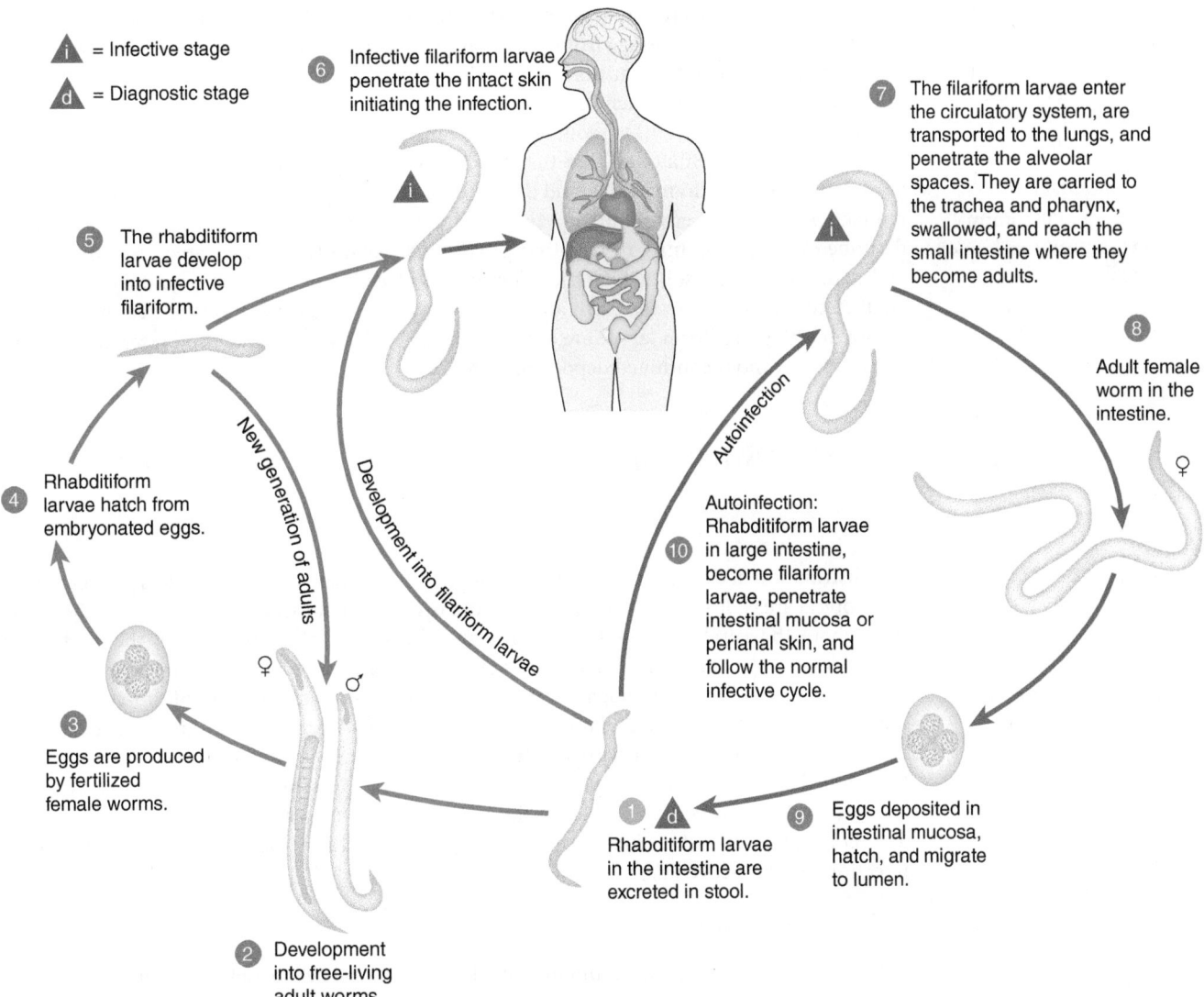

i = Infective stage

d = Diagnostic stage

⑥ Infective filariform larvae penetrate the intact skin initiating the infection.

⑤ The rhabditiform larvae develop into infective filariform.

④ Rhabditiform larvae hatch from embryonated eggs.

③ Eggs are produced by fertilized female worms.

② Development into free-living adult worms.

New generation of adults

Development into filariform larvae

⑦ The filariform larvae enter the circulatory system, are transported to the lungs, and penetrate the alveolar spaces. They are carried to the trachea and pharynx, swallowed, and reach the small intestine where they become adults.

⑧ Adult female worm in the intestine.

Autoinfection

⑩ Autoinfection: Rhabditiform larvae in large intestine, become filariform larvae, penetrate intestinal mucosa or perianal skin, and follow the normal infective cycle.

① **d** Rhabditiform larvae in the intestine are excreted in stool.

⑨ Eggs deposited in intestinal mucosa, hatch, and migrate to lumen.

The *Strongyloides* life cycle is more complex than that of most nematodes with its alternation between free-living and parasitic cycles, and its potential for autoinfection and multiplication within the host. Two types of cycles exist:

Free-living cycle: The rhabditiform larvae passed in the stool ① (see "Parasitic cycle" below) can either molt twice and become infective filariform larvae (direct development) ⑥ or molt four times and become free-living adult males and females ② that mate and produce eggs ③ from which rhabditiform larvae hatch ④. The latter in turn can either develop ⑤ into a new generation of free-living adults (as represented in ②), or into infective filariform larvae ⑥. The filariform larvae penetrate the human host skin to initiate the parasitic cycle (see below) ⑥.

Parasitic cycle: Filariform larvae in contaminated soil penetrate the human skin ⑥, and are transported to the lungs where they penetrate the alveolar spaces; they are carried through the bronchial tree to the pharynx, are swallowed and then reach the small intestine ⑦. In the small intestine they molt twice and become adult female worms ⑧. The females live threaded in the epithelium of the small intestine and by parthenogenesis produce eggs ⑨, which yield rhabditiform larvae. The rhabditiform larvae can either be passed in the stool ① (see "Free-living cycle" above), or can cause autoinfection ⑩. In autoinfection, the rhabditiform larvae become infective filariform larvae, which can penetrate either the intestinal mucosa (internal autoinfection) or the skin of the perianal area (external autoinfection); in either case, the filariform larvae may follow the previously described route, being carried successively to the lungs, the bronchial tree, the pharynx, and the small intestine where they mature into adults; or they may disseminate widely in the body. To date, occurrence of autoinfection in humans with helminthic infections is recognized only in *Strongyloides stercoralis* and *Capillaria philippinensis* infections. In the case of *Strongyloides*, autoinfection may explain the possibility of persistent infections for many years in persons who have not been in an endemic area and of hyperinfections in immunodepressed individuals.

FIGURE 54-12. *Strongyloides* **life cycle.**

rhabditiform larvae that work their way out to the gastrointestinal (GI) lumen. After these larvae are passed in the stool, they molt in the soil to become larger, infectious filariform larvae, which can penetrate human skin just like hookworms—or be ingested on soil-contaminated food. After transport from the skin to the lung (Figure 54–11D) via the vascular system, they are coughed up and swallowed, then mature into adults in the small bowel. In the second, or **autoinfective cycle**, the rhabditiform larva's passage from the colon to the outside world is delayed by constipation or other factors, allowing it to transform into an infective filariform larva while still within the body of its host. This larva may then invade the internal mucosa (internal autoinfection) or perianal skin (external autoinfection) without an intervening soil phase. Thus, S stercoralis—unlike any of the other intestinal nematodes—has the capacity to multiply within the human body. The worm burden may increase dramatically, and the infection may persist indefinitely, without the need for reinfection from the environment—and with potentially dire consequences to the host, as described later. In the third, or **free-living cycle**, the rhabditiform larvae are passed in the stool and deposited on the soil, where they develop into free-living adult males and females. These adults feed on bacteria in the earth and may propagate several generations of free-living worms before infective filariform larvae are again produced. This cycle creates a soil reservoir that may persist even without continued deposition of feces.

* Complexity: direct cycle resembles hookworm, except larvae develop in human gut

* Further complexity: development of filariform stage in gut produces human autoinfection

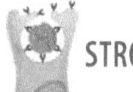

STRONGYLOIDIASIS

EPIDEMIOLOGY

The distribution of S stercoralis parallels that of the hookworms, although it is less prevalent in all but tropical areas. It infects 90 million individuals worldwide, including hundreds of thousands throughout the rural areas of Puerto Rico and the southeastern sections of the continental United States. Like hookworm infection, S stercoralis is generally acquired by direct contact of skin with soil-dwelling larvae, although infection may also follow ingestion of filariform-contaminated food. Transformation of the rhabditiform larvae to the filariform stage within the gut can result in seeding of the perianal area with infectious organisms. These larvae may continue to autoinfect the original host over and over again for years or decades. Thus, individuals who currently reside in low-prevalence areas may still harbor the infection long after leaving highly endemic regions—an epidemiological factor that separates strongyloidiasis from the other intestinal nematode infections we have covered.

Like hookworm but may persist for years in travelers and migrants

PATHOGENESIS AND IMMUNITY

Invasion of the intestinal epithelium may accelerate epithelial cell turnover, alter intestinal motility, and induce acute and chronic inflammatory lesions, ulcerations, and abscess formation, all of which may play a role in the malabsorptive syndrome that frequently characterizes clinical disease. Steroid- or malnutrition-related immunosuppression of the GALT appears to accelerate the metamorphosis of rhabditiform to filariform larvae within the bowel lumen, enhancing the frequency and intensity of autoinfection. T lymphocytes are important for maintaining control of auto-infection, although in many cases the immune system is unable to permanently clear the infection. and so the loss of T-lymphocyte function may trigger catastrophic hyperinfection.

Damage may cause malabsorption

* Immunosuppression enhances autoinfection by accelerating larval development

STRONGYLOIDIASIS: CLINICAL ASPECTS

MANIFESTATIONS

Patients with strongyloidiasis often have no symptoms at all. They may present with a history of "ground itch," or with the pulmonary disease seen in both ascariasis and, less often, in hookworm infection. The intestinal infection itself is usually asymptomatic. With heavy worm loads, however, the patient may complain of epigastric pain and tenderness, often aggravated by eating. In fact, peptic ulcer-like pain associated with peripheral eosinophilia strongly suggests strongyloidiasis. In severe infections, the biliary and pancreatic ducts, the entire small bowel, and the colon may be involved. With widespread involvement of the intestinal mucosa, vomiting, diarrhea, paralytic ileus, and malabsorption may be seen.

Pulmonary, intestinal manifestations like hookworm, Ascaris

Sometimes, rhabditiform larvae remain on the perianal skin after a bowel movement, and develop into infectious filariform larvae which penetrate the skin and continue the life cycle. This external autoinfection produces transient, raised, red, serpiginous lesions over the buttocks, abdomen, and lower back caused by larval invasion of the perianal area, called **larva currens**. If the patient is not treated, these lesions may recur at irregular intervals over a period of decades; they are particularly common after recovery from a febrile illness. Over 25% of British and American servicemen imprisoned in Southeast Asia during World War II continued to demonstrate such lesions before diagnosis and treatment some 40 years after exposure.

Massive **hyperinfection** with strongyloidiasis may occur in immunosuppressed patients, especially in those receiving glucocorticoid therapy, which reduces the GALT's T-lymphocyte–mediated cellular immune response that usually keeps *Strongyloides* under control. Because the original infection may have happened years earlier, and because autoinfection is often asymptomatic, patients and physicians often fail to appreciate the presence of these infections. This can have catastrophic consequences if immunosuppressive medications are initiated before the infection is cured. In these tragic cases of hyperinfection, larvae cause severe enterocolitis and disseminate throughout the body to organs including the heart, lungs, and central nervous system. The larvae may carry enteric bacteria with them, producing Gram-negative bacteremia and occasionally Gram-negative meningitis that may result in death. Surprisingly, this phenomenon has been unusual in patients with acquired immunodeficiency syndrome (AIDS), even in areas where strongyloidiasis is highly endemic. Immunodeficiency due to another retrovirus, human T-lymphotropic virus-1 (HTLV-1), has a stronger association with *Strongyloides* hyperinfection.

DIAGNOSIS

The diagnosis of strongyloidiasis is sometimes made by finding rhabditiform larvae in the stool. Preferably, only fresh specimens should be examined to avoid the confusion induced by the hatching of hookworm eggs with the release of their look-alike larvae. The number of larvae passed in the stool varies from day to day, often requiring the examination of several specimens before the diagnosis of strongyloidiasis can be made. When absent from the stool, larvae may sometimes be found in duodenal aspirates or jejunal biopsy specimens. If the pulmonary system is involved, the sputum should be examined for the presence of larvae. Agar plate culture methods may recover organisms that go undetected by microscopic examination. Diagnosing autoinfection is best accomplished with a blood test: serology via enzyme-linked immunosorbent assays for antibodies to excretory–secretory or somatic antigens is the preferred method, because rhabditiform larvae are challenging to detect in stool. Serology carries a strong positive predictive value. Unfortunately, serology's negative predictive value is less reliable. On the other hand, during hyperinfection time is of the essence and a more rapid and reliable technique is essential. Fresh and stained specimens from the sputum or bronchoalveolar fluid should be inspected with a microscope, because these may teem with filariform larvae. Whereas eosinophilia is common in autoinfection, it is usually *absent* in hyperinfection; indeed, it is the lack of these cells that seems to predispose patients to hyperinfection in the first place.

TREATMENT AND PREVENTION

All infected patients should be treated to prevent the buildup of the worm burden by autoinfection and the serious consequences of hyperinfection. The drug of choice for uncomplicated strongyloidiasis is two doses of oral ivermectin, another contrast with the other intestinal nematodes which respond best to albendazole. In strongyloides hyperinfection syndrome, supportive treatment and antibacterials are essential to address sepsis; ivermectin therapy must be extended for at least 1 week, and potentially as long as 6 months, if the underlying immunosuppression cannot be removed. The cure rate is less than 100%, and stools should be checked after therapy to see whether retreatment is indicated. Patients who have resided in an endemic area at any time in their lives should be assessed for *S stercoralis* both before corticosteroid treatment or immunosuppressive therapy. Medical personnel caring for patients with hyperinfection syndromes should wear gowns and gloves because stool, saliva, vomitus, and body fluids may contain infectious filariform larvae.

Autoinfection lesions over buttocks, abdomen, back

✻ May persist for decades

✻ Hyperinfection in immunosuppressed, uncommon in AIDS

✻ Rule out strongyloidiasis before immunosuppression

✻ Subclinical autoinfection: serology, eosinophilia, rhabditiform larvae in stool or duodenal aspirates

✻ Symptomatic or hyperinfection: filariform larvae in sputum, no eosinophilia

✻ Treat autoinfection to prevent hyperinfection

✻ Outcomes poor in hyperinfection

 Which of the gastrointestinal helminth infections described earlier could be prevented with improved disposal of human waste?

KEY CONCLUSIONS

- Embryonation in the soil is a common theme for most of these worms.
- Gastrointestinal helminths are usually well tolerated by the human host.
- Some have larvae that migrate through tissue, causing temporary side effects.
- Symptoms caused by adults in the gut increase with the number of adult worms: a handful of adults are usually harmless, whereas hundreds may cause true illness.
- Of the common GI helminths discussed here, only strongyloides may persist in the human host indefinitely.
- Infections with all the GI helminths can be treated medically.

CASE STUDY

A Worm in the Throat!

This 4-year-old boy, who resides in the rural Southeastern United States, likes to play barefooted in the summer. He is brought to the physician's office with a 3-day history of fever, cough, and mild wheezing. On initial examination, the physician is startled to observe two small worm-like objects in the posterior oropharynx.

QUESTIONS

1. Which of the following is the LEAST likely cause?
   A. *Ascaris*
   B. *Trichuris*
   C. *Necator*
   D. *Ancylostoma*

2. Stool examination is the usual initial diagnostic approach in all of the following, EXCEPT:
   A. *Enterobius*
   B. *Trichuris*
   C. *Ascaris*
   D. *Necator*

3. Which of the following can multiply within the human host (autoinfection)?
   A. *Ascaris*
   B. *Ancylostoma*
   C. *Trichuris*
   D. *Strongyloides*

ANSWERS

1. **(B)**

2. **(A)**

3. **(D)**

 Think ▸▸ Apply 54-2: **All except for enterobiasis, which is usually spread directly from anus to hand to mouth. The others involve transmission via feces deposited on the ground.**

chapter 55

Tissue Nematodes

Toxocara canis • Baylisascaris procyonis • Trichinella spiralis • Ancylostoma braziliense • Wuchereria bancrofti •

Brugia malayi • Onchocerca volvulus • Loa Loa • Dracunculus medinensis

> *The message is not so much that the worms will inherit the Earth, but that all things play a role in nature, even the lowly worm.*
>
> —Gary Larson

OVERVIEW

The nematodes discussed in this chapter cause disease through their presence in the tissues and lymphohematogenous system of the human body. Some migrate through the human gastrointestinal tract on their way there, but because this is a temporary part of their life cycle, they are not considered to be "intestinal" nematodes.

Four of them—*Toxocara canis, Baylisascaris procyonis, Trichinella spiralis,* and *Ancylostoma braziliense*—are **zoonotic**, meaning natural parasites of domestic and wild animals. Although they are capable of infecting humans, they cannot complete their life cycle in the human host. Humans, therefore, serve only as "accidental hosts," injured bystanders rather than major participants in the life cycle of these parasites.

The remaining four major tissue nematodes—*Wuchereria bancrofti, Brugia malayi, Onchocerca volvulus,* and *Loa loa*—are members of a single superfamily (Filarioidea). All are **anthroponotic**, meaning they use humans as their definitive host. The thin, thread-like adults live for years in the subcutaneous tissues and lymphatic vessels, where they discharge their live-born offspring called "microfilariae." These progeny circulate in the blood or migrate in the subcutaneous tissues until they are ingested by a specific blood-sucking insect. Within this insect, they transform into filariform larvae capable of infecting another human when the vector again takes a blood meal. We will also touch briefly on *Dracunculus medinensis,* the guinea worm, which is on the verge of eradication.

Table 55–1 summarizes these nematodes, diseases they cause, their definitive host, and usual routes of human infection.

● TOXOCARA

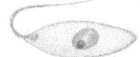 TOXOCARA CANIS: PARASITOLOGY AND LIFE CYCLE (FIGURE 55–1)

T canis is a large intestinal ascarid of canines, including dogs, foxes, and wolves. Occasionally, a related organism found in cats (*Toxocara cati*) can behave in a similar fashion. (Note: Do not confuse this worm with the similar-sounding protozoan *Toxoplasma gondii*. Both derive their name from the Latin root "toxo" meaning "poison" or "harm.") Each female worm discharges approximately 200,000 thick-shelled eggs daily into the fecal stream. After reaching the soil, these eggs embryonate for a minimum of 2 to 3 weeks. Thereafter, the eggs are infectious to canines,

TABLE 55–1	General Characteristics of Tissue Nematodes		
PARASITE	**DISEASE**	**NATURAL DEFINITIVE HOST**	**USUAL SOURCE OF HUMAN INFECTION**
Toxocara canis	Toxocariasis (visceral or ocular larva migrans)	Dog	Ingestion of ova from canine stools
Baylisascaris procyonis	Eosinophilic CNS or ocular disease	Raccoon	Ingestion of ova from raccoon stools
Trichinella spiralis	Trichinosis	Pig	Ingestion of improperly cooked pork
Ancylostoma braziliense	Cutaneous larva migrans	Cat	Soil contaminated with dog or cat feces
Wuchereria bancrofti, Brugia malayi	Lymphatic filariasis (elephantiasis)	Human	Mosquito
Onchocerca volvulus	Onchocerciasis (river blindness, dermatitis)	Human	*Simulium* fly
Loa loa (eye worm)	Loiasis (Calabar swellings)	Human	*Chrysops* fly
Dracunculus medinensis (guinea worm)	Dracunculiasis	Human	Drinking water contaminated by *cyclops*

humans, and other mammals that ingest them. The eggs may remain infectious in the soil for months to years. When eaten by a puppy, the larvae exit from the eggshell, penetrate the intestinal mucosa, and migrate through the liver to the right side of the heart and from there to the lung. Here, like the offspring of *Ascaris lumbricoides*, they burst into the alveolar airspaces and are

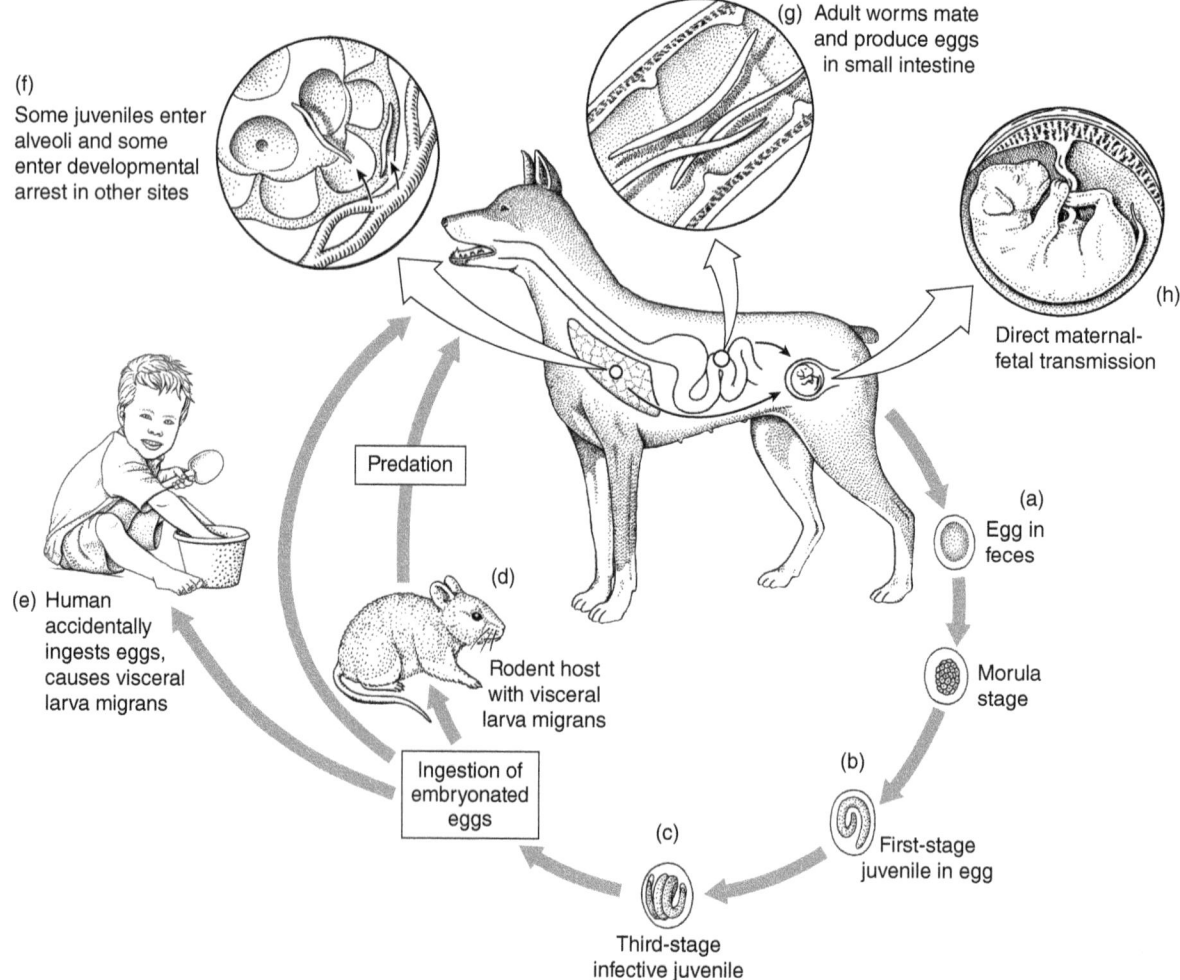

FIGURE 55-1. Life cycle of *Toxocara canis*. (Reproduced with permission from Roberts RL, Janovy J, Nadler S: *Foundations of Parasitology*, 9th ed. New York, NY: McGraw Hill; 2013.)

coughed up and swallowed; thereafter, they mature in the small bowel. However, in fully grown dogs, the life cycle is different: most of the migrating larvae pass through the pulmonary capillaries and reach the systemic circulation. These larvae eventually are filtered out and encyst in the dog's tissues, where they lie dormant for months or longer. Hormonal changes and/or diminished immunity in the pregnant female stimulate the larvae to resume development, migrate across the placenta, and infect the unborn pups. Larvae may also pass to the newborn puppies in their mother's milk. Approximately 4 weeks after birth, both the puppies and the lactating mother begin to pass large numbers of eggs in their stools, shed by the adult worms that inhabit their intestinal tract. These eggs embryonate in the soil for 2 to 3 weeks before becoming infectious. The mother may then be superinfected by ingesting the eggs from the soil or eating visceral cysts in an intermediate host such as a rodent.

Cycle in canines resembles ascariasis in humans, but with tissue cysts

✳ Infected puppies, lactating mothers excrete numerous ova

Eggs embryonate in soil

Think of the life cycle of human toxocariasis as the same as human ascariasis, but with a key difference: When humans ingest infectious eggs, the liberated larvae are small enough to pass through the pulmonary capillaries and reach the systemic circulation. Only rarely do larvae break into the alveoli, get coughed up, and swallowed to reach the intestine to mature into adults, which is what happens in human ascariasis. Instead, larvae in the systemic circulation continue to grow there. Thus, humans are intermediate rather than definitive hosts of *T canis*. When their size exceeds the diameter of the vessel through which they are passing, they penetrate its wall and enter the tissue. The larvae induce a T_H2-type CD4+ response characterized by eosinophilia and IgE production.

✳ Transmission to humans by ingestion of eggs in soil

Like ascaris, but larvae invade tissues and encyst instead of returning to GI tract via lung

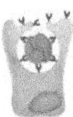

TOXOCARIASIS

EPIDEMIOLOGY

T canis is a cosmopolitan parasite. The infection rate in the 50 million dogs inhabiting the United States is very high; over 80% of puppies and 20% of older animals are parasitized. "Man's best friend" deposits more than 3500 tons of feces daily in the streets, yards, and parks of America, and there is a real health risk. In some areas, between 10% and 30% of soil samples taken from public parks have contained viable *Toxocara* eggs. Moreover, serologic surveys of humans indicate that 4% to 20% of the population has ingested these eggs at some time. The incidence of infection appears to be higher in the Southeastern United States; presumably the warm, humid climate prolongs survival of the eggs, thereby increasing exposure. Indeed, seroprevalence rates of more than 50% have been noted in some developing nations. Puppies in the home increase the risk of infection. Clinical manifestations occur predominantly among children 1 to 6 years of age; many have a history of geophagia, suggesting that disease transmission results from direct ingestion of eggs in the soil. Most infections are subclinical, but the incidence of overt disease is likely underreported.

Eggs deposited soil by domestic dogs

Children often infected

Infection more common than disease

TOXOCARIASIS: CLINICAL ASPECTS

MANIFESTATIONS

The larvae of *Toxocara* that reach the systemic circulation may invade any tissue of the human body, where they can induce necrosis, bleeding, eosinophilic granulomas, and subsequent fibrosis. The liver, lungs, heart, skeletal muscle, brain, and eye are involved most frequently. The severity of clinical manifestations is related to the number and location of these lesions and the degree to which the host has become sensitized to larval antigens. Children with more intense infection may have fever and an enlarged, tender liver. Those who are seriously ill may develop a skin rash, an enlarged spleen, asthma, recurrent pulmonary infiltrates, abdominal pain, sleep and behavioral changes, focal neurologic defects, and seizures. This illness, called "visceral larva migrans," often persists for weeks to months. Death may result from respiratory failure, cardiac arrhythmia, or brain damage. In older children and adults, these systemic manifestations are uncommon, although eye invasion by larvae ("ocular larva migrans") is more common. Typically, unilateral strabismus, loss of red reflex (leukocoria), or decreased visual acuity causes the patient to consult

Any tissue invaded by larvae

✳ Organ invasion causes hypersensitivity

✳ Ocular invasion produces granulomatous endophthalmitis

an ophthalmologist. Examination reveals granulomatous endophthalmitis, a reaction to larvae that are often already dead; it is sometimes mistaken for malignant retinoblastoma, and unnecessary enucleations have been performed.

DIAGNOSIS

* Usually a clinical diagnosis

Serodiagnosis using EIA

Tissue biopsy provides confirmation

Stool examination for eggs is not helpful because the parasite seldom reaches adulthood in humans. A presumptive diagnosis may be made based on the clinical picture: eosinophilic leukocytosis, elevated serum levels of IgE, and elevated antibody titers to blood group antigens, particularly the group A antigen. An enzyme immunoassay (EIA) using larval antigens has been developed, providing clinicians with a reasonable but imperfect negative and positive predictive value. A western blot procedure is somewhat more sensitive but is not widely available. Unfortunately, many patients with related ocular infections remain seronegative; some demonstrate elevated antibody titers within the ocular fluids. Definitive diagnosis requires demonstration of the larva in a liver biopsy specimen or at autopsy.

TREATMENT AND PREVENTION

* Corticosteroids in serious disease

Disposal of pet feces, deworming

Reduction of the exuberant host immune response is the main goal of treatment. Corticosteroid treatment may be lifesaving if the patient has serious pulmonary, myocardial, or central nervous system (CNS) involvement. Anthelmintic therapy using albendazole is often administered after steroids are started, although the efficacy of this drug remains uncertain. Prevention requires control of indiscriminate defecation by dogs and repeated deworming of household pets. Deworming must begin when the animal is 3 weeks of age and should be repeated every 3 months during the first year of life and twice a year thereafter.

● BAYLISASCARIS

* Raccoon roundworm mimics *Toxocara*, but can be lethal

Another nematode that shares clinical and epidemiologic similarities with *Toxocara* has been increasingly recognized. *B procyonis* (raccoon roundworm) has predominantly affected children playing in wooded areas that are frequented by raccoons. Raccoons tend to defecate in dedicated areas called "latrines" which may teem with infective eggs. When these eggs area accidentally ingested, they may cause a disease that mimics toxocariasis. Unfortunately, this organism has a predilection for neural and eye tissue, and can lead to devastating eosinophilic meningoencephalitis and retinitis. The diagnostic and therapeutic approaches are like those for *Toxocara*, but the clinical outcome may be fatal, especially when therapy is delayed.

● TRICHINELLA

TRICHINELLA SPIRALIS: PARASITOLOGY AND LIFE CYCLE

Intestinal parasites of many flesh-eating mammals

Adult *Trichinella* live in the duodenal and jejunal mucosa of carnivores throughout the world, particularly swine, rodents, bears, canines, felines, and marine mammals. Originally thought to be members of a single species, it is now clear that arctic, temperate, and tropical strains of *Trichinella* demonstrate significant epidemiologic and biologic differences, and they have been reclassified into eight distinct species. Only two species, *T spiralis* and the arctic species *T nativa*, display a high level of pathogenicity for humans. (Note: Do not confuse the tissue roundworm *T spiralis* with the similar-sounding protozoan *Trichomonas vaginalis*; both derive their name from the Latin root "trich," meaning "hairy," based on their appearance under the microscope.)

Within the host intestinal tissue, the tiny (1.5 mm) male copulates with his larger (3.5 mm) mate and, apparently spent by the effort, dies. Within 1 week, the inseminated female begins to discharge offspring. Unlike those of most nematodes, these progeny undergo intrauterine embryonation and are released as second-stage larvae. The viviparous birthing continues for the next 4 to 16 weeks, resulting in the generation of some 1500 larvae, each measuring 6 by 100 μm.

From their submucosal position, the larvae find their way into the vascular system and pass from the right side of the heart through the pulmonary capillary bed to the systemic circulation, where they are distributed throughout the body. Larvae that end up in tissue other than skeletal muscle disintegrate and die. Those finding their way to striated muscle continue to grow, molt, and gradually encapsulate over a period of several weeks. Calcification of the cyst wall begins 6 to

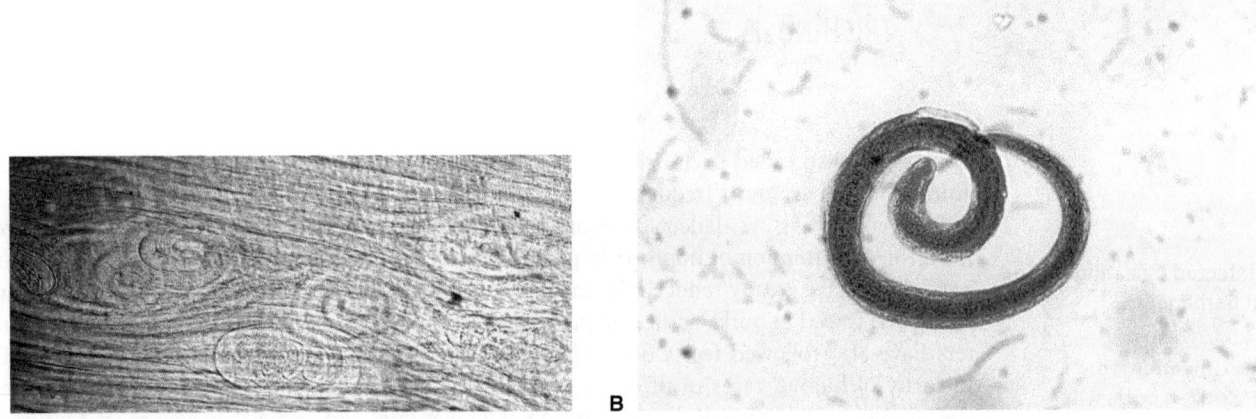

FIGURE 55-2. *Trichinella spiralis* larvae. A. Coiled larvae in a "squash prep" of deltoid muscle biopsy, in which a small sliver of muscle is squashed under the cover slip and examined without further fixation. **B.** Coiled larva from a muscle digest. (A, Used with permission from Paul Pottinger MD. B. Reproduced with permission from Connor DH, Chandler FW, Schwartz DQ, et al: *Pathology of Infectious Diseases*. Stamford CT: Appleton & Lange; 1997.)

18 months later, but the contained larvae may remain viable for 5 to 10 years (**Figure 55-2**). The muscles invaded most frequently are the extraocular muscles of the eye, the tongue, the deltoid, pectoral, and intercostal muscles, the diaphragm, and the gastrocnemius. If a second animal feeds on the infected flesh of the original host, the encysted larvae are freed by gastric digestion, penetrate the columnar epithelium of the intestine, and mature just above the lamina propria. This cycle is summarized in **Figure 55-3**.

✳ Larvae reach striated muscle, encapsulate but viable

✳ Eating infected flesh spreads disease

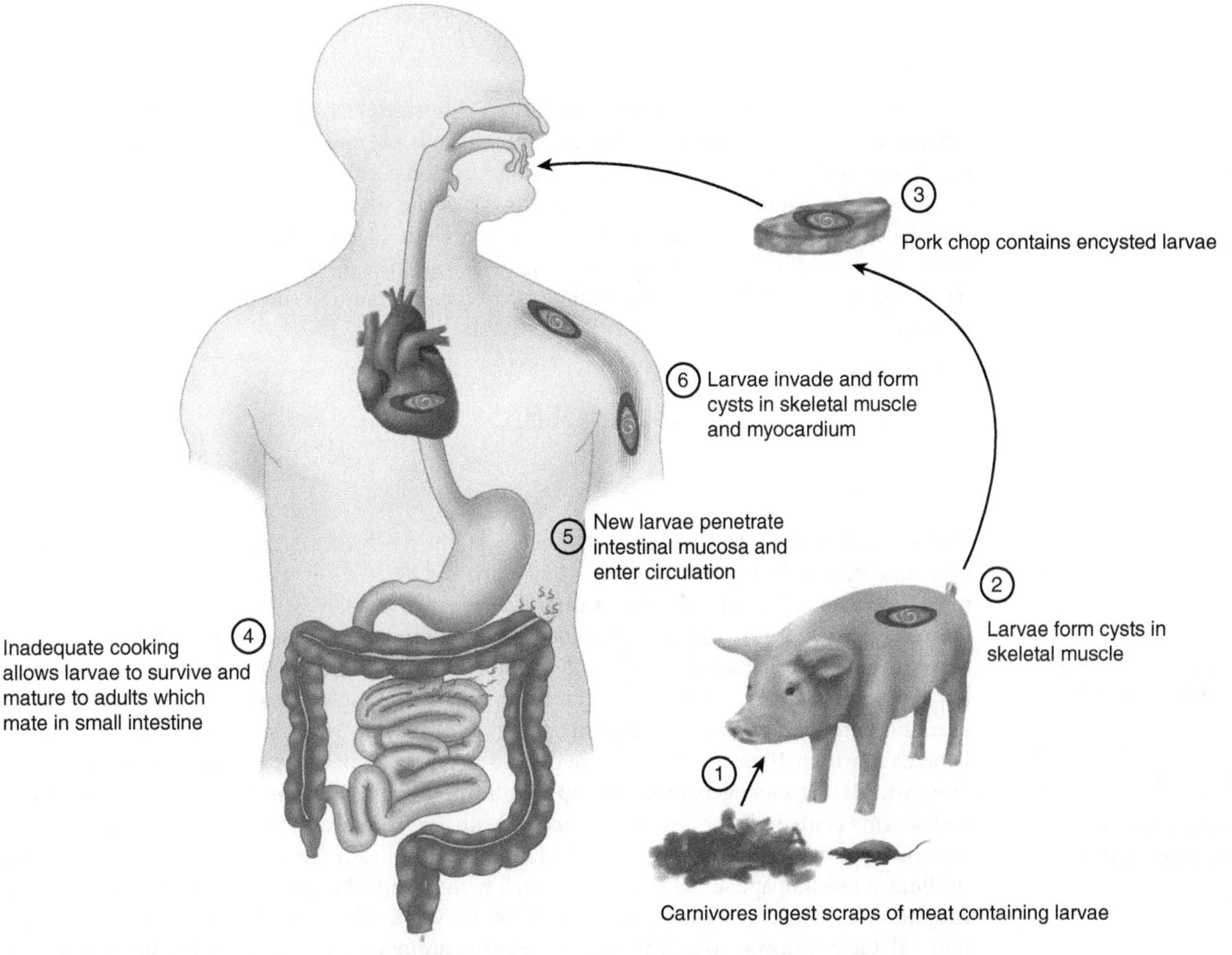

③ Pork chop contains encysted larvae

⑥ Larvae invade and form cysts in skeletal muscle and myocardium

⑤ New larvae penetrate intestinal mucosa and enter circulation

② Larvae form cysts in skeletal muscle

④ Inadequate cooking allows larvae to survive and mature to adults which mate in small intestine

① Carnivores ingest scraps of meat containing larvae

FIGURE 55-3. Trichinosis. *Trichinella spiralis* larvae ingested by pig (1) eventually end up as human cysts (6).

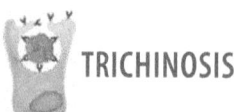 **TRICHINOSIS**

EPIDEMIOLOGY

Trichinosis, also called trichinellosis, is widespread in carnivores worldwide. Among domestic animals, swine are most frequently involved. They acquire the infection by eating dead rats or garbage containing cyst-laden scraps of uncooked meat. Human infection, in turn, results largely from the consumption of improperly prepared pork products. In the United States, agricultural regulations have greatly reduced the incidence of trichinosis, and most pig-associated outbreaks have been traced to pork sausage prepared in the home or in small, unlicensed butcheries. Clusters have also followed feasts on wild pig in California and Hawaii. At present, however, the majority of human cases in the United States, particularly those in Alaska and other western states, have been attributed to consumption of wild animal meat, especially bear meat. Outbreaks among Alaskan and Canadian Inuit populations have followed the ingestion of raw *T nativa*-infected walrus meat. Outbreaks in Europe have involved horse meat or wild boar flesh. In other areas of the world, infection is commonly acquired from wild animals ("sylvatic sources"), including wild boar, bush pigs, and warthogs.

Human infections occur worldwide. In the United States, the prevalence of cysts found in the diaphragms of patients at autopsy has declined substantially. This decline has been attributed to decreased consumption of pork and pork products; federal guidelines for the commercial preparation of such foodstuffs; the widespread practice of freezing pork, which kills all but arctic strains of *T nativa*; and legislation requiring the thorough cooking of any meat scraps to be used as hog feed. Nevertheless, it is estimated that many Americans carry live *Trichinella* in their musculature and that more acquire it annually. Fortunately, most have a small number of larvae and are asymptomatic. Only a handful of clinically recognized cases are reported annually to federal officials.

PATHOGENESIS AND IMMUNITY

The pathologic lesions of trichinosis are related almost exclusively to the presence of larvae in striated muscle, heart, and CNS. Invaded muscle cells enlarge, lose their cross-striations, and undergo basophilic degeneration. Intense inflammation surrounds the involved area, consisting of neutrophils, lymphocytes, and eosinophils. With the development of specific IgG and IgM antibodies, eosinophil-mediated destruction of circulating larvae begins, production of new larvae is slowed, and the expulsion of adult worms is hastened. A vasculitis demonstrated in some patients has been attributed to deposition of circulating immune complexes in the walls of the vessels.

TRICHINOSIS: CLINICAL ASPECTS

MANIFESTATIONS

One or two days after the host ingests tainted meat, the newly matured adults penetrate the intestinal mucosa, producing nausea, abdominal pain, and diarrhea. In mild infections, these symptoms may be overlooked, except in a careful retrospective analysis; in more serious infections, they may persist for several days and render the patient prostrate. Diarrhea persisting for a period of weeks has been characteristic of *T nativa* outbreaks after ingestion of walrus meat by the Inuit population of northern Canada. Larval invasion of striated muscle begins approximately 1 week later and initiates the more characteristic phase of the disease, which may last for about 6 weeks. Patients in whom 10 or fewer larvae are deposited per gram of tissue are usually asymptomatic; those with 100 or more generally develop significant disease; and those with 1000 to 5000 have a very stormy course that occasionally ends in death. Fever, muscle pain, muscle tenderness, and weakness are the most prominent manifestations of trichinosis. Patients may also display eyelid swelling, a maculopapular skin rash, and small hemorrhages beneath the conjunctiva of the eye and the nails of the digits. Hemoptysis and pulmonary consolidation are common in severe infections. If there is myocardial involvement, electrocardiographic abnormalities, tachycardia, or

---

Swine infected by eating rats or meat in garbage

✱ Human infection from undercooked pork, wild animals

Declining due to meat inspection, cooking, freezing pork

Infections usually subclinical

✱ Larvae in striated muscle, heart, CNS

Eosinophil-mediated larvae destruction

Abdominal pain, diarrhea as adults penetrate gut wall

✱ Symptoms depend on extent of larval muscle invasion

Complications: hemoptysis, heart failure, coma, death

congestive heart failure may be seen. CNS invasion is marked by encephalitis, meningitis, and polyneuritis. Delirium, psychosis, paresis, and coma can follow.

DIAGNOSIS

Trichinosis presents in a protean fashion, which can delay diagnosis and impact clinical outcomes. The most consistent laboratory abnormality is an eosinophilic leukocytosis during the second week of illness, which persists for the remainder of the clinical course. Eosinophils typically range from 15% to 50% of the white cell count, and in some patients, this may induce extensive damage to the cardiac endothelium. In severe or terminal cases, the eosinophilia may disappear altogether. Serum levels of IgE and muscle enzymes are elevated in most clinically ill patients.

* Eosinophilia up to 50% starting in second week

There are a number of valuable serologic tests, including indirect fluorescent antibody and enzyme-linked immunosorbent assay. Significant antibody titers are generally absent before the third week of illness but may then persist indefinitely.

Antibody after 2 weeks

Biopsy of the deltoid or gastrocnemius muscles during the third week of illness often reveals encysted larvae (**Figure 55–2B**).

* Muscle biopsy reveals larvae

TREATMENT

Patients with severe edema, pulmonary manifestations, myocardial involvement, or CNS disease are treated with corticosteroids. The value of specific anthelmintic therapy remains controversial. The mortality rate of symptomatic patients is 1%, rising to 10% if the CNS is involved. Mebendazole and albendazole halt the production of new larvae, but in severe infection, the destruction of tissue larvae may provoke a hazardous hypersensitivity response in the host. This may be moderated by initiating corticosteroids before treating with antihelminthics.

* Corticosteroids in severe cases

* Antihelminthic therapy with caution

PREVENTION

Control of trichinosis requires adherence to feeding regulations for pigs, and limiting contact between domestic pigs and wild animals, particularly rodents, who might be carrying *Trichinella* larvae in their tissues. Domestically, care should be taken to cook pork to an internal temperature of at least 76.6°C, or freeze it at −15°C for 3 weeks before cooking. *Trichinella nativa* in the flesh of arctic animals may survive freezing for a year or more. All strains may survive apparently adequate cooking in microwave ovens due to the variability in the internal temperatures achieved.

* Prevention via thorough cooking

● *ANCYLOSTOMA BRAZILIENSE*

Cutaneous larva migrans, or "creeping eruption," is an infection of the skin caused by the larvae of a number of animal and human parasites, most commonly the dog and cat hookworm *A braziliense*. Adult worms live and copulate in the intestines of infected animals. Eggs discharged in animal feces onto warm, moist, sandy soil then develop into filariform larvae capable of penetrating mammalian skin on contact, just as with human hookworm infection. These parasites are common in tropical areas worldwide; in the United States, parasite transmission is particularly common in the beach areas of the southern Atlantic and Gulf states.

Larvae of dog and cat hookworms

* Filariform larvae penetrate, migrate in skin

However, these species are not well adapted to human hosts, and larvae rarely make it across the lung to reach the human intestines. Rather, they may migrate within the skin for a period of weeks to months. Clinically, the patient notes a pruritic, raised, red, serpiginous, irregularly linear lesion 10 to 20 cm long. Skin excoriation from scratching increases the likelihood of secondary bacterial infection. Some patients develop transient, migratory pulmonary infiltrations associated with peripheral eosinophilia, probably reflecting pulmonary migration of larvae. Larvae are rarely found in either sputum or skin biopsies, and the diagnosis must be established on skin pattern recognition (**Figure 55–4**).

Adult forms do not develop in humans

* Intensely itchy, linear rash

Cutaneous larva migrans respond well to albendazole or ivermectin. Antihistamines and antibiotics may be helpful in controlling pruritus and secondary bacterial infection, respectively.

 In toxocariasis, baylisascariasis, trichinosis, and dog hookworm, which form is responsible for human symptoms: adult worms or larvae?

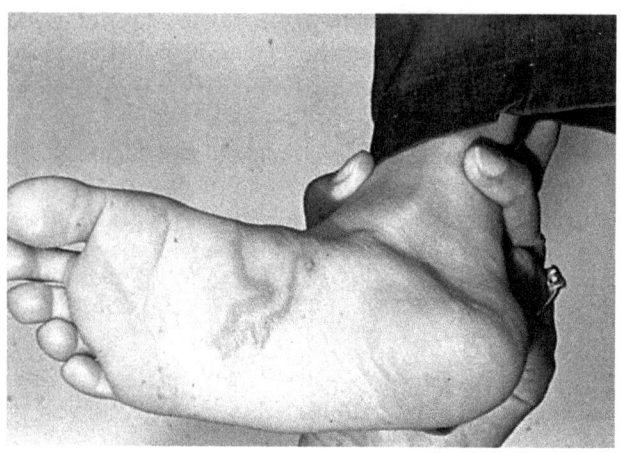

FIGURE 55–4. **Creeping eruption caused by infection with *Ancylostoma braziliense* larva.** (Reproduced with permission from Roberts RL, Janovy J, Nadler S: *Foundations of Parasitology*, 9th ed. New York, NY: McGraw Hill; 2013.)

● LYMPHATIC FILARIA

Lymphatic filariasis encompasses a group of diseases produced by certain members of the super-family Filarioidea ("thread like") that inhabit the human lymphatic system. Their presence induces an acute inflammatory reaction, chronic lymphatic blockade, and, in some cases, grotesque lymphedematous swelling of the extremities and genitalia. When the skin becomes rough and thickened over time, this is called **elephantiasis**.

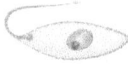 ### *WUCHERERIA* AND *BRUGIA*: PARASITOLOGY AND LIFE CYCLE

The two agents most commonly responsible for lymphatic filariasis are *W bancrofti* and *B malayi*. Both are thread-like worms whose adults lie coiled in the lymphatic vessels, male and female together, for the duration of their decade-long lifespan. The female *W bancrofti* measures 100 mm in length, and the male 40 mm. *B malayi* adults are approximately half these sizes. The gravid females produce large numbers of embryonated eggs. At oviposition, the embryos uncoil to their full length (200-300 μm) to become microfilariae ("small threads"). The shell of the egg elongates to accommodate the embryo and is retained as a thin, flexible sheath. Although the offspring of the two species resemble each other, they may be differentiated on the basis of length, staining characteristics, and internal structure (**Table 55–2**). The microfilariae eventually reach the blood (**Figure 55–5**). In most *W bancrofti* and *B malayi* infections, they accumulate in the pulmonary vessels during the day. At night, possibly in response to changes in oxygen tension, they spill out into the peripheral circulation, where they are found in greatest numbers between 9 PM and 2 AM. A Polynesian strain of *W bancrofti* displays a different periodicity, with the peak concentration of organisms occurring in the early evening. Periodicity has an important

✱ Adult worms live in lymphatic vessels for a decade

Microfilariae develop from ova

✱ Microfilariae circulate in peripheral blood each night

TABLE 55–2	Differentiation of Microfilariae				
PARASITE	**LOCATION**	**SHEATH**	**SIZE (MM)**	**NUCLEI OF TAIL**	**PERIODICITY**
Wuchereria bancrofti	Blood	Yes	360	None	Usually nocturnal
Brugia malayi	Blood	Yes	220	Two	Nocturnal
Loa loa	Blood	Yes	275	Continuous	Diurnal
Onchocerca volvulus	Skin	No	300	None	None

 Think ▸▸ Apply 55-1: **The larvae of these animal parasites cause symptoms in humans, when they migrate through our tissues.**

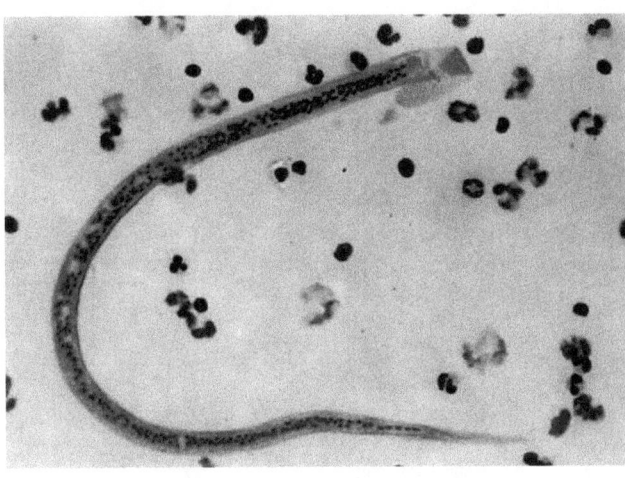

FIGURE 55-5. **Microfilaria of *Wuchereria bancrofti* in blood film.** (Reproduced with permission from Connor DH, Chandler FW, Schwartz DQ, et al: *Pathology of Infectious Diseases*. Stamford CT: Appleton & Lange; 1997.)

epidemiologic consequence, because it happens in response to the species of mosquito that serves as vector and intermediate host: to improve their chances of being taken up during the blood meal of a mosquito, the different filarial species enter the bloodstream during the nighttime when that mosquito is most likely to bite. Presumably, they do not spend all their time in the peripheral blood because doing so would increase their odds of being cleared via the spleen and liver.

Once ingested by a mosquito during the blood meal, the microfilariae enter its thoracic muscles and transform first into rhabditiform and then into filariform larvae. The latter actively penetrate the human skin at the feeding site when the mosquito takes its next meal. Within the new host, the parasite migrates to the lymphatic vessels, undergoes a series of molts, and reaches adulthood in 6 to 12 months (**Figure 55-6**). Bancroftian filariasis is exclusive to humans, whereas certain strains of brugian filariasis can also infect domestic and wild animals. The life cycle is illustrated in **Figure 55-7**.

Adult filarial worms have a fascinating feature: They carry endosymbiotic bacteria of the genus *Wolbachia* in their gut. These bacteria are beneficial to the worm in ways that are not yet fully understood. However, adult worms seem much healthier when their *Wolbachia* are healthy, and when *Wolbachia* are not present they are less able to reproduce. This observation has implications for disease treatment and control, as described below.

Wuchereria and Brugia worms contain Wolbachia bacteria.

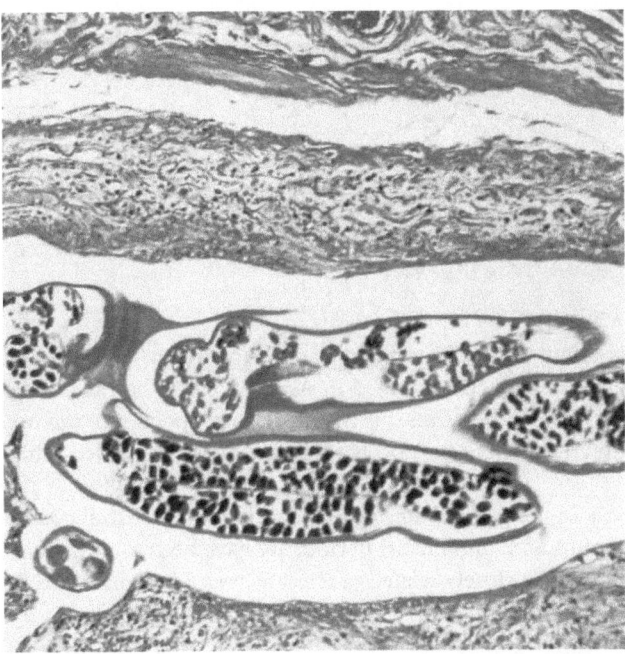

FIGURE 55-6. **Lymphatic filariasis.** These dilated lymphatics are filled with a gravid adult *W bancrofti* female. Eggs and developing microfilaria are within the paired uterine tubes. Note the surrounding thickened fibrous tissue. (Reproduced with permission from Connor DH, Chandler FW, Schwartz DQ, et al: *Pathology of Infectious Diseases*. Stamford CT: Appleton & Lange; 1997.)

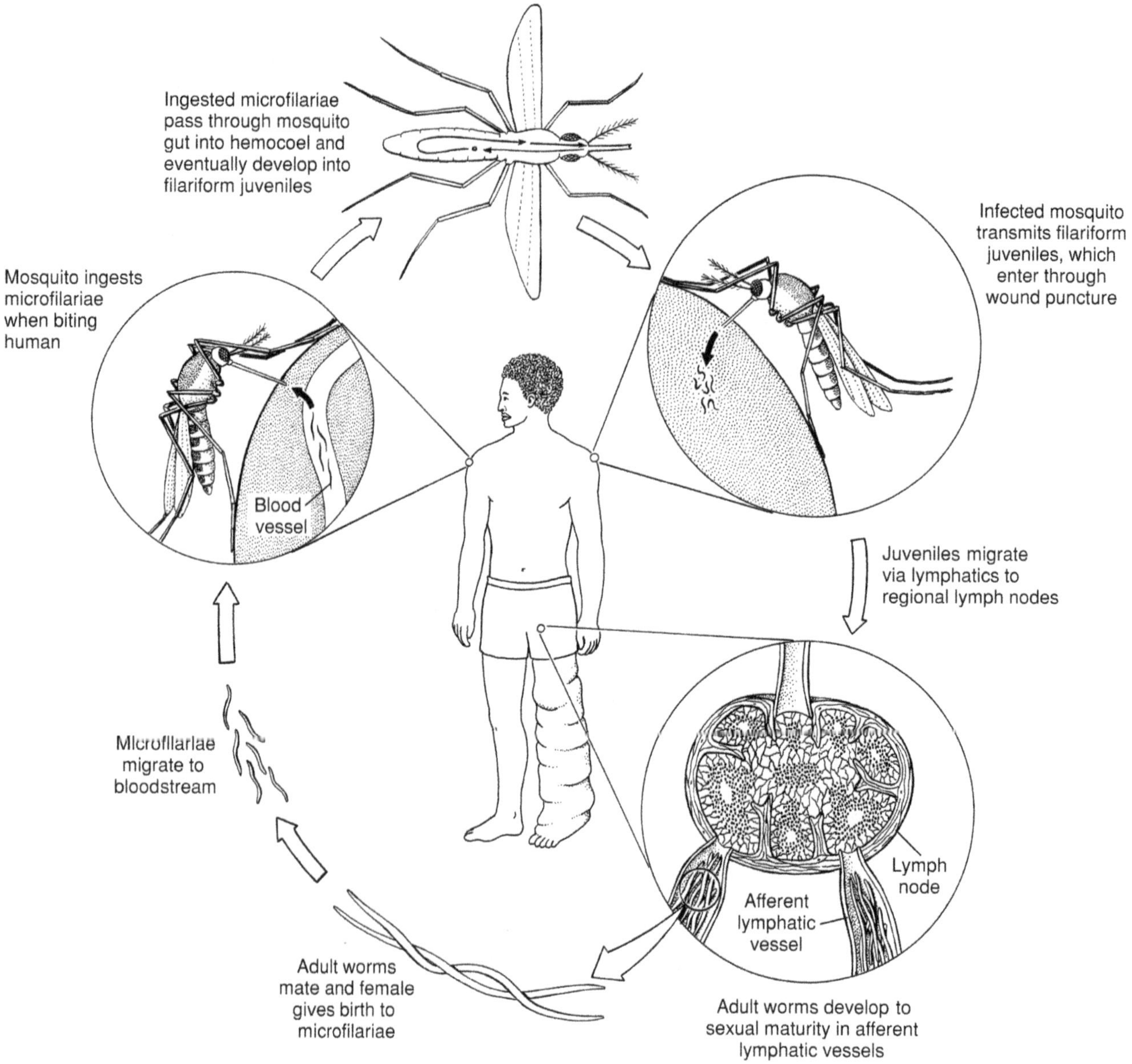

Ingested microfilariae
pass through mosquito
gut into hemocoel and
eventually develop into
filariform juveniles

Infected mosquito
transmits filariform
juveniles, which
enter through
wound puncture

Mosquito ingests
microfilariae
when biting
human

Blood
vessel

Juveniles migrate
via lymphatics to
regional lymph nodes

Microfilariae
migrate to
bloodstream

Lymph
node

Afferent
lymphatic
vessel

Adult worms
mate and female
gives birth to
microfilariae

Adult worms develop to
sexual maturity in afferent
lymphatic vessels

FIGURE 55–7. Life cycle of *Wuchereria bancrofti* and *Brugia malayi*. (Reproduced with permission from Roberts RL, Janovy J, Nadler S: *Foundations of Parasitology*, 9th ed. New York, NY: McGraw Hill; 2013.)

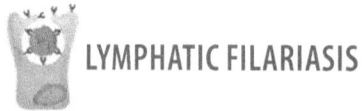

LYMPHATIC FILARIASIS

EPIDEMIOLOGY

Lymphatic filariasis currently infects about 120 million people in Africa, Latin America, the Pacific Islands, and Asia; most of these cases are concentrated in Asia. *W bancrofti*, transmitted primarily by mosquitoes of the genera *Anopheles* or *Culex*, is the more cosmopolitan of the two species; it is found in patchy distribution throughout the poorly sanitized, densely crowded urban areas of all three continents.

Primarily in Asia and other tropical areas

B malayi, transmitted by mosquitoes of the genus *Mansonia*, is confined to the rural coastal areas of Asia and the South Pacific. Strains with an unusual periodicity have been found in animals. In the eastern Indonesian archipelago, a closely related species, *B timori*, is transmitted by night-feeding anopheline mosquitoes.

PATHOLOGY AND PATHOGENESIS

Pathologic changes, which are confined primarily to the lymphatic system, can be divided into acute and chronic lesions. In acute disease, the presence of molting adolescent worms and dead or dying adults stimulates dilatation of the lymphatics, hyperplastic changes in the vessel endothelium, lymphatic infiltration by lymphocytes, plasma cells, and eosinophils, and thrombus formation (ie, acute lymphangitis). These developments are followed by granuloma formation, fibrosis, and permanent lymphatic obstruction. Repeated infections eventually result in massive lymphatic blockade. The skin and subcutaneous tissues become edematous, thickened, and fibrotic. Dilated lymphatics may rupture, spilling lymph into the tissues or body cavities, including the ureters. Bacterial and fungal superinfections of the skin often supervene and contribute to tissue damage.

✳ Lymphatic blockade with repeated infections

LYMPHATIC FILARIASIS: CLINICAL ASPECTS

MANIFESTATIONS

Individuals who enter endemic areas as adults and reside therein for months to years often present with acute lymphadenitis, urticaria, eosinophilia, and elevated serum IgE levels; they seldom go on to develop lymphatic obstruction. A significant proportion of indigenous populations present with asymptomatic microfilaremia. Some of these spontaneously clear their infection, whereas others go on to experience "filarial fevers" and lymphadenitis 8 to 12 months after exposure. The fever is typically low grade; in more serious cases, however, temperatures as high as 40°C, chills, muscle pains, and other systemic manifestations may be seen. Classically, lymphadenitis is first noted in the femoral area as an enlarged, red, tender lump. The inflammation spreads centrifugally down the lymphatic channels of the leg. The lymphatic vessels become enlarged and tender, the overlying skin warm, red, and edematous. In Bancroftian filariasis, the lymphatic vessels of the testicle, epididymis, and spermatic cord are frequently involved, producing a painful orchitis, epididymitis, and funiculitis; inflamed retroperitoneal vessels may simulate an acute abdomen. Epitrochlear, axillary, and other lymphatic vessels are involved less frequently. These acute manifestations last a few days and resolve spontaneously, only to recur periodically over a period of weeks to months.

Lymphadenitis, urticaria, eosinophilia early findings

Acute manifestations recur

With repeated infection, permanent lymphatic obstruction develops in the involved areas. Edema, ascites, pleural effusion, hydrocele, and joint effusion may result. The lymphadenopathy persists and the palpably swollen lymphatic channels may rupture, producing an abscess or draining sinus. Rupture of intraabdominal vessels may give rise to chylous ascites or urine. In patients heavily and repeatedly infected over a period of decades, elephantiasis may develop. Such patients may continue to experience acute inflammatory episodes. Recurrent streptococcal and staphylococcal skin infections are common sequels to this condition, which in turn lead to more lymphatic damage, perpetuating a cycle of pain and suffering.

✳ Lymphedema, recurrent inflammation triggered by adult worms in lymphatics

In southern India, Pakistan, Sri Lanka, Indonesia, Southeast Asia, and East Africa, an aberrant form of filariasis is sometimes seen. This form, termed tropical eosinophilia syndrome or tropical pulmonary eosinophilia, is characterized by an intense eosinophilia, elevated levels of IgE, high titers of filarial antibodies, the absence of microfilariae from the circulating blood, and a chronic clinical course marked by massive enlargement of the lymph nodes and spleen in children or chronic cough, nocturnal bronchospasm, and pulmonary infiltrates in adults. Untreated, it may progress to interstitial pulmonary fibrosis. Microfilariae have been found in the tissues of such patients, and the clinical manifestations may be terminated with antifilarial treatment. It is believed that this syndrome is precipitated by the removal of circulating microfilariae by an IgG-dependent, cell-mediated immune reaction. Microfilariae are trapped in various tissue sites, where they incite an eosinophilic inflammatory response, granuloma formation, and fibrosis.

✳ Tropical pulmonary eosinophilia caused by microfilariae in tissues (not found in blood)

DIAGNOSIS

Eosinophilia is usually present during the acute inflammatory episodes, but definitive diagnosis requires the presence of microfilariae in the blood or lymphatic, ascitic, or pleural fluid. They are sought in Giemsa- or Wright-stained thick and thin smears. The major distinguishing features of these and other microfilariae are listed in Table 55–2. Because the appearance of the microfilariae is usually periodic, specimen collection must be properly timed. If the parasitemia is below the threshold of detection, the specimen may be concentrated before it is examined. If this procedure proves fruitless, the patient may be retested after being challenged with the antifilarial agent diethylcarbamazine (DEC). This drug stimulates the migration of the microfilariae from the pulmonary to the systemic circulation and enhances the possibility of their recovery. Once found, the microfilariae can be differentiated from those produced by other species of filariae. A number of serologic tests have been used for the diagnosis of microfilaremic disease, but until recently they have lacked adequate sensitivity and specificity; IgG4 testing is the most specific for filarial infection, although cross-reactivity to other tissue parasites is well described, and these tests are of little diagnostic significance in individuals indigenous to the endemic area, because many people have experienced a prior filarial infection. Circulating filarial antigens can be found in most microfilaremic patients and also in some seropositive nonmicrofilaremic individuals. Antigen detection may thus prove to be a specific indicator of active disease, although the test is not widely available. Tropical eosinophilia is diagnosed as described previously.

TREATMENT AND PREVENTION

DEC eliminates the microfilariae from the blood and may injure or even kill some of the adult worms, resulting in long-term suppression of the infection or parasitologic cure in some cases. Frequently, the dying microfilariae stimulate an allergic reaction in the host. This response is occasionally severe, requiring antihistamines and corticosteroids. This phenomenon is even more common among patients coinfected with onchocerciasis (see later), and thus coinfection with that condition should be ruled out before DEC is dosed in endemic areas. However, DEC use in lymphatic filariasis is generally safe, so much so that it is sometimes added to cooking salt in highly endemic areas or dosed intermittently on a mass scale; the idea is to suppress microfilaremia, which benefits the individual patient and the entire community by reducing transmission pressure. Ivermectin has a similar effect on microfilariae, and it can temporarily clear microfilaremia after the administration of a single dose. Albendazole seems to have beneficial effects on both microfilariae and adult worms. The antibiotic doxycycline has been demonstrated to kill endosymbiotic *Wolbachia* bacteria, and with prolonged administration, alone or in combination with other agents such as albendazole, may ultimately help to kill the adult worms. The tissue changes of elephantiasis are often irreversible, but the enlargement of the extremities may be ameliorated with pressure bandages or plastic surgery. Treatment and prevention of bacterial superinfection are essential, and can be augmented by access to proper shoe gear plus soap and water. Control programs combine mosquito control with mass treatment of the entire population.

● *ONCHOCERCA*

Onchocerciasis, or "river blindness," is produced by the skin filaria *O volvulus*. The disease is characterized by subcutaneous nodules, thickened pruritic skin, and—in some cases—blindness.

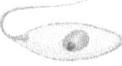 *ONCHOCERCA VOLVULUS*: PARASITOLOGY AND LIFE CYCLE

The 40 to 60 cm long, thread-like female adults lie with their diminutive male partners in coiled masses within fibrous subcutaneous and deep tissue nodules. The female gives birth to more than 2000 microfilariae each day of her 15-year lifespan. These progeny lose their sheaths soon after leaving the uterus, exit from the fibrous capsule, and migrate for up to 2 years in the subcutaneous tissues, skin (**Figure 55–8**), and eye. In contrast to the microfilariae of lymphatic filariasis that travel in the bloodstream, the microfilariae of onchocerciasis migrate through the subcutaneous tissues to the skin, where ultimately they die or are ingested by black flies of the genus *Simulium*. Unlike stealthy blood-sucking mosquitoes, flies feed on humans by taking a bite of skin—if an *O volvulus* larva happens to be in the hunk of skin taken by the fly, the life cycle will continue. After transformation into filariform larvae in the fly, they are transmitted to another human host. There they molt repeatedly over 6 to 12 months before reaching adulthood and becoming encapsulated. Like the worms of lymphatic filariais, adult *O volvulus* parasites appear to harbor endosymbiotic *Wolbachia* bacteria. The name "river blindness" derives from the association of the infection with exposure to turbulent, fast-moving streams, where the vector *Simulium* fly breeds. The *Onchocerca* life cycle is illustrated in **Figure 55–9**.

Eosinophilia during acute episodes

✳ Search for microfilariae in blood

✳ Killing microfilariae with DEC may stimulate allergic response

✳ Killing adult worms' endosymbiotic *Wolbachia*

✳ Treatment of complications improves quality of life

✳ Adults in subcutaneous tissue, skin, eye

✳ Transmitted by bite of *Simulium* fly

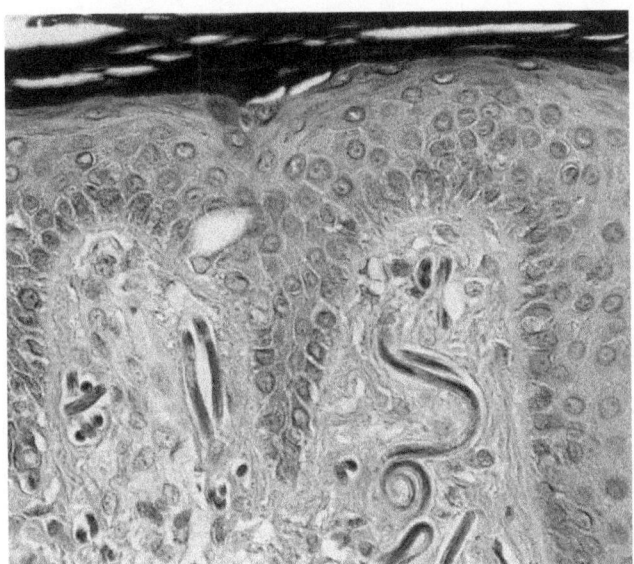

FIGURE 55–8. Onchocercal dermatitis. *Onchocerca volvulus* microfilaria are concentrated in the dermal papillae, which makes them particularly available when the vector *Simulium* flies bite and feed. (Reproduced with permission from Connor DH, Chandler FW, Schwartz DQ, et al: *Pathology of Infectious Diseases*. Stamford CT: Appleton & Lange; 1997.)

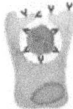 ## ONCHOCERCIASIS

EPIDEMIOLOGY

Onchocerciasis infects approximately 37 million persons, rendering approximately 500,000 of them blind. Most of the afflicted live in sub-Saharan Africa, over half of these in Nigeria and the Congo. Foci of infection are also found in Yemen, Saudi Arabia, and Latin America from southern Mexico through the northern half of South America. It has been suggested that the disease was introduced into South America by West Africans enslaved and transported there for the purpose of mining gold in the mountain streams of Venezuela and Colombia. The Central American foci probably date from Napoleon III's use of Sudanese troops to support his invasion of Mexico in 1862. Onchocerciasis persists on the high slopes of the Sierra, where coffee plantations lie along the rapidly flowing streams that serve as breeding places for *Simulium* species.

Most cases in tropical Africa

 ## ONCHOCERCIASIS: CLINICAL ASPECTS

MANIFESTATIONS

The subcutaneous nodules that harbor the adult worms can be located anywhere on the body, generally over bony prominences. In Mexico and Guatemala, where flies typically bite the upper part of the body, they are concentrated on the head; in South America and Africa, they are found primarily on the trunk and legs. Although nodules may number in the hundreds, most infected persons have fewer than 10. The nodules are firm, movable, and measure 1 to 3 cm in diameter. Unless the nodule is located over a joint, pain and tenderness are unusual.

Of greater consequence to the patient are the effects of the presence of microfilariae in the tissues. An immediate hypersensitivity reaction to antigens released by dead or dying parasites results in acute and chronic inflammatory reactions. In the skin, this manifests as a papular or erysipelas-like rash with severe itching. In time, due to the trauma of repeated scratching, the skin thickens and lichenifies. As subepidermal elastic tissue is lost, wrinkles and large skinfolds or "hanging groins" may form. In parts of Africa, fibrosing, obstructive lymphadenitis may result in elephantiasis. The most devastating lesions, however, are caused by invasion of the eye. Iritis and chorioretinitis can lead to decreased visual acuity and, in time, total blindness. Even if the anterior eye alone is infected, scarring and opacification of the cornea may cause irreversible blindness when the optic disk atrophies due to lack of light perception. In Central America, eye lesions may be seen in up to 30% of infected patients. In certain communities in West Africa, 85% of the population has ocular lesions, and 50% of the adult male population is blind. *O volvulus* microfilariae

Adult worms cause multiple subcutaneous nodules

✳ Microfilariae cause hypersensitivity reactions: pruritus, eye damage

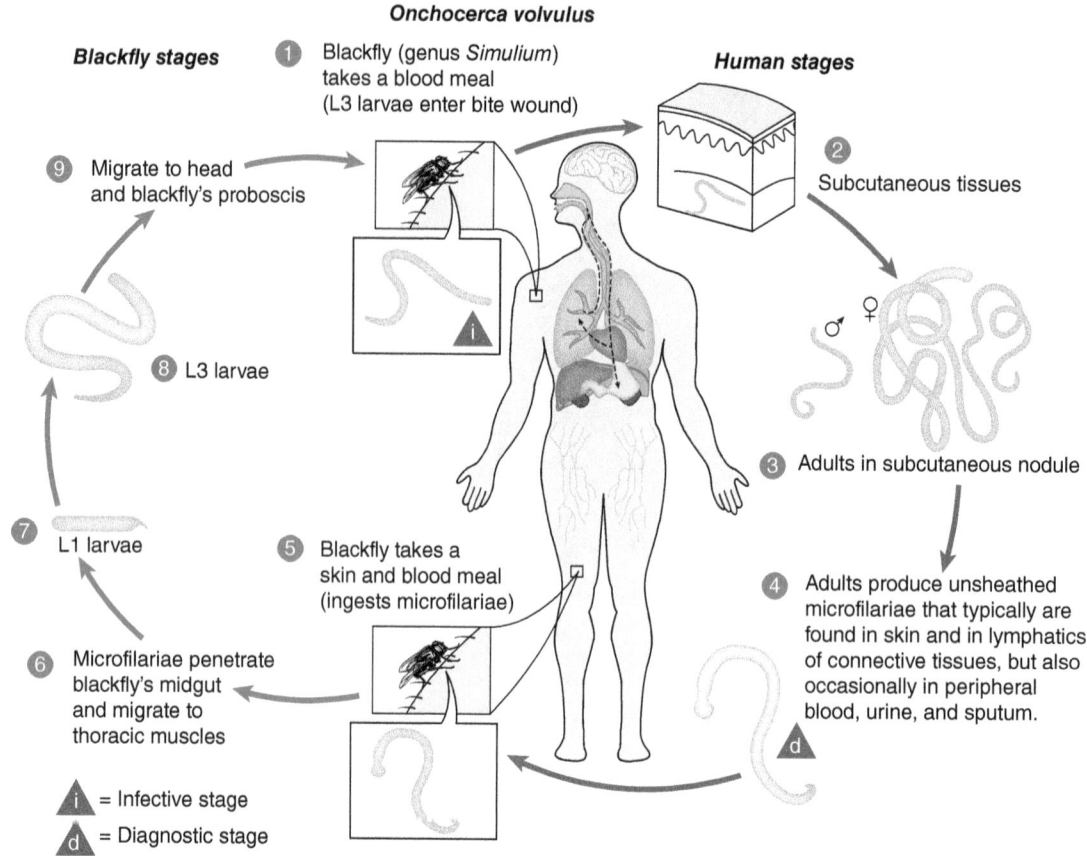

During a blood meal, an infected blackfly (genus *Simulium*) introduces third-stage filarial larvae onto the skin of the human host, where they penetrate into the bite wound ❶. In subcutaneous tissues the larvae ❷ develop into adult filariae, which commonly reside in nodules in subcutaneous connective tissues ❸. Adults can live in the nodules for approximately 15 years. Some nodules may contain numerous male and female worms. Females measure 33 to 50 cm in length and 270 to 400 μm in diameter, whereas males measure 19 to 42 mm by 130 to 210 μm. In the subcutaneous nodules, the female worms are capable of producing microfilariae for approximately 9 years. The microfilariae, measuring 220 to 360 μm by 5 to 9 μm and unsheathed, have a life span that may reach 2 years. They are occasionally found in peripheral blood, urine, and sputum but are typically found in the skin and in the lymphatics of connective tissues ❹. A blackfly ingests the microfilariae during a blood meal ❺. During a skin and blood meal, the microfilariae migrate from the blackfly's midgut through the hemocoel to the thoracic muscles ❻. There the microfilariae develop into first-stage larvae ❼ and subsequently into third-stage infective larvae ❽. The third-stage infective larvae migrate to the blackfly's proboscis. ❾ and can infect another human when the fly takes a blood meal ❶.

FIGURE 55–9. **Life cycle of *Onchocerca volvulus*.**

❊ Important cause of blindness

may trigger autoimmunity that is responsible for an unusual form of epilepsy called "nodding syndrome," although this is not proven.

DIAGNOSIS

Patients from endemic areas who present with subcutaneous nodules, unexplained pruritus, or ocular changes should be ruled out for onchocerciasis. The diagnosis is confirmed by demonstrating the microfilariae in thin skin snips taken from an involved area (**Figure 55–10**). When the eye is involved, the organism may sometimes be seen in the anterior chamber with the help of a slit lamp. Topical DEC can be applied safely to a patch of skin, which will yield a local wheal and flare when microfilariae die and release antigens. Previously, a technique called the "Mazzotti test" was performed, in which DEC was administered in a low dose to patients, who were then observed for a flare of their pruritus due to rapid microfilariae death and resultant inflammatory reactions. However, this practice is generally discouraged for safety concerns, especially when skin snips can be obtained.

❊ Microfilariae seen in skin samples

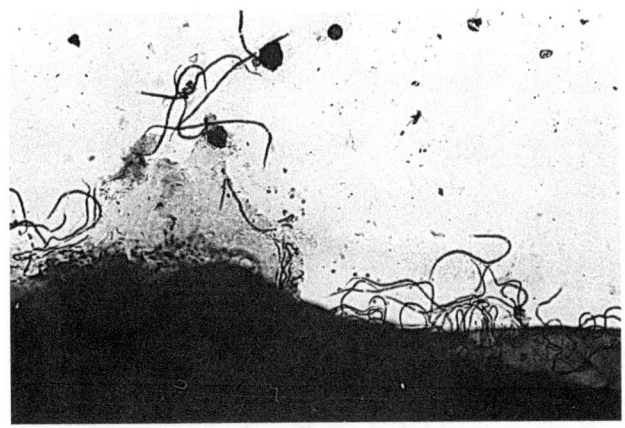

FIGURE 55–10. Skin snip from a patient with onchocerciasis, dropped into a vial of saline. Note microfilariae emerging from the specimen into surrounding solution. (Reproduced with permission from Roberts RL, Janovy J, Nadler S: *Foundations of Parasitology*, 9th ed. New York, NY: McGraw Hill; 2013.)

TREATMENT AND PREVENTION

Traditionally, DEC has been used to kill the microfilariae. Treatment was begun with very small doses to prevent rapid parasite destruction and the attendant allergic consequences. This consideration was particularly important when the eye was involved, because a treatment-induced inflammatory reaction can damage the eye further. This hypersensitivity reaction, sometimes called a "Mazzotti reaction," can have grave consequences for the patient.

Ivermectin is a safer and more effective microfilaricide than DEC and does not appear to induce the severe allergic manifestations seen with the latter agent. However, because it does not kill the adult worm, periodic retreatment is necessary. Mass treatment or chemoprophylaxis with ivermectin has been a major achievement. The manufacturer of this drug has pledged a virtually unlimited, cost-free supply of ivermectin to governments that administer it on a mass scale to endemic populations. This improves symptoms and may reduce parasitism in biting *Simulium* flies, helping to interrupt the transmission cycle. Mass ivermectin administration has allowed communities to reclaim large areas of arable land in Africa previously abandoned because of disease burden. However, because ivermectin does not fully cure the individual patient, retreatment is required. Furthermore, ivermectin carries a risk of perversely facilitating the entry of *L loa* worms (see later) into the CNS of patients coinfected with that parasite, thus posing challenges for mass drug administration in areas endemic for both infections.

The finding that doxycycline is toxic to endosymbiotic *Wolbachia* has led to interest in an approach similar to that being adopted in lymphatic filariasis, in which doxycycline is combined with ivermectin or albendazole. The goal is to simultaneously kill microfilariae with the antihelminthic while gradually killing—or at least rendering sterile—the adult worms with the antibiotic. Unfortunately, prolonged courses of doxycycline are not practical to administer on a mass scale, and thus this approach is generally reserved for individual patients.

Progress has been substantial, although no fully satisfactory methods of control have yet been developed. There is no effective vaccine. Application of insecticides to the vector's breeding waters must be sustained for decades to disrupt transmission permanently, because the parasite is so long-lived within humans. A World Health Organization-funded *Simulium* larva control program using aerial insecticides has succeeded in interrupting transmission of onchocerciasis in parts of the savanna regions of West Africa.

* DEC treatment may cause hypersensitivity

* Ivermectin clears microfilariae, but retreatment necessary

Risky if *Loa loa* coinfection

* Targeting *Wolbachia* may kill or sterilize adults

> How does the approach to onchocerciasis differ between treating individual patients and controlling the infection in an entire community?

● LOA LOA

Loiasis is a filarial disease of West Africa produced by the eye worm, *L loa*. Biting deer flies of the genus *Chrysops* serve as vectors. The female produces sheathed microfilariae, which are found in the bloodstream during daytime hours—because that is the time when the flies bite their victims (**Figure 55–11**). Unlike onchocerciasis, and more similar to lymphatic filariasis, it is the adult worm rather than the microfilariae that cause clinical illness. The long-lived adults migrate continuously through the subcutaneous tissues of humans at a maximum rate of about 1 cm/hour.

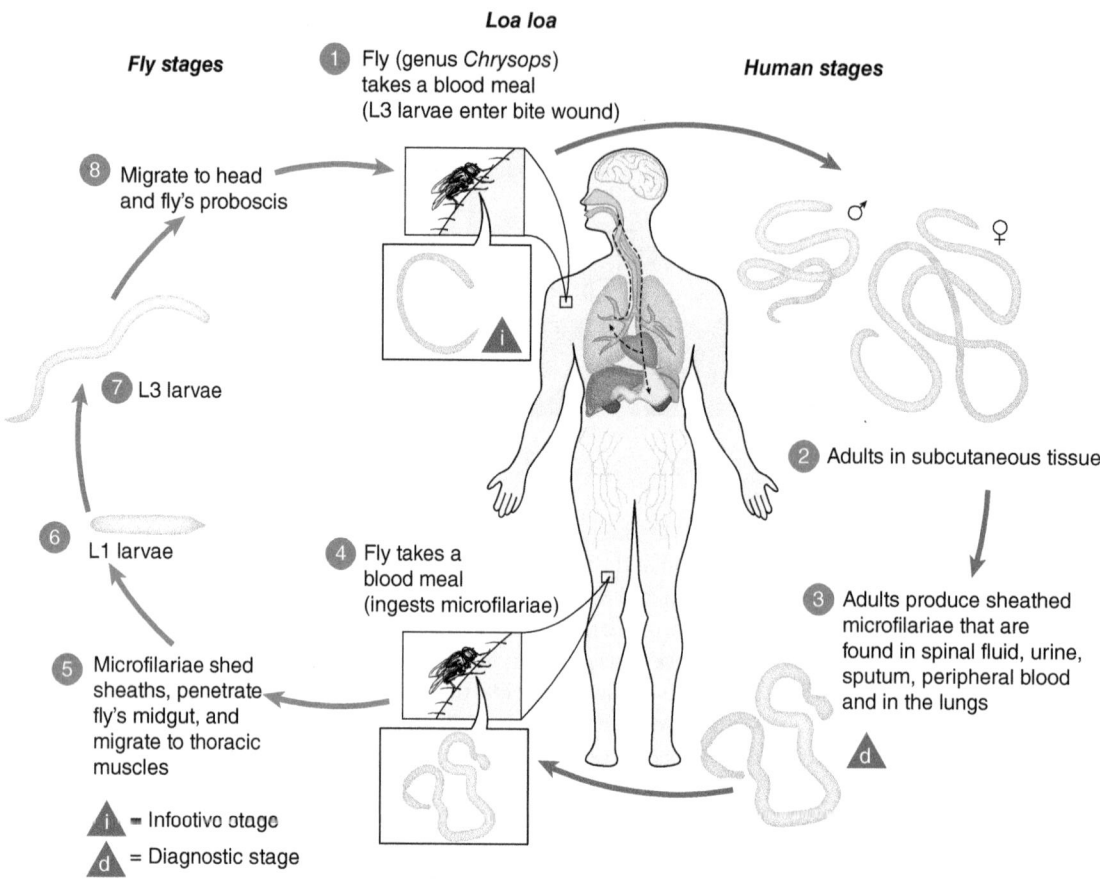

Loa loa

Fly stages

1. Fly (genus *Chrysops*) takes a blood meal (L3 larvae enter bite wound)

Human stages

8. Migrate to head and fly's proboscis

7. L3 larvae

6. L1 larvae

5. Microfilariae shed sheaths, penetrate fly's midgut, and migrate to thoracic muscles

4. Fly takes a blood meal (ingests microfilariae)

2. Adults in subcutaneous tissue

3. Adults produce sheathed microfilariae that are found in spinal fluid, urine, sputum, peripheral blood and in the lungs

i = Infective stage

d = Diagnostic stage

FIGURE 55–11. Life cycle of *Loa loa*.

* **Adults migrate through subcutaneous tissues producing Calabar swellings**

Microfilariae generally harmless

Adult worm in eye, microfilaria in blood or tissue

Treatment options limited

* **Natural history usually benign**

During migration, they may produce localized areas of allergic inflammation termed "Calabar swellings." These may appear as egg-sized lesions or swollen extremities which persist for 2 to 3 days and may be accompanied by fever, itching, urticaria, and pain, before they resolve fully and spontaneously. Occasionally, the adult worms may cross under the conjunctiva of the eye, producing tearing, pain, and alarm (**Figure 55–12**). However, in contrast to onchocerciasis, this phenomenon is harmless and does not threaten the patient's sight.

The diagnosis is usually made by asking patients whether they have noticed a worm wriggling across their eye—a memorable experience. If in doubt, the diagnosis is confirmed by recovering the adult worm from the eye or by isolating the characteristic microfilariae from the blood or Calabar swellings. Eosinophilia is common. DEC destroys microfilariae, but is less effective in killing the adults, and must be administered cautiously to avoid marked allergic reactions. Albendazole slowly decreases microfilarial levels without producing allergic reactions, possibly by preferential action on the adult worms. In some cases, symptoms persist for years, in spite of treatment, until the adults are removed while they cross the eye, or until they die of old age. As described above, ivermectin is contraindicated in patients with loiasis: for unknown reasons, ivermectin may ironically make things worse by facilitating adult *L loa* entry into the CNS, thus causing dangerous meningoencephalopathy. Thus, perhaps the most important medical reason to diagnose Loiasis is to avoid giving ivermectin to patients who are coinfected with *O volvulus*. Unfortunately, *L loa* adults do not harbor endosymbiotic *Wolbachia* bacteria, making doxycycline ineffective.

 Think ▸▸ Apply 55-2: **For individual patients, the goal is cure via killing the adult worms with prolonged courses of doxycycline. Because this is not practical on a massive scale, control strategies for entire communities involve periodic mass drug administration of ivermectin to kill the microfilariae—thus easing symptoms and interrupting the transmission cycle.**

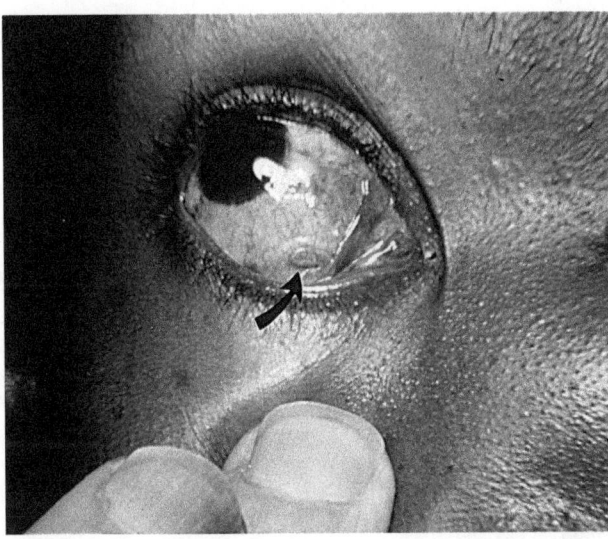

FIGURE 55–12. Adult female *L loa* coiled under the conjunctival epithelium (*arrow*) of the eye of a patient from the Congo. (Reproduced with permission from Roberts RL, Janovy J, Nadler S: *Foundations of Parasitology*, 9th ed. New York, NY: McGraw Hill; 2013.)

OTHER FILARIAL WORMS

Other microfilarial parasites have been detected in humans, including species of *Mansonella*. These are transmitted to people during the bite of the *Culicoides* midge. For generations, these worms were felt to be harmless to patients, and their importance in parasitology was limited to distinguishing them from "pathogenic" microfilariae found in the blood. However, this opinion may be changing. It is now believed that *M perstans* may cause a wide variety of problems, including fever, fatigue, headache, arthralgias, CNS disturbances, and occasionally migration across the eye, as seen in loiasis. Like most other microfilarial infections, their adults contain endosymbiotic *Wolbachia*, and treatment with doxycycline may accelerate clearance of the adult parasites; whether this will lead to widespread clinical benefit is unclear.

Other microfilariae of unclear significance

DRACUNCULUS

The guinea worm, *Dracunculus medinensis*, deserves inclusion here as an example of successful control of a parasitic infection. Guinea worms are transmitted when humans drink water contaminated with infected, tiny copepods of the *Cyclops* family. Larval *Dracunculus* worms exit *Cyclops* in the human gut, then migrate to the loose connective tissues and mate. The female may grow to more than 60 cm in length. Eventually she migrates to the skin, where her uterus protrudes into the environment, releasing young into the water when the patient bathes. These exit sites are exquisitely painful, often become secondarily infected, and may cause orthopedic injury if an ankle or knee joint is involved. Pulling on the uterus too quickly leads to worm injury and death, making the situation worse; only painstaking, gradual removal over time may succeed. Prevention of this painful and disfiguring condition has been achieved to a tremendous degree by simply filtering the water before it is consumed, as well as by applying larvicides to the water supply. Currently, only a few nations including Chad are still believed to have ongoing transmission. However, the discovery that dogs are also parasitized poses a barrier to full global eradication of this parasite.

Near eradication of guinea worm by filtering water supply

KEY CONCLUSIONS

- Tissue nematode infections may be acquired via ingestion, skin penetration, or the bite of arthropod vectors. Know their route of transmission summarized in Table 55–1.
- In lymphatic filariasis and loiasis, the *adult* worms cause symptoms, whereas in the other worms covered here the *larval* forms are harmful to the patient.
- Care must be exercised when treating some of these infections, because killing their larvae may elicit a brisk allergic reaction.
- The adult worms of lymphatic filariasis, onchocerciasis, and loiasis are relatively resistant to antihelminthic treatment; because they harbor endosymbiotic Wolbachia bacteria, the first two (but not *L loa*) may respond to prolonged courses of antibacterials such as doxycycline.
- For the vector-borne tissue invasive nematodes, strategies may differ when treating individual patients (goal of killing the adult worms) versus interrupting transmission in communities (goal of killing the microfilariae).

CASE STUDY

A Toddler Who Loves Dogs

This 2-year-old boy loves to go to the public park and play with other people's pets. He also has a history of pica (eating dirt). Over the last week, he has developed fever and wheezing, along with some vague complaints of abdominal discomfort. Physical findings include wheezes and a moderately enlarged, tender liver.

Laboratory findings: white blood cell count of 29,000/mm³ with 40% eosinophils and a mild anemia. Imaging findings: scattered interstitial pulmonary infiltrates;

QUESTIONS

1. What worm is the most likely cause of this child's illness?
   A. *Trichinella*
   B. *Toxocara*
   C. *Baylisascaris*
   D. *Ancylostoma*

2. *Ancylostoma* infections are acquired by:
   A. Mosquito transmission
   B. Black fly bites
   C. Deer fly bites
   D. Direct larval penetration of skin

3. Skin snips are used to diagnose:
   A. *Loa*
   B. *Wuchereria*
   C. *Brugia*
   D. *Onchocerca*

ANSWERS

1. **(B)**

2. **(D)**

3. **(D)**

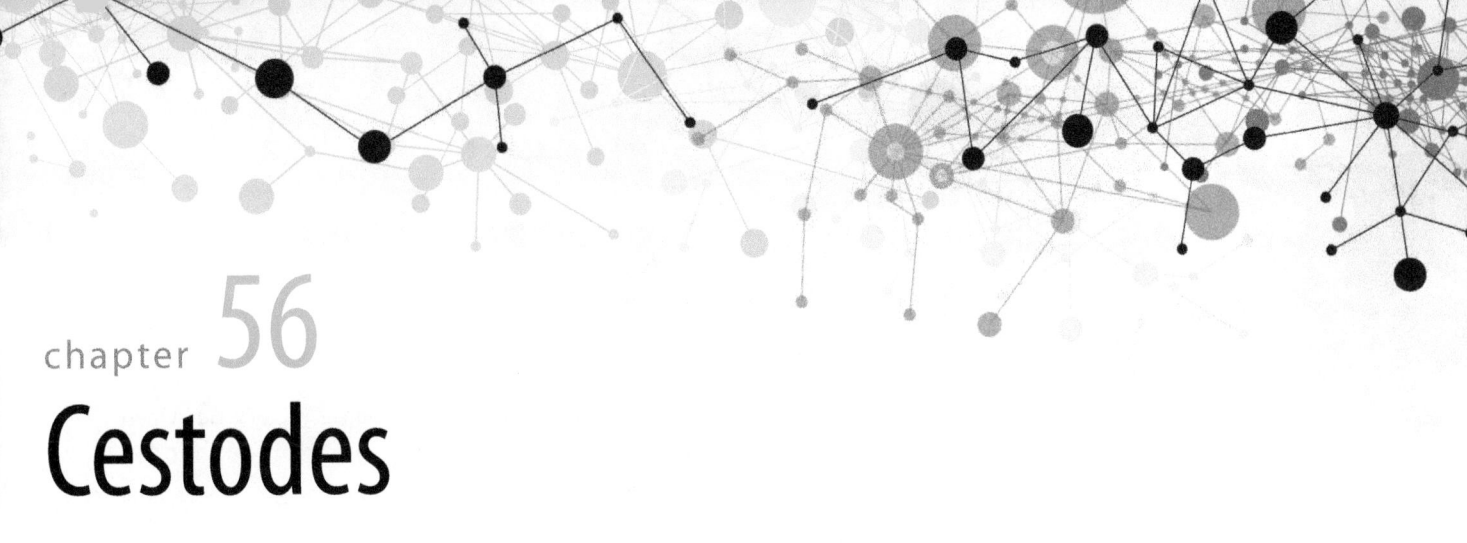

chapter 56

Cestodes

Taenia saginata · Taenia solium · Dibothriocephalus latus · Echinococcus granulosus · Echinococcus multilocularis

Hymenolepis nana

Only kings, presidents, editors, and people with tapeworms have the right to use the editorial "we."

—Mark Twain

OVERVIEW

Cestodes are long, ribbon-like helminths that have gained the common appellation of "tapeworm" from their superficial resemblance to sewing tape. Although improvements in sanitation have dramatically reduced their prevalence in the United States, they continue to inhabit the bowels of many of its citizens. In some parts of the world, people take purgatives regularly to rid themselves of these large, repulsive intestinal parasites. Ironically, when a human serves as the definitive host for tapeworms (when they harbor adult worms), it is usually of little medical consequence to that person; the intestinal form of these creatures rarely causes serious harm. In contrast, clinical disease is a greater concern when people serve as *intermediate* hosts (harbor larvae), because it is the presence of cysts in tissue that is most dangerous. Life cycles and characteristics of the six most important tapeworms infecting humans are summarized in **Table 56–1.**

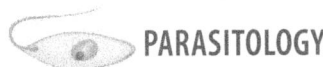 PARASITOLOGY

MORPHOLOGY

Like all helminths, tapeworms lack vascular and respiratory systems. In addition, they are devoid of both gut and body cavities. Nutrients are absorbed across their surface cuticle, and the internal organs are embedded in solid parenchyma. The adult is divided into three distinct parts: The "head" or scolex; a generative "neck"; and a long, segmented body called the strobila. The scolex typically measures less than 2 mm in diameter and is equipped with muscular sucking disks used to attach the worm to the intestinal mucosa of its host. (In one genus, *Dibothriocephalus*, the disks are replaced by two grooves called bothria.) As a further aid in attachment, the scolex of some species possesses a retractable protuberance, or rostellum, armed with a crown of chitinous hooks. Immediately posterior to the scolex is the neck from which individual segments, or proglottids, are generated one at a time to form the chain-like strobila. Each proglottid is a self-contained hermaphroditic reproductive unit joined to the remainder of the colony by a common cuticle, nerve trunks, and excretory canals. Its male and female gonads mature and self-fertilize as the segment is pushed farther and farther from the neck by the formation of new proglottids. When the segment reaches gravidity, it releases its eggs by rupturing, disintegrating, or passing them through its uterine pore.

Nutrients absorbed from host

✳ Divided into scolex, neck, segmented strobila

Proglottids hermaphroditic units releasing eggs

TABLE 56–1	Intestinal and Tissue Tapeworms					
STAGE	**TAENIA SAGINATA**	**TAENIA SOLIUM**	**DIPHYLLOBOTHRIUM LATUM**	**ECHINOCOCCUS GRANULOSUS**	**ECHINOCOCCUS MULTILOCULARIS**	**HYMENOLEPIS NANA**
Adult						
Definitive host	Humans	Humans	Humans, cats, dogs, bears	Dogs, wolves	Foxes	Humans, rodents
Location	Gut lumen^a	Gut lumen^a	Gut lumen^a	Gut lumen	Gut lumen	Gut lumen^a
Length (m)	4-6	2-4	3-10	0.005	0.005	0.02-0.04
Attachment device	Disks	Disks, hooklets	Grooves	Disks, hooklets	Disks, hooklets	Disks, hooklets
Mature segment	Elongated	Elongated	Broad	Elongated	Elongated	Broad
Egg						
Distinguishing characteristic	Radial striations	Radial striations	Operculated	Radial striations	Radial striations	Polar filaments
Larval development in humans	No	Yes	No	Yes	Yes	Yes
Larva						
Intermediate host	Cattle	Swine, humans	Copepods, fishes	Herbivores, humans	Field mice, humans	Humans, rodents
Location	Tissue	Tissue^a	Tissue	Tissue^a	Tissue^a	Gut mucosa^a
Form	Cysticercus	Cysticercus	Procercoid (copepod) Plerocercoid (fish)	Hydatid cyst	Hydatid cyst	Cysticercoid

^aSite of human infection.

● BEEF TAPEWORM

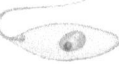 *TAENIA SAGINATA*: PARASITOLOGY AND LIFE CYCLE

Taenia saginata inhabits the human jejunum, where it may live for up to 25 years and grow to a maximum length of 10 m. Its 1 mm scolex lacks hooklets but possesses the four sucking disks typical of most cestodes (**Figure 56–1A**). The creamy white strobila consists of 1000 to 2000 individual proglottids. The terminal segments are longer (20 mm) than they are wide (5 mm), and contain testes and a large uterus with 15 to 20 lateral branches; these characteristics are useful in differentiating them from those of the closely related pork tapeworm, *Taenia solium* (see later). When fully gravid, strings of six to nine terminal proglottids, each containing approximately 100,000 eggs, break free from the remainder of the strobila. These muscular segments may crawl unassisted through the anal canal or be passed intact with the stool. Proglottids reaching the soil may remain motile for a time, perhaps in order to move away from human feces and into fresh grass that will entice a cow during grazing. Eventually, the proglottids disintegrate, releasing their distinctive ova. These eggs are 30 to 40 μm in diameter, spherical, and possess a thick, radially striated shell which appear very similar to those of *T solium* (**Figure 56–1B**). In appropriate environments, the embryo may survive in the egg for months. If ingested by cattle or certain other herbivores, the embryo is released, penetrates the intestinal wall, and is carried by the vascular system to the striated muscles of the tongue, diaphragm, and hindquarters. Here it transforms into a white, ovoid (5 by 10 mm) cysticercus (*Cysticercus bovis*). When present in large numbers, cysticerci impart a spotted or "measly" appearance to the flesh. Humans are infected when they ingest inadequately cooked meat containing these larval forms, which evaginate into scolices, attach to the jejunal epithelium, and begin to grow into a full-sized adult tapeworm, thus completing the life cycle.

✳ *T saginata* inhabits human jejunum

Gravid proglottids passed in stool

Eggs ingested by herbivore intermediates

Transform into larvae forming cysts in cow

✳ Humans infected by eating inadequately cooked meat

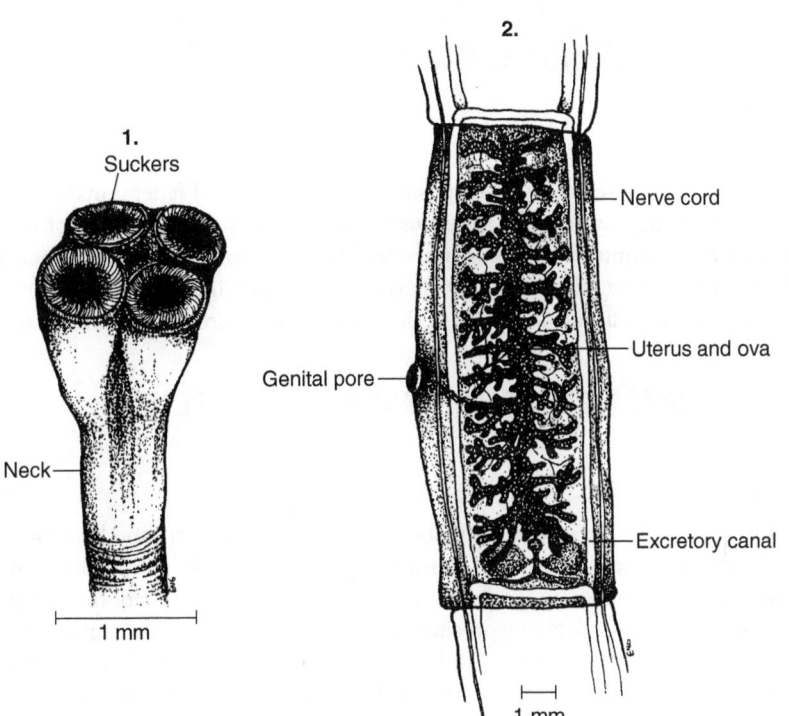

FIGURE 56–1. **Tapeworm structures.**
A. *Taenia saginata.* **B.** *Taenia solium.*
(1, 3) scolices; (2, 4) gravid proglottids;
(5) ova (indistinguishable between
species).

1.
Suckers

Neck

1 mm

2.

Nerve cord

Genital pore

Uterus and ova

Excretory canal

1 mm

A

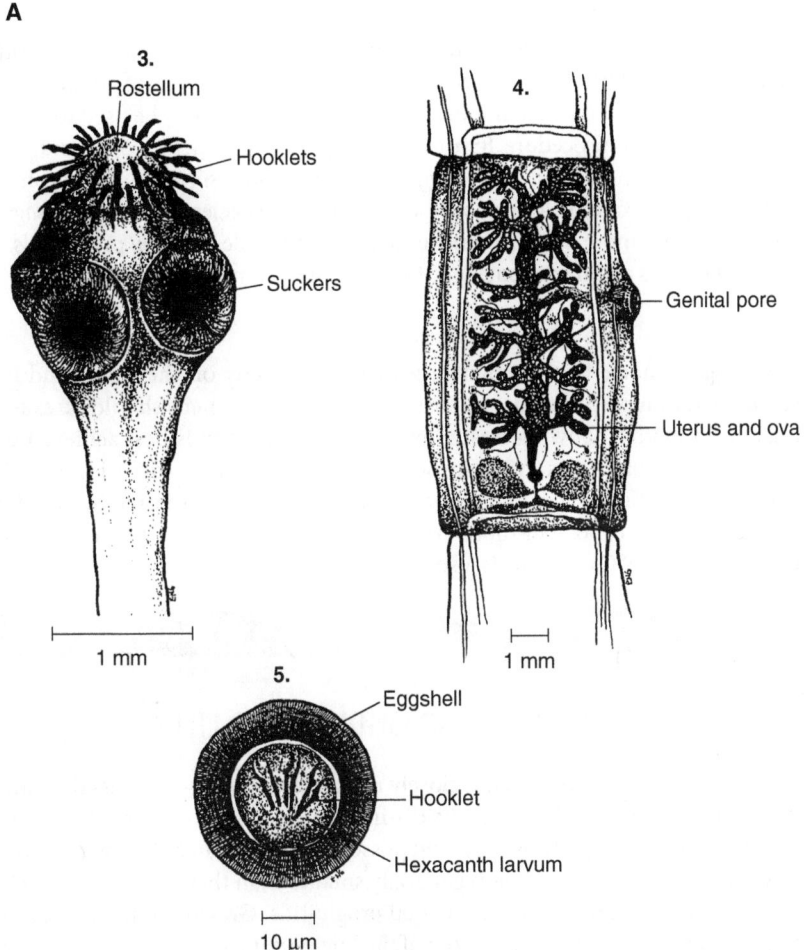

3.
Rostellum

Hooklets

Suckers

1 mm

4.

Genital pore

Uterus and ova

1 mm

5.
Eggshell

Hooklet

Hexacanth larvum

10 μm

B

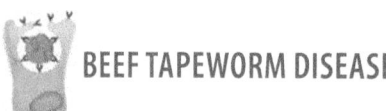

BEEF TAPEWORM DISEASE

EPIDEMIOLOGY

In the United States, sanitary disposal of human feces and federal inspection of meat have nearly interrupted transmission of *T saginata*. At present, fewer than 1% of examined carcasses are infected. In countries where sanitary facilities are less comprehensive and undercooked or raw beef is eaten, *T saginata* is highly prevalent. Examples include Kenya, Ethiopia, the Middle East, the former Yugoslavia, and parts of the former Soviet Union and South America.

Disease rare in the United States

BEEF TAPEWORM DISEASE: CLINICAL ASPECTS

MANIFESTATIONS

Most persons infected with beef tapeworm are asymptomatic and become aware of the infection only through the spontaneous passage of proglottids. The proglottids may be observed on the surface of the stool or appear in the underclothing or bedsheets of the alarmed host. Passage may occur irregularly and can be precipitated by excessive alcohol consumption. Some patients report epigastric discomfort, nausea, abdominal irritability, diarrhea, and weight loss. Occasionally, the proglottids may obstruct the appendix, biliary duct, or pancreatic duct.

✳ Symptoms usually mild

DIAGNOSIS

The diagnosis of beef tapeworm disease is made by finding eggs or proglottids in the stool. Eggs may also be distributed on the perianal area secondary to rupture of proglottids during passage. The adhesive cellophane tape technique described for pinworm can be used to recover the worms from this area. With this procedure, 85% to 95% of infections are detected, in contrast to only 50% to 75% by stool examination. Because the eggs of *T solium* and *T saginata* are morphologically identical, it is necessary to examine a proglottid to identify the species correctly—*T saginata* proglottids are motile and have more uterine branches than the immotile *T solium* proglottids. As discussed below, the implications and management of these two infections may be substantially different.

✳ Cellophane tape technique, stool examination detect eggs, proglottids

TREATMENT AND PREVENTION

The drug of choice is praziquantel, which acts directly on the worm and is highly effective in single-dose oral preparations. To ensure cure, fecal specimens should be examined again approximately 3 months following treatment. Ultimately, control is best achieved through the sanitary disposal of human feces. Meat inspection is helpful; the cysticerci are readily visible. In areas where the infection is common, thorough cooking is the most practical method of control. Internal temperatures of 56°C or more for 5 minutes or longer destroy the cysticerci. Salting or freezing for 1 week at −15°C or below is also effective.

✳ Sewage waste disposal, meat inspection, adequate cooking

● PORK TAPEWORM

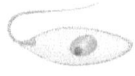

TAENIA SOLIUM: PARASITOLOGY AND LIFE CYCLE

Like the beef tapeworm, which it closely resembles, *T solium* inhabits the human jejunum, where it may survive for decades. It can be distinguished from its close relative only by careful scrutiny of the scolex and proglottids; *T solium* possesses a rostellum armed with a double row of hooklets (**Figure 56–1B3**). The strobila is generally smaller than that of *T saginata*, seldom exceeding 5 m in length or containing more than 1000 proglottids. Gravid segments measure 6 by 12 mm and thus appear less elongated than those of the bovine parasite (**Figure 56–1B4**). Typically, the uterus has only 8 to 12 lateral branches. Although the eggs appear morphologically identical to those of *T saginata*, they are infective only to swine and—perhaps reflecting a genetic proximity we might prefer to overlook—humans. Unlike *T saginata*, both pigs and people may become intermediate hosts when they ingest food contaminated with viable eggs (**Figure 56–2**). Humans with tapeworms may be autoinfected when gravid proglottids are carried backward into the stomach

T solium* strobila shorter than *T saginata

✳ Humans worms by eating undercooked pork cysts

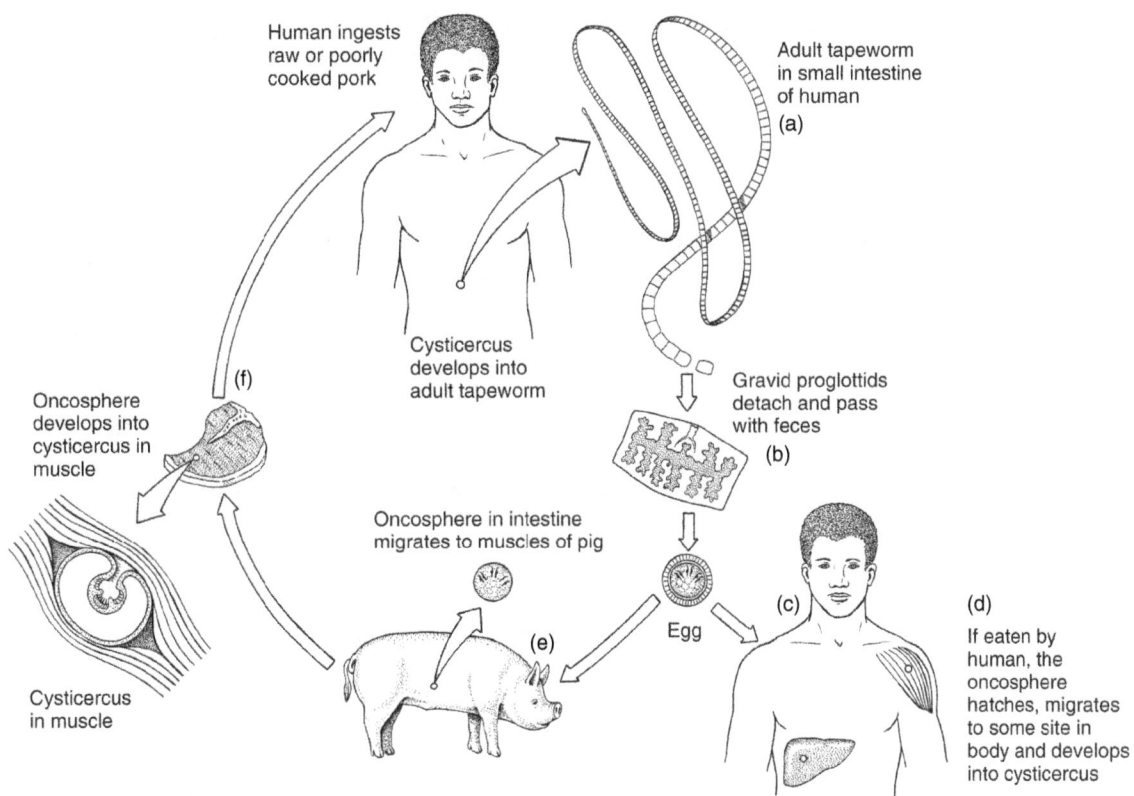

FIGURE 56–2. Pork tapeworm life cycle. (Reproduced with permission from Roberts RL, Janovy J, Nadler S: *Foundations of Parasitology*, 9th ed. New York, NY: McGraw Hill; 2013.)

during the act of vomiting, initiating the release of the contained eggs. Autoinfection probably also results when eggs are transported from the perianal area to the mouth on contaminated fingers. The pork tapeworm life cycle is illustrated in Figure 56–2.

Regardless of the route of entry, an egg reaching the stomach of an appropriate intermediate host hatches, releasing an embryo called a "hexacanth," because it has six hooklets. The embryo penetrates the intestinal wall and may be carried by the lymphohematogenous system to any tissue in the body. There it develops into a 1 cm, white, opalescent cysticercus over 3 to 4 months (**Figure 56–3**). The cysticercus may remain viable in pigs for up to 5 years, eventually infecting

✴ Complexity: cysts just like swine when eggs consumed from human stool

✴ Difference from beef tapeworm: tissue cysticerci develop in swine and humans

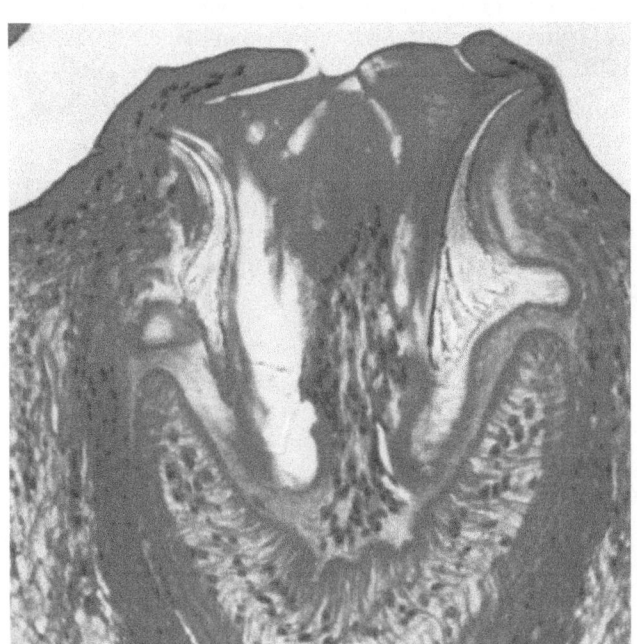

FIGURE 56–3. Cysticercosis of muscle. This section shows a cysticercus with the hooklets of a worm scolex. (Reproduced with permission from Connor DH, Chandler FW, Schwartz DQ, et al: *Pathology of Infectious Diseases*. Stamford CT: Appleton & Lange; 1997.)

* Mantra of *T solium:* "Eat a cyst in pork, get a worm … Eat an egg in human stool, get a cyst"

humans when they ingest undercooked "measly" flesh. In the human gut, the scolex everts, attaches to the mucosa, and develops into a new adult worm, thereby completing the cycle. When humans eat eggs, we serve as accidental, dead-end hosts, because the cysts will never be eaten by another person. However, these cysts may cause seizures if they form in the brain.

In summary, humans will acquire pork tapeworms if they consume undercooked pork; they will acquire cysticercosis if they consume tapeworm eggs from human feces.

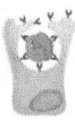

PORK TAPEWORM DISEASE

EPIDEMIOLOGY

T solium rarely found in the U.S. swine

Although infected swine are still occasionally found in the United States, most human disease is diagnosed in immigrants from endemic areas. Although pork tapeworm disease is widely distributed throughout the world, it is particularly common in South and Southeast Asia, Africa, Latin America, and Eastern Europe.

PORK TAPEWORM DISEASE: CLINICAL ASPECTS

MANIFESTATIONS

Gut tapeworms well tolerated

* Manifestations reaction to cysts in tissue

The signs and symptoms of infection with the *adult* worm are mild and similar to those of *T saginata* taeniasis. However, clinical manifestations are totally different when humans serve as *intermediate* hosts. Cysticerci develop in the subcutaneous tissues, muscles, heart, lungs, liver, eye, and brain (**Figure 56–4**). As long as their number is small and the cysticerci remain viable, tissue reaction is moderate and the patient is typically asymptomatic. The death of the larvae, however, may lead to a marked inflammatory reaction, fever, muscle pains, and eosinophilia.

* CNS invasion called neurocysticercosis

Multiple small cysts form

* Meningoencephalitis, eosinophilia, focal neurologic signs, epilepsy

The most important and dramatic clinical presentation of lesions in the central nervous system (CNS) is called neurocysticercosis. During the acute invasive stage, patients may experience fever, headache, and eosinophilia. In heavy infections, a meningoencephalitic syndrome with cerebrospinal fluid (CSF) eosinophilic pleocytosis may be present. Established cysts can be found in the cerebrum, ventricles, subarachnoid space, spinal cord, and eye. Cerebral cysts are usually small, often measuring 2 cm or less in diameter; racemose (clustered) lesions may be threefold larger. Parenchymal infections can induce focal neurologic abnormalities, personality changes, intellectual impairment, and/or seizures; in many endemic areas, cysticercosis is the leading cause of epilepsy. Subarachnoid lesions and cysticerci located within the fourth ventricle may obstruct the flow of CSF, producing increased intracranial pressure with associated headache, vomiting, visual disturbances, or psychiatric abnormalities. Multiple lesions have a

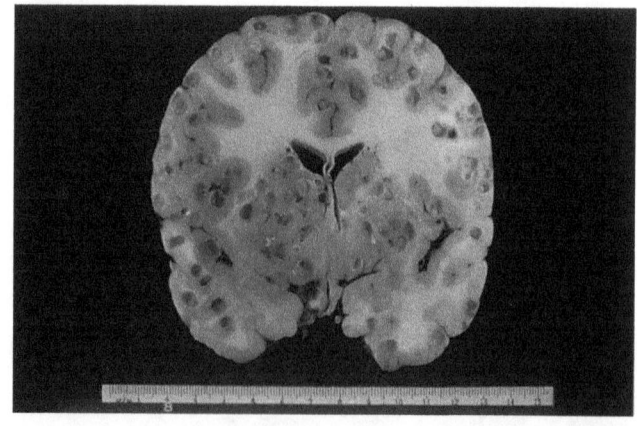

FIGURE 56–4. **Cysticercosis of brain.** This brain from a 16-year-old girl shows multiple cysticercal cysts primarily at the junction of white and gray matter. (Reproduced with permission from Connor DH, Chandler FW, Schwartz DQ, et al: *Pathology of Infectious Diseases.* Stamford CT: Appleton & Lange; 1997.)

predilection for the basal cisterns. Spinal involvement produces cord compression or meningeal inflammation. Eye lesions incite pain and visual disturbances.

DIAGNOSIS

Infection with the adult worm is diagnosed as described for *T saginata*. Cysticercosis is suspected when an individual who has been in an endemic area presents with neurologic manifestations or subcutaneous nodules. Radiographs of the soft tissues may reveal dead, calcified cysticerci. Viable lesions may be detected as low-density masses by computed tomography (CT) or magnetic resonance imaging (MRI). Brain cysticerci typically are 5 to 10 mm in diameter (Figure 56–4). Subarachnoid lesions are often larger, may be lobulated, and are often "isodense," making them difficult to identify radiographically. The lesions may resemble brain malignancy, which is managed differently, and thus it is important to confirm the diagnosis. This can be done by demonstrating the larva in a biopsy sample of a subcutaneous nodule or by detecting specific antibodies in the circulating blood. Serum and CSF enzyme immunoassays and western blot testing for specific anticysticercal antibodies have a sensitivity of 80% to 95%. The presence of IgG antibodies alone may reflect the presence of past or inactive disease.

* Adult worm diagnosed from proglottids, eggs in stool

Cysticercosis diagnosed by imaging, biopsy, serology

TREATMENT AND PREVENTION

Infection with the adult worm is treated with praziquantel, as described for *T saginata*. Symptomatic neurocysticercosis requires a different approach. For patients who present with seizures, antiepileptic medications are the most important priority; treatment of brain parenchymal lesions can then be attempted with albendazole and corticosteroids (to help minimize the inflammatory response to dying cysticerci). However, seizure control—not antiparasitic medication—is the first priority. Mechanical blockage of the brain's ventricles is another feared complication. Intraventricular, subarachnoid, and eye lesions appear relatively refractory to chemotherapy; surgery, CSF shunts, and corticosteroids may help ameliorate symptoms. Tapeworm acquisition can be prevented by adequately cooking pork before ingestion. Egg ingestion can be prevented by proper hand hygiene among food service workers after using the toilet.

* Antiepileptic medications with or without antiparasitics, corticosteroids

Surgery occasionally needed

 Is it possible for someone who consumes no pork to develop neurocysticercosis?

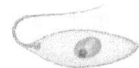 **FISH TAPEWORM**

 DIBOTHRIOCEPHALUS LATUS: **PARASITOLOGY AND LIFE CYCLE**

This parasite was formerly called *Diphyllobothrium latum*. The adult *D latus* attaches to the human ileal mucosa with the aid of two sucking grooves (bothria) located in an elongated fusiform scolex (**Figure 56–5**). In lifespan and overall length, it resembles the *Taenia* species discussed previously. The 3000 to 4000 proglottids, however, are uniformly wider than they are long, accounting for this cestode's species designation as well as one of its common names, the "broad tapeworm." The gravid segments contain a centrally positioned, rosette-shaped uterus unique among the tapeworms of humans. Over 1 million oval (55 by 75 μm) operculated eggs are released daily into the stool (Figure 56–5).

Dibothriocephalus latus **has broad proglottids**

 Think ▸▸ Apply 56-1: **Yes. Neurocysticercosis happens when humans ingest eggs from the feces of other humans, who in turn harbor an adult worm (taeniasis) they acquired by eating undercooked pork. "Eat a cyst, get a worm . . . eat an egg, get a cyst."**

FIGURE 56–5. *Dibothriocephalus latus.* **A.** Structure of scolex. **B.** Structure of egg. **C.** Scolex from a human case. **D.** Ova in stool stained with iodine. (C and D, Reproduced with permission from Connor DH, Chandler FW, Schwartz DQ, et al: *Pathology of Infectious Diseases.* Stamford CT: Appleton & Lange; 1997.)

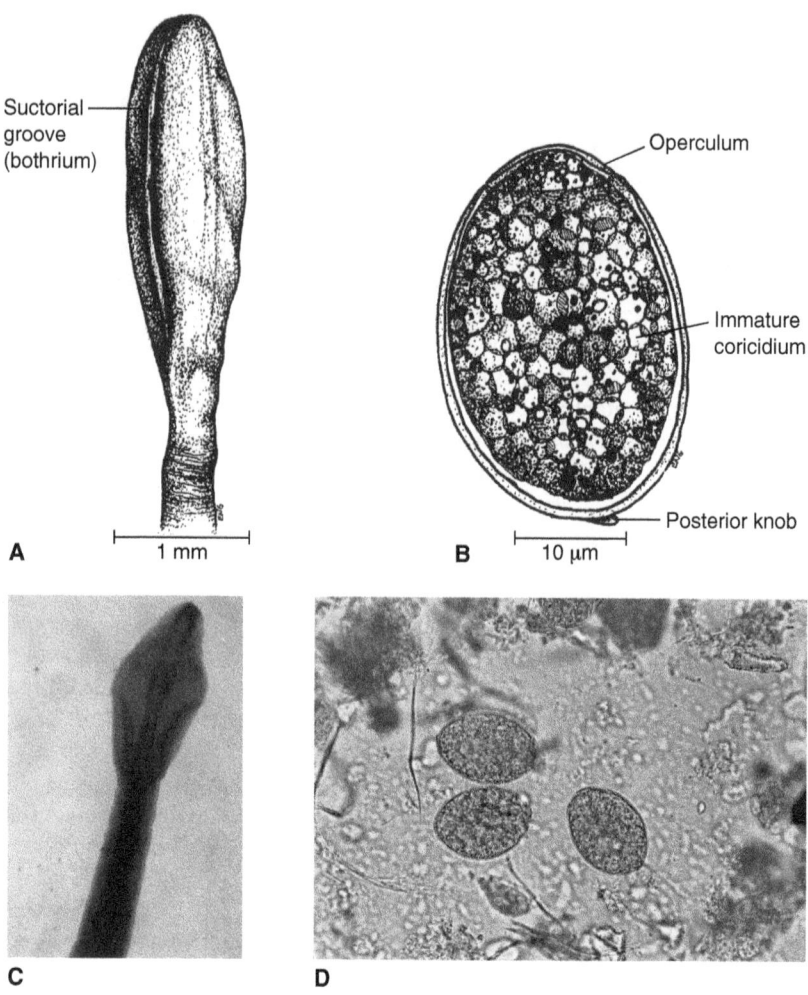

On reaching fresh water the eggs hatch, releasing ciliated, free-swimming larvae called coracidia. If ingested within a few days by small freshwater crustaceans of the genera *Cyclops* or *Diaptomus,* they develop into procercoid larvae. When the parasitized crustacean is then ingested by a freshwater or anadromous marine fish (eg, salmon), the larvae migrate into the musculature of the fish and develop into infectious plerocercoid larvae. Humans are infected when they eat improperly prepared freshwater fish containing such forms. The life cycle is illustrated in **Figure 56–6.**

Eggs release motile coracidia into water

✳ Humans infected eating undercooked fish

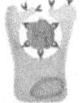 **FISH TAPEWORM DISEASE**

EPIDEMIOLOGY

Fish tapeworms are found wherever raw, pickled, or undercooked freshwater fish from fecally contaminated lakes and streams are eaten by humans. Other fish-eating mammals like cats, dogs, and bears may serve as reservoir hosts. Human infections have been described in the Baltic and Scandinavian countries, Russia, Switzerland, Italy, Japan, China, the South Pacific, Chile, and Argentina. The worm, possibly brought to North America by Scandinavian immigrants, is now found in Alaska, Canada, the midwestern states, California, and Florida. In the Pacific Northwest and Pacific Rim, a closely related species *Dibothriocephalus nihonkaiense* seems comparatively hardy in cold conditions and is able to form infectious plerocercoid larvae in anadromous salmon. Human cases have been traced to the ingestion of fish freshly taken from Alaskan waters. The increasing popularity of raw fish dishes, such as Japanese sushi and sashimi, may lead to increased prevalence of this disease in the United States—although freezing the fish before consumption is usually fatal to the cysts. Among native Americans, infection has been acquired by eating salted

Worldwide distribution

Worm in Alaska, Canada, Midwest, California, Florida

✳ Eating raw fish increases risk

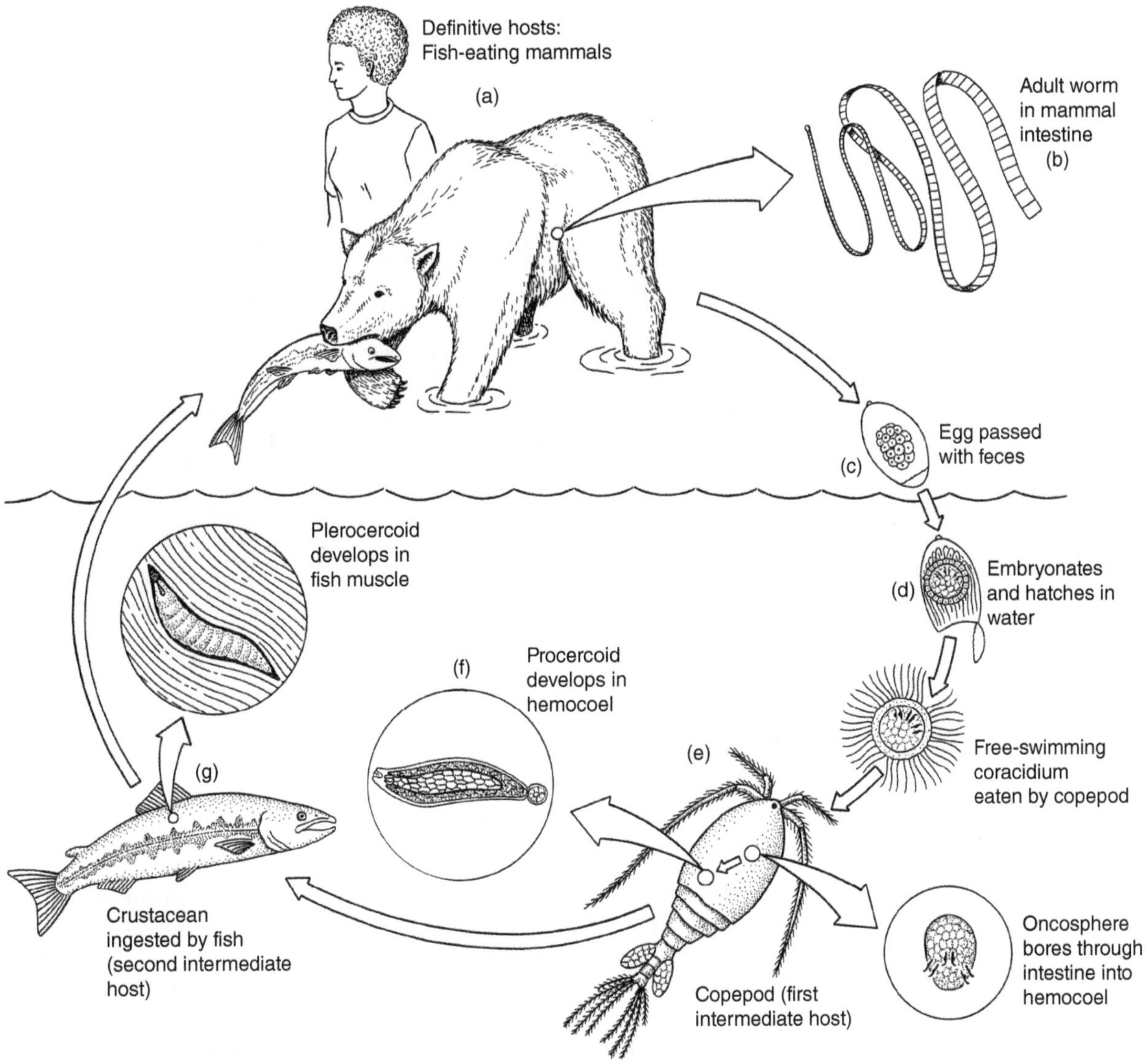

FIGURE 56–6. **Life cycle of *Dibothriocephalus latus*.** (Reproduced with permission from Roberts RL, Janovy J, Nadler S: *Foundations of Parasitology*, 9th ed. New York, NY: McGraw Hill; 2013.)

fish. Even when fish is appropriately cooked, individuals may become infected by sampling the flesh during the process of preparation.

FISH TAPEWORM DISEASE: CLINICAL ASPECTS

MANIFESTATIONS

Most infected patients are asymptomatic. On occasion, however, they may complain of epigastric pain, abdominal cramping, vomiting, and weight loss. Moreover, the presence of several adult worms within the gut has been known to precipitate intestinal or biliary obstruction. Forty percent of fish tapeworm carriers demonstrate low serum levels of vitamin B_{12}, apparently because of the competition between the host and the worm for this ingested nutrient. Studies have shown that a worm located high in the jejunum may take up 80% to 100% of vitamin B_{12} given by mouth. Approximately 0.1% to 2% of patients develop macrocytic anemia. They tend to be elderly, to have impaired production of intrinsic factor, and to have worms located high in the jejunum. In many, folate absorption is also diminished. Lysolecithin, a tapeworm product, may also contribute to anemia. Neurologic manifestations of vitamin B_{12} deficiency may occur, sometimes in the absence of anemia. They include numbness, paresthesias, loss of vibration sense, and, rarely, optic atrophy with central scotoma.

Occasional intestinal obstruction

✳ Vitamin B_{12} deficiency due to consumption by worm

DIAGNOSIS

* Eggs demonstrated in stool

The diagnosis should be suspected among patients with a compatible dietary history, ill-defined GI symptoms, or B₁₂ deficiency. It is confirmed by finding eggs in the stool. Because *D latus* produces large numbers of ova, identification is usually accomplished without the need for concentration techniques.

TREATMENT AND PREVENTION

* Fish noninfectious if cooked or frozen

Treatment is the same as described for *T saginata* tapeworm infections, using praziquantel. When anemia or neurologic manifestations are present, parenteral administration of vitamin B₁₂ is also indicated. Personal protection can be accomplished by thorough cooking of all salmon and freshwater fish. Devotees of raw fish may choose to freeze their favorite dish at −10°C for 48 hours before serving, as this is also effective in killing the plerocercoids. Ultimately, control of *Dibothriocephalus* infection is accomplished by prohibiting the discharge of untreated sewage into lakes and streams, although animal reservoir hosts are not addressed via this technique.

● ECHINOCOCCUS

Echinococcosis, or "hydatid disease," is a tissue infection of humans caused by larvae of *Echinococcus granulosus* and *E multilocularis*. The former is a more common cause of human disease.

ECHINOCOCCUS GRANULOSUS

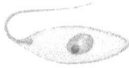 **PARASITOLOGY AND LIFE CYCLE**

Adult in canines

* Herbivores, humans intermediate hosts

Larvae reach portal or systemic circulation

* Cysts in tissues

Cycle completed in canines

The adult *E granulosus* tapeworm inhabits the small bowel of dogs, wolves, and other canines, where it survives for a scant 12 months. The scolex possesses four sucking disks and a double row of hooklets. The entire strobila, however, measures only 5 mm in length, and contains just three proglottids: one immature, one mature, and one gravid. The latter segment splits open either before or after passage in the stool, releasing eggs that appear identical to those of *T saginata* and *T solium*. A number of mammals may serve as intermediates, including sheep, goats, camels, deer, caribou, moose, and—most importantly—humans. When one of these hosts ingests eggs, they hatch, releasing embryos that penetrate the intestinal mucosa and are then carried via the portal blood to the liver. There, many are trapped in the hepatic sinusoids. The rest traverse the liver and are carried to the lung, where they may lodge. A few pass through the pulmonary capillaries, enter the systemic circulation, and are carried to the brain, heart, bones, kidneys, and other organs. Many of the larvae are phagocytosed and destroyed by host immune cells. The survivors form a cyst wall composed of an external laminated cuticle and an internal germinal membrane. The cyst fills with fluid and slowly expands, reaching a diameter of 1 cm over the next 5 to 6 months (**Figure 56–7**). However, they may grow substantially larger in subsequent months and years, in some cases reaching diameters greater than 10 cm. In time, secondary "brood capsules" arise from the germinal layer and form within the original hydatid, or break through the cyst surface to form new "daughter cysts." Within these brood capsules and daughter cysts, new protoscolices develop from the germinal lining. Degenerated protoscolices and germinal membranes fall to the bottom of the cyst to form hydatid "sand." When hydatid-containing tissues of the intermediate host are ingested by a canine, scolices are released in the intestine where they develop into adult worms. The life cycle is illustrated in **Figure 56–8**.

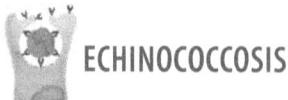 **ECHINOCOCCOSIS**

EPIDEMIOLOGY

There are two major epidemiologic forms of *E granulosus*-induced echinococcosis: Pastoral and sylvatic. The more common pastoral form has its highest incidence in Australia, New Zealand, South and East Africa, the Middle East, Central Europe, and South America, where domestic

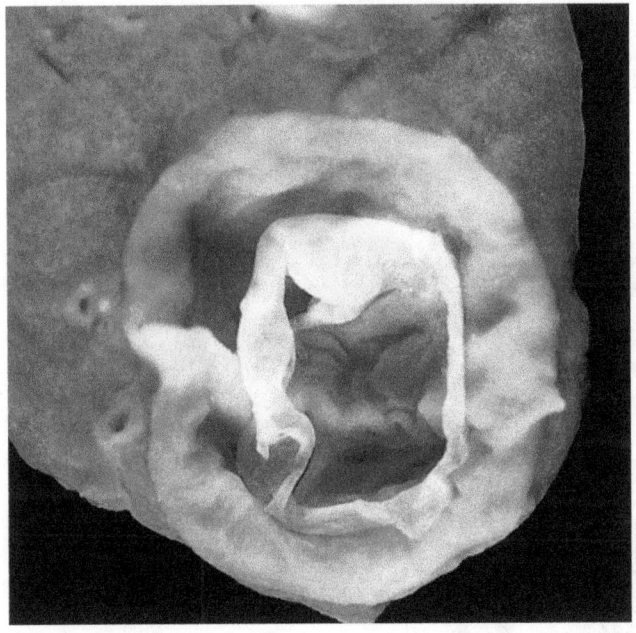
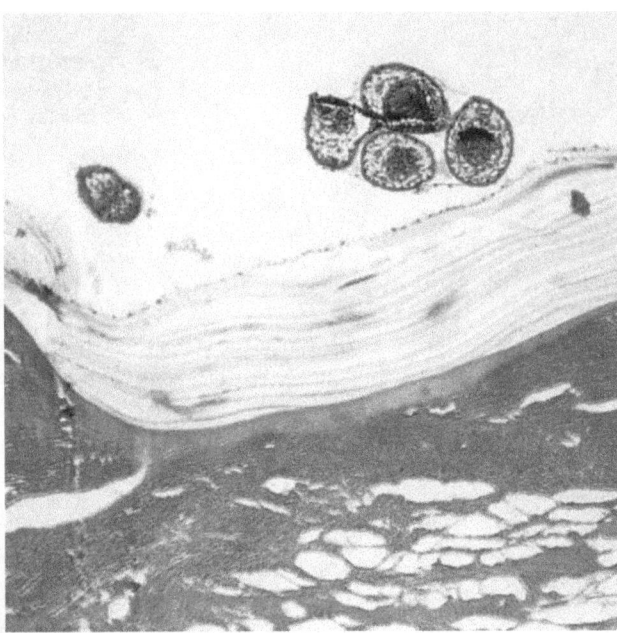

A   **B**

FIGURE 56–7. Echinococcosis. A. Echinococcal cyst in lung with white lining membrane. **B.** Echinococcal cyst wall with lung parenchyma below and five scolices above. (Reproduced with permission from Connor DH, Chandler FW, Schwartz DQ, et al: *Pathology of Infectious Diseases.* Stamford CT: Appleton & Lange; 1997.)

herbivores such as sheep, cattle, and camels are raised by people in close contact with domestic dogs. Although approximately 200 human cases are reported each year in the United States, most were acquired internationally. Indigenous cases have been reported, however, particularly among Basque sheep farmers in western states and Native Americans in the southwest. Animal husbandry practices that permit dogs to feed on the raw viscera of slaughtered sheep perpetuate cycle. Transmission also depends on suboptimal hand hygiene, in that shepherds become infected while handling their dogs: microscopic eggs are transferred from dog feces to their fur, where they are transferred onto their masters' hands and later ingested. Sylvatic echinococcosis, in contrast, is found principally in Alaska and western Canada, where wolves act as the definitive hosts and moose or caribou are the intermediates. In two counties in California, a second sylvatic cycle involving deer and coyotes has been described. When hunters kill these wild deer and feed their offal to accompanying dogs, a pastoral cycle may be established.

✳ **Hand-to-mouth infection of humans after dog contact**

Maintained by dogs feeding on sheep viscera

Sylvatic cycle in Alaska and western Canada

 ## ECHINOCOCCOSIS: CLINICAL ASPECTS

MANIFESTATIONS

The enlarging *E granulosus* cysts produce tissue damage by mechanical means. The clinical presentation depends on their number, location, and rate of growth. Typically, a latent period of 5 to 20 years occurs between acquisition of infection and subsequent diagnosis. Intervals as long as 75 years have been reported.

The majority of cysts are found in the liver and/or in the lung. One-fifth of all patients show involvement of multiple sites. Many patients are asymptomatic when the lesion is discovered on routine imaging or physical examination. Occasionally, the patient may present with hemoptysis, pain in the right upper quadrant of the abdomen, or a tender hepatic mass. Significant morbidity is uncommon, and death rare. However, hydatid cysts may reach enormous size. They may eventually rupture, inducing fever, pruritus, urticaria, and—at times—anaphylactic shock. Germinal tissue or brood capsules may also spread to other areas, leading to dissemination of the infection. Rupture of pulmonary lesions also induces cough, chest pain, and hemoptysis. Liver cysts may break through the diaphragm or rupture into the bile duct or peritoneal cavity. Most patients who

✳ **Disease caused by mechanical effects of cysts**

✳ **Many asymptomatic**

Cysts may attain large size

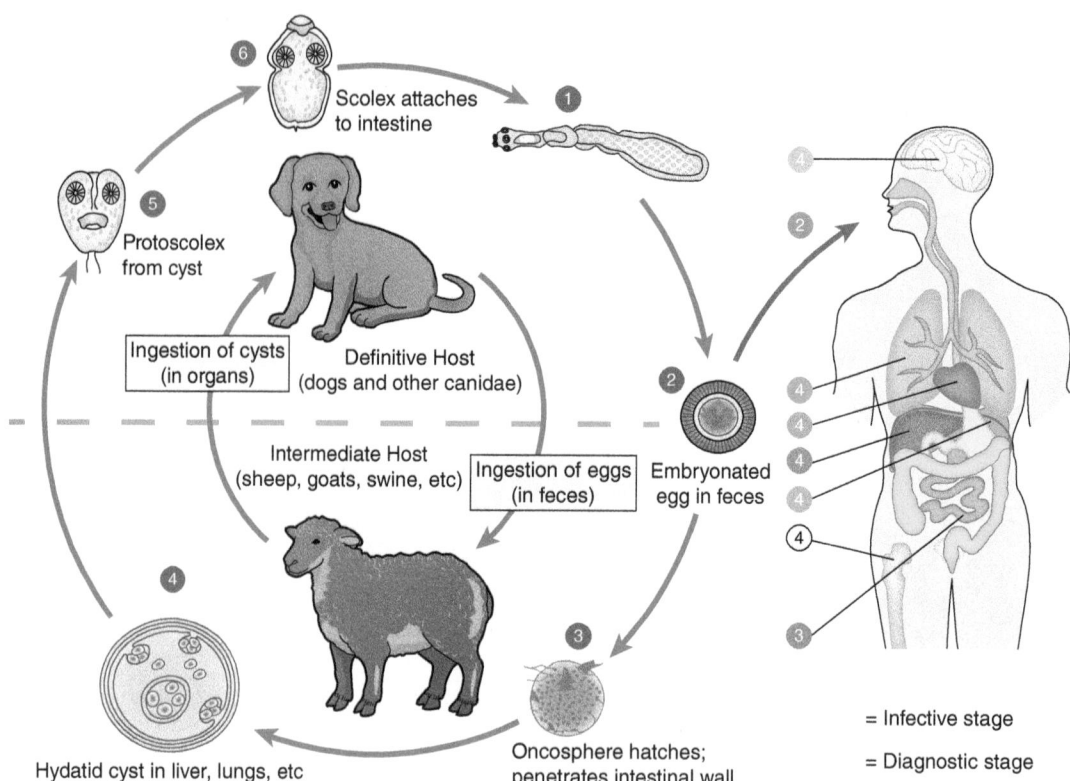

The adult *Echinococcus granulosus* (3-6 mm long) ❶ resides in the small bowel of the definitive hosts, dogs, or other canids. Gravid proglottids release eggs ❷ that are passed in the feces. After ingestion by a suitable intermediate host (under natural conditions: sheep, goat, swine, cattle, horses, and camel), the egg hatches in the small bowel and releases an oncosphere ❸ that penetrates the intestinal wall and migrates through the circulatory system into various organs, especially the liver and lungs. In these organs, the oncosphere develops into a cyst ❹ that enlarges gradually, producing protoscolices and daughter cysts that fill the cyst interior. The definitive host becomes infected by ingesting the cyst-containing organs of the infected intermediate host. After ingestion, the protoscolices ❺ evaginate, attach to the intestinal mucosa ❻, and develop into adult stages ❶ in 32 to 80 days. The same life cycle occurs with *E multilocularis* (1.2-3.7 mm), with the following differences: The definitive hosts are foxes, and to a lesser extent dogs, cats, coyotes, and wolves; the intermediate host are small rodents; and larval growth (in the liver) remains indefinitely in the proliferative stage, resulting in invasion of the surrounding tissues. With *E vogeli* (up to 5.6 mm long), the definitive hosts are bush dogs and dogs; the intermediate hosts are rodents; and the larval stage (liver, lungs, and other organs) develops both externally and internally, resulting in multiple vesicles. *E oligarthrus* (up to 2.9 mm long) has a life cycle that involves wild felids as definitive hosts and rodents as intermediate hosts. Humans become infected by ingesting eggs ❷, with resulting release of oncospheres ❸ in the intestine and the development of cysts ❹, ❹, ❹, ❹, ❹, ④ in various organs.

FIGURE 56–8. Life cycle of *Echinococcus* species.

develop symptoms, however, present with a tender, palpable hepatic mass. Intrabiliary extrusion of calcified cysts may mimic the signs of acute cholecystitis; complete obstruction results in jaundice. Bone cysts may produce pathologic fractures. Lesions in the CNS may manifest with blindness or seizures. Cardiac lesions have been associated with conduction disturbances, ventricular rupture, and embolic metastases. It has been suggested that circulating antigen–antibody complexes may deposit in the kidney, initiating membranous glomerulonephritis.

✳ Rupture leads to hypersensitivity, dissemination

DIAGNOSIS

In *E granulosus*-infected patients, chest X-rays may demonstrate pulmonary lesions as slightly irregular, round masses of uniform density, often devoid of calcification. In contrast, more than one-half of hepatic lesions display a smooth, calcific rim. CT, ultrasonography, and MRI may reveal either a simple fluid-filled cyst or daughter cysts with hydatid sand. Endoscopic retrograde cholangiography has been valuable for determining cyst location and possible communication with the biliary tree. Because of the potential for an allergic reaction or spread of infection, diagnostic aspiration may be contraindicated. Nevertheless, in select cases, ultrasonically guided

✳ Radiologic, scanning appearance characteristic

percutaneous drainage, followed by the introduction of hypertonic saline to kill protoscolices and germinal layer, has proved safe and useful both diagnostically and therapeutically (see PAIR later). In patients with ruptured pulmonary cysts, scolices may be demonstrated in the sputum.

In some cases, confirmation of the diagnosis before drainage requires serologic testing. Unfortunately, current options are not totally satisfactory. Indirect hemagglutination and latex agglutination tests are positive in 90% of patients with hepatic lesions and 60% of those with pulmonary hydatid cysts. Polymerase chain reaction assay has been shown to be capable of detecting picogram quantities of *Echinococcus* genomic DNA in fine-needle biopsy material from patients with suspected echinococcosis.

✻ Cyst puncture perilous

Serology needs improved sensitivity

TREATMENT AND PREVENTION

For years, the only definitive therapy available was surgical extirpation. Patients with pulmonary hydatid cysts of the sylvatic type and small calcified hepatic lesions underwent surgery only when they became symptomatic or the cysts increased dramatically in size over time. However, for uncomplicated lesions, **P**uncture, **A**spiration, **I**njection of scolicide, and **R**easpiration (PAIR) can be used in lieu of surgery. The scolicide of choice is probably hypertonic saline, although other chemicals have been used. If performed properly, this technique is safer and better tolerated than open surgery. Presently, it is recommended that high-dose albendazole be administered before and for several weeks (or years in the case of *E multilocularis* infection) after surgery and/or aspiration. Infected dogs should be dewormed, and infected carcasses and offal burned or buried. Hands should be carefully washed after contact with potentially infected dogs.

✻ Treatment may include PAIR with concomitant albendazole

 A shepherd is shocked to learn that he has hydatid disease, because he is a lifelong vegetarian who has never consumed undercooked animal organ meat. How do you explain this?

ECHINOCOCCUS MULTILOCULARIS

Echinococcus multilocularis is found primarily in subarctic and arctic regions in North America, Europe, and Asia. The adult worms are found in the gut of foxes and, to a lesser extent, coyotes. Their larvae grow in the tissues of mice and voles, the rodent prey of canines. Domestic dogs may acquire adult tapeworms by killing and ingesting these larva-infected sylvatic rodents. Humans are infected with larval forms through the ingestion of eggs passed in the feces of their domestic dogs or ingestion of egg-contaminated vegetation, for instance when eating berries sprayed with an invisible layer of fox stool. Unlike the larval forms of *E granulosus*, those of *E multilocularis* bud *externally*, producing proliferative, multilocular cysts that slowly but progressively invade and destroy the affected organs and adjacent tissues.

Foxes definitive hosts

Larvae bud externally; produce multilocular cysts

The clinical course in humans is characterized by epigastric pain, obstructive jaundice, and, less frequently, metastasis to the lung and brain, closely mimicking liver cancer. As with *E granulosus*, medical treatment of *E multilocularis* often fails to achieve cure. Patients with multilocular infection may require surgical management. The prognosis is grim if not diagnosed early.

● *HYMENOLEPIS*

Like *Echinococcus* species, and in contrast to the cow, pig, and fish tapeworms, the adult *Hymenolepis nana* worm is very small, perhaps 4 cm in length. Rodents are the most common definitive hosts, but humans may become infected. In fact, the so-called "dwarf tapeworm" is the only tapeworm that can be transmitted directly from human to human. Eggs are ingested via the fecal–oral route. They then release embryos that penetrate the intestinal wall. The resulting cysts mature in

 Think ▸▸ Apply 56-2: Presumably, he acquired hydatid disease from accidental ingestion of the feces of his sheepdog, which in turn was infected while eating livestock offal filled with cysts. Dogs get worms by eating cysts; humans get cysts by consuming eggs in dog stool.

Can be transmitted directly from human to human

the intestinal wall, then reenter the gut lumen to develop into adult worms again. Endemic areas include parts of Asia, Europe, Central and South America, and Africa. Occasionally, it is found in institutionalized persons in North America. Most persons are asymptomatic, but heavy worm burdens may be associated with diarrhea, abdominal cramping, and anorexia. Finding characteristic eggs in the stool makes the diagnosis. Treatment is similar to that for other tapeworms, but may need to be prolonged to fully eradicate cysts in the intestinal wall.

KEY CONCLUSIONS

- The clinical manifestations of tapeworm infections depend on whether humans are definitive hosts (harboring intestinal tapeworms) or intermediate hosts (harboring tissue-invasive cysts).
- Generally, intestinal worms are well tolerated, whereas tissue cysts are more dangerous.
- Treatment of taeniasis is straightforward and effective using praziquantel.
- Treatment of cystic disease is more complex and hazardous.
- Breaking the cycle of cestode infection requires knowledge of their transmission modes.

CASE STUDY

Seizures on the Tennis Court

A 26-year-old professional tennis player from Mexico suddenly developed a left-sided epileptic seizure, lasting for 5 minutes, while competing in an international tournament. He had no history of such occurrences and had been well before this episode.

Physical examination was normal, but brain MRI imaging revealed a round, calcified 3 cm lesion in the right parietal lobe.

QUESTIONS

1. Which of the following is most likely responsible for this patient's condition?
    A. *Taenia saginata*
    B. *Taenia solium*
    C. *Echinococcus granulosus*
    D. *Dibothriocephalus latus*

2. Vitamin B$_{12}$ deficiency, with macrocytic anemia is associated with which of the following parasites?
    A. *Echinococcus multilocularis*
    B. *Dibothriocephalus latus*
    C. *Taenia saginata*
    D. *Taenia solium*

3. Which is the most common definitive host for transmission of echinococcosis?
    A. Pig
    B. Cow
    C. Fish
    D. Dog

ANSWERS

1. (B)

2. (B)

3. (D)

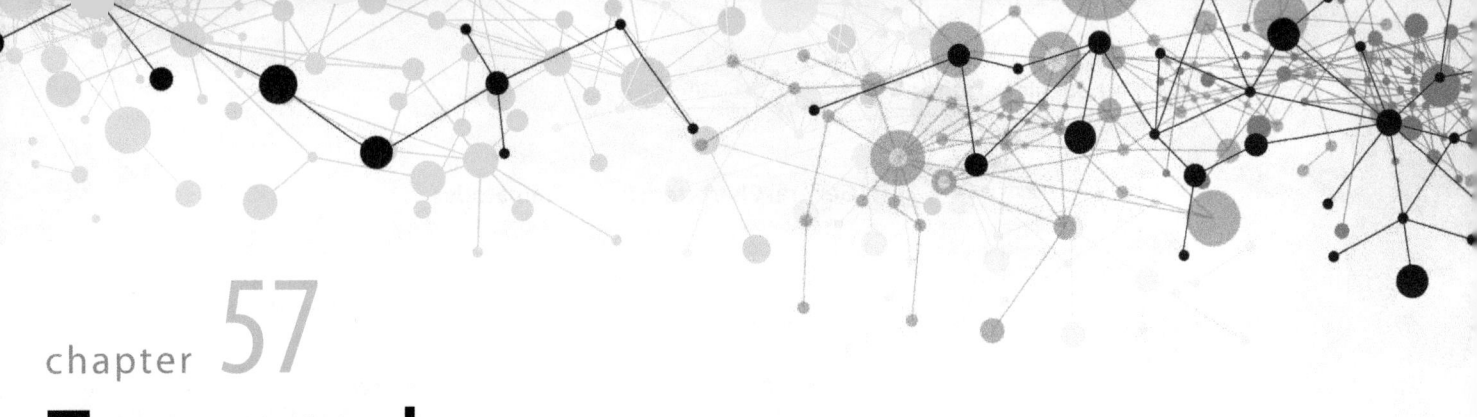

chapter 57

Trematodes

Paragonimus westermani · *Clonorchis sinensis* · *Schistosoma haematobium* · *Schistosoma japonicum* · *Schistosoma mansoni*

> *Sometimes the patient with schistosomiasis experiences no trouble whatever; in other instances the suffering is very great.*
>
> —Sir Patrick Manson, 1898

OVERVIEW

Trematodes are flatworms, also called "platyhelminths" or "flukes." They are divided into two major categories: the *hermaphrodites* and the *schistosomes* (**Table 57–1**). Of the many relationships that have developed between humans and helminths over millennia, perhaps the most destructive to our health and productivity is that forged by the trematodes. Typically, the adults live for decades within human tissues (for the hermaphrodites) and vasculature (for the schistosomes), where they resist immunologic attack and damage vital organs. Physicians and public health officers must understand trematode life cycles in order to make a meaningful difference in the lives of people impacted by these parasites.

GENERAL FEATURES OF TREMATODES

Morphologically, trematodes are bilaterally symmetric, vary in length from a few millimeters to several centimeters, and possess two deep suckers from which they derive their name ("body with holes"). One surrounds the oral cavity, and the other is located on the ventral surface of the worm. These organs are used for both attachment and locomotion; movement is accomplished in a characteristic inchworm fashion.

The digestive tract begins at the oral sucker and continues as a muscular pharynx and esophagus before bifurcating to form bilateral ceca that end blindly near the posterior extremity of the worm. Undigested food is vomited through the oral cavity. The excretory system consists of a number of hollow, ciliated "flame" cells that excrete waste products into interconnecting ducts terminating in a posterior pore.

Trematodes are divided into two major categories, based on their reproductive systems: the *hermaphrodites* and the *schistosomes* (Table 57–1). The adult hermaphrodites contain both male and female gonads and produce operculated eggs (defined as having a lid). In contrast, the schistosomes have separate sexes, and the fertilized female deposits nonoperculated eggs. However, the two groups have similar life cycles. In both cases, eggs are excreted from the human host and—if they reach fresh water—hatch to release ciliated larvae called **miracidia.** These larvae find and penetrate a snail host specific for the trematode species. In this intermediate snail host, they are transformed by a process of asexual reproduction into thousands of tail-bearing larvae called **cercariae,** which are released from the snail over a period of weeks. The cercariae swim in fresh water, searching vigorously for their next host. In the case of schistosomal cercariae, this host is the human: When they contact the skin surface, they attach, discard their tails, and invade, thereby completing their life cycle. The cercariae of the hermaphroditic flukes, in contrast, encyst in or on an aquatic plant or animal, where they undergo a second transformation to become infective **metacercariae.** Their cycle is completed when this second intermediate host is ingested by a human.

Flukes move through tissue and vasculature with inchworm locomotion

✳ Hermaphrodites and Schistosomes

Snails release motile cercariae in water

✳ Cercariae infect human skin

✳ Hermaphroditic cercariae encyst on aquatic plant or animal, transform into metacercariae

TABLE 57–1	General Characteristics of Trematodes	
CHARACTERISTIC	**SCHISTOSOMES**	**HERMAPHRODITES**
Genus	*Schistosoma*	*Paragonimus, Clonorchis, Opisthorchis, Fasciola, Fasciolopsis, Heterophyes/Metagonimus*
Adult location in human body		
	Bloodstream	Tissue or intestines
Morphology		
Adult	Oral and ventral suckers	Oral and ventral suckers
	Blind gastrointestinal tract	Blind gastrointestinal tract
	Slender, worm like	Flat, leaf like
Egg	Nonoperculated	Operculated
Biology		
Sexes	Separate	Hermaphroditic
Intermediates	One	Two
Lifespan	Long	Long

Of the many trematodes that infect humans, only the five of greatest medical importance are discussed here: the hermaphroditic lung (*Paragonimus* spp.) and liver (*Clonorchis sinensis*) flukes; and the blood flukes, all of which are members of the genus *Schistosoma* (*S mansoni, S haematobium,* and *S japonicum*). Basic features of these and other hermaphroditic tissue and intestinal flukes are listed in **Table 57–2.**

TABLE 57–2	Hermaphroditic Trematodes					
	PARAGONIMUS	**CLONORCHIS**	**OPISTHORCHIS**	**FASCIOLA**	**FASCIOLOPSIS**	**HETEROPHYES/ METAGONIMUS**
Distribution						
Geographic	Asia, Africa, Central America	Japan, China, Taiwan, Vietnam	Asia, Eastern Europe	Worldwide	East and Southeast Asia	Asia, former USSR, Mediterranean
Infected population (in millions)	3	20	4	2	10	Unknown
Adult worms						
Reservoir hosts	Domestic and wild animals	Cats, dogs	Domestic and wild animals	Sheep and other herbivores	Pigs	Fish-eating mammals
Location in body	Lungs, CNS	Biliary tract	Biliary tract	Biliary tract	Small intestine	Small intestine
Length (mm)	7-12	10-25	10	20-30	20-75	1-2
Lifespan (years)	4-6	20-30	20-30	10-15	0.5	1
Eggs						
Characteristics	Operculated	Operculated	Operculated	Operculated	Operculated	Operculated
Size (μm)	80-100	26-30	26-30	130-150	130-150	26-30
Location[a]	Sputum, stool	Bile, stool	Bile, stool	Bile, stool	Stool	Stool
Larvae						
First intermediate	Snail	Snail	Snail	Snail	Snail	Snail
Second intermediate	Freshwater crab and crayfish	Freshwater fish	Freshwater fish	Watercress and other aquatic plants	Water chestnut and other aquatic plants	Freshwater fish

CNS, central nervous system.
[a]Diagnostic specimens.

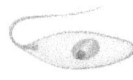

• PARAGONIMUS

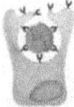

PARAGONIMUS SPECIES: PARASITOLOGY AND LIFE CYCLE

Several *Paragonimus* species may infect humans. *Paragonimus westermani*, which is widely distributed in East Asia, is the species most frequently involved. The short, plump (10 by 5 mm), reddish-brown adults are characteristically found encapsulated in the pulmonary parenchyma of their definitive host. The adults are often, but not always, found in pairs in these capsules, where they usually cross-fertilize each other. Here they deposit operculated, golden-brown eggs, which are distinguished by their size (50 by 90 μm) and prominent periopercular shoulder (**Figure 57–1**). Eggs may be released into a bronchiole before the capsule of human fibrous tissue is complete, or when a capsule erodes into a bronchiole. The eggs are then coughed up and spat out or swallowed and passed in the stool. In either case, if they reach fresh water, they embryonate for several weeks before the ciliated miracidia emerge through the open opercula. After invasion of an appropriate snail host, 3 to 5 months pass before cercariae are released. These larval forms invade the gills, musculature, and viscera of certain crayfish or freshwater crabs; over 6 to 8 weeks, the cercariae transform into metacercariae. When the raw or undercooked flesh of the second intermediate host is ingested by humans, the metacercariae encyst in the duodenum and burrow through the gut wall into the peritoneal cavity. Most then continue their migration through the diaphragm and reach maturity in the lungs 5 to 6 weeks later (**Figure 57–2**). However, some are retained in the intestinal wall and mesentery or wander to other foci such as the liver, pancreas, kidney, skeletal muscle, or subcutaneous tissue. Young worms migrating through the neck and jugular foramen may encyst in the brain, a common ectopic site. Paragonimiasis is a zoonosis: in addition to humans, other carnivores may serve as definitive hosts, including the rat, cat, dog, and pig. Immature ectopic adults in the striated muscles of the pig may infect humans after ingestion of undercooked pork.

* Adults encapsulate in lung

Capsule erodes into bronchiole, eggs coughed up; continue if eggs reach water with snail

* Crayfish, freshwater crabs second intermediate hosts

Other carnivores also definitive hosts

PARAGONIMIASIS (LUNG FLUKE INFECTION)

EPIDEMIOLOGY

There are thought to be millions of human infections worldwide. Although most are concentrated in the Far East (eg, Korea, Japan, China, Taiwan, the Philippines, and Indonesia), paragonimiasis has been described in India, Africa (*Paragonimus africanus*), and Latin America (*Paragonimus mexicanus*). *Paragonimus kellicotti*, a parasite of mink, is widely distributed in eastern Canada and the United States but rarely produces human infection. Approximately 1% of recent Vietnamese immigrants to the United States were once found to be infected with *P westermani*. Infection of the snail host, which is typically found in small mountain streams located away from human habitation, is probably maintained by animal hosts other than humans. Human disease occurs when food shortages or local customs expose individuals to infected crabs. When these crustaceans are prepared for cooking, juice containing metacercariae may be left behind on the working surface and contaminate other foods subsequently prepared in the same area. Fresh crab juice, which has been used to treat infertility in Cameroon and measles in Korea, may also transmit the disease. In Southeast Asia, crabs are eaten after they have been lightly salted, pickled, or immersed briefly in wine ("drunken crab"), practices seldom lethal to the metacercariae. This has occurred in the United States as well. Children living in endemic areas may be infected while handling or ingesting crabs during the course of play.

Infected snails found in mountain streams

* Humans infected by ingesting undercooked infected crustaceans

PARAGONIMIASIS (LUNG FLUKE INFECTION): CLINICAL ASPECTS

MANIFESTATIONS

During their migration from the gut to the lungs, larvae may cause tender, raised subcutaneous nodules, which migrate slowly along the abdominal wall. Adult worms in the lung elicit an eosinophilic inflammatory reaction and, eventually, the formation of a 1 to 2 cm fibrous capsule that

FIGURE 57–1. **Trematode eggs. A.** Structure of *Paragonimus* and *Clonorchis* adults and ova. **B.** Structure of *Fasciola* and *Schistosoma* adults and ova. **C.** Two *C sinensis* eggs in stool. The left egg has an open operculum to hatch a transparent miracidium. **D.** Mature *S mansoni* egg in stool with lateral spine. **E.** Mature *S haematobium* egg in urine with terminal spine. **F.** Mature *S japonicum* egg in stool with diminutive spine. (C and D, Reproduced with permission from Connor DH, Chandler FW, Schwartz DQ, et al: *Pathology of Infectious Diseases.* Stamford CT: Appleton & Lange; 1997. E and F, Used with permission from Paul Pottinger, M.D.)

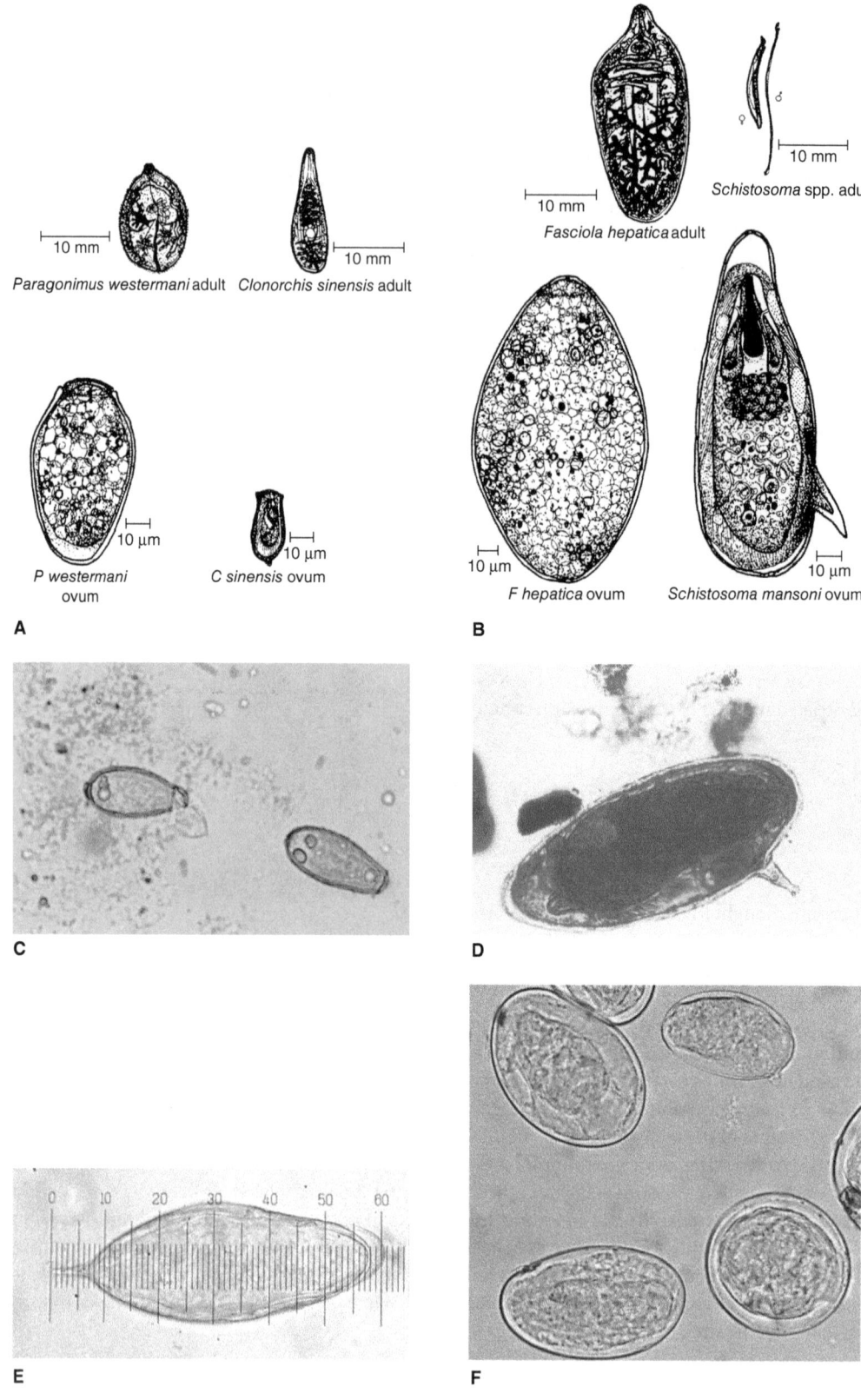

Paragonimus westermani adult   *Clonorchis sinensis* adult

P westermani ovum   *C sinensis* ovum

Fasciola hepatica adult

Schistosoma spp. adult

F hepatica ovum   *Schistosoma mansoni* ovum

A

B

C

D

E

F

Multiple lung cysts may form

surrounds and encloses one or more parasites. An infected patient may harbor more than 20 such lesions. With the onset of oviposition, the capsule swells and erodes into a bronchiole, resulting in expectoration of the brownish eggs, blood, and an inflammatory exudate. Secondary bacterial infection of the evacuated cysts is common, producing a clinical picture of chronic bronchitis or bronchiectasis. When cysts rupture into the pleural cavity, chest pain and effusion can result.

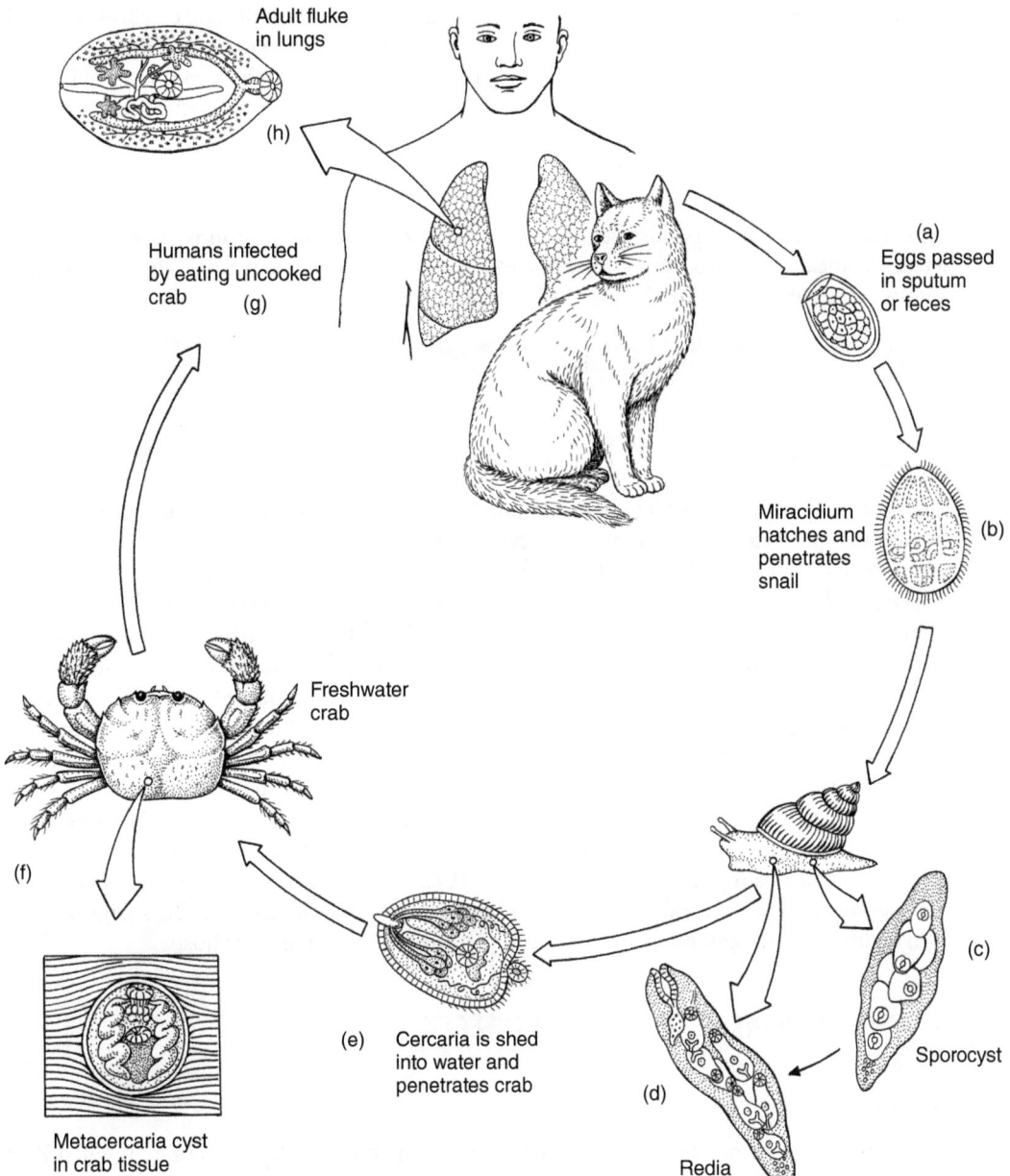

Adult fluke
in lungs

(h)

(a)
Eggs passed
in sputum
or feces

Humans infected
by eating uncooked
crab
(g)

Miracidium
hatches and
penetrates
snail

(b)

Freshwater
crab

(c)

(f)

Sporocyst

Metacercaria cyst
in crab tissue

(e) Cercaria is shed
into water and
penetrates crab

(d)

Redia

FIGURE 57–2. Life cycle of *Paragonimus westermani*. (Reproduced with permission from Roberts RL, Janovy J, Nadler S: *Foundations of Parasitology*, 9th ed. New York, NY: McGraw Hill; 2013.)

Early in infection, chest X-rays demonstrate small segmental infiltrates; these are gradually replaced by round nodules that may cavitate. Eventually, cystic rings, fibrosis, and calcification occur, producing a picture closely resembling that of pulmonary tuberculosis (TB). This confusion is compounded by the frequent coexistence of the two diseases.

Adult flukes in the intestine and mesentery produce pain, bloody diarrhea, and occasionally palpable abdominal or cutaneous masses; the latter is more characteristic of a related Chinese fluke, *P skrjabini*. In approximately 1% of the cases of paragonimiasis in Southeast Asia, more commonly in children, parasites lodge in the brain and produce a variety of neurologic manifestations, including epilepsy, paralysis, homonymous hemianopsia, optic atrophy, and papilledema.

※ Chronic pulmonary abscess resembles TB

DIAGNOSIS

Eggs are usually absent from the sputum during the first 3 months of overt infection; however, repeated examinations eventually demonstrate them in more than 75% of infected patients. When a pleural effusion is present, it should be checked for eggs. Stool examination is frequently helpful, particularly in children who swallow their expectorated sputum. Approximately 50% of patients

✳ Eggs in sputum, pleural fluid, feces

✳ Serology for diagnosis, monitor treatment

with brain lesions demonstrate calcification on X-ray films of the skull. The cerebrospinal fluid in such cases shows elevated protein levels and eosinophilic leukocytosis. A diagnosis in these cases, however, often depends on the detection of circulating antibodies via immunoblot technique. Their presence usually correlates well with acute disease and eventually disappears with successful therapy.

TREATMENT AND PREVENTION

Lung fluke infection responds well to praziquantel therapy. Brain lesions may require anti-seizure medications, and a short course of corticosteroids before praziquantel is initiated. Control requires adequate cooking of shellfish before ingestion.

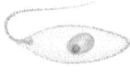 **● CLONORCHIS**

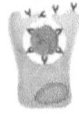 ### CLONORCHIS SINENSIS: PARASITOLOGY AND LIFE CYCLE

✳ Adults survive decades in biliary tract

Eggs discharged in bile ducts appear in feces

✳ Snails first intermediate host; fish the second

Metacercariae migrate to biliary system

Flukes of the genera *Fasciola, Opisthorchis,* and *Clonorchis* all may infect the human biliary tract and at times produce manifestations of ductal obstruction (Table 57–2). *Clonorchis sinensis,* the "Chinese liver fluke," is discussed here. The small, slender (5 by 15 mm) adult survives up to 50 years in the biliary tract of its host by feasting on its rich mucosal secretions. A cone-shaped anterior pole, a large oral sucker, and a pair of deeply lobular testes arranged one behind the other in the posterior third of the worm distinguish it from other hepatic parasites (Figure 57–4H). Approximately 2000 tiny (15 by 30 µm) fertilized ovoid eggs are discharged daily and travel down the bile duct and into the fecal stream. The urn-shaped eggshells have a discernible shoulder at their opercular rim and a tiny knob on the broader posterior pole (Figure 57–4A). On reaching fresh water, they are ingested by their intermediate snail host, where they transform into cercariae (**Figure 57–3A**). These cercariae are released into the water, where they swim until they penetrate the tissues of freshwater fish, in which they encyst to form metacercariae. If the latter host is ingested by a fish-eating mammal, the larvae are released in the duodenum, ascend the common bile duct, migrate to the second-order bile ducts, and mature to adulthood over 30 days (**Figure 57–4**).

In addition to humans, rats, cats, dogs, and pigs may serve as definitive hosts.

CLONORCHIASIS (LIVER FLUKE INFECTION)

EPIDEMIOLOGY

Clonorchiasis is endemic in Southeast Asia, particularly in Korea, Japan, Taiwan, the Red River Valley of Vietnam, the Southern Chinese province of Guangdong, and Hong Kong. In previous years, parasite transmission was perpetuated by the practice of fertilizing commercial fish ponds

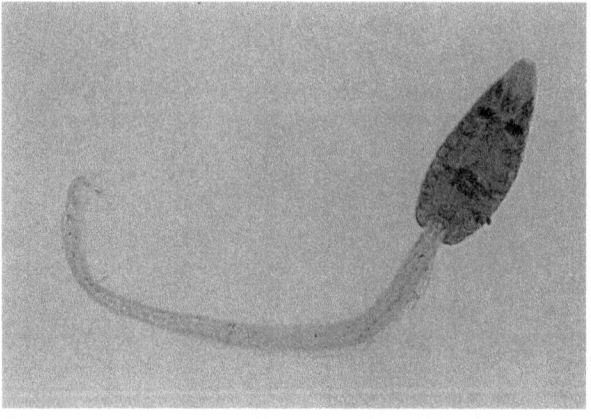

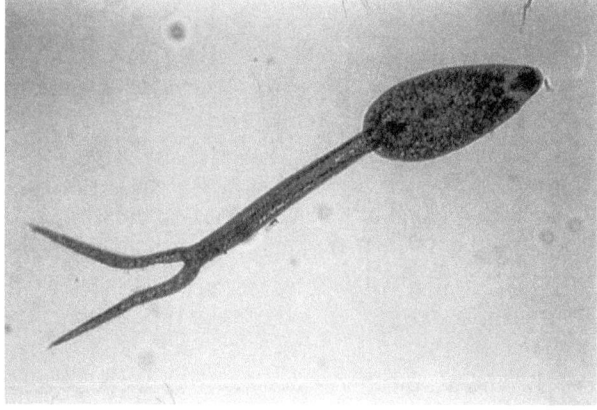

A   B

FIGURE 57–3. Trematode cercarial larvae. A. *Clonorchis sinensis.* **B.** *Schistosoma mansoni.* (Reproduced with permission from Connor DH, Chandler FW, Schwartz DQ, et al: *Pathology of Infectious Diseases.* Stamford CT: Appleton & Lange; 1997.)

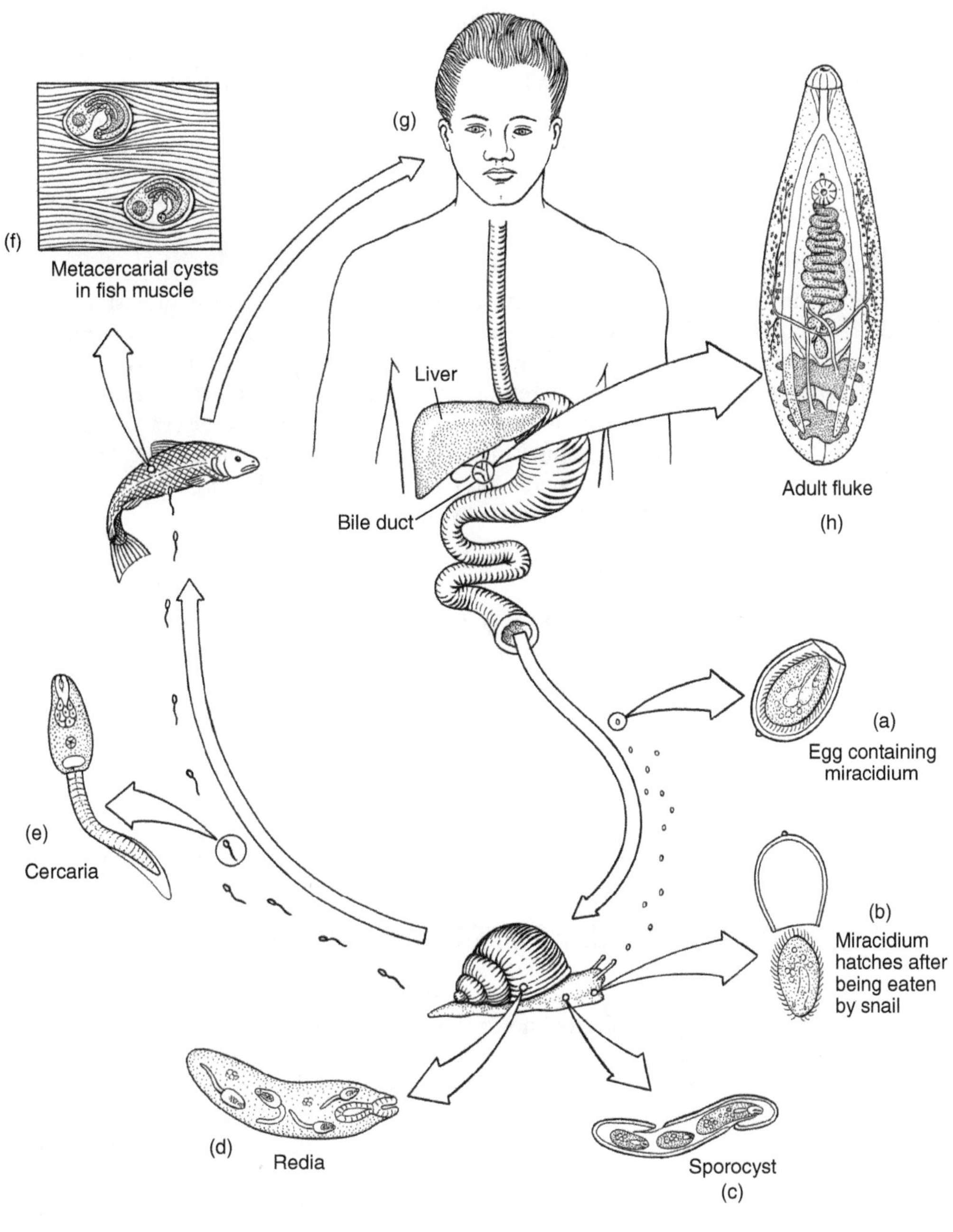

FIGURE 57–4. Life cycle of *Clonorchis*. (Reproduced with permission from Roberts RL, Janovy J, Nadler S: *Foundations of Parasitology*, 9th ed. New York, NY: McGraw Hill; 2013.)

(f)
Metacercarial cysts
in fish muscle

(g)

Liver

Bile duct

Adult fluke
(h)

(a)
Egg containing
miracidium

(b)
Miracidium
hatches after
being eaten
by snail

(e)
Cercaria

(d) Redia

Sporocyst
(c)

with human feces. Improvements in the disposal of human waste have diminished acquisition of the disease in many areas. However, the extremely long lifespan of these worms is reflected in a much slower decrease in the overall infection prevalence. In some villages in southern China, virtually the entire adult population may be infected. A survey of stool specimens from immigrants from Hong Kong to Canada showed an infection rate of more than 15% overall and 23% in adults between 30 and 50 years of age. Clonorchiasis is acquired by eating raw, frozen, dried, salted, smoked, or pickled fish. Commercial shipment of such products outside of the endemic area may result in the acquisition of worms far from their original source.

✳ Endemic in Southeast Asia

✳ Human transmission related to waste disposal

✳ Eating uncooked fish infects humans

CLONORCHIASIS (LIVER FLUKE INFECTION): CLINICAL ASPECTS

MANIFESTATIONS

Migration of the larvae from the duodenum to the bile duct may produce fever, chills, mild jaundice, eosinophilia, and liver enlargement. The adult worm induces epithelial hyperplasia, adenoma formation, and periductal inflammation. In light infection, clinical disease seldom results.

Light infection usually asymptomatic

❋ Hepatic, biliary manifestations from worm loads, including cholangiocarcinoma

However, numerous reinfections may produce worm loads of 500 to 1000, resulting in the formation of bile stones and sometimes bile duct carcinoma (cholangiocarcinoma) in patients with severe, long-standing infections. Calculus formation may be accompanied by asymptomatic biliary carriage of *Salmonella enterica* serovar Typhi. Dead worms may obstruct the common bile duct and induce secondary bacterial cholangitis, which may, in turn, be accompanied by bacteremia and endotoxic shock. Occasionally, adult worms are found in the pancreatic ducts, where they can produce ductal obstruction and acute pancreatitis.

DIAGNOSIS

Eggs in feces, duodenal aspirates

❋ Eosinophilia common in acute disease

Definitive diagnosis of clonorchiasis requires the recovery and identification of the distinctive egg from the stool or duodenal aspirates. In mild infections, repeated examinations may be required. Because most patients are asymptomatic, any individual with clinical manifestations of disease in whom *Clonorchis* eggs are found should be evaluated for the presence of other causes of illness. In acute symptomatic clonorchiasis, there is usually leukocytosis, eosinophilia, elevation of alkaline phosphatase levels, and abnormal computed tomography and ultrasonographic liver scans. Cholangiograms may reveal dilatation of the intrahepatic ducts, small filling defects compatible with the presence of adult worms, and occasionally cholangiocarcinoma.

TREATMENT AND PREVENTION

❋ Praziquantel or albendazole

Manage complications

Praziquantel is the treatment of choice, although albendazole has also been found to be effective. Patients with acute obstructive cholangitis due to a worm or stone in the large collecting ducts should be managed as for any other cause of obstruction, including consideration of antibiotics for secondary infection and correction of the obstruction (eg, via endoscopic retrograde pancreatography cholangiopancreatography [ERCP]). Prevention requires thorough cooking of freshwater fish and appropriate sanitary disposal of human feces.

● SCHISTOSOMA

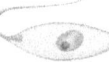 ### SCHISTOSOMA SPECIES: PARASITOLOGY AND LIFE CYCLE

The schistosomes are a group of closely related flukes that inhabit the vascular system of a number of animals. Of the five species known to infect humans, *S mansoni*, *S haematobium*, and *S japonicum* are of primary importance. The remaining two species are found in limited areas of West Africa (*S intercalatum*) and Southeast Asia (*S mekongi*), and are not discussed here in detail.

❋ Separate sexes, different morphology

❋ *S japonicum*—small intestines veins

❋ *S mansoni*—portal colon veins, rectum

❋ *S haematobium*—bladder veins, pelvic organs

The adult worms can be distinguished from the hermaphroditic trematodes by the anterior location of their ventral sucker, by their cylindric bodies, and by their reproductive systems (ie, separate sexes). Adult specimens of different species are differentiated from one another only with difficulty. The 1 to 2 cm male possesses a deep ventral groove, or "schist." Within this canal it carries the longer, more slender female in lifelong copulatory embrace. The schistosome life cycle (**Figure 57–5**) begins after mating in the hepato-portal circulation when the conjoined couple uses their suckers to ascend the mesenteric vessels against the flow of blood. Guided by unknown stimuli, *S japonicum* enters the superior mesenteric vein, eventually reaching the venous radicals of the small intestine and ascending colon; *S mansoni* and *S haematobium* are directed to the inferior mesenteric system. The destination of the former is the descending colon and rectum; the latter, however, passes through the hemorrhoidal plexus to the systemic venous system, ultimately coming to rest in the venous plexus of the bladder and other pelvic organs.

Eggs deposited submucosally, rupture to lumina, pass outside

On reaching the submucosal venules, the worms begin to lay eggs. Each pair deposits 300 (*S mansoni*, *S haematobium*) to 3000 (*S japonicum*) eggs daily for the remainder of its 4- to 35-year lifespan. Enzymes secreted by the enclosed miracidium diffuse through the shell and digest the surrounding tissue. Ova lying immediately adjacent to the mucosal surface rupture into the lumen of the bowel (*S mansoni*, *S japonicum*) or bladder (*S haematobium*) and are passed to the outside in the excreta. Here, with appropriate techniques, they may be readily observed and differentiated. The eggs of *S mansoni* are oval, possess a sharp lateral spine, and measure 60 by 140 μm. Those of

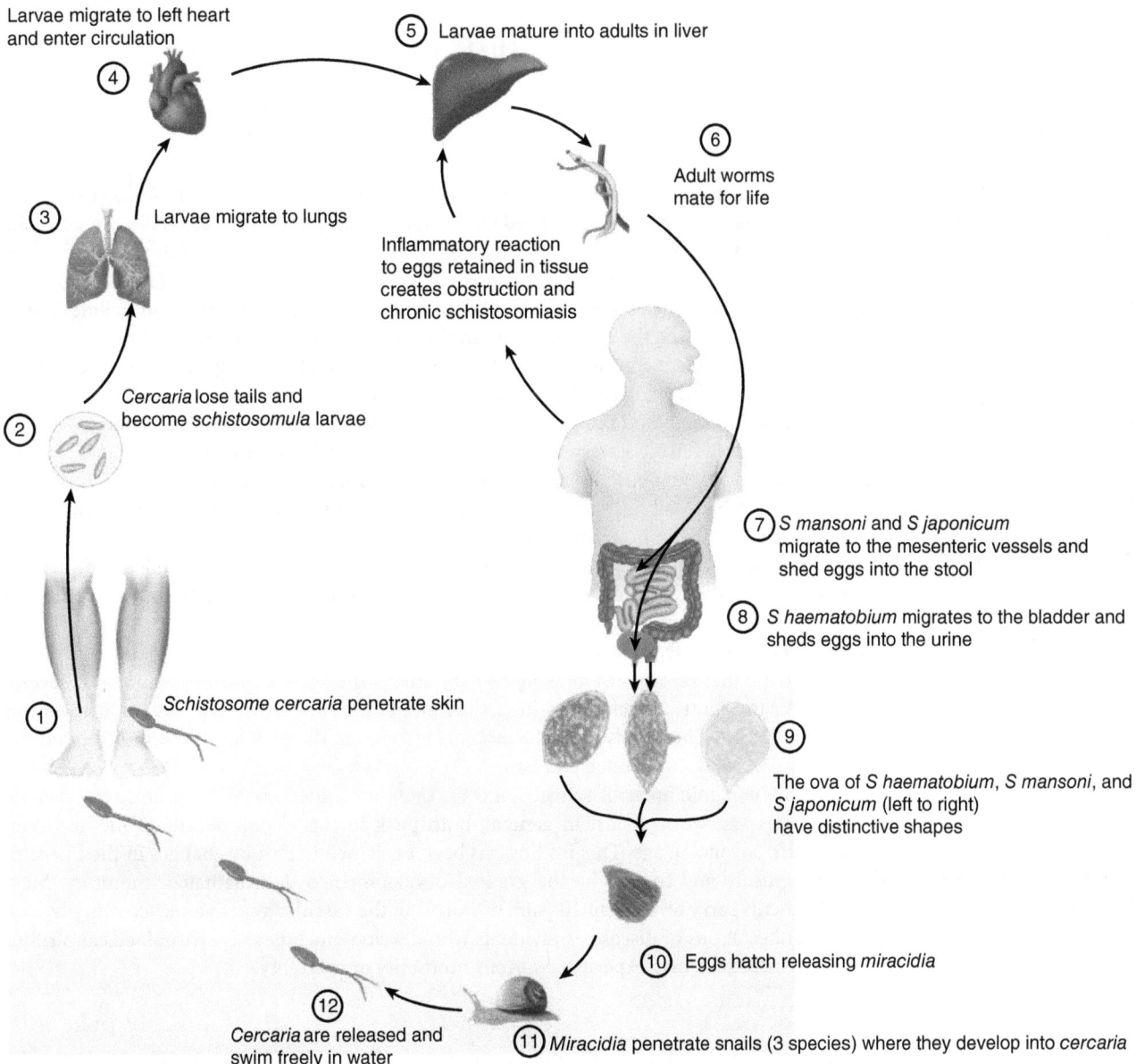

Larvae migrate to left heart
and enter circulation

④

⑤ Larvae mature into adults in liver

Larvae migrate to lungs

③

⑥ Adult worms
mate for life

Inflammatory reaction
to eggs retained in tissue
creates obstruction and
chronic schistosomiasis

Cercaria lose tails and
become *schistosomula* larvae

②

① *Schistosome cercaria* penetrate skin

⑦ *S mansoni* and *S japonicum*
migrate to the mesenteric vessels and
shed eggs into the stool

⑧ *S haematobium* migrates to the bladder and
sheds eggs into the urine

⑨ The ova of *S haematobium*, *S mansoni*, and
S japonicum (left to right)
have distinctive shapes

⑩ Eggs hatch releasing *miracidia*

⑫ *Cercaria* are released and
swim freely in water

⑪ *Miracidia* penetrate snails (3 species) where they develop into *cercaria*

FIGURE 57–5. Life cycle of schistosomes.

S haematobium differ primarily in the terminal location of their spine. The eggs of *S japonicum*, in contrast, are more nearly circular, measuring 70 by 90 μm. A minute lateral spine can be visualized only with care (Figure 57–1D-F).

The miracidia hatch quickly when the eggs are deposited in fresh water. On finding a snail host appropriate for their species, they invade and are transformed over 1 to 2 months into thousands of forked-tailed cercariae (Figure 57–3B). When released from the snail, these infectious larvae swim about vigorously for a few days. Cercariae coming in contact with human skin during this time attach, discard their tails, and penetrate. During a 1- to 3-day sojourn in the skin, the cercaria with three outer membrane layers develop into schistosomula with seven outer layers, a change that is thought to be critical to the survival of the parasite within the human body. These schistosomula enter small venules and find their way through the right side of the heart to the lung. After a delay of several days, the parasites enter the systemic circulation. Those surviving passage through the pulmonary and intestinal capillary beds return to the portal vein, where they mature to sexually active adults over 1 to 3 months and find a mate of the opposite sex, thus completing the life cycle. Schistosomiasis is primarily a human condition, but may be zoonotic in exceptional circumstances, as demonstrated by the presence of *S japonicum* infection in cattle and water buffalo in southern China.

**Eggs hatch to form miracidia,
which invade snails**

✷ Cercariae from snail traverse
human skin, develop into
schistosomula that invade
vascular system

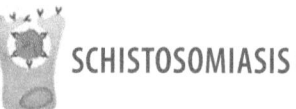

SCHISTOSOMIASIS (BLOOD FLUKE INFECTION)

EPIDEMIOLOGY

The widespread distribution and extensive morbidity of schistosomiasis make it the single most important helminthic infection in the world today. Currently, more than 200 million people—roughly 1 in 40 of all humans—are infected worldwide. Of these, roughly 200,000 die annually. The continued transmission of the parasite depends on the disposal of infected human urine and excrement into fresh water, the presence of appropriate snail hosts, and the exposure of humans to water infested with cercariae. The construction of modern sanitation and water purification facilities would break this cycle but exceed the economic resources of many endemic nations. Paradoxically, several massive land irrigation projects launched for the express purpose of speeding economic development have resulted in the dispersion of infection to previously uninvolved areas. *Schistosoma mansoni*, the most widespread of the blood flukes, is the only one present in the Western Hemisphere. Perhaps originally introduced during slavery, *S mansoni* is now found in Venezuela, Brazil, Surinam, Puerto Rico, the Dominican Republic, St. Lucia, and several other Caribbean islands.

Because a suitable snail host is lacking, transmission of *S mansoni* does not occur within the continental United States; however, many thousands of individuals residing in the United States have acquired schistosomiasis elsewhere. In the Eastern Hemisphere, the prevalence of *S mansoni* infection is highest in the Nile Delta and tropical Africa. Isolated foci are also found in East and South Africa, Yemen, Saudi Arabia, and Israel.

Schistosoma haematobium is largely confined to Africa and the Middle East, where its distribution overlaps that of *S mansoni*. *S japonicum* affects the agricultural populations of several Southeast Asian countries, including China, the Philippines, and Sulawesi (it was eradicated from Japan in the 1990s). The closely related *S mekongi* is found in the Mekong and Mun River valleys of Vietnam, Thailand, Cambodia, and Laos.

Within the endemic areas of schistosomiasis, there are wide variations in both age-specific infection rates and worm loads. In general, both peak in the second decade of life and then decrease with advancing age. This finding has been explained in part by changes in the intensity of water exposure and in part by the gradual development of IgE-mediated immunity. Most infected patients carry fewer than 10 pairs of worms in the vascular system and, accordingly, lack clinical manifestations of disease. Individuals who develop much heavier worm loads as a result of repeated infections may experience serious morbidity or mortality.

PATHOGENESIS

There are three major clinicopathologic stages in schistosomiasis. The first stage is initiated by the penetration and migration of the schistosomula. The second or intermediate stage begins with oviposition and is associated with a complex of clinical manifestations. The third or chronic stage is characterized by granuloma formation and scarring around retained eggs.

IMMUNITY

The major clinicopathologic manifestations of schistosomiasis result from the host's cell-mediated immune response to the presence of retained eggs. Not all eggs are excreted into the environment, and those left behind in tissue serve as antigenic stimuli for our immune system, which walls them off in eosinophilic granulomas ("Splendore-Hoeppli reactions"). With time, the intensity of this reaction is muted; granulomas formed in the later stages of infection are smaller and less damaging than those formed early. The mechanisms responsible for this modulation are not fully understood. Present evidence suggests that both suppressor T-lymphocyte activity and antibody blockade are involved. The correlation in humans between human leukocyte antigen (HLA) types A1 and B5 and the development of hepatosplenomegaly suggests that the extent of the immunoregulation is influenced, at least in part, by the genetic background of the host.

As evidenced by their prolonged survival, the adult worms are remarkably well tolerated by their hosts. In part, this tolerance may be attributable to the formation of IgG4 blocking antibodies early in the course of infection. Tolerance may also reflect the ability of the developing parasites to disguise themselves by adsorbing host molecules, including immunoglobulins, blood group glycolipids, and histocompatibility complex antigens. Nevertheless, as mentioned earlier,

---

Sidebar notes (left margin):

✳ Most important helminthic infection

✳ Stopped by modern waste disposal

Spread by irrigation projects

Distribution varies with species, depends on snail host

Age-related susceptibility with peak in second decade

✳ Major disease manifestations from cell-mediated immune response to eggs

the prevalence and intensity of human infection begin to abate during adolescence, despite continuing exposure to infective cercariae. It has been suggested that schistosomula penetrating the skin after the primary infection are coated with specific antibodies, bound to eosinophils, and destroyed before they can reach the portal system. Although protection is not complete, a 60% to 80% kill rate is highly effective in controlling the intensity of parasitism. This condition, in which adult worms from a primary infection can survive in a host resistant to reinfection, is termed **concomitant immunity.** Eventually, production of blocking antibodies wanes whereas production of protective IgE antibodies active against adult worms increases, leading to a decrease in the host's total worm population.

Blocking antibodies, adsorption of host molecules provide antigenic disguise

Concomitant immunity reduces new infections

SCHISTOSOMIASIS (BLOOD FLUKE INFECTION): CLINICAL ASPECTS

EARLY STAGE

Within 24 hours of penetrating the skin, a large proportion of the schistosomula die. In *S mansoni* and *S haematobium* infections, immediate and delayed hypersensitivity to parasitic antigens results in an intensely pruritic papular skin rash, which increases in severity with repeated exposures to cercariae. As the viable schistosomula begin their migration to the liver, the rash disappears and the patient experiences fever, headache, and abdominal pain for 1 to 2 weeks.

Of note, a related condition happens in North America when certain schistosoma species adapted to aquatic birds mistakenly invade the skin of swimmers; unable to penetrate deeper into the human vascular systems, these cercariae remain trapped in the skin. The parasites die there without causing serious harm, but not before causing a localized pruritic, inflammatory reaction called cercarial dermatitis, or "swimmer's itch."

✳ Local and systemic hypersensitivity reactions produce rash

✳ Avian schistosomiasis causes swimmer's itch in North America

INTERMEDIATE STAGE

One to two months after primary exposure, once the sexually mature adult worms begin to lay eggs (oviposition), patients with severe *S mansoni* or *S japonicum* infections may experience an acute febrile illness that bears a striking resemblance to serum sickness. This happens because of relative egg antigen excess, with formation of soluble immune complexes that deposit in host tissues. Indeed, high levels of such complexes have been demonstrated in the peripheral blood and correlate well with the severity of illness. This symptom complex is commonly termed **Katayama syndrome.** In addition to fever and chills, patients experience cough, urticaria, arthralgia, lymphadenopathy, splenomegaly, abdominal pain, and diarrhea. Sigmoidoscopic examination reveals an inflamed colonic mucosa and petechial hemorrhages; occasionally, patients with *S japonicum* infection develop clinical manifestations of encephalitis. Typically, leukocytosis, marked peripheral eosinophilia, and elevated levels of IgM, IgG, and IgE immunoglobulins are present. It is more common and severe in visitors to endemic areas, in whom it may persist for 3 months or more. If untreated, it occasionally results in death.

✳ Katayama syndrome: prolonged febrile period with circulating immune complexes

Intestinal inflammation and encephalitis occur acutely

CHRONIC STAGE

Approximately one-half of all deposited eggs reach the lumen of the bowel or bladder and are shed from the body. Retained eggs induce inflammation and scarring, initiating the final and most morbid phase of schistosomiasis. Soluble antigens excreted by the eggs stimulate the formation of T-lymphocyte–mediated eosinophilic granulomas. Early in the infection, the inflammatory response is vigorous, producing lesions more than 100-fold larger than the inciting egg itself. With time, the host's inflammatory response moderates, leading to a significant decrease in granuloma size. Fibroblasts stimulated by factors released by both retained eggs and the granulomas lay down scar tissue, rendering the earlier, granuloma-induced vascular obstruction permanent. The severity of tissue damage is directly related to the total number of eggs retained.

In *S haematobium* infection, the bladder mucosa becomes thickened, papillated, and ulcerated. Hematuria and dysuria result; repeated hemorrhages produce anemia. In severe infections, the muscular layers of the bladder are involved, with loss of bladder capacity and contractibility. Vesicoureteral reflux, ureteral obstruction, and hydronephrosis may follow. Progressive obstruction may lead to renal failure and uremia. Calcification of the bladder wall is occasionally seen, and approximately 10% of patients harbor urinary tract calculi. Secondary bacterial infections are

✳ Inflammatory, fibrotic reactions to retained eggs cause chronic disease

***S haematobium* bladder lesions with hemorrhage, obstruction**

Urinary carriage may cause *Salmonella* bacteremia

❋ Bladder squamous cell carcinoma a serious complication

common. Chronic *Salmonella* bacteriuria with recurrent bouts of bacteremia has been reported in Egypt, where squamous cell bladder carcinoma is frequently seen as a late complication of disease. Other urogenital organs may also be involved, including the spermatic cord, testes, fallopian tubes, ovaries, and vagina.

 Most bladder cancer originates from transitional cells; why is bladder cancer due to *S haematobium* different?

In *S mansoni* and *S japonicum* infections, the bowel mucosa is congested, thickened, and ulcerated. Patients experience abdominal pain, diarrhea, and blood in the stool. Eggs deposited in the larger intestinal veins may be carried by the portal blood flow back to the liver, where they lodge in the presinusoidal capillaries. The resulting inflammatory reaction leads to the development of periportal fibrosis and hepatic enlargement. The frequency and severity with which the liver is involved appear to be genetically determined and associated with the patient's HLA type. In contrast to cirrhosis, in most cases of schistosomiasis liver function is well preserved. Infected persons who subsequently acquire hepatitis B or C viruses develop chronic active hepatitis more frequently than those without schistosomiasis. Presinusoidal obstruction of blood flow can result in portal hypertension and serious manifestations of portal obstruction. Eggs that are carried around the liver in the portosystemic collateral vessels may lodge in the small pulmonary arterioles, where they produce interstitial scarring, pulmonary hypertension, and right ventricular failure. Immune complexes shunted to the systemic circulation may induce glomerulonephritis. Occasionally, eggs may be deposited in the central nervous system, where they may cause epilepsy or paraplegia.

Some differences between the clinical presentation of *S mansoni* and that of *S japonicum* have been noted. Manifestations of the latter disease typically occur earlier in the course of the infection and tend to be more severe. When involvement of the central nervous system develops, it is more likely to occur in the brain than in the spinal cord. On the other hand, immune complex nephropathy and recurrent *Salmonella* bacteremia are more commonly seen in hepatosplenic *S mansoni* infections. The latter phenomenon is apparently related to the ability of *Salmonella* to parasitize the gut and integument of the adult fluke, providing a persistent bacterial focus within the portal system of the infected patient. This focus cannot be eradicated without treatment of the schistosomal infection.

❋ Portal hypertension develops without cirrhosis

Hepatitis B or C superinfection may progress to hepatitis

Elimination of *Salmonella* requires eradication of parasite

DIAGNOSIS

Definitive diagnosis of schistosomiasis requires the recovery of the characteristic eggs in urine, stool, or biopsy specimens. In *S haematobium* infections, eggs are most numerous in urine samples obtained at midday, especially the last drops voided. When examination of the sediment yields negative results, eggs may sometimes be recovered by filtering the urine through a fine membrane. Cystoscopy with biopsy of the bladder mucosa may be required for the diagnosis of mild infection. Eggs of *S mansoni* and *S japonicum* are passed in the stool. Concentration techniques such as formalin–ether or gravity sedimentation are necessary when the ova are scanty. Results of rectal biopsy may be positive when those of repeated stool examinations are negative.

Because dead eggs may persist in tissue for a long time after the death of the adult worms, active infection is confirmed only when the eggs are shown to be viable. This may be performed by observing the eggs microscopically for movement of flame cell cilia or by hatching them in water and watching for motile miracidia to emerge. Quantitation of egg output may be useful in estimating the severity of infection and in following response to treatment.

Conventional serologic tests detect circulating antibodies with sensitivities exceeding 90% but cannot distinguish active from prior infection. Enzyme immunoassay (EIA)-based reagent strip (dipstick) tests, capable of detecting circulating, genus-specific, adult worm antigens in blood and

❋ *S haematobium* eggs in urine

❋ *S mansoni* and *S japonicum* eggs in stool and rectal biopsy

Determination of egg viability, output useful

 Think ▸▸ Apply 57-1: This cancer is caused by a prolonged cycle of injury, at locations where eggs lodge in the bladder wall, or where they exit into the urine, triggering inflammation, repair, and scar. Over time, the squamous cells involved may become dysplastic or malignant; in effect, this is a cancer triggered by inflammation.

urine, are rapid, simple, and sensitive. They are particularly helpful in the diagnosis of Katayama syndrome in those returning from endemic areas. Moreover, because antigen levels drop rapidly after successful therapy, these tests may prove helpful in distinguishing active from inactive disease.

EIA detection of antigens in blood and urine

TREATMENT

No specific therapy is available for the treatment of schistosomal dermatitis or Katayama syndrome. Antihistamines and corticosteroids may be helpful in ameliorating their more severe manifestations. The maturing organisms seem resistant to antiparasitic medications, thus no immediate postexposure prophylaxis after water exposure is possible. In the late stage of schistosomiasis, therapy is directed at interrupting egg deposition by killing or sterilizing the adult worms.

Several anthelmintic agents may be used for the chronic stage. Praziquantel, which is active against all three species of schistosomes, is the agent of choice. Use of this drug is relatively contraindicated in early pregnancy. Unfortunately, reports suggest decreased efficacy of this single-dose oral agent in areas where it has been used in mass therapy programs; in this setting, repeat dosing is an option, although *S mansoni* infections acquired in such areas may be treated with oxamniquine (not available in the United States). Artemisinin derivatives have worked well in experimental settings, and may be useful in select cases; fostering *Plasmodium* resistance in patients coinfected with malaria is a real concern.

✳ **Praziquantel drug of choice for schistosomiasis**

✳ **It kills adult worms, but not immature forms**

PREVENTION

Controlling this deadly disease has proved both difficult and expensive. Programs aimed at interrupting transmission by the provision of pure water supplies and the sanitary disposal of human feces are often beyond the economic reach of nations most seriously affected. Similarly, measures to deny snails access to newly irrigated lands are expensive. Chemical molluscicides have been effective in limited trials, but less successful when used over large areas for prolonged periods. Mass therapy of the infected human population has until recently been severely limited by the toxicity of older agents, or by unanticipated consequences, such as the unsanitary injection of tartrate emetic in Egypt, an antiparasitic drug that provided little benefit in terms of schistosomiasis but perversely transmitted Hepatitis C to thousands of patients. Oral praziquantel has proved to be more suitable for this purpose, albeit at the risk of selecting drug resistance. Furthermore, without other control measures, discontinuation of mass therapy can result in a rapid rebound of active disease.

Sanitary disposal of feces limited by economic status

Molluscicides effective, but large-scale application difficult

In 2009, a report of an extensive controlled study in an area of Southeastern China that was hyperendemic for *S japonicum* yielded remarkable results. These included removal of cattle from snail-infested grasslands, providing mechanized equipment to farmers, improving sanitation of drinking water, building lavatories and latrines, providing boats with fecal matter containers, and implementing intensive health education programs. Infection rates fell dramatically in the intervention villages as compared to nonintervention areas. Thus, a multipronged approach such as this offers the best hope for lasting control.

Multipronged approach is necessary

Currently, there is intense interest in developing a vaccine suitable for human use. A vaccine made from irradiated *S bovis* cercariae, which was developed for cattle, appears to confer a significant degree of protection against infection. Although a similar live vaccine would not be practical for human populations, the success of the animal vaccine has provided clues to potential immunoprotective mechanisms in human schistosomiasis. Monoclonal antibodies have been used to identify a number of schistosomula and adult antigens thought to be capable of inducing protective immunity; more than a dozen antigens are now in various stages of investigation as vaccine candidates.

Vaccines under development

KEY CONCLUSIONS

- Trematode (fluke) infections come in two groups: tissue hermaphrodites and schistosomes.
- Hermaphrodites are acquired by eating larval parasites; schistosomes are acquired via transcutaneous invasion while people bathe in contaminated water, making it more challenging to control.
- For the hermaphrodites, most clinical illness is caused by adult parasites in visceral organs.
- For the schistosomes, disease is more complex: distinct illnesses happen at the time of initial skin invasion (cercarial dermatitis), at the time of oviposition (Katayama syndrome), and in response to long-egg burden (portal hypertension, granulomatous visceral injury, bladder cancer).

CASE STUDY

The Risks of Adventurous Tourism

A 35-year-old American adventurer returned from a 3-week tour of rural areas in Southeast Asia, which involved hiking forays and sharing meals with local residents. One month after his return to the United States, he developed fever and chills, accompanied by cough, urticaria, arthralgia, abdominal pain, and diarrhea.

Laboratory studies demonstrated leukocytosis and marked eosinophilia, with elevated immunoglobulin levels.

Sigmoidoscopic examination revealed mucosal inflammation and petechial hemorrhages.

QUESTIONS

1. Which of the following is the most likely cause of this man's symptoms?
   A. Paragonimiasis
   B. Schistosomiasis
   C. Clonorchiasis
   D. Fascioliasis

2. Which of the following is *not true* regarding Paragonimus infection?
   A. Ingestion of crayfish and freshwater crabs is risky.
   B. Chest X-ray can mimic tuberculosis.
   C. Praziquantel is effective treatment.
   D. Biliary tract involvement is prominent.

3. Perpetuation of transmission in *Clonorchis* infections is primarily due to which of the following?
   A. Wading in fresh water
   B. Refusal to treat with albendazole
   C. Lack of careful handwashing
   D. Use of human waste as fertilizer

ANSWERS

1. (B)

2. (D)

3. (D)

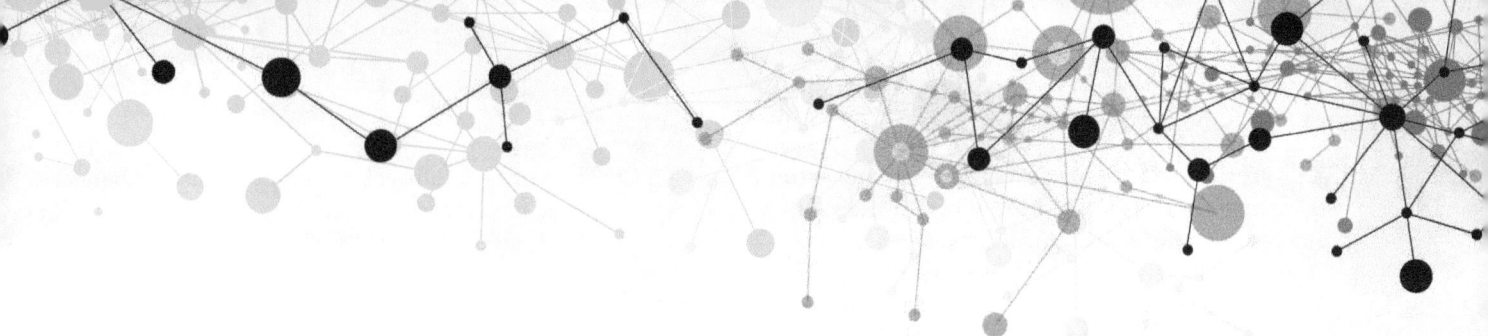

Practice Questions in USMLE Format

VIRAL DISEASES

V.1 Which one of the following contains lipid in its virion?

A. Adenovirus
B. Parvovirus
C. Picornavirus
D. Coronavirus
E. Retrovirus

V.2 A 30-year-old man has had fever and a sore throat for a week. On examination he has bilateral cervical lymphadenopathy. Which of the following is *least* likely to cause these clinical findings?

A. Epstein-Barr virus
B. Varicella-zoster virus
C. Coxsackie A virus
D. Adenovirus
E. Parainfluenza virus

V.3 Which one of the following is *true* regarding temperate viruses? Temperate viruses:

A. Undergo both productive and nonproductive infections and only establish latent infections
B. Lead to a productive infection called lytic infection
C. Undergo both productive and nonproductive infections and can establish both latent and lytic infections
D. Enter the cells and persist indefinitely with no virus production, called nonproductive responses

V.4 Which one of the following is *true* concerning viral capsids?

A. Viruses acquire host proteins as their capsids.
B. Capsids are virus-specific proteins, which protect their genome and provide shape to viruses.
C. Capsid protein subunits form a helix with the core proteins to mainly provide helical symmetry.
D. Capsids are lipid bilayer membranes containing proteins and/or glycoproteins.

V.5 A young man has returned from a short trip to Mexico where he was bitten by a dog. Eight weeks after returning he developed excessive salivation, aversion to drinking water, and hallucinations and died in cardiac arrest. Which of the following measures might have prevented this death if implemented upon his return?

A. Interleukin 2 infusions
B. Acyclovir prophylaxis
C. Specific vaccine administration
D. Gamma globulin therapy
E. Ciprofloxacin prophylaxis

V.6 Which one of the following statements is *true* regarding the interaction of viruses and cell surface receptors?

A. When receptor sites are occupied the viral infection will be lytic.
B. The interaction can be prevented by neutralizing antibodies to the virus surface protein.
C. The interaction directs host DNA polymerase to synthesize RNA genomes for viral assembly.
D. The interaction determines whether the purified genome of a virus is infectious.

V.7 A transplant patient has developed seizures and an MRI reveals a lesion in the temporal lobe. A biopsy of the area shows multinucleated giant cells with intranuclear inclusions. Which of the following is the most probable etiologic agent?

A. Poliovirus
B. Herpes simplex virus type 1
C. Listeria monocytogenes
D. Toxoplasma
E. Parvovirus

V.8 A 28-year-old woman has developed fever and extreme fatigue over 2 days. She is short of breath and radiographs reveal pulmonary infiltrates. A genetic and biochemical analysis of a virus isolated from her throat that reveals the genome to be composed of eight unequally sized segments of single-stranded RNA, each of which is complementary to viral mRNA in infected cells. Which one of the following statements about this virus is *true*?

A. Several proteins are encoded by each segment of the viral genome.

B. Purified RNA extracted from the virus is infectious because it can interact with the receptor on the host cell.

C. The virus particle contains a virion-associated RNA-dependent RNA polymerase that can copy the RNA genome into its complementary strand.

D. The virus cannot undergo high frequency recombination via reassortment of its RNA segments.

E. The genome can integrate easily into the host chromosome because of being segmented.

V.9 Which of the following statements is *most* characteristic of poliovirus?

A. The genome is double-stranded DNA.

B. Intestinal replication is extensive.

C. Congenital infections are frequent.

D. A skin test can identify previous exposure.

E. Amantadine chemoprophylaxis is effective.

V.10 An emergency room worker suffered a needle stick while caring for an accident victim. The employee health service recommended immediate prophylaxis with zidovudine (ZDV or AZT). This drug's inhibition of reverse transcription is achieved by termination of:

A. Viral RNA elongation

B. Viral RNA transcription

C. Viral DNA integration

D. Viral DNA elongation

E. Viral DNA replication

V.11 An 8-year-old boy has an illness which begins with fever and malaise. Later a rash appears on his cheeks, which makes them look as if he had been slapped. The virus causing this syndrome has also been linked to aplastic crises in persons with sickle cell disease. Which of the following is most likely?

A. Herpes simplex

B. Parvovirus B19

C. Rubella

D. Rubeola

E. Varicella-zoster

V.12 Each year there are discussions about new formulations of the vaccine for influenza A virus. Why?

A. Because mutations occur mainly in the envelope proteins, hemagglutinin, and neuraminidase.

B. The half-life of the vaccine is a few months and degrades quickly in host cells.

C. The hemagglutinin envelope protein changes but not the neuraminidase protein.

D. Mutations predominantly take place in the matrix protein that interacts with the host cell receptor.

E. Because the vaccine is comprised of several drugs that are active against the virus for one season.

V.13 A 10-month-old infant is brought to the hospital by his mother with a fever, dry cough, and shortness of breath. He has become more restless with a worsening cough over the past day. There is no relevant past medical history and he is up-to-date with his immunization schedule. On examination, a diagnosis of acute bronchiolitis is made. Which one of the following viruses is *most* likely involved?

A. Influenza virus

B. Measles virus

C. Parainfluenza virus

D. Adenovirus

E. Respiratory syncytial virus

V.14 A 28-year-old woman presents with a fever and painful genital ulcers. A culture of the lesions is positive for herpes simplex virus. Which of the following is most characteristic of this infection?

A. Type 1 virus is most common.

B. It is rare if there is a high antibody titer.

C. The initial infection is by the fecal–oral route.

D. It may be reactivated by stress.

E. The brain and visceral organs are typically involved.

V.15 A virus is isolated from the stool of a patient with diarrhea. Detailed analysis reveals that its genome is composed of multiple pieces of double-stranded RNA. Which one of the following statements about this virus is *true*?

A. Each RNA segment encodes a different protein.

B. The virus uses host-encoded RNA-dependent RNA polymerase.

C. The virion contains a lipid bilayer capsid protein.

D. The genome integrates into the host chromosome.

E. This virus has oncogenic potential and further tests should be performed.

V.16 Coxsackieviruses appear worldwide particularly in young persons. Their epidemiology and pathogenesis most closely resembles:

A. Adenoviruses

B. Influenza A

C. Polioviruses

D. Hepatitis A

E. Mumps

V.17 A 35-year-old man was addicted to intravenous drug use and has been a carrier for hepatitis B virus surface antigen (HBsAg) for 10 years. He suddenly develops acute fulminant hepatitis. Which one of the following laboratory tests would contribute *most* to a diagnosis?

A. Antibody to HBsAg
B. HBeAg
C. Antibody to HBcAg
D. Antibody to hepatitis C virus antigen
E. Antibody to hepatitis delta antigen

V.18 In counseling parents about childhood immunizations there are a number of differences between the viral vaccines. Regarding the rubella vaccine all of the following statements are true *except*:

A. Antibodies are induced, which neutralize circulating virus.
B. Induced antibodies prevent reinfection and limit spread.
C. The immunogenic component is killed virus.
D. Vaccine use has reduced both childhood and congenital rubella.
E. Vaccine is often combined with other vaccines.

V.19 A 45-year-old man presented with an acute onset of fever, nausea, and pain in the right upper abdominal quadrant. He had jaundice and dark urine several days earlier. If the correct diagnosis is hepatitis A, then which one of the following statements is *true*?

A. It was parenterally transmitted.
B. Antibody to hepatitis A can be detected during early illness.
C. The patient is most likely to develop chronic hepatitis.
D. The patient is likely to become a chronic carrier.
E. It is the most common sexually transmitted form of hepatitis in the United States.

V.20 A 30-year-old woman is seen with a painful lesion on the vulva and complains of fever, headache, and stiff neck. On pelvic examination, she has several tender ulcers of approximately 4 mm in diameter. She was diagnosed with aseptic meningitis. The *most likely* etiologic agent and the antiviral used for her treatment are:

A. Human papillomavirus infection and ribavirin
B. Cytomegalovirus infection and ganciclovir
C. Herpes simplex virus infection and acyclovir
D. Varicella-zoster virus infection and zidovudine
E. Hepatitis B virus infection and interferon

V.21 Which one of the following statements about retrovirus replication is *true*? By using reverse transcriptase retroviral:

A. Positive stranded RNA is converted to double-stranded DNA, which integrates into the host chromosome after transcription and replication.
B. Positive sense RNA is converted to double-stranded DNA, which integrates into the host chromosome before transcription and replication.

C. Negative sense RNA is converted to DNA, which integrates into the host chromosome before replication.
D. Double-stranded DNA is converted to circular DNA, which integrates into the viral chromosome after transcription and replication.

V.22 While vacationing in the Caribbean, a man was bitten by *Aedes aegypti* mosquito. He developed fever and severe pain in the back, head, muscles, and joints. An erythematous rash is also seen on his body. The *most likely* diagnosis is:

A. Eastern equine encephalitis
B. St. Louis encephalitis
C. Dengue fever
D. Western equine encephalitis
E. Yellow fever

V.23 A 40-year-old man develops ataxia, slurred speech, and dementia. At autopsy the brain shows widespread neuronal degeneration, a spongy appearance due to many vacuoles between the cells, no inflammation, and no evidence of virus particles. Mice injected with homogenized brain tissue develop similar disease after 6 months. The *most likely* agents of this disease are:

A. Virus-like particles with nucleic acid in their core
B. Herpes-like incomplete viruses
C. Prions resulting from a conformationally rearranged protein
D. Double-stranded DNA virus
E. Single-stranded RNA virus

V.24 A 64-year-old man with chronic lymphocytic leukemia develops progressive deterioration of mental and neuromuscular function. At autopsy the brain shows enlarged oligodendrocytes whose nuclei contain naked, icosahedral virus particles. The *most likely* diagnosis is:

A. Herpes encephalitis
B. Progressive multifocal leukoencephalopathy
C. Rabies encephalitis
D. Creutzfeldt-Jakob disease
E. Subacute sclerosing panencephalitis

V.25 Which one of the following infections peaks mainly in adults?

A. Shingles
B. Rotavirus
C. Respiratory syncytial virus
D. Mumps virus
E. Western equine encephalitis virus

V.26 You have a 25-year-old female patient in your office who had just discovered that her sex partner is HIV positive. She is on birth control pills, so they have not been using condoms. Before she left him this week, they have had sex about 10 to 15 times. You got a blood test done for HIV that came back negative. She is also negative for other sexually transmitted diseases. Which one of the following statements is *true* for this patient?

A. Since the HIV test came back negative, she is not infected and there is no need to test her again.

B. The risk of HIV transmission through heterosexual route is so remote that this patient should not be concerned anymore.

C. She needs to be tested again in 6 months and if negative, she is probably uninfected.

D. She should be tested again in 6 months and if negative, she is definitely uninfected and need not be tested again.

E. Since she is using birth control pills, she should not be concerned because HIV is inactivated by birth control pills.

V.27 You have decided to do a 6-month clinical rotation in a teaching hospital situated in the Indian subcontinent and will be accompanied by your spouse and a 1-year-old child. Your child is up-to-date with all the routine immunizations. In addition, you will take other recommended immunizations before traveling. Which one of following statements is *true* about a viral disease that may affect one of you?

A. Rotavirus infections are more common in infants than adults.

B. Norwalk-like viruses causing diarrhea are seen generally in women.

C. The incubation period for astroviruses is very long because they are DNA viruses and establish latent infection.

D. Viruses of diarrhea are not a major concern in the Indian subcontinent.

E. Enteroviruses that are the major cause of diarrhea can be prevented by boiling the drinking water.

V.28 A 10-year-old girl has developed fever and loss of appetite. By the time she is seen by her physician, she has tender swelling in the area of both parotid glands. What are other features typical of this infection and its agent?

A. It is maintained in domestic animals.

B. It is preventable by immunization.

C. Progression to the central nervous system is common.

D. Recurrences are common.

E. A helical DNA virus is the cause.

V.29 A young woman presents with malaise, fever, and loss of appetite. On examination her sclera reveals jaundice. Initial testing reveals negative tests for HBs antigen and anti-HBs antibody. Which of the following tests would be most useful in establishing a diagnosis of infection with hepatitis B virus?

A. Delta antigen

B. Anti-HBc antibody

C. Anti-HBe antibody

D. HBe antigen

E. Alanine aminotransferase (ALT)

Answers

V.1 (E), **V.2** (B), **V.3** (C), **V.4** (B), **V.5** (C), **V.6** (B), **V.7** (B), **V.8** (C), **V.9** (B), **V.10** (D), **V.11** (B), **V.12** (A), **V.13** (E), **V.14** (D), **V.15** (A), **V.16** (C), **V.17** (E), **V.18** (C), **V.19** (B), **V.20** (C), **V.21** (B), **V.22** (C), **V.23** (C), **V.24** (B), **V.25** (A), **V.26** (C), **V.27** (A), **V.28** (B), **V.29** (B)

BACTERIAL DISEASES

B.1 Five post office workers have all come down with a similar respiratory illness characterized by low-grade fever, chills, cough, dyspnea on exertion, and generalized malaise. A chest radiograph taken on one of them shows mediastinal edema and a sputum Gram stain shows WBCs and large Gram-positive rods. A blood culture also shows Gram-positive rods. This infection was most likely acquired by:

A. Inhalation of vegetative bacteria

B. Inhalation of conidia

C. Inhalation of spores

D. Traumatic inoculation of vegetative bacteria

E. Traumatic inoculation of spores

B.2 A young girl in the former Soviet Republic of Georgia has a severe sore throat and multiple white plaques in the back of her throat. She is acutely ill and has a heart murmur. She has had only one set of her childhood immunizations because the supplies in the village where she lives had run out. The manifestations in her throat and heart are due to a toxin which:

A. Stimulates adenylate cyclase

B. Inserts into sarcolemmal membranes

C. Inhibits protein synthesis

D. Inhibits acetylcholine release

E. Stimulates cytokine release

B.3 Over half the persons attending a banquet developed a vague febrile illness 2 to 5 days later. Most of those who sought medical aid had the same organism isolated from their bloodstream. Food histories incriminate dairy products but it appears certain they were kept refrigerated right up to the serving time. Which of the following is most likely to be the cause?

A. *Escherichia coli* O:157:H7
B. *Salmonella enterica*
C. *Salmonella* serotype Typhi
D. *Clostridium perfringens*
E. *Listeria monocytogenes*

B.4 A newborn was delivered at home without medical assistance. The umbilical cord was cut with kitchen shears. The baby initially did fine but in the third week of life began to have involuntary muscle contractions. The infant now has generalized muscle contractions and difficulty breathing. The abnormal muscle spasms are due to a toxin which:

A. Stimulates neuromuscular synapses
B. Stimulates neurotransmission in the spinal cord
C. Blocks postsynaptic inhibition in the spinal cord
D. Blocks acetylcholine release in the spinal cord
E. Blocks acetylcholine release at neuromuscular junctions

B.5 An emergency call to a neighbor leads to an entire family with apparent paralysis of ocular and respiratory muscles. They had just embarked on a project of home canning and had consumed one of their own products (green beans) the evening before. It is most likely they consumed a toxin which:

A. Stimulates neuromuscular synapses
B. Stimulates neurotransmission in the spinal cord
C. Blocks postsynaptic inhibition in the spinal cord
D. Blocks acetylcholine release in the spinal cord
E. Blocks acetylcholine release at neuromuscular junctions

B.6 A woman has been in the hospital for 3 weeks due to complications following surgery for colon cancer. Five days into a course of ceftriaxone for suspected pneumonia she developed diarrhea. Colonoscopy revealed multiple plaques on the mucosa which are composed of fibrin and WBS. Stool examinations for *Salmonella*, *Shigella*, *Campylobacter*, and amoebas are negative. The diarrhea and plaques are most likely produced by:

A. Endotoxin from clostridial spores
B. Exotoxin from clostridial spores
C. Exotoxin from clostridial cells
D. Exotoxin from *E coli* cells
E. Endotoxin from *E coli* cells

B.7 Two isolates of *Neisseria gonorrhoeae* have been obtained from a woman with disseminated gonococcal infection (DGI). One is from the cervix, the other from the blood. Detailed studies of these isolates show that antibody directed against the pili of the cervical isolate neutralize its binding to epithelial cells but the same antibodies have no effect on the blood isolate. The most likely explanation for these observations is:

A. She is infected with two strains from different partners.
B. The cervical isolate has a plasmid which was lost in the blood.
C. A translational frame shift has shut off the pili of the blood isolate.
D. Recombination between pilin genes has altered the pili.
E. The cervical isolate has a transposon lacking in the blood isolate.

B.8 A young woman has been identified as a sexual partner of a man recently diagnosed with gonococcal urethritis. She is in good health with no genital pain or discharge. The best way to determine if she has gonorrhea is:

A. Pilin serology
B. Opa serology
C. Gram stain
D. Vaginal culture
E. Cervical culture

B.9 Most cases of meningococcal meningitis occur between the ages of 6 months and 5 years (peak 18 months). The best explanation for this age distribution is:

A. This is the age when exposure is most likely.
B. The T-cell-dependent immune response is poorly developed at this age.
C. Antimeningococcal antibody is less likely to be present at this age.
D. Maternal antibody persists through this period.
E. Maternal antibody is not protective.

B.10 A small college has adopted an aggressive immunization policy which includes use of the newest Hib, meningococcal, and pneumococcal vaccines. Despite this, an outbreak of meningitis has developed on campus with clear evidence of transmission between roommates. Which of the following would have the greatest potential to produce an outbreak under these circumstances?

A. *Haemophilus influenzae*, type b
B. *Haemophilus influenzae*, type a
C. *Neisseria meningitidis*, group A
D. *Neisseria meningitidis*, group B
E. *Streptococcus pneumoniae*, type 24

B.11 An outbreak of diarrhea has spread through a day-care center caring for 3- to 5-year-old children. No food is served in the center. Which of the following organisms is most likely to be spread directly from child to child by the fecal–oral mechanism?

A. *Shigella*
B. *Salmonella* serotypes
C. *Salmonella* serotype Typhi
D. Enterotoxigenic *E coli*
E. *Listeria*

B.12 If an *E coli* is introduced into the urinary bladder by mechanical disruption of the perineal flora, which of the following characteristics would give it the best chance to produce pyelonephritis?

A. Alpha hemolysin
B. CFA pili
C. P (gal–gal) pili
D. Type 1 pili
E. LPS endotoxin

B.13 An elderly man with an enlarged prostate has frequent and painful urination. Suddenly he develops fever and chills. Examination reveals hypotension (blood pressure 55/10 mm Hg) and a blood culture is positive for *Klebsiella pneumoniae*. The fever, chills, and hypotension likely derive from the bacterial:

A. Alpha toxin
B. Outer membrane
C. Capsule
D. Endoplasmic reticulum
E. Polysaccharide capsule

B.14 A child has had abdominal pain and diarrhea for 2 days. A stained preparation of the stool demonstrates polymorphonuclear leukocytes. Which of the following is *least likely* to produce these findings?

A. *Vibrio cholerae*
B. *Shigella sonnei*
C. *Shigella dysenteriae*
D. *Salmonella* serotype Typhimurium
E. *Campylobacter jejuni*

B.15 A 6-month-old infant presents with fever, hoarseness, and difficult breathing. Examination reveals a red, swollen, epiglottis. The laboratory reports that a blood culture is growing Gram-negative coccobacilli. Immunity to infection with this organism is provided by antibodies directed against:

A. Cytotoxic T cells
B. M protein
C. Polyribitol phosphate
D. Surface pili
E. Outer membrane proteins

B.16 A 3-month-old infant was admitted to the hospital with a 10-day history of repetitive coughing and choking spells. His white blood cell count was 30,000/mm³ (normal <10,000/mm³) with 70% lymphocytes. The child's chest radiograph was clear. The most sensitive method for making a diagnosis is:

A. Sputum culture on blood agar
B. Nasopharyngeal culture on special medium
C. "Cough plate" culture on special medium
D. Sputum Gram stain
E. Sputum acid-fast stain

B.17 A 56-year-old man has had a cough with hemoptysis for 6 weeks and has lost 25 pounds. His chest X-ray reveals a right upper lobe cavity. His sputum shows multiple slender acid-fast bacilli. The primary mechanism of injury to his lung is:

A. Lipopolysaccharide endotoxin
B. Protein exotoxin
C. Pore-forming toxin
D. Delayed type hypersensitivity
E. Immune complex deposition

B.18 The characteristic of the organism which causes tuberculosis which best distinguishes it from other genera is:

A. Thick peptidoglycan
B. High cell wall lipid content
C. Impermeable outer membrane
D. Injection secretion system
E. Lancefield carbohydrate

B.19 As part of an annual evaluation, a 30-year-old medical resident's tuberculin skin test shows 16 mm induration. She has always had negative tests in the past including one a year earlier. She is afebrile, feels well, and her chest X-ray is clear. The best course of action at this point is:

A. Sputum acid-fast stain
B. Sputum TB culture
C. Bronchoalveolar lavage (BAL) with culture
D. 4 drug TB therapy
E. Isoniazid chemoprophylaxis
F. Rifampin chemoprophylaxis

B.20 An immunocompromised patient reported chest pains and weight loss. Sputum showed branching, filamentous Gram-positive rods which were weakly acid-fast. This organism was most probably acquired from:

A. Oropharyngeal flora
B. Family member
C. Domestic pet
D. Insect vector
E. Soil

B.21 A 9-year-old boy returned home after attending summer camp in Rhode Island. Upon his return he had complaints of recurrent fever, muscle aches, severe headaches, and fatigue. The patient also had an annular (ring-like) rash on his left arm and later developed a facial palsy. In order to consider a diagnosis of Lyme disease what additional history would be most helpful?

A. Food consumption
B. Swimming in lakes or streams
C. Sexual contact
D. Hiking locales
E. Illness of friends

B.22 A sexually active, 30-year-old male patient has a history of genital ulcer which healed several weeks ago. He now presents with a maculopapular rash over his entire body, extending to the palms, soles, and face. Examination of one of the skin lesions by what method would be most likely to demonstrate the causative agent of this infection?

A. Gram stain
B. Darkfield microscopy
C. Modified acid-fast stain
D. Acid-fast stain
E. Culture

B.23 A 40-year-old man has dysuria and copious amounts of pus coming from the urethra. He has been with multiple sexual partners in the past 2 months. A Gram stain of the pus shows many Gram-negative diplococci both in and outside neutrophils. He is also discovered to have a positive fluorescent treponemal antibody (FTA-ABS) test but a negative nontreponemal (RPR) test. What best describes his disease(s) state?

A. Gonorrhea (active)
B. Syphilis (active)
C. Gonorrhea (active) and syphilis (active)
D. Gonorrhea (active) and syphilis (previous)
E. Gonorrhea (previous) and syphilis (previous)

B.24 A 29-year-old man presents with a 2-day history of burning on urination and a thin, watery urethral discharge. He had unprotected sex with a new female partner 4 weeks ago. A Gram stain reveals 50% polymorphonuclear (PMN) and 50% mononuclear leukocytes. No microorganisms were visible and a culture for gonococci was negative. Transmission to another sexual partner would be by acquisition of:

A. Elementary body
B. Reticulate body
C. Outer membrane protein
D. Pili
E. Invasin

B.25 A purified polysaccharide vaccine was successful in preventing invasive meningococcal disease in military populations but not in children under 2 years of age. The most probable explanation for this involves:

A. Maternal IgG transfer at birth
B. CD4+ T-cell function
C. Bone marrow stem cells
D. Maturation of T-cell–dependent responses
E. Maturation of T-cell–independent responses

B.26 Plague continues to exist in many parts of the world. Select the combination from the list that most favors this persistence?

A. Fleas and deer
B. Ticks and wild rodents
C. Fleas and wild rodents
D. Mosquitoes and urban rats
E. Fleas and urban rats

B.27 A number of residents of a migratory worker camp in Arizona have developed fever and night sweats that seem to come and go each day. For some it has been going on more than a month. There are no signs which point to any organ system but most had eaten from a large supply of cheese brought by one of them from Mexico. The best way to establish a diagnosis in these workers is:

A. Blood culture
B. Gram stain
C. Sputum culture
D. CSF culture
E. Serology

B.28 A 30-year-old man presents with fever, headache, and a decline in mental status. He was previously healthy and had received the standard immunizations in school. A lumbar puncture reveals more than 100 white blood cells per milliliter of cerebrospinal fluid (CSF). If a CSF Gram stain reveals Gram-negative diplococci, which of the following actions would best prevent spread of the infection to others in the family?

A. Penicillin chemoprophylaxis
B. Rifampin chemoprophylaxis
C. Polysaccharide vaccine
D. Wearing masks
E. Handwashing

B.29 A 25-year-old student has developed diarrhea with 8 to 10 stools a day. He was healthy 2 days earlier and has no known immune deficits. If the infection developed while traveling in a developing country and the stool contains neither red or white blood cells, the diarrhea is most likely due to:

A. Shiga toxin (Stx)
B. A protein synthesis inhibiting toxin
C. An ADP-ribosylating toxin
D. A pore-forming toxin
E. An invading bacterium

B.30 An 8-year-old boy has been listless and irritable for a week. The mother says he had a sore throat 3 weeks ago but did not see a physician because the family lacks healthcare coverage and "it wasn't that bad." Examination reveals arthritis in two joints and a heart murmur. His antistreptolysin O (ASO) titer is elevated. His cardiac findings are most likely due to antibody stimulated by:

A. Pyrogenic exotoxin
B. M protein
C. Streptolysin O
D. Lipoteichoic acid
E. Fibronectin

B.31 A man presents to urgent care with a history of fever, a shaking chill, and the production of reddish-colored sputum. The X-ray shows consolidation of the right middle lobe of the lung, and a Gram stain of the sputum shows numerous neutrophils and lancet-shaped Gram-positive diplococci. External to the cell wall of this organism_____is typically found:

A. Flagella
B. Pili
C. Lipopolysaccharide
D. Polysaccharide
E. Exotoxin

B.32 Twelve hours after birth a newborn is lethargic and feeding poorly. A blood culture reveals Gram-positive cocci in short chains which are catalase negative. The cell wall of this organism most certainly contains:

A. Pili
B. Flagella
C. Lipopolysaccharide
D. Outer membrane
E. Peptidoglycan

B.33 A teenage boy has developed a tender, painful, lump in his axilla. The lesion eventually came to a "point" and drained purulent material. A Gram stain of the pus revealed WBCs and Gram-positive cocci. Which of the following would be the most probable source of this infection?

A. Resident microbiota
B. Food
C. Insect bite
D. Swimming pool
E. Pet

B.34 An elderly woman recovering from surgery had been in the hospital receiving intravenous fluids for 6 days. On the fifth hospital day she developed a low-grade fever. Physical examination and radiographs revealed no obvious source but a 3 of 3 blood cultures taken were positive for Gram-positive cocci which were catalase positive and coagulase negative. When her IV line was removed, the fever went away. What virulence feature of the organism facilitated this episode?

A. Pili adherent to epithelial cells
B. Pili adherent to plastic
C. Polysaccharide adherent to epithelial cells
D. Polysaccharide adherent to plastic
E. Pore-forming toxin

B.35 A transient man is seen in the emergency room for fever, chills, and a productive cough. The episode began suddenly with a severe shaking chill. A Gram stain of his sputum shows Gram-positive cocci in pairs and his chest X-ray shows consolidation of the right middle lobe. Which feature of the bacterium was most important in the *initiation* of this infection?

A. Pili adhering to tracheal mucosa
B. Polysaccharide interference with complement
C. Catalase generating superoxide ions
D. Superantigen generation of cytokines
E. Cell injury by pore-forming toxin

B.36 A 5-year-old girl has a sore throat. She is febrile and has a scant exudate on one tonsillar pillar. The most sensitive way to detect whether this infection is due to group A streptococci is:

A. Throat culture
B. Streptococcal group A antigen detection
C. Streptococcal M protein antigen detection
D. Gram stain
E. ASO titer

B.37 A few days after birth, a newborn developed an umbilical infection from which Gram-positive cocci in clusters were isolated. The next day he appeared "sunburned" and the superficial layers of his skin peeled away. Except for elevated WBC count routine, hematologic and chemistry tests were normal. The cutaneous findings, in this case, are most likely due to:

A. Endotoxin
B. Pyrogenic exotoxin
C. Exfoliatin
D. Peptidoglycan
E. Coagulase

B.38 A major difference between the structure of the Gram-positive and Gram-negative cell wall is that the Gram-negative wall contains:

A. Peptidoglycan
B. Pili
C. Flagella
D. Outer membrane
E. Capsule

B.39 During a urinary tract infection, a 30-year-old woman developed hypotension, shock, and purpura. Gram-negative rods were discovered in the bloodstream. The shock state is most due to the action of:

A. Lipopolysaccharide (LPS) lipid A
B. LPS side chains
C. Peptidoglycan
D. Cytoplasmic membrane
E. Pyrogenic exotoxin

B.40 A research microbiologist is said to have caused a fatal pneumonia by sending bacterial spores through the mail. These spores are:

A. Structures for sexual reproduction
B. Packets of toxin
C. Concentrated peptidoglycan
D. Concentrated endotoxin
E. Inert survival forms

B.41 The bacterial structure most likely to be acquired by one bacterial cell from another using the conjugation mechanism is:

A. Circular chromosome
B. Bacteriophage
C. Plasmid
D. DNA fragment
E. Transposon

B.42 A bacterial strain has acquired a set of genes by transduction. The process entered the lysogenic cycle and the bacterial cells have gone through a cycle of reproduction. In the daughter cells these genes will be found in:

A. Bacteriophage
B. Plasmid
C. Chromosome
D. Transposon
E. Cytosol

B.43 A human cell has been brought in contact with a bacterial A/B toxin. The cell type is known to be susceptible to the toxin. The most important determinant of the type of physiologic effect of the toxin on the cell is:

A. Surface-binding receptors
B. Ribosomal receptor sites
C. Endocytotic vacuole
D. Type of enzymatic reaction
E. Function of target protein

B.44 Which of the following biologic substances functions commonly as the *receptor* for bacterial adherence?

A. Ribosome
B. Fibronectin
C. Cholesterol
D. Polysaccharide
E. Pili

B.45 A 12-year-old girl woke up saying it hurt to swallow. Her mother took her to a physician who said it looked like a viral pharyngitis and performed a rapid strep antigen test which was negative. Three weeks later she became listless and irritable. Physical examination revealed a febrile girl with arthritis in two joints and a heart murmur. Her antistreptolysin O (ASO) titer was elevated. Her cardiac findings are most likely due to antibody directed against:

A. Pyrogenic exotoxin
B. Streptolysin O
C. Sarcolemmal membranes
D. Lipoteichoic acid
E. Adhesive pili

B.46 A young woman has developed fever and hypotension 3 days into her menstrual cycle. Laboratory findings include leukocytosis and an elevated blood urea nitrogen. Blood cultures were negative but a vaginal culture grew Gram-positive cocci which were catalase and coagulase positive. The systemic findings are most likely due to production of:

A. Endotoxin
B. A/B toxin
C. Superantigen exotoxin
D. Pore-forming toxin
E. Peptidoglycan
F. Coagulase

Answers

B.1 (C), B.2 (C), B.3 (E), B.4 (C), B.5 (E), B.6 (C), B.7 (D), B.8 (E), B.9 (C), B.10 (D), B.11 (A), B.12 (C), B.13 (B), B.14 (A), B.15 (C), B.16 (B), B.17 (D), B.18 (B), B.19 (F), B.20 (E), B.21 (D), B.22 (B), B.23 (D), B.24 (A), B.25 (E), B.26 (C), B.27 (A), B.28 (B), B.29 (C), B.30 (B), B.31 (D), B.32 (E), B.33 (A), B.34 (D), B.35 (B), B.36 (A), B.37 (C), B.38 (D), B.39 (A), B.40 (E), B.41 (C), B.42 (C), B.43 (E), B.44 (B), B.45 (C), B.46 (C)

FUNGAL DISEASES

F.1 A young Phoenix woman has developed fever, cough, and after 1 month of illness has an infiltrate in the upper lobe of her right lung. A sputum specimen digested with KOH was negative but the culture grew a mold with alternating arthroconidia.

This infection was most likely acquired by inhalation of:

A. Spherules
B. Yeasts
C. Sexual, macroconidia
D. Asexual, arthroconidia
E. Asexual chlamydoconidia

F.2 A young woman who recently moved to Arizona has developed fever and malaise which have lasted for 3 weeks. Her chest radiograph is clear and her physician has diagnosed "valley fever." Which of the following tests, using a specific preparation of the infecting agent, would raise the greatest concerns about her disease disseminating outside the lung?

A. Positive skin test
B. High levels of IgG antibody
C. Absent IgM antibody
D. Absent IgG antibody
E. High levels of capsular antigen

F.3 A young woman has developed fever and diffuse pulmonary infiltrates 1 week after undergoing a bone marrow transplant. She is on immunosuppressive therapy. Material collected in a bronchoalveolar lavage has demonstrated septate branching hyphae and she was placed on amphotericin B. The target of this therapy is:

A. Cell wall mannoprotein
B. Nucleic acids
C. Cytoplasmic membrane
D. Mitotic spindle fibers
E. Cell wall glucan

F.4 You are asked to evaluate the antifungal therapy of a patient with an enlarged liver and spleen. The laboratory finding shows that culture of a lymph node biopsy yielded a small (4 mm) yeast at 35°C, which at 25°C grew as a mold with tuberculate macroconidia. The patient most probably acquired this infection in:

A. Semitropical regions of North and South America
B. Ohio and Mississippi River valleys
C. Arid deserts of America and Africa
D. Lower Sonoran life zone
E. Worldwide

F.5 A 75-year-old man presents with headache and confusion. He has a low-grade fever and 10 lymphocytes in his cerebrospinal fluid (CSF). Cultures of sputum, urine, blood, and CSF yielded no pathogens. For which of the following fungal agents would detection of circulating antigen be a useful diagnostic test?

A. *Candida albicans*
B. *Aspergillus fumigatus*
C. *Histoplasma capsulatum*
D. *Coccidioides immitis*
E. *Cryptococcus neoformans*

F.6 A diabetic patient has developed fever and swelling around the eye. Material taken from the adjacent nasal sinus shows large nonseptate hyphae. Which of the following agents is the most probable cause?

A. Candida
B. Aspergillus
C. Trichophyton
D. Rhizopus
E. Sporothrix

F.7 Human-to-human transmission is most likely to occur with:

A. *Coccidioides immitis*
B. *Epidermophyton floccosum*
C. *Cryptococcus neoformans*
D. *Aspergillus flavus*
E. *Histoplasma capsulatum*

F.8 A 25-year-old woman suffers from vaginal discharge and itching. A Gram smear of the discharge demonstrates abundant yeast cells. Culture of the vaginal discharge yielded yeast cells, which readily formed germ tubes (hyphae) when incubated in serum. The feature of this organism which facilitates its initial binding to vaginal epithelial cells is:

A. Mannoprotein
B. Hyphae
C. Ergosterol
D. Conidia
E. Chlamydoconidia

F.9 Skin scrapings have been collected from the advancing edge of a ring-like lesion on the arm of a child. Which of the following observations is diagnostic of dermatophyte infection in a direct KOH preparation?

A. Arthroconidia
B. Chlamydoconidia
C. Macroconidia
D. Septate hyphae
E. Nonseptate hyphae

F.10 A 27-year-old man has experienced malaise over a 2-week period. On examination he has fever and is short of breath. A chest radiograph shows bilateral diffuse pulmonary infiltrates and a bronchoalveolar massage revealed delicate 5-8 mm cystic structures, some of which were folded and had nuclei. He improved with trimethoprim/sulfamethoxazole therapy. The most likely etiologic agent is:

A. *Candida*
B. *Aspergillus*
C. *Pneumocystis*
D. *Ascaris*
E. *Coccidioides*

Answers

F.1 (D), **F.2** (B), **F.3** (C), **F.4** (B), **F.5** (E), **F.6** (D), **F.7** (B), **F.8** (A), **F.9** (D), **F.10** (C)

PARASITIC DISEASES

P.1 A traveler developed diarrhea 2 weeks after returning from a trip to Moscow and St. Petersburg, Russia. The diarrhea has lasted for over 3 weeks and his stools are greasy and foul-smelling. Which of the following is the most probable etiologic agent?

A. Toxoplasma
B. Giardia
C. Trichinella
D. Entamoeba
E. Toxocara

P.2 A 45-year-old African man suffers from chronic fatigue and weakness. At a routine examination at his village clinic he was found to be profoundly anemic. Which of the following agents is most likely to be responsible?

A. *Diphyllobothrium latum*
B. *Strongyloides stercoralis*
C. *Ascaris lumbricoides*
D. *Enterobius vermicularis*
E. *Ancylostoma duodenale*

P.3 An Indonesian man has vague complains of epigastric pain and abdominal tenderness. An evaluation for a peptic ulcer was negative. A diagnosis of strongyloidiasis has been suggested. The best way to confirm this diagnosis is:

A. Finding eggs in the feces
B. Finding adult worms in the feces
C. Finding larval worms in the feces
D. X-ray evidence of pneumonia

P.4 A man who moved to the United States from Ethiopia 10 years ago has been well but over the past year has lost significant weight. He reports a healthy appetite and no change in his food consumption. If he has a tapeworm, it was acquired by ingesting tissue containing:

A. Cysticerci
B. Cercariae
C. Copepods (crustaceans)
D. Hydatid cysts
E. Microfilariae

P.5 A child presents with a prolapsed rectum, a history of diarrhea and a fondness for eating dirt. She is anemic and looks malnourished. A stool examination reveals barrel-shaped eggs with "plugs" at either end. She is most likely infected with:

A. *Ascaris lumbricoides*
B. *Enterobius vermicularis*
C. *Trichuris trichiura*
D. *Necator americanus*
E. *Strongyloides stercoralis*

P.6 At a party, a student consumed sushi which contained fish from Canada. If a parasite becomes established from this raw fish consumption, which of the following problems is most likely?

A. Diarrhea
B. Formation of hydatid cysts
C. Formation of cercaria that will infect other hosts
D. Formation of oocysts
E. Vitamin B_{12} deficiency

P.7 A 29-year-old woman has persistent vaginal discharge and itching. Which one of the following would establish a diagnosis of trichomoniasis?

A. Vaginal clue cells seen by cytology
B. Visualization of organisms by KOH

C. Stool for ova and parasites (O and P)
D. Visualization of motile organisms in vaginal fluid
E. White blood cells with no organisms seen in vaginal fluid

P.8 A man just returned from a mission around the world that included visits to poverty-stricken rural regions of Thailand, India, Kenya, Nigeria, and Brazil. He recalls numerous evenings when he was bitten by mosquitoes. He took chloroquine during the trip and is still taking it. He now presents with fever and chills, and on examination he has an enlarged spleen. A blood smear reveals ring-shaped structures within erythrocytes. This infection was most likely acquired by the bite of:

A. *Anopheles* mosquito
B. Tsetse fly
C. Sand fly
D. *Aedes* mosquito
E. Reduviid (kissing, triatomine) bug

P.9 An immigrant from Bolivia complains of abdominal pain and cramping. Two months prior he passed numerous bloody stools. On examination he has right upper quadrant pain and hepatomegaly. If this is a liver abscess, which of the following might have caused it?

A. Ascaris
B. Entamoeba
C. Balantidium
D. Taenia
E. Acanthamoeba

P.10 Which one of the following can complete its entire life cycle in the human host?

A. *Toxoplasma gondii*
B. *Cryptosporidium parvum*
C. *Plasmodium falciparum*
D. *Trypanosoma cruzi*
E. *Trypanosoma brucei*

P.11 Which of the following parasites primarily infects macrophages?

A. Plasmodium falciparum
B. Trypanosoma cruzi
C. Trichomonas vaginalis
D. Leishmania donovani
E. Echinococcus granulosus

P.12 A man returned 4 weeks ago from Tanzania, East Africa, where he was on a safari. Earlier, he had an ulcer on the back of his neck. He now has headaches, fevers, and decreased level of consciousness. Which one of the following could *most readily* explain his symptoms?

A. *Plasmodium vivax*
B. *Trypanosoma brucei rhodesiense*
C. *Toxoplasma gondii*
D. *Trypanosoma cruzi*
E. *Leishmania donovani*

P.13 **Which one of the following may explain the chronicity of infection caused by African trypanosomes?**

A. Antigenic variation

B. Inhibition of macrophage phagosome–lysosome fusion

C. Resistance to complement lysis

D. Ingestion of neutrophils

E. Formation of tissue cysts

P.14 **Which one of the following may explain the long latency of infection caused by *Toxoplasma gondii*?**

A. Antigenic variation

B. Intraerythrocytic survival

C. Resistance to complement lysis

D. Ingestion of neutrophils

E. Formation of tissue cysts

P.15 **A young man noticed deterioration of vision after storing his contact lenses in tap water. An ophthalmologist diagnosed severe retinitis. Examination of the water and vitreous fluid would most likely reveal which of the following?**

A. Babesia

B. Entamoeba

C. Naegleria

D. Acanthamoeba

E. Cryptosporidium

Answers

P.1 (B), **P.2** (E), **P.3** (C), **P.4** (A), **P.5** (C), **P.6** (E), **P.7** (D), **P.8** (A), **P.9** (B), **P.10** (B), **P.11** (D), **P.12** (B), **P.13** (A), **P.14** (E), **P.15** (D)

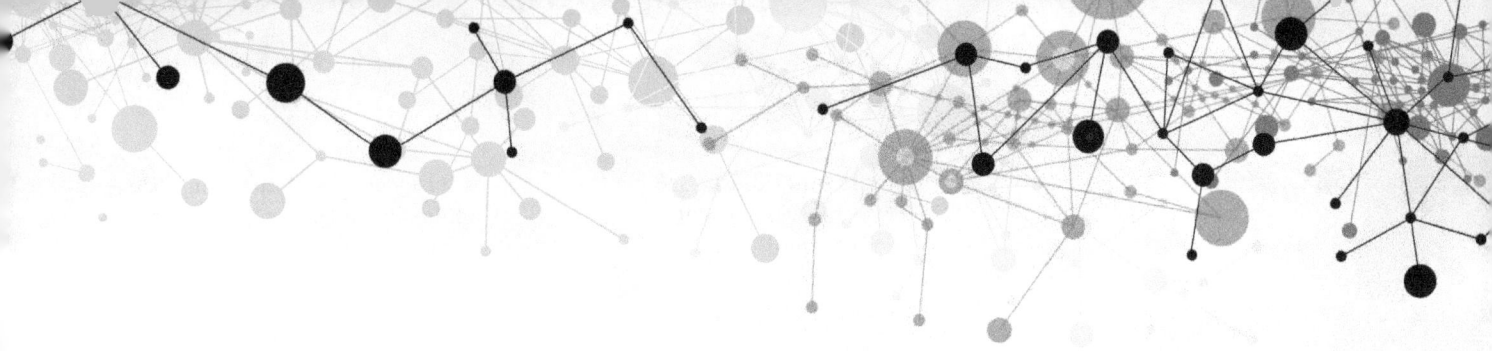

Index

Page numbers followed by italic *f* or *t* denote figures or tables, respectively.

9 781260 464283